McDonald's   Fifth Edition

VETERINARY ENDOCRINOLOGY AND REPRODUCTION

McDonald's   Fifth Edition

VETERINARY ENDOCRINOLOGY AND REPRODUCTION

Edited by M. H. PINEDA, D.V.M., Ph.D.

Professor Emeritus of Physiology
Department of Veterinary Physiology and Pharmacology
Iowa State University

With the editorial assistance of **MICHAEL P. DOOLEY, Ph.D.**

Iowa State Press
A Blackwell Publishing Company

Iowa State Press
2121 State Avenue, Ames, Iowa 50014

ORDERS: 1-800-862-6657

OFFICE: 1-515-292-0140

FAX: 1-515-292-3348

WEB SITE: www.iowastatepress.com

Printed on acid-free paper in the United States of America

First edition, 1969
Second edition, 1975
Third edition, 1980
Fourth edition, 1989
Fifth Edition, 2003

International Standard Book Number: 0-8138-1106-6

Library of Congress Cataloging-in-Publication Data

McDonald's veterinary endocrinology and reproduction /
  edited by M.H. Pineda with the editorial assistance of
  Michael P. Dooley — 5th ed.

  p. cm.
  Rev. ed. of: Veterinary endocrinology and reproduction.
4th ed. 1989.
  Includes bibliographical references and index.
  ISBN 0-8138-1106-6 (alk. paper)
  1. Veterinary endocrinology. 2. Domestic animals—
Reproduction.

  I. Pineda, M.H. II. Dooley, Michael P. III. Veterinary endocrinology and reproduction
  SF768.3.M335 2002
  6336.089'4—dc21

    98-009931

The last digit is the print number: 9 8 7 6 5 4 3 2 1

To my father

who had mastered the art of breeding and rearing animals. Although he lacked an understanding of the sciences of endocrinology and reproduction, few people possessed his intuition concerning reproduction of farm animals.

Dr. McDonald's dedication to his father as it appeared in the first, second, third, and fourth editions.

Preface

The foundations for the understanding of the reproductive processes of domestic species that were established in the previous four editions of this textbook have been maintained and updated in this fifth edition. The authors contributing chapters to this new edition of *Veterinary Endocrinology and Reproduction* have incorporated and emphasized the new developments and progress made in many areas of endocrinology, physiology, and biology of reproduction. These include, but are not restrictive to, advanced biochemical, cellular, and molecular components. Designing a book to serve as a textbook for the teaching of curricular courses on endocrinology and reproduction for the use of students in colleges of veterinary medicine, as well as to serve as a guide for veterinary practitioners, implies an ipso facto medical orientation to the coverage of the subjects. However, we have emphasized, as much as possible the basic aspects, concepts, and mechanisms of action participating in the reproductive processes. After all, the basic physiological concepts provide the foundation needed for a successful treatment of a reproductive failure and for the management of reproductive activities of our domestic species that, depending on the species and circumstances, may be addressed to either increase or reduce their fertility. By design, Dr. L. E. McDonald originally included the reproductive process of the bovine, canine, equine, feline, ovine, and porcine species in the first, second, and third editions; the reproductive process of the caprine species was added in the fourth edition. We have maintained this emphasis in the fifth edition, though we recognize the increasing importance of other species. Hence, for this fifth edition we have incorporated a new Chapter 18, contributed by Dr. P. A. Martin, on the reproduction of South American camelids: alpacas, llamas, guanacos, and vicuñas. Dr. T. J. Reimers rewrote Chapters 1 and 2, Dr. T. J. Rosol collaborated with Dr. Capen in updating Chapter 4, Drs. P. A. Martin and M. H. Crump rewrote Chapters 5 and 6, Dr. G. C. Althouse collaborated with Dr. Hopkins in updating Chapter 13, and Dr. M. P. Dooley, assistant editor for this fifth edition, co-authored Chapter 11.

Many references were deleted from each of the chapters, in an attempt to maintain an equilibrium between the number of new references added and those deleted. This process is always difficult for an author of any chapter, though necessary to maintain the correct number of pages for each chapter and to keep the price of the book within reasonable limits. Notwithstanding, we endeavored to provide the reader with a number of selected references to serve as a solid support for the concepts, statements of fact, mechanisms, and hypothesis regarding the endocrine control and the environmental effects on the reproductive activities of the animal species that form the body of the book. For those readers interested in a given subject, references that were deleted may be found in the references listed for each chapter from the previous first, second, third, and fourth editions. Graduate students and researchers interested in the reproductive processes of a particular species of those covered in this textbook, will find that the references given in each chapter are comprehensive and were carefully selected to be those from well-designed studies that provided the most authoritative information. This careful and comprehensive selection of references is not commonly found in other textbooks.

The continuing contributions of Drs. R. A. Bowen, C. C. Capen, M. H. Crump, L. E. Evans, S. M. Hopkins, and S. L. Martin and the new contributions of Drs. G. C. Althouse, M. P. Dooley, S. M. Hopkins, P. A. Martin, T. J. Reimers, and T. J. Rosol strengthen this textbook.

Finally, this preface would not be complete if we do not acknowledge the pioneering effort of Dr. L. E. McDonald, editor for the first, second, third, and fourth editions of this textbook. Thus, in recognition to his contribution to the education of students of Veterinary Medicine and in his honor, the title of this textbook has now been changed to: *McDonald's Veterinary Endocrinology and Reproduction*.

M. H. Pineda
Editor for the fifth edition

Acknowledgments

I am fortunate to have been assisted in the editorial assembling of this textbook by Dr. Michael P. Dooley, the assistant editor and by colleagues, students of veterinary medicine, and graduate students from the College of Veterinary Medicine at Iowa State University. Each contributed and helped me to eliminate errors, improve the text, and keep consistency between chapters. Also, the contribution of all of the authors and their cooperation to the process of revision and editorial work is acknowledged and greatly appreciated. I must state here, however, that none but me is to be held responsible for the shortcomings that may have remained unnoticed or the errors that may have remained uncorrected. Perhaps it is proper to say ex post facto hic et nunc, paraphrasing Dr. Samuel Johnson on completion of his dictionary in 1755, "In this work, when it shall be found that much was omitted, let it not be forgotten that much likewise was performed."

I express my appreciation to Dr. Richard L. Engen, former Chair of the Department of Veterinary Physiology and Pharmacology, for his continued support during the writing and editing of this textbook. Likewise, I shall recognize and express my sincere thanks to Ms. Kim Adams and Vernice Hoyt for the excellent secretarial assistance and perhaps more importantly, for their understanding and patience in times of crises.

I shall recognize and thank Mr. Carroll C. Cann, formerly from Lea & Febiger, with whom the preparation for the 5th Edition was begun. I also would like to recognize and thank Mr. David M. Rosenbaum, Publisher, and Ms. Gretchen Van Houten, Publishing Director, from Iowa State Press for their continued assistance during the preparation and publication of this textbook.

And last, but not least, I thank Rosa Amelia, my wife of 47 years now, for her support, enduring patience and understanding. For that, I dedicate the fifth edition of this book to her.

M. H. Pineda
Editor for the fifth edition

Contributors

GARY C. ALTHOUSE, DVM, MS, PhD,
  Diplomate, ACT
Associate Professor of Reproduction and Swine
  Production Medicine
Department of Clinical Studies – New Bolton
  Center
School of Veterinary Medicine
University of Pennsylvania
Kennett Square, Pennsylvania

R.A. BOWEN, DVM, PhD
Professor of Physiology and Biophysics
College of Veterinary Medicine and
  Biomedical Sciences
Colorado State University
Fort Collins, Colorado

C.C. CAPEN, DVM, MSc, PhD
Distinguished University Professor
Department of Veterinary Biosciences
College of Veterinary Medicine
The Ohio State University
Columbus, Ohio

M.H. CRUMP, DVM, MS, PhD
Associate Professor of Physiology - Emeritus
Department of Biomedical Sciences
College of Veterinary Medicine
Iowa State University
Ames, Iowa

MICHAEL P. DOOLEY, MS, PhD

L.E. EVANS, DVM, MS PhD
Professor of Clinical Sciences
Department of Veterinary Clinical Sciences
College of Veterinary Medicine
Iowa State University
Ames, Iowa

S.M. HOPKINS, DVM, Diplomate, ACT
Professor, Department of Veterinary Diagnostic
  and Production Animal Medicine
College of Veterinary Medicine
Iowa State University
Ames, Iowa

P.A. MARTIN, DVM, MS, PhD
Associate Professor of Physiology
Department of Biomedical Sciences
College of Veterinary Medicine
Iowa State University
Ames, Iowa

S.L. MARTIN, DVM, MSc
Professor - Emeritus
Department of Veterinary Clinical Sciences
College of Veterinary Medicine
The Ohio State University
Columbus, Ohio

M.H. PINEDA, DVM, MS, PhD
Professor Emeritus of Physiology
Department of Biomedical Sciences
Iowa State University
Ames, Iowa

THOMAS J. REIMERS, MS, PhD
Professor of Endocrinology, Emeritus
College of Veterinary Medicine
Cornell University
Ithaca, New York

THOMAS J. ROSOL, DVM, PhD
Professor of Veterinary Pathobiology & Senior
  Associate Vice President for Research
Department of Veterinary Biosciences
College of Veterinary Medicine
The Ohio State University
Columbus, Ohio

Contents

Introduction

T. J. REIMERS

1

EXTRACELLULAR COMMUNICATION

Animals are incredibly complex multicellular organisms requiring many very simple to very sophisticated control mechanisms to maintain a state of physiologic and biochemical equilibrium. These control mechanisms require equally sophisticated communications networks and strategies. Classically, communications among cells, tissues, and organs within an individual were considered to be generated and mediated by either the nervous system or the endocrine system. The nervous system communicated physically, using electrochemical signals between the brain and other organs, such as a muscle group, or signals from one organ to another, as in a reflex arc. In contrast, the endocrine system communicated via chemical blood-borne mes-

sengers, for instance between the pituitary gland and the adrenal cortex. Whereas communication via the nervous system is very rapid, endocrine communication is slower.

This simple dual-component classification of extracellular communication has been modified significantly in the past 20 years. It is much more complicated. Whereas it is customary and convenient to categorize cardiovascular, respiratory, reproductive, gastrointestinal, nervous, and endocrine functions into discrete physiological systems, anatomic and functional components of these systems overlap to lesser or greater degrees. For example, one cannot describe normal and abnormal function of the heart and blood vessels without including major aspects of the respiratory and nervous systems. Likewise, the nervous system is significantly dependent on hormones from the endocrine system for normal function. Conversely, the adrenal medulla, considered a component of the endocrine system, is highly integrated with the nervous system.

Endocrinology is the study of communication within a living organism by means of hormones. Hormones are the chemical messengers of the endocrine system. The discipline of endocrinology includes the study of hormones; the anatomy and physiology of the cells, tissues, and organs that produce these hormones; the way that hormones are transported and act on target cells; and the clinical abnormalities of hormonal deficiencies and overproduction.

In the classical sense, a hormone was described as a chemical messenger secreted from a

1

ductless gland, emptied directly into the circulation, and transported by the blood, i.e., hemocrine communication (Fig. 1-1A), some distance to alter the function of a target organ. By today's definition, this blood-borne communication is but one manifestation of the endocrine system. In addition, the concept that ductless glands are the sole sources of hormones has gone by the wayside because hormones also are secreted throughout the body by nonglandular tissues whose major functions are primarily nonendocrine.

Components of the endocrine system that communicate by routes other than blood vessels are characterized as autocrine, paracrine, neurocrine, and solinocrine. In autocrine communication, hormones are secreted locally into the extracellular space only to return to self-regulate the very cells that released them (Fig. 1-1B).

Paracrine communication involves secretion of hormones from a cell directly into the surrounding extracellular space; the hormones then interact with adjacent or nearby cells without being transported by blood (Fig. 1-1C). Paracrine communication delivers very high concentrations of the hormone to its target site. Neurocrine communication, involving secretion of peptides or other neurotransmitter molecules by neurons, is a specialized form of paracrine function in which the chemical messenger is transferred to a target cell via a synapse or neuromuscular junction.

Finally, several hormones, e.g., gastrin, somatostatin, vasoactive intestinal peptide, calcitonin, secretin, and serotonin, are secreted directly into the lumen of the gastrointestinal, respiratory, and reproductive tracts. This type of communication is called solinocrine (Fig. 1-1D).

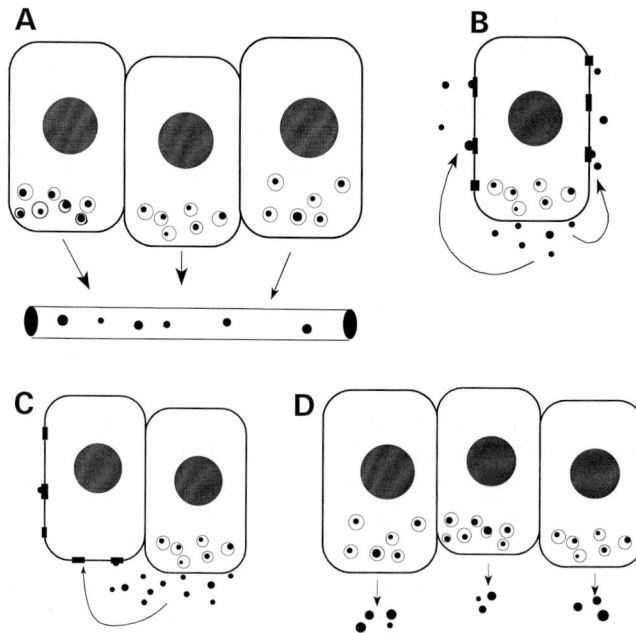

Fig. 1-1. Schematic representations of hormonal communications. **A.** In hemocrine communication, a chemical messenger is secreted from a ductless gland directly into the circulation and transported by the blood some distance to a target organ whose function is altered as a result. **B.** In autocrine communication, hormones are secreted locally into the extracellular space and return to self-regulate the very cells that released them. **C.** Paracrine communication involves secretion of hormones from a cell directly into the surrounding extracellular space. These hormones then interact with adjacent or nearby cells without being transported by blood. **D.** In solinocrine type of communication, hormones are secreted directly into the lumen of the gastrointestinal, respiratory, and reproductive tracts. ● = hormone, ○ = secretory vesicle, ■ = receptor.

FUNCTIONS OF HORMONES

Nearly all complex physiologic and metabolic processes are regulated by the endocrine system and the hormones that comprise it. A single hormone can affect a single function, e.g., erythropoietin on hemoglobin synthesis by erythrocytes, but this one-on-one action is very rare. Rather, actions of the endocrine system on other physiologic and metabolic processes are very complex, involving single hormones having multiple actions, e.g., thyroxine on enzyme synthesis, erythropoiesis, bone turnover, carbohydrate, and lipid metabolism, or multiple hormones having single actions, e.g., regulation of lactation by prolactin, placental lactogen, corticosteroids, thyroxine, sex steroids, and oxytocin, and multiple hormones producing multiple actions, such as reproductive steroids, oxytocin, and corticosteroids on pregnancy, fetal development, and parturition.

Reproduction depends on the effects of hormones on gametogenesis as well as development of sexual characteristics and elicitation of behaviors that culminate in the fertilization of an oocyte by a spermatozoon and the production of offspring. Many hormones play important functions for the maintenance of pregnancy, including growth of the embryo and fetus, development of the reproductive tract for pregnancy, and initiation of parturition. Once birth has occurred, the newborn must independently adapt quickly to the extrauterine environment, respond to stressors, and maintain homeostasis in every physiological function. Hormones and the nervous system are vital for maintenance of the animal's internal environment. Hormones and their actions are essential for pre- and postnatal growth and development. Hormones are also important in timing the cessation of growth. For example, hormone-mediated closure of the epiphyses of long bones after maturity is necessary for proper adult body conformation.

Maintenance of an animal's internal environment requires metabolic energy generated from nutrients processed by enzymes regulated by hormones. Production, storage, and utilization of energy require complex endocrine-regulated ingestive, digestive, anabolic, catabolic, and excretory processes.

CHARACTERISTICS OF THE ENDOCRINE SYSTEM

The players of the endocrine system are hormones–including proteins, smaller peptides, amino acid derivatives, and lipids. The protein hormones include prolactin and growth hormone. Glycoprotein hormones include thyrotropin or thyroid-stimulating hormone (TSH), luteinizing hormone (LH), and follicle-stimulating hormone (FSH). Peptide hormones include insulin, insulin-like growth factor-1 (IGF-1), and adrenocorticotropin (ACTH). Triiodothyronine (T_3) and catecholamines such as epinephrine and norepinephrine are examples of hormones that are derivatives of amino acids. The large category of lipidic hormones includes the subcategories of steroids, e.g., progestogens, estrogens, androgens, glucocorticoids, and mineralocorticoids, and eicosanoids, e.g., prostaglandins, thromboxanes, and leukotrienes.

Whatever the chemical nature of hormones, they all have several characteristics in common. First, they are present in the blood and other extracellular fluids in low concentrations. The range of hormone concentrations from 10^{-11} to 10^{-9} M in extracellular fluids is in contrast to concentrations of other chemicals like nonhormonal amino acids, peptides, and lipids that are present in the range from 10^{-5} to 10^{-3} M. Despite their low concentrations, development and refinements of the radioimmunoassay and other modern quantitative techniques allow routine measurements of hormones in small samples of serum, plasma, or urine for research, clinical diagnostic procedures, and therapeutic monitoring.

The second common characteristic of hormones is the existence of mechanisms that direct hormones to their target cells and tissues. These mechanisms are necessary because hormones are in low concentrations in extracellular fluids. Cells have high-affinity receptors to capture or bind hormones from the extracellular fluid. These receptors can reside on the external surface of the cell membrane, e.g., gonadotropin receptors, or be located inside the cell, such as those in the cytoplasm or nucleus, e.g., estradiol receptors. The principal target tissue(s) for a hormone has the greatest concentration of the receptor specific for that hormone. Some hormones are concentrated in target cells because of the proximity of the source of hormone to the target cell, allowing direct diffusion of the hormone from its source to an adjacent target cell. For example, testosterone, synthesized by Leydig cells of the testis, diffuses only a short distance to Sertoli cells and to the adluminal compartment of the seminiferous epithelium to promote spermatogenesis. Still other hormones are produced within their target cells. Dihydrotestosterone, the hormonally active form of testosterone in the male, is produced by androgen-sensitive target cells such as those of the prostate. Similarly, thyroxine (T_4) is converted to T_3 within cells of the pituitary gland to play a major role in the regulation of TSH secretion.

One anatomic feature that efficiently directs hormones to their target tissues is the so-called portal circulation. Portal circulation consists of blood flowing from capillaries in one organ to a vein and then to capillaries in another organ. The hepatic portal circulation is structured so that insulin, secreted into capillaries of the endocrine pancreas, is carried by the hepatic portal vein to capillaries of the liver, where it exerts its major actions. In that way, insulin does not circulate great distances to the heart and then to the liver. Likewise, releasing hormones for hormones of the anterior pituitary gland pass from capillaries in the hypothalamus to the hypophyseal portal vessels and then to the capillaries of the pituitary gland.

HORMONE SYNTHESIS AND SECRETION

Hormones are synthesized like any other protein, peptide, amino acid, and lipid. Synthesis of peptide and protein hormones begins with transcription of DNA in the nucleus to yield messenger RNA (mRNA), which encodes a prohormone on the rough endoplasmic reticulum (Fig. 1-2). The latter consists of polyribosomes attached to membranous cisternae. Amino acids are then polymerized into a polypeptide prohormone by the process of translation. Newly synthesized prohormones are released into the cisternae of the endoplasmic reticulum where they

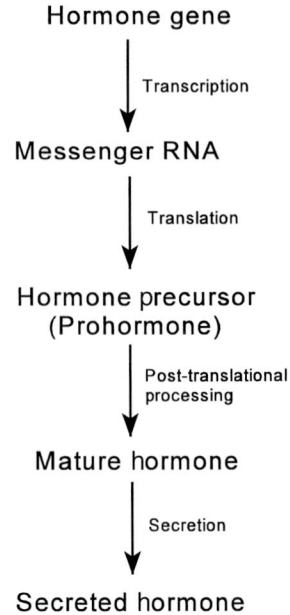

Hormone gene

↓ Transcription

Messenger RNA

↓ Translation

Hormone precursor (Prohormone)

↓ Post-translational processing

Mature hormone

↓ Secretion

Secreted hormone

Fig. 1-2. Steps involved in synthesis and secretion of protein and peptide hormones. (Adapted from: W. W. Chin, *In*: Principles and Practice of Endocrinology and Metabolism, edited by K. L. Becker. Philadelphia, PA, J. B. Lippincott Co., 1990, p. 15).

are carried to the Golgi complex. There, the proteins are processed and packaged into secretory granules or vesicles by budding from the endoplasmic reticulum and Golgi membranes. The immature granules undergo maturation, and upon receiving an appropriate extracellular stimulus, the granules and vesicles migrate to and fuse with the plasma membrane of the cell. The processed hormone is then released into the extracellular fluid.

For peptide hormones, the initial synthetic product is a large protein (prohormone) that is cleaved step-by-step into several peptides, more than one of which may have hormonal activity. For example, adrenocorticotropin (ACTH) is a 39-amino acid peptide derived from a much larger precursor (235 amino acids) called proopiomelanocortin (POMC; Fig. 1-3). Other peptides with hormonal activity derived from POMC include melanocyte-stimulating hormone, beta-endorphin, and beta-lipotropin. Parathyroid hormone (PTH) is synthesized as part of a larger precursor by the chief cells of the

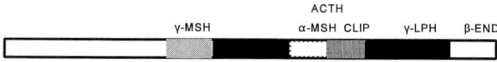

Fig. 1-3. Schematic representation of proopiomelanocortin (POMC). Adrenocorticotropin (**ACTH**) is a 39-amino acid peptide derived from the much larger POMC precursor. Other peptides with hormonal activity derived from POMC include alpha-melanocyte-stimulating hormone (**α-MSH**), beta-endorphin (**β-END**), and gamma-lipotropin (**γ-LPH**). Adrenocorticotropin consists of the peptide **α-MSH** and the corticotropin-like intermediate lobe peptide (**CLIP**). (Adapted from: J. F. Habener, *In*: Williams Textbook of Endocrinology, edited by J. D. Wilson and D. W. Foster. Philadelphia, PA, W.B. Saunders Co., 1992, p. 13).

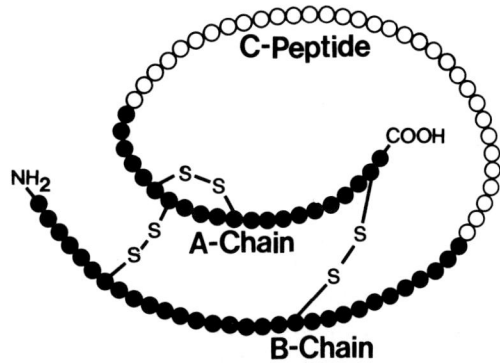

Fig. 1-4. Schematic representation of the proinsulin molecule showing the relationship between the **A** and **B chains** of insulin and with **C-peptide**.

parathyroid gland. The precursor (preproPTH), a polypeptide of 113 amino acids, is synthesized on ribosomes of chief cells. PreproPTH is reduced in the endoplasmic reticulum to proPTH, with 90 amino acids. An N-terminal hexapeptide then is cleaved within the Golgi region to form native PTH with 84 amino acids and a molecular weight of 9,500 daltons. Other prohormones include proinsulin (Fig. 1-4), proglucagon, progastrin, and procalcitonin.

An outdated notion that hormones are synthesized only in specific glands has been challenged often. For example, the complete amino acid sequence of pancreatic glucagon is found within the sequence of a larger gastrointestinal form of glucagon called enteroglucagon, glicentin, or glucagon-like immunoreactivity (see Chapter 5, Fig. 5-9). Thyroxine, a prohormone, is converted to the hormone T_3 in the liver, kidney, brain, and pituitary gland. Finally, estrogens are produced from androgen precursors, primarily androstenedione in females and testosterone in males, by enzymes present in peripheral nonendocrine tissues.

Characteristics of a true endocrine gland that separate it from other organs that also produce hormones are that endocrine glands synthesize the hormone at faster rates, efficiently process prohormones, and have mechanisms for releasing the hormone in a controlled manner. Usually, only small amounts of hormones are stored by endocrine glands. Therefore, secretion is determined ultimately by the rate of hormone synthesis. One significant exception to this rule is the thyroid gland, in which thyroglobulin represents the storage form of the iodothyronines. Canine thyroglobulin is a protein with a molecular weight of 660,000 daltons. Thyroglobulins from humans, pigs, sheep, goats, and cattle are physically similar. Thyroid follicles store abundant iodothyronines as thyroglobulin, providing a mechanism to delay hypothyroidism should synthetic mechanisms fail.

HORMONE TRANSPORT

Once hormones are secreted in a hemocrine manner, they must be transported by the circulatory system to target tissues. Water-soluble hormones, such as proteins and peptides, do not require additional carrier proteins for transport. On the other hand, the insoluble hormones such as iodothyronines and steroids require carrier proteins.

Cortisol circulates in the blood in an unbound form or bound to a specific corticosteroid-binding globulin (CBG, transcortin) or to plasma albumin. Corticosteroid-binding globulin is a glycoprotein with a molecular weight of 51,700 daltons. Progesterone, prednisolone (a synthetic steroid used therapeutically), and aldosterone also bind to CBG. Human CBG binds about 70% of the plasma cortisol, but this proportion varies greatly among other animal species.

Carrier proteins have significant effects on the clearance rates of hormones. Upon secretion of T_4 and T_3, both iodothyronines become reversibly bound to several liver-derived proteins.

Less than 1% of iodothyronines are normally circulating in blood in the unbound form. Consequently, total concentrations of bound + unbound T_3 and T_4 in blood not only depend on secretion, but also depend on concentrations of their binding proteins in plasma because the unbound fractions are vulnerable to metabolism and excretion. In humans, iodothyronines are bound with high affinity primarily to thyronine-binding globulin (TBG), and the plasma half-life of T_4 is about 7 days. In contrast, dogs have only about 15% of the TBG as humans, and cats apparently have none. Dogs and cats rely on low-affinity carrier proteins such as albumin and prealbumin to bind T_3 and T_4. As a result, the half-life of T_4 in dogs is shortened significantly at 10 to 16 hours.

Transport of hormones in blood from the endocrine gland to target tissues is not without its problems. Deficiencies of carrier proteins in humans have been documented. However, these deficiencies rarely lead to disease because feedback mechanisms usually compensate adequately. Abnormalities in transport may appear during endocrine function tests but are not usually associated with endocrine dysfunction.

FEEDBACK CONTROL OF HORMONE PRODUCTION

Synthesis and secretion of most hormones are under feedback control, sometimes in a very complicated manner. In endocrinology, feedback control means regulation of hormonal secretion from an endocrine gland by an effect of the circulating hormone that the gland itself produces. This effect may be direct or mediated by another hormone, a metabolite produced by the hormone's action, or a physical factor. The result of this type of regulation can generate more hormone (positive feedback) or less hormone (negative feedback). A classic example of this process involves the hypothalamus-pituitary-thyroid axis (Fig. 1-5). In the euthyroid (normally functioning thyroid gland) animal, thyrotropin-releasing hormone (TRH) from the hypothalamus and TSH from the pituitary gland are secreted in a state of equilibrium. When iodothyronine concentrations in the blood are inadequate, e.g., primary hypothyroidism, TRH

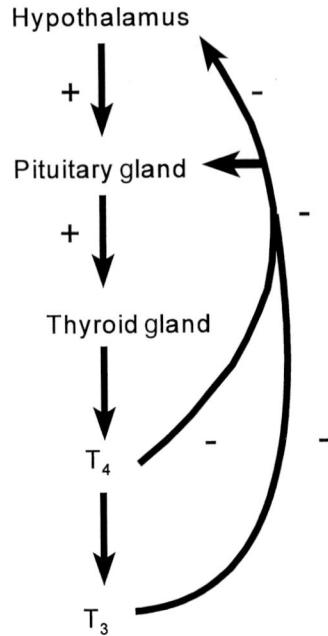

Fig. 1-5. Schematic representation of negative feedback of **T_3** and **T_4** on the hypothalamo-pituitary-thyroid axis.

secretion from the hypothalamus increases to stimulate TSH secretion from the pituitary, and TSH stimulates the thyroid gland to produce more T_4 and T_3. The increased blood concentrations of iodothyronines feed back negatively on the hypothalamus and pituitary gland so that secretions of TRH and TSH are reduced. Secretion of TSH is controlled at the level of the adenohypophysial thyrotrope (TSH-secreting cell) by a complex association: (a) hypothalamic TRH stimulates synthesis and secretion of TSH; (b) TSH stimulates the secretion of iodothyronines by the thyroid gland; and (c) T_3 interacting locally with nuclear receptors decreases TSH synthesis and secretion from the pituitary. The exact mechanism by which iodothyronines inhibit TSH secretion and antagonize TRH action remains undetermined. Conversion of T_4 to T_3 within the pituitary gland itself via a special enzymatic system plays a major role in regulation of TSH secretion.

Glucocorticoids also affect ACTH secretion by similar negative feedback mechanisms in the pituitary and/or hypothalamus. However, the frequent secretory bursts of glucocorticoids measured in blood (see the following section) do not occur because of decreasing adrenal secretion of glucocorticoids that stimulates increased ACTH secretion. Rather, the pattern of ACTH secretion is controlled intrinsically by the central nervous system or pituitary gland independently of feedback control by corticosteroids.

Some hormones are under feedback control by metabolites and physical factors as well as other hormones. Ionized calcium negatively controls PTH secretion, glucose negatively controls glucagon and positively controls insulin secretion, and the volume of extracellular fluid negatively controls aldosterone production by feedback mechanisms.

Late in the estrous cycle, increasing concentrations of the ovarian steroid estradiol exert a positive feedback influence on the pituitary gland to cause an increase in the frequency and amplitude of the pulsatile release of LH. The increased LH concentrations lead to a further increase in estradiol secretion that leads to the ovulatory surge of LH (Fig. 1-6).

A few hormones are produced without feedback regulation. Those produced by the placenta, such as equine chorionic gonadotropin, progesterone, and estrogens, appear not to be regulated by classic feedback mechanisms. Likewise, hormones produced by ectopic glands are free of feedback control.

PATTERNS OF HORMONES IN BLOOD

Given the extremely well-regulated nature of hormone synthesis, secretion, and transport as previously described, one might expect hormone concentrations in blood and other tissues to vary little from moment to moment except during stress or after eating or other activities. Rather, concentrations of some hormones in blood change significantly minute by minute or

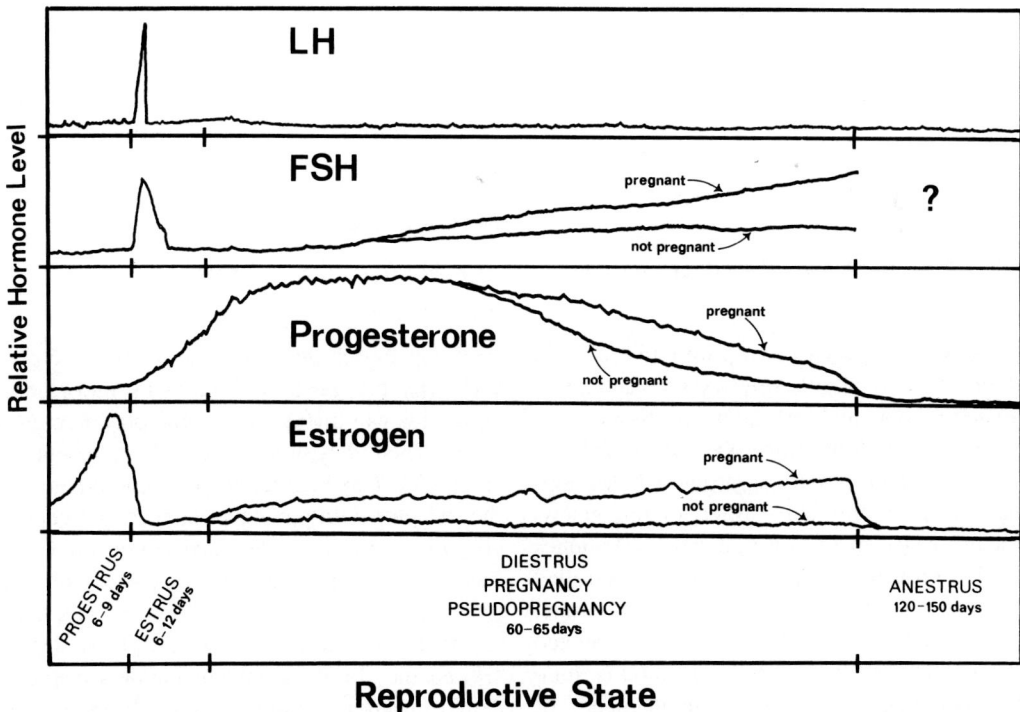

Fig. 1-6. Changes in **LH**, **FSH**, **progesterone**, and **estrogen** in bitches during the estrous cycle and pregnancy. (Modified from: P. W. Concannon, *In*: Current Veterinary Therapy IX, edited by R. W. Kirk. Philadelphia, PA, W. B. Saunders Co., 1986, p. 1215).

at least several times within an hour. An example of this rapid change is the pulsatile secretion and release of testosterone whereby each secretory pulse of testosterone is preceded by a pulse of LH. Secretion of glucocorticoids from the adrenal cortex is pulsatile rather than at a constant rate. In sheep, the number of pulses of cortisol in a 24-hour period varies with the time of adaptation to the experimental environment. In the horse, secretory pulses of ACTH in pituitary venous blood generally last 10 minutes or less and occur every 15 to 25 minutes.

Beside pulsatile secretion of glucocorticoids and other hormones, there are also circadian secretory patterns that last approximately 24 hours. In mares, the highest concentrations of cortisol in serum or plasma occur between 0700 and 0900 hours (7:00 to 9:00 AM) daily, and the lowest concentrations occur from 1900 to 2300 hours (7:00 to 11:00 PM). Similar patterns have been described in other animals.

Longer intervals between dramatic changes in hormone concentrations are associated with the estrous cycle. Changes in progesterone, estrogen, and gonadotropin concentrations in blood vary with the length of the estrous cycle (Fig. 1-6). These intervals are extended by pregnancy or pseudopregnancy. Thyroxine concentrations in blood also change seasonally, responding to changes in ambient temperature.

GENERAL PRINCIPLES OF HORMONE ACTION

An outdated description proposed that each hormone had a unique, single source and a single action in a single or few target tissues. For example, growth hormone was responsible for growth, and progesterone promoted development of the reproductive tract for pregnancy. Today, it is well known that many hormones regulate growth and that pregnancy is controlled by more than progesterone alone. Furthermore, growth hormone has actions not directly related to growth, and progesterone has actions quite different from its role in the maintenance of pregnancy.

A revolutionary concept regarding hormone action arose in the 1960s and 1970s when hor-

mone receptors were identified. The existence of hormone receptors on target cells allows for an understanding of hormone specificity and selectivity of response. With external or cell membrane receptors and internal or cytosolic receptors, target cells can attract preferentially and bind to the exact hormones they need for normal function.

All hormone receptors are proteins and have two functional domains—one that binds the hormone (recognition domain) and the other that regulates post-binding biochemical events (coupling domain). The goodness or tightness of binding of the hormone to the recognition domain is measured as the affinity for binding the hormone or the K-value. A perfect-fitting hormone has a K-value of 1. Other molecules have K-values from 0 to 1.

In general, receptors for neurotransmitters, peptides, and proteins are located within the cell membrane, whereas receptors for steroids, vitamin D, and iodothyronines reside within the cytoplasm or nucleus. Binding of catecholamines, peptides, and protein hormones to their receptors initiates a sequence of intracellular signals that regulate intracellular function. For steroids and iodothyronines, binding to the intracellular receptors is the signal. The coupling domain binds to specific regions of DNA on chromosomes to initiate intracellular changes or regulate other cellular functions.

Intracellular Action of Steroid Hormones

Being lipophilic, steroid hormones such as estrogens, progestagens, androgens, and glucocorticoids can diffuse across the plasma membrane, where they bind to intracellular receptors (Fig. 1-7). This interaction causes activation of the receptor with resultant changes in receptor conformation. The steroid-receptor complex then binds to a specific region on the cell's DNA to promote the transcriptional process with help from a protein acceptor molecule. These DNA regions may be short polynucleotide sequences called promotor elements and hormone response elements that are located 'upstream' from the 5′ transcription initiation site of the gene being regulated (Fig. 1-8). Promotor ele-

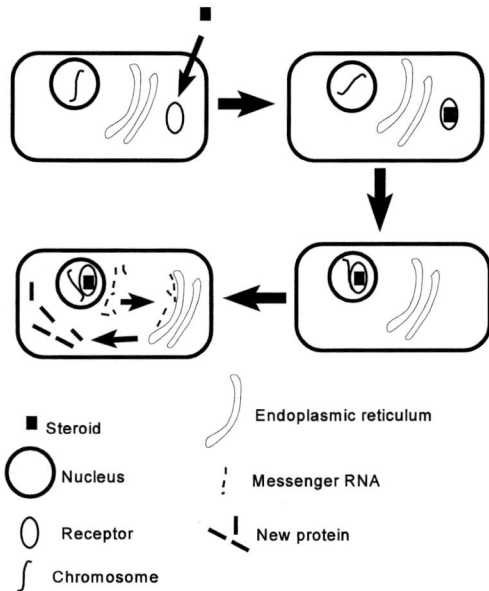

Fig. 1-7. Representation of the interaction between steroid hormones and target cells. Steroid hormones diffuse across the plasma membrane, where they bind to intracellular receptors. The steroid-receptor complex then binds to a specific region on the cell's DNA to promote the transcription and synthesis of new proteins.

Intracellular Action of Iodothyronines

Figure 1-9 illustrates current concepts on the interaction of T_3 with target cells. Intracellular saturable binders of T_3 have been identified in nuclei, mitochondria, and membranes of many animal tissues. Whereas steroid hormones must be transported by a cytosolic receptor to the nucleus upon entering the target cell, free T_3 probably enters the cell and initially interacts with a nuclear receptor. In kidney and liver, most nuclear-associated T_3 comes from the blood, having been deiodinated previously elsewhere. In contrast, nearly half of T_3 in the pituitary gland is derived from local monodeiodination of T_4, rather than having been obtained from the blood after deiodination elsewhere. The nuclear receptor is a protein associated with DNA composed of a single polypeptide chain with a molecular weight of 50,000 to 70,000 daltons.

The exact biochemical interaction of the T_3-receptor complex with DNA is unknown, but it does involve modification of transcriptional events in the nucleus, resulting in an increase in specific messenger RNA (mRNA) that codes for

ments seem to modify the abundance of gene products, i.e., proteins, by specifying the site on DNA where RNA polymerase attaches, whereas hormone response elements affect the frequency of transcript initiation.

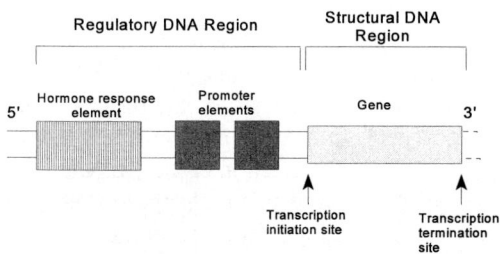

Fig. 1-8. Representation of DNA including the regulatory and structural gene regions. The hormone response element and promoter elements are located 'upstream' of the gene being regulated. Promoter elements appear to modify the abundance of gene products (i.e., proteins) by specifying the site on DNA where RNA polymerase attaches, whereas hormone response elements affect the frequency of transcript initiation.

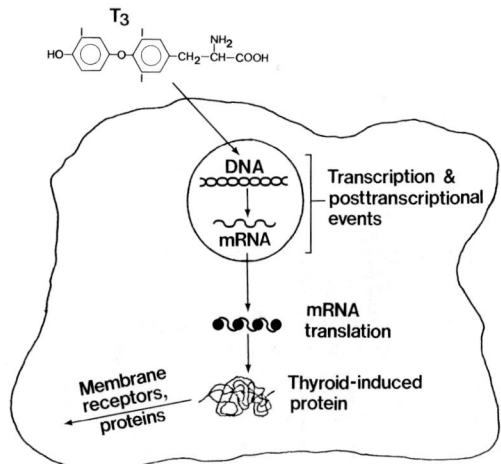

Fig. 1-9. Current concepts of interactions between T_3 and target cells. Unbound T_3 enters the cell and binds to a nuclear receptor protein. The T_3-receptor complex controls transcriptional and/or posttranscriptional events that code for synthesis of specific proteins. (Reprinted with permission from: H. H. Samuels, *In*: Molecular Basis of Thyroid Hormone Action, edited by J. H. Oppenheimer and H. H. Samuels. New York, NY, Academic Press, Inc., 1983, p. 62).

the synthesis of specific structural and enzymatic proteins regulated by iodothyronines. These proteins may be transported elsewhere to regulate other tissues; they may be soluble enzymes that regulate metabolic function of the target cell; or they may be membrane-associated proteins such as receptors for other hormones.

Intracellular Action of Protein and Polypeptide Hormones

Proteins are lipophobic and do not pass readily through the lipid-rich plasma membrane as do steroids and iodothyronines. Rather, they have receptors in the plasma membrane and rely on intracellular messengers to transmit signals (signal transduction) to modify cellular functions. Second messengers for hormones that bind to cell surface receptors include cyclic AMP (cAMP), calcium, phosphatidylinositides, and other unknown factors.

Cyclic AMP (3′,5′-adenylic acid) is derived from ATP (adenosine triphosphate) through the action of adenylate cyclase (Fig. 1-10) and is degraded by phosphodiesterase. Concentrations of cyclic AMP increase or decrease in response to many hormones, including ACTH, LH, FSH, calcitonin, and PTH. Interaction of a hormone with its receptor causes activation or inactivation of adenylate cyclase, a process mediated by a family of stimulatory and inhibitory regulatory proteins. These regulatory proteins are located within the plasma membrane and adenylate cyclase is on the inner surface of the membrane. Therefore, the initial steps in signal transduction are as follows: (a) hormone binds to receptor on the outer surface of the plasma membrane; (b) receptor binding activates intramembranous regulatory proteins; (c) stimulatory regulatory proteins increase adenylate cyclase activity; and (d) adenylate cyclase catalyzes formation of cyclic AMP from ATP.

Other events within the cytoplasm continue the signal transduction process. Cyclic AMP next binds to a protein kinase, an enzyme con-

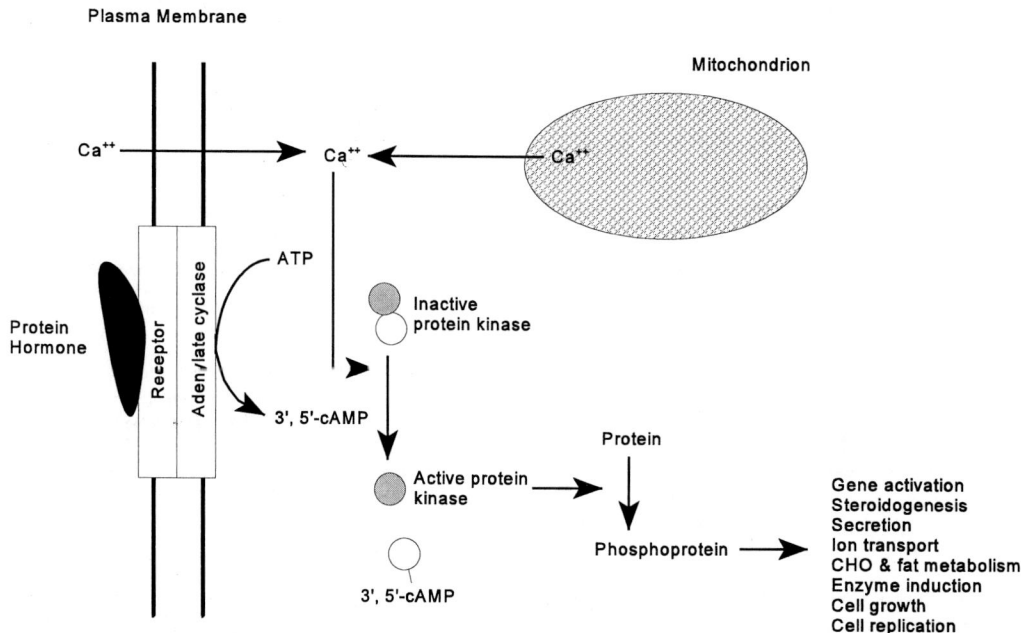

Fig. 1-10. Mechanisms of action of a peptide hormone in a target cell. The signal transduction process is initiated by binding of the peptide to a receptor on the plasma membrane. Second messengers, including 3′,5′-cAMP (cyclic AMP) and ionized calcium, activate intracellular enzymes, leading to phosphorylation of certain proteins that influence such processes as gene activation, steroidogenesis, and secretion. (Modified from: J. F. Habener, *In*: Williams Textbook of Endocrinology, edited by J. D. Wilson and D. W. Foster. Philadelphia, PA, W. B. Saunders Co., 1992, p. 26).

sisting of two regulatory units and two catalytic units. Kinases are enzymes that catalyze the conversion of inactive proenzymes to active enzymes. Cyclic AMP binds to the regulatory units, which leads to dissociation of the catalytic units from the regulatory units. The now-activated catalytic units promote the transfer of the γ-phosphate of ATP to a serine or threonine residue in certain proteins by a process called protein phosphorylation. Protein phosphorylation ultimately leads to diverse processes such as gene activation and inactivation, steroidogenesis, secretion, ion transport, carbohydrate and fat metabolism, enzyme induction, and cell growth and replication.

Some hormone and target cells use ionized calcium or phosphatidylinositides or both as intracellular messages. Other hormones can alter concentrations of ionized calcium in the cytoplasm by changing the permeability of the cell to calcium. Several types of calcium channels in the plasma membrane increase the influx of ionized calcium into the cell. ATP-dependent mechanisms that extrude ionized calcium from the cells or transfer ionized calcium between the cytoplasm and intracellular pools, like those in mitochondria and endoplasmic reticulum, participate in the process (Fig. 1-10). Changes in ionized calcium within the cell regulate a protein called calmodulin. Occupancy of calmodulin's four calcium-binding sites markedly changes its conformation, which leads to regulation of protein kinases and other enzymes as well as changes in structural elements of cells, e.g., mitotic apparatus, endocytosis, and cell motility. Calmodulin is also a component of the enzyme phosphorylase b kinase that converts inactive phosphorylase a to active phosphorylase b. Therefore, like cyclic AMP, ionized calcium regulates several critical metabolic enzymes regulated by protein phosphorylation.

Under certain conditions, calcium can be considered a tertiary messenger because there are other signals between hormone binding to the receptor and intracellular fluxes of ionized calcium. These signals are metabolites of phosphatidylinositol-4,5-diphosphate, a minor plasma membrane phospholipid, that is hydrolyzed by phospholipase C to inositol-1,4,5-P_3 and 1,2-diacylglycerol. These intracellular messengers activate protein kinase C to phosphorylate proteins and promote release of calcium from intracellular stores to activate other protein kinases and cellular changes, as previously described.

QUANTIFICATION OF HORMONES IN BIOLOGICAL FLUIDS

Modern methods of hormone quantification for diagnosis of endocrine diseases, research, and therapeutic monitoring began in the 1950s and 1960s with the discovery and development of the radioimmunoassay. The radioimmunoassay is a type of *in vitro* competitive protein-binding assay in which radioactively labeled and nonradiolabeled ligand, e.g., hormone, compete for a limited number of binding sites on a binding protein. Radioimmunoassays for hormones use specific antisera as the binding proteins and radiolabeled hormones to measure corresponding nonradiolabeled hormones in biologic specimens such as serum, plasma, and urine. Two research groups–one at the Bronx Veterans Administration Hospital in New York City and the other at the University of Washington School of Medicine–were studying metabolism of radiolabeled insulin in human patients with and without diabetes mellitus. Development of a protein-binding assay technique was not the specific aim of their studies. The two research groups simultaneously discovered that serum from diabetic patients who were injected routinely with insulin contained substances that bound the radiolabeled insulin. Whereas both groups suggested that these substances were antibodies produced by the injection of insulin, only Berson and Yalow characterized the substances adequately to prove they were antibodies. They also showed that binding of radiolabeled insulin decreased when nonradiolabeled insulin was added to the serum *in vitro*. These researchers recognized the potential of developing an assay system, prepared high-affinity antisera, and studied kinetics and specificity of antibodies to insulin.

The basic principle of all hormone radioimmunoassays, illustrated in Figure 1-11, is competitive inhibition of binding of radiolabeled

$$Ab + H + H^* \longleftrightarrow Ab\text{-}H + Ab\text{-}H^* + H^*_{excess}$$

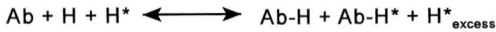

Fig. 1-11. The basic principle of all hormone radioimmunoassays. There is competitive inhibition of binding of radiolabeled hormone (**H***) to antibody (**Ab**) by unlabeled hormone (**H**) present in unknown specimens and standard solutions.

hormone (H*) to antibody (Ab) by unlabeled hormone (H) present in unknown specimens and standard solutions. The labeled and unlabeled hormones are chemically similar. After appropriate incubation, the antibody-bound radiolabeled and unlabeled hormones are separated from the unbound radiolabeled and unlabeled hormones, and the radioactivity in one or the other fraction is quantified with a radiation detector such as a gamma counter or liquid scintillation counter (Fig. 1-12). The amount of radiolabeled hormone bound to the antibody is inversely proportional to the amount of hormone in standard solutions and unknown samples. In other words, the nonradioactive hormone in the standard solutions and unknown samples competes with the radiolabeled hormone for a limited number of binding sites on the antibody molecules. A standard inhibition curve is generated from the standard solutions and used to determine the concentration of the hormone in the unknown samples.

Radioimmunoassays have several advantages over other quantitative procedures for hormones: (a) small sample volumes are needed;

(b) one can assay many samples at a time; and (c) little if any sample preparation is required. Radioimmunoassays can provide excellent specificity, accuracy, sensitivity, and precision. In addition, most reagents are fairly stable, and there is rapid turnaround of results. A few disadvantages include acquiring, handling, and disposal of radioactive materials, expensive radiation detection equipment, limited availability of reagents for animal hormones, and limited shelf life of reagents because of chemical and radioactive deterioration.

Radioimmunoassays must be validated rigorously to prove that they generate reliable results by measuring what they are supposed to measure. The four criteria for assay validity are specificity, accuracy, precision, and sensitivity. Specificity is defined as freedom from interference by substances other than the one intended to be measured. Accuracy is the extent to which a set of measurements of a substance agrees with the exact amount of the substance that is present. Precision is the extent to which a given set of measurements of the same sample agrees with the mean. Finally, sensitivity is defined as the smallest amount of unlabeled hormone that can be distinguished from having no hormone in the sample.

ABNORMAL HORMONE SECRETION

In the last 20 years, the radioimmunoassay and other immunoassay technologies have

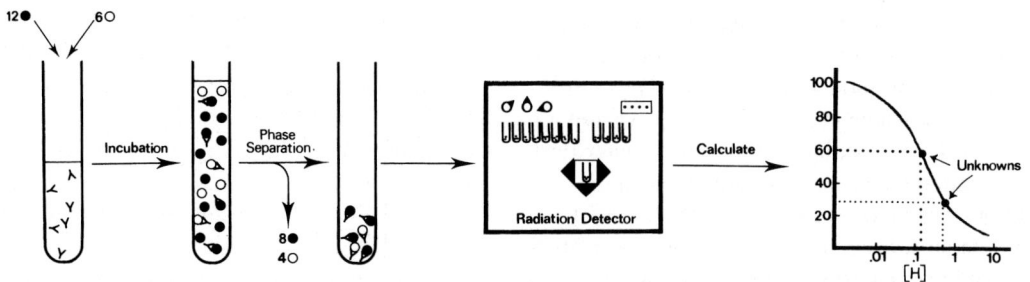

Fig. 1-12. Processes in a radioimmunoassay. After appropriate incubation, the antibody-bound radiolabeled (●) and unlabeled (○) hormone is separated from the unbound radiolabeled and unlabeled hormone and radioactivity in one or the other fraction is quantified with a radiation detector, such as a gamma counter or liquid scintillation. The amount of radiolabeled hormone bound to the antibody is inversely proportional to the amount of hormone in standard solutions and unknown samples. A standard inhibition curve is generated from data obtained from standard solutions and used to determine the concentration of the hormone in the unknown samples.

greatly changed the way abnormal hormone secretion, i.e., endocrine disease, is diagnosed and monitored. Many laboratories now provide immunoassay services for veterinary medical applications.

If an endocrine gland fails to develop properly, is destroyed by disease, synthesizes a biochemically defective hormone, or is damaged by therapy (iatrogenic), primary hypofunction results. Primary hypothyroidism is often the result of an autoimmune process whereby the thyroid gland is invaded by immune cells and the hormone-secreting cells are destroyed. Secondary hypothyroidism can be due to insufficient secretion of TSH, but it should be distinguished from 'hypothyroxinemia', which can be produced by concurrent disease, e.g., hyperadrenocorticism, malnutrition, and certain drugs. In dogs, panhypopituitarism can occur as a result of a developmental defect whereby hormone-secreting cells of the anterior pituitary gland fail to differentiate completely, leading to multiple deficiencies (see Chapter 2, Fig. 2-6). Initially, young puppies will express the condition as pituitary dwarfism because there is a lack of growth hormone secretion. Retarded growth is aggravated by secondary hypothyroidism from lack of TSH secretion, secondary hypoadrenocorticism caused by reduced ACTH secretion, and hypogonadism owing to diminished FSH and LH secretion.

Hyperfunction of endocrine glands causes the expression of several common endocrine diseases in dogs and cats. Hyperadrenocorticism is caused by excessive production of cortisol by the adrenal cortex. In the primary form, an adenoma or carcinoma of the adrenal cortex is formed, producing cortisol that is not controlled by ACTH (Cushing's syndrome). Secondary hyperadrenocorticism (Cushing's disease) results from excessive secretion of ACTH by the pituitary gland, causing morphologic and functional hyperplasia of the adrenal cortex.

Primary hyperparathyroidism is due to excessive autonomous secretion of parathyroid hormone. This excess leads to demineralization of bone, hypercalcemia, renal calculi, and calcification of soft tissues, e.g., nephrocalcinosis. Hyperthyroidism is one of the most common endocrinopathies in cats and is related to the excessive secretion of iodothyronines by proliferative lesions of the follicular cells of the thyroid gland (see Chapter 3, Fig. 3-25). Hyperinsulinemia in dogs and ferrets is caused by neoplasia of the pancreatic beta cells, leading to hypoglycemia.

Occasionally, iatrogenic endocrine diseases occur. An iatrogenic disease is an unfavorable response to therapy caused by the therapeutic effort itself. A common iatrogenic endocrine disease is caused by inappropriate or excessive treatment of animals with glucocorticoids. The disease shows the same manifestations as Cushing's syndrome, which is the spontaneous disease.

REFERENCES

1. Apriletti, J. W., David-Inouye, Y., Baxter, J. D., et al. (1983): Physiochemical characterization of the intranuclear thyroid hormone receptor. *In*: Molecular Basis of Thyroid Hormone Action, edited by J. H. Oppenheimer and H. H. Samuels. New York, NY, Academic Press, Inc., p. 67.
2. Arnaud, C. D. (1983): Hormonal regulation of calcium homeostasis. *In*: Assay of Calcium-regulating Hormones, edited by D. D. Bikle. New York, NY, Springer-Verlag, p. 1.
3. Beato, M., Herrlich, P., and Schütz, G. (1995): Steroid hormone receptors: Many actors in search of a plot. Cell *83*:851.
4. Becker, K. L., Nylén, E. S., and Snider, Jr., R. H. (1990): Endocrinology and the endocrine patient. *In*: Principles and Practice of Endocrinology and Metabolism, edited by K. L. Becker. Philadelphia, PA, J. B. Lippincott Co., p. 2.
5. Benjamin, S. A., Stephens, L. C., Hamilton, B. F., et al. (1996): Associations between lymphocytic thyroiditis, hypothyroidism, and thyroid neoplasia in Beagles. Vet. Pathol. *33*:486.
6. Berson, S. A. and Yalow, R. S. (1959): Quantitative aspects of reaction between insulin and insulin-binding antibody. J. Clin. Invest. *38*:1996.
7. Birnbaumer, L., Codina, J., Mattera, R., et al. (1985): Regulation of hormone receptors and adenylyl cyclases by guanine nucleotide binding N proteins. Recent Prog. Hormone Res. *41*:41.
8. Bondy, P. K. (1985): Disorders of the adrenal cortex. *In*: Williams Textbook of Endocrinology, edited by J. D. Wilson and D. W. Foster. Philadelphia, PA, W. B. Saunders Co., p. 816.
9. Bottoms, G. D., Roesel, O. F., Rausch, F. D., et al. (1972): Circadian variation in plasma cortisol and corticosterone in pigs and mares. Am. J. Vet. Res. *33*:785.
10. Chin, W. W. (1990): Biosynthesis and secretion of peptide hormones. *In*: Principles and Practice of Endocrinology and Metabolism, edited by K. L. Becker. Philadelphia, PA, J. B. Lippincott Co., p. 15.

11. Concannon, P. W. (1986): Clinical and endocrine correlates of canine ovarian cycles and pregnancy. *In*: Current Veterinary Therapy IX, edited by R. E. Kirk. Philadelphia, PA, W. B. Saunders Co., p. 1215.
12. Crantz, F. R. and Larsen, P. R. (1980): Rapid thyroxine to 3,5,3'-triiodothyronine conversion and nuclear 3,5,3'-triiodothyronine binding in rat cerebral cortex and cerebellum. J. Clin. Invest. *65*:935.
13. Darlington, D. N. and Dallman, M. F. (1990). Feedback control in endocrine systems. *In*: Principles and Practice of Endocrinology and Metabolism, edited by K. L. Becker. Philadelphia, PA, J. B. Lippincott Co., p. 38.
14. Dillmann, W. H. (1985): Mechanism of action of thyroid hormones. Med. Clin. North Am. *69*:849.
15. Feldman, E. C. and Nelson, R. W. (1996): Canine and Feline Endocrinology and Reproduction, 2nd ed. Philadelphia, PA, W. B. Saunders Co., p. 38.
16. Ferguson, D. C. (1995): Free thyroid hormone measurements in the diagnosis of thyroid disease. *In*: Current Veterinary Therapy XII, edited by J. D. Bonagura and R. W. Kirk. Philadelphia, PA, W. B. Saunders Co., p. 360.
17. Ghinea, N. and Milgrom, E. (1995): Transport of protein hormones through the vascular endothelium. J. Endocrinol. *145*:1.
18. Granner, D. K. (1990): Hormonal action. *In*: Principles and Practice of Endocrinology and Metabolism, edited by K. L. Becker. Philadelphia, PA, J. B. Lippincott Co., p. 26.
19. Habener, J. F. (1992): Genetic control of hormone formation. *In*: Williams Textbook of Endocrinology, edited by J. D. Wilson and D. W. Foster. Philadelphia, PA, W. B. Saunders Co., p. 9.
20. Holst, J. J. (1983): Gut glucagon, enteroglucagon, gut glucagon-like immunoreactivity, glicentin–current status. Gastroenterology *84*:1602.
21. Horton, R. J. (1990): Testicular steroid transport, metabolism, and effects. *In*: Principles and Practice of Endocrinology and Metabolism, edited by K. L. Becker. Philadelphia, PA, J. B. Lippincott Co., p. 937.
22. Ingbar, S. H. (1985): The thyroid gland. *In*: Williams Textbook of Endocrinology, edited by J. D. Wilson and D. W. Foster. Philadelphia, PA, W. B. Saunders Co., p. 682.
23. Johnson, A. L. (1986): Serum concentrations of prolactin, thyroxine and triiodothyronine relative to season and the estrous cycle in the mare. J. Anim. Sci. *62*:1012.
24. Johnson, A. L. and Malinowski, K. (1986): Daily rhythm of cortisol, and evidence for a photo-inducible phase for prolactin secretion in nonpregnant mares housed under non-interrupted and skeleton photoperiods. J. Anim. Sci. *63*:169.
25. Kahl, S., Bitman, J., and Rumsey, T. S. (1984): Extrathyroidal thyroxine-5'-monodeiodinase activity in cattle. Domestic Anim. Endocrinol. *1*:279.
26. Kendall, J. W. and Allen, R. G. (1990): Adrenocorticotropin and related peptides, and their disorders. *In*: Principles and Practice of Endocrinology and Metabolism, edited by K. L. Becker. Philadelphia, PA, J. B. Lippincott Co., p. 140.
27. Larsen, P. R. and Silva, J. E. (1983): Intrapituitary mechanisms in the control of TSH secretion. *In*:

28. Mangelsdorf, D. J. and Evans, R. M. (1995): The RxR heterodimers and orphan receptors. Cell *83*:841.
29. Mangelsdorf, D. J., Thummel, C., Beato, M., et al. (1995): The nuclear receptor superfamily: The second decade. Cell *83*:835.
30. McDonald, L. E. and Capen, C. C. (1989): Introduction. *In*: Veterinary Endocrinology and Reproduction, 4th ed., edited by L. E. McDonald and M. H. Pineda. Philadelphia, PA, Lea & Febiger, p. 1.
31. McDonald, L. E. (1982): Hormones influencing metabolism. *In*: Veterinary Pharmacology and Therapeutics, 5th ed., edited by N. H. Booth and L. E. McDonald. Ames, IA, Iowa State University Press, p. 553.
32. McKnight, S. L. and Kingsbury, R. (1982): Transcriptional control signals of a eukaryotic protein-coding gene. Science *217*:316.
33. McNatty, K. P., Cashmore M., and Young, A. (1972): Diurnal variation in plasma cortisol levels in sheep. J. Endocrinol. *54*:361.
34. Means, A. R. and Chafouleas, J. G. (1982): Calmodulin in endocrine cells. Annu. Rev. Physiol. *44*:667.
35. Mercken, L., Simons, M.-J., Swillens, S., et al. (1985): Primary structure of bovine thyroglobulin deduced from the sequence of its 8,431-base complementary DNA. Nature *316*:647.
36. Midgley, A. R., Jr., Niswender, G. D., and Rebar, R. W. (1969): Principles for the assessment of radioimmunoassay methods (precision, accuracy, sensitivity, specificity). *In*: Karolinska Symposia on Research Methods in Reproductive Endocrinology, 1st Symposium, edited by A. Diczfalusy. Karolinska Institutet, Stockholm, Sweden, p. 163.
37. Norman, A. W. and Litwack, G. (1987): Hormones. Orlando, FL, Academic Press, Inc., p. 492.
38. Odell, W. D. (1983): Introduction and general principles. *In*: Principles of Competitive Protein-binding Assays, edited by W. D. Odell and P. Franchimont. New York, NY, John Wiley & Sons, p. 1.
39. Rasmussen, H. (1986): The calcium messenger system. N. Engl. J. Med. *314*:1094.
40. Redekopp, C., Irvine, C. H. G., Donald, R. A., et al. (1986): Spontaneous and stimulated adrenocorticotropin and vasopressin pulsatile secretion in the pituitary venous effluent of the horse. Endocrinology *118*:1410.
41. Samuels, H. H. (1983): Identification and characterization of thyroid hormone receptors and action using cell culture techniques. *In*: Molecular Basis of Thyroid Hormone Action, edited by J. H. Oppenheimer and H. H. Samuels. New York, NY, Academic Press, Inc., p. 35.
42. Seal, U. S. and Doe, R. P. (1966): Corticosteroid-binding globulin: Biochemistry, physiology, and phylogeny. *In*: Steroid Dynamics, edited by G. Pincus, T. Nakao, and J. F. Tait. New York, NY, Academic Press, Inc., p. 63.
43. Setchell, B. P. (1993): Male reproduction. *In*: Reproduction in Domestic Animals, World Animal Science B9, edited by G. J. King. Amsterdam, The Netherlands, Elsevier Science Publishers BV, p. 83.

Molecular Basis of Thyroid Hormone Action, edited by J. H. Oppenheimer and H. H. Samuels. New York, NY, Academic Press, Inc., p. 351.

44. Silva, J. E. and Larsen, P. R. (1978): Contributions of plasma triiodothyronine and local thyroxine monodeiodination to triiodothyronine to nuclear triiodothyronine receptor saturation in pituitary, liver, and kidney of hypothyroid rats. J. Clin. Invest. *61*:1247.
45. Van Cauter, E. (1990): Endocrine rhythms. *In:* Principles and Practice of Endocrinology and Metabolism, edited by K. L. Becker. Philadelphia, PA, J. B. Lippincott Co., p. 45.
46. Verschueren, C. P., Selman, P. J., de Vijlder, J. J. M., et al. (1991): Characterization of and radioimmunoassay for canine thyroglobulin. Domestic Anim. Endocrinol. *8*:509.
47. Visser, T. J., Van Der Does-Tobe, I., Docter, R., et al. (1975): Conversion of thyroxine into tri-iodothyronine by rat liver homogenate. Biochem. J. *150*:489.
48. Wilson, J. D. and Foster, D. W. (1992): Introduction. *In*: Williams Textbook of Endocrinology, edited by J. D. Wilson and D. W. Foster. Philadelphia, PA, W. B. Saunders Co., p. 1.
49. Yalow, R. S. and Berson, S. A. (1959): Assay of plasma insulin in human subjects by immunological methods. Nature *184*:1648.
50. Yaniv, M. (1982): Enhancing elements for activation of eukaryotic promoters. Nature *297*:17.

References Added in Proof

51. Barzon, L., Bonaguro. R., Palu, G., et al. (2000): New perspectives for gene therapy in endocrinology. Europ. J. Endocrinol. *143*:447.
52. Houseknecht, K. L., Baile, C. A., Matteri, R. L., et al.(1998):The biology of leptin: A review. J. Anim. Sci. *76*:1405.
53. Hull, K. L. and Harvey, S. (2000): Growth hormone: Roles in male reproduction. Endocrine *13*:243.
54. Lucy, M. C., Bilby, C. R., Kirby, C. J., et al. (1999): Role of growth hormone in development and maintenance of follicles and corpora lutea. J. Reprod. Fertil. *54* (Suppl.):49.
55. Perone, M. J. and Castro, M. G. (1997): Prohormone and proneuropeptide synthesis and secretion. Histol. Histopathol. *12*:1179.
56. Sapolsky, R. M., Romero, L. M., and Munck, A. U. (2000): How do glucocorticoids influence stress responses? Integrating permissive, suppressive, stimulatory, and preparative actions. Endocrine Rev. *21*:55.
57. Turzillo, A. M. and Nett, T. M. (1999): Regulation of GnRH receptor gene expression in sheep and cattle. J. Reprod. Fertil. *54* (Suppl.):75.

The Pituitary Gland

T. J. REIMERS

2

INTRODUCTION

The Greek origin of the word pituitary is *ptuo*, meaning to spit, and the Latin origin of the word pituitary is *pituita*, meaning mucus. Ancient scholars thought that the brain produced mucus secreted by the pituitary gland through the nose. Despite this rhinorrheal attribution, the pituitary gland once was considered the "Master Gland of the Body". This title was bestowed on it because the hormones it secreted affected almost all other endocrine glands of the body and because the pituitary gland seemed to be at the physical and functional apex of the endocrine system. However, as alluded to in Chapter 1, endocrinology has become less provincial

in the past 30 years because of significant research discoveries. In the 1960s and 1970s, important functional connections between the nervous system and pituitary gland were discovered and investigated. The pituitary gland is now known to be controlled by chemical and electrochemical messengers emanating from the brain and other organs and glands.

Despite descendance of master gland status in the 1960s and 1970s, the pituitary gland remains a major controlling participant in the endocrine system. Only the adrenal cortex can match the plethora of hormones produced by the pituitary gland. However, the adrenal cortex produces only closely related steroids, whereas the pituitary gland produces many polypeptide hormones ranging from small peptides to large full-fledged proteins, like luteinizing hormone (LH), follicle-stimulating hormone (FSH), prolactin, and growth hormone, each consisting of approximately 200 amino acids.

MORPHOLOGY

Anatomy

The pituitary gland is also called the hypophysis, a term derived from Greek: *hypo* meaning under and *physis* meaning growth. It is found ventral to the brain in a dorsal concavity of the sphenoid bone called the *sella turcica* or hypophyseal fossa. The sphenoid bone surrounds the pituitary gland bilaterally and ventrally. It is covered by the dura mater, a tough fibrous membrane lining the *sella turcica* and forming the outer layer of the brain. The pituitary stalk or *infundibulum* rises dorsally from the pituitary to connect with the hypothalamus. The hypothalamus forms the floor of the third ven-

17

tricle of the brain and is the site where hypothalamic-releasing hormones enter the primary plexus of the hypophyseal portal system. The pituitary gland is subdivided anatomically into the adenohypophysis and neurohypophysis.

The adenohypophysis has three parts: the *pars distalis*, the *pars tuberalis*, and the *pars intermedia*. The *pars distalis* of the anterior pituitary is the largest part of the adenohypophysis and contains five populations of cells: **thyrotropes, gonadotropes, lactotropes**, and **corticotropes**, which secrete the "tropic" hormones that regulate function of other endocrine glands, and **somatotropes**, which regulate other nonendocrine organs and tissues. The tropic hormones are thyrotropin or thyroid-stimulating hormone (TSH), luteinizing hormone (LH), follicle-stimulating hormone (FSH), prolactin, adrenocorticotropin (ACTH), and growth hormone (GH) or somatotropin (STH).

The *pars tuberalis* is an upward extension of the adenohypophysis and is attached to the *infundibulum*. The *pars intermedia* forms the junction between the *pars distalis* and *pars nervosa* and is the source of melanocyte-stimulating hormone (MSH), particularly important in amphibians in which MSH regulates skin pigmentation. In cattle, pigs, and rats, ACTH produced by the *pars intermedia* is cleaved into α-MSH and corticotropin-like intermediate lobe peptide, or CLIP (see Chapters 1, Fig. 1-3 and 6, Fig. 6-2). The *pars intermedia* of the dog and horse is a significant source of ACTH, and tumors of the *pars intermedia* can lead to spontaneous hyperadrenocorticism in these species.

The neurohypophysis consists of two parts, the *infundibulum* or pituitary stalk and the *pars nervosa* (also called posterior or neural lobe). Hormones produced in the hypothalamus and stored in and released from the neurohypophysis are nonapeptides—with an intramolecular disulfide bond connecting two cysteine residues—and include oxytocin, arginine vasopressin, lysine vasopressin, and arginine vasotocin.

Blood circulation to, within, and from the pituitary gland is complex and plays a major role in regulation of the gland by the hypothalamus and neurohypophysis. The pituitary gland receives both arterial and venous blood. The arterial sources are two paired arteries originating from the internal carotid arteries–the superior and inferior hypophyseal arteries. Venous blood enters the adenohypophysis from two capillary beds. The first is from the median eminence of the hypothalamus (Fig. 2-1). The second is from the lower *infundibulum* and neurohypophysis. Venous blood from the median eminence is collected into two long parallel veins coursing down the *infundibulum* and draining into capillaries of the *pars distalis*. Blood in the primary capillary bed of the posterior pituitary reaches the adenohypophysis via short portal vessels. This unique circulatory architecture constitutes the hypophyseal portal system and forms the endocrine link of the hypothalamus, higher brain centers, and neurohypophysis with the adenohypophysis. High concentrations of hypothalamic hormones affecting adenohypophyseal function are present in the portal blood. The fact that 80 to 90% of the blood supply for the adenohypophysis comes from the portal circulation emphasizes its functional significance. Blood for the neurohypophysis comes from the inferior hypophyseal arteries. Venous blood leaves the pituitary gland through venous sinuses to enter the internal jugular veins.

Despite the proximity of the brain and neurohypophysis to the adenohypophysis, the adenohypophysis receives no direct innervation, except for a few sympathetic fibers that enter along the blood vessels. These fibers seem not to affect hormone synthesis or release directly. Rather, they may affect hypophyseal endocrine function by influencing blood flow. In contrast, the neurohypophysis possesses a rich supply of nerves. Fibers originating from the paraventricular, supraoptic, and other hypothalamic nuclei (Fig. 2-2) enter the neurohypophysis via the *infundibulum*. These fibers contain oxytocin, vasopressin, or vasotocin in nonmammalian species. The fibers also contain their respective carrier proteins called neurophysins.

Embryology

The adenohypophysis and neurohypophysis develop from different embryologic structures (Fig. 2-3). The neurohypophysis, including the

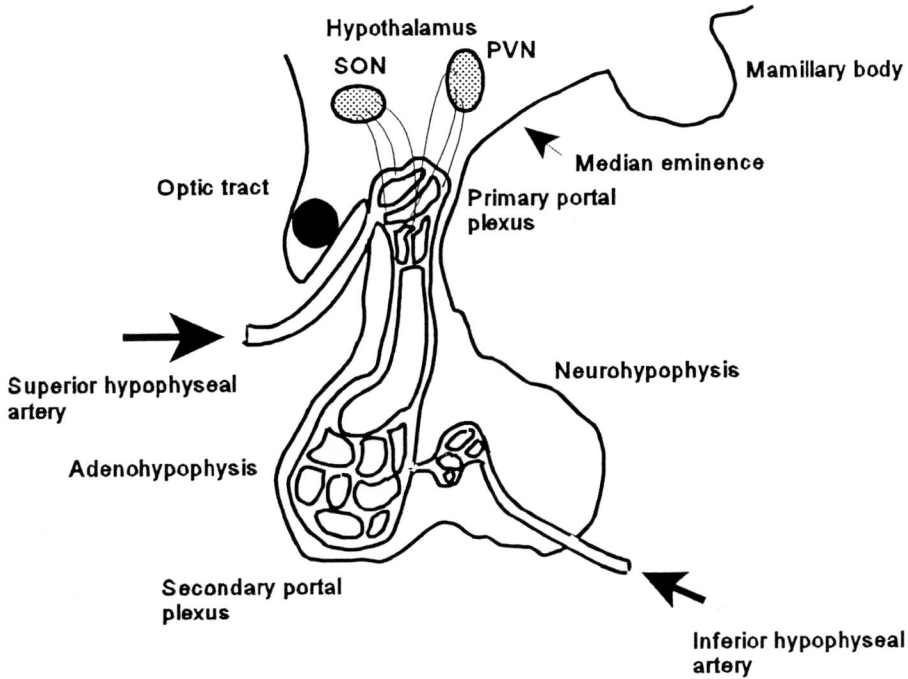

Fig. 2-1. Hypophyseal portal system supplying blood to the anterior pituitary gland. Releasing hormones secreted by neurons in the supraoptic (**SON**) and paraventricular (**PVN**) nuclei of the hypothalamus are released into the primary capillary plexus of the portal system and are transported along the pituitary stalk to the adenohypophysis, where they exert control of the hormone-secreting cells.

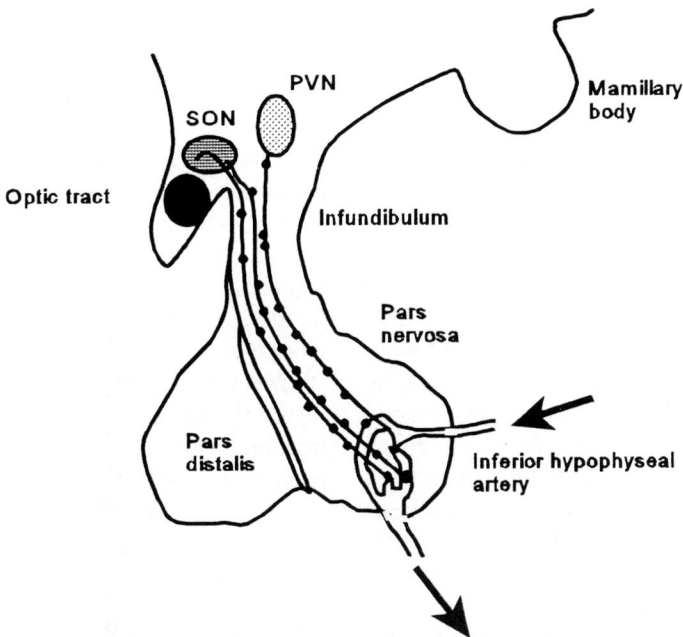

Fig. 2-2. Innervation of the *pars nervosa* of the pituitary gland. Unmyelinated axons originating from cell bodies in the paraventricular (**PVN**), supraoptic (**SON**), and other hypothalamic nuclei enter the neurohypophysis via the *infundibulum*. These fibers transport oxytocin and vasopressin bound to neurophysins, which are released into capillaries draining the neurohypophysis.

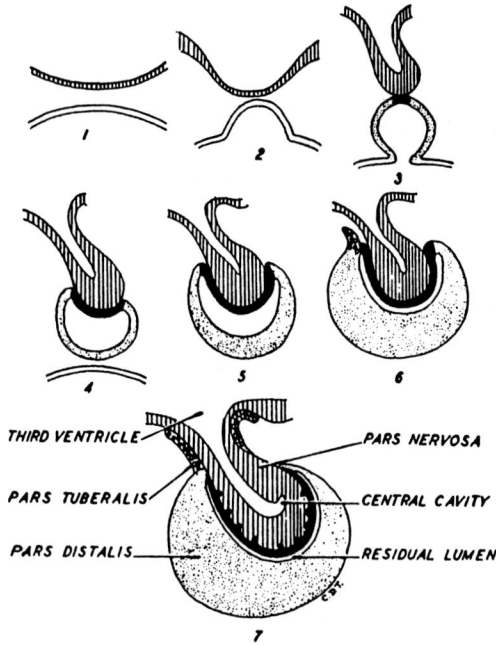

Fig. 2-3. Embryonic development of the mammalian hypophysis. The adenohypophysis, consisting of the *pars distalis*, *pars intermedia* (solid black), and *pars tuberalis*, arises from evagination of the ectodermal roof of the oropharynx, commonly called Rathke's pouch (sketches 1–3). The neurohypophysis, including the infundibulum and the neural lobe, is a specialized extension from the wall of the diencephalon of the developing brain (sketches 1–7). Rathke's pouch enlarges quickly, flattens against the infundibular extension from the brain, and encircles it (sketches 4–6). (Reprinted with permission from: C. D. Turner, General Endocrinology, 3rd ed. W. B. Saunders Co., Philadelphia, PA, 1960, p. 46).

infundibulum and the neural lobe, is a specialized extension from the wall of the diencephalon of the developing brain. The adenohypophysis arises from an evagination of the ectodermal roof of the oropharynx, i.e., a mouth cavity, commonly called Rathke's pouch, named after its discoverer. Rathke's pouch enlarges quickly, flattens against the infundibular extension from the brain, and encircles it. The adenohypophysis surrounds the neurohypophysis to varying degrees in different animal species. The anterior wall of Rathke's pouch thickens to become the *pars distalis*; the back wall remains thin and becomes the *pars inter-*

media. The pouch's connection to the oropharynx elongates into a slender stalk and vanishes. The *pars intermedia* forms from the craniopharyngeal duct near the point that fuses with the *pars nervosa*. This embryonic development results in a total neurologic connection of the neurohypophysis with the hypothalamus but in an almost total lack of innervation to the adenohypophysis.

HYPOTHALAMIC CONTROL OF PITUITARY GLAND FUNCTION

Every hormone produced by the adenohypophysis is regulated by at least one hormone synthesized in hypothalamic nuclei and released into the blood of the hypophyseal portal system to be transported to the *pars distalis*. Hypothalamic hormones were discovered in the 1960s and 1970s by demonstrating that disruption of the anatomic connection between the hypothalamus and pituitary gland greatly affected adenohypophyseal function. Furthermore, extracts of the median eminence and hypothalamus exerted major effects on pituitary hormone secretions both *in vivo* and *in vitro*. Hypothalamic hypophysiotropic substances that stimulate pituitary function originally were called releasing factors after the initial designation of corticotropin-releasing factor (CRF). Now, CRF and other releasing factors are considered true hormones, secreted for hemocrine communication. All hypophysiotropic hormones except dopamine (prolactin release-inhibiting hormone) are peptides. They have been sequenced and synthesized and are available for investigational and therapeutic purposes (Fig. 2-4). The synthetic stimulatory hypophysiotropic hormones are thyrotropin-releasing hormone (TRH), gonadotropin-releasing hormone (GnRH), corticotropin-releasing hormone (CRH), and growth hormone-releasing hormone (GHRH). In addition, cells in the supraoptic and paraventricular hypothalamic nuclei secrete vasopressin and oxytocin, hormones discussed in the Hormones of the Neurohypophysis section of this chapter. Arginine vasopressin (AVP) also is involved in the control of secretion of ACTH.

Corticotropin-releasing hormone (CRH)

Ser-Glu-Glu-Pro-Pro-Ile-Ser-Leu-Asp-Leu-Thr-Phe-His-Leu-Leu-Arg-Glu-Val-Leu-Glu-Met-Ala-Arg-Arg-Glu-Gln-Leu-Ala-Gln-Gln-Ala-His-Ser-Asn-Arg-Lys-Leu-Met-Glu-Ile-Ile-NH₂

Thyrotropin-releasing hormone (TRH)

pGlu-His-Pro-NH₂

Gonadotropin-releasing hormone (GnRH)

pGlu-His-Trp-Ser-Tyr-Gly-Leu-Arg-Pro-Gly-NH₂

Growth hormone-releasing hormone (GHRH)

Tyr-Ala-Asp-Ala-Ile-Phe-Thr-Asn-Ser-Tyr-Arg-Lys-Val-Leu-Gly-Gln-Leu-Ser-Ala-Arg-Lys-Leu-Leu-Gln-Asp-Ile-Met-Ser-Arg-Gln-Gln-Gly-Glu-Ser-Asn-Gln-Glu-Arg-Gly-Ala

Somatotropin release-inhibiting factor (SRIF) or Somatostatin

Ala-Gly-Cys-Lys-Asn-Phe-Phe-Trp-Lys-Thr-Phe-Thr-Ser-Cys

Arginine vasopressin (AVP)

Cys-Tyr-Phe-Gln-Asn-Cys-Pro-Arg-Gly-NH₂

Oxytocin

Cys-Tyr-Ile-Gln-Asn-Cys-Pro-Leu-Gly-NH₂

Fig. 2-4. Amino acid sequences of hypophysiotropic peptides produced by the hypothalamus.

It originally was believed that pituitary hormones were regulated only by stimulatory hypothalamic factors. Now, it is recognized that some pituitary hormones also are under control of inhibiting hormones secreted by the hypothalamus. Prolactin, growth hormone, and TSH are regulated by both releasing and inhibitory hormones. To complicate the hypothalamo-pituitary functional relationship even more, it must be recognized that actions of individual hypophysiotropic hormones are not limited to a single pituitary hormone. For example, TRH not only stimulates release of TSH, but it also induces the release of prolactin and growth hormone. Gonadotropin-releasing hormone stimulates release of both LH and FSH. Finally, it should be emphasized that releasing hormones do more than stimulate release of pituitary hormones. They also regulate pituitary cell differentiation, proliferation, and hormone synthesis.

PITUITARY PROTEIN HORMONES

Adrenocorticotropin

Adrenocorticotropin is a 39-amino acid peptide derived from a much larger precursor called proopiomelanocortin (POMC, MW 28,500 daltons; see Fig. 1-3). The first 18 amino acids of ACTH have the full biologic activity of the whole molecule, and the first 24 amino acids are the same in all species of animals. Other peptides with hormonal activity derived from POMC include β-endorphin, β-lipotropin, and α-melanocyte-stimulating hormone (α-MSH). The role of these three peptides in mammals is not thoroughly understood. Beta-endorphin and β-lipotropin may act to regulate prolactin secretion.

Secretion of ACTH is regulated by hypothalamic CRH and AVP. Arginine vasopressin is a weak regulator of ACTH; it acts synergistically with CRH to stimulate secretion of ACTH. After binding to its receptor on corticotropes, i.e., pituitary ACTH-secreting cells, there is an accumulation of cyclic AMP that serves as the second messenger. Cyclic AMP induces the immediate release of ACTH and transcription of the gene for POMC. Depending on the animal species, cortisol or corticosterone from the adrenal cortex feeds back negatively to regulate CRH and ACTH secretion (see Chapter 6, Fig. 6-6). In addition, ACTH regulates CRH secretion via short-loop feedback to the hypothalamus.

Corticotropin-releasing hormone stimulates the release of ACTH in a pulsatile manner. Also, a circadian rhythm with the highest pulse frequency of ACTH release in blood occurs just before and during the hour after awakening in the morning. This is followed by a progressive decline in ACTH release throughout the remainder of the day. Studies to examine pulsatile and circadian secretion of ACTH require frequent collection of blood samples for analysis of hormone concentrations. These studies must be done with great care because hemorrhage, even minor, is a potent stimulus for secretion of ACTH and cortisol. Furthermore, handling of animals during blood sampling causes significant elevations in serum cortisol concentrations, even after previous adaptation. Many other internal and external stress stimuli increase ACTH and cortisol secretion in prenatal and postnatal domestic animals. These include hypoxemia, hypotension, hypoglycemia, ambient temperature, surgery, trauma, and pain.

Adrenocorticotropin stimulates the cortex of the adrenal gland to secrete the steroid hormone cortisol in most mammals or corticosterone in rodents and lagomorphs. In birds, ACTH stimulates secretion of androgens and mineralocorticoids. In mammals, the adrenal secretion of mineralocorticoids is not under the control of ACTH. Adrenocorticotropin acts on the two inner zones (*zonae fasciculata* and *reticularis*) of the adrenal cortex to increase cortisol or corticosterone secretion. The adrenal cortex responds to ACTH morphologically, by hypertrophy of cells in the *zonae fasciculata* and *reticularis*, and functionally, by increased production of glucocorticoids. Whether ACTH or ACTH-related peptides of proopiomelanocortin directly modulate aldosterone secretion is unresolved, although various stresses that stimulate ACTH secretion also cause aldosterone secretion to increase.

Synthesis of adrenocortical steroids requires: (a) cleavage of the side chain from the 27-carbon cholesterol to form a 21-carbon steroid called pregnenolone; (b) various hydroxylations of pregnenolone; (c) oxidation of the 3β-hydroxyl to a 3-ketone; and (d) a shift of the double bond from carbons 5 and 6 to carbons 4 and 5. Side-chain cleavage of cholesterol is usually the rate-limiting step in steroidogenesis. Four major sources of cholesterol are available to the cell to meet its metabolic needs: Hydrolysis of intracellular cholesterol ester, *de novo* cholesterol synthesis, direct delivery into the cell by passive diffusion of monomolecular cholesterol, or uptake of cholesterol associated with plasma lipoproteins (Fig. 2-5). Uptake of lipoproteins by adrenal cells, conversion of a cholesterol ester to cholesterol, and side-chain cleavage of cholesterol are all stimulated by ACTH. These actions of ACTH are mediated by specific high-affinity receptors on the plasma membrane of the adrenal cortical cell. The intracellular bio-

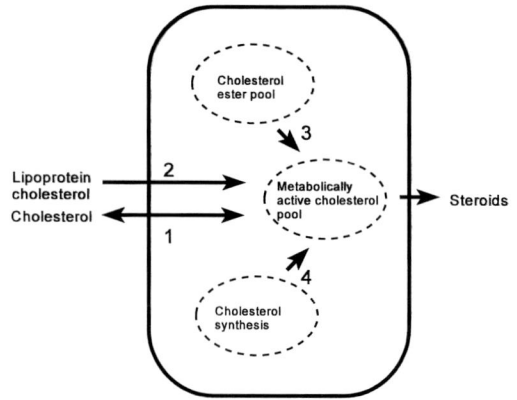

Fig. 2-5. Sources of cholesterol for a steroid-producing cell. The metabolically active cholesterol pool may arise from passive diffusion of monomolecular cholesterol across the cell membrane (*1*), from cholesterol that enters the cell associated with lipoproteins (*2*), from hydrolysis of stored cholesterol esters (*3*), and from *de novo* synthesis of cholesterol (*4*). (Modified from: J. M. Andersen and J. M. Dietschy, J. Biol. Chem. *253*:9024, 1978).

chemical events stimulated by hormones involve activation of adenylate cyclase, accumulation of cyclic AMP, increased protein kinase activity, and phosphorylation of regulatory proteins.

Prolactin

Prolactin is a single-chain polypeptide hormone with a molecular weight of about 23,000 daltons. Its structure is similar in many species with only a few amino acid substitutions. Prolactin is produced by widely dispersed pituitary gland cells called lactotropes or mammotropes, named because of the hormone's indispensable role in lactation. Prolactin is prevalent in all vertebrates from fish to humans. It plays a major role in many reproductive and nonreproductive events including regulation of metamorphosis in amphibians, osmoregulation in teleost fish, proliferative effects on male accessory organs, regulation of parental behavior in several species, stimulation of the brood patch in the sparrow, and stimulation of crop milk formation in pigeons. In rodents, prolactin is important in maintaining structure and function of corpora lutea of the female. Thus, in some old and new literature, prolactin is called luteotropic hormone (LTH). In addition, prolactin stimulates development of receptors for LH on Leydig cells. Hence, prolactin indirectly stimulates secretion of testosterone.

Although prolactin is the most versatile pituitary hormone as to function and species distribution, its role in differentiation and maintenance of the mammary gland and secretion of milk are of primary importance. The stimulus for let-down of milk is provided by suckling. Neurogenic impulses are carried to the brain and to secretory neurons in the hypothalamus that release hypophysiotropic hormones. These hypophysiotropic hormones are relayed to the pituitary gland via the hypophyseal portal system. In the pituitary gland, prolactin secretion is stimulated or inhibited by these hormones.

Whereas all other pituitary hormones are affected primarily by hypophysiotropic hormones that are stimulatory, prolactin is under inhibitory control by dopamine, secreted by the hypothalamus and released into the long vessels of the portal circulation, and by the neurohypophysis, where dopamine is released into the short portal vessels. Surgical disconnection of the pituitary gland from the hypothalamus causes severe reduction in concentrations of most pituitary hormones in blood because of removal of hypothalamic-releasing hormones on the gland. In contrast, pituitary stalk transection initiates a prolonged tonic increase in prolactin secretion. Likewise, posterior lobectomy of male rats produces a significant elevation in prolactin concentrations in blood.

Like other pituitary hormones, prolactin is released in a pulsatile manner. This pulsatility seems independent of any regulation by dopamine because secretion of prolactin from the pituitary gland maintained in culture is also pulsatile. Unlike other pituitary endocrine cells, pituitary lactotropes require constant inhibition by dopamine to keep prolactin secretion under control. Other prolactin-inhibiting factors have been reported to exist–γ-aminobutyric acid and GnRH-associated peptide, for example.

Many naturally occurring compounds that release prolactin also have been described, including TRH, vasoactive intestinal peptide (VIP, so-called because it is produced by cells of the small intestine and the nervous system and because it is a potent vasodilator), serotonin, β-endorphin, somatostatin, gastrin, GnRH, vasopressin, oxytocin, and angiotensin II. Thyrotropin-releasing hormone and VIP have gained considerable credit as prolactin-releasing hormones. Both are directly secreted into the hypophyseal portal blood and directly stimulate prolactin release from the pituitary gland. In addition, VIP is synthesized by the adenohypophysis and is present in lactotropes. Thus, VIP is a hemocrine and autocrine regulator of prolactin secretion.

Prolactin is synthesized, processed, packaged, stored, and released by lactotropes. Dopamine, TRH, and VIP affect both synthesis and release of prolactin. Receptors for these three substances are membrane-bound, and the receptor-ligand interaction is mediated intracellularly by the second messengers–cyclic AMP, ionized calcium, and phosphoinositides. The primary mechanism of dopamine action may be inhibition of cyclic AMP production. Vasoactive intestinal peptide stimulates adenylate cyclase activity and production of cyclic AMP. Calcium, phosphoinositides, and to a lesser extent, cyclic AMP may be involved in the action of TRH on the release of prolactin.

Physiological actions of prolactin are mediated through specific cell-surface receptors in cells of the mammary gland, liver, ovary, testis, and prostate. Intracellular second messengers for prolactin include ionized calcium, polyamines (derivatives of the amino acid arginine), and prostaglandins. The primary action of prolactin on target cells does not appear to involve cyclic AMP. The main site of action is the mammary gland. During pregnancy, insulin, cortisol, triiodothyronine (T_3), estrogen, progesterone, growth hormone, and prolactin play roles in the development of the milk secretory apparatus. Estrogen and progesterone inhibit lactation during pregnancy. However, after parturition, estrogen and progesterone concentrations in blood decrease rapidly, allowing prolactin to initiate lactation. Its effects on lactation include regulation of transcription of genes that encode for milk proteins, such as casein, and stimulation of epithelial cell proliferation in mammary tissue.

Growth Hormone

Growth hormone, or somatotropin, is a single-chain, nonglycosylated protein with a molecular weight of about 22,000 daltons secreted by the pituitary gland. Its pulsatile secretion is regulated by a hypothalamic growth hormone-releasing hormone (GHRH) and growth hormone release-inhibiting factor, or somatostatin, represented by the acronym SRIF (Fig. 2-4). Growth hormone-releasing hormone controls growth hormone synthesis and release by affecting transcription of mRNA; its intracellular second messenger is cyclic AMP. Ionized calcium, diacylglycerol, and inositol triphosphate are also likely to be involved as intracellular mediators.

Somatostatin appears to reduce growth hormone secretion independently of GHRH and by blocking GHRH action. Although the mechanism is not known completely, SRIF may block adenylate cyclase activation caused by GHRH or by inhibiting fluxes in ionized calcium initiated by GHRH. Secretions of GHRH and SRIF are controlled by neuropeptides and neurotransmitters from higher brain centers.

Growth hormone has several major actions involving metabolism, growth, and cellular differentiation. Growth hormone increases lipolysis in adipose cells, glycogenolysis and protein synthesis in liver and muscle cells, and chondrogenesis in bone. It also interacts with membrane receptors of the liver to cause the release of growth-stimulatory peptides called somatomedins. Somatomedins are single-chain proteins that closely resemble proinsulin (see Fig. 1-4). They circulate in blood complexed with binding proteins. Other growth promoters, such as insulin-like growth factors 1 and 2 (IGF-1 and IGF-2) are important participants in tissue growth and organ development. Insulin-like growth factor 1, previously known as somatomedin C, is an important mediator of growth hormone action and is produced by many cells, particularly those of the liver. It also feeds back on the pituitary gland to regulate growth hormone secretion. Blood concentrations of IGF-1 are low in growth-hormone deficiency, i.e., dwarfism, and high in growth hormone excess, i.e., acromegaly. Plasma concentrations of growth hormone and IGF-1 are highly correlated with body size. Large-breed dogs had the highest mean concentrations of IGF-1; concentrations decreased with decreasing body size. Within a single type of dog, Standard Poodles had six times the mean plasma concentration of IGF-1 as Toy Poodles. Insulin-like growth factor 2 is secreted by cells of the central nervous system and is involved mainly with fetal tissue development.

There is considerable species specificity for the actions of growth hormone. Humans respond only to growth hormone purified from human or monkey pituitary glands. Most domestic animals respond best to exogenous growth hormone from their own species. However, the laboratory rat responds to exogenous growth hormone purified from pituitary glands of most other species except fish.

Growth hormone plays a central role in lactation and increases both the soft and osseous tissue masses of the body. Concentrations of growth hormone in blood are high during rapid growth in several species including cattle, swine, and poultry. Growth of the long bones continues as long as the epiphyseal growth plates do not close. In domestic animals, closure of epiphyseal plates after puberty results in cessation of skeletal growth under normal conditions.

Protein metabolism is influenced markedly by growth hormone. Growth hormone stimulates protein synthesis by gene activation and mRNA, ribosomal RNA, and transfer RNA production by liver cells. Prolonged administration of growth hormone to dogs and several other species can induce a permanent hyperglycemia; therefore, growth hormone is diabetogenic. The high blood glucose concentrations stimulate the beta cells of the pancreatic islets to produce insulin until they are eventually exhausted and undergo degeneration.

Growth hormone injected into growing and lactating animals leads to improved nutrient utilization. Pharmacologic doses of growth hormone injected into growing pigs and lambs increase nitrogen retention, improve feed efficiency, increase muscle mass, reduce carcass lipid content, and increase carcass protein content. In high-producing dairy cows, exogenous growth hormone, such as genetically engineered bovine somatotropin (BST), increases milk production 10 to 15% without affecting feed intake, enhances the ability of the mammary tissue to synthesize milk components, and preferentially "partitions" nutrients to the mammary gland and takes these nutrients away from other organs.

PITUITARY GLYCOPROTEIN HORMONES

The three hormones TSH, LH, and FSH are chemically closely related. They are all glycoproteins and consist of two noncovalently bound polypeptide chains called alpha (α) and beta (β) subunits. Within a species, the α subunit is essentially identical for all three hormones, and the differences are minor among species. In contrast, the β subunit, which is also well conserved, is different and accounts for the hormones' biologically specific activities. Each subunit is produced by a separate gene. These polypeptide hormones consist of significant sugar constituents including D-mannose, D-galactose, L-fucose, D-glucosamine, D-galactosamine, and sialic acid. Approximately 16% of the molecular weight is carbohydrate. The α subunit has 92 amino acids in humans and 96 in other species.

Full hormonal activity of these glycoproteins is expressed only by the combined α and β subunits. Hybrids of α and β subunits within and among species have been produced, e.g., TSH α and LH β; LH α and TSH β. In all cases, hormonal activity is dictated by the particular β subunit in the hybrid.

Thyrotropin

Thyrotropin, or thyroid-stimulating hormone (TSH), appears to have only one physiological function–stimulation of the thyroid gland. A few other cell types, e.g., adipocytes, specifically bind TSH, but the physiologic significance of this binding is not known. Bovine TSH is a glycoprotein with a molecular weight of about 28,500 daltons. The molecular weight of the β subunit of TSH is about 18,000 daltons and consists of 110 amino acids. However, multiple forms of biologically active TSH may exist, rep-

resenting different stages of hormone synthesis. Nearly all steps in synthesis and secretion of thyroxine (T_4) and 3,5,3'-triiodothyronine (T_3) are enhanced by TSH. The adenylate cyclase-cyclic AMP system is the intracellular mediator of TSH.

The primary regulator of TSH secretion is feedback by T_3 on the pituitary gland to inhibit TSH synthesis and on the hypothalamus to inhibit TRH synthesis. Conversion of T_4 to T_3 via a special enzymatic system within the pituitary gland plays a major role in regulation of TSH secretion. Within the pituitary gland, production of TSH is regulated at the transcriptional level by T_3 and affects mRNAs for both α and β subunits. Triiodothyronine causes a rapid reduction in transcription of mRNA by a direct action on its nuclear receptor in the promoter regions of the α and β subunit genes. Administration of T_3 to hypothyroid mice rapidly suppressed levels of mRNA encoding for TSH in the thyrotropes. The suppressive action of T_3 on the gene for the β subunit was faster and greater than for the α subunit.

Hypothalamic TRH, which rapidly increases transcription of mRNAs for α and β subunits, is synthesized by peptidergic neurons in the supraoptic and paraventricular nuclei of the hypothalamus and is stored in the median eminence. Lactotropes and thyrotropes of the pituitary gland contain receptors for TRH. Hence, TRH stimulates the *in vivo* secretion of prolactin as well as the secretion of TSH.

Gonadotropins

The gonadotropins LH and FSH are presented together because of their biochemical similarities and close functional relationships. Like TSH, both LH and FSH are glycoproteins consisting of α and β subunits associated by noncovalent bonds. The α subunit is common to both hormones, whereas the specific hormone activity is associated with the β subunit. Combination of both subunits is required for biologic activity. Each gonadotropin is a glycosylated globular protein with a molecular weight of about 28,000 daltons.

Synthesis of gonadotropins by the pituitary gonadotropes consists of transcription of DNA to mRNA, translation of mRNA to prohormone, extensive posttranslational processing and modification including incorporation and modification of oligosaccharides, folding of each subunit into its three-dimensional structure, and formation of the two-subunit complex. The α and β subunits of LH and FSH are encoded by different genes on separate chromosomes. In the pituitary gland, the gonadotropes are often close to the lactotropes, suggesting paracrine communication between them.

Secretion of gonadotropins is regulated by gonadal steroids, i.e., estrogens, androgens, progesterone, and at least one peptide, i.e., inhibin, interacting with hypothalamic GnRH secretion. Inhibin is a glycoprotein with two polypeptide subunits synthesized by Sertoli cells of the testis, granulosa cells of the ovary, the placenta, pituitary gonadotropes, and the brain. Inhibin feeds back negatively on the hypothalamus and pituitary gland to specifically reduce secretion of FSH.

The gonadotropes have specific membrane receptors for GnRH. The intracellular messengers include ionized calcium, inositol triphosphate, and diacylglycerol. Although not completely understood, the proposed mechanism of action of GnRH on the gonadotrope involves increased influx of ionized calcium, increased turnover of phosphatidylinositol to form inositol triphosphate and diacylglycerol, release of calcium from intracellular stores, release of gonadotropin-containing granules near the plasma membrane, movement of more granules toward the plasma membrane, and enhanced gonadotropin synthesis.

Gonadotropes are bihormonal: They synthesize both LH and FSH. Because of this, there must be some mechanism whereby the two gonadotropins can be secreted individually. In Rhesus monkeys and sheep, the frequency and amplitude of exogenous GnRH administered in a pulsatile fashion significantly affects the output of LH and FSH from the pituitary gland. The frequency and amplitude of GnRH secretory pulses determine the relative proportions of LH and FSH secreted by the gonadotropes.

The roles of LH and FSH in reproduction are described in detail in subsequent chapters of this book. Although males do not have corpora lutea, the currently accepted terminology uses LH, standing for luteinizing hormone, for both sexes. Occasionally, readers will see LH in male animals referred to as interstitial cell-stimulating hormone (ICSH).

HORMONES OF THE NEUROHYPOPHYSIS

Arginine Vasopressin and Oxytocin

The *pars nervosa* contains capillaries, small neuroglial cells called pituicytes, and nonmyelinated axons that extend to the *pars nervosa* from neurons in the supraoptic and paraventricular nuclei of the hypothalamus. These axonic fibers contain secretory granules of neurohypophyseal hormones. The hormones secreted by cells in these hypothalamic nuclei in most mammalian species are oxytocin and arginine vasopressin (AVP; Fig. 2-4). Arginine vasopressin is also called antidiuretic hormone or ADH. Oxytocin and AVP are both nonapeptides with a sulfhydryl bond between two cysteine residues at positions 1 and 6. Pigs and other members of the suborder Suina produce lysine vasopressin, which contains lysine instead of arginine in position 8 (Fig. 2-4). Oxytocin and AVP are released into the capillary blood in the *pars nervosa*. In addition, AVP is secreted by cells in the hypothalamic nuclei and released into the primary hypophyseal portal capillary complex and thus reaches the anterior pituitary gland.

Cell bodies of the neurons producing AVP and oxytocin are located in the paraventricular and supraoptic nuclei at the base of the hypothalamus (Fig. 2-2). Cells of both nuclei synthesize both hormones, but the hormones are synthesized by different cells within the nuclei. Cells of the hypothalamic nuclei initially synthesize prohormones, the products of single genes, with a molecular weight of about 21,000 daltons. In the Golgi apparatus, these proteins are glycosylated and packaged as neurosecretory granules. The prohormone-containing granules are transported down the long neuronal axons to their terminals in the *pars nervosa*. During transport, these prohormones are cleaved to yield AVP or oxytocin, with a molecular weight of 1,100 daltons, and their binding proteins, called neurophysins, with a molecular weight of about 10,000 daltons. The binding protein for oxytocin is designated neurophysin I, and that for AVP is designated neurophysin II. Both neurophysins are similar in structure. The hormone-neurophysin complex stabilizes the hormone within the neurosecretory granules.

Release of the hormone and neurophysin from neurosecretory granules is initiated by electrical signals from sensory receptors monitoring the osmolarity of extracellular fluid. Action potentials generated in the osmoreceptors cause an influx of calcium into the axonal terminals, and AVP is released by exocytosis through fusion of the granule's membrane with the neuron's plasma membrane and release of the granular material. Upon release into the blood, AVP and neurophysin II probably dissociate from each other. Hydration of the body or injection of saline solution into the blood going to the hypothalamus inhibits release of AVP, leading to resorption of less water from the glomerular filtrate. Excess water is excreted from the body as diluted urine. Dehydration or injection of hypertonic electrolyte solutions into the hypothalamus stimulates release of AVP, causing increased water resorption in the distal tubules and decreased glomerular filtration, resulting in less urine being produced.

Vasopressin is transported by blood to the kidney, where it binds to specific receptors in the distal part of the nephron and collecting ducts. The major effect of AVP is to increase reabsorption of water from the glomerular filtrate. The AVP-receptor complex activates adenylate cyclase, resulting in increased levels of cyclic AMP. Cyclic AMP activates protein kinases and increases phosphorylation of proteins in cells of the renal distal tubules. Under the influence of AVP, there is a significant uptake of water from the tubular fluid; water moves through small pores across the luminal surface of the cell membrane.

Like AVP, oxytocin is stored as neurosecretory granules and is released from axonal terminals by calcium-dependent exocytosis. The primary stimuli for oxytocin release from storage sites in the neurohypophysis are distention of the reproductive tract, particularly in the pregnant female, stimulation of the mammary gland by the young, or audiovisual contact with the offspring.

Oxytocin has specific effects on contraction of smooth muscle of the uterus and cells of the mammary gland. In veterinary medicine, oxytocin is used for inducing parturition in some species, or to increase uterine contractions at parturition, and for the treatment of retained placenta, metritis, and in some cases agalactia (absence of milk flow from the udder).

DISORDERS OF PITUITARY FUNCTION

As discussed previously in this chapter, the mammalian anterior pituitary secretes six major hormones–prolactin, growth hormone, ACTH, LH, FSH, and TSH. A deficiency of any of these can occur, such as in secondary hypothyroidism or secondary hypoadrenocorticism. In panhypopituitarism, secretion of all hormones from the anterior pituitary is abnormally low or absent. In young dogs, most of the clinical manifestations are associated with diminished growth hormone secretion and dwarfism (Fig. 2-6). Juvenile panhypopituitarism occurs most frequently in German Shepherd dogs, but it also has been reported in a few other breeds. Pituitary dwarfism in German Shepherds usually is caused by a failure of Rathke's pouch to differentiate into the hormone-secreting cells of the *pars distalis*. In their place develop multiple large and small cysts in the *sella turcica*, which are distended with amorphous mucoidal material. Few differentiated, tropic endocrine cells are present in the *sella turcica* of dwarfs. Basal growth hormone and IGF-1 concentrations in plasma of dwarf dogs are greatly reduced, and growth hormone concentrations do not increase after injection of clonidine (an α-adrenergic antagonist), a standard dynamic test for growth hormone secretory capacity.

Affected pups appear normal at birth and usually are indistinguishable from littermates up to about 2 months of age. Subsequently, the slower growth rate relative to their littermates, the retention of puppy hair coat, and a lack of primary guard hairs (coarse hairs covering the underfur) are indicative of dwarfism (Fig. 2-7).

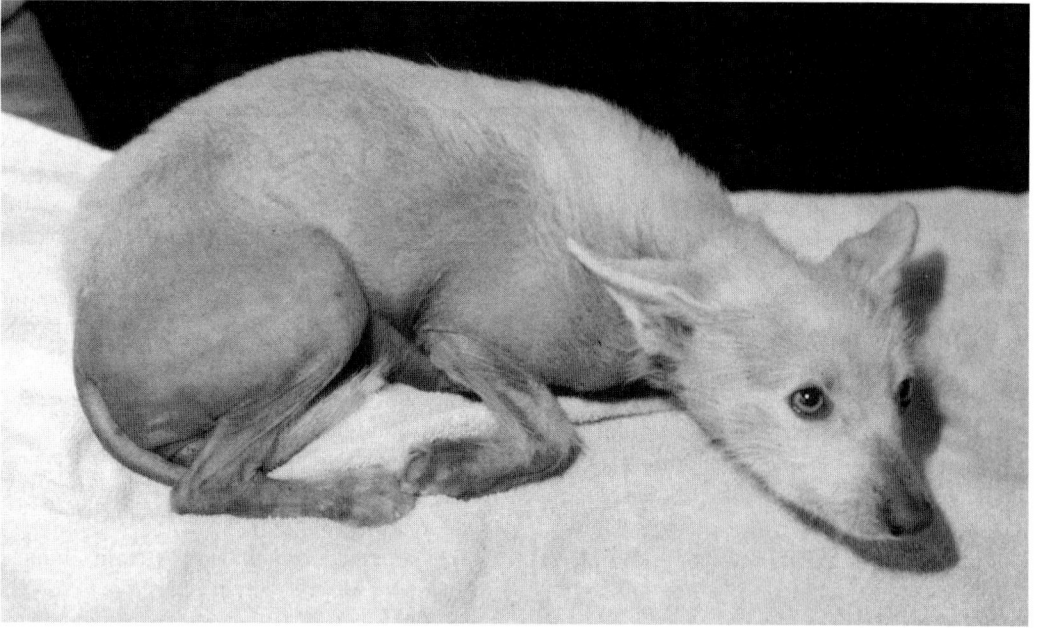

Fig. 2-6. Panhypopituitarism in a white German Shepherd dog. Note the failure of somatic maturation and large areas of alopecia. (Courtesy of Dr. Danny Scott, Department of Clinical Sciences, College of Veterinary Medicine, Cornell University, Ithaca, NY).

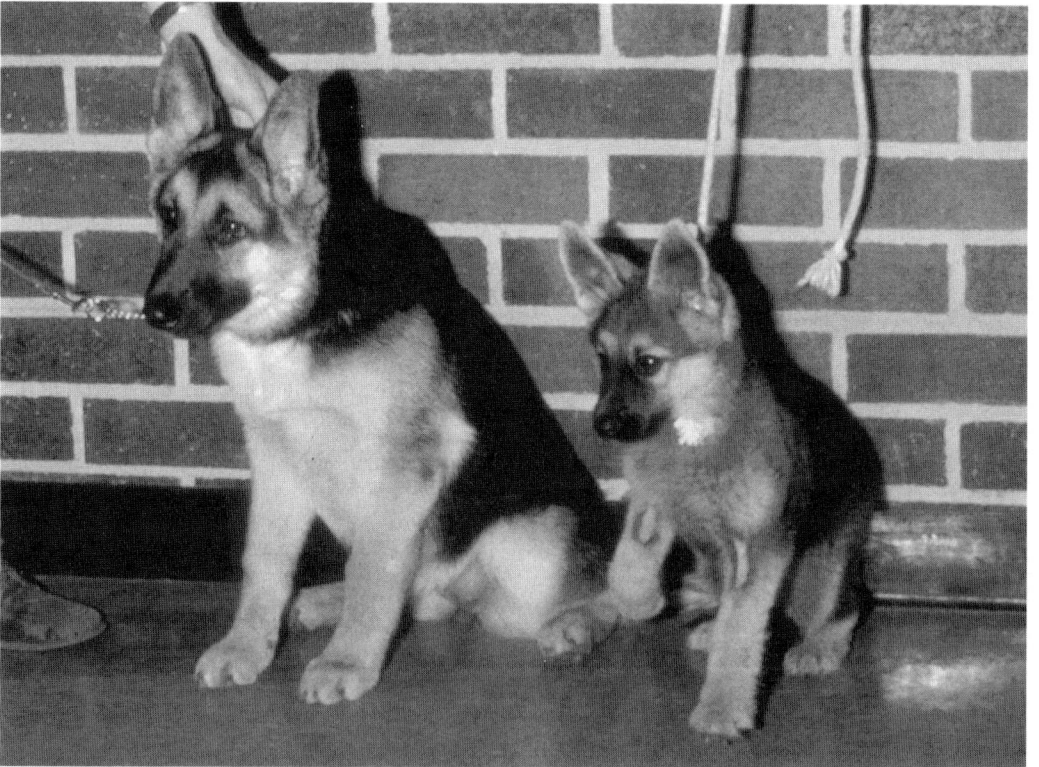

Fig. 2-7. Pituitary dwarfism in a German Shepherd (**right**) along with an unaffected littermate. (Courtesy of Dr. Danny Scott, Department of Clinical Sciences, College of Veterinary Medicine, Cornell University, Ithaca, NY).

A bilaterally symmetric alopecia develops gradually and often progresses to complete alopecia except for the head and tufts of hair on the legs. There is progressive hyperpigmentation of the skin until it is uniformly brown-black over most of the body. Adult German Shepherd dogs with juvenile-onset panhypopituitarism vary in weight from only 2 kg up to nearly half the normal size of 35 to 55 kg, apparently depending upon whether there was a partial or a complete failure of adenohypophyseal development during embryogenesis.

Permanent dentition is delayed or completely absent in growth hormone-deficient dogs. Closure of epiphyseal plates is delayed as long as 4 years depending on the severity of hormonal deficiency. The testes and penis remain small in males that have reached the age of sexual maturity; the ovarian cortex is hypoplastic and estrus is irregular or absent in females. Clinical manifestations of growth hormone deficiency are worsened by concomitant secondary hypoadrenocorticism, hypothyroidism, and hypogonadism.

Acromegaly is a disease caused by excess growth hormone secretion. Its clinical manifestations include an overgrowth of connective tissue, increased growth of bone, coarsening of facial features, and enlargement of viscera (Fig. 2-8). The most common cause of the disease in cats appears to be growth hormone-secreting tumors of somatotropes. In dogs, the most common type of acromegaly is due to somatotropic hyperplasia induced by progesterone and progestagens, which are progesterone-like compounds. Stimulation of growth hormone secretion by these hormones is dose related–the greater the dose of progestagen, the higher the growth hormone concentration in plasma.

Functional tumors arising in the pituitary gland often are derived from corticotropes in either the *pars distalis* or the *pars intermedia*, leading to hyperadrenocorticism or excess cortisol secretion from the adrenal cortex. These neoplasms are encountered most frequently in dogs and horses. They develop in adult to geriatric dogs and have been reported in several breeds, but Boxers, Boston Terriers, and

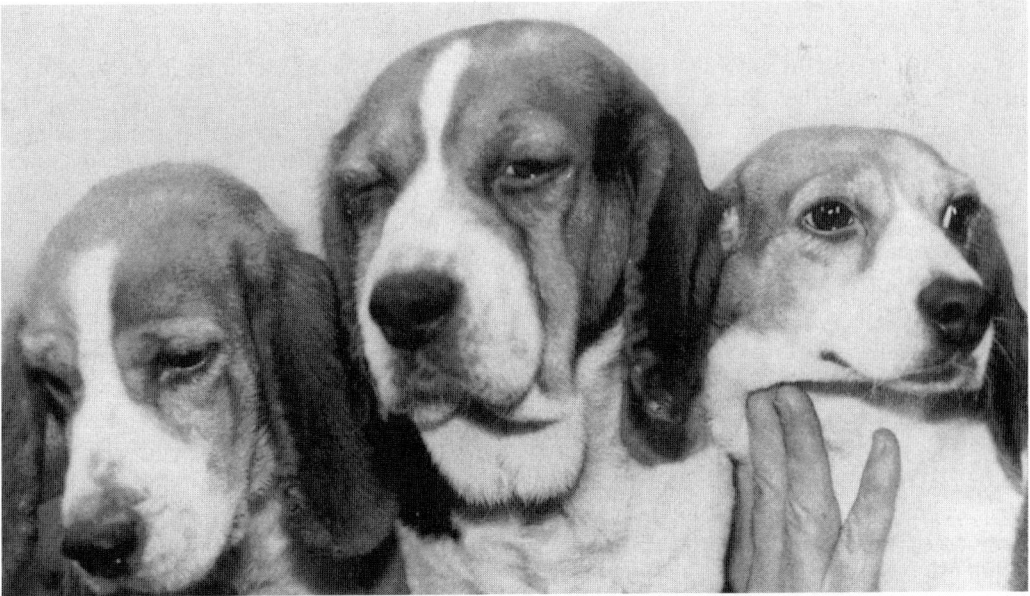

Fig. 2-8. Acromegaly in a Beagle dog (**center**) compared with unaffected littermates (**left** and **right**). Note the coarseness of facial features and marked thickening and folding of the skin of the face. (Courtesy of Dr. Patrick Concannon, Department of Physiology, College of Veterinary Medicine, Cornell University, Ithaca, NY).

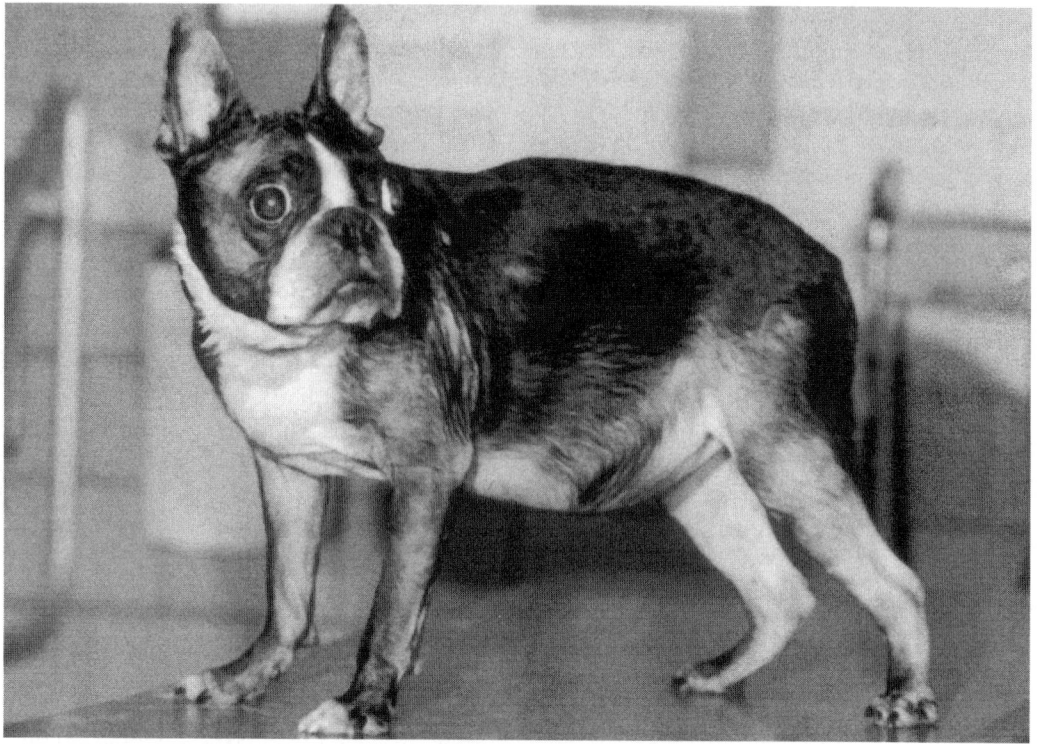

Fig. 2-9. Hyperadrenocorticism in a Boston Terrier with an ACTH-secreting pituitary tumor. Long-term secretion of excessive cortisol resulted in alopecia and muscle wasting, evident from the pendulous abdomen. (Courtesy of Dr. John Randolph, Department of Clinical Sciences, College of Veterinary Medicine, Cornell University, Ithaca, NY).

Dachshunds appear to have the highest incidence (Fig. 2-9). The clinical manifestations and lesions that develop are the result of long-term overproduction of ACTH by the tumor and cortisol by bilaterally hyperplastic adrenal cortices. These changes are the result of the combined gluconeogenic, lipolytic, protein catabolic, and anti-inflammatory actions of adrenocortical hormones on many organ systems of the body.

Adenomas derived from cells of the *pars distalis* are the most common type of ACTH-secreting pituitary tumor in horses, ponies, and donkeys. These tumors develop in older animals, with females affected more frequently than males. Affected animals often develop a strikingly excessive growth of hair (hirsutism) because of a failure of seasonal shedding of hair (Fig. 2-10). Hair over most of the trunk and extremities is long, up to 4 or 5 inches, abnormally thick, wavy, and often matted. Other clinical manifestations and sequelae associated with tumors of the *pars distalis* are polyuria, polydipsia, hyperphagia, muscle weakness, laminitis, diabetes mellitus, dullness, intermittent fever, and excessive sweating.

Diabetes insipidus is a disorder characterized by chronic excretion of large volumes of dilute urine that is accompanied by extreme thirst caused by hyperosmolarity of body fluids and dehydration. Central diabetes insipidus is caused by inadequate production of AVP by the posterior pituitary gland. Nephrogenic diabetes insipidus is produced by several disorders that interfere with the interaction between AVP and its receptors in target cells of the kidney. Central diabetes insipidus results mainly from destruction of the supraoptic and paraventricular nuclei of the hypothalamus, where AVP is produced, or by destruction of the axons carrying AVP to ax-

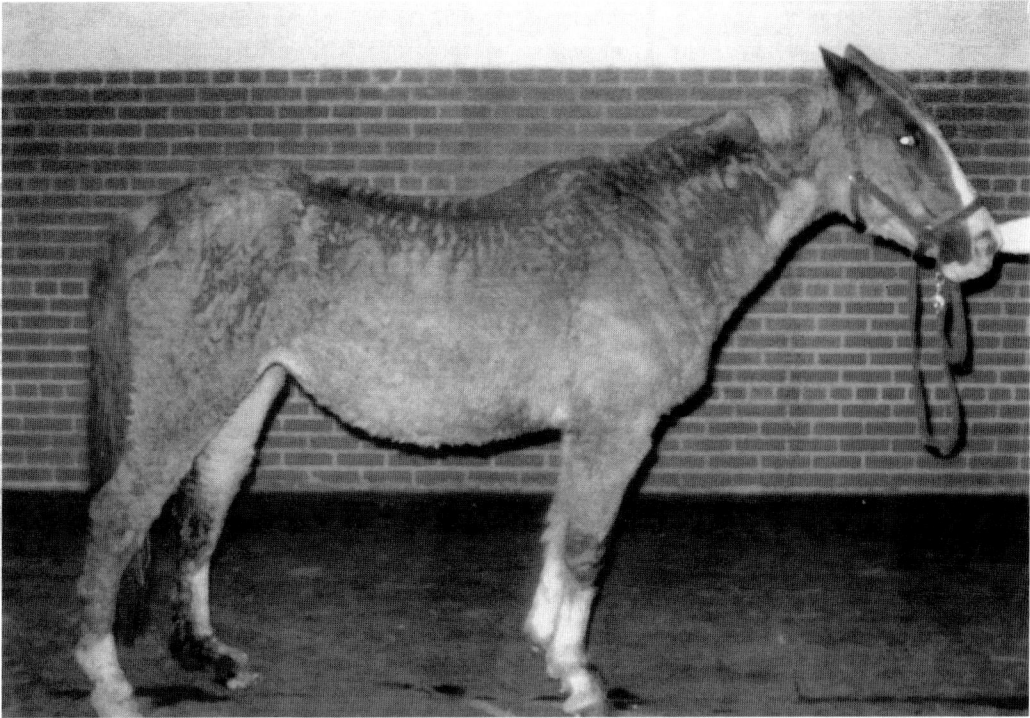

Fig. 2-10. A horse with a pituitary adenoma resulting in hirsutism from a failure of seasonal shedding of hair. (Courtesy of Dr. Dorothy Ainsworth, Department of Clinical Sciences, College of Veterinary Medicine, Cornell University, Ithaca, NY).

onal terminals in the *pars nervosa*. The lesions responsible for this disruption of AVP secretion include large pituitary neoplasms, a dorsally expanding cyst or inflammatory granuloma, and traumatic injury to the skull.

PITUITARY-LIKE HORMONES OF THE PLACENTA

Since Halban suggested that the placenta had an endocrine function in 1905, many articles have been published on the production of peptide, protein, and steroid hormones by this organ. Most of the placental protein and peptide hormones are structurally and functionally similar to hormones produced by the pituitary gland and hypothalamus. Several placental hormones are useful therapeutic agents for veterinary medicine.

Placental Lactogen

Placental lactogen is a protein hormone so-named because it has lactogenic properties in bioassays and prolactin-like activity in radioreceptor assays. Ovine placental lactogen (oPL), a protein with a molecular weight of 20,000 to 23,000 daltons, has an amino acid composition similar to ovine prolactin and ovine growth hormone. Using immunocytochemical methods, oPL has been localized in secretory granules of mononucleate and binucleate cells of the trophoblastic component of the placenta. The binucleate trophoblastic cells migrate across the fetomaternal junction and fuse to form a syncytium that is closely associated with the maternal blood circulation. After the sixth week of pregnancy, concentrations of oPL in the circulation of the ewe increase steadily, reach their highest concentrations between 120 and 140 days of gestation, and decline before parturition. Concentrations of oPL in the blood of the fetus remain relatively constant until about 120 days of gestation and then decline until parturition.

During the first half of pregnancy, maternal blood concentrations of oPL may be governed in part by changes in the number of binucleate cells in the placenta. Maternal blood concentrations also are affected by the number of fetuses present–concentrations are greater in ewes carrying twins or triplets than in ewes with one fetus. Ovine PL concentrations in blood also are influenced by metabolic state, e.g., fasting.

Caprine and bovine placental lactogens have molecular weights of 20,000 to 25,000 and 30,000 to 34,000 daltons, respectively. Bovine PL has been localized in the binucleate cells of the fetal placenta. Although not totally understood, placental lactogens appear to plays roles in regulating mammary gland function, fetal growth, maternal intermediary metabolism, and ovarian steroidogenesis.

Gonadotropins

Chorionic (i.e., placental) gonadotropins are used commonly in veterinary medicine to duplicate the biological effects of LH and FSH. Human chorionic gonadotropin (hCG) for medical use is obtained from the urine of pregnant women. It closely mimics the effects of LH and has some FSH activity. In female animals, injected hCG promotes maturation of ovarian follicles, ovulation, and formation of corpora lutea. In males, it stimulates testicular interstitial cells to produce testosterone. It is used clinically to treat ovarian follicular cysts, nymphomania (constant or frequent heat), cryptorchidism, and male infertility, and to induce or hasten ovulation. It is used also in dynamic diagnostic tests to determine if remnant testicular tissue is present in castrated male dogs and cats and if remnant ovarian tissue is present in ovariohysterectomized females.

Like TSH, LH, and FSH, hCG is a glycoprotein consisting of two nonidentical α and β subunits. The α subunit of hCG is a single chain of 92 amino acids, whereas the β subunit consists of 145 amino acids. Both subunits are required for biologic activity because portions of both subunits bind to cellular receptors. Using immunocytochemical techniques, hCG and its subunits have been localized primarily in syncytiotrophoblast of the placenta.

The placenta of the mare also produces a gonadotropin called equine chorionic gonado-

tropin (eCG) or pregnant mare's serum gonadotropin (PMSG). Chorionic gonadotropins have been identified in horses, donkeys, zebras, and their hybrids. Horse CG is a glycoprotein consisting of two noncovalently associated subunits. However, their amino acid sequences are not the same among species like other α subunits. The α subunit consists of 96 amino acids. The β subunit consists of 149 amino acids and is identical with the β subunit of horse LH.

Equine CG is synthesized by the endometrial cups of the uterus, which in mares begin to develop about day 36 of pregnancy. The endometrial cups are formed when trophoblastic cells from the chorion attach to the endometrial epithelium and migrate into the endometrium. The cups begin to degenerate by day 60 of gestation but persist until about day 120 of pregnancy.

In horse mares, eCG appears in maternal blood on about day 40 of pregnancy. Blood concentrations increase rapidly to peak values between days 55 and 65 and then decline to very low concentrations by day 125. Concentrations in blood parallel formation and degeneration of the endometrial cups. Equine CG has high FSH-like activity and is administered to cows to induce superovulation for embryo transfer.

Other Endocrine Activities

Beside lactogens and gonadotropins, the placenta also produces peptides with GnRH-, TRH-, GHRH-, CRH-, and ACTH-like activities. Much more research remains to be done to determine functions and regulatory processes for all of the placental hormones.

REFERENCES

1. Andersen, J. M. and Dietschy, J. M. (1978): Relative importance of high- and low-density lipoproteins in the regulation of cholesterol synthesis in the adrenal gland, ovary, and testis of the rat. J. Biol. Chem. *253*:9024.
2. Arey, L. B. (1965): Developmental Anatomy. Philadelphia, PA, W. B. Saunders Co., p. 230.
3. Barinaga, M., Yamonoto, G., Rivier, C., et al. (1983): Transcriptional regulation of growth hormone gene expression by growth hormone-releasing factor. Nature *306*:84.
4. Bauman, D. E., Eisemann, J. H., and Currie, W. B. (1982): Hormonal effects on partitioning of nutrients for tissue growth: Role of growth hormone and prolactin. Fed. Proc. *41*:2538.

5. Ben-Jonathan, N. (1985): Dopamine: A prolactin-inhibiting hormone. Endocrine Rev. *6*:564.

6. Bondy, P. K. (1985): Disorders of the adrenal cortex. *In*: Williams Textbook of Endocrinology, 7th ed., edited by J. D. Wilson and D. W. Foster. Philadelphia, PA, W. B. Saunders Co., p. 816.

7. Buonomo, F. C. and Baile, C. A. (1990): The neurophysiological regulation of growth hormone secretion. Domestic Anim. Endocrinol. *7*:435.

8. Capen, C. C. and Martin, S. L. (1989): The pituitary gland. *In*: Veterinary Endocrinology and Reproduction, 4th ed., edited by L. E. McDonald and M. H. Pineda. Philadelphia, PA, Lea & Febiger, p. 19.

9. Chin, W. W., Shupnik, M. A., Ross, D. S., et al. (1985): Regulation of the α and thyrotropin β-subunit messenger ribonucleic acids by thyroid hormones. Endocrinology *116*:873.

10. Clarke, I. J., Cummins, J. T., Findlay, J. K., et al. (1984): Effects on plasma luteinizing hormone and follicle-stimulating hormone of varying the frequency and amplitude of gonadotropin-releasing hormone pulses in ovariectomized ewes with hypothalamo-pituitary disconnection. Neuroendocrinology *39*:214.

11. Concannon, P., Altszuler, N., Hampshire, J., et al. (1980): Growth hormone, prolactin, and cortisol in dogs developing mammary nodules and an acromegaly-like appearance during treatment with medroxyprogesterone acetate. Endocrinology *106*:1173.

12. De Silva, M., Kiehm, D. J., Kaltenbach, C. C., et al. (1986): Comparison of serum cortisol and prolactin in sheep blood sampled by two methods. Domestic Anim. Endocrinol. *3*:11.

13. DeBold, C. R., Sheldon, W. R., DeCherney, G. S., et al. (1984): Arginine vasopressin potentiates adrenocorticotropin release induced by ovine corticotropin-releasing factor. J. Clin. Invest. *73*:533.

14. Dickson, W. M. (1984): Endocrine glands. *In*: Dukes' Physiology of Domestic Animals, 10th ed., edited by M. J. Swenson. Ithaca, NY, Cornell University Press, p. 761.

15. Driefuss, J. J. (1975): A review of neurosecretory granules: Their contents and mechanisms of release. Ann. N. Y. Acad. Sci. *248*:184.

16. Dumont, J. E., Willems, C., Van Sande, J., et al. (1971): Regulation of the release of thyroid hormones: Role of cyclic AMP. Ann. N. Y. Acad. Sci. *185*:291.

17. Eigenmann, J. E., Zanesco, S., Arnold, U., et al. (1984): Growth hormone and insulin-like growth factor I in German Shepherd dwarf dogs. Acta Endocrinol. *105*:289.

18. Eigenmann, J. E. (1985): Growth hormone and insulin-like growth factor in the dog: Clinical and experimental investigations. Domestic Anim. Endocrinol. *2*:1.

19. Eipper, B. A. and Mains, R. E. (1980): Structure and biosynthesis of pro-adrenocorticotropin/endorphin and related peptides. Endocrine Rev. *1*:1.

20. Etherton, T. D., Wiggins, J. P., Evock, C. M., et al. (1987): Stimulation of pig performance by porcine growth hormone: Determination of the dose-response relationship. J. Anim. Sci. *64*:433.

21. Everett, J. W. (1956): Functional corpora lutea maintained for months by autografts of rat hypophysis. Endocrinology *58*:786.

22. Evock, C. M., Etherton, T. D., Chung, C. S., et al. (1988): Pituitary porcine growth hormone (pGH) and a recombinant pGH analog stimulate pig growth performance in a similar manner. J. Anim. Sci. *66*:1928.

23. Feldman, E. C. and Nelson, R. W. (1996): Canine and Feline Endocrinology and Reproduction, 2nd ed. Philadelphia, PA, W. B. Saunders Co., p. 9.

24. Fink, G. (1988): Gonadotropin secretion and its control. *In*: The Physiology of Reproduction, edited by E. Knobil and J. Neill. New York, NY, Raven Press, p. 1349.

25. Ghinea, N. and Milgrom, E. (1995): Transport of protein hormones through the vascular endothelium. J. Endocrinol. *145*:1.

26. Halmi, N. S., Peterson, M. E., Colurso, G. J., et al. (1981): Pituitary intermediate lobe in dogs: Two cell types and high bioactive adrenocorticotropin content. Science *211*:72.

27. Heinrichs, M., Baumgartner, W., Capen, C. C. (1990): Immunocytochemical demonstration of pro-opiomelanocortin-derived peptides in pituitary adenomas of the *pars intermedia* in horses. Vet. Pathol. *27*:419.

28. Ingbar, S. H. (1985): The thyroid gland. *In*: Williams Textbook of Endocrinology, 7th ed., edited by J. D. Wilson and D. W. Foster. Philadelphia, PA, W. B. Saunders, p. 682.

29. Kendall, J. W. and Allen, R. G. (1990): Adrenocorticotropin and related peptides and their disorders. *In*: Principles and Practice of Endocrinology and Metabolism, edited by K. L. Becker. Philadelphia, PA, J. B. Lippincott Co., p. 140.

30. Larsen, P. R., Silva, J. E., and Kaplan, M. M. (1981): Relationships between circulating and intracellular thyroid hormones: Physiological and clinical implications. Endocrine Rev. *2*:87.

31. Leong, D. A., Frawley, L. S., and Neill, J. D. (1983): Neuroendocrine control of prolactin secretion. Annu. Rev. Physiol. *45*:109.

32. Leung, P. C. K. and Steele, G. L. (1992): Intracellular signaling in the gonads. Endocrine Rev. *13*:476.

33. Lilly, M. P., Engeland, W. C., and Gann, D. S. (1983): Responses of cortisol secretion to repeated hemorrhage in the anesthetized dog. Endocrinology *112*:681.

34. Love, S. (1993): Equine Cushing's disease. Br. Vet. J. *149*:139.

35. Mahesh, V. B. and Brann, D. W. (1992): Interaction between ovarian and adrenal steroids in the regulation of gonadotropin secretion. J. Steroid Biochem. Mol. Biol. *41*:495.

36. McDonald, L. E. (1982): Hormones influencing metabolism. *In*: Veterinary Pharmacology and Therapeutics, 5th ed., edited by N. H. Booth and L. E. McDonald. Ames, IA, Iowa State University Press, p. 553.

37. Muir, L. A., Wien, S., Duquette, P. F., et al. (1983): Effects of exogenous growth hormone and diethylstilbestrol on growth and carcass composition of growing lambs. J. Anim. Sci. *56*:1315.

38. Muller, G. H. and Jones, S. R. (1973): Pituitary dwarfism and alopecia in a German Shepherd with a cystic Rathke's cleft. J. Am. Anim. Hosp. Assoc. *9*:567.

39. Murai, I. and Ben-Jonathan, N. (1987): Posterior pituitary lobectomy abolishes the suckling-induced rise in

prolactin (PRL): Evidence for a PRL-releasing factor in the posterior pituitary. Endocrinology *121*:205.

40. Murphy, B. D. and Martinuk, S. D. (1991): Equine chorionic gonadotropin. Endocrine Rev. *12*:27.

41. Neill, J. D. (1988): Prolactin secretion and its control. *In*: The Physiology of Reproduction, edited by E. Knobil and J. Neill. New York, NY, Raven Press, p. 1379.

42. Nicoll, C. S. (1974): Physiological actions of prolactin. *In*: Handbook of Physiology, Vol. IV, Sec. 7, Part 2, edited by R. O. Greep and E. B. Astwood. Washington, DC, American Physiological Society, p. 253.

43. Norman, A. W. and Litwack, G. (1987): Hormones. Orlando, FL, Academic Press, Inc. p. 210.

44. Peters, L. L., Hoefer, M. T., and Ben-Jonathan, N. (1981): The posterior pituitary: Regulation of anterior pituitary prolactin secretion. Science *213*:659.

45. Peterson, M. E., Krieger, D. T., Drucker, W. D., et al. (1982): Immunocytochemical study of the hypophysis in 25 dogs with pituitary-dependent hyperadrenocorticism. Acta Endocrinol. *101*:15.

46. Peterson, M. E., Taylor, R. S., Greco, D. S., et al. (1990): Acromegaly in 14 cats. J. Vet. Intern. Med. *4*:192.

47. Pierce, J. G. (1988): Gonadotropins: Chemistry and biosynthesis. *In*: The Physiology of Reproduction, edited by E. Knobil and J. Neill. New York, NY, Raven Press, p. 1335.

48. Pierce, J. G. and Parsons, T. F. (1981): Glycoprotein hormones: Structure and function. Annu. Rev. Biochem. *50*:465.

49. Pohl, C. R., Richardson, D. W., Hutchinson, J. S., et al. (1983): Hypophysiotropic signal frequency and the functioning of the pituitary-ovarian system in the Rhesus monkey. Endocrinology *112*:2076.

50. Rapoport, B. and Seto, P. (1985): Bovine thyrotropin has a specific bioactivity 5- to 10-fold that of previous estimates for highly purified hormone. Endocrinology *116*:1379.

51. Reeves, W. B. and Andreoli, T. E. (1992): The posterior pituitary and water metabolism. *In*: Williams Textbook of Endocrinology, 8th ed., edited by J. D. Wilson and D. W. Foster. Philadelphia, PA, W. B. Saunders Co., p. 311.

52. Reichlin, S. (1992): Neuroendocrinology. *In*: Williams Textbook of Endocrinology, 8th ed., edited by J. D. Wilson and D. W. Foster. Philadelphia, PA, W. B. Saunders Co., p. 135.

53. Reimers, T. J., Cummings, J. F., Summers, B. A., et al. (1984): The neuroendocrine control of the secretion of adrenocorticotropin by the fetal sheep. *In*: Fetal Neuroendocrinology, edited by F. Ellendorff, P. D. Gluckman, and N. Parvizi. Ithaca, NY, Perinatology Press, p. 241.

54. Rillema, J. A., Etindi, R. N., Ofenstein, J. P., et al. (1988): Mechanisms of prolactin action. *In*: The Physiology of Reproduction, edited by E. Knobil and J. Neill. New York, NY, Raven Press, p. 2217.

55. Rose, J. C., Meis, P. J., and Morris, M. (1981): Ontogeny of endocrine (ACTH, vasopressin, cortisol) responses to hypotension in lamb fetuses. Am. J. Physiol. *3*:E656.

56. Scott, D. W. and Concannon, P. W. (1983): Gross and microscopic changes in the skin of dogs with progestagen-induced acromegaly and elevated growth hormone levels. J. Am. Anim. Hosp. Assoc. *19*:523.

57. Shupnik, M. A. (1996): Gonadotropin gene modulation by steroids and gonadotropin-releasing hormone. Biol. Reprod. *54*:279.

58. Simpson, E. R. and MacDonald, P. C. (1981): Endocrine physiology of the placenta. Annu. Rev. Physiol. *43*:163.

59. Stewart, J. K., Clifton, D. K., Koerker, D. J., et al. (1985): Pulsatile release of growth hormone and prolactin from the primate pituitary *in vitro*. Endocrinology *116*:1.

60. Swennen, L. and Denef, C. (1982): Physiological concentrations of dopamine decrease adenosine 3'5'-monophosphate levels in cultured rat anterior pituitary cells and enriched populations of lactotrophs: Evidence for a causal relationship to inhibition of prolactin release. Endocrinology *111*:398.

61. Talamantes, F. and Ogren, L. (1988): The placenta as an endocrine organ: Polypeptides. *In*: The Physiology of Reproduction, edited by E. Knobil and J. Neill. New York, NY, Raven Press, p. 2093.

62. Thorner, M. O., Vance, M. L., Horvath, E., et al. (1992): The anterior pituitary. *In*: Williams Textbook of Endocrinology, 8th ed., edited by J. D. Wilson and D. W. Foster. Philadelphia, PA, W. B. Saunders Co., p. 221.

63. Tuggle, C. K. and Trenkle, A. (1996): Control of growth hormone synthesis. Domestic Anim. Endocrinol. *13*:1.

64. Van der Kolk, J. H., Wensing, T., Kalsbeek, H. C., et al. (1995): Laboratory diagnosis of equine pituitary *pars intermedia* adenoma. Domestic Anim. Endocrinol. *12*:35.

65. Vandesande, F. and Dierickx, K. (1975): Identification of the vasopressin-producing and of the oxytocin-producing neurons in the hypothalamic magnocellular neurosecretory system of the rat. Cell Tissue Res. *164*:153.

66. Wildt, L., Häusler, A., Marshall, G., et al. (1981): Frequency and amplitude of gonadotropin-releasing hormone stimulation and gonadotropin secretion in the Rhesus monkey. Endocrinology *109*:376.

67. Wilson, B., Raghupathy, E., Tonoue, T., et al. (1968): TSH-like actions of dibutyryl-cAMP on isolated bovine thyroid cells. Endocrinology *83*:877.

68. Zimmerman, E. A. and Silverman, A. J. (1983): Vasopressin and adrenal cortical interactions. Prog. Brain Res. *60*:493.

References Added in Proof

69. Parvizi, N. (2000): Neuroendocrine regulation of gonadotropins in the male and the female. Anim. Reprod. Sci. *60-61*:31.

70. Perone, M. J. and Castro, M. G. (1997): Prohormone and proneuropeptide synthesis and secretion. Histol. Histopathol. *12*:1179.

71. Wittkowski, W., Bockmann, J., Kreutz, M. R., et al. (1999): Cell and molecular biology of the *pars tuberalis* of the pituitary. Int. Rev. Cytol *185*:157.

The Thyroid Gland

C. C. CAPEN AND S. L. MARTIN

3

INTRODUCTION

THE thyroid gland is unique in that it has a follicular structure and is the only tissue of the body which is able to accumulate iodine in large quantities and incorporate it into hormones. The metabolism of iodine is so closely related to thyroid function that the two must be considered together. The enlargement of the thyroid in the iodine-deficient animal has long served as a classic example of how an organ hypertrophies in order to compensate for a deficiency of a nutrient until a balance has again been achieved. This compensatory hypertrophy and hyperplasia has been recognized for many centuries, even back to the time of the Ebers Papyrus (at least 1500 B.C.) and man has learned to compensate for an iodine deficiency by eating iodine-rich foods such as seaweed.

Thyroid hormones have many functions in the body and, in general, regulate growth, differentiation, and the metabolism of lipids, proteins, and carbohydrates. The advent of radioactive iodine stimulated extensive research into thyroid function. The affinity of the thyroid gland for elemental iodine and its isotopes has permitted definitive studies on the distribution, synthesis, and metabolism of thyroid hormones; triiodothyronine (T_3) and tetraiodothyronine (thyroxine, T_4).

STRUCTURE AND FUNCTION OF THE THYROID GLAND

Anatomy

In most animal species there are two thyroid lobes located on the lateral surfaces of the trachea. In pigs, the main lobe of the thyroid is on the midline in the ventral cervical region with dorso-lateral projections from each side. In the dog, the right lobe of the thyroid is situated slightly cranial to the left lobe and almost touches the caudal aspect of the larynx. The lobes are situated superficially on the lateral surfaces of the trachea. Each lobe of the thyroid

35

gland is about 2 cm by 1 cm by 0.5 cm in the average size adult dog and the combined weight of the two lobes is about 1 g. Because these lobes are relatively small and located beneath the *sternocephalicus* muscle, they are not readily palpable except when enlarged. The major supply of blood is via the cranial thyroid artery (a branch of the common carotid) and the principal venous drainage is via the caudal thyroid vein, which enters the internal jugular vein.

Lymph drainage from the cranial pole of the thyroid lobes is to the retropharyngeal lymph nodes in dogs. Lymph flow from the caudal aspects of each thyroid lobe is more variable but it often bypasses any lymph nodes before entering the brachiocephalic trunk. Efferent lymphatics usually enter directly into the cervical lymphatic trunk or internal jugular vein. This explains the frequent occurrence of pulmonary metastases from a thyroid carcinoma in dogs prior to development of secondary foci in the regional lymph nodes. Small efferent lymphatics may pass through the caudal cervical lymph nodes located along the ventral surface of the trachea before entering the cranial mediastinum.

The vascular supply to the thyroid fluctuates considerably depending upon the activity of the gland. Considering its size, it receives one of the richest supplies of blood of any organ of the body when expressed as blood flow per unit of tissue. The thyroid has a rich supply of sympathetic nerves associated with blood vessels which enter the gland at the hilus on the medial aspect of each lobe. These nerves are thought to regulate the blood supply to the organ, because transplantation does not affect the function of the thyroid. Only thyrotropin or thyroid-stimulating hormone (TSH) and the supply and availability of iodine affect the rate of synthesis of thyroid hormone.

Development of the Thyroid Gland

The thyroid gland originates as a thickened plate of epithelium in the floor of the pharynx and in the adult animal consists of follicular cells, parafollicular or C-cells, colloid, and interstitial connective tissues. The thyroid is intimately related to the aortic sac in its development and this association frequently leads to the formation of accessory thyroid parenchyma in the mediastinum. Branched cell cords develop from the pharyngeal plate and migrate dorsolaterally, but remain attached to the pharyngeal area by the narrow thyroglossal duct (for reference, see Chapter 4, Fig. 4-5). The cell cords expand laterally and upward, and these extensions form the anteromedial two-thirds of the adult lobes. The more medial portion remains close to the aortic sac and forms a transitory isthmus. The ultimobranchial bodies fuse with the lateral extensions of the cell cords and deliver the C-cells to the developing thyroid. These C-cells originate from the neural crest and are the secretory cells within each of the thyroid lobes that synthesize and release calcitonin. A portion of the thyroglossal duct may persist postnatally and form a cyst due to the accumulation of proteinic material secreted by the lining epithelium. Thyroglossal duct cysts are present in the ventral aspect of the anterior cervical region in dogs and the epithelium of the duct may undergo neoplastic transformation and give rise to papillary carcinomas.

Accessory Thyroid Tissue

Accessory thyroid tissue is common in the dog and may be located anywhere from the larynx to the diaphragm. About 50% of adult dogs have 1 to 5 or more accessory nodules of thyroid tissue embedded in the fat on the intrapericardial aorta (Fig. 3-1). These nodules are usually 1 to 2 mm in their greatest dimension. This accessory thyroid tissue is completely lacking in C-(parafollicular) cells, which secrete calcitonin, but their follicular structure and function are the same as that of the main thyroid lobes. The existence of accessory thyroids in the dog was recognized early, but many investigators appear to have been unaware of their frequent occurrence. Attempts to induce hypothyroidism in the dog by surgical thyroidectomy usually are not successful because the accessory thyroids readily respond to an increase in endogenous TSH secretion and undergoes sufficient hypertrophy and hyperplasia of follicular cells to sustain adequate thyroid hormone production. This accessory thyroid tissue may undergo neoplastic transformation in the adult dog.

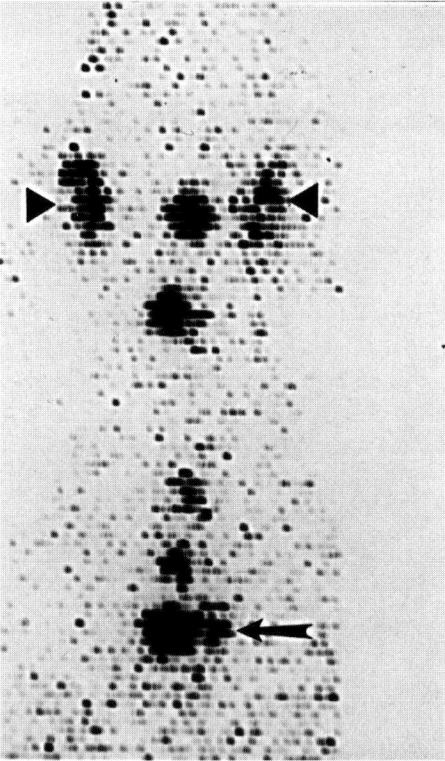

Fig. 3-1. Scan of the cervical region of a dog following the administration of radioactive iodine illustrating uptake of iodine not only by the thyroid lobes (arrowheads) but also by accessory (functional) thyroid tissue in the anterior mediastinum near the base of the heart (arrow). [Courtesy of Dr. Victoria Voith (1970): Accessory thyroids in the dog, Ohio State University, Columbus, Ohio (Thesis)].

The findings of cysts derived from remnants of the ultimobranchial body and the presence of calcitonin-immunoreactive cells in the wall of the ultimobranchial tubule, as well as thyroglobulin-positive staining in adjacent follicles support the premise that the ultimobranchial body contributes to the formation of follicles in certain areas of the thyroid lobes.

Histology of the Thyroid Gland

The basic structure of the thyroid is unique for an endocrine gland. The thyroid gland contains follicles ranging from 20 to 250 μm in size and are filled with a colloid produced by the cells lining the follicle (Fig. 3-2). The follicular cells are cuboidal to columnar and their secretory polarity is directed toward the lumen of the follicle (Fig. 3-3). An extensive network of inter- and intrafollicular capillaries provides the follicular cells with an abundant supply of blood. Follicular cells have long profiles of microfilaments and tubules formed by rough endoplasmic reticulum and a large Golgi apparatus in their cytoplasm for the synthesis and packaging of substantial amounts of proteins, primarily thyroglobulin, released into the follicular lumen. The interface between the luminal side of follicular cells and the colloid is modified by numerous microvillar projections (Fig. 3-3).

During folliculogenesis an intracytoplasmic cavity develops initially in individual cells. Thyroidal follicles appear to grow during development of the thyroid gland by proliferation of component cells and coalescence of adjacent colloid-containing microfollicles within the follicular cell. *In vitro* studies suggest folliculogenesis is stimulated by TSH and that microfilament integrity and phosphorylation of tyrosine are essential to thyroid cell responses. These are potential intracellular loci, where TSH and intercellular contact may regulate adhesion of follicular cells to extracellular matrix and influence thyroid cell behavior.

The volumetric fractions of the histologic components of the rat thyroid: Follicular cells, C-cells, colloid, and interstitial tissue change considerably during development from birth to 120 days of age. During the first 4 months of life, the absolute volumes occupied by follicular cells, C-cells, colloid, and stroma increased 13.3, 30.8, 39, and 34 times, respectively in the rat.[21] Morphometrically, volume and numerical densities of follicles vary during a 24-hour period in rats and reflect changes in the subcellular organelles of follicular cells.

The majority of the epithelial cells and the most important functional cells of the thyroid are the follicular cells (Fig. 3-4). Depending on the intensity of stimulation by pituitary TSH, they vary in height, ranging between cuboidal (low TSH) to columnar (high TSH) in appearance.

The histologic appearance of the thyroid is dramatically influenced by the level of circulating TSH from the adenohypophysis.[20] Thy-

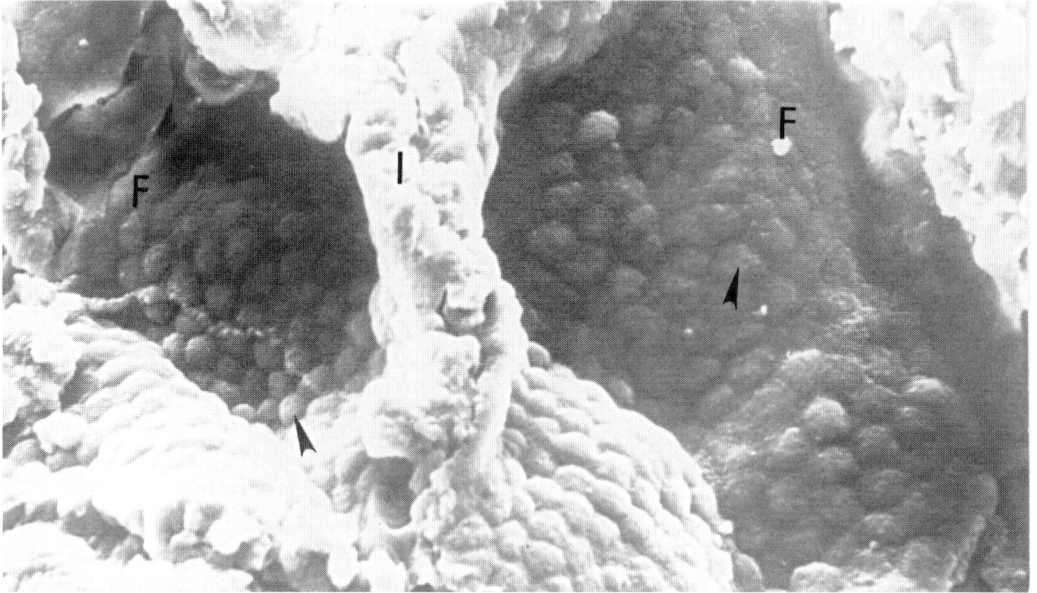

Fig. 3-2. Scanning electron micrograph of the thyroid gland of a dog with 2 opened follicles (**F**). The luminal aspect of individual follicular cells has numerous microvillar projections (**arrowheads**). (**I** = interfollicular space with connective tissue and capillaries)

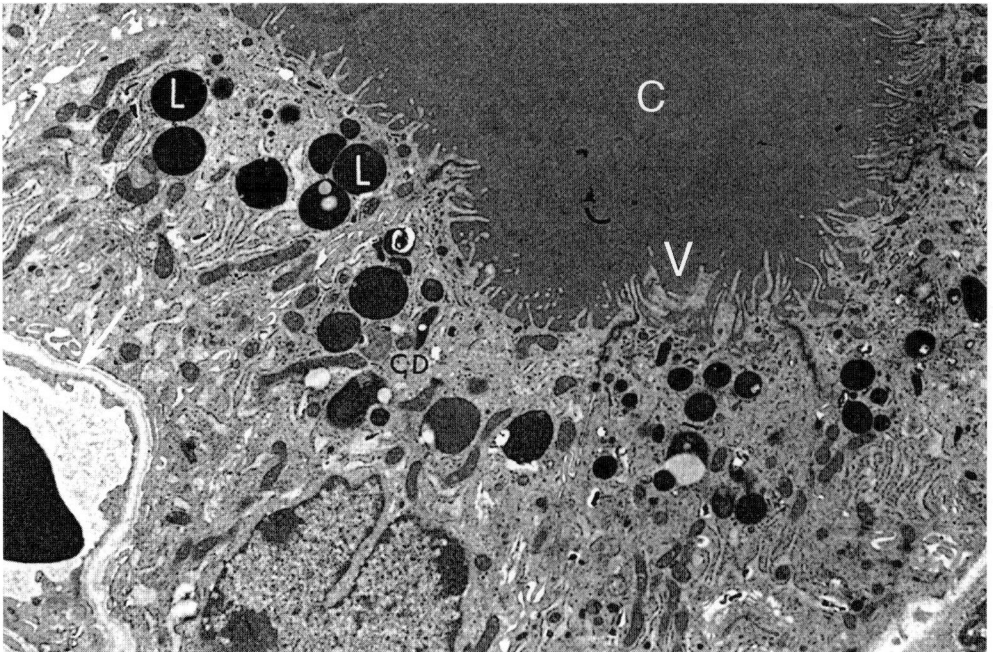

Fig. 3-3. Electron micrograph of normal thyroid follicular cells with long microvilli (**V**) extending into the colloid-filled lumen (**C**) of the follicle. Pseudopods from the apical membrane engulf a portion of the colloid to form a colloid droplet (**CD**). Numerous lysosomes (**L**) in the apical cytoplasm contribute proteolytic enzymes that hydrolyze the thyroglobulin and release the thyroid hormones, which enter intrafollicular capillaries located at the base of the follicular cells (**arrow**).

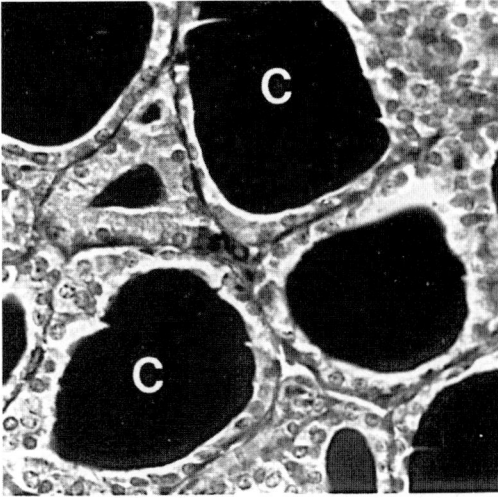

Fig. 3-4. Normal rat thyroid gland illustrating basic histologic structure of colloid-filled (**C**) follicles of varying size lined by cuboidal thyroid follicular cells (thyrocytes). An extensive network of capillaries is present between the thyroid follicles. Periodic acid-Schiff reaction.

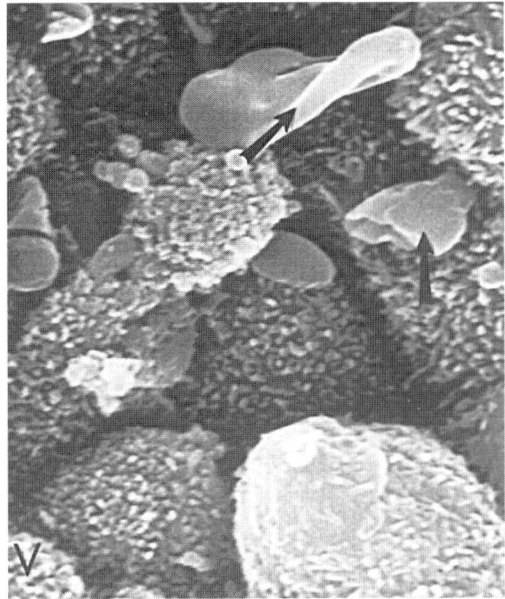

Fig. 3-5. Scanning electron micrograph of apical surface of hypertrophied thyroid follicular cell 4 hours post-TSH stimulation. Numerous elongated microvilli (**V**) and cytoplasmic projections (**arrows**) extend into the follicular lumen to engulf colloid as part of the initial stages of thyroid hormone secretion in response to TSH.

rotropin binds to receptors on the basilar aspect of thyroid follicular cells, activates adenylate cyclase with the resultant accumulation of cyclic AMP, and increases the rate of biochemical reactions responsible for the biosynthesis and secretion of thyroid hormones.[123]

One of the initial structural responses of follicular cells to TSH is the graded formation of numerous cytoplasmic pseudopodia. The extent of pseudopod formation is dependent upon the level of TSH and results in the increased endocytosis of colloid and release of the preformed thyroid hormone that is stored within the follicular lumen (Fig. 3-5).

If the secretion of TSH is sustained (hours or days), thyroid follicular cells become more columnar and the follicular lumens become smaller and appear as slit-like spaces due to the increased endocytosis of colloid (Fig. 3-6). Numerous periodic acid-Schiff (PAS)-positive colloid droplets are present in the luminal aspect of the hypertrophied follicular cells. Stimulation by TSH not only elicits a highly macropinocytotic response among different follicular cells as a function of the levels of TSH, but, progressively increases the recruitment and responsiveness of the follicular cells.

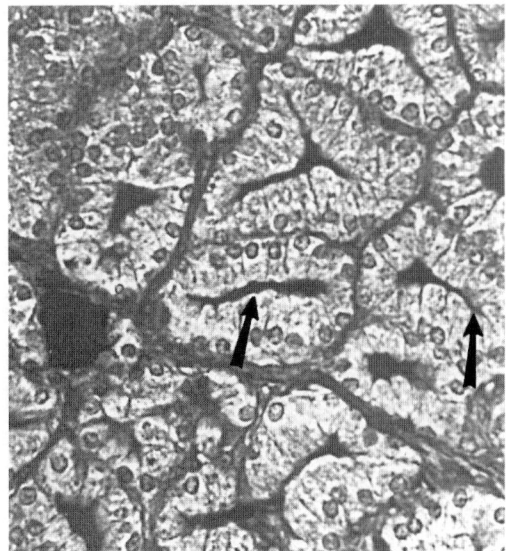

Fig. 3-6. Histologic appearance of thyroid follicular cells 8 hours post-TSH stimulation. The follicular cells are columnar and many follicles are nearly depleted of colloid and partially collapsed (**arrow**). Periodic acid-Schiff reaction.

Diffuse thyroid hyperplasia, clinically called goiter, is caused by iodine deficiency in the diet. Before the widespread addition of iodized salt to the diet, this condition (Fig. 3-7) was common in animals and humans in many of the goitrogenic areas throughout the world. Marginally iodine-deficient diets containing certain goitrogenic compounds may result in hypothyroidism with follicular cell hypertrophy and hyperplasia and clinical evidence of goiter. These goitrogenic substances include thiouracil, sulfonamides, complex anions, and a number of plants from the family *Brassicacceae,* amongst many others.

In response to long-term stimulation of follicular cells by TSH, as occurs with chronic iodine deficiency, both of the lateral lobes of the thyroid are uniformly enlarged (Fig. 3-7). These enlargements may be extensive and result in prominent swelling in the cranial cervical area. The affected lobes are firm and dark red in appearance because of the extensive interfollicular capillary network that develops due to the influence of long-term stimulation by TSH. These thyroid enlargements are the result of intense hypertrophy and hyperplasia of follicular cells, often with the formation of papillary projections into the lumens of follicles or multiple layers of cells lining the follicles (Fig. 3-8). Endocytosis of follicular colloid usually proceeds at a rate greater than colloid synthesis, resulting in the progressive depletion of colloid. Thyroid follicles become smaller than normal and there may be a partial collapse of follicles due to the lack of colloid (Fig. 3-8). The hypertrophic follicular cells are columnar with a deeply eosinophilic cytoplasm and small hyperchromatic nuclei that often are situated in the basilar part of the cell.

The converse of what has just been described occurs in follicular cells as a response to an increase in the circulating levels of thyroid hormones, after the administration of thyroxine, or in patients with a large space-occupying lesion that markedly decreases the ability of the pituitary to secrete TSH. As a result of decreased

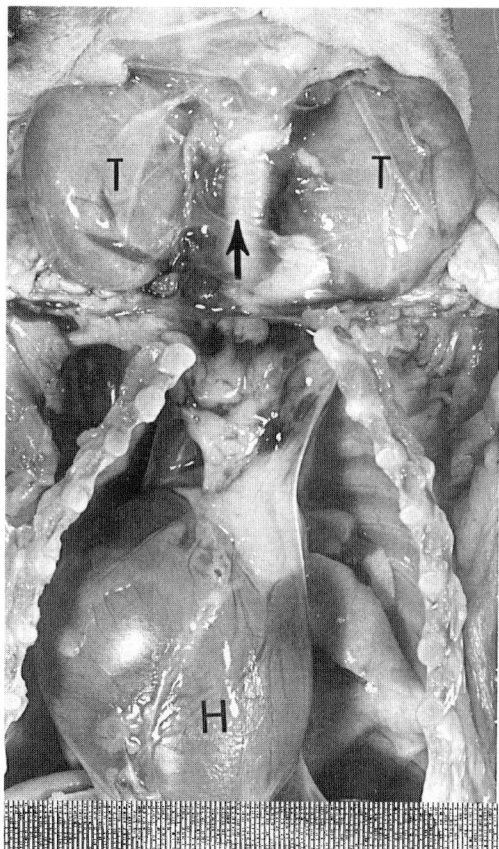

Fig. 3-7. Diffuse hyperplastic goiter in a pup resulting in prominent symmetrical enlargements of both lobes (**T**) of the thyroid gland. The hyperplastic thyroid lobes were freely movable from the trachea (**arrow**) in the cervical region. (**H** = heart).

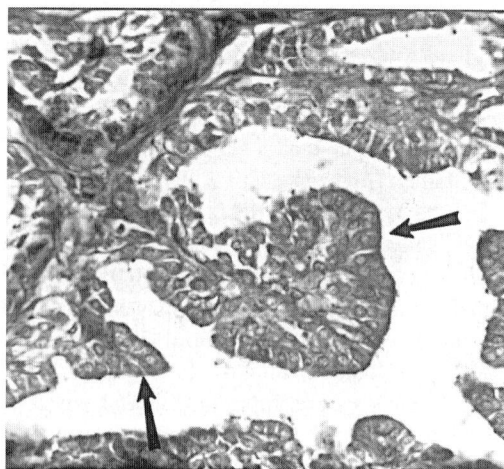

Fig. 3-8. Histopathology of diffuse hyperplastic goiter in a pup illustrating the papillary projections (**arrows**) into follicular lumens and partial collapse of follicles due to the increased endocytosis of colloid. Hematoxylin and eosin.

levels of TSH, the thyroid follicles become enlarged and distended with densely staining colloid due to the decreased rate of TSH-mediated endocytosis of colloid. The luminal surface of the follicular cell is flattened. Follicular cells lining the involuted follicles are low cuboidal and there are few endocytotic vacuoles at the interface between the colloid and follicular cells (Fig. 3-9). A long-standing decreased secretion of TSH results in widely-separated and short microvilli extending into the colloid-filled lumen.

The thyroid stroma is exceptionally rich in blood vessels that form extensive interfollicular capillary plexuses lying in close proximity to the basement membranes of follicular cells. There is also a network of lymphatic vessels within the gland. The stroma encloses a number of nerve fibers, some of which are parasympathetic, but most are sympathetic. These nerves terminate on blood vessels or are found in apposition to follicular cells.

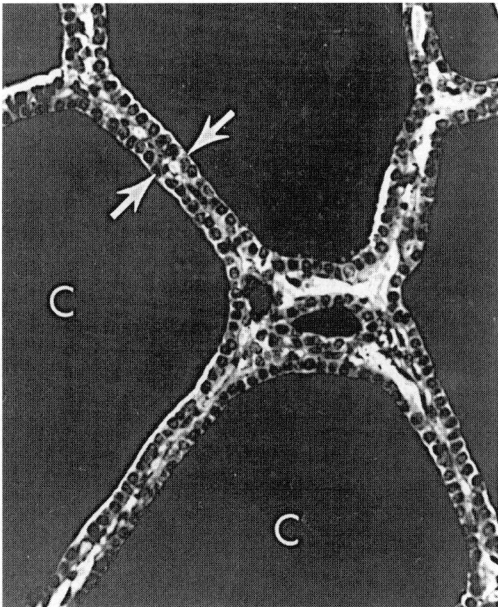

Fig. 3-9. Histologic response of thyroid follicular cells (thyrocytes) to long-term administration of exogenous thyroxine. The follicular cells (**arrows**) are cuboidal in response to the decreased secretion of TSH and the thyroid follicles are distended by the dense colloid (**C**). Periodic acid-Schiff reaction.

Much less numerous in the thyroid gland are cells concerned with the secretion of calcitonin. Calcitonin (CT) is a peptide hormone of the mammalian thyroid that has been shown to be secreted by C-cells. These parafollicular or light cells, comprise a second endocrine cell population in the mammalian thyroid gland. The C-cells are distinct from the follicular cells that secrete thyroid hormones (T_3 and T_4). Within the thyroid gland, these C-cells are either situated within the follicular wall immediately beneath the basement membrane or as small groups of cellbetween thyroid follicles. The C-cells do not border the follicular colloid directly and their secretory polarity is oriented toward the interfollicular capillaries. The distinctive feature of C-cells, as compared to thyroid follicular cells, is the presence of numerous small membrane-limited secretory granules in the cytoplasm that contain calcitonin.

Synthesis of Thyroid Hormone

The biosynthesis of thyroid hormones is also unique among endocrine glands because the final assembly of hormones occurs extracellularly within the follicular lumen. Essential raw materials, such as iodide (I⁻) from the plasma, are efficiently trapped by follicular cells, transported rapidly against a concentration gradient to the lumen, and oxidized by a peroxidase in microvillar membranes to form iodine (I_2, Fig. 3-10). The assembly of thyroid hormones within the follicular lumen is made possible by a unique protein called thyroglobulin which is synthesized by follicular cells.

Thyroglobulin is a high molecular weight glycoprotein (600,000 to 750,000 daltons) synthesized in successive subunits on the ribosomes of the endoplasmic reticulum of follicular cells. The constituent amino acids (tyrosine and others) and carbohydrates (*i.e.,* mannose, fructose, galactose) come from the circulation. The recently synthesized thyroglobulin leaves the Golgi apparatus and is packaged into apical vesicles and extruded into the follicular lumen.[83] The amino acid tyrosine, an essential component of thyroid hormones, is incorporated within the molecular structure of thyroglobulin.

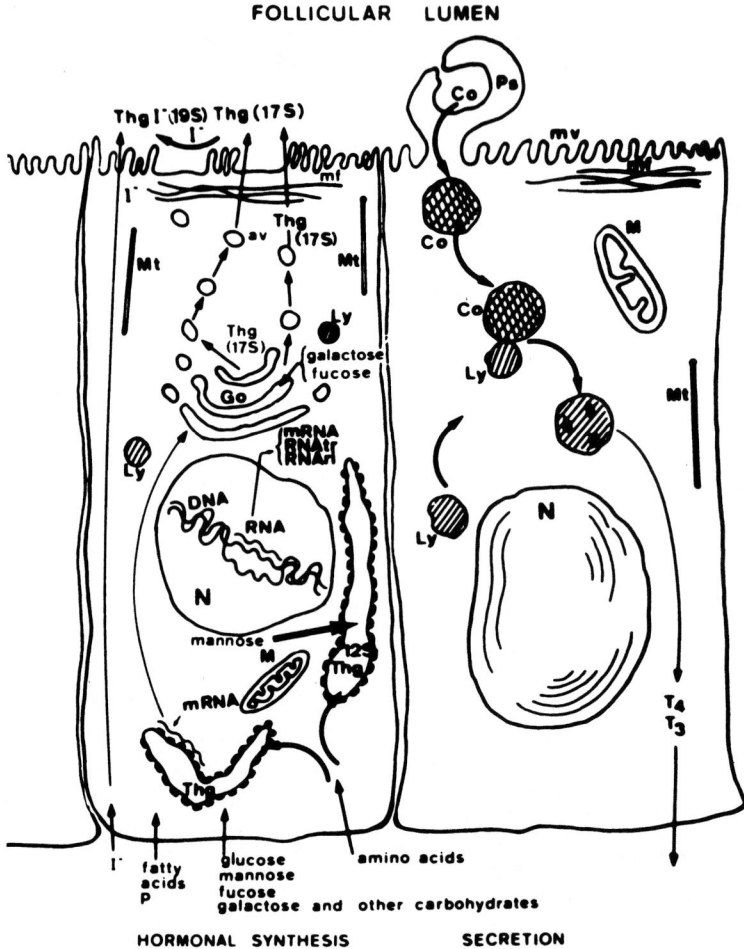

Fig. 3-10. Thyroid follicular cells (thyrocytes) illustrating the two-way traffic of materials between the capillaries and the lumen of the thyroid follicle. Raw materials, such as iodine, are concentrated by follicular cells and rapidly transported into the lumen (left side of drawing). Amino acids (tyrosine and others) and sugars are assembled by follicular cells into thyroglobulin (**Thg**), packaged into apical vesicles (**av**) and released into the lumen of the thyroid follicle. The iodination of tyrosyl residues to form thyroid hormones occurs within the thyroglobulin molecule while in the follicular lumen. Elongation of microvilli (**mv**) and endocytosis of colloid by follicular cells occurs in response to TSH stimulation (right side of drawing). The intracellular colloid droplets (**Co**) fuse with lysosomal bodies (**Ly**) and active thyroid hormone is enzymatically cleaved from thyroglobulin and free T_4 and T_3 are released into the circulation. (**M** = mitochondria;. **mf** = microfilaments; **Mt** = microtubules; **N** = nucleus; **Ps** = pseudopod. (Reprinted with permission from: P. A. Bastenie, A. M. Ermans, M. Bonnyns, et al. In: Molecular Pathology, edited by R. A. Good. Springfield, Il, Charles C. Thomas, 1975).

Iodine is bound to tyrosyl residues in thyroglobulin at the apical surface of follicular cells to form successively monoiodotyrosine (MIT) and diiodotyrosine (DIT, Fig. 3-11). The resulting MIT and DIT combine to form the two biologically active iodothyronines (thyroxine-T_4 and triiodothyronine-T_3) secreted by the thyroid gland (Fig. 3-12).

The extracellular storage of thyroglobulin in the follicular lumen is essential for maintaining constant blood levels of thyroid hormones in vertebrates under conditions of varied intake of iodine and varying metabolic demands for T_4 and T_3. Storage of large amounts of thyroglobulin is made possible by compaction or the tight packing of thyroglob-

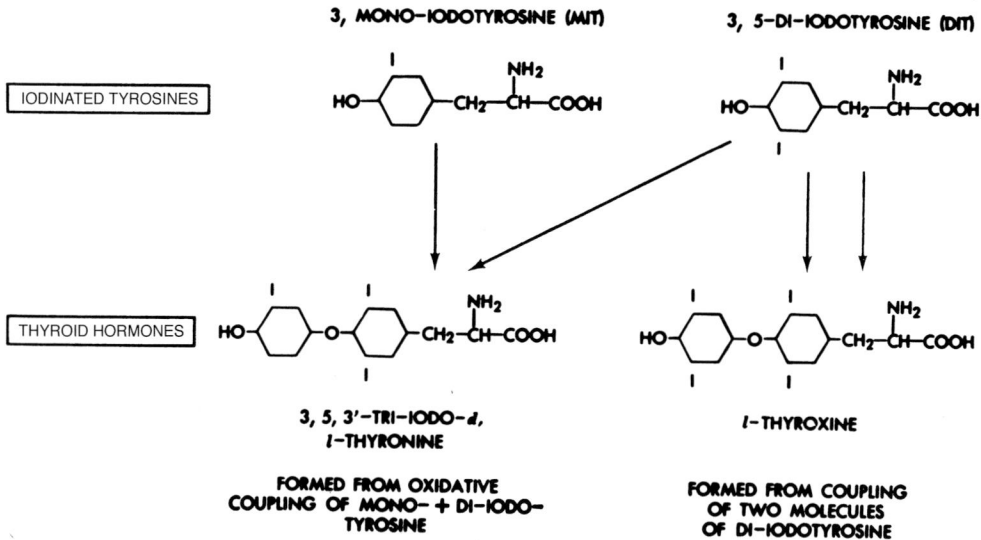

FORMATION OF THYROID HORMONES FROM IODINATED TYROSINES

Fig. 3-11. Formation of thyroid hormones (3,5,3'-triiodothyronine and l-thyroxine) from iodinated tyrosines (**MIT** and **DIT**) within the follicular lumen of the thyroid gland. (Reprinted with permission from: R.W. Rawson, The Thyroid Gland, CIBA Clinical Symposia, CIBA Corp., Summit, N.J., 1965).

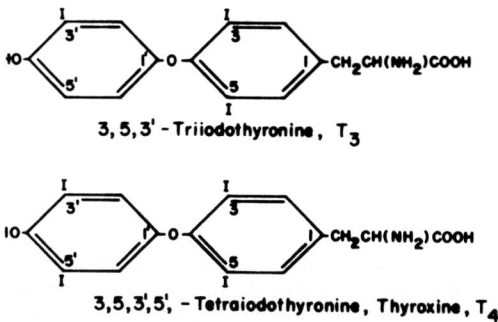

Fig. 3-12. Triiodothyronine (T_3) and tetraiodothyronine (T_4) are the two biologically active iodothyronines secreted by the thyroid gland. They have similar biologic actions and differ by the presence of an additional molecule of iodine at the 5' position on the outer phenolic ring of the thyroxine molecule.

ulin molecules in the follicular lumen.[50] Protein concentrations as high as 100 to 400 mg/ml have been reported in colloid collected from the lumens of single thyroid follicles by micropuncture techniques. The luminal content of follicles is composed of discrete 20 to 120 μm in diameter globules which, by scanning electron microscopy, revealed a unique cobblestone-like surface pattern from impressions of microvilli of the apical plasma membranes of thyroid follicular cells (thyrocytes). The thyroglobulin in isolated globules is highly iodinated, ~ 55 iodine atoms per 12S (S = sedimentation coefficient) subunit, suggesting that a covalent nondisulfide cross-linking occurs during iodination of thyroglobulin and that this process involves the formation of intermolecular dityrosine bridges.[50]

The active transport of iodide has been shown to be associated with a sodium-iodide ($Na^+ - I^-$) symporter (NIS). Transport of iodide ion across the thyroid cell membrane is linked to the transport of Na^+. The ion gradient generated by the Na^+-K^+ ATPase appears to be the driving force for the active co-transport of iodide. The transporter protein is present in the basolateral membrane of thyroid follicular cells (thyrocytes) and is a large protein containing 643 amino acids with 12 transmembrane domains. Other tissues such as the salivary gland, gastric mucosa, and lactating mammary gland also have the capacity to actively transport iodide, albeit at a much lower level than the thyroid. The NIS gene is complex (16 exons, 14 introns) and its expression in the thyroid is up-regulated by TSH.

The functionally active iodine transport system in the thyroid gland has important clinical applications in the evaluation, diagnosis, and treatment of several thyroid disorders, including cancer. Radioiodine is used to ablate residual tumor tissue as well as recurrent and metastatic thyroid cancer.[67] The NIS and active transport of iodide can be selectively inhibited by chemicals such as perchlorate and thiocyanate; thereby, effectively blocking the ability of the gland to synthesize thyroid hormones.

Secretion of Thyroid Hormone

The secretion of thyroid hormones from stores within luminal colloid is initiated by elongation of microvilli on follicular cells and formation of pseudopods. These elongated cytoplasmic projections (see Figs. 3-5 and 3-10) are increased by pituitary TSH and extend into the follicular lumen to indiscriminatingly phagocytize a portion of adjacent colloid. Colloid droplets within follicular cells fuse with the numerous lysosomal bodies that contain proteolytic enzymes (Fig. 3-10). Triiodothyronine and thyroxine are released from the thyroglobulin molecule and secreted into adjacent capillaries. The biogically inactive iodinated tyrosines, MIT and DIT released from the colloid droplets are enzymatically deiodinated and under normal conditions the iodide generated is either recycled to the lumen of the thyroid follicle to iodinate new tyrosyl residues or released into the circulation. The structural and functional characteristics of the thyroid gland suggests that the phylogenetically oldest endocrine gland has evolved a unique structure adapted to perform vital metabolic functions.

Negative feedback control of thyroid hormone secretion is accomplished by the coordinated response of the adenohypophysis and hypothalamic nuclei to circulating levels of T_4 and T_3 (Fig. 3-13). A decrease in the thyroid hormone concentration in plasma is sensed by groups of neurosecretory neurons in the hypothalamus that synthesize and release a small tri-peptide called

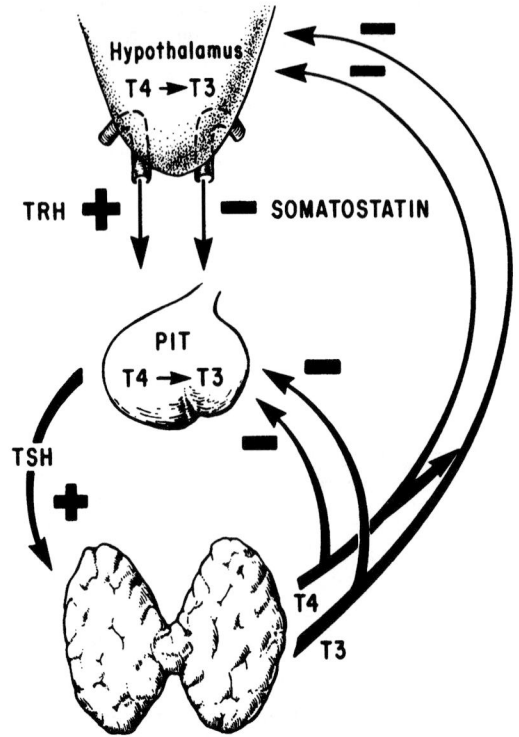

Fig. 3-13. Hypothalamic-pituitary-thyroid axis. Thyroid-stimulating hormone (**TSH**) from the pituitary stimulates the secretion of both and tetraiodothyronine (**T_4**) and triiodothyronine (**T_3**). These act at the pituitary (**PIT**) level to control secretion of TSH by a negative feedback mechanism. In addition, **T_4** is converted to the more potent **T_3** within the pituitary by a monodeiodinase. Secretion of TSH is stimulated by thyrotropin-releasing hormone (**TRH**) from the hypothalamus and inhibited by somatostatin and to a lesser extent by dopamine. Thus, hypothalamic factors interact at the pituitary level to determine the rate of TSH secretion. Thyroid hormone acts at the hypothalamus to stimulate the secretion of somatostatin (this effect acts as a negative signal to the pituitary). Within the hypothalamus, T_4 is also deiodinated to T_3 and this conversion may play a role in feedback control. (Reproduced with permission from: S. Reichlin, Neuroendocrinology. In: Williams Textbook of Endocrinology, 8th edition, Chapter 5, edited by J. D. Wilson and D. W. Foster. Philadelphia, PA, W. B. Saunders Co., p. 169, 1992).

thyrotropin-releasing hormone (TRH; MW 361 daltons, see Chapter 2, Fig. 2-4) into the hypophyseal portal circulation.[48] Thyrotropin-releasing hormone binds to receptors on the plasma membrane of thyrotrophic basophils in the adenohypophysis and activates adenylate cyclase, resulting in the formation of 3',5' cyclic adenosine monophosphate (cyclic AMP). The intracellular accumulation of cyclic AMP in thyrotrophic basophils results in the contraction of microfilaments and peripheral movement and discharge of the TSH-containing secretory granules into the pituitary capillaries. Thyroid stimulating hormone (TSH) is conveyed to the thyroid follicular cells where it binds to receptors on the basilar aspect of the cell, activates adenylate cyclase, and increases the rate of the biochemical reactions concerned with the synthesis and secretion of thyroid hormones.

Pseudopods appear to engulf thyroglobulin that is located at some distance from the apical surface and may provide a mechanism of selective **macropinocytosis** by which newly synthesized thyroglobulin delivered to the follicle lumen is prevented from immediate reuptake.[35] This process, termed endocytosis, results in the formation of colloid droplets in the cytoplasm of follicular cells. Small clathrin-containing coated vesicles, also appear to be involved in the uptake and transport of iodinated thyroglobulin from the follicular lumen to the lysosomal compartment of thyroid follicular cells. The process of 'micropinocytosis' of colloid is receptor-mediated and may be a major pathway of thyroglobulin uptake in the normal thyroid gland when the demands for thyroid hormone secretion are low. During the vesicular transport ("transcytosis") of thyroglobulin through the cytoplasm of follicular cells the molecule does not undergo cleavage and its electrophoretic mobility remains unchanged. Thyroglobulin may be released in small quantities as an intact molecule into the circulation by this TSH-regulated transepithelial vesicular transport. Clearance of thyroglobulin from the circulation occurs primarily in the Kupffer cells of the liver.

Microtubules and microfilaments in the cytoplasm beneath the apical plasma membrane of follicular cells are involved with the movement of colloid droplets into close proximity to the lysosomal bodies. The membranes of the colloid droplets and lysosomes fuse resulting in the local release of enzymes that break down the colloid and release thyroid hormones into the cytosol (Fig. 3-10).

Thyroperoxidase is the most important enzyme in the synthetic pathway of thyroid hormones. In humans, thyroperoxidase is a membrane-bound, heme-containing protein composed of 933 amino acids with a transmembrane domain. Thyroperoxidase oxidizes iodide ion (I^-) taken up by follicular cells into reactive iodine (I_2) which binds to the tyrosine residues in thyroglobulin. Iodine is incorporated not only into newly synthesized thyroglobulin recently delivered to the follicular lumen but also into molecules already stored in the lumen. Thyroperoxidase also functions as a "coupling" enzyme to combine monoiodotyrosine (MIT) and diiodotyrosine (DIT) to form triiodothyronine (T_3) or 2 molecules of DIT to form tetraiodothyronine (T_4) or thyroxine (Fig. 3-11).

The follicular cells of the thyroid are involved, concurrently with the synthesis of MIT, DIT, T_3, and thyroxine (T_4) in the luminally directed processes of thyroglobulin synthesis and exocytosis, as well as the basally directed processes of colloid endocytosis with breakdown and eventual release of active thyroid hormones into the interfollicular capillaries (Fig. 3-10). The incorporation of amino acids into peptides and the synthesis of the carbohydrate chains of thyroglobulin starts in the endoplasmic reticulum and is completed in the Golgi apparatus of the thyrocyte.

There are marked differences in thyroid morphology and function between the canine breeds of European origin and the Basenji, which originated in Africa. At the same level of iodine intake, thyroidal turnover of iodine in the Basenji is 2 to 3 times faster than in European breeds. The corresponding differences in thyroid morphology in the Basenji include smaller follicles with more widespread and uniform vacuolation of the colloid, a taller follicular epithelium, and ultrastructural features of follicular cells that more closely resemble those of a TSH-stimulated gland in European breeds, such as the Beagle.

Iodine Metabolism

Iodine metabolism and thyroid function should be viewed as an integrated system composed of metabolic subsystems for uptake and transport of iodide, iodine incorporation into the hormones of the thyroid gland (e.g., T_3 and T_4), and factors which regulate the overall function of the thyroid gland. This integrated system is controlled by feedback mechanisms involving the hypothalamus and pituitary gland (Fig. 3-13), and also by the intake of iodine. The function of the system is to provide a carefully regulated supply of T_3 and T_4 to animal cells, which in turn influences the rates of many metabolic processes. There is sufficient flexibility in the system to accommodate day-to-day variations in iodine intake and to sustain a near normal metabolic rate, even with short-term dietary iodine deficiency.

The daily maintenance requirement of iodine is about 140 μg for a 10- to 15-kg adult dog. *Ad libitum* consumption of most commercially manufactured dry dog foods provides the average dog with a daily iodine intake of at least 500 μg, and some foods provide as much as 1,500 μg per day. Most of the iodine in the diet is reduced to iodide in the gastrointestinal tract and absorption of iodide is essentially complete within 2 hours after ingestion. Iodide is cleared from the plasma by the thyroid gland, the parotid salivary gland, and by the gastric mucosa. A small amount of iodide is normally lost in the feces (about 20 to 25 μg per day at the usual levels of intake), possibly via secretion into the colon.

The principal features of iodine metabolism in the dog, for a daily iodide intake slightly in excess of the normal requirement, are as follows. The dietary intake of 160 μg is augmented by 65 μg of recycled iodide; approximately 50 μg of this recycled iodide is released by the thyroid gland and 15 μg is derived from the peripheral degradation of T_3 and T_4. Two-thirds of this combined input of 225 μg is excreted, chiefly in the urine. The thyroid clears about one-third of the iodide input, to achieve a net daily uptake of about 75 μg of iodide.

At the usual levels of iodine intake, the concentration of inorganic iodide in the dog is about 5 to 10 μg per 100 ml of plasma. In man, plasma iodide concentration is usually about 0.5 μg/100 ml. The principal reasons for the higher level of iodide concentration in the dog

are the higher intake relative to body weight, proportionately greater recycling of iodide from the thyroid and from the peripheral degradation of thyroid hormones, and lower fractional clearance of iodide by the kidney. Another pertinent difference in iodide metabolism between dogs and humans is that in addition to free iodide and the iodine incorporated in the circulating thyroid hormone, canine plasma contains a significant amount of nonhormonal iodine that is bound to plasma proteins. This iodine (usually present in a concentration of 1 μg or more per 100 ml of plasma) appears to be incorporated during the synthesis of plasma proteins, principally albumin. The total iodine content of the normal canine thyroid is about 1,000 μg. Two-thirds of the iodine is in the form of MIT and DIT, and about one-fourth is in the form of T_3 and T_4, all of which are incorporated in thyroglobulin molecules in the follicular colloid.

Thyroid Hormone Metabolism

Data primarily from the dog will be utilized to discuss the metabolism of thyroid hormone because more is known about this domestic animal species and clinically significant disorders of thyroid function are common in canine patients. In dogs, T_4 in the plasma is bound to albumin and several globulin fractions, whereas T_3 is bound to albumin and one globulin fraction. The overall binding affinity of the plasma proteins for T_4 is lower in the dog than in man. Most importantly, the affinity of the canine inter-α globulin fraction for T_4 is much less than that of the thyroxine-binding globulin (TBG) in man. Partly as a result of this weaker binding, the total T_4 concentration is lower, the unbound or free fraction of circulating T_4 is higher, and hormone turnover is more rapid in the dog than in man.

About 40% of the extrathyroidal T_4 in the dog is in the plasma. Most of the remaining T_4 (60%) is taken up by the liver and equilibrates rapidly with the plasma. The total plasma-equivalent space of distribution of T_4 is about 12% of body weight. By comparison, T_3 enters peripheral tissues more readily than T_4, partly because it is less firmly bound to plasma proteins, and may reach a total distribution volume equal to 65% of body weight. Largely owing to the great difference in their respective volumes of distribution, the ratio of T_4 to T_3 in canine plasma is about 20:1, even though they are produced in a ratio of about 2:1 in the thyroid gland. The average total T_4 concentration in the dog is about 1.8 μg per 100 ml of plasma and the average total T_3 level is 84 ng per 100 ml. These values represent measurements made between 11 AM and noon. The time of measurement is important because there appears to be diurnal oscillations in plasma levels of T_3 and T_4. Peak concentration usually occurs at about midday and the minimum at about midnight.

An equivalent of 100% of the total extrathyroidal T_4 and T_3 is metabolized and must be replaced each day in dogs. About 45% of the turnover of T_4 is via deiodination and 55% is via fecal excretion; whereas for T_3 70% is via deiodination and 30% is via fecal excretion. Both the overall rates of turnover via deiodination and the loss of hormone in the feces are much higher in the dog than in man. Fecal wastage substantially reduces the efficiency of hormone utilization, but it also explains in part the remarkable tolerance of the dog to an excess of thyroid hormone. The radiothyroidectomized hypothyroid dog converts a substantial amount

of administered T_4 to T_3. This extrathyroidal mechanism for production of T_3 is important because the ratio of T_4 to T_3 in thyroglobulin is approximately 3.6:1, while the ratio of the daily production rates, based on plasma concentration and turnover of the two hormones, is 2:1.

Biologic Action of Thyroid Hormones

Thyroxine and triiodothyronine once released into the circulation act on many different target cells in the body. The overall functions of thyroxine and triiodothyronine are similar, though much of the biologic activity is the result of monodeiodination to 3,5,3'-triiodothyronine (T_3) prior to interacting with receptors in target cells (Fig. 3-14 and 3-15). Under conditions of protein starvation, liver and kidney diseases, febrile illness, and in neonatal animals, thyroxine is preferentially monodeiodinated by a 5-deiodinase to 3, 3',5'-triiodothyronine which is called "reverse T_3," (Fig. 3-14). Because the reverse T_3 formed by target cells is biologically inactive, monodeiodination to form reverse T_3 provides a mechanism to attenuate the overall metabolic effects of thyroid hormones.

Thyroxine stimulates oxygen utilization and heat production by many different cells of the body. It causes increased utilization of carbohydrates, increased protein catabolism and excre-

MONODEIODINATION OF THYROXINE

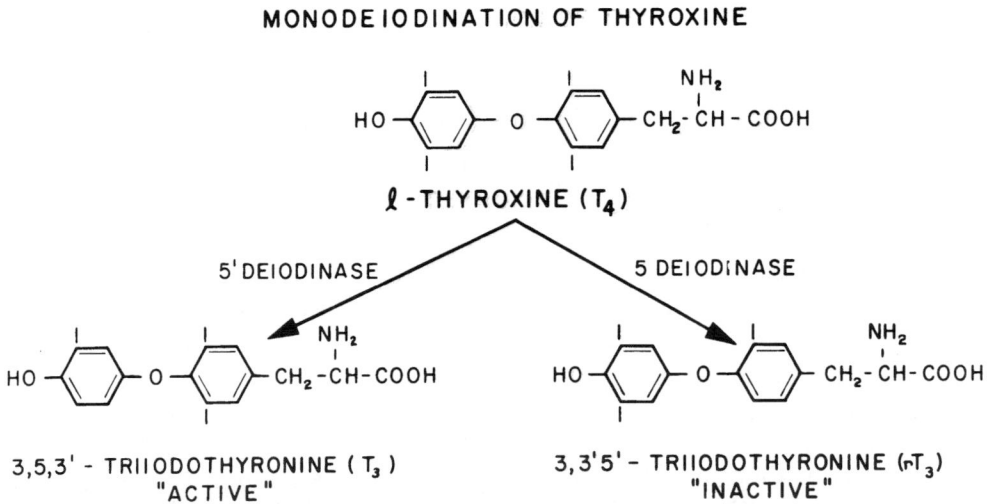

Fig. 3-14. Depending upon the metabolic need for the actions of thyroid hormone monodeiodination of thyroxine by 5' deiodinase forms active **T_3** (left) or by 5-deiodinase forms inactive (reverse) **T_3** (**rT_3**; right).

tion of nitrogen, oxidation of fats, and loss in body weight. In addition, the administration of thyroxine will increase the heart rate by a direct effect on heart muscle cells.

Normal function of the central nervous system is dependent upon the normal output of thyroid hormones in animals and humans. During periods when thyroxine levels are deficient, the central nervous system fails to function in the normal fashion and the animal is lethargic, dull, and mentally deficient. The content of myelin in the fiber tracts is decreased, cortical neurons are smaller and fewer, and vascularity of the central nervous system (CNS) is reduced. The neuronal dysfunction caused by thyroxine deficiency is reversible in the adult animal but not in the young growing animal. The neurons in the young growing animal are permanently damaged by thyroid hormone deficiency. On the other hand, excess secretion of thyroid hormone stimulates CNS activity and affected animals are nervous, jumpy, irritable, and hyperactive.

The subcellular mechanism of action of thyroid hormones appears to resemble that of steroid hormones in that free hormone enters into target cells and binds to a cytosol-binding protein (Fig. 3-15). Thyroxine (T_4) is mono-deiddinated to T_3 prior to interacting with the target cell. Free triiodothyronine (T_3) also binds to receptors on the inner mitochondrial membrane to activate mitochondrial energy metabolism or to a nuclear receptor (see Chapter 1, Fig. 1-9) and increases transcription of the genetic message to facilitate new protein synthesis. The overall physiological effects of thyroid hormones are to:

1. increase the basal metabolic rate,

2. make more glucose available to meet the elevated metabolic demands of an animal by increasing glycolysis, gluconeogenesis, and glucose absorption from the intestine,

3 stimulate the synthesis of enzymes or structural proteins,

4. increase lipid metabolism, including the conversion of cholesterol into bile acids and other substances, activation of lipoprotein lipase, and by increasing the sensitivity of adipose tissue to metabolic hormones that stimulate lipolysis,

THYROID HORMONE-RESPONSIVE CELL

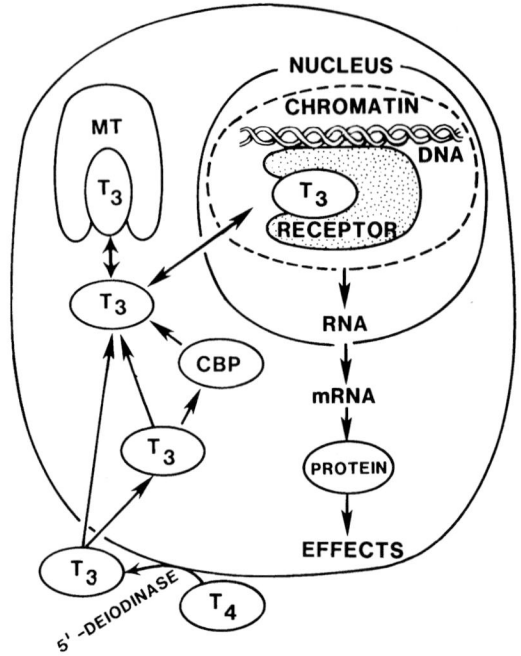

Fig. 3-15. Mechanism of action of thyroid hormones in target cells. Free triiodothyronine (**T_3**) primarily enters target cells because most of the thyroxine (**T_4**) undergoes monodeiodination in the liver or elsewhere in the periphery to form T_3. In the target cell, free T_3 either binds to cytosolic binding proteins (**CBP**), to nuclear receptors in target cells, or to high affinity receptors on the inner mitochondrial (**MT**) membrane and activates oxidative phosphorylation. In the nucleus, T_3 increases the transcription of **mRNA** which is released into the cytoplasm to direct the synthesis of new proteins. The increased synthesis of enzymes or new structural proteins results in the multiple biologic effects attributed to the activity of thyroid hormones.

5. stimulate heart rate, cardiac output, and blood flow, and

6. increase neural transmission, cerebration, and neuronal development in young animals.

DISORDERS OF THYROID FUNCTION

The levels of T_4 and T_3 normal in the blood of domestic species are shown in Table 3-1.

Hypothyroidism

Hypothyroidism is a well-recognized clinical entity in dogs. Although the disease may occur in many purebred and mixed breed dogs, certain breeds (Doberman Pinschers, Golden Retriev-

Table 3-1 Serum Thyroxine (T₄) and Triiodothyronine (T₃) Levels in Domestic Animals

Species	T_4 (nmol/L)*	T_3 (nmol/L)**
Bovine	**54.0 – 110.7** **(82.4)**	0.63 – 2.61 (1.42 ± 0.90)
Caprine	38.6 – 54.4 (44.4 ± 6.1)	1.35 – 2.92 (2.24 ± 0.45)
Equine	**11.6 – 36.0** **(20.0 ± 3.5)**	0.48 – 2.43 (1.18 ± 0.70)
Ovine	38.0 – 79.2 (56.8 ± 14.5)	0.97 – 2.30 (1.53 ± 0.43)
Porcine	21.9 – 60.2 (42.7 ± 10.3)	0.66 – 2.15 (1.38 ± 0.56)
Llama	**131.6 – 286.4** **(185.8 ± 50.3)**	**1.35 – 4.06** **(2.27 ± 0.94)**
Cat	**1.3 – 32.3** **(12.9 ± 6.5)**	**0.23 – 1.59** **(0.99 ± 0.32)**
Dog	**7.7 – 46.4** **(29.7 ± 10.3)**	**1.26 – 2.13** **(1.65 ± 0.28)**

Data shown as range with mean ± standard deviation in parentheses.
*T_4 – μg/dl × 12.87 = nmol/L
**T_3 – ng/dl × 0.01536 = nmol/L
Adapted from: M. Reap et al.,[93] (non-bold values) or Clinical Biochemistry of Domestic Animals, 5th ed., edited by J. J. Kaneko, J. W. Harvey, and M. L. Bruss. San Diego, CA, Academic Press, 1997, pp. 894 & 899 (**bold values**).

ers, and Beagles) appear to be more commonly affected than other breeds.

Clinical hypothyroidism usually is the result of primary diseases of the thyroid gland, especially idiopathic follicular atrophy also termed "follicular collapse" (Fig. 3-16) and lymphocytic thyroiditis (Fig. 3-17). In cases of "follicular collapse" there is a progressive loss of follicular cells and replacement by adipose connective tissue with a minimal inflammatory response.

Lymphocytic thyroiditis in dogs closely resembles Hashimoto's disease in humans and appears to be genetically conditioned, at least in certain breeds. Though the mechanisms for the disease are not well-established for the dog, it seems that a polygenic pattern of inheritance similar to that observed in the human disease also occurs in dogs. The immunologic basis for the development of chronic lymphocytic thyroiditis in both man and dog appears to be through the production of autoantibodies di-rected against thyroglobulin, a microsomal antigen (thyroperoxidase), and a second colloid antigen. In cases of lymphocytic thyroiditis, the thyroid gland consists of either a diffuse or nodular infiltration of lymphocytes, plasma cells, and macrophages (Fig. 3-17). Many of the remaining thyroid follicles are small and lined by tall columnar follicular cells, reflecting the long-standing stimulation of the thyroid gland by TSH; an attempt to compensate for the low blood levels of thyroid hormones. Ultrastructurally, numerous lymphocytes and macrophages are observed within the follicular basement membrane extending between follicular cells into the lumens of follicles (Fig. 3-18).

Hypothyroidism secondary to long-standing pituitary or hypothalamic lesions that prevent the release of either TSH or TRH is infrequent in the dog. In affected animals, the thyroid gland is only slightly reduced in size and is composed of colloid-distended follicles lined by flattened follicular cells (Fig. 3-19) due to a lack of TSH-

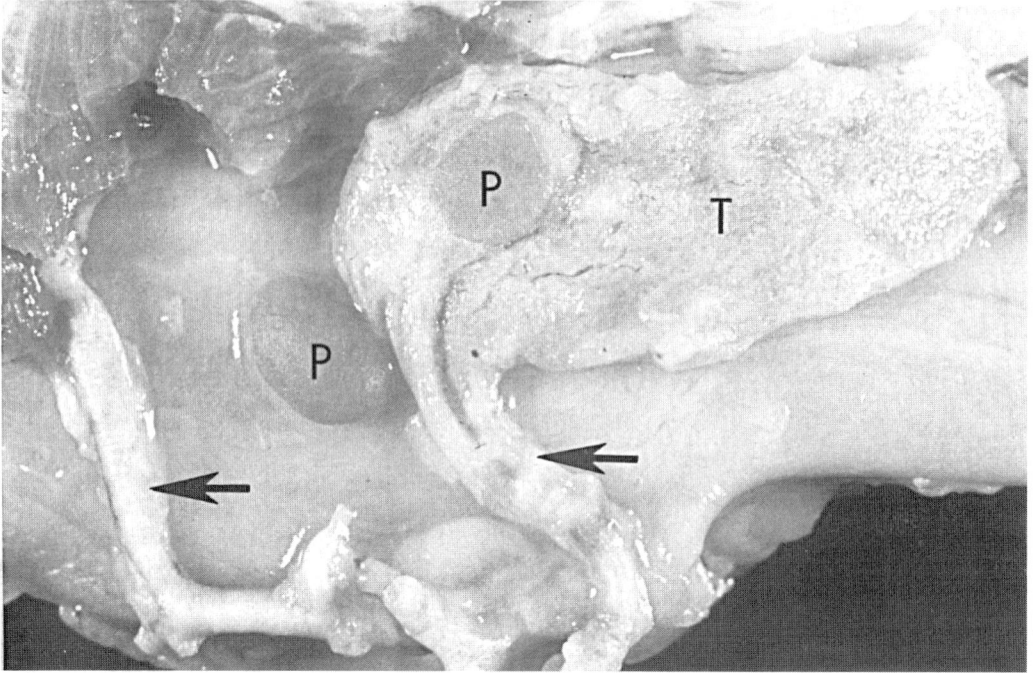

Fig. 3-16. Follicular collapse in a dog with hypothyroidism. The thyroid gland (**T**) is reduced in size compared to the adjacent parathyroid glands (**P**) and is lighter in color due to the replacement by adipose connective tissue. Branches of the cranial thyroid artery (**arrows**) are prominent due to atherosclerosis resulting from severe hyperlipidemia.

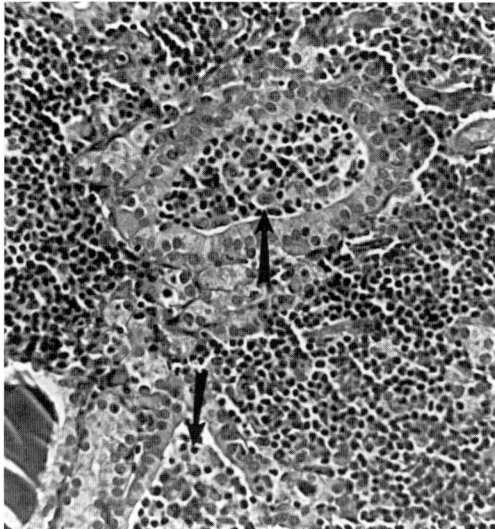

Fig. 3-17. Lymphocytic thyroiditis in a dog with hypothyroidism. Large focal accumulations of lymphocytes and plasma cells are present between the few remaining small thyroid follicles. Numerous lymphocytes and macrophages (**arrow**) are present within the lumen of a thyroid follicle.

induced endocytosis of colloid and secretion of thyroid hormones.

Clinical disturbances associated with hypothyroidism vary among affected animals and not every sign is seen in each patient. Many clinical signs associated with hypothyroidism are due to a reduction in basal metabolic rate. A gain in body weight without an associated change in appetite occurs frequently. The weight gain may vary from slight to striking obesity. The animal usually is less active and the owner may observe a reluctance to play or take walks. The inactivity also contributes to the weight gain.

Dogs with hypothyroidism may have difficulty in maintaining normal body temperature and are often "heat seekers." They will lie on or near sources of heat, such as registers, radiators, and electric blankets, and be reluctant to venture outdoors in cold weather. Excessive shivering may be observed and the skin frequently feels cool.

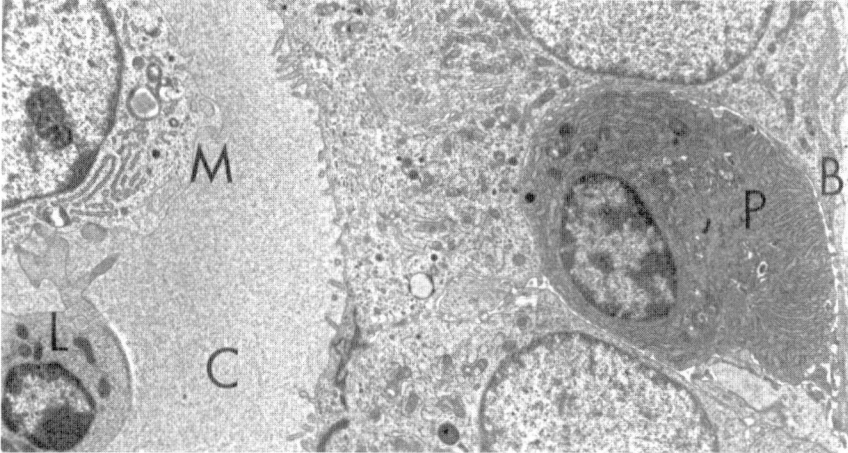

Fig. 3-18. Immune-mediated lymphocytic thyroiditis in a dog with hypothyroidism. A plasma cell (**P**) is migrating between follicular cells from the basement membrane (**B**) of the follicle into the colloid (**C**) in the follicular lumen. Lymphocytes (**L**) and macrophages (**M**) are present in the colloid. The continuous release of antigens from the colloid into the interstitial tissues in an animal with defective immune surveillance results in the progressive destruction of thyroid follicles, subnormal circulating levels of thyroid hormones, and the clinical syndrome of hypothyroidism.

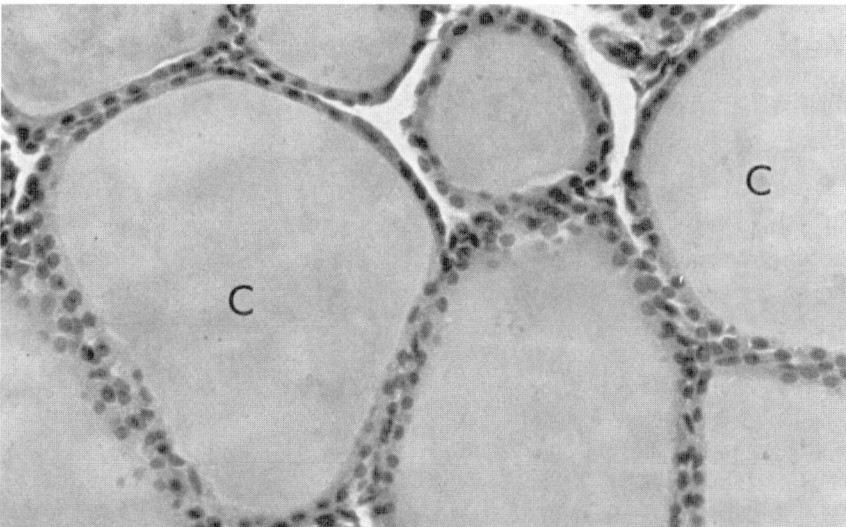

Fig. 3-19. Histologic appearance of the canine thyroid in TSH deficiency caused by a large nonfunctional pituitary tumor. Thyroid follicles are distended by the continued accumulation of colloid (**C**), and the follicular epithelium is flattened. Note the complete absence of endocytotic vacuoles about the periphery of the colloid.

In long-standing and severe hypothyroidism in dogs, myxedema may develop and produce a characteristic appearance (Fig. 3-20). There is accumulation of mucin and acid mucopolysaccharides combined with protein in the dermis and subcutis. This material binds considerable amounts of water and produces a marked thickening of the skin. Myxedema is obvious around the face and head where accentuation of the normal skin folds causes a sad or "tragic" appearance (Fig. 3-20).

Other manifestations of hypothyroidism are the failure of hair regrowth after clipping for either cosmetic or therapeutic purposes and

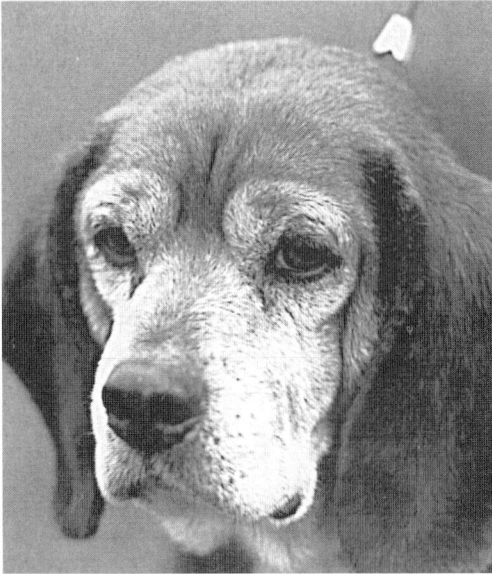

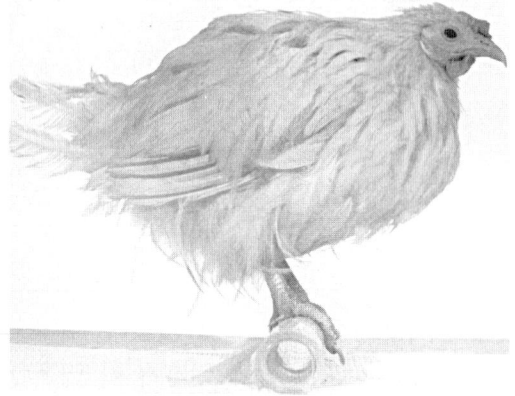

Fig. 3-21. Hypothyroidism in the inbred strain (OS) of chicken resulting from immune-mediated thyroiditis and progressive destruction of the thyroid gland.

Fig. 3-20. Myxedema in a dog with long-standing and severe hypothyroidism. The thickening of skin folds of the face and eyelids results in a "tragic" facial expression.

abnormalities in reproduction including lack of libido and reduction in sperm count in males or abnormal or absent estrous cycles with reduced conception rates in females. In addition, a change in attitude often is observed by the owner. The affected animal often appears dull and less active (Fig. 3-20).

Hypothyroidism is encountered only sporadically in other animal species. Hypothyroidism is reported infrequently in cats and the clinical signs include prolonged periods of apathy, poor hair growth, severe seborrhea, and myxedema of the face with a blunted serum T_4 increase in response to exogenous TSH administration. Hypothyroid chickens are small, moderately obese with increased accumulations of abdominal fat, have a small, dry comb, and an abnormally silky plumage (Fig. 3-21). Feathers from chickens with hypothyroidism (Fig. 3-22; Left) are long, silky, and with reduced numbers of hooklets on the distal barbules to grasp the proximal barbule necessary for normal feather structure (Fig. 3-22; Right).

The diagnosis of hypothyroidism is based on the history, clinical signs, and demonstration of

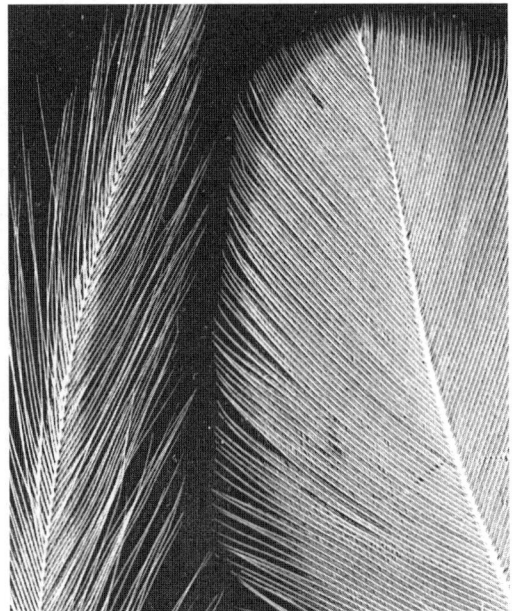

Fig. 3-22. Abnormal feather (**left**) from a hypothyroid (OS strain) chicken compared to a control (**right**). In the hypothyroid animal, the feathers are long and silky with reduced hooklets on the distal barbules necessary to grasp the proximal barbule.

lowered levels of circulating thyroid hormones. At present, the most sensitive and clinically available method for measurement of blood T_4 and T_3 levels is radioimmunoassay (RIA;

see Chapter 1 for review). The normal blood level of total T_4 in the dog is between 1.5 and 3.4 µg/dl and for total T_3 between 48 and 154 ng/dl. In dogs with hypothyroidism the total T_4 level usually is below 0.8 µg/dl and total T_3 is below 50 ng/dl. When the hormonal levels are borderline, clearer separation of dogs with hypothyroidism from normal dogs can be made by challenging the thyroid gland of the patient with an injection of TSH and evaluating the elevation in total T_4 in a second blood sample taken 4 to 8 hours later.

The serum cholesterol is elevated (400 to 900 mg/dl and above) in many hypothyroid dogs. The decreased rate of lipid metabolism with diminished intestinal excretion of cholesterol and conversion of lipids into bile acids and other compounds frequently results in hypercholesterolemia. Atherosclerosis of coronary and cerebral vessels may occur in animals with severe hypothyroidism and long-standing hyperlipidemia (Fig. 3-23). This occasionally results in hemorrhage and ischemic necrosis of the myocardium due to occlusion of the vessel lumen by numerous lipid-laden macrophages in the tunica media and adventitia.

The treatment of hypothyroidism involves the oral administration of synthetic thyroxine or triiodothyronine on a daily basis.

Hyperthyroidism

Among domestic animal species, disturbances of growth resulting from the production of excess thyroid hormone is most common in adult cats and often related to adenomas composed of hyperactive follicular cells. These neoplastic cells release both T_4 and T_3 at an uncontrolled rate resulting in markedly elevated blood levels of both hormones.

Cats with hyperthyroidism have elevated levels of total serum thyroxine and triiodothyronine. Normal serum levels of T_4 in cats, as measured by radioimmunoassay, are approximately 1.5 to 4.5 µg/dl and serum T_3 levels are 60 to 100 ng/dl. In hyperthyroid cats the total levels of T_4 in the serum range from 5.0 to over 50 µg/dl and total levels of T_3 in the serum range from 100 to 1,000 ng/dl (Fig. 3-24). Hyperthyroidism is associated with weight loss[88] in spite of a normal or increased appetite (Fig. 3-25) and with restlessness and increased activity.

There has been a dramatic increase in the incidence in feline hyperthyroidism since the

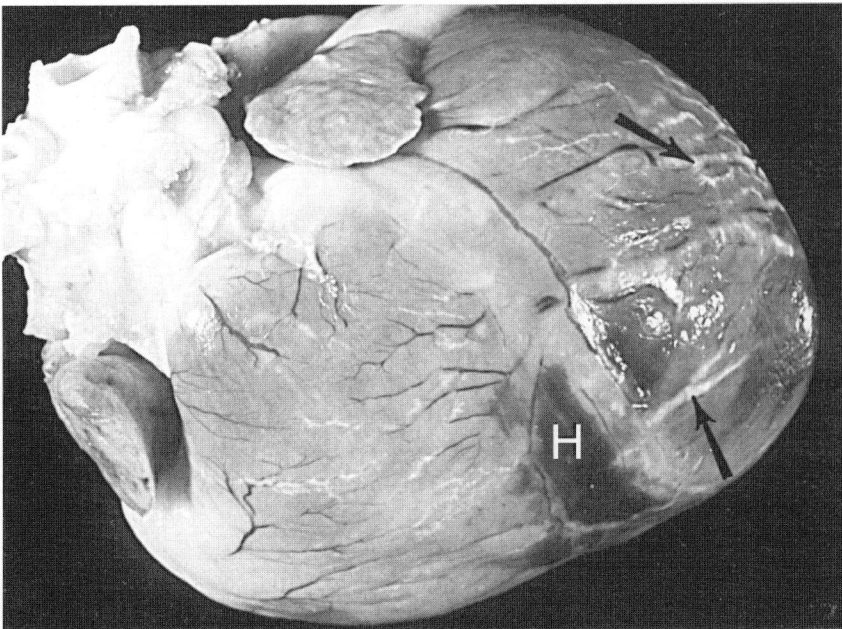

Fig. 3-23. Coronary atherosclerosis (**arrows**) with areas of ischemic necrosis and hemorrhage of myocardium (**H**) in a dog with marked hyperlipidemia associated with severe hypothyroidism.

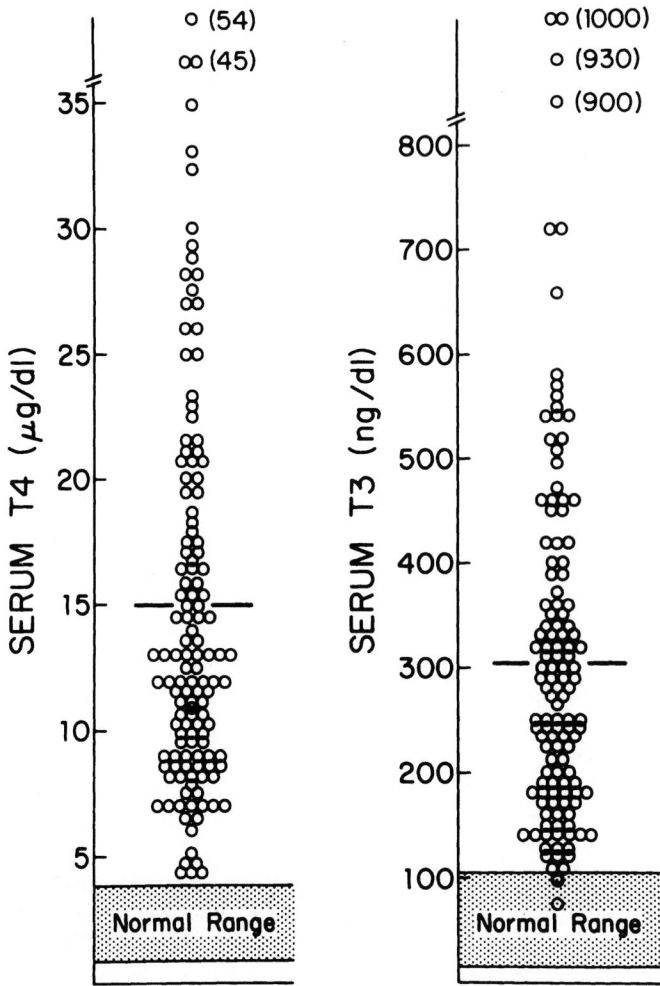

Fig. 3-24. Serum thyroid hormone levels in cats with hyperthyroidism. There is a marked elevation of serum thyroxine (mean = 15 µg/dl) and triiodothyronine (mean = 300 ng/dl) in cats with hyperthyroidism. (From: M. E. Peterson, et al.,[88] 1983).

late 1970s, and now it is one of the two most common endocrine diseases in adult-age cats. The increased incidence of the disease is likely due to:

1.   the larger number of older cats receiving veterinary medical care,

2.   improved assays for thyroid hormones,

3.   the detailed characterization of this syndrome and increased awareness of its occurrence in adult cats by veterinary clinicians, and

4.   autonomous proliferation of follicular cells.

Dogs have a very efficient enterohepatic excretory mechanism for thyroid hormones that is difficult to overload, either from endogenous production by a tumor or by exogenous administration of thyroid hormones. Hence, thyroid tumors in the dog only occasionally secrete sufficient amounts of thyroid hormone to overload the highly efficient enterohepatic excretory pathways for thyroid hormones and produce clinical signs of hyperthyroidism. The clinical signs of hyperthyroidism in dogs with functional thyroid tumors include polyuria and polydipsia (Fig. 3-26) and weight loss, despite increased appetite and

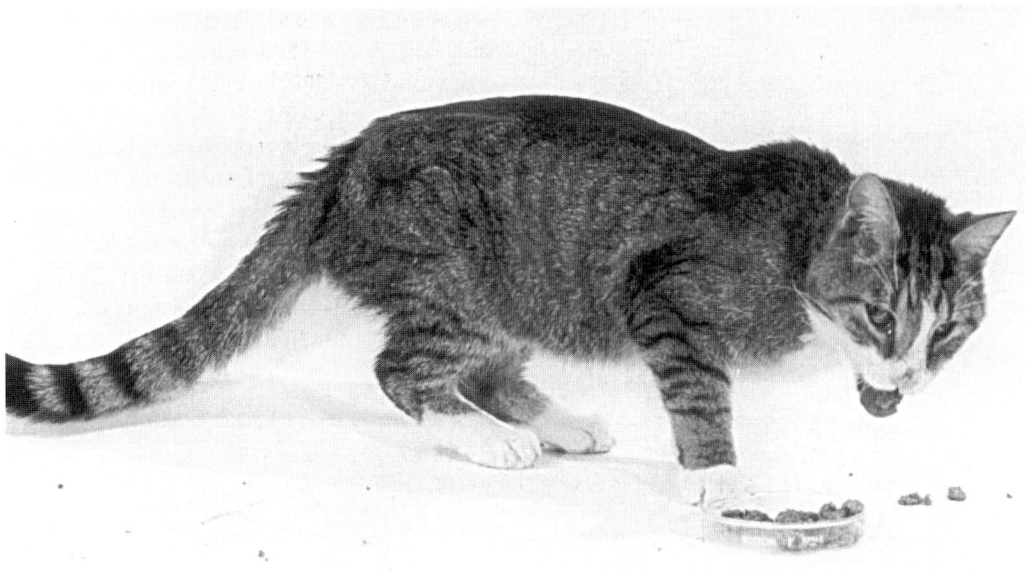

Fig. 3-25. Hyperthyroidism in a cat caused by a functional tumor derived from thyroid follicular cells that secreted thyroid hormones at an uncontrolled rate resulting in markedly elevated blood levels of T_4 and T_3. This cat had lost considerable body weight in spite of an increased appetite owing to the gluconeogenic effects of the long-standing elevation of thyroid hormones.

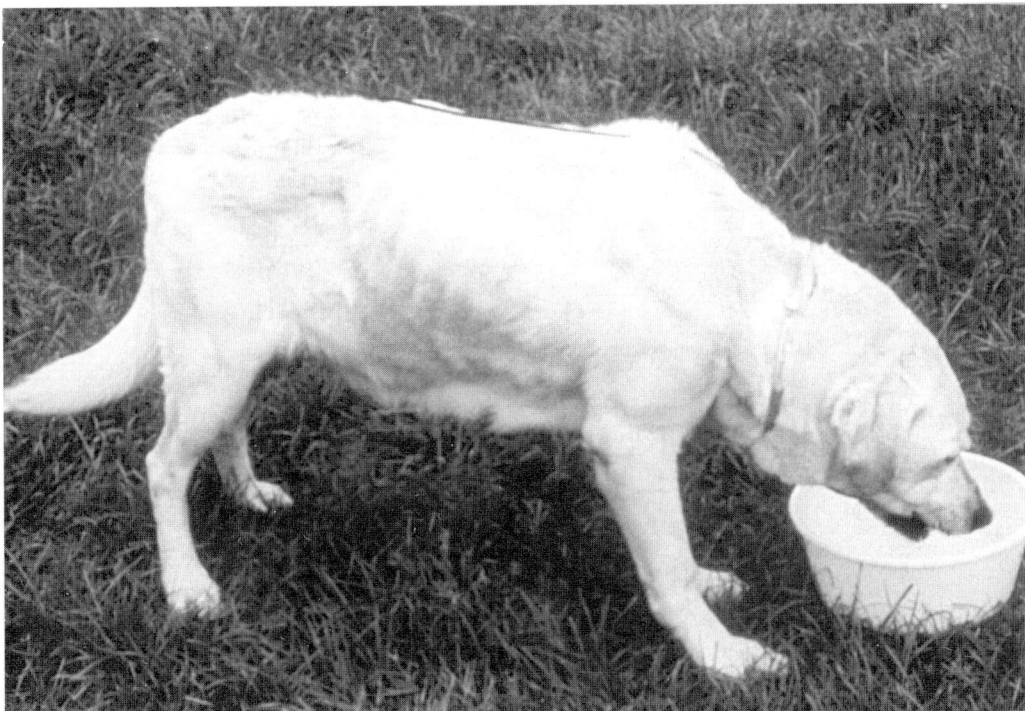

Fig. 3-26. Hyperthyroidism associated with a carcinoma of the thyroid gland of a dog was accompanied by severe weight loss, muscle atrophy, and polydipsia.

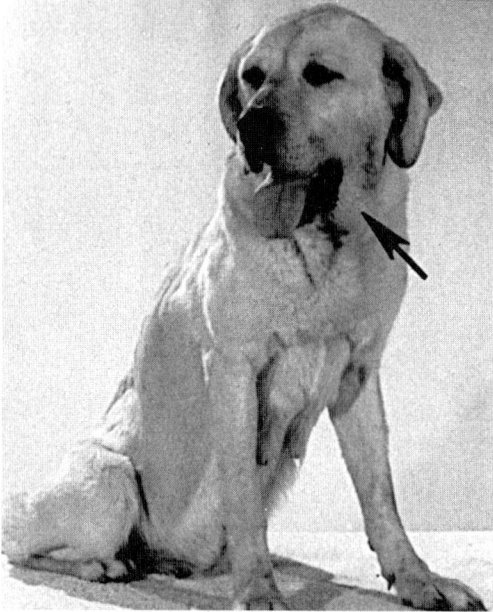

Fig. 3-27. Hyperthyroidism in a 7.5-year-old, female Labrador Retriever with a functional carcinoma in the thyroid gland (**arrow**) arising at the base of the tongue from ectopic thyroid tissue.

polyphagia, leading to muscle atrophy and weakness (Fig. 3-27). The levels of T_3 and T_4 in the serum of dogs with clinical hyperthyroidism are only mildly elevated: 300-400 ng/dl and 5-7 µg/dl, respectively. As compared to dogs, cats are very sensitive to phenol and phenol-derivatives. They have a poor ability to conjugate phenolic compounds such as T_4 with glucuronic acid and to excrete the T_4-glucuronide into the bile (Fig. 3-28). In cats, the capacity for conjugation of T_3 with sulfate is also limited and can easily be overloaded.

Hyperplasia of Thyroid Follicular Cells ("Goiter")

"Goiter" is a clinical term for a non-neoplastic and non-inflammatory enlargement of the thyroid gland which develops in mammals, birds, and submammalian vertebrates. The major pathogenic mechanisms responsible for the development of thyroid hyperplasia include iodine-deficient diets, goitrogenic compounds that interfere with hormone synthesis, dietary

Thyroxine Metabolism

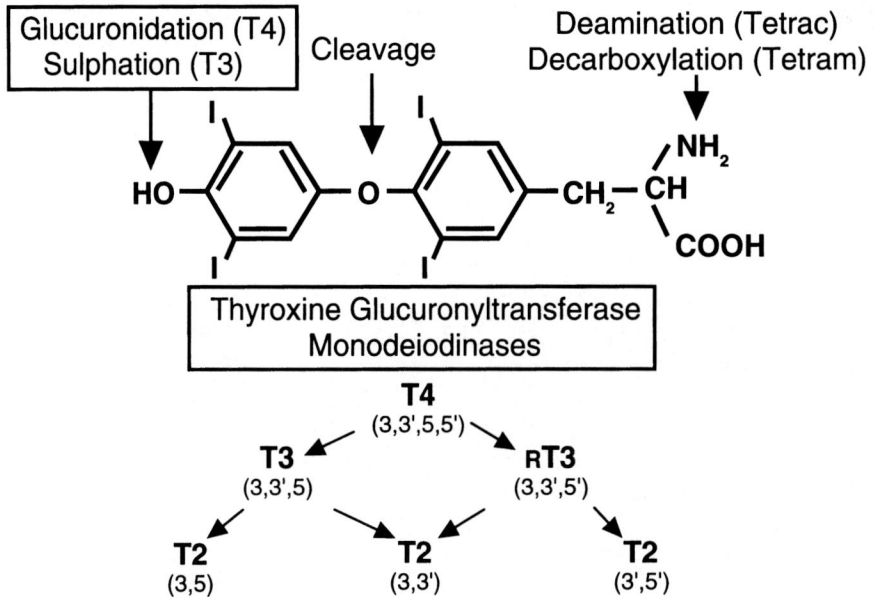

Fig. 3-28. Degradation of thyroid hormones. Thyroxine is conjugated with glucuronic acid in a reaction catalyzed by UDP-glucuronyl transferase and T_4-glucuronide is excreted in the bile. Triiodothyronine is conjugated with sulfate and T_3-sulfate is excreted in the bile.

iodide-excess, and genetic defects in the biosynthesis of thyroid hormones (Fig. 3-29). All of these seemingly divergent factors result in deficient thyroxine and triiodothyronine synthesis and decreased blood levels of thyroid hormones. This is sensed by the hypothalamus and pituitary gland and leads to an increased secretion of TSH, which results in hypertrophy and hyperplasia of follicular cells in the thyroid gland (Fig. 3-29). The following subtypes of goiters are recognized: diffuse hyperplastic, colloid, iodide-excess, multifocal hyperplastic, and congenital dyshormonogenetic. A full description of the pathophysiology and clinical symptoms of these forms of goiter is beyond the scope of this chapter. Interested readers may find pertinent reference to diseases of the thyroid gland in the bibliography supplied with this chapter.

Diffuse Hyperplastic Goiter

Diffuse thyroid hyperplasia due to iodine deficiency in the diet was common in many goitrogenic areas throughout the world before the widespread addition of iodized salt to animal and human diets. Although iodine-deficient goiter still occurs worldwide in domestic animals, the outbreaks are sporadic and fewer animals are affected. Marginally iodine-deficient diets containing certain goitrogenic substances may result in severe thyroid hyperplasia and clinical evidence of goiter. Goitrogenic substances include thiouracil, propylthiouracil, sulfonamides, complex anions such as perchlorate [CLO_4], pertechnetate [TcO_4^-], perrhenate [ReO_4^-], and tetrafluoroborate [BF_4]. In addition, a number of plants from the genus *Brassica* contain thioglycosides which after digestion release thiocyanate (Fig. 3-30) and isothiocyanate. A particularly potent thioglycoside, goitrin (L-5-vinyl-2 thiooxazolidone), from plants is excreted in milk. Young animals born to females on iodine-deficient diets are more likely to develop severe thyroid hyperplasia and have clinical signs of hypothyroidism including palpable enlargement of the thyroid gland (Fig. 3-7).

Iodine deficiency may be conditioned by other antithyroid compounds present in animal feeds and in particular situations, these can be responsible for a high incidence of goiter. Hyperplastic goiter in ruminants is associated with prolonged low-level exposure to thiocyanates produced by the ruminal degradation of cyanogenic glucosides of plants such as white clover (*Trifolium*), couch grass, and linseed meal, and by degradation of glucosinolates of *Brassica* crops. These goitrogenic chemicals in plants become clinically significant when the dietary intake of iodine is low and can result in goiter due to TSH-mediated hypertrophy and hyperplasia of follicular cells. *Leucaerna leucocephala* and other legumes of this genus are native or cultivated in many subtropical areas and contain the toxic amino acid mimosine.

Goiter in adult animals is usually of little clinical significance and the general health of the animal is not impaired, except for occasional local pressure influences. However, goiter is of significance as a disease of the newborn, although the drastic losses of animals in endemic areas are now controlled by the prophylactic use of iodized salt. Congenital hypothyroidism in domestic animals may be associated with iodine-deficient hyperplastic goiter, even though the dam shows no evidence of thyroid dysfunction. Gestation often is significantly prolonged, particularly for animals with large goiters, and there is increased incidence of dystocia (difficult birth) with retention of the fetal placenta. Foals affected with iodine-deficient goiter have moderately enlarged thyroids, are weak at birth, and frequently die within a few days after birth. Calves with goiter are born partially or completely hairless and are either born dead or die soon after birth. Newborn goitrous pigs, goats, and lambs frequently have myxedema and hair loss. The mortality rate is high in these species, with the majority of offspring born dead or dying within a few hours of birth. Enlarged thyroid glands are readily palpable or visible in kids and lambs, but are not apparent in piglets because of the combination of short neck and myxedema. Asphyxiation may result from the pressure exerted by the enlarged thyroid gland, however, young goitrous animals that are treated promptly and survive usually do not show permanent harmful effects.

Mechanisms of Goitrogenesis

Goitrogenic compounds
- Complex anions
  KSCN⁻
  KCLO₄⁻
  TcO₄⁻
- Thiouracil, PTU
- Sulfonamides
- Plant goitrins
  Genus Brassicae

Deficient dietary iodine

Excess dietary iodine

Genetic defects "Congenital Goiter"
- Defective Thyroglobulin synthesis (O,B,C)
- Iodination Defect (H)
- Coupling Defect
- (↓) I⁻ uptake (NIS)
- (↓) 2I⁻ $\overset{O}{\rightarrow}$ I₂ (TPO)

Inadequate Thyroxine Synthesis or Release

+

Increased Thyroxine Demand
- Young animal
- Pregnancy
- Stress
- Severe Infection
- Puberty

→ **Decreased Blood T₄/T₃**

+

(↑) Hypothalamic TRH (Releasing Hormone)

+

(↑) Pituitary TSH

+

Defective Homeostasis (Exophthalmic Goiter) ──LATS──→ **Thyroid Gland Hypertrophy and Hyperplasia Follicular Cells**

(↑) Thyroid hormone synthesis & secretion

Hypothyroid   **Euthyroid**   **Hyperthyroid**

Clinical Status

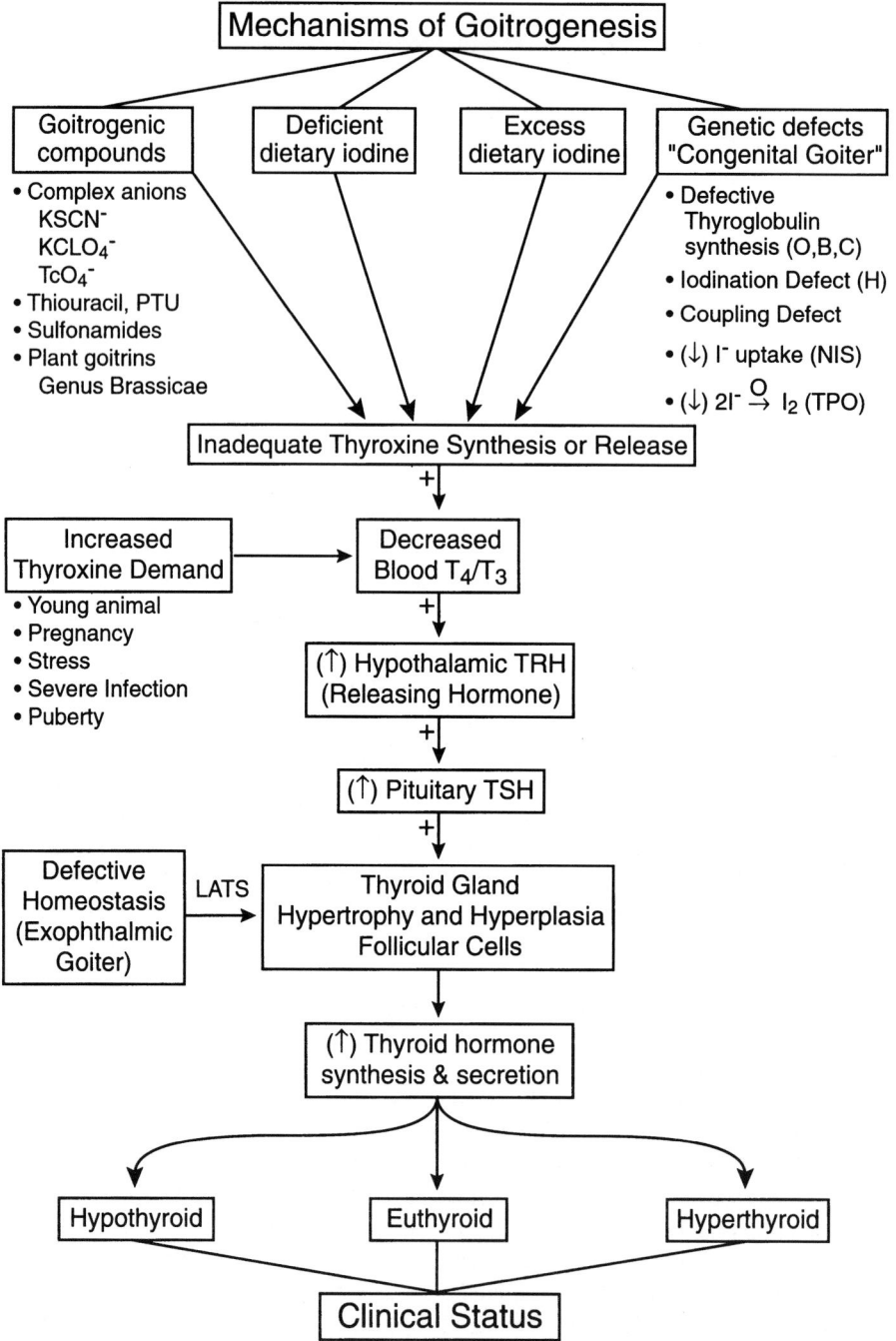

Fig. 3-29. Mechanisms of goitrogenesis. Multiple pathogenic factors (goitrogenic compounds, deficient and excess dietary iodine intake, and genetic defects) result in inadequate thyroxine/triiodothyronine synthesis and leads to long-term stimulation of thyroid follicular cells resulting in hypertrophy and hyperplasia due to the increased pituitary secretion of thyroid-stimulating hormone (**TSH**). (**LATS** = Long Acting Thyroid Stimulator, an autoantibody that binds to the TSH receptor to stimulate the synthetic and secretory activity of follicular cells; **NIS** = Sodium Iodine Symporter; **PTU** = propylthiouracil; **TPO** = thyroperoxidase; **H** = human; **O** = ovine; **B** = bovine; **C** = caprine; **KClO₄⁻** = potassium perchlorate; **TcO₄⁻** = pertechnetate; **KSCN⁻** = potassium thiocyanate; **TRH** = thyrotropin-releasing hormone).

MECHANISM OF ACTION OF GOITROGENS
ON THYROID HORMONE SYNTHESIS AND SECRETION

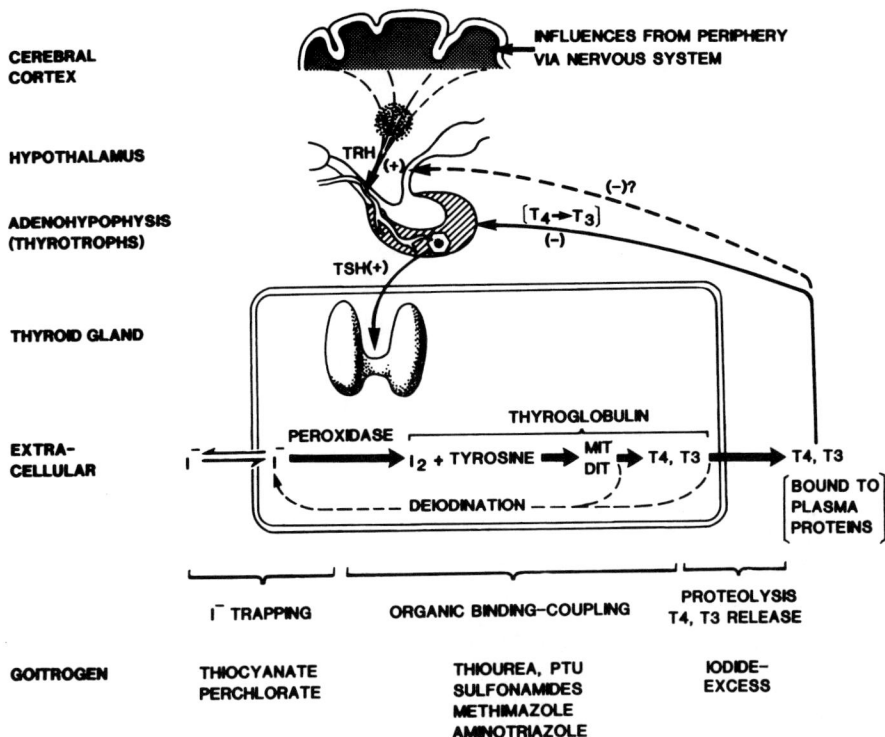

Fig. 3-30. Mechanism of action of goitrogens on thyroid hormone synthesis and secretion. (**DIT** = diiodotyrosine; **MIT** = monoiodotyrosine; **PTU** = propylthiouracil **TRH** = Thyrotropin releasing hormone; **TSH** = Thyroid-stimulating hormone).

Colloid Goiter

Colloid goiter represents the involutionary phase of diffuse hyperplastic goiter in young-adult and adult animals. The markedly hyperplastic follicular cells continue to produce colloid but endocytosis of colloid is decreased due to diminished pituitary TSH levels in a feedback response to the return of blood levels of T_4 and T_3 to the normal range. Both thyroid lobes are diffusely enlarged but are more translucent and lighter in color than in animals with hyperplastic goiter. The differences in macroscopic appearance are the result of less vascularity in colloid goiter and the development of macrofollicles distended with colloid (Figs. 3-31 and 3-32). The interface between the colloid and luminal surface of follicular cells is smooth (Fig. 3-33) and lacks the characteristic endocytotic vacuoles of actively secreting follicular cells.

Iodide-Excess Goiter

Although seemingly paradoxical, an excess of iodide in the diet also results in thyroid hyperplasia in animals and man. Foals of mares fed dry seaweed containing excessive iodide may develop thyroid hyperplasia and clinically evident goiter. Due to the concentration of iodide by the placenta and by the mammary gland, the thyroid glands of the young are exposed to higher blood iodide levels than the dam. High blood levels of iodide interfere with one or more steps of thyroxinogenesis, leading to lowered blood levels of thyroid hormones and a compensatory increase in pituitary TSH secretion. Excess iodine appears to block the release of T_3 and T_4 from the follicular cell by interfering with the proteolysis of phagocytized colloid droplets by lysosomal bodies, as well as affecting other steps in hormonal synthesis.

Multifocal ("Nodular") Hyperplasia ("Goiter")

Nodular hyperplasia in the thyroid glands of older horses, cats, and dogs appears as multiple nodules of varying size (Fig. 3-34). The affected

lobes are moderately enlarged and irregular in contour. Multinodular goiter in most animals, with the exception of cats, is endocrinologically inactive and encountered as an incidental lesion at necropsy. However, older cats with hyperthyroidism often develop a thyroid gland with multinodular hyperplasia (Fig. 3-34). Nodular goiter consists of multiple foci of hyperplastic

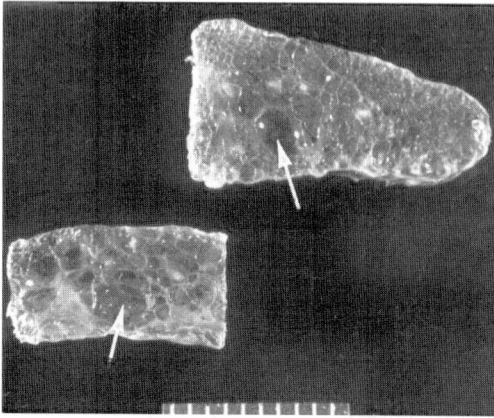

Fig. 3-31. Colloid goiter with macroscopically visible follicles filled with colloid (**arrows**). The scale represents 1 cm.

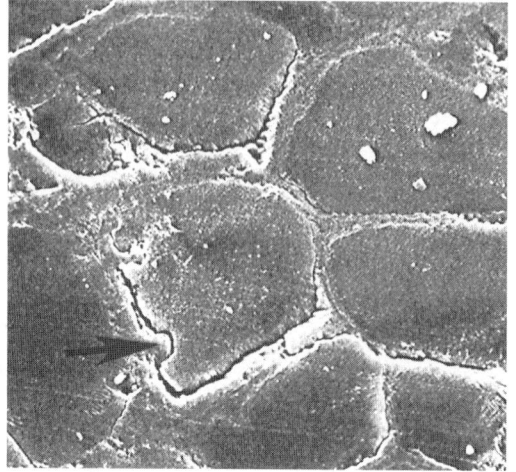

Fig. 3-32. Scanning electron micrograph of enlarged thyroid with colloid goiter illustrating large involuted follicles distended with colloid and remnants of papillary projections of hyperplastic follicular cells (**arrow**).

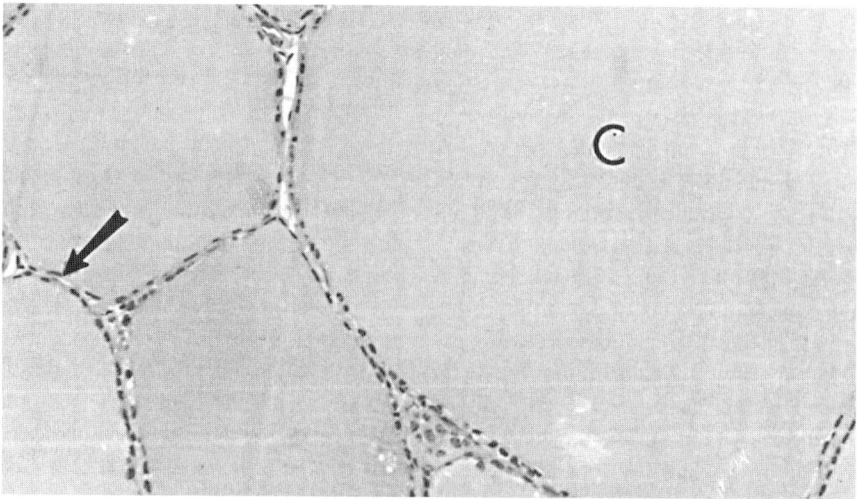

Fig. 3-33. Colloid goiter illustrating large distended thyroid follicles lined by flattened atrophic follicular cells (**arrow**). Distention of follicles with colloid (**C**) occurs due to diminished TSH-mediated endocytosis in the hyperplastic thyroid gland following the return of blood levels of T_4 and T_3 to the normal range.

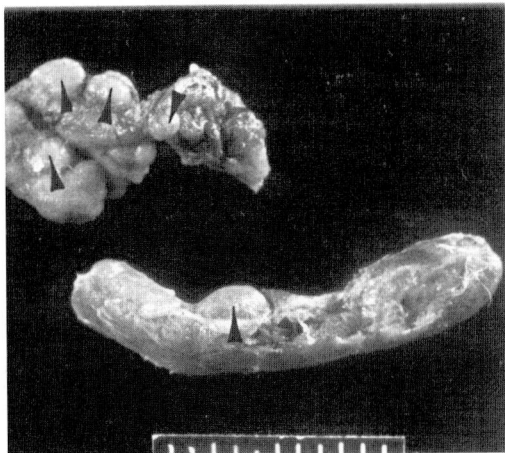

Fig. 3-34. Multinodular follicular cell hyperplasia (**arrowheads**) in the thyroid lobes from a cat with hyperthyroidism.

follicular cells that are not encapsulated but are sharply demarcated from the adjacent thyroid parenchyma.

Congenital Dyshormonogenetic Goiter

Congenital dyshormonogenetic goiter has been documented in several animal species and is characterized by the inability of the animal to synthesize and secrete adequate amounts of thyroid hormones prior to or at birth.

Congenital goiter (Fig. 3-29) is inherited as an autosomal recessive gene in sheep, Afrikander cattle, and Saanen dwarf goats. The subnormal growth rate, absence of normal wool development or a rough, sparse, hair coat, myxedematous swellings of the subcutis, weakness, and sluggish behavior suggest that the affected young are clinically hypothyroid. Most lambs with congenital goiter die shortly after birth or are highly sensitive to the effects of adverse environmental conditions.

Although thyroidal uptake and turnover of ^{131}I are greatly increased compared with euthyroid controls, circulating levels of T_4 and T_3 are consistently low in these animals. The lack of a defect in the mechanisms related to iodide transport, iodide organification or the dehalogenation of thyroxine, the absence of normal 19S thyroglobulin in animals with goitrous thyroids,

and relatively minute amounts of thyroglobulin-related antigens (0.01% of normal), suggests an impairment of thyroglobulin biosynthesis in animals with congenital goiter.

The levels of protein-bound iodine in animals with inherited congenital goiter are markedly elevated. This appears to be the result of the iodination of albumin and other plasma proteins by the thyroid gland in response to long-term stimulation by TSH. However, the concentration of thyroglobulin-mRNA sequences in tissues from affected animals are considerably reduced (1-2% of normal).

COMPARATIVE PATHOBIOLOGY OF THE THYROID GLAND

The basic functions of the hypothalamic-pituitary-thyroid axis are similar in animals and humans. However, species differences must be considered before attempting to use animal data related to the effects of drugs and chemicals on thyroid function for assessment of human risk. Long-term alterations of the pituitary-thyroid axis by various xenobiotic chemicals or pathophysiological disturbances, such as those caused by iodine deficiency and partial thyroidectomy, are more likely to predispose laboratory rodents, rats and mice, to a higher incidence of hyperplasia and tumors of follicular cells than in the human thyroid.[17] This appears to be particularly true for male rats which have higher circulating levels of TSH than females.

The plasma half-life of T_4 is shorter in rats (12-24 hours) than in humans and monkeys (5-9 days). This is related in part to differences between these species in the transport proteins for T_4 and T_3,[32] because rodents, birds, amphibians, or fish do not synthesize the high affinity protein (thyroxine-binding globulin - TBG which binds T_4).

Although T_4 is the principal secretory product of the thyroid gland, it functions primarily as a prohormone and undergoes a single deiodination of the phenolic ring in extrathyroidal tissues to form the metabolically more active T_3.[104] Triiodothyronine is bound to TBG and albumin in humans, monkeys, and dogs, but is bound only to albumin in mice, rats, and chickens.

Many xenobiotic chemicals and drugs disrupt one or more steps in the synthesis and secretion of thyroid hormones or enhance the catabolism of thyroid hormones (Fig. 3-35), especially those which increase the cytochrome p450 thyroxine-metabolizing enzymes of the liver. In long-term studies using laboratory rodents this results in subnormal levels of T_4 and T_3 which are associated with a compensatory increase in the secretion of pituitary TSH. Rats and mice are particularly sensitive to the decreased availability of T_4 and T_3 and respond with hypertrophy and hyperplasia of follicular cells and in long-term studies there is increased incidence of thyroid tumors. These tumors develop as an indirect response to the hormonal imbalance.

In the indirect or secondary mechanism of thyroid oncogenesis in rodents, the specific xenobiotic chemical or physiologic perturbation evokes a stimulus, such as the chronic hypersecretion of TSH, that promotes the development of nodular proliferative lesions derived from follicular cells. Compounds acting by this indirect mechanism usually have little or no evidence for mutagenicity or for producing DNA damage.

By comparison, there is little, if any, increase in the incidence of thyroid cancer in humans who have markedly altered changes in thyroid function and elevated TSH levels. The relative resistance to the development of thy-

Disruption of Hypothalamic, Pituitary, Thyroid Triad by Xenobiotic Chemicals

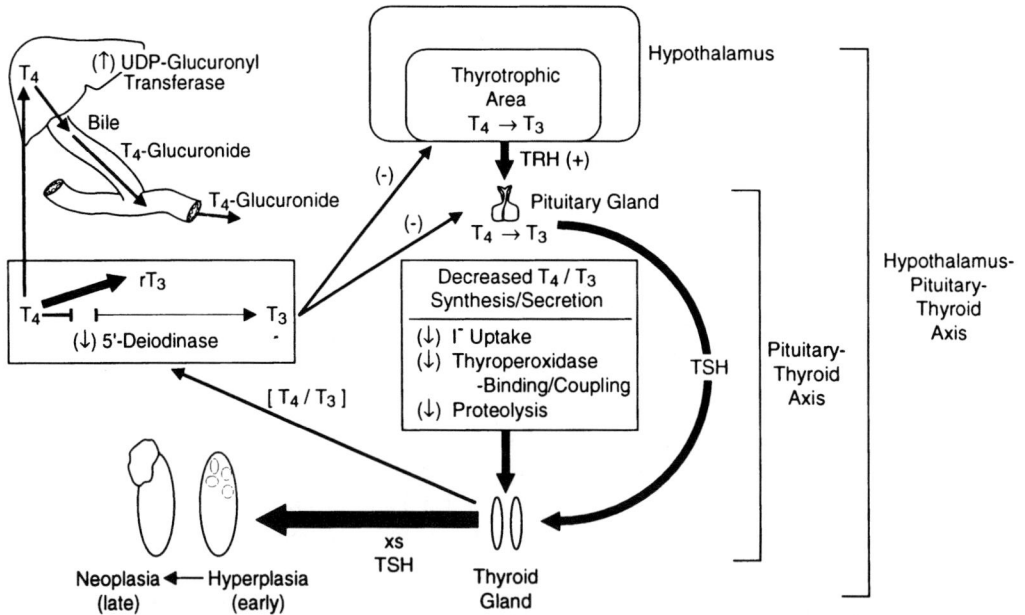

Fig. 3-35. Multiple sites of disruption of the hypothalamic-pituitary-thyroid triad by xenobiotic chemicals. Chemicals can exert direct effects by disrupting thyroid hormone synthesis or secretion and may indirectly influence the thyroid through an inhibition of 5'-deiodinase or by inducing hepatic microsomal enzymes (e.g., T_4-UDP-glucuronyl transferase). All of these mechanisms can lower circulating levels of thyroid hormones (T_4 and T_3) resulting in a release from negative feedback inhibition leading to the increased secretion of thyroid-stimulating hormone (**TSH**) by the pituitary gland. The chronic hypersecretion of TSH predisposes the sensitive rodent thyroid gland to develop an increased incidence of focal hyperplastic and neoplastic (adenomas) lesions by a secondary (epigenetic) mechanism of oncogenesis due to hormonal imbalances. (**TRH** = thyrotropin-releasing hormone; **rT₃** = inactive or reverse triiodothyronine; **xs** = excess).

roid cancer in humans with elevated plasma TSH levels is in marked contrast to the response of the thyroid gland of rats or mice to chronic TSH stimulation. Hence, laboratory rodents are not good models for safety assessment of a new drug or chemical projected for use in humans, particularly when the factor affects thyroid function.

The rate of secretion of the thyroid hormones T_3 and T_4 is seldom measured *in vitro* due to the lack of follicular organization and the reduced ability of follicular cells growing in monolayer culture to concentrate and efficiently iodinate thyroglobulin. The *in vitro* testing of thyroid function usually is restricted to the evaluation of specific phases of thyroid hormone synthesis, including iodide-trapping, thyroid peroxidase synthesis and activity, TSH-receptor expression, and the expression, secretion, and iodination of thyroglobulin.

The phagocytic activity of thyroid follicular cells can be quantitated by a sensitive nonradioactive assay using a follicular cell line (FRTL-5) from normal rat thyroid. This *in vitro* assay permits the rapid discrimination of the number of functionally active follicular cells after exposure to xenobiotic chemicals.

THYROID FUNCTION TESTS

Thyroid function tests are frequently used for the diagnosis of thyroid diseases in animals. In hypothyroid animals there is a reduced rate of metabolism. The most direct indicator of hypothyroidism is the measurement of basal oxygen consumption to determine the magnitude of the reduction in metabolic activity. However, valid and satisfactorily reproducible measurements of oxygen consumption cannot be used in clinical conditions because a long and painstaking training of the animal is required to achieve the relaxation of mental and physical activity that is necessary for accurate measurement of the basal metabolic rate.

Other tests of the functional integrity of the thyroid and which can be used clinically include: (a) determination of serum cholesterol levels in dogs; (b) thyroidal uptake of radioiodine; and (c) radioimmunoassays for thyroid hormones.

Serum Cholesterol

The levels of cholesterol in the serum of dogs is a clinical variable that can be used as an index of the peripheral action of thyroid hormones. A differential diagnosis, particularly with respect to liver and pancreatic diseases and diabetes mellitus is mandatory. Fasting levels of cholesterol in excess of 600 mg/100 ml are commonly observed in hypothyroid dogs.[17] Furthermore, these elevated levels of serum cholesterol are responsible for the secondary lesions of hypothyroidism including atherosclerosis with infarction (Fig. 3-23), as well as renal glomerular, hepatic, and corneal lipidosis.

Thyroidal Uptake of Radioiodine

The test for thyroidal uptake of radioiodine is primarily based on the amount of radioiodine taken up by the thyroid. Clinical measurements of iodine uptake are dependent upon the functional integrity of the gland, the endogenous output of TSH, and the dietary intake of iodine. The increased uptake and turnover of radioiodine due to iodine deficiency (Fig. 3-36) can be

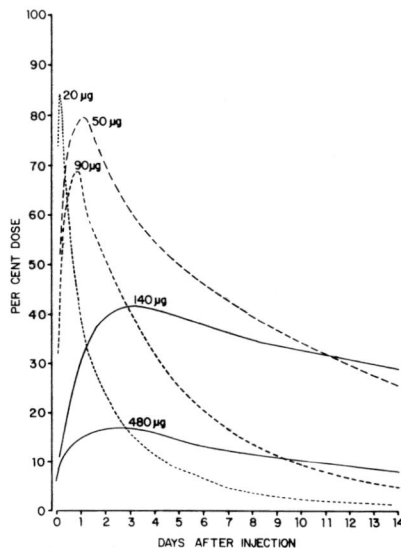

Fig. 3-36. Influence of iodine intake on thyroidal uptake and turnover of radioiodine. Each curve represents the averaged data for five adult Beagles maintained at the designated level of iodine intake for periods ranging from 5 months (at 480 µg per day) to 1 year (at 20 µg per day). (Reproduced with permission from: C. C. Capen, B. E. Belshaw, and S. L. Martin,[17] 1975).

distinguished from that of functional thyroid tumors by repetition of the tracer studies after a week or more following feeding of a diet that provides a daily dose of iodine that is slightly in excess of the normal requirement.

Radioimmunoassay of Thyroid Hormones

The most sensitive and accurate method for measurement of circulating levels of total thyroxine and triiodothyronine is the radioimmunoassay (see Chapter 1). The normal blood levels of total T_4 (Fig. 3-37) and T_3 (Fig. 3-38) in dogs range between 1.5 to 3.6 µg/dl and 48 and 154 ng/dl, respectively.[4] Hypothyroid dogs usually have a blood level of T_4 below 1.0 µg/dl (Fig. 3-37) and T_3 is below 50 ng/dl (Fig. 3-38). When hormonal levels are borderline, clearer separation of dogs with hypothyroidism from euthyroid dogs can be accomplished by a systemic injection of TSH. In the euthyroid dog the T_4 level will at least double 8 hours after IV or IM administration of TSH (Fig. 3-39). The increase in serum levels of T_3 after TSH injection is more variable in normal dogs than for T_4 (Fig. 3-40), but in dogs with pri-

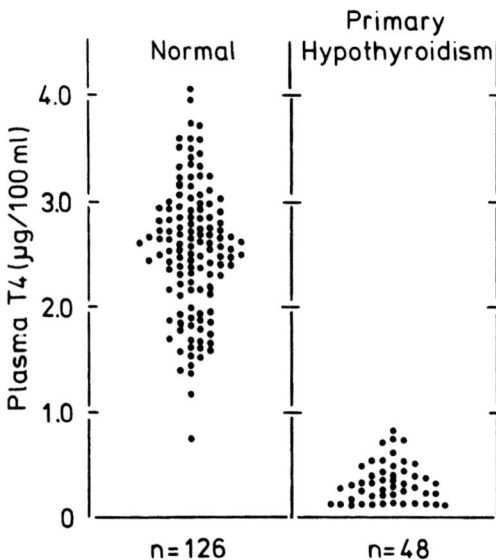

Fig. 3-38. Plasma total triiodothyronine (T_3) values in 126 normal dogs and 48 dogs with primary hypothyroidism determined by radioimmunoassay. (Reproduced with permission from: B. E. Belshaw and A. Rijnberk,[4] 1979).

mary hypothyroidism, the T_4 and T_3 levels do not change significantly after injection of TSH (Figs. 3-39 and 3-40). Serum levels for T_4 and T_3 in domestic animals are summarized in Table 3-1.

There are two additional considerations in the measurement of serum levels of T_4 and T_3. First, there are diurnal variations in circulating thyroid hormone concentrations in the dog, and for any of the above methods, the best separation between normal and hypothyroid dogs is obtained by measurements made before noon, when concentrations of TSH in normal dogs usually are at their peak. The second consideration is that the serum T_4 concentration declines in response to a dietary deficiency of iodine in the dog, while serum T_3 levels remain within the normal range.

Normal serum levels of T_4 in cats, as determined by radioimmunoassay, are approximately 1.5 to 4.5 µg/dl and serum T_3 levels are 60 to 100 ng/dl (Fig. 3-24). Serum T_4 levels in cats with hyperthyroidism range from 5.0 to over 50 µg/dl and serum T_3 levels range from 100 to 1,000 ng/dl (Fig. 3-24).

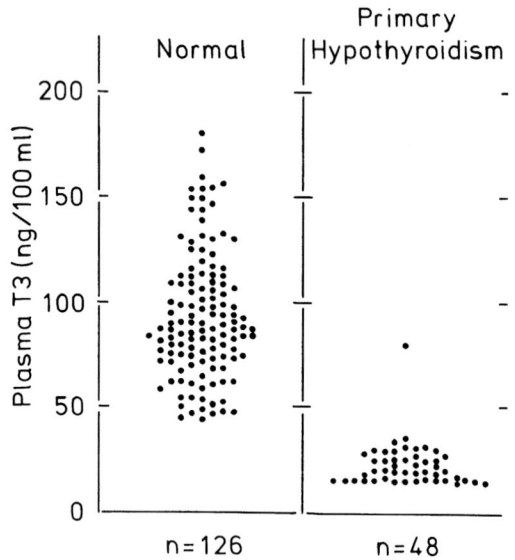

Fig. 3-37. Plasma total thyroxine (T_4) values in 126 normal dogs and 48 dogs with primary hypothyroidism as determined by radioimmunoassay. (Reproduced with permission from: B. E. Belshaw and A. Rijnberk,[4] 1979).

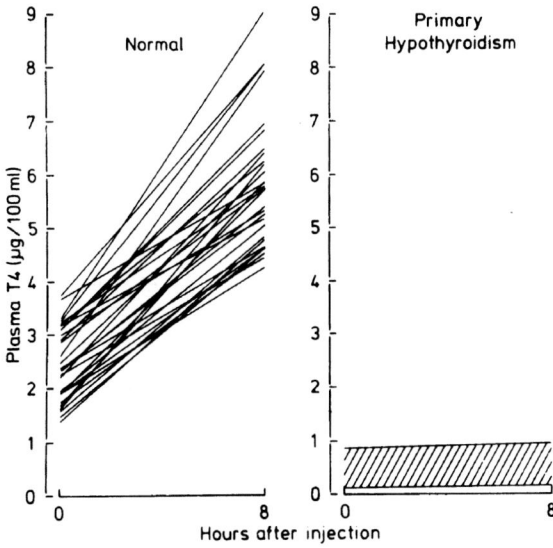

Fig. 3-39. Plasma total thyroxine (T_4) responses to TSH stimulation in 30 normal dogs and 28 dogs with primary hypothyroidism as determined by radioimmunoassay. Only the highest and lowest response lines are shown for the hypothyroid dogs. (Reproduced with permission from: B. E. Belshaw and A. Rijnberk,[4] 1979).

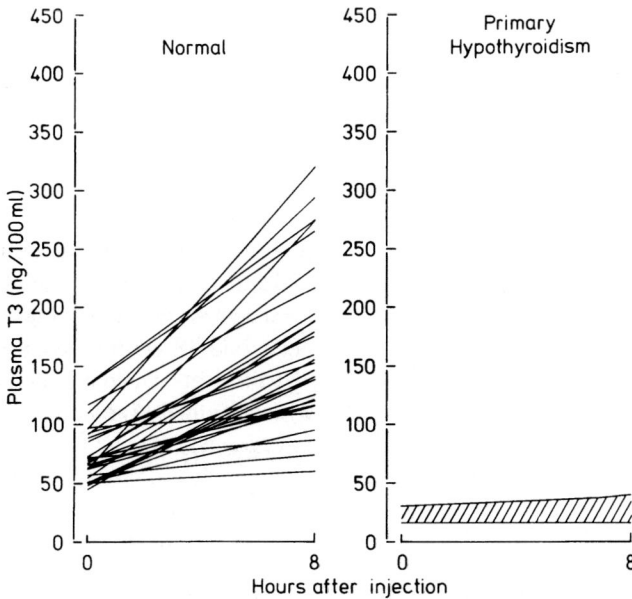

Fig. 3-40. Plasma total triiodothyronine (T_3) responses to TSH stimulation in 30 normal dogs and 28 dogs with primary hypothyroidism as determined by radioimmunoassay. Only the highest and lowest response lines are shown for the hypothyroid dogs. (Reproduced with permission from: B. E. Belshaw and A. Rijnberk,[4] 1979).

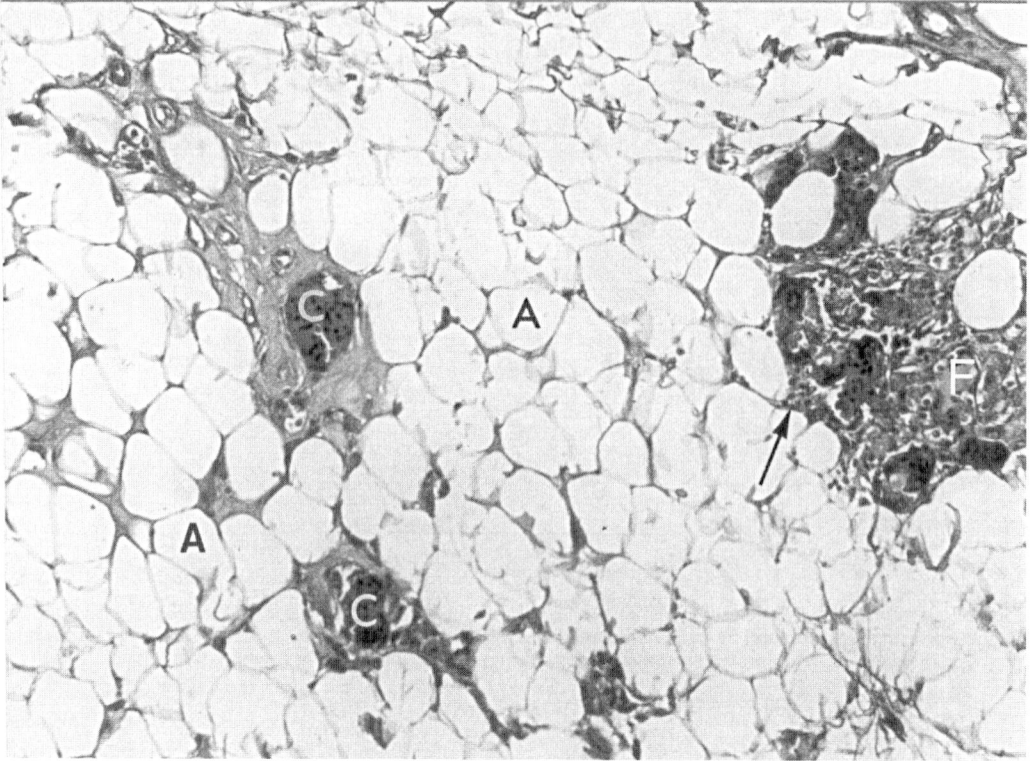

Fig. 3-41. Idiopathic atrophy ("follicular collapse") of the thyroid from a dog with hypothyroidism. There is extensive loss of follicular epithelium and replacement by adipose connective tissue (**A**). Only a few viable follicles (**F**) remain, together with small nests of parafollicular or C-cells (**C**).

It is also possible to use radioimmunoassay to measure free (unbound) thyroxine in the circulation; however, the assay is technically more difficult than the measurement of total T_4. There are several reported advantages of measuring free T_4 over total T_4 including:

1. higher correlation with thyroid secretory rate,

2. slower decrease of circulating levels in non-thyroidal illnesses, and

3. less overlap of levels of thyroxine in hypothyroid and euthyroid patients.

Thyroid Biopsy

The removal of the caudal one-fourth of either lobe of the thyroid for histologic examination is a simple surgical procedure that is without significant risk, even if the dog is hypothyroid. In most cases of primary hypothyroidism, there is either a marked loss of thyroid follicles ("follicular collapse") with replacement by adipose connective tissue (Fig. 3-41) or multifocal lymphocytic thyroiditis which develops on an immunologic basis (Fig. 3-17). Histologic examination of a biopsy of the thyroid gland is a useful and reliable aid in the diagnosis of thyroid disease in animals when the results of serum assays for T_4 and T_3 are equivocal or a nodular enlargement is palpated within the thyroid area.

REFERENCES

1. Avvedimento, V. E., Monticelli, A., Tramontano, D., et al. (1985): Differential expression of thyroglobulin gene in normal and transformed thyroid cells. Europ. J. Biochem. *149*:467.
2. Belshaw, B. E., Barandes, M., Becker, D. V., et al. (1974): A model of iodine kinetics in the dog. Endocrinology *95*:1078.
3. Belshaw, B. E. and Becker, D. V. (1971): Necrosis of follicular cells and discharge of thyroidal iodine in-

duced by administering iodide to iodine-deficient dogs. J. Clin. Endocrinol. Metab. *36:*466.

4. Belshaw, B. E. and Rijnberk, A. (1979): Radio-immunoassay of plasma T$_4$ and T$_3$ in the diagnosis of primary hypothyroidism in dogs. J. Am. Anim. Hosp. Assoc. *15:*17.

5. Bernier-Valentin, F., Kostrouch, Z., Rabilloud, R., et al. (1990): Coated vesicles from thyroid cells carry iodinated thyroglobulin molecules. First indication for an internalization of the thyroid prohormone via a mechanism of receptor-mediated endocytosis. J. Biol. Chem. *265:*17373.

6. Birchard, S. J., Peterson, M. E., and Jacobson, A. (1984): Surgical treatment of feline hyperthyroidism: Results of 85 cases. J. Am. Anim. Hosp. Assoc. *20:*705.

7. Björkman, U., Ekholm, R., and Ericson, L. E. (1978): Effects of thyrotropin on thyroglobulin exocytosis and iodination in the rat thyroid gland. Endocrinology *102:*460.

8. Bone, E., Kohn, L. D., and Chomczynski, P. (1986): Thyroglobulin gene activation by thyrotropin and cAMP in hormonally depleted FRTL-5 thyroid cells. Biochem. Biophys. Res. Commun. *141:*1261.

9. Brandi, M. L., Rotella, C. M., Mavilia, C., et al. (1987): Insulin stimulates cell growth of a new strain of differentiated rat thyroid cells. Mol. Cell. Endocrinol. *54:*91.

10. Brent, G. A. (1994): The molecular basis of thyroid hormone action. N. Engl. J. Med. *331:*847.

11. Brix, K. and Herzog, V. (1994): Extrathyroidal release of thyroid hormones from thyroglobulin by J774 mouse macrophages. J. Clin. Invest. *93:*1388.

12. Broussard, J. D., Peterson, M. E., and Fox, P. R. (1995): Changes in clinical and laboratory findings in cats with hyperthyroidism from 1983 to 1993. J. Am. Vet. Med. Assoc. *206:*302.

13. Capen, C. C. (1980): Criteria for the development of animal models of diseases of the endocrine system. Am. J. Pathol. *101:*S141.

14. Capen, C. C. (1983): Chemical injury of the thyroid: Pathologic and mechanistic considerations. *In:* Proc. of the 1983 Toxicology Forum Annual Winter Meeting, Arlington, VA, p. 260.

15. Capen, C. C. (1994): Mechanisms of chemical injury of the thyroid gland. In: Receptor-mediated Biological Processes: Implications for Evaluating Carcinogens. Proc. of the Barton Creek Conference on Carcinogenesis and Risk Assessment, edited by H. L. Spitzer, et al. Progress in Clinical and Biological Research Series, Washington, D.C., Wiley-Liss/ISLI Press, p. 193.

16. Capen, C. C. (1997): Mechanistic data and risk assessment of selected toxic end points of the thyroid gland. Toxicol. Pathol. *25:*39.

17. Capen, C. C., Belshaw, B. E., and Martin, S. L. (1975): Endocrine diseases. *In:* Textbook of Veterinary Internal Medicine—Diseases of the Dog and Cat, Section X, Chapter 50, edited by S. J. Ettinger. Philadelphia, PA, W. B. Saunders Co., p. 1351.

18. Capen, C. C. and Martin, S. L. (1989): The effects of xenobiotics on the structure and function of thyroid follicular and C-cells. Toxicol. Pathol. *17:*266.

19. Carrasco, N. (1993): Iodide transport in the thyroid gland. Biochim. Biophys. Acta *1154:*65.

20. Collins, W. T. and Capen, C. C. (1980): Ultrastructural and functional alterations of the rat thyroid gland produced by polychlorinated biphenyls compared with iodide excess and deficiency, and thyrotropin and thyroxine administration. Virchows Arch. *33:*213.

21. Conde, E., Martin-Lacave, I., Gonzalez-Campora, R., et al. (1991): Histometry of normal thyroid glands in neonatal and adult rats. Am. J. Anat. *191:*384.

22. Consiglio, E., Acquaviva, A. M., Formisano, S., et al. (1987): Characterization of phosphate residues on thyroglobulin. J. Biol. Chem. *262:*10304.

23. Curran, P.G. and DeGroot, L. J.: (1991): The effect of hepatic enzyme-inducing drugs on thyroid hormones and the thyroid gland. Endocrine Rev. *12:*135.

24. Dai, G., Levy, O., and Carrasco, N. (1996): Cloning and characterization of the thyroid iodide transporter. Nature, London, England *379:*458.

25. Damante, G., Chazenbalk, G., Russo, D., et al. (1989): Thyrotropin regulation of thyroid peroxidase messenger ribonucleic acid levels in cultured rat thyroid cells: Evidence for the involvement of a nontranscriptional mechanism. Endocrinology *124:*2889.

26. De Grandi, P. B., Kraehenbuhl, J. P., and Campiche, M. A. (1971): Ultrastructural localization of calcitonin in the parafollicular cells of the pig thyroid gland with cytochrome c-labeled antibody fragments. J. Cell Biol. *50:*446.

27. De Sandro, V., Chevrier, M., Boddaert, A., et al. (1991): Comparison of the effects of propylthiouracil, amiodarone, diphenylhydantoin, phenobarbital, and 3-methylcholanthrene on hepatic and renal T4 metabolism and thyroid gland function in rats. Toxicol. Appl. Pharmacol. *111:*263.

28. De Vijlder J. J. M., van Voorthuizen W. F., van Dijk, J. E., et al, (1978): Hereditary congenital goiter with thyroglobulin deficiency in a breed of goats. Endocrinology *102:*1214.

29. Delverdier, M., Cabanie, P., Roome, N., et al. (1991): Quantitative histology of the rat thyroid. Anal. Quant. Cytol. Histol. *13:*110.

30. Di Jeso, B. and Gentile, F. (1992): TSH-induced galactose incorporation at the NH$_2$ terminus of thyroglobulin secreted by FRTL-5 cells. Biochem. Biophys. Res. Commun. *189:*1624.

31. Dixon, R. M., Graham, P. A., and Mooney, C. T. (1996): Serum thyrotropin concentrations: A new diagnostic test for canine hypothyroidism. Vet. Rec. *138:*594.

32. Döhler, K-D., Wong, C. C., and von zur Mühlen, A. (1979): The rat as model for the study of drug effects on thyroid function: Consideration of methodological problems. Pharmacol. Ther. B. *5:*305.

33. Doliger, S., Delverdier, M., Moré, J., et al. (1995): Histochemical study of cutaneous mucins in hypothyroid dogs. Vet. Pathol. *32:*628.

34. Ericson, L. E. and Engström, G. (1978): Quantitative electron microscopic studies on exocytosis and endocytosis in the thyroid follicle cell. Endocrinology *103:*883.

35. Ericson, L. E., Ring, K. M., and Öfverholm, T. (1983): Selective macropinocytosis of thyroglobulin in rat thyroid follicles. Endocrinology *113:*1746.

36. Ferguson, D. C. (1994): Update on diagnosis of canine hypothyroidism. Vet. Clin. North Am., Small Anim. Pract. *24*:515.

37. Foti, D. and Rapoport, B. (1990): Carbohydrate moieties in recombinant human thyroid peroxidase: Role in recognition by antithyroid peroxidase antibodies in Hashimoto's thyroiditis. Endocrinology *126*:2983.

38. Gerber, H., Peter, H. J., Bachmeier, C., et al. (1987): Progressive recruitment of follicular cells with graded secretory responsiveness during stimulation of the thyroid gland by thyrotropin. Endocrinology *120*:91.

39. Gerber, H., Peter, H., Ferguson, D. C., et al. (1994): Etiopathology of feline toxic nodular goiter. Vet. Clin. North Am., Small Anim. Pract. *24*:541.

40. Gerber, H., Studer, H., and von Grünigen, C. (1985): Paradoxical effects of thyrotropin on diffusion of thyroglobulin in the colloid of rat thyroid follicles after long term thyroxine treatment. Endocrinology *116*:303.

41. Giraud, A., Franc, J-L., Long, Y., et al. (1992): Effects of deglycosylation of human thyroperoxidase on its enzymatic activity and immunoreactivity. J. Endocrinol. *132*:317.

42. Gosselin, S. J., Capen, C. C., Krakowka, S., et al. (1981): Lymphocytic thyroiditis in dogs: Induction with local graft-versus-host reaction. Am. J. Vet. Res. *42*:1856.

43. Gosselin, S. J., Capen, C. C., and Martin, S. L. (1981): Histopathologic and ultrastructural evaluation of thyroid lesions associated with hypothyroidism in dogs. Vet. Pathol. *18*:299.

44. Gosselin, S. J., Capen, C. C., Martin, S. L., et al. (1981): Induced lymphocytic thyroiditis in dogs: Effect of intrathyroidal injection of thyroid autoantibodies. Am. J. Vet. Res. *42*:1565.

45. Gosselin, S. J., Martin, S. L., Capen, C. C., et al. (1980): Biochemical and immunological investigations of hypothyroidism in dogs. Can. J. Comp. Med. *44*:158.

46. Graves, P. N. and Davies, T. F. (1990): A second thyroglobulin messenger RNA species (rTg- 2) in rat thyrocytes. Mol. Endocrinol. *4*:155.

47. Guptill, L., Scott-Moncrieff, J. C. R., Janovitz, E. V., et al. (1995): Response to high-dose radioactive iodine administration in cats with thyroid carcinoma that had previously undergone surgery. J. Am. Vet. Med. Assoc. *207*:1055.

48. Hammarström, S., Sterling, K., Milch, P. O., et al. (1977): Thyroid hormone action: The mitochondrial pathway. Science *197*:996.

49. Harach, H. R. (1988): Solid cell nests of the thyroid. J. Pathol. *155*:191.

50. Herzog, V., Berndorfer, U., and Saber, Y. (1992): Isolation of insoluble secretory product from bovine thyroid: Extracellular storage of thyroglobulin in covalently cross-linked form. J. Cell Biol. *118*:1071.

51. Hoge, W. R., Lund, J. E., and Blakemore, J. C. (1974): Response to thyrotropin as a diagnostic aid for canine hypothyroidism. J. Am. Vet. Med. Assoc. *10*:167.

52. Holzworth, J., Theran, P., Carpenter, J. L., et al, (1980): Hyperthyroidism in the cat: Ten cases. J. Am. Vet. Med. Assoc. *176*:345.

53. Isozaki, O., Tsushima, T., Emoto, N., et al. (1991): Methimazole regulation of thyroglobulin biosynthesis and gene transcription in rat FRTL-5 thyroid cells. Endocrinology *128*:3113.

54. Jernigan, A.D. (1989): Idiosyncrasies of feline drug metabolism. *In:* Proc. 12th Annual Kal Kan Symposium for the Treatment of Small Animal Diseases. Vernon, CA, Veterinary Learning Systems Co., Inc., p. 65.

55. Johnson, L. A., Ford, H. C., Tarttelin, M. F., et al. (1992): Iodine content of commercially-prepared cat foods. N. Z. Vet. J. *40*:18.

56. Kalina, M. and Pearse, A. G. E. (1971): Ultrastructural localization of calcitonin in C-cells of dog thyroid: An immunocytochemical study. Histochemie *26*:1.

57. Kameda, Y. (1972): The accessory thyroid glands of the dog around the intrapericardial aorta. Arch. Histol. Jpn. *34*:375.

58. Kaminsky, S.M., Levy, O., Salvador, C., et al. (1994): Na$^+$-I$^-$ symport activity is present in membrane vesicles from thyrotropin-deprived non-I = transporting cultured thyroid cells. Proc. Nat. Acad. Sci., USA *91*:3789.

59. Kaptein, E. M., Hays, M. T., and Ferguson, D. C. (1994): Thyroid hormone metabolism: A comparative evaluation. Vet. Clin. North Am., Small Anim. Pract. *24*:431.

60. Kowalski, K., Babiarz, D., and Burke, G. (1972): Phagocytosis of latex beads by isolated thyroid cells: Effects of thyrotropin, prostaglandin E$_1$, and dibutyryl cyclic AMP. J. Lab. Clin. Med. *79*:258.

61. Laurberg, P. (1978): Non-parallel variations in the preferential secretion of 3,5,3'-triiodothyronine (T$_3$) and 3,3',5'-triiodothyronine (rT$_3$) from dog thyroid. Endocrinology *102*:757.

62. Lee, N. T., Kamikubo, K., Chai, K-J., et al. (1991): The deoxyribonucleic acid regions involved in the hormonal regulation of thyroglobulin gene expression. Endocrinology *128*:111.

63. Leer, L. M., Ossendorp, F. A., and de Vijlder, J. J. M. (1990): TSH action on iodination in FRTL-5 cells. Hormone Metab. Res. Suppl. *23*:43.

64. Many, M-C., Denef, J-F., Haumont, S., et al. (1985): Morphological and functional changes during thyroid hyperplasia and involution in C3H mice: Effects of iodine and 3,5,3'-triiodothyronine during involution. Endocrinology *116*:798.

65. Martin, S. L. and Capen, C. C. (1979): Hypothyroidism and the skin. *In:* Symposium on Skin and Internal Diseases, Vol. 9, edited by G. H. Muller. Philadelphia, PA, W. B. Saunders, Co., p. 29.

66. Martin-Lacave, I., Conde, E., Moreno, A., et al. (1992): Evidence of the occurrence of calcitonin cells in the ultimobranchial follicle of the rat postnatal thyroid. Acta Anat. *144*:93.

67. Mazzaferri, E. L. (1996): Radioiodine and other treatments and outcomes. *In:* Werner and Ingbar's The Thyroid: A Fundamental and Clinical Text, 7th edition, edited by L. E. Braverman and R. D. Utiger. Philadelphia, PA, J. B. Lippincott Co., p. 922.

68. McLoughlin, M. A., DiBartola, S. P., Birchard, S. J., et al. (1993): Influence of systemic nonthyroidal illness on serum concentration of thyroxine in hyperthyroid cats. J. Am. Anim. Hosp. Assoc. *29*:227.

69. Merryman, J. I., Buckles, E. L., Bowers, G., et al. (1998): Overexpression of c-*Ras* in hyperplasia and adenomas of the feline thyroid gland: An immunohistochemical analysis of 34 cases. Vet. Pathol. *35*:445.

70. Mizejewski, G. J., Baron, J., and Poissant, G. (1971): Immunologic investigations of naturally occurring canine thyroiditis. J. Immunol. *107*:1152.

71. Mizukami, Y., Matsubara, F., and Matsukawa, S. (1985): Cytochemical localization of peroxidase and hydrogen-peroxide-producing NAD(P)H-oxidase in thyroid follicular cells of propylthiouracil-treated rats. Histochemistry *82*:263.

72. Mooney, C. T., Little, C. J., and Macrae, A. W. (1996): Effect of illness not associated with the thyroid gland on serum total and free thyroxine concentrations in cats. J. Am. Vet. Med. Assoc. *208*:2004.

73. Mori, M., Naito, M., Watanabe, H., et al. (1990): Effects of sex difference, gonadectomy, and estrogen on N-Methyl-N-nitrosourea-induced rat thyroid tumors. Cancer Res. *50*:7662.

74. Murray, L. A. and Peterson, M. E. (1997): Ipodate treatment of hyperthyroidism in cats. J. Am. Vet. Med. Assoc. *211*:63.

75. Nachreiner, R. F. and Refsal, K. R. (1992): Radioimmunoassay monitoring of thyroid hormone concentrations in dogs on thyroid replacement therapy: 2,674 cases (1985-1987). J. Am. Vet. Med. Assoc. *201*:623.

76. Nilsson, M., Engström, G., and Ericson, L. E. (1986): Graded response in the individual thyroid follicle cell to increasing doses of TSH. Mol. Cell. Endocrinol. *44*:165.

77. Öfverholm, T. and Ericson, L. E. (1984): Intraluminal iodination of thyroglobulin. Endocrinology *114*:827.

78. Oppenheimer, J. H. (1979): Thyroid hormone action at the cellular level. Science *203*:971.

79. Oppenheimer, J. H., Schwartz, H. L., Surks, M. I., et al. (1976): Nuclear receptors and the initiation of thyroid hormone action. Recent Prog. Hormone Res. *32*:529.

80. Ossendrop, F. A., Leer, L. M., Bruning, P. F., et al. (1989): Iodination of newly synthesized thyroglobulin by FRTL-5 cells is selective and thyrotropin dependent. Mol. Cell. Endocrinol. *66*:199.

81. Ozaki, A., Sagartz, J. E., and Capen, C. C. (1995): Phagocytic activity of FRTL-5 rat thyroid follicular cells as measured by ingestion of fluorescent latex beads. Exp. Cell Res. *219*:547.

82. Pammenter, M., Albrecht, C., Liebenberg, W., et al. (1978): Afrikander cattle congenital goiter: Characteristics of its morphology and iodoprotein pattern. Endocrinology *102*:954.

83. Pelletier, G., Puviani, R., and Dussault, J. H. (1976): Electron microscope immunohistochemical localization of thyroglobulin in the rat thyroid gland. Endocrinology *98*:1253.

84. Peter, H. J., Gerber, H., Studer, H., et al. (1985): Pathogenesis of heterogeneity in human multinodular goiter: A study on growth and function of thyroid tissue transplanted onto nude mice. J. Clin. Invest. *76*:1992.

85. Peterson, M. E. (1983): Diagnosis and treatment of feline hyperthyroidism. *In:* Proc. 6th Annual Kal Kan Symposium for the Treatment of Small Animal Diseases, edited by E. van Marthens. Vernon, CA, Veterinary Learning Systems Co., Inc., p. 63.

86. Peterson, M. E. (1984): Feline hyperthyroidism. Vet. Clin. North Am., Small Anim. Pract. *14*:809.

87. Peterson, M. E. and Becker, D. V. (1995): Radioiodine treatment of 524 cats with hyperthyroidism. J. Am. Vet. Med. Assoc. *207*:1422.

88. Peterson, M. E., Kintzer, P. P., Cavanagh, P. G., et al. (1983): Feline hyperthyroidism: Pretreatment clinical and laboratory evaluation of 131 cases. J. Am. Vet. Med. Assoc. *183:*103.

89. Peterson, M. E., Livingston, P., and Brown, R. S. (1987): Lack of circulating thyroid stimulating immunoglobulins in cats with hyperthyroidism. Vet. Immunol. Immunopathol. *16*:277.

90. Ramsey, I. and Herrtage, M. E. (1997): Distinguishing normal, sick and hypothyroid dogs using total thyroxine and thyrotropin concentrations. Canine Pract. *22*:43.

91. Rand, J. S., Levine, J., Best, S. J., et al. (1993): Spontaneous adult-onset hypothyroidism in a cat. J. Vet. Intern. Med. *7*:272.

92. Reader, S. C., Davison, B., Ratcliffe, J. G., et al. (1985): Measurement of low concentrations of bovine thyrotrophin by iodide uptake and organification in porcine thyrocytes. J. Endocrinol. *106*:13.

93. Reap, M., Cass, C., and Hightower, D. (1978): Thyroxine and triiodothyronine levels in ten species of animals. Southwestern Vet. *31:*31.

94. Rijnberk, A. (1971): Iodine metabolism and thyroid disease in the dog. University of Utrecht, Utrecht, The Netherlands (Thesis).

95. Rijnberk, A., de Vijlder J. J., van Dijk, J. E., et al. (1977): Congenital defect in iodothyronine synthesis. Clinical aspects of iodine metabolism in goats with congenital goitre and hypothyroidism. Br. Vet. J. *133:*495.

96. Rogers, W. A., Donovan, E. F., and Kociba, G. J. (1975): Lipids and lipoproteins in normal dogs and in dogs with secondary hyperlipoproteinemia. J. Am. Vet. Med. Assoc. *166:*1092.

97. Rojko, J. L., Hoover, E. A., and Martin, S. L. (1978): Histopathologic interpretation of cutaneous biopsies from dogs with various dermatologic disorders. Vet. Pathol. *15:*579.

98. Romagnoli, P. and Herzog, V. (1991): Transcytosis in thyroid follicle cells: Regulation and implications for thyroglobulin transport. Exp. Cell Res. *194*:202.

99. Sagartz, J. E., Ozaki, A., and Capen, C. C. (1995): Phagocytosis of fluorescent beads by rat thyroid follicular cells (FRTL-5): Comparison with iodide trapping as an index of functional activity of thyrocytes *in vitro*. Toxicol. Pathol. *23*:635.

100. Saito, K., Kaneko, H., Sato, K., et al. (1991): Hepatic UDP-glucuronyltransferase(s) activity toward thyroid hormones in rats: Induction and effects on serum thyroid hormone levels following treatment with various enzyme inducers. Toxicol. Appl. Pharmacol. *111*:99.

101. Santisteban, P., Kohn, L. D., and Di Lauro, R. (1987): Thyroglobulin gene expression is regulated by insulin and insulin-like growth factor I, as well as thyrotropin, in FRTL-5 thyroid cells. J. Biol. Chem. *262*:4048.

102. Scarlett, J. M. (1994): Epidemiology of thyroid diseases of dogs and cats. Vet. Clin. North Am., Small Anim. Pract. *24*:477.

103. Scott-Moncrieff, J. C., Nelson, R. W., Bruner, J. M., et al. (1998): Comparison of serum concentrations of thyroid-stimulating hormone in healthy dogs, hypothyroid dogs, and euthyroid dogs with concurrent disease. J. Am. Vet. Med. Assoc. *212*:387.

104. Sharifi, J. and St. Germain, D. L. (1992): The cDNA for the type I iodothyronine 5'-deiodinase encodes an enzyme manifesting both high K_m and low K_m activity. J. Biol. Chem. *267*:12539.

105. Sinha, N., Lal, B., and Singh, T. P. (1991): Pesticides induced changes in circulating thyroid hormones in the freshwater catfish *Clarias batrachus.* Comp. Biochem. Physiol. *100*C:107.

106. Slater, M. R., Komkov, A., Robinson, L. E., et al. (1994): Long-term follow-up of hyperthyroid cats treated with iodine-131. Vet. Radiol. Ultrasound *35*:204.

107. Smanik, P.A., Liu, W., Furminger, T.L., et al. (1996): Cloning of the human sodium iodide symporter. Biochem. Biophys. Res. Commun. *226*:339.

108. Smith, P., Wynford-Thomas, D., Stringer, B. M. J., et al. (1986): Growth factor control of rat thyroid follicular cell proliferation. Endocrinology *119*:1439.

109. Sundick, R. S., Herdegen, D. M., Brown, T. R., et al. (1987): The incorporation of dietary iodine into thyroglobulin increases its immunogenicity. Endocrinology *120*:2078.

110. Taurog, A. (1996): Hormone synthesis: Thyroid iodine metabolism. *In:* Werner and Ingbar's The Thyroid: A Fundamental and Clinical Text, 7th edition, edited by L. E. Braverman and R. D. Utiger. Philadelphia, PA, J. B. Lippincott Co., p. 47.

111. Thacker, E. L., Davis, J. M., Refsal, K. R., et al. (1995): Isolation of thyroid peroxidase and lack of autoantibodies to the enzyme in dogs with autoimmune thyroid disease. Am. J. Vet. Res. *56*:34.

112. Thake, D. C., Cheville, N. F., and Sharp, R. K. (1971): Ectopic thyroid adenomas at the base of the heart of the dog: Ultrastructural identification of dense tubular structures in endoplasmic reticulum. Vet. Pathol. *8*:421.

113. Tice, L. W. and Wollman, S. H. (1974): Ultrastructural localization of peroxidase on pseudopods and other structures of the typical thyroid epithelial cell. Endocrinology *94*:1555.

114. Toda, S. and Sugihara, H. (1990): Reconstruction of thyroid follicles from isolated porcine follicle cells in three-dimensional collagen gel culture. Endocrinology *126*:2027.

115. Uchiyama, Y., Oomiya, A., and Murakami, G. (1986): Fluctuations in follicular structures of rat thyroid glands during 24 hours: Fine structural and morphometric studies. Am. J. Anat. *175*:23.

116. Van Herle A. J., Vassart, G., and Dunmont, J. E. (1979): Control of thyroglobulin synthesis and secretion. N. Engl. J. Med. *301*:239 and *301*:307.

117. Van Voorthuizen, W. F., Dinsort, C., Flavell R. A. et al. (1978): Abnormal cellular localization of thyroglobulin deficiency. Proc. Natl. Acad. Sci., USA *75*:74.

118. Weetman, A. P. and McGregor, A. M. (1994): Autoimmune thyroid disease: Further developments in our understanding. Endocrine Rev. *15*:788.

119. Weiss, S. J., Philp, N. J., and Grollman, E. F. (1984): Iodide transport in a continuous line of cultured cells from rat thyroid. Endocrinology *114*:1090.

120. Whur, P., Herscovics, A., and Leblond, C. P. (1969): Radioautographic visualization of the incorporation of galactose-³H and mannose-³H by rat thyroids *in vitro* in relation to the stages of thyroglobulin synthesis. J. Cell Biol. *43*:289.

121. Wick, G., Brezinschek, H. P., Hala, K., et al. (1989): The obese strain of chickens: An animal model with spontaneous autoimmune thyroiditis. Adv. Immunol. *47*:433.

122. Wolff, J. and Williams, J. A. (1973): The role of microtubules and microfilaments in thyroid secretion. Recent Prog. Hormone Res. *29*:229.

123. Wynford-Thomas, D., Smith, P., and Williams, E. D. (1987). Proliferative response to cyclic AMP elevation of thyroi d epithelium in suspension culture. Mol. Cell. Endocrinol. *51*:163.

124. Yap, A. S., Keast, J. R., and Manley, S. W. (1994): Thyroid cell spreading and focal adhesion formation depend upon protein tyrosine phosphorylation and actin microfilaments. Exp. Cell Res. *210*:306.

125. Zarrilli, R., Formisano, S., and DiJeso, B. (1990): Hormonal regulation of thyroid peroxidase in normal and transformed rat thyroid cells. Mol. Endocrinol. *4*:39.

126. Zbinden, G. (1988): Hyperplastic and neoplastic responses of the thyroid gland in toxicological studies. The Target Organ and the Toxic Process. Arch. Toxicol. *12* (Suppl.):98.

References Added in Proof

127. Dixon, R. M. and Mooney, C. T. (1999): Evaluation of serum free thyroxine and thyrotropin concentrations in the diagnosis of canine hypothyroidism. J. Small Anim. Pract. *40*:72.

128 Dixon, R. M., Reid, S. W., Mooney, C. T. (1999): Epidemiological, clinical, haematological and biochemical characteristics of canine hypothyroidism. Vet. Rec. *145*:481.

129. Frank, N., Sojka, J. E., Latour, M. A., et al. (1999): Effect of hypothyroidism on blood lipid concentrations in horses. Am. J. Vet. Res. *60*:730.

130. Hulbert, A. J. (2000): Thyroid hormones and their effects: A new perspective. Biol. Rev. Camb. Philos. Soc. *75*:519.

131. Nilsson, M. (1999): Molecular and cellular mechanisms of transepithelial iodide transport in the thyroid. Biofactors *10*:277.

The Calcium Regulating Hormones: Parathyroid Hormone, Calcitonin, and Cholecalciferol

C. C. CAPEN AND T. J. ROSOL

4

INTRODUCTION

Calcium is an essential mineral component of the skeleton and plays a central role in maintaining the homeostasis of vertebrate animals. Ionized calcium is involved in a wide variety of physiological processes including muscular contraction, blood coagulation, enzyme activity, neural excitability, hormone secretion, and cell adhesion. The levels of calcium in the body are influenced by a variety of endocrine factors. These include parathyroid hormone synthesized and released by the chief cells of the parathyroid glands, calcitonin secreted by the parafollicular or C-cells of the thyroid gland, and calcitriol (1,25-dihydroxycholecalciferol; 1,25-dihydroxyvitamin D), the bioactive vitamin D metabolite derived from cholecalciferol (vitamin D_3). Disruption of the normal regulation of calcium balance in animals results in hypercalcemia or hypocalcemia[70] and can lead to metabolic disease and death.

Pathological effects associated with abnormal levels of calcium in the body include calcification of vital organs and other soft tissues, rickets, osteoporosis, and reproductive disorders such as parturient hypocalcemia and paresis in dairy cattle and puerperal tetany in bitches.

CALCIUM METABOLISM

Approximately 99% of the calcium of the body is present in the inorganic matrix of bone as hydroxyapatite (Fig. 4-1). Most of the remaining calcium is sequestered in the plasma membrane and endoplasmic reticulum of cells. Extracellular fluid contains 0.1% of the body's calcium mass with a total calcium concentration of about 2.5 mmol/L. Approximately 50% of the extracellular calcium (1.2 mmol/L) is in the ionized form (Ca^{2+}), which is the biologically active form of calcium. Neonatal animals have slightly greater concentrations of extracellular calcium compared to adult animals. There is very little calcium in the cytosol, approximately 100 nM, which is predominantly in the ionized form.

Vertebrates, such as the marine fishes, originally evolved in an environment with a high concentration of Ca^{2+}. Sea water contains approximately 10 mmol/L Ca^{2+}, but the extracellular fluids of marine fishes contain less than 2 mmol/L Ca^{2+}. Therefore, fishes had to limit and regulate Ca^{2+} absorption from the intestinal tract, skin, or gills and develop mechanisms to efficiently excrete Ca^{2+}. Evolutionarily, this was probably conducive to the development of hormones such as calcitonin and stanniocalcin which reduce the concentration of Ca^{2+} in the serum. Fishes lack parathyroid glands which have the primary role of reducing the loss of body Ca^{2+} and maintaining serum Ca^{2+}. Phylogenetically, parathyroid glands first appear in amphibians which spend most of their life cycle on land, in an environment low in Ca^{2+}. In terrestrial vertebrates, both the parathyroid glands and the kidneys are important regulators of total body calcium. Because there is less need for promoting the excretion of calcium or lowering serum Ca^{2+} in land animals, hormones such as calcitonin are less critical for the maintenance of calcium homeostasis.

Functions of Calcium

Calcium serves two primary functions in the body:

1. structural integrity of bones and teeth, and

2. as a messenger or regulatory ion.

There is a 10,000-fold concentration gradient of Ca^{2+} between the extracellular fluid (1.2 mmol/L) and the cytoplasm (100 nM). This gradient permits Ca^{2+} to function as a signaling ion to activate intracellular processes. The lipid bilayer of the cell membrane has a low permeability to Ca^{2+}; therefore, influx of Ca^{2+} into the cytoplasm is controlled by a heterogeneous group of calcium channels regulated by membrane potential, cell membrane receptors, or intracellular secondary messengers. Influx of Ca^{2+} into cells can:

1. regulate cellular function by interactions with intracellular calcium-binding proteins (e.g., calmodulin) and calcium-sensitive protein kinases, and

2. stimulate biologic responses such as neurotransmitter release, contraction, and secretion.

Calcium in the Body

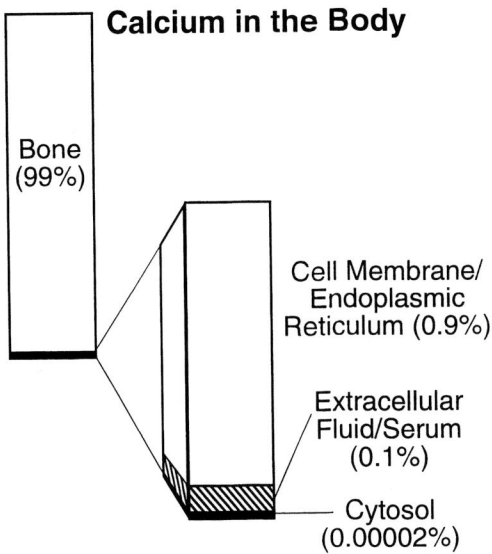

Bone (99%)

Cell Membrane/ Endoplasmic Reticulum (0.9%)

Extracellular Fluid/Serum (0.1%)

Cytosol (0.00002%)

Fig. 4-1. Distribution of calcium in the body. (From: T. J. Rosol et al.,[234] 1995).

Extracellular Calcium

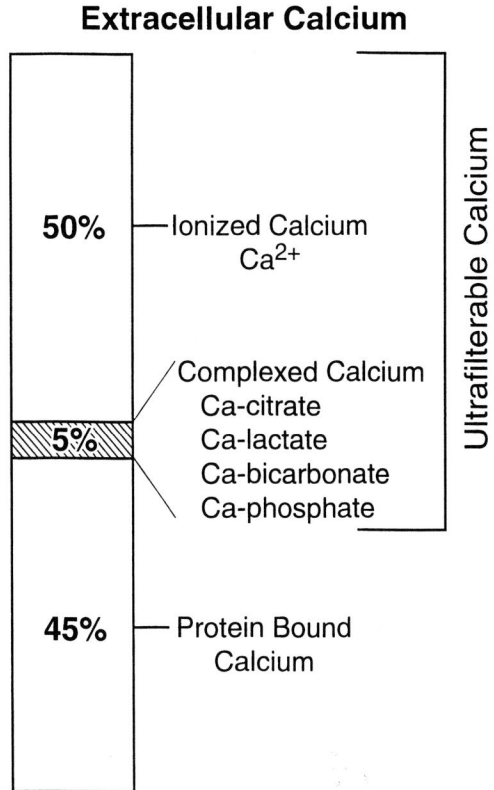

50% — Ionized Calcium Ca^{2+}

5% Complexed Calcium Ca-citrate Ca-lactate Ca-bicarbonate Ca-phosphate

45% — Protein Bound Calcium

Ultrafilterable Calcium

Fig. 4-2. Calcium (Ca) fractions in the extracellular fluid. (From: T. J. Rosol et al.,[234] 1995).

Ionized calcium also plays an important role in cell adhesion and blood coagulation. In addition, Ca^{2+} may regulate cellular function by binding to a G-protein-linked Ca^{2+}-sensing receptor in the cell membrane, such as in parathyroid chief cells or renal epithelial cells.[37]

Maintenance of low levels of intracellular Ca^{2+} is indispensable for cellular viability. If cellular calcium homeostasis fails due to anoxia, or to an energy-deprived state, or perturbed membrane integrity, cell viability is threatened due to uncontrolled entry of Ca^{2+} through the plasma membrane or from extracellular stores.[249]

Forms of Calcium

Extracellular and serum calcium exists in three forms (Fig. 4-2):

1. ionized,
2. complexed to anions such as citrate, bicarbonate, phosphate, or lactate (5% of total calcium), and
3. protein-bound.

The protein-bound fraction of Ca^{2+} is dependent on the pH of the serum and is principally bound to negatively-charged sites on albumin

with smaller amounts bound to globulins. As the pH of serum becomes more acidic, the $[Ca^{2+}]$ will increase due to the competition of hydrogen ions $[H^+]$ for binding to the negatively-charged sites on serum proteins. The ionized and complexed Ca^{2+} compose the ultrafilterable fraction of Ca^{2+} and represent the fraction that is present in the glomerular filtrate. The concentration of ionized Ca^{2+} in the serum is approximately 1.25-1.6 mmol/L (5.0 - 6.4 mg/dl) in most domestic animals.

Renal Handling of Calcium

The kidney normally reabsorbs 98% or more of the filtered calcium. This high degree of reabsorption is an important mechanism to maintain the balance of calcium in the body. If necessary, the kidneys excrete large amounts of calcium in the urine. Ionized and complexed calcium enters the glomerular filtrate by convection and is reabsorbed by the renal tubules. The kidneys reabsorb approximately 40-fold more calcium than is absorbed by the intestinal tract due to the high degree of blood flow and ultrafiltration in the glomerulus. Reduction of glomerular filtration impairs the ability of the kidneys to excrete calcium.

About 70% of filtered calcium is reabsorbed in the proximal convoluted tubules by diffusion and convection with water uptake between the epithelial cells (Fig. 4-3). The thick ascending loop of Henle also absorbs about 20% of the filtered calcium, but the precise mechanism is unclear. Much of the calcium reabsorption appears to be passive, but an active component[239] may also be present in the distal convoluted tubule, which reabsorbs approximately 10% of the filtered calcium. The principal stimulator of calcium reabsorption in the distal convoluted tubule is parathyroid hormone. Reabsorption of calcium in the distal convoluted tubule is an active transcellular process requiring the presence of calcium channels in the luminal cell membrane, intracellular calcium-binding proteins, such as calbindins, a Ca^{2+}-ATPase, and Na^+/Ca^{2+} exchanger in the basolateral cell membranes. Renal epithelial cells express the Ca^{2+}-sensing receptor on their cell membranes and the distribution of the receptor overlaps with the localization of PTH receptors, so the kidneys may partially autoregulate the renal reabsorption of calcium based on concentration of Ca^{2+} in the blood.

Measurements of calcium excretion in animals include calcium and calcium:creatine (Ca/Cr) ratio in the urine, fractional calcium excretion, and 24-hour calcium excretion. Urinary calcium excretion correlates with dietary absorbance in normal, adult animals. The concentration of calcium in urine is usually < 4 mg/dl (1.0 mmol/L) and is of little value as a diagnostic tool due to large fluctuations in the volume of normal urine. Horses excrete larger amounts of calcium in the urine and urine [Ca] is typically much higher than 4 mg/dl (1.0 mmol/L). The Ca/Cr ratio of the urine is a better indicator of calcium excretion because it corrects for errors in timing of urine collections, urine concentration or dilution, and differences in lean body mass.[272] Calculation of fractional calcium excretion requires measurement of urine and serum Ca and Cr concentrations and is an indication of renal calcium reabsorption at the time of analysis as well as the degree of excretory renal function. Fractional calcium excretion is best measured in a fasting animal to eliminate the role of dietary calcium on renal calcium excretion. Measurement of calcium excretion in a fasted animal is an indirect measurement of bone resorption since calcium released from bone and the obligate renal calcium loss are the major sources of urinary calcium when there is little gastrointestinal absorption of calcium. The 24-hour calcium excretion is a good measurement of daily calcium loss and may be used to investigate calcium balance.

Calcium Reabsorption in the Nephron

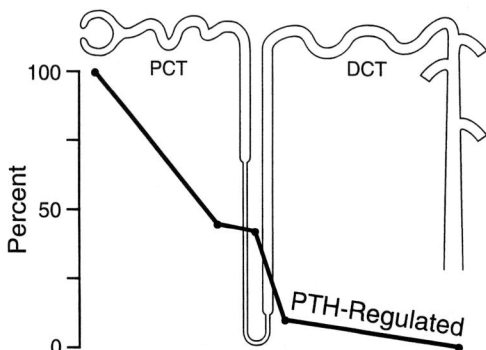

Fig. 4-3. Calcium reabsorption in the nephron. Most of the filtered calcium is passively reabsorbed in the proximal convoluted tubule (**PCT**). Active regulation of calcium reabsorption by parathyroid hormone (**PTH**) occurs in the epithelial cells lining the distal convoluted tubule (**DCT**). (From: T. J. Rosol et al.,[234] 1995).

Intestinal Absorption of Calcium

There are two components of calcium absorption from the intestinal tract, namely saturable or transcellular transport and nonsaturable or intercellular (paracellular) transport.[96] The percentage of intestinal absorption of calcium is proportional to dietary intake. Low-calcium diets are associated with absorption rates of up to 95% whereas high-calcium diets have absorption rates of about 40%. However, high-calcium diets may increase serum calcium concentrations due to the presence of nonsaturable intestinal absorption. In contrast, diets deficient in calcium are associated with normal serum calcium concentrations due to compensation by bone resorption stimulated by parathyroid hormone, renal calcium reabsorption, and increased synthesis of 1,25-dihydroxyvitamin D.

Saturable transport is a carrier-mediated, vitamin D-dependent process and occurs predominantly in the duodenal segment of the small intestine, and to a lesser degree in the cecum and colon. Saturable transport requires influx of calcium into intestinal epithelial cells via Ca^{2+} channels, movement and buffering in the cytoplasm, and basolateral exit by a Ca^{2+}-ATPase. The active form of vitamin D (1,25-dihydroxyvitamin D) stimulates transcellular transport of Ca^{2+}. One function of 1,25-dihydroxyvitamin D in the intestinal epithelial cell is to increase the expression of calbindin, an intracellular calcium-binding protein. In contrast, nonsaturable calcium transport occurs throughout the small intestine and is the main mechanism for calcium absorption in animals deficient in vitamin D. Nonsaturable Ca^{2+} transport is dependent on the luminal $[Ca^{2+}]$. As the dietary intake of calcium increases, much of the calcium in the intestinal lumen is unavailable for nonsaturable absorption due to precipitation of calcium salts or complexes formed with other anions.

Fractional intestinal calcium absorption is approximately 20-40% in adult animals and can exceed 60% during increased demand for calcium. Fractional absorption is increased during pregnancy, lactation, growth, and when animals are fed low-calcium diets. The blood concentration of 1,25-dihydroxyvitamin D is the primary adaptive influence on calcium absorption. Factors which increase intestinal calcium absorption, directly or indirectly, due to stimulation of 1,25-dihydroxyvitamin D synthesis, include: parathyroid hormone, growth hormone, testosterone, estrogen, and furosemide. Factors that reduce intestinal absorption of calcium, include: glucocorticoids, thyroid hormones, chronic acidosis, and luminal conditions that induce the complexation of Ca^{2+}, such as high concentrations of phosphate, phytates, oxalate, fatty acids, pH > 6.1, and other anions.

Bone and Calcium Balance

There are two sources of Ca^{2+} in bone that can enter the circulation:

1. readily mobilizable calcium salts in the extracellular fluid, and

2. hydroxyapatite crystals that require digestion by osteoclasts before Ca^{2+} can be released from bone.

The nature and regulation of the readily mobilizable calcium in bone is poorly understood; however, it is present in small amounts and likely plays a role in the fine regulation of serum calcium concentration. If there is a significant need for calcium from bone it must come from osteoclastic resorption of hydroxyapatite crystals. In adult animals there is a stable balance between calcium deposition associated with bone formation and calcium release, associated with osteoclastic bone resorption. In young animals, bone has a positive calcium balance due to the relative excess of bone formation, a condition that results in excessive bone resorption. Humoral hypercalcemia of malignancy, osteolytic bone metastases, and primary hyperparathyroidism are associated with bone resorption and the release of calcium from bone which contributes to the development of hypercalcemia.

Calcium Ion-sensing Receptors in the Cell Membrane

The concentration of ionized calcium in serum and extracellular fluid can regulate cellular function by interacting with a recently identified Ca^{2+}-sensing receptor in the plasma membrane of various cells.[36, 69] The cell membrane Ca^{2+} receptor is coupled to G-protein and this 7-transmembrane domain receptor is unique because the ligand for this receptor is an ion. The Ca^{2+} receptor plays an important role in the regulation of extracellular Ca^{2+} homeostasis and is present on parathyroid chief cells, thyroid C-cells, renal epithelial cells, brain, and placenta amongst other tissues. The Ca^{2+} receptor is responsible for sensing serum Ca^{2+} concentration and modifying parathyroid hormone secretion, calcitonin secretion, and calcium transport by renal epithelial cells. Mutations in one or both of the Ca^{2+}-sensing receptor genes in humans results in familial hypocalciuric hypercalcemia or neonatal severe hypercalcemia, respectively, due to an inadequate ability to sense the extracellular Ca^{2+} concentration and coordinate the appropriate cellular response.

PHOSPHATE METABOLISM

About 90% of phosphate in the mammalian body is present as hydroxyapatite $[Ca_{10}(PO_4)_6(OH)_2]$ in the mineralized matrix of bone, with most of the remaining 10% occurring intracellularly in soft tissues. Phosphate is the major intracellular anion existing in inorganic form, primarily as HPO_4^{2-} and $H_2PO_4^-$, and in organic compounds such as phospholipids, nucleic acids, phosphoproteins, and ATP. Although phosphate plays an integral role in metabolic processes such as energy metabolism, delivery of O_2 to tissues, muscle contraction, and skeletal integrity, the available fluorometric and ion-sensitive methods to measure intracellular phosphate are inadequate. Rapid translocation between intracellular and serum phosphate pools can dramatically change serum phosphate concentrations. In nonruminant animals on normal diets and with adequate amounts of vitamin D, the kidneys are the major regulators of the phosphate concentration in the serum.[288]

Serum Phosphate

Methods for the colorimetric determination of inorganic orthophosphate rely on the formation of a complex of phosphate ion with molybdate. Although inorganic phosphate is measured, it is often expressed as elemental phosphorus (P_i). Because the atomic weight of phosphorus is 31, 3.1 mg of P_i/dl serum is equivalent to 1 mmol/L phosphorus or 1 mmol/L phosphate. Serum P_i ranges from 2.5-6.0 mg/dl (0.8-1.9 mmol/L) in adult animals. Most of the inorganic phosphate (80%) in the serum is in the dibasic form, HPO_4^{2-}, and the remaining 20% is primarily in the monobasic form, $H_2PO_4^-$. This results in an average valence of serum inorganic phosphate of -1.8 and the milliequivalence of serum phosphate can be estimated by the following calculation: 1 mmol/L phosphate = 1.8 mEq/L phosphate.

For the accurate determination of phosphate in serum, it is important to prevent hemolysis of blood samples which will artificially increase the serum phosphate due to the release of intracellular stores. Phosphate circulates as a free anion, bound to Na^+, Mg^{2+}, or Ca^{2+}; or bound to protein (10-20% of total serum phosphate). Serum phosphate is an unreliable indicator of body stores and may be higher in growing animals than in adults, especially the giant dog breeds, because growth hormone increases renal phosphate reabsorption. Feeding of high carbohydrate diets or glucose infusions will decrease serum phosphate due to an intracellular shift of phosphate in response to increased glycolysis and to the need for phosphorylated intermediates. High meat diets may increase serum phosphate due to their high phosphate content.

Intestinal Absorption of Phosphate

Approximately 60-70% of dietary phosphate is absorbed from the intestine by active transport utilizing a Na/phosphate cotransporter and by passive diffusion. In ruminants the transporter may be coupled to H^+ rather than Na^+. Phosphate absorption takes place principally in the forestomachs in ruminants, from the duodenum and jejunum in monogastric animals, and from the large intestine in horses.[13] The active form of vitamin D, 1,25-dihydroxyvitamin D, increases intestinal phosphate absorption in all species. Low dietary levels of phosphate result in adaptive changes in the intestine and a net increase in phosphate absorption. In addition, increased renal production of 1,25-dihydroxyvitamin D and adaptation of the kidney to increase renal phosphate reabsorption compensates for low levels of dietary phosphate.

The source of dietary phosphorus affects its bioavailability. Some diets contain substances or nutrients which antagonize phosphate absorption, including aluminum and magnesium. Diets high in calcium and fat raise the requirement for phosphorus. Most phosphorus in concentrate sources is in the organic form of phytate which is poorly utilized in nonruminants. Ruminant species have phytase in the rumen which releases the phosphate from the sugar moiety, but nonruminants do not produce this enzyme. However, the addition of microbial phytase to concentrate diets increases the bioavailability of phosphorus for nonruminants. The digestibility of phytates from different foodstuffs varies for ruminants.

In ruminants, large amounts of endogenous phosphate reenter the gastrointestinal tract due to salivary secretions. Parotid saliva in ruminants contains phosphate at levels of 16-40 mmol/L and the total phosphate secretion by the salivary glands is significantly greater than the supply of phosphate in the diet. This endogenous salivary secretion of phosphate is complemented by intestinal phosphate absorption and results in greater phosphate absorption in the gastrointestinal tract in ruminants when compared to monogastric animals. Phosphate anions buffer volatile fatty acids and are nutrients for microorganisms in the rumen. High fiber diets increase saliva production and the total salivary secretion of phosphate. This increased endogenous salivary secretion of phosphate not only leads to increased intestinal absorption, but also to increased fecal losses and results in the net loss of phosphate. Ruminants fed a high roughage diet use this endogenous fecal loss of phosphate as the principle mechanism to regulate phosphate excretion. In contrast, ruminants on concentrate diets excrete more phosphate in the urine due to the reduced flow of saliva and the reduction in endogenous fecal loss of phosphate. Therefore, the quantity of saliva and the regulation of the phosphate concentration in saliva are important determinants of phosphate excretion in ruminants.

Renal Excretion of Phosphate

Renal excretion of phosphate is regulated by the glomerular filtration rate and the maximal rate of tubular reabsorption. The majority of renal phosphate reabsorption occurs in the proximal convoluted tubules of the kidney with small amounts reabsorbed from the distal elements of the nephron. The rate of reabsorption of renal phosphate is dependent on the availability of Na^+ and is regulated by the need of the animal for phosphate. Reabsorption is increased with growth, lactation, pregnancy, and low phosphate diets and is decreased during periods

of slow growth, renal failure, or excess intake of dietary phosphorus.[163, 252] The major hormonal regulator of the reabsorption of phosphate is parathyroid hormone, which decreases the rate of tubular reabsorption and increases the renal excretion of phosphate. Other hormones which inhibit Na/P_i cotransport include calcitonin, atrial natriuretic peptide, epidermal growth factor, transforming growth factors α and β, and parathyroid hormone-related protein. In contrast, insulin, growth hormone, and insulin-like growth factor-1 stimulate Na/P_i cotransport by renal epithelial cells.

PARATHYROID HORMONE

Parathyroid glands are present in all air-breathing vertebrates. Phylogenetically, the parathyroid first appears in amphibians, coincidentally with the transition from an aquatic to a terrestrial life. It has been suggested that the appearance and development of parathyroid glands may have arisen from the need to protect against the development of hypocalcemia and the necessity to maintain skeletal integrity in terrestrial animals, which often are in a relatively low-calcium, high-phosphorus environment.

Macroscopic Anatomy of the Parathyroid Glands

The parathyroid glands in our domestic species and in most other animal species consist of two pairs of glands, the internal and the external parathyroids, situated in the anterior cervical region (Fig. 4-4). Embryologically, both parathyroid glands are of entodermal origin. The external parathyroid is derived from the third (III) and the internal parathyroid is derived from the fourth (IV) pharyngeal pouches, in close association with the primordia of the thymus (Fig. 4-5).

In the dog and cat, both the external and internal parathyroids are close to the thyroid gland. The external parathyroid is 2 to 5 mm in length and is found within the loose connective tissue cranial and slightly lateral to the anterior pole of the thyroid. The internal parathyroid is smaller, flatter, and situated on the medial surface of the thyroid beneath the fibrous capsule. The blood supply to the internal and external glands is separate in the dog, with the external parathyroid being supplied by a branch from the cranial thyroid artery and the internal parathyroid by minute ramifications from the arterial supply to the thyroid.

In other species, such as cattle and sheep, the external parathyroid gland is located a considerable distance and cranial to the thyroid gland in the loose connective tissue along the common carotid artery (Fig. 4-4), while the internal parathyroid is situated on the dorsal and medial surface of the thyroid. The horse has an upper parathyroid gland located near the thyroid and a larger, lower parathyroid gland located a considerable distance from the thyroid in the caudal cervical region near the bifurcation of the bicarotid trunk and at the level of the first rib (Fig. 4-4). Pigs have only a single pair of parathyroids found cranial to the thyroid and embedded in the thymus in young animals or in the adipose connective tissue of adult pigs. Rats also have a single pair of parathyroid glands located close to the thyroid.

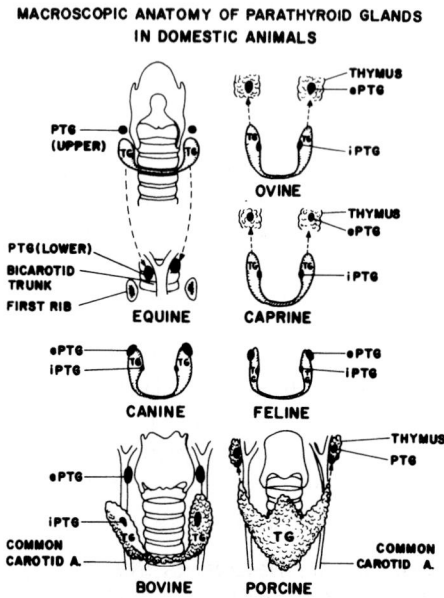

Fig. 4-4. Anatomic location of the parathyroid glands (**PTG**) in relation to the thyroid gland (**TG**) and related structures in several species of domestic animals (**A** = artery; **e** = external; **I** = internal). (Modified from: H. Grau and H. D. Dellmann,[114] 1958).

Functional Cytology of the Parathyroid Glands

Chief Cells

The parathyroid glands of man and animals contain a single, basic type of secretory cell termed chief cells, which secrete and release parathyroid hormone. Oxyphil and transitional cells, which may not have an active function in the biosynthesis of parathyroid hormone are also found in the parathyroid glands of some animal species (Fig. 4-6). Chief cells (Fig. 4-7) display various stages of secretory activity such as resting, involuted, or inactive in man and most animal species. Inactive chief cells are cuboidal and have uncomplicated interdigitations between contiguous cells. The relatively

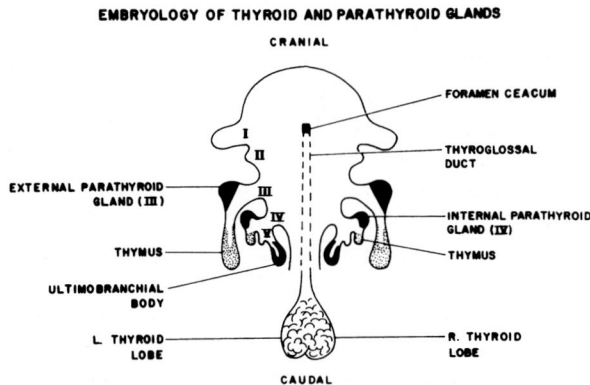

Fig. 4-5. Embryological origin of the parathyroid glands and relationship to primordia for the thyroid gland and ultimobranchial body (L = left; R = right).

Water-Clear Cell

↑

Transitional Water-Clear Cell

Vacuolated Chief Cell

Hyperactive Chief Cell

↑

Stimulation
Low Ca⁺⁺
(Excess Pi)

| **Chief Cell** |

Normal
Secretory
Cycle

Involution   Synthesis

Inactive

Secretion   Packaging

Active

Advancing Age

Suppression
High Ca⁺⁺

Transitional Oxyphil Cell

Inactive Chief Cell

Oxyphil Cell

Atrophic Chief Cell

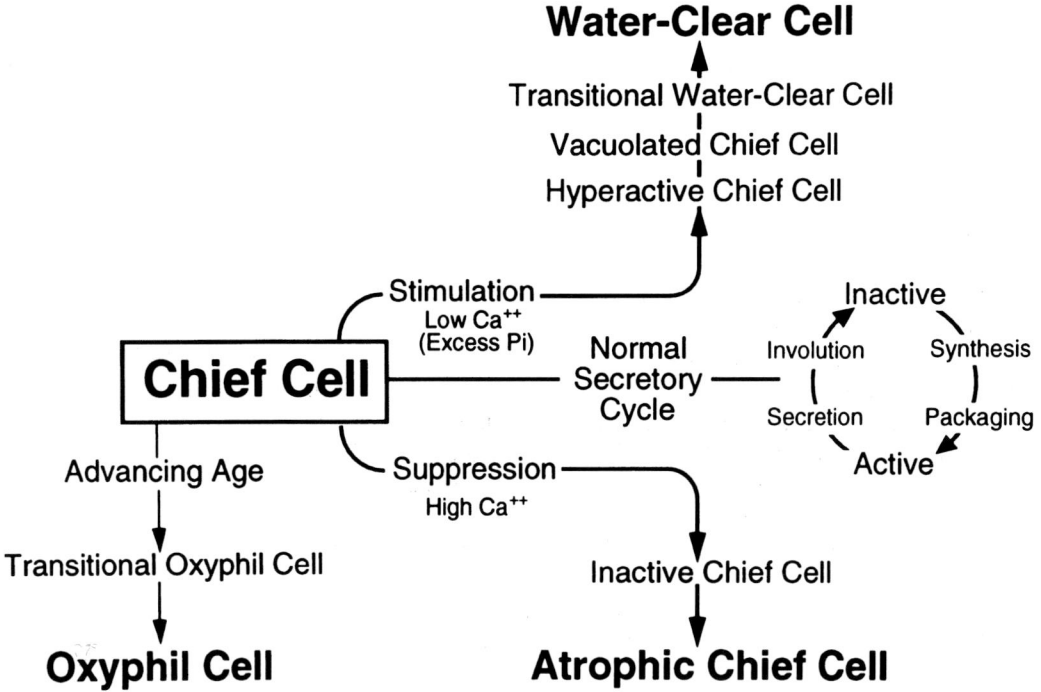

Fig. 4-6. Functional cytology of the parathyroid glands under normal and pathologic conditions (**Ca⁺⁺** = ionized calcium; **Pᵢ** = phosphorus).

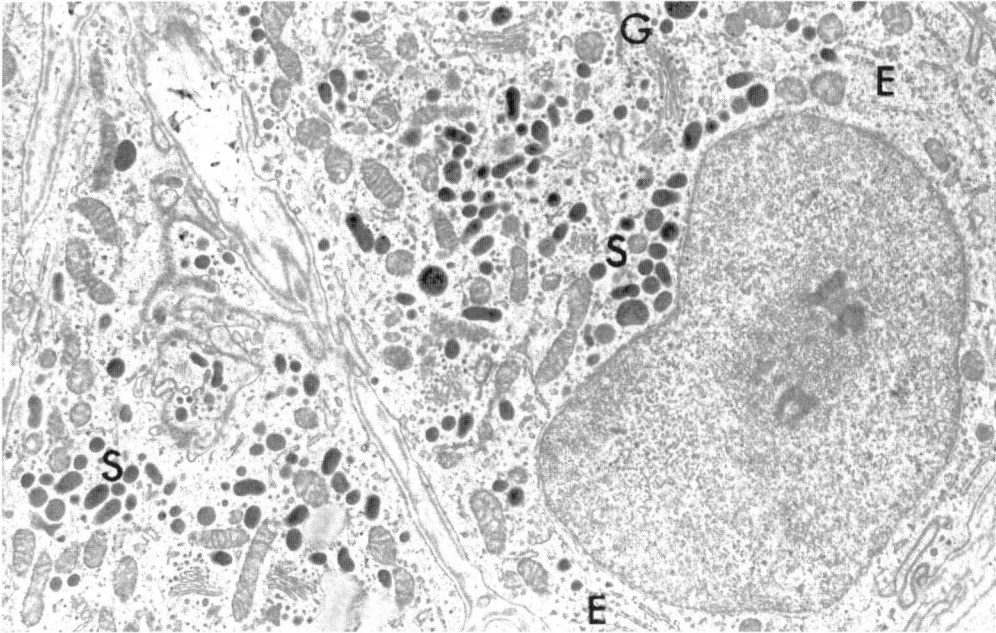

Fig. 4-7. Active chief cell from the parathyroid gland of a cow. The cytoplasm contains many PTH-containing secretory granules (**S**) and well-developed organelles such as rough endoplasmic reticulum (**E**) and Golgi apparatus (**G**). Glutaraldehyde and osmium tetroxide fixation, uranyl acetate and lead hydroxide staining. Magnification 11,300 x. (From: C. C. Capen,[44] 1971).

electron-transparent cytoplasm contains poorly developed organelles and few secretory granules. The Golgi apparatus is small, composed of straight or curved stacks of agranular membranes, and is associated with few prosecretory granules and vesicles. Granular endoplasmic reticulum, ribosomes, and small mitochondria are dispersed throughout the cytoplasm. The cytoplasm of cells of the bovine parathyroid glands has numerous lipid bodies and lipofuscin droplets whereas the cytoplasm of human and feline parathyroid glands has aggregations of glycogen granules.

Chief cells in the active stage of the secretory cycle (Fig. 4-7) occur less frequently in the parathyroid glands of most species. The cytoplasm of the active chief cell has an increased electron-density due to the close proximity of organelles, secretion granules, the overall density of the cytoplasmic matrix, and the loss of glycogen particles and lipid bodies (Fig. 4-7).

Oxyphil Cells and Transitional Forms

Oxyphil cells are not present in the fetal parathyroid gland of the human, first appear in late childhood, and increase in number with advancing age, often forming nodules in the parathyroids of older individuals. They are absent in the parathyroid glands of the rat, chicken, and many species of lower animals.

Oxyphil cells are observed either singly or in small groups interspersed between chief cells. Oxyphil cells are larger than chief cells and their abundant cytoplasmic area is filled with numerous large, often abnormal-shaped, mitochondria. Glycogen particles and free ribosomes are interspersed between the mitochondria. Granular endoplasmic reticula, Golgi apparatuses, and secretory granules are poorly developed in oxyphil cells of normal parathyroid glands, suggesting that oxyphil cells do not have an active function in the biosynthesis of parathyroid hormone.

Cells with cytoplasmic characteristics intermediate between those of chief and oxyphil cells are also observed. These transitional cells also have numerous mitochondria, and granular endoplasmic reticula, Golgi apparatuses, and secretory granules. The significance of oxyphil cells in the pathophysiology of the parathyroid glands has not been completely elucidated. Oxyphil cells are not altered in response to short-term hypocalcemia or hypercalcemia in animals, but both oxyphil and transitional cells may increase in numbers in humans in response to long-term stimulation of the parathyroid glands.

Synthesis of Parathyroid Hormone

The ribosomes of the rough endoplasmic reticulum in chief cells synthesize a biosynthetic precursor of parathyroid hormone called pre-proparathyroid hormone (pre-proPTH). Pre-proparathyroid hormone (Fig. 4-8) is composed of 115 amino acids and contains a hydrophobic signal or leader sequence of 25 amino acids that facilitate the penetration and subsequent discharge of the peptide into the cisternal space of the rough endoplasmic reticulum (Fig. 4-7). Within 1 minute or less of its synthesis, pre-proPTH is converted to proparathyroid hormone (proPTH) by the proteolytic cleavage of the NH_2-terminal sequence of 25 amino acids (Figs. 4-8 and 4-9).

The intermediate precursor, proPTH, is composed of 90 amino acids (Fig. 4-8) and is conveyed within membranous channels of the endoplasmic reticulum to the Golgi apparatus (Fig. 4-10). Enzymes with trypsin-like and carboxypeptidase B-like activity within membranes of the Golgi apparatus cleave a hexapeptide from the NH_2-terminal, biologically active end of the molecule forming active parathyroid hormone (Figs. 4-8 and 4-9). Active PTH is packaged into membrane-limited, macromolecular aggregates in the Golgi apparatus for subsequent storage in chief cells (Fig. 4-10). Under certain conditions of increased demand, newly synthesized PTH may be released directly from chief cells without being packaged into secretory granules (Fig. 4-9).

The biologically active parathyroid hormone is a straight chain polypeptide consisting of 84 amino acid residues with a molecular weight of approximately 9,500 daltons (Fig. 4-8). The complete amino acid sequence has been reported for bovine and porcine PTH. There are seven differences in amino acid residues be-

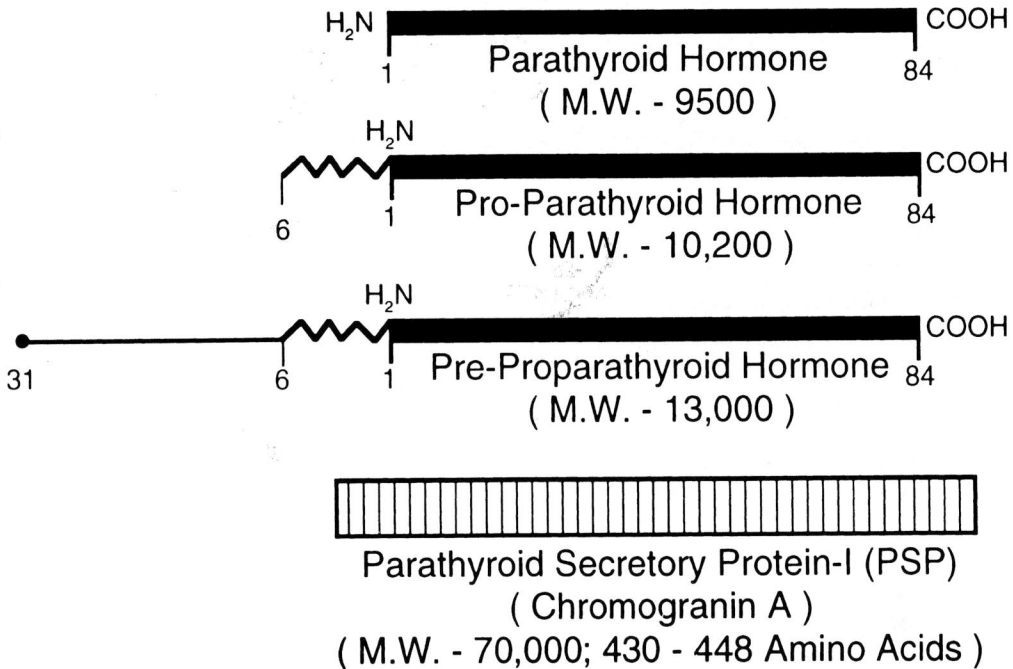

Fig. 4-8. Chemistry of parathyroid hormone and related peptides synthesized by chief cells. Active parathyroid hormone is derived from larger biosynthetic precursor molecules. Pre-proparathyroid hormone (115 amino acids) is the initial translational product from ribosomes of the chief cell and is rapidly converted to pro-parathyroid hormone in the rough endoplasmic reticulum. Pro-parathyroid hormone (90 amino acids) is converted enzymatically to active parathyroid hormone (84 amino acids) in the Golgi apparatus as the hormone is packaged into secretory (storage) granules. Parathyroid secretory protein (PSP-1) is a high molecular weight molecule synthesized by chief cells that is incorporated into storage granules with active parathyroid hormone. The PSP-1 is co-secreted with active parathyroid hormone (PTH) in response to changes in blood calcium and probably functions as a binding protein during intracellular transport and secretion of PTH into the extracellular space (M. W. = molecular weight of the protein in daltons).

tween PTH molecules from these two species. Molecular fragments of PTH are formed in the peripheral circulation and at the target cells of the hormone. The immunoheterogeneity created by the multiple circulating fragments of PTH caused significant problems in the development and application of highly specific radio-immunoassays for the clinical diagnosis of parathyroid-related problems in human and animal patients. The plasma half-life of PTH is 18 to 22 minutes.

Secretion of Parathyroid Hormone

In the early phases of secretory activity, the endoplasmic reticulum of chief cells aggregates into large lamellar arrays and free ribosomes

The active hormone (PTH) is cleaved enzymatically from proparathyroid hormone by an enzyme with trypsin- and carboxypeptidase ß-like activity and packaged into mature secretory or storage granules. As the Golgi apparatus subsequently involutes, acid phosphatase activity appears in the membranes of portions of the Golgi complex, and acid phosphatase-positive lysosomal bodies are formed. During the involuting phase, the packaged parathyroid hormone is displaced from the Golgi region to the periphery of the cell where it is stored prior to secretion. As the Golgi apparatus continues to involute, glycogen particles and lipid bodies accumulate in the cytoplasm, and the chief cell returns to the inactive or resting stage (Fig. 4-11). *In vitro* studies indicate that it is during the secreting and involuting phases that the concentration of calcium exerts an effect on chief cells. Low levels of intra- and extracellular cal-

Circulation   **Parathyroid Chief Cell**   ECF

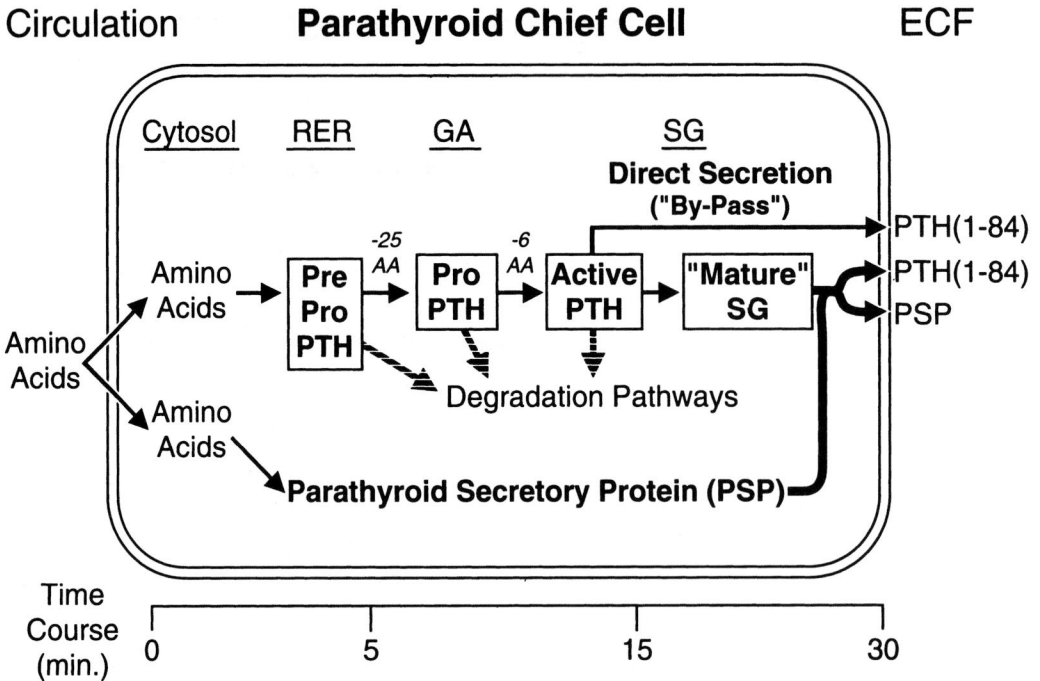

Fig. 4-9. Synthesis of parathyroid hormone (**PTH**) in the cytosol of the chief cell. Pre-proparathyroid hormone (**pre-proPTH**), the product from ribosomes of the rough endoplasmic reticulum (**RER**) is rapidly converted to proparathyroid hormone (**proPTH**) by the cleavage of a 25-amino acid (**AA**) N-terminal fragment. Enzymatic removal of a **6-AA** fragment from ProPTH results in the biologically active PTH in the Golgi apparatus. A major portion of the biosynthetic precursors and active PTH that is synthesized is degraded within the chief cell. Parathyroid secretory protein (**PSP**) may function as a binding protein for PTH during intracellular storage of hormone in secretory granules (**SG**) and during release of PTH into the extracellular space. During periods of high demand, the active hormone **PTH (1-84)** may be secreted directly into the perivascular space.

cium speed up the rate of secretion and shorten the resting phase; conversely, high intra- and extracellular levels of calcium suppress the rate of PTH secretion and lengthen the resting phase of the secretory cycle.

The time-course of the secretory cycle of parathyroid chief cells, as determined by electron microscopic autoradiography, indicated that as early as 2 minutes after intravenous injection of ^{3}H-tyrosine in rats, the label was mainly located over the rough endoplasmic reticulum. Five to 10 minutes after injection, much of the label was present in the Golgi apparatus, after 20 to 30 minutes the labeled tyrosine had migrated into the secretory granules, and by 45 to 60 minutes the radio-labeled content of the cells had decreased, suggesting the release of synthesized material from chief cells. The rapid uptake and release of ^{3}H-tyrosine are consistent with the hypothesis that the turnover of parathyroid hormone is rapid and that chief cells store relatively small amounts of pre-formed hormone, but that chief cells are capable of rapidly responding to fluctuations in the concentration of calcium in blood by altering the rates of synthesis and secretion of PTH.

Storage of Parathyroid Hormone

Secretory Granules

The secretory granules that develop by sequential accumulation and condensation of finely granular material within cisternae of the Golgi apparatus are concentrated in the vicinity of the Golgi apparatus and occasionally are observed in the process of becoming detached from the membranes of the Golgi complex. These secretory ("storage") granules have been demonstrated ultrastructurally within chief

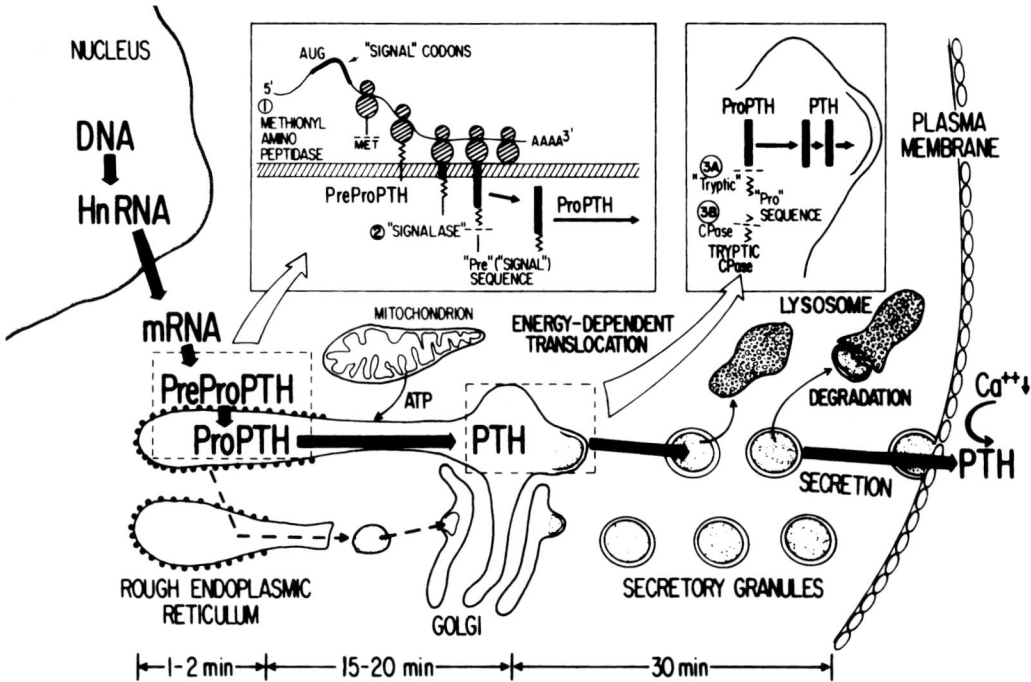

Fig. 4-10. Subcellular compartmentalization, transport, and cleavage of precursors of parathyroid hormone (**PTH**). The hydrophobic sequence on the amino-terminal end of pre-proparathyroid hormone (**pre-proPTH**) facilitates the penetration of the leading portion of the nascent peptide into the lumen of the endoplasmic reticulum. Cleavage of a peptide fragment results in the **ProPTH** that is transported to the Golgi apparatus and converted by carboxypeptidase (**CPase**) to biologically active PTH. Lysosomes engulf the excess secretory granules that form in chief cells under normal conditions. (From: J. F. Habener and J. T. Potts, Jr.,[121] 1978).

cells of the parathyroid glands in man and all of the other animal species that have been examined.

The secretory granules of chief cells are composed of fine, dense particles that are usually round to oval in shape and range from 100 to 300 nm in their greatest diameter (Fig. 4-12). The granules are electron-dense and are surrounded by a delicate, closely-applied limiting membrane. The number of granules within chief cells varies considerably between species, with bovine parathyroid cells having consistently more secretory granules than man and other animals. Chief cells have relatively few storage granules when compared to other endocrine cells concerned with the biosynthesis of polypeptide hormones, e.g., the calcitonin-secreting C-cells of the thyroid gland (Fig. 4-13). The secretory granules that form, migrate peripherally in chief cells and their limiting membrane then fuses with the plasma membrane of the cell. An internal cy-

toskeleton composed of microtubules and contractile filaments are important in the control of the peripheral movement of secretory granules and liberation of secretory products from chief cells (Fig. 4-13). Secretory granules are extruded from chief cells into the perivascular space.

Chromogranin A

In addition to parathyroid hormone, secretory granules in chief cells (Fig. 4-7) also contain chromogranin A (CGA), a parathyroid secretory peptide (molecular weight of approximately 49,000 daltons) first isolated from secretory granules of the bovine adrenal medulla. Chromogranin A comprises up to 50% of the total protein secreted by the parathyroid gland and is a major component of secretory granules of cells of the adrenal medulla, pituitary, parathyroid, thyroid C-cells, pancreatic islets, endocrine cells of the gastrointestinal tract, and sympathetic nerves.

SECRETORY CYCLE OF CHIEF CELLS
IN THE PARATHYROID GLAND

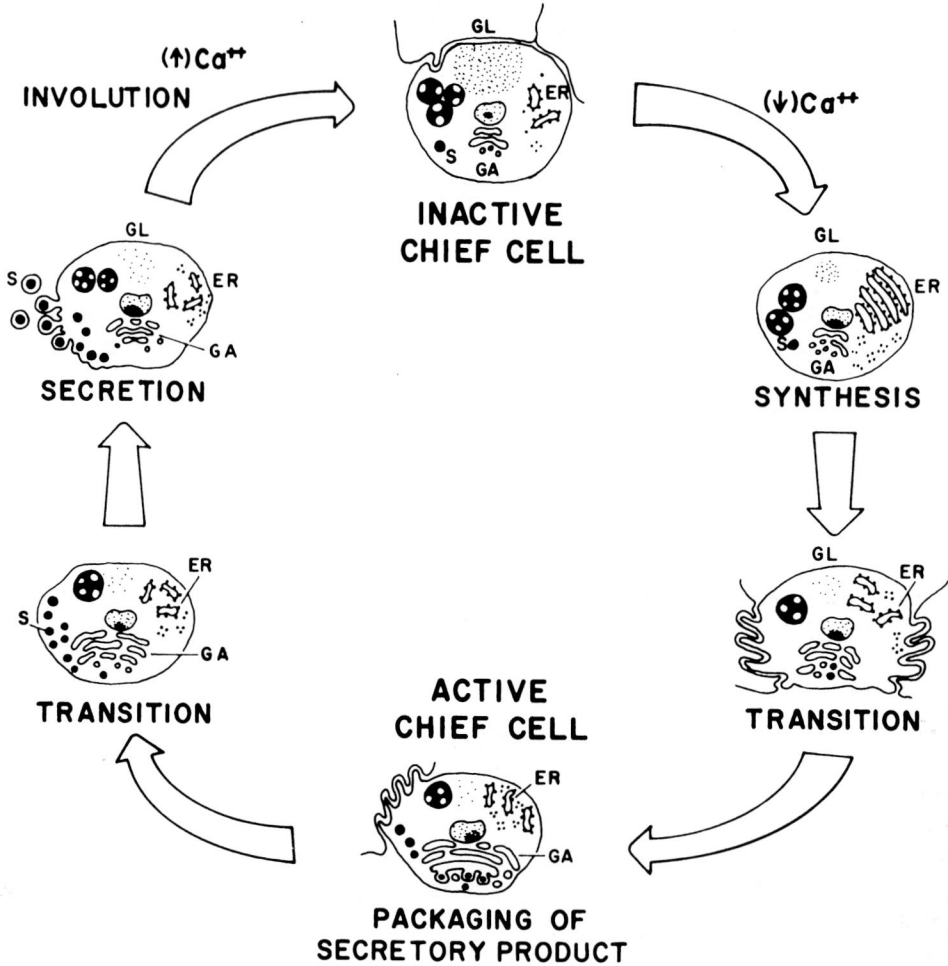

Fig. 4-11. Diagram illustrating the synthetic and secretory phases of the secretory cycle of chief cells of the parathyroid gland. In response to a reduction in the concentration of calcium in the extracellular fluid, chief cells are stimulated to enter the active phase and synthesize pro-PTH. The pro-PTH synthesized on ribosomes associated with the endoplasmic reticulum is transported to the Golgi apparatus where it is packaged into secretory granules for storage and converted to PTH. Secretory granules are discharged from chief cells by exocytosis into the perivascular space where the granules rapidly break up and the PTH molecules enter the circulation. (Modified from: S. I. Roth and C. C. Capen,[238] 1974).

Chromogranin A shares considerable homology between species. Immunologic cross-reactivity to mammalian proteins has been observed in reptiles, amphibians, fish, and *Drosophila* tissues. Chromogranin A is synthesized as a pre-protein and is directed to the internal cavity of the rough endoplasmic reticulum by the N-terminal pre-region of the peptide and cleaved by a signal peptidase.

Although the functions of CGA are still under investigation, several roles have been postulated. Chromogranin A is suspected to play an important role in the maturation of secretory granules. Inside the Golgi apparatus, CGA is involved in

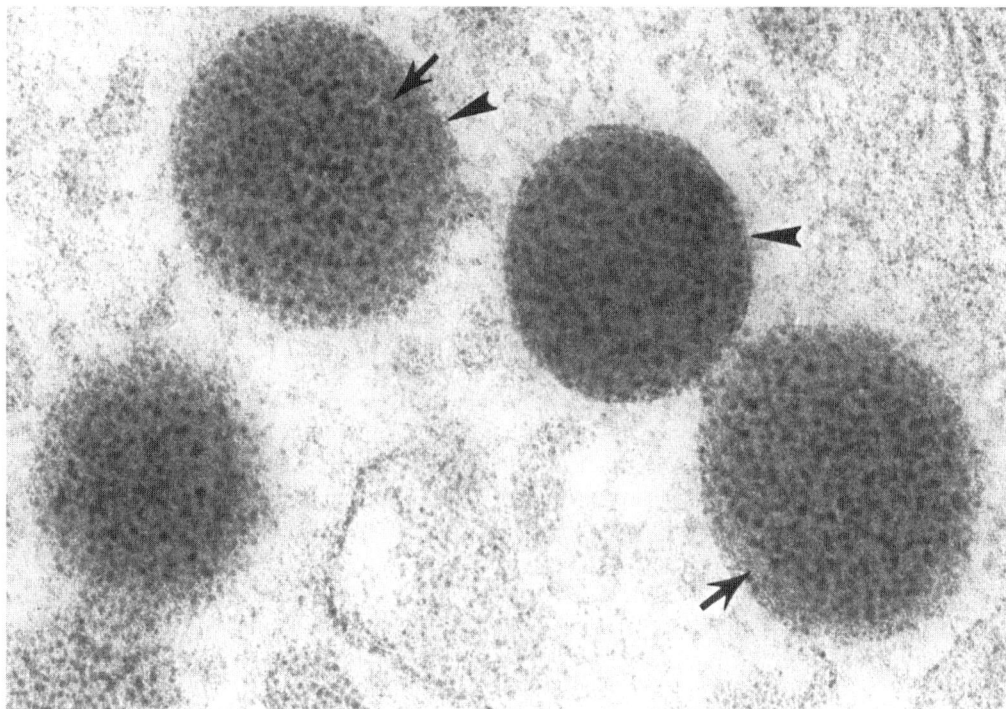

Fig. 4-12. Electron micrograph of the secretory granules composed of numerous small dense particles (**arrows ➤**) and surrounded by a closely applied limiting membrane (**arrow heads ➤**) within a chief cell. These granules are believed to contain active PTH and parathyroid secretory protein. Magnification 82,500 ×.

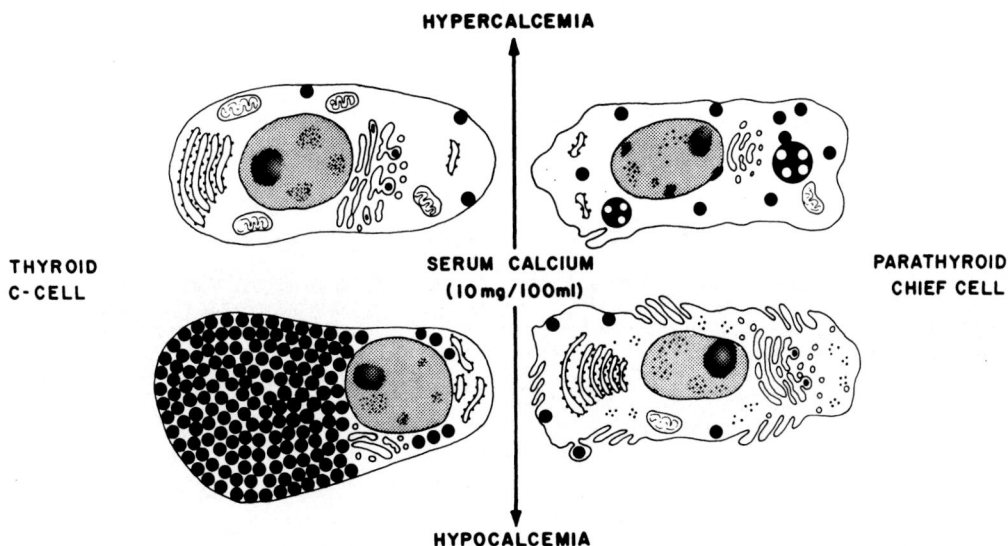

Fig. 4-13. Responses of C-cells of the thyroid gland and chief cells of the parathyroid glands to hyper- and hypocalcemia. Hypocalcemia induces the accumulation of secretory granules in C-cells whereas chief cells are nearly degranulated and there is increased development of synthetic and secretory organelles. In response to hypercalcemia, the C-cells are degranulated and secretory organelles develop, whereas the chief cells are predominantly in the involutionary or inactive stages of the secretory cycle.

the packaging of the contents of newly formed vesicles. Chromogranin A precipitates as it diffuses into the trans-Golgi network and secretory products such as parathyroid hormone become entrapped in the growing CGA conglomerate and are subsequently packaged into secretory granules. Chromogranin A has a large calcium-binding capacity which may enhance the stability of secretory vesicles. As granules mature, they accumulate up to 40 mM of calcium, which also may serve as a route of Ca^{2+} secretion. Chromogranin A-calcium complexes are important in maintaining the integrity of the secretory granule; the absence of calcium causes dissociation of protein complexes and results in osmotic lysis of the vesicle. In summary, the intragranular functions of CGA include hormone packaging, stabilization of the granule against osmotic gradients, and the excretion of intracellular calcium.

During the process of secretion, the contents of secretory granules are extruded into the pericapillary space. The pH and calcium concentration of the extracellular fluid promote the dissociation of CGA complexes and solubilization of bound calcium and other contents of the granule. Once solubilized, extracellular peptidases cleave CGA into biologically active peptides which act as paracrine or autocrine regulators of endocrine secretion.[81]

Secretion of Parathyroid Hormone

To release their contents, the secretory granules migrate peripherally and their limiting membrane fuses with the plasma membrane of the chief cell. An internal cytoskeleton composed of microtubules and contractile filaments may play an important role in the peripheral migration of secretory granules and secretion of PTH by chief cells. Secretory granules appear to be extruded from chief cells by exocytosis into the perivascular space (Figs. 4-10, 4-12, and 4-14). The release of insulin from secretory granules in the cells of the pancreatic islet (see Chapter 5, Fig. 5-3) has been termed **emiocyto-**

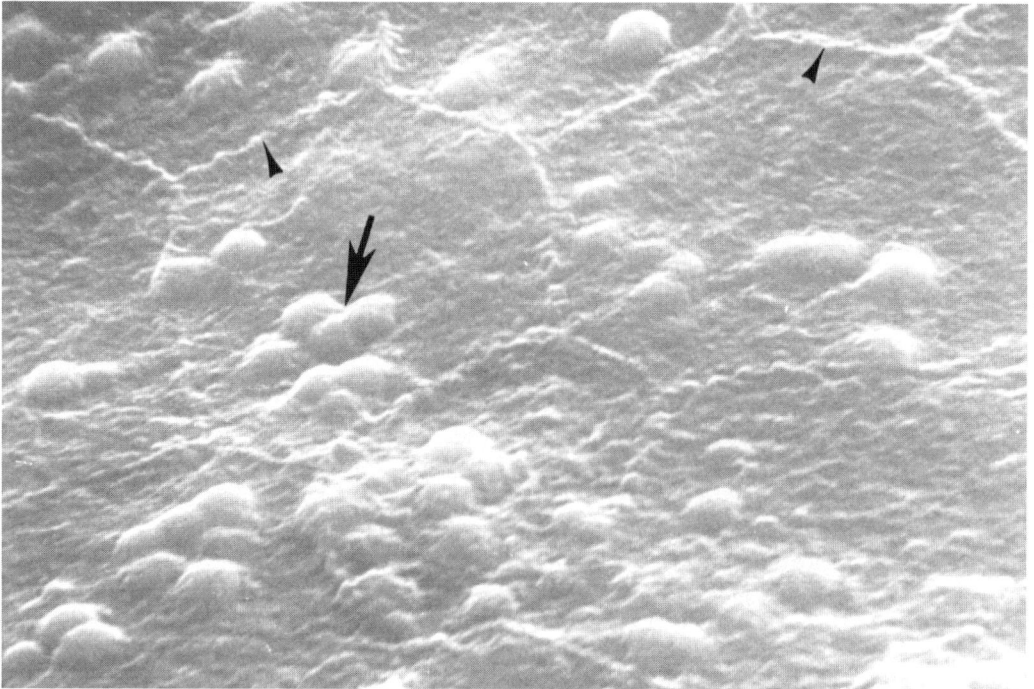

Fig. 4-14. Scanning electron micrograph of the surface of active chief cells. Exocytosis of secretory granules (**arrow ➤**) appear as the budding of the cell into the perivascular space. Chief cells are polyhedral and distinct cell boundaries can be visualized (**arrow heads ➤**). Glutaraldehyde and osmium tetroxide fixation, uranyl acetate and lead citrate staining. Magnification 3,000 ×.

sis. Similar terminology may be applicable to the release of the contents of secretory granules from chief cells.

Control of Parathyroid Hormone Secretion

Secretory cells in the parathyroid gland store small amounts of pre-formed hormone and respond to minor fluctuations in calcium concentration by rapidly altering the rate of release of stored hormone and more slowly, by altering the rate of hormonal synthesis and release. The parathyroid glands have a unique mechanism for feedback control due to the cellular response to the concentration of calcium and to a lesser extent of magnesium ions in the serum and perivascular space.

The influence of serum levels of ionized calcium and interaction with the Ca^{2+}-sensing re-ceptors on chief cells results in the formation of an inverse sigmoidal-type of relationship be-tween serum Ca^{2+} and PTH concentrations (Fig. 4-15). The serum $[Ca^{2+}]$ that results in half maximal PTH secretion is defined as the serum calcium 'set point' and this is stable for an individual animal. The sigmoidal-type of relationship between serum $[Ca^{2+}]$ and PTH secretion permits the chief cells to respond rapidly to a reduction in serum $[Ca^{2+}]$. Ionized calcium binds to the Ca^{2+}-sensing receptor and results in an increase in the intracellular Ca^{2+} concentration of chief cells and a reduction in the secretion of PTH. This makes the parathyroid chief cells unique, because increased intracellular Ca^{2+} concentrations typically serve as a stimulus for secretion in most cell types. The major inhibitors of PTH synthesis and secretion are increased serum levels of $[Ca^{2+}]$ and 1,25-

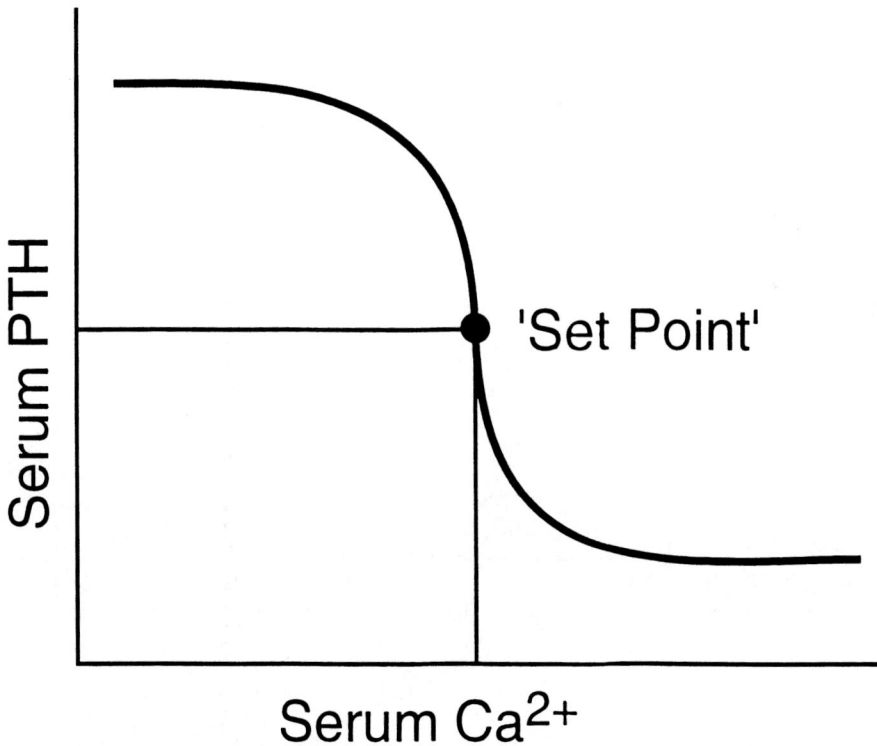

Fig. 4-15. The "set-point" for ionized calcium (**Ca²⁺**) is defined as the concentration of ionized calcium at which the concentration of parathyroid hormone (**PTH**) in serum is half-maximal. The sigmoidal relationship between concentrations of Ca²⁺ and PTH enables the parathyroid glands to rapidly respond to a minor reduction in serum calcium and increase PTH secretion to restore the concentration of calcium in the serum to normal levels. In most animals, the concentration of calcium in the serum is maintained above the "set-point" concentration. (From: T. J. Rosol et al.,[234] 1995).

dihydroxyvitamin D. Inhibition of PTH synthesis by 1,25-dihydroxyvitamin D completes an important endocrine feedback loop between the parathyroid chief cells and the renal epithelial cells because PTH stimulates renal production of 1,25-dihydroxyvitamin D (Fig. 4-16).

If the blood calcium level is elevated by the intravenous infusion of calcium, there is a rapid and pronounced reduction in circulating levels of immunoreactive parathyroid hormone; however, a small percentage of the PTH secretion is nonsuppressible. Therefore, there are always low concentrations of circulating PTH in the blood, even under extreme conditions of hypercalcemia. Conversely, if the blood calcium is lowered by infusion of ethylenediaminetetraacetic acid (EDTA), there is a brisk and substantial increase in the level of immunoreactive PTH. The concentration of blood phosphate has no direct regulatory influence on the synthesis and secretion of PTH; however, certain disease conditions with hyperphos-phatemia in animals and man are associated clinically with hyperparathyroidism. An elevated blood phosphorus level may lead indirectly to parathyroid stimulation by virtue of its ability to lower blood levels of calcium. If the blood level of phosphorus is elevated significantly by the simultaneous infusion of phosphate and calcium in amounts sufficient to prevent the accompanying reduction of blood calcium by phosphate, plasma levels of immunoreactive PTH remain within the normal range (Fig. 4-17).

Magnesium ion $[Mg^{2+}]$ has an effect on secretory rate of parathyroid hormone similar to that of calcium, but the effect is not equipotent to that of calcium. The reduced potency of $[Mg^{2+}]$ compared to Ca^{2+} may be due to reducing binding affinity of $[Mg^{2+}]$ for the Ca^{2+}-sensing membrane receptors on chief cells. The more potent effects of Ca^{2+} in the control of PTH secretion, together with its preponderance over Mg^{2+} in the extracellular fluid, suggest a

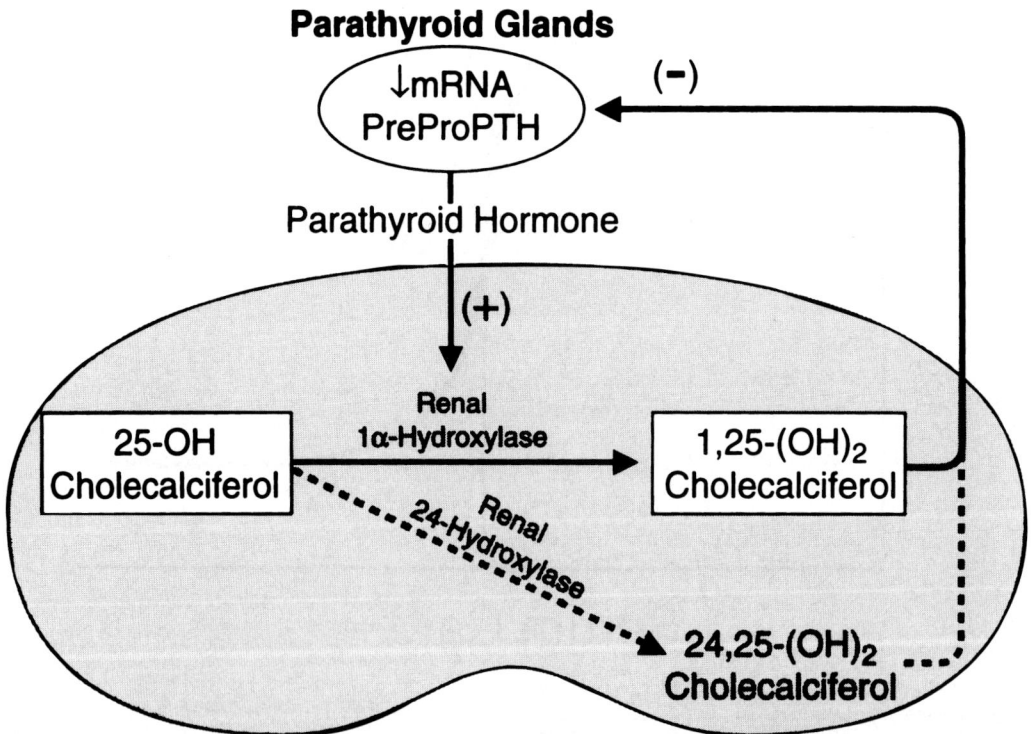

Fig. 4-16. Negative feedback exerted by vitamin D metabolites on the parathyroid chief cell to regulate the rate of parathyroid hormone secretion.

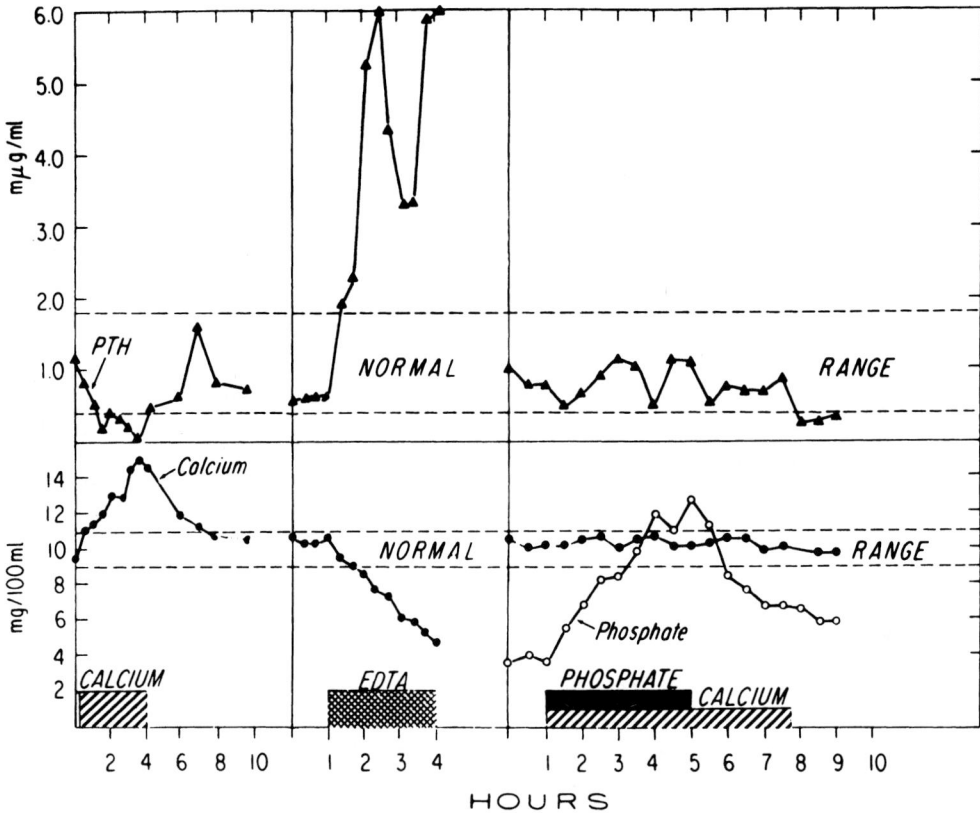

Fig. 4-17. Concentration of plasma immunoreactive parathyroid hormone (**PTH**) in response to hypercalcemia induced by **calcium** infusion, hypocalcemia produced by ethylenediaminetetraacetic acid (**EDTA**) infusion, and hyperphosphatemia with normocalcemia in a cow. (From: G. D. Aurbach and T. J. Potts, Jr.,The parathyroids. *In:* Advances in Metabolic Diseases, edited by R. Levine and R. Luft. New York, NY, Academic Press, Inc., p. 45, 1964).

secondary role for magnesium in the control of the parathyroid gland.

Calcium ion not only controls the rate of biosynthesis and secretion of parathyroid hormone (Fig. 4-18), but also other metabolic and intracellular degradative processes occur within chief cells. An increase of calcium ions in extracellular fluids rapidly inhibits uptake of amino acids, synthesis of proPTH and conversion to PTH, and secretion of stored PTH by chief cells, and also increases the intracellular degradation of PTH. The shifting of the percentage of flow of proparathyroid hormone from the degradative pathways to the secretory route (Figs. 4-9 and 4-18) represents a key adaptive response of the parathyroid gland to a low calcium diet. During periods of long-term calcium restriction, the enhanced synthesis and secretion of PTH is accomplished by an increase in the capacity of the synthetic pathway in individual, hypertrophied chief cells and through hyperplasia to form active chief cells.

In response to increased demand, newly synthesized PTH may be released from the cell and bypass the storage pool of mature secretory granules in the cytoplasm of the chief cell. This bypass secretion (Figs. 4-9 and 4-18) can only be stimulated by a low circulating concentration of calcium ion and not by the other secretagogues for PTH (Figs. 4-17 and 4-18). Lysosomal enzymes degrade the PTH stored in secretory granules of chief cells during periods of prolonged exposure to a high-calcium environment.

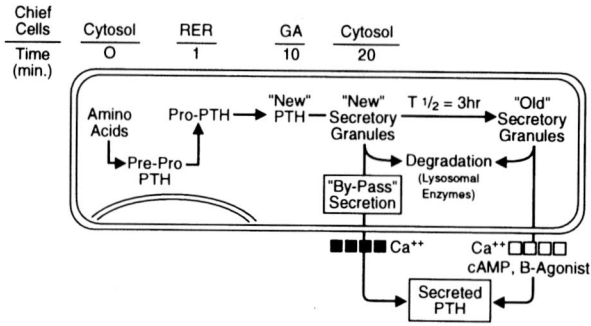

Fig. 4-18. Bypass secretion of parathyroid hormone (PTH) in response to the demand signaled by a decrease in the calcium ion concentration in the blood. Recently synthesized and processed active **PTH** may be released directly from the chief cell and does not enter the storage pool of mature ("old") secretory granules in the cytoplasm of the chief cell. Release of PTH from the storage pool is stimulated by cyclic adenosine monophosphate (**cAMP**) and beta (ß)-agonists (e.g., epinephrine, norepinephrine, and isoproterenol) as well as by low concentrations of calcium ion in the blood. Secretion from the pool of recently synthesized PTH can only be stimulated by a decrease in the calcium ion concentration (**RER** = rough endoplasmic reticulum; **GA** = Golgi apparatus). (Redrawn from: D. V. Cohn and R. R. MacGregor,[76] 1981).

Biologic Effects of Parathyroid Hormone

Parathyroid hormone is the principal hormone involved in the minute-to-minute, fine regulation of blood calcium in mammals. It exerts its biologic actions by directly influencing the function of target cells, primarily in the bone (Figs. 4-19 and 4-20) and kidney (Fig. 4-16), and secondarily in the intestine (Fig. 4-21) to maintain plasma calcium at a level sufficient to ensure the optimal functioning of a wide variety of body cells.

In general, the most important biologic effects of PTH are to:

1. elevate the blood concentration of calcium,

2. decrease the blood concentration of phosphorus,

3. increase the urinary excretion of phosphorus by a decreased rate of tubular reabsorption,

4. increase the tubular reabsorption of calcium,

5. increase the rate of skeletal remodeling and the net rate of bone resorption,

6. increase the numbers of osteoclasts on bone surfaces and the rate of osteolysis,

7. increase the urinary excretion of hydroxyproline,

8. activate adenylyl cyclase in target cells, and

9. accelerate the formation of the principal active vitamin D metabolite (1,25-dihydroxycholecalciferol; 1,25-dihydroxyvitamin D) through a tropic effect of PTH on the 1α-hydroxylase in mitochondria the epithelial cells lining the convoluted tubules of the kidney.

Parathyroid hormone mobilizes calcium from skeletal reserves into the extracellular fluids. The administration of PTH to an animal causes an initial decline in serum calcium followed by a sustained increase in circulating levels of calcium. This transitory decrease in blood calcium is considered to be the result of the sequestration of calcium-phosphate in bone and soft tissues. The subsequent increase in blood calcium results from the interaction of parathyroid hormone with osteoblasts and osteoclasts in the bone.

The response of bone to parathyroid hormone is biphasic. The immediate effects are the result of increasing the activity of existing osteocytes and osteoclasts. This rapid effect of PTH depends upon the continuous presence of hormone and results in an increased flow of calcium to the bone surface through the coordinated action of osteocytes and the activation of endosteal lining cells which are inactive osteoblasts. This osteocyte-osteoblast "pump" (Fig. 4-19) facilitates the

movement of calcium from bone to the extracellular fluid for the fine adjustment of the calcium
concentration in the blood.

The later effects of parathyroid hormone on
bone are of a greater magnitude of response and

OSTEOCYTE-OSTEOBLAST PUMP

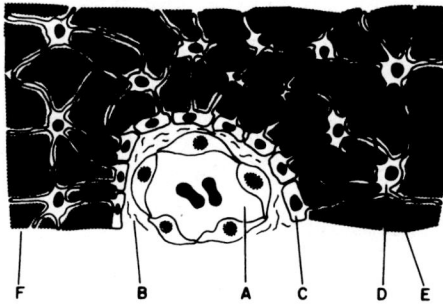

Fig. 4-19. The osteocyte-osteoblast "pump" is formed
by the fusion of processes of endosteal lining cells (**C**;
inactive osteoblasts) with the osteocytes (**D**) embedded in cortical bone (**F**). This functional cellular syncytium provides a mechanism for the transcellular
transport of calcium from the bone-fluid compartment
around osteocytes (**E**) to the extracellular fluid compartment (**B**) and transfer to the adjacent capillary (**A**).

are not dependent upon the continuous presence
of PTH. Osteoclasts appear to be primarily responsible for the long-term actions of PTH on
increasing bone resorption and overall bone remodeling. This is interesting, in light of studies
which provided evidence for the presence of receptors for PTH on osteoblasts but had failed to
demonstrate receptors on osteoclasts (Fig.
4-20 and 4-21).

Bone resorption is a complex, multistep, process that involves the activation of multiple
genes and the action of multiple hormones.[298,306]
Most hormones and cytokines involved in the
regulation of bone, including parathyroid hormone, calcitriol, interleukin-1 beta, tumor
necrosis factor (TNF), interleukin-6, and prostaglandin E2, act via receptors on osteoblasts. Additionally, three members of the TNF ligand and
receptor signaling system that appear to play a
critical role in the regulation of bone resorption
(RANKL, RANK, osteoprotegerin) have recently been identified and cloned.[296, 300, 301] In
the presence of permissive concentrations of
macrophage colony-stimulating factor (M-
CSF), these newly identified TNF superfamily

Cellular Control of Bone Resorption

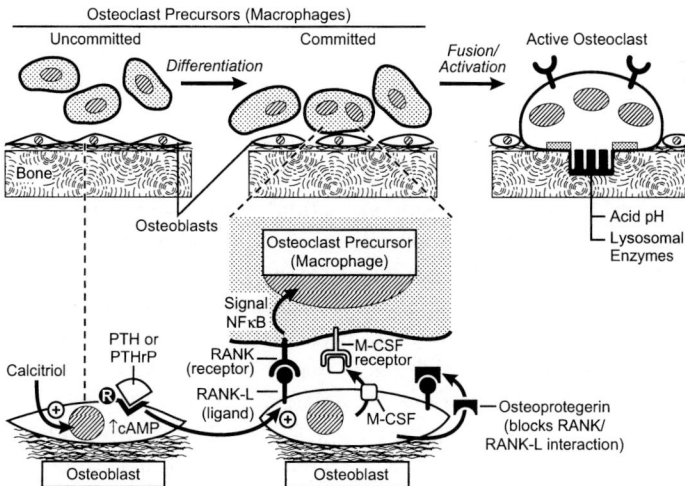

Fig. 4-10. Cellular control of bone resorption. Specific receptors for parathyroid hormone (**PTH**) are present on osteoblasts but not on osteoclasts. RANK-L or osteoclast differentiation factor is produced by cells of the osteoblast
lineage, serves as a common mediator for osteoclastic bone resorption, and its expression is up-regulated by
osteotrophic factors such as PTH, PTHrP and calcitriol. Rank-L=Receptor Activator NF-Kappa B Ligand. M-CSF
= Macrophage Colony – Simulating Factor; R=Receptor for either PTH or PTHrP.

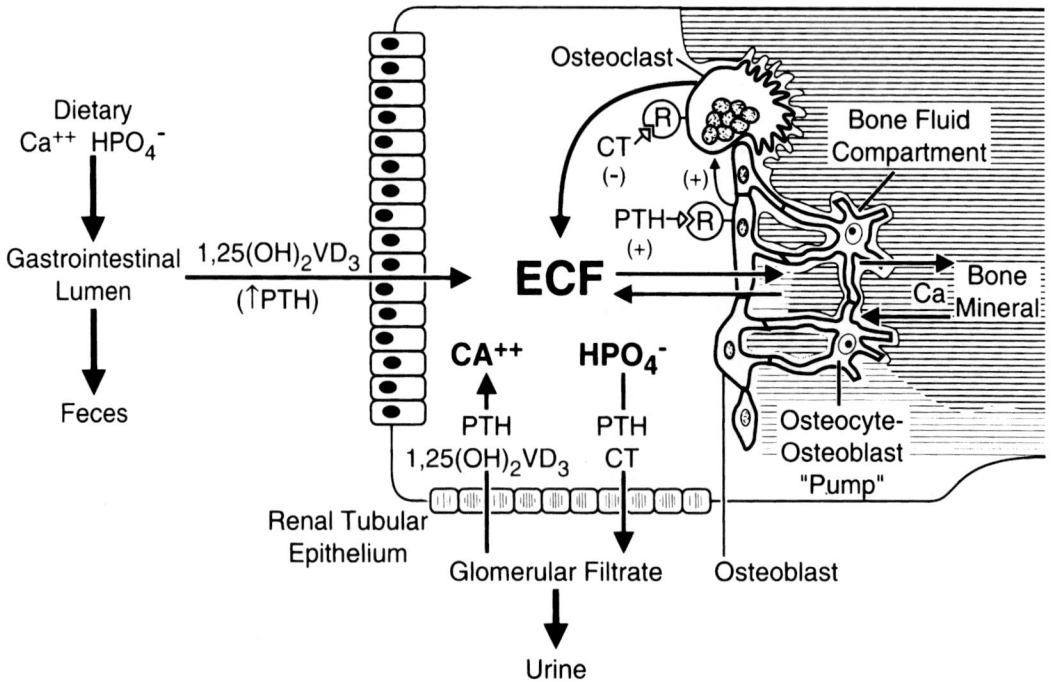

Fig. 4-21. Interrelationship of parathyroid hormone (**PTH**), calcitonin (**CT**), and 1,25-dihydroxycholecalciferol (**1,25(OH)$_2$VD$_3$**) on the regulation of calcium (**Ca**) and phosphorus in extracellular fluids.

molecules constitute a common pathway for regulation of osteoclast formation and function by cells of the osteoblast lineage, thereby, mediating the biologic effects of many upstream hormones and cytokines (Fig. 4-20).[304]

The receptor ligand referred to as RANK ligand or RANKL is a membrane-bound protein on osteoblasts that serves as a common mediator for osteoclastic bone resorption. This ligand was initially termed osteoclast differentiation factor or osteoprotegrin ligand and is produced by osteoblast lineage cells and stimulates differentiation of cells of the osteoclast lineage, enhances the functional activity of mature osteoclasts, and prolongs osteoclast life by inhibiting apoptosis.[296, 298, 306] Targeted deletion of this receptor ligand in mice leads to osteopetrosis, shortened bones, impaired tooth eruption, and immunologic abnormalities. The expression of RANK ligand by osteoblasts and/or stromal cells is up-regulated by osteotrophic factors such as calcitriol, PTH, and interleukin-11.[304] This molecule is identical to the TNF-related

activation-induced cytokine or the receptor activator of NF-kappa B ligand reported to to stimulate T-cell growth and dendritic cell function in the immunology literature.[296]

The membrane receptor for the RANK ligand on cells of the osteoclast lineage is also identical to a receptor of similar name identified previously on immune cells.[296] This receptor has also been referred to as osteoclast differentiation and activation receptor. Binding of the RANK ligand to the RANK receptor activates signal transduction pathways in osteoclasts, leading to increased functional activity. Osteoclast precursors also express the membrane receptor for the RANK ligand and mice made deficient for this receptor by targeted gene deletion develop severe osteopetrosis due to decreased osteoclast function. Furthermore, these mice fail to develop peripheral lymph nodes.[296]

Osteoprotegerin, also called 'decoy receptor', is a novel member of the TNF receptor superfamily that is produced by cells of the osteoblast lineage and is a negative regulator of bone resorption.[300,301] When soluble osteoprotegerin binds to the RANK receptor, it prevents the RANK ligand from binding and activating the receptor. Overexpression of osteoprotegerin in transgenic mice leads to osteopetrosis associated with decreased osteoclast formation and function. In contrast, targeted gene ablation in mice results in severe osteoporosis and arterial mineralization.[296]

These findings clearly indicate a role for the microenvironment within bone marrow and identify the regulatory factors that influence osteoclast differentiation and function. Osteoclast formation appears to be determined by the ratio of RANK ligand to osteoprotegerin (RANKL:OPG) and alterations in this ratio may be a major cause of bone loss in metabolic disorders such as estrogen-deficiency or glucocorticoid- excess.[300,301]

Osteoblasts normally are flat and cover bone surfaces (Figs. 4-20 and 4-21). The initial binding of PTH to osteoblasts lining bone surfaces appears to cause the cells to contract, thereby exposing the underlying mineral to osteoclasts (Fig. 4-20). If the increase in PTH is sustained, the size of the active osteoclast pool in bone is increased by the activation of osteoprogenitor cells in the cell envelope of the endosteal bone. The plasma membrane of osteoclasts in intimate contact with the resorbing bone surface is modified to form a series of membranous projections referred to as the brush "ruffled" border (Figs. 4-20 and 4-21). This area of active bone resorption is isolated from the extracellular fluids by adjacent transitional "sealing" zones, thereby localizing the lysosomal enzymes and acidic environment to the immediate area undergoing dissolution (Figs. 4-20 and 4-21). The mineral and also organic components such as hydroxyproline released from bone are phagocytized by osteoclasts and transported across the cell in transport vesicles to be released into the extracellular fluid compartment.

Parathyroid hormone-induced changes in osteoblasts are evident within 1 hour after PTH administration to thyroparathyroidectomized rats. Changes in the shape of osteoblasts associated with PTH (Fig. 4-21) may be related to calcium entry into the cell and alteration in microtubule and microfilament function. Parathyroid hormone appears to inhibit microfilament function and cellular changes in shape are blocked by drugs which prevent the assembly of microtubules. Thus, PTH-induced changes require a balance between microfilament and microtubular function. The increase in the calcium/phosphate ratio in the mitochondria of the lining cells of bone in young rats is associated with an increase in mitochondrial granules; cellular changes which are evident within 5 minutes after the injection of PTH. In addition to alterations in microfilaments, microtubules and mitochondrial granules, PTH increases endocytosis in lining cells of bone.

A long-term increase in the secretion of PTH also may result in the formation of greater numbers of osteoblasts and an increase in bone formation and resorption. However, because bone resorption by osteoclasts usually is greater than bone formation by osteoblasts, there is a net negative balance in skeletal mass.

The major physiological effect of PTH is exerted on bone cells on the endosteal surfaces and in the Haversian cell envelope. In cases of hyperparathyroidism, the activation of osteoprogenitor cells occurs in the periosteal bone cell envelope as well, leading to the formation of metabolically active regions on the periosteal surface. This process results in the characteristic subperiosteal areas of bone resorption which are seen radiographically in both primary and secondary hyperparathyroidism (Fig. 4-22).

Parathyroid hormone has a direct and rapid effect on renal tubular function. Five to 10 minutes after PTH administration the reabsorption of phosphate is decreased, causing phosphaturia. The site of action of PTH on the tubular reabsorption of phosphate has been localized by micropuncture methods to the proximal convoluted tubule of the nephron (Fig. 4-23). In addition, PTH leads to the increased urinary excretion of potassium, sodium, bicarbonate, cyclic adenosine monophosphate, and amino acids.

Although the effect of PTH on the tubular reabsorption of phosphate has been considered to be of importance, the capability of PTH to en-

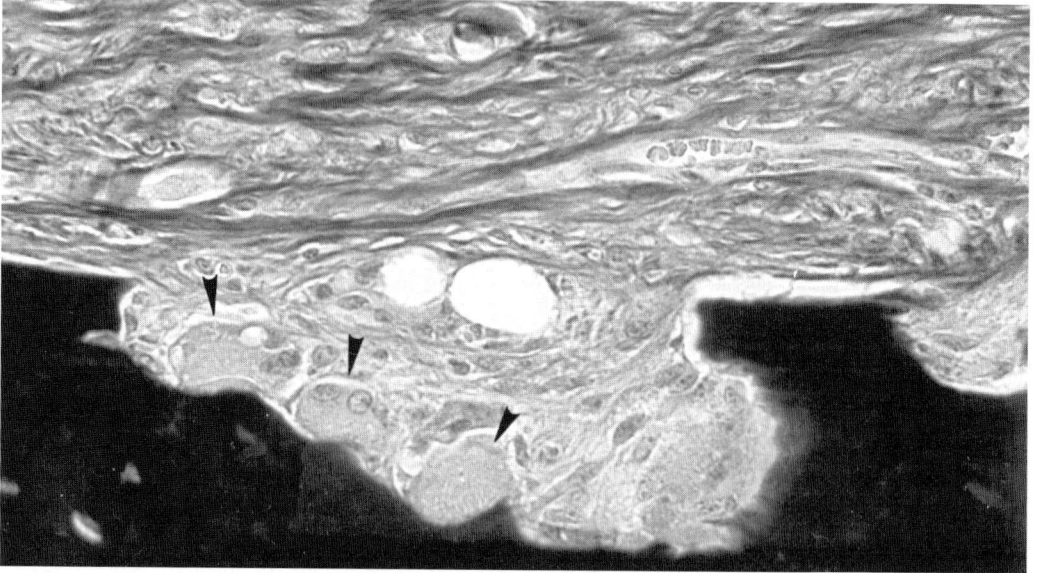

Fig. 4-22. Subperiosteal activation of osteoclasts (**arrow heads** ➤) in response to a long-term increase in PTH secretion in an animal with hyperparathyroidism. The resultant increase in bone resorption may disrupt the tendinous insertions of muscles elevating the periosteum and result in bone pain. Hematoxylin and eosin staining, magnification 315 ×.

DISTRIBUTION OF ADENYLATE CYCLASE-LINKED HORMONE RECEPTORS IN THE NEPHRON

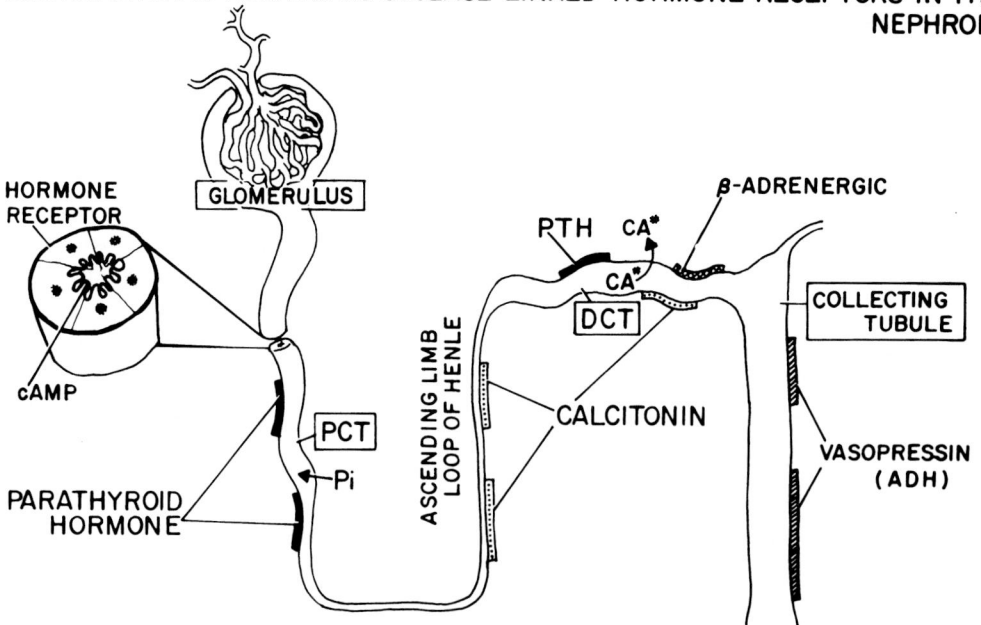

Fig. 4-23. Distribution of target cells for parathyroid hormone (**PTH**) and calcitonin in the kidney nephron. The parathyroid hormone-mediated inhibition of the tubular reabsorption of phosphorus (**P**$_i$) occurs in the epithelial cells lining the proximal convoluted tubule (**PCT**), whereas the increased reabsorption of calcium caused by PTH occurs in the renal epithelia of the distal convoluted tubule (**DCT**). Target cells for calcitonin are situated along the ascending limb of the loop of Henle and the DCT and hormonal stimulation diminishes the tubular reabsorption of phosphorus, causing phosphaturia (**ADH** = antidiuretic hormone; **cAMP** = cyclic adenosine monophosphate).

hance the renal reabsorption of calcium is of considerably more importance in the maintenance of calcium homeostasis. This effect of PTH upon tubular reabsorption of calcium appears to be due to a direct action on cells of the distal convoluted tubule of the kidney nephron. The urinary excretion of magnesium and ammonia, and the titratable acidity of the urine also are decreased by PTH. The other important effect of PTH on the kidney is the regulation of the conversion of 25-hydroxycholecalciferol to 1,25-dihydroxycholecalciferol and other metabolites of vitamin D (see Fig. 4-16). The role of PTH as a tropic hormone in the metabolic activation of cholecalciferol will be discussed further in the section of this chapter on vitamin D metabolites.

Parathyroid hormone promotes the absorption of calcium from the gastrointestinal tract in animals under a variety of experimental conditions.[199] This effect is not as rapid as the action of PTH on the kidney and is not observed in vitamin D-deficient animals. This increased intestinal calcium transport may be due to a direct effect of PTH on the absorptive cells lining the intestine, however it is more likely an indirect effect of PTH

due to the stimulation of the renal synthesis of the biologically active metabolite of vitamin D.

Under normal conditions, PTH is secreted continuously from chief cells. Parathyroid hormone, a peptide chain of 84 amino acids, is cleaved in the liver and possibly elsewhere into the biologically active portion, an amino-terminal fragment comprised of approximately one-third of the PTH molecule, and a larger, carboxy-terminal fragment that is biologically inactive. The kidney is a major organ for the degradation of PTH (Fig. 4-24). Biologically active PTH is degraded in the peritubular capillaries by specific proteases on the surface of renal tubular cells. In addition, both the biologically active (NH_2-1–34) and inactive (34–84 COOH) fragments of the PTH are absorbed and degraded by lysosomal enzymes within cells of the renal tubule (Fig. 4-24).

Parathyroid Hormone Receptor

The receptor for the N-terminal portion of PTH has been cloned and sequenced.[1, 243] The receptor for N-terminal PTH is a 7-transmembrane domain receptor that is expressed in renal epithelial cells, osteoblasts, and dermal fibroblasts, and

METABOLIC DEGRADATION OF PARATHYROID HORMONE BY THE KIDNEY

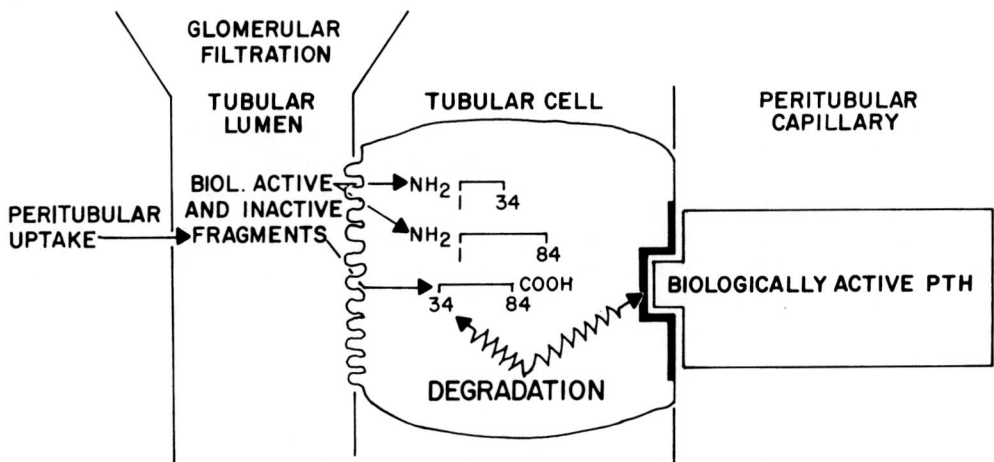

Fig. 4-24. Degradation of parathyroid hormone by the kidney. Biologically active parathyroid hormone (**PTH**) is degraded by specific proteases on the surface of renal tubular epithelial cells. Biologically active (**NH2 - 1–34**) and inactive (**34–84 - COOH**) fragments are degraded by lysosomal enzymes within the renal tubular cell.

is also found on cells that are not associated with the actions of PTH. Binding of PTH to the receptor results in increased levels of cytoplasmic cAMP and Ca^{2+} by stimulation of the adenylate cyclase and phosphatidyl inositol pathways.

Assays for Parathyroid Hormone

Parathyroid hormone has a half-life of less than 5 minutes and is rapidly removed from the circulation by endopeptidases in hepatic Kupffer cell membranes or by glomerular filtration.[7] Some C-terminal peptide is released into the circulation by Kupffer cells and is then cleared by the kidney. As a result, the C-terminal PTH fragment has a biological half-life that is longer than that of intact PTH and is present in the serum in higher concentrations (50 to 90% of total PTH), especially in cases of hyperparathyroidism.

The multiple forms of PTH and PTH fragments in the circulation made the development of specific and sensitive radioimmunoassays for this hormone difficult. Early immunoassays for PTH were single-site radioimmunoassays for C-terminal peptides. These assays were suboptimal because both the biologically active and inactive forms of PTH were measured. Nevertheless, the assay was clinically useful to diagnose and monitor hyperparathyroidism in patients with normal renal function. Mid-region and C-terminal RIAs measure both intact PTH (active) and C-terminal PTH (inactive) which renders them less clinically relevant. In addition, conditions that reduce the glomerular filtration rate, such as renal failure, result in a large increase in the serum concentration of C-terminal PTH.

Concentrations of intact PTH in the serum are best measured by two-site immunoradiometric assay or N-terminal radioimmunoassay. Serum levels of intact PTH can be measured in dogs, cats and horses with assays developed for human PTH due to the cross-reactivity of the antisera with PTH from these species.

Mechanism of Action of Parathyroid Hormone

The calcium-mobilizing and phosphaturic activities of parathyroid hormone are mediated through the intracellular accumulation of 3',5'-adenosine monophosphate (cAMP) or Ca^{2+} in target cells. Binding of PTH to receptors on target cells results in activation of the receptor, binding of the receptor to stimulatory or inhibitory G proteins, and stimulation of adenyl (adenylyl) cyclase or the hydrolysis of phosphatidylinositol (Fig.4-25). Receptors for PTH also bind a parathyroid-like factor, called parathyroid hormone-related protein (PTHrP). This factor is discussed on the next section of this chapter. Stimulation of adenylyl cyclase stimulates the conversion of ATP to cAMP in target cells. The accumulation of cAMP functions as an intracellular mediator or second messenger of parathyroid hormone action in target cells to increase the permeability of the cell membrane for calcium ions. The cytosolic Ca^{2+} concentration may also be increased by the actions of inositol triphosphate to release Ca^{2+} from intracytoplasmic stores or by stimulation of Ca^{2+} transport through transmembrane channels. The resultant increase in cytosolic calcium, in combination with cAMP accumulation, initiates biochemical reactions in bone cells and renal epithelial cells to transduce the intracellular functions attributed to stimulation by PTH.

In addition, PTH contributes to the regulation of the rate of formation of the active form of vitamin D by the mitochondria in epithelial cells of the renal tubules. The active metabolites of vitamin D make bone cells more sensitive to the direct effect of PTH ("permissive effect") and greatly enhance the gastrointestinal absorption of calcium, thereby amplifying the effect of PTH on the concentration of calcium in the plasma.

PARATHYROID HORMONE-RELATED PROTEIN (PTHrP)

Parathyroid hormone-related protein (PTHrP) was identified in 1987 as an important PTH-like factor that plays a central role in the pathogenesis of humoral hypercalcemia of malignancy. Parathyroid hormone-related protein (PTHrP) is a 139-173 amino acid peptide, originally isolated from human and animal tumors associated with humoral hypercalcemia of malignancy (Fig. 4-26). The PTHrP peptide shares 70% sequence homology with first 13 amino acids of intact PTH. The N-terminal region of PTHrP (amino acids 1-34) binds and stimulates PTH receptors in bone and kidney cells with equal affinity as PTH. However, PTHrP is not strictly a calcium-regulating hormone and the other actions of PTHrP are listed in Figure 4-26. Since its discovery, it has been determined that PTHrP is widely produced in many tissues in adult animals including endocrine glands, smooth, skeletal, and cardiac muscles, brain, lymphocytes, lactating mammary gland, kidney, prostate gland, lung, skin, and bone. The function of PTHrP in most of these tissues is poorly understood, but likely is an autocrine or paracrine regulatory factor. Circulating concentrations of PTHrP in normal animals and humans are low (<1 pM)[40,234] and the PTH/PTHrP receptor is often expressed on the same or adjacent cells in tissues that synthesize PTHrP.

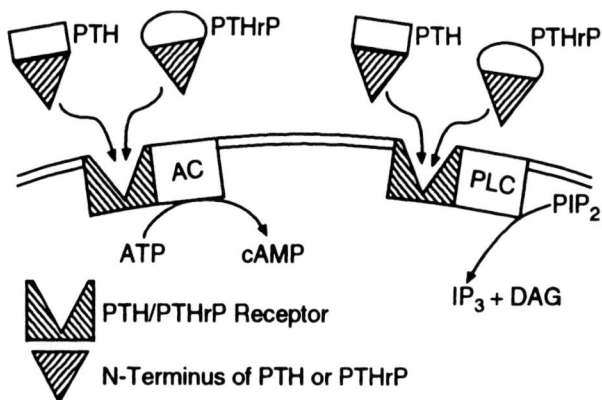

Fig. 4-25. Mechanism of action of parathyroid hormone (**PTH**) and parathyroid hormone-related protein (**PTHrP**). The biologically active N-terminal ends of PTH and PTHrP bind to **PTH/PTHrP** receptors on the surface of the target cell. The receptor-hormone complexes are coupled to the catalytic subunit of adenylyl cyclase (**AC**) or to phospholipase C (**PLC**) by a nucleotide regulatory protein (G-protein). This results in the conversion of **ATP** to cyclic adenosine monophosphate (**cAMP**) by AC or phosphatidylinositol to inositol triphosphate (IP_3) and diacylglycerol (**DAG**) by PLC. The IP_3 that forms stimulates the release of Ca^{2+} from intracellular stores. Both cAMP and Ca^{2+} serve as second messengers for polypeptide hormones such as PTH and PTHrP and result in the expression of the biological responses induced by these hormones. (From: T. J. Rosol and C. C. Capen,[233] 1992).

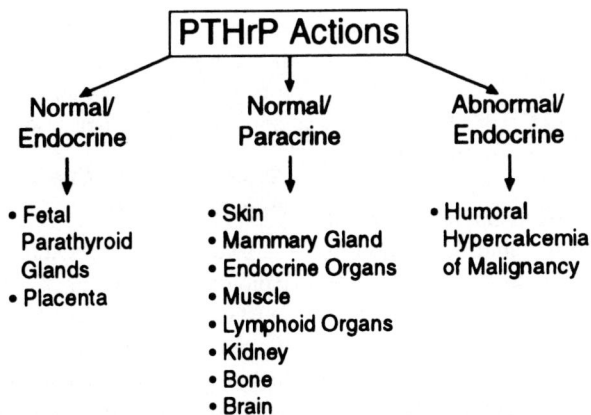

Fig. 4-26. Spectrum of paracrine and endocrine actions of parathyroid hormone-related protein (**PTHrP**) under normal and abnormal conditions. (From: T. J. Rosol and C. C. Capen,[233] 1992).

Role of Parathyroid Hormone-related Protein in the Fetus

Fetal Calcium Balance

The fetus maintains higher concentrations of serum calcium compared to the dam. Because the fetal parathyroid glands produce low levels of PTH, the mechanism of maintaining increased serum concentrations of calcium was unknown until the finding[61] that PTHrP influences calcium balance in the fetus and is the major hormone secreted by the chief cells of the fetal parathyroid glands. The PTHrP produced by the placenta also stimulates the uptake of calcium by the fetus.

Fetal Bone Development

Parathyroid hormone-related peptide plays a role in the differentiation of many tissues during gestation and is especially important in the growth and development of bone. Growth of cartilage at the epiphyseal plate is regulated by the actions or PTHrP which stimulates chondrocyte proliferation, inhibits apoptosis, and inhibits the maturation of chondrocytes from the proliferative zone to the hypertrophic zone,[266] responses which are dependent on the translocation of PTHrP to the nucleus and nucleolus.[130]

Role of Parathyroid Hormone-related Protein in Adult Animals

Skin

Epidermal keratinocytes produce PTHrP which plays a role in their proliferation or differentiation. However, keratinocytes do not contain the classic PTH/PTHrP receptor, which suggests that keratinocytes have an alternate PTHrP receptor.[207]

Mammary Gland

The greatest concentration of PTHrP is found in milk (10-100 nmol/L) and is 10,000 to 100,000-fold greater than in the serum.[224,230] The function of PTHrP in the mammary gland and in milk is poorly understood at present. However, over-expression of PTHrP in the mammary gland during glandular development prior to lactation results in glandular hypoplasia due to a reduction in the morphogenesis and branching of the mammary ducts.

Biologically active PTHrP produced by alveolar epithelial cells during lactation results in the high concentration of PTHrP in milk and this PTHrP may play a role in stimulating the transport of calcium by alveolar epithelial cells from serum to milk, although this has not been confirmed in all species.[14,213] Synthesis of PTHrP by the mammary gland abruptly ceases when suckling stops and the gland undergoes involution. The PTHrP peptide is enzymatically cleaved in milk, but the N-terminal PTHrP fragment retains biologic activity.

Although circulating concentrations of PTHrP may be minimally increased in lactating dams, no relationship has been demonstrated between PTHrP and the pathogenesis of parturient hypocalcemia and paresis in lactating dairy cattle.[229] Hence PTHrP from the mammary gland likely plays a minor role in the systemic calcium balance of lactating animals but may have physiological functions in suckling neonates, such as regulation of growth or differentiation of the gastrointestinal tract.

Smooth Muscle

Smooth muscle, including blood vessels, uterus, urinary bladder, gastrointestinal tract, and the oviduct of the hen produce PTHrP. In general, PTHrP expression is increased when smooth muscle is stretched and PTHrP induces relaxation of smooth muscle and attenuation of contraction. With progressive distension of the uterus during pregnancy or during descent of the ovum in the hen's oviduct, PTHrP likely functions as a paracrine regulator of vascular tone causing vasodilation and modulating vasoconstriction by other vasoactive compounds.

Assays for Parathyroid Hormone-related Protein

Two-site immunoradiometric and N-terminal radioimmunoassays are available for the measurement of human PTHrP. These assays can be used to measure PTHrP in the dog and cat due to the high degree of sequence homology in PTHrP between species. However, an N-terminal RIA for human PTHrP has not proven useful to measure circulating PTHrP in a small number of horses.[236] The PTHrP concentrations are best measured in fresh or frozen plasma using EDTA as an antico-agulant and with the addition of protease inhibitors, such as aprotinin and leupeptin.[211]

Canine Parathyroid Hormone-related Protein

Canine PTHrP cDNA has been cloned and sequenced.[237] The PTHrP gene is complex, with multiple promoters, up to nine exons, and alternate splicing of the exons which encode the C-terminal peptides. The canine PTHrP gene is more closely related to the human PTHrP gene; as compared to PTHrP genes in rats, mice, and chickens.

CALCITONIN

Although the appearance of calcitonin in primitive elasmobranch fish precedes the first appearance of PTH in amphibians, calcitonin (CT), also called thyrocalcitonin (TCT), was discovered after PTH. Early experiments to test the McLean-Urist hypothesis of a negative feedback control of blood calcium by parathyroid hormone involved the perfusion of the parathyroid-thyroid complex of dogs with alternating low and high concentrations of calcium. However, the results were difficult to explain based on the concept that a single hormone controlled the concentration of calcium in the blood. First, the fall in systemic calcium following perfusion of the thyroid-parathyroid complex was more rapid and of greater magnitude than would be expected due to the inhibition of PTH secretion. Second, thyroparathyroidectomy performed following the last low-calcium perfusion resulted in a continued progressive rise in blood calcium, rather than the expected fall in levels of blood calcium following the removal of the source of PTH (Fig. 4-27). These results and subsequent experiments led to the hypothesis that a second calcium-regulating hormone secreted by the parathyroid-thyroid complex in response to hypercalcemia was responsible for the reduction of the plasma concentration of calcium.

Conflicting views on the source and role of calcitonin in mammals were resolved by definitive studies in the goat whose parathyroid glands, unlike those of the dog, can be perfused independent of the thyroid gland. The presence of a calcium-lowering hormone within the mammalian thyroid gland was further confirmed by the demonstration that a thyroid extract would produce a similar fall in plasma calcium (Fig. 4-28). It is now well-established that calcitonin is of thyroidal origin in mammals and that calcitonin and thyrocalcitonin are one and the same hormone.

C (Parafollicular)-Cells in Thyroid or Ultimobranchial Glands

Calcitonin is secreted by a second population of endocrine cells in the mammalian thyroid gland called C-cells (see Chapter 3, Fig. 3-41). These cells are distinct from the follicular cells of the thyroid gland that are responsible for the secretion of thyroxine (T_4) and triiodothyronine (T_3). The C-cells of the mammalian thyroid gland are situated within the follicular wall immediately beneath the basement membrane or between follicular cells (Fig. 4-29). These C-cells do not border the follicular colloid directly and their secretory polarity is oriented toward the interfollicular capillaries (Fig. 4-29). The distinctive feature of the C-cell of the thyroid gland is the presence of numerous small membrane-limited secretory granules in the cytoplasm (Fig. 4-29).

Calcitonin-secreting cells are derived from cells of the neural crest. Primordial C-cells migrate ventrally from the neural crest and become incorporated within the last pharyngeal (branchial) pouch of the developing embryo. The C-cells displace caudally with the ultimobranchial body to the point of fusion with the midline primordia that gives rise to the thyroid gland (Fig. 4-30). The ultimobranchial body fuses with and is incorporated into the thyroid hilus in mammals, and the C-cells subsequently are distributed throughout the gland. Although C-cells are found throughout the thyroid gland in man and most other adult mammals, they often remain more numerous near the hilus and the point of fusion with the ultimobranchial body. In submammalian species, the C-cells and calcitonin activity remain segregated in the ultimobranchial glands (bodies) which are anatomically distinct from the thyroid and the parathyroid glands (Fig. 4-31). The avian ulti-

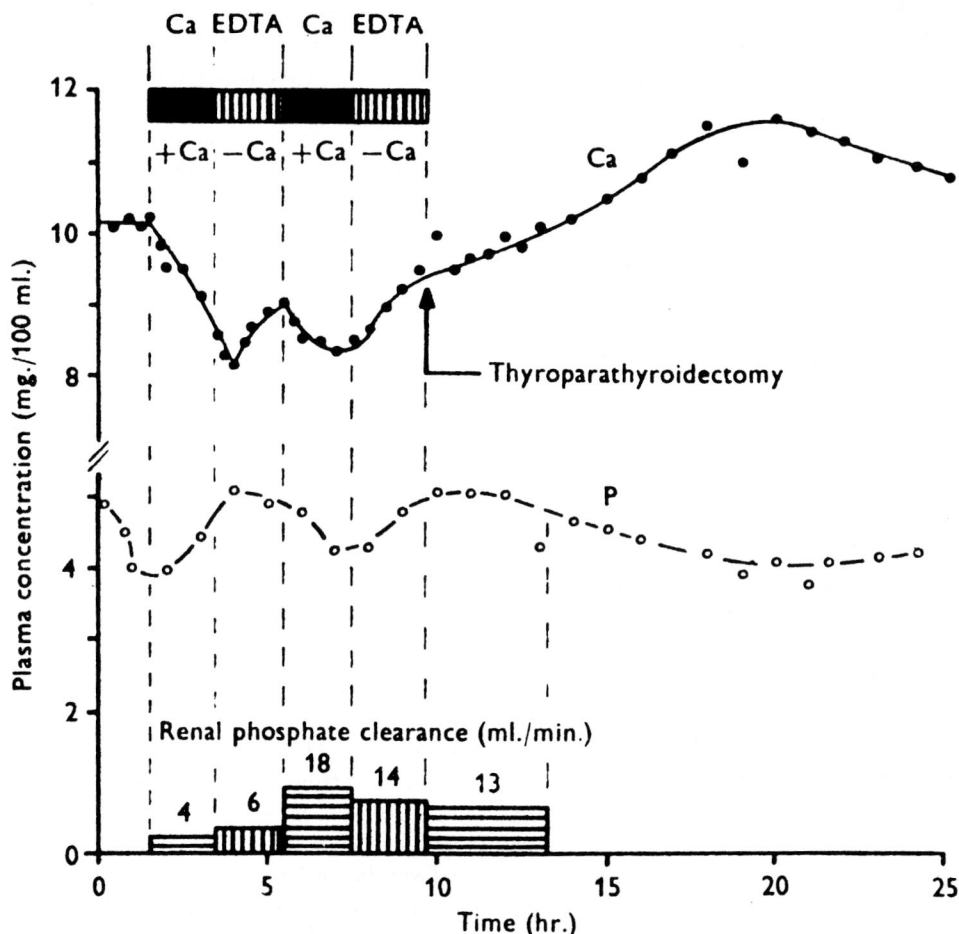

Fig. 4-27. Experiment of Copp and associates that led to the discovery of calcitonin. Perfusion of the thyroid-parathyroid complex in dogs with high calcium concentration in blood resulted in a more rapid and greater decline in peripheral calcium concentration than was expected only by the inhibition of PTH secretion. Thyroidectomy (**thyroparathyroidectomy**) following the last low calcium infusion resulted in a progressive hypercalcemia rather than the expected decline in blood calcium following removal of the source of PTH. (From: D. H. Copp, E. C. Cameron, B. A. Cheney, et al., Evidence for calcitonin—a new hormone from the parathyroid that lowers blood calcium. Endocrinology *70*:638, 1962).

mobranchial gland contains a network of stellate cells with long cytoplasmic processes which support the C-cells.[294]

Synthesis of Calcitonin

Calcitonin is a polypeptide hormone composed of 32 amino acid residues arranged in a straight chain with a 1–7 disulfide linkage.[69] The amino acid sequence of porcine, canine, bovine, equine, ovine, salmon, and human calcitonin, as well as for other animal species, has been determined. Calcitonin is synthesized as part of a larger biosynthetic precursor molecule[283] called pre-procalcitonin (Fig. 4-32). It is transported to the Golgi apparatus where it is converted to procalcitonin and then to calcitonin prior to packaging in membrane-limited secretory granules. Depending upon the need for calcitonin, a proportion of the precursors and active hormone undergo degradation prior to release from C-cells. Under certain pathologic conditions, C-cells derived from the neural crest may secrete other humoral factors including serotonin, bradykinin, ACTH, and prostaglandins (Fig. 4-32).

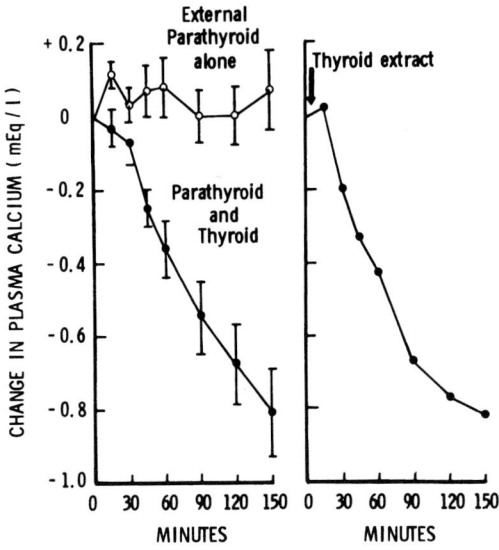

Fig. 4-28. Evidence to support the thyroidal rather than parathyroidal origin of calcitonin in mammals. Hypercalcemic perfusion of the external parathyroid gland of the goat has no effect on systemic levels of calcium in the plasma; however, when the thyroid gland was simultaneously perfused with a hypercalcemic solution there was a striking fall in the concentration of calcium in the plasma. Administration of thyroidal extracts to animals produced a similar hypocalcemic response. (From: G. V. Foster et al.,[102] 1972).

The calcitonin gene is expressed differently in thyroid (C-cells) than in neural tissues.[146, 255] In C-cells of the mammalian thyroid the mRNA encodes primarily for pre-procalcitonin with a molecular weight of 17,400 daltons, whereas in neural tissues there is alternative RNA processing and encoding for pre-procalcitonin gene-related peptide (CGRP). This CGRP is a neuropeptide composed of 37 amino acids with a molecular weight of 15,900 daltons and participates in nociception, ingestive behavior, and modulation of the nervous and endocrine systems.

The structure of calcitonin differs considerably between species. The molecular structure of calcitonin for five selected species (Fig. 4-33) share only 9 of the 32 amino acid residues. However, the amino terminal portion of the calcitonin molecule is similar in all species. It consists of a seven-member ring enclosed by an intrachain (1-7) disulfide bridge. The complete sequence of 32 amino acids and the disulfide bond are essential for full biologic activity. It is surprising that on a weight basis, salmon calcitonin is more potent in lowering blood calcium

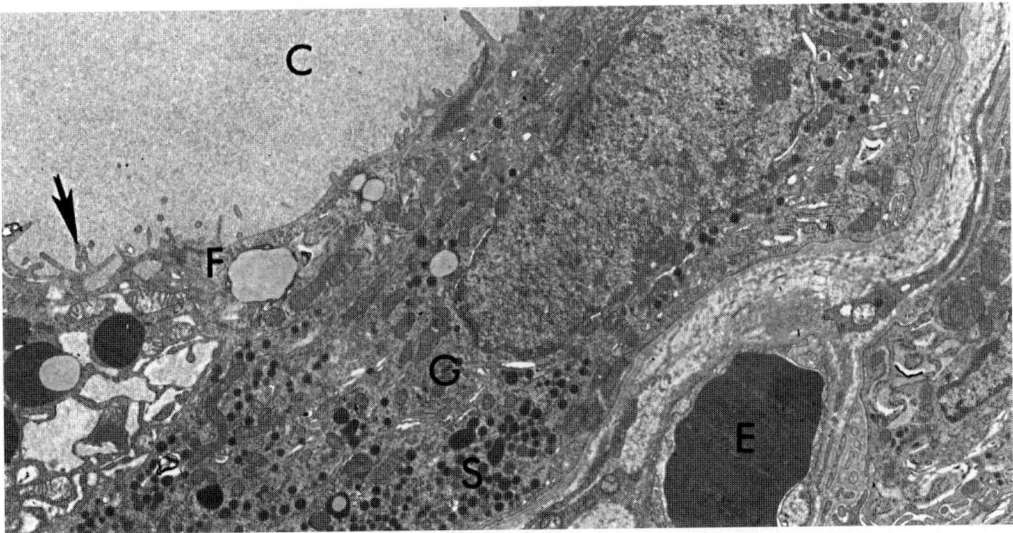

Fig. 4-29. Electron micrograph of a C-cell in the wall of a thyroid follicle. The calcitonin-secreting cell is wedged between several follicular cells (**F**) and the associated capillary. The C-cell has a prominent Golgi apparatus (**G**) and many calcitonin-filled granules (**S**) are evident in the cytoplasm. Follicular cells (**F**) line the follicle and extend microvilli (arrow) into the colloid (**C**). The secretory polarity of the C-cell is directed toward the interfollicular capillary (**E**) rather than toward the follicle lumen as for the follicular cells. Glutaraldehyde and osmium tetroxide fixation, uranyl acetate and lead hydroxide staining. Magnification 7,700 3.

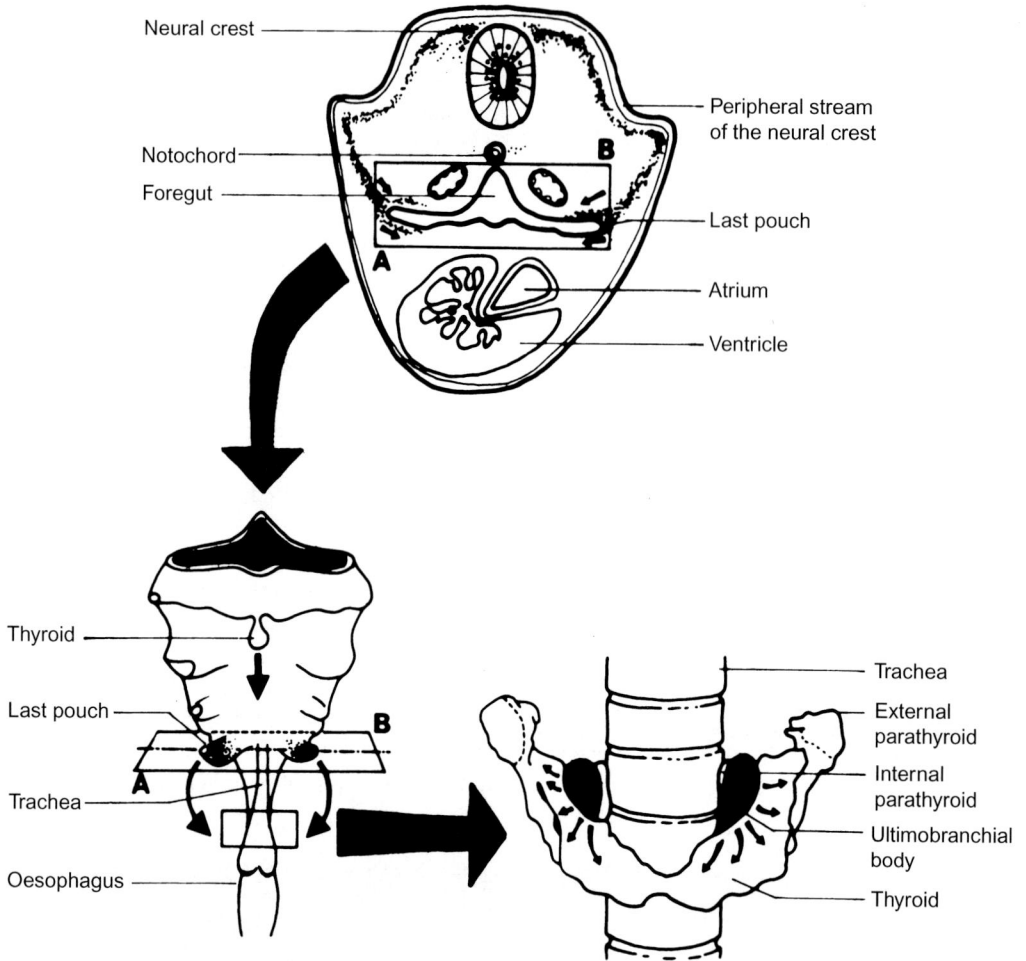

Fig. 4-30. Schematic representation of the neural crest origin of calcitonin-secreting C-cells. During embryological development, primordial cells from the neural crest migrate ventrally to become incorporated in the last pharyngeal pouch. The ultimobranchial body fuses with primordia of the mammalian thyroid gland and C-cells are distributed throughout the gland. (From: G. V. Foster et al.,[102] 1972).

than any of the other calcitonins when administered to mammals, including man. The reason for the greater biologic potency of salmon calcitonin in mammals is uncertain but probably is related to an increased resistance to metabolic degradation and longer half-life or to a greater affinity for receptor sites in bone and other target tissues.[123]

Regulation of Calcitonin Secretion

The concentration of ionized calcium in plasma and extracellular fluids is the principal physiologic stimulus for the secretion of calcitonin by C-cells. Calcitonin is secreted continuously under conditions of normocalcemia, but the rate of secretion of calcitonin increases greatly in response to an elevation in blood calcium. Magnesium ion has a similar effect on calcitonin secretion but this effect has been observed only under experimental conditions and for nonphysiologic levels of magnesium.

Under normal conditions, C-cells store substantial amounts of calcitonin in their cytoplasm in the form of membrane-limited secretory granules (Fig. 4-29). The C-cell response to hypercalcemia is rapid and stored hormone is discharged into interfollicular capillaries (Fig. 4-13). If the hypercalcemic stimulus is sustained,

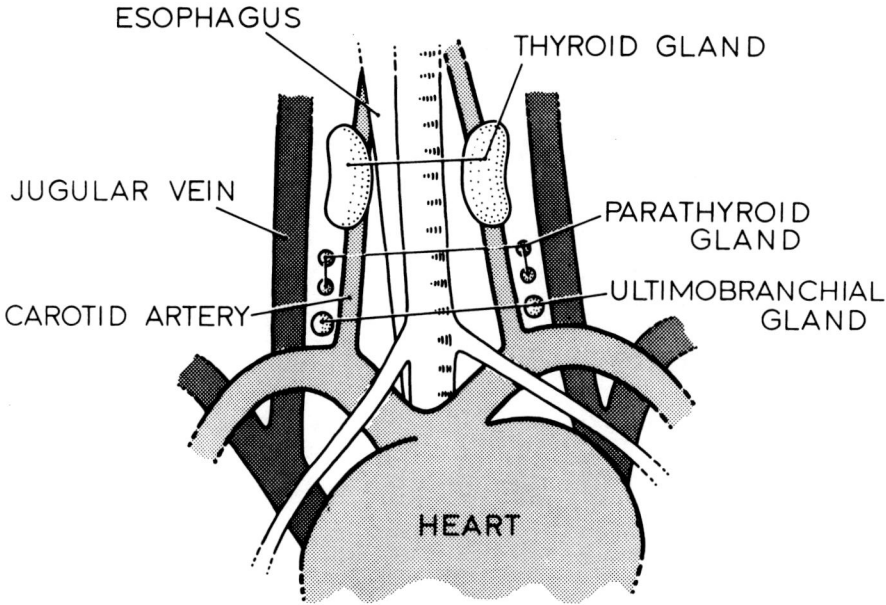

Fig. 4-31. Calcitonin-secreting C-cells in submammalian vertebrates remain in an anatomically distinct endocrine organ. In the chicken, the ultimobranchial gland is situated along the carotid artery and caudal to the 2 pairs of parathyroid glands and to the thyroid gland.

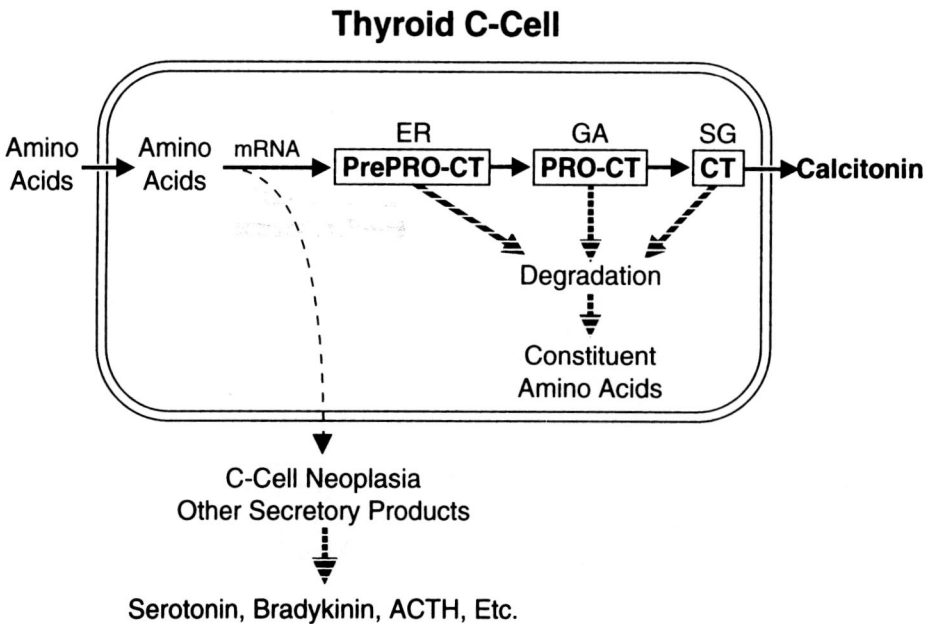

Fig. 4-32. Biosynthesis of calcitonin in C-cells of the thyroid gland. Preprocalcitonin (**PrePRO-CT**) and procalcitonin (**PRO-CT**) are biosynthetic precursors that undergo post-translational processing to form biologically active calcitonin (**CT**). Some of these precursor molecules and biologically active calcitonin may undergo enzymatic degradation to the constituent amino acids (**AA**) prior to secretion from the C-cell. Under certain disease conditions, C-cells may secrete other neuroendocrine products, including serotonin, bradykinin, and ACTH (**ER** = endoplasmic reticulum; **GA** = Golgi apparatus; **mRNA** = messenger ribonucleic acid; **SG** = secretory granule).

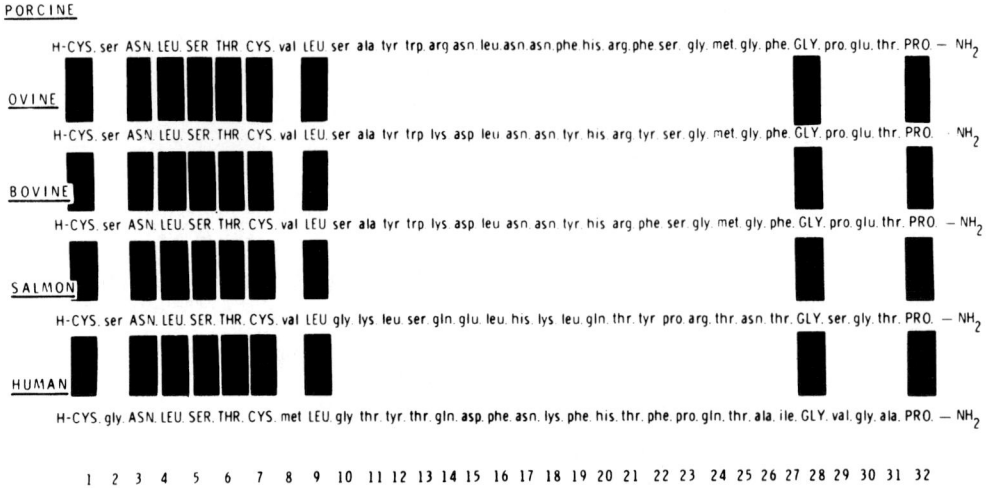

PORCINE

H-CYS. ser. ASN. LEU. SER. THR. CYS. val. LEU. ser. ala. tyr. trp. arg. asn. leu. asn. asn. phe. his. arg. phe. ser. gly. met. gly. phe. GLY. pro. glu. thr. PRO. — NH₂

OVINE

H-CYS. ser. ASN. LEU. SER. THR. CYS. val. LEU. ser. ala. tyr. trp. lys. asp. leu. asn. asn. tyr. his. arg. tyr. ser. gly. met. gly. phe. GLY. pro. glu. thr. PRO. — NH₂

BOVINE

H-CYS. ser. ASN. LEU. SER. THR. CYS. val. LEU. ser. ala. tyr. trp. lys. asp. leu. asn. asn. tyr. his. arg. phe. ser. gly. met. gly. phe. GLY. pro. glu. thr. PRO. — NH₂

SALMON

H-CYS. ser. ASN. LEU. SER. THR. CYS. val. LEU. gly. lys. leu. ser. gln. glu. leu. his. lys. leu. gln. thr. tyr. pro. arg. thr. asn. thr. GLY. ser. gly. thr. PRO. — NH₂

HUMAN

H-CYS. gly. ASN. LEU. SER. THR. CYS. met. LEU. gly. thr. tyr. thr. gln. asp. phe. asn. lys. phe. his. thr. phe. pro. gln. thr. ala. ile. GLY. val. gly. ala. PRO. — NH₂

1 2 3 4 5 6 7 8 9 10 11 12 13 14 15 16 17 18 19 20 21 22 23 24 25 26 27 28 29 30 31 32

Fig. 4-33. Sequence of the 32 amino acids of calcitonin molecules from 5 species. The 9 amino acid residues shared by the calcitonin molecules from the 5 species are indicated by heavy vertical bars. (From: G. V. Foster et al.,[102] 1972).

this is followed by the increased development of cytoplasmic organelles concerned with the synthesis and secretion of calcitonin (Fig. 4-13). The endoplasmic reticulum with attached ribosomes is hypertrophied and the Golgi apparatus is enlarged and associated with prosecretory granules in the process of synthesis of calcitonin. Hyperplasia of C-cells occurs in response to long-term hypercalcemia. When the blood calcium is lowered, the stimulus for calcitonin secretion is diminished and numerous secretory granules accumulate in the cytoplasm of C-cells (Fig. 4-13). The storage of large amounts of preformed hormone in C-cells and the rapid release of calcitonin in response to moderate elevations in blood calcium probably are a reflection of the physiologic role of calcitonin as an emergency hormone to protect against the development of hypercalcemia. Gastrointestinal hormones may also be important in triggering the early release of calcitonin to prevent the development of hypercalcemia following the ingestion of a high calcium meal (Fig. 4-34).

Biologic Effects of Calcitonin

The administration of calcitonin or stimulation of endogenous secretion results in the development of varying degrees of hypocalcemia and hypophosphatemia in animals. The effects of

calcitonin on plasma calcium and phosphorus are most evident in young or older animals with increased rates of skeletal turnover. Calcitonin exerts its function by interacting with target cells located in bone and kidney, and to a lesser extent in intestinal cells. The actions of PTH and CT on bone resorption are antagonistic (Fig. 4-21) but they synergize to decrease the renal tubular reabsorption of phosphorus (Fig. 4-23). The hypocalcemic effects of calcitonin are primarily the result of the decreased entry of calcium from the skeleton into plasma due to a temporary inhibi-

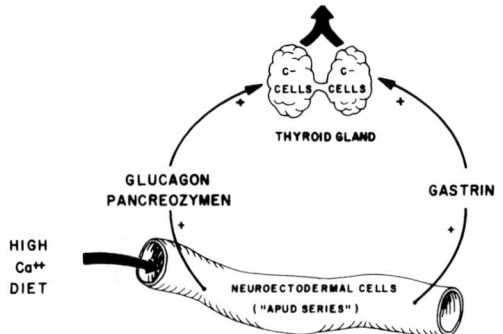

Fig. 4-34. The gastrointestinal hormone-thyroid C-cell axis provides a mechanism for rapid release of calcitonin from the **C-cells** of the thyroid in response to a high calcium diet and before there is a significant elevation in the blood level of calcium (**APUD** = Amine Precursor Uptake Decarboxylase).

tion of PTH-stimulated resorption of bone.[106] Hypophosphatemia develops from a direct action of calcitonin on increasing the rate of movement of phosphate out of plasma into soft tissue and bone, as well as from the inhibition of bone resorption by blockage of osteoclastic osteolysis (Fig. 4-21). Osteoclasts have receptors for calcitonin, however the action of calcitonin is not dependent on vitamin D. Calcitonin acts in vitamin D-deficient animals and after the administration of large doses of vitamin D.

The effects of calcitonin on bone formation are less dramatic. Initially there appears to be an increase in the rate of bone formation, but the long-term administration of calcitonin appears to lead to reductions in bone resorption and formation. Calcitonin-secreting C-cell neoplasms in bulls and humans are associated with low rates of skeletal turnover and densely mineralized bone. Unfortunately, calcitonin has not proven to be an effective therapeutic agent to induce a long-term increase in bone formation in human patients with post-menopausal osteoporosis.

Physiologic Significance of Calcitonin

Calcitonin and parathyroid hormone act in concert to provide a negative feedback mechanism to maintain the concentration of calcium in extracellular fluids within narrow limits. Under normal conditions, parathyroid hormone is the major factor concerned with the minute-to-minute regulation of blood levels of calcium and protect against the development of hypocalcemia. Calcitonin functions more as an emergency hormone to:

1. prevent the development of "physiologic" hypercalcemia during the rapid, postprandial absorption of calcium (Fig. 4-35) and

2. protect against excessive losses of calcium and phosphorus from the maternal skeleton during pregnancy.[12]

In hibernating vertebrates, the alternating secretion of CT and PTH permits the cyclic withdrawal of calcium from the skeleton to maintain plasma calcium homeostasis during hibernation and ensure adequate bone structure after arousal.

Assays for Calcitonin

Serum levels of calcitonin are best measured by radioimmunoassay. However, the low degree of homology of calcitonin between species and the low degree of cross-reactivity of antibodies to calcitonin among species have precluded the development of radioimmunoassays for each species. Additionally, there is relatively little clinical need to measure calcitonin in clinical veterinary medicine due to the low incidence of calcitonin-secreting neoplasms and metabolic disorders resulting from abnormal levels of calcitonin.

CHOLECALCIFEROL (VITAMIN D₃)

The third major hormonal factor involved in the regulation of calcium metabolism and skeletal remodeling are the various metabolites of vitamin D (calciferol). The vitamin D family includes vitamin D_3 or cholecalciferol, vitamin D_2, also referred to as ergocalciferol or irradiated ergosterol, and 1,25 dihydroxycholecalciferol (calcitriol; 1,25 dihydroxyvitamin D). Due to their biological actions, these compounds, which have long been considered to be vitamins, can equally be considered hormones (Table 4-1). Cholecalciferol is ingested in small

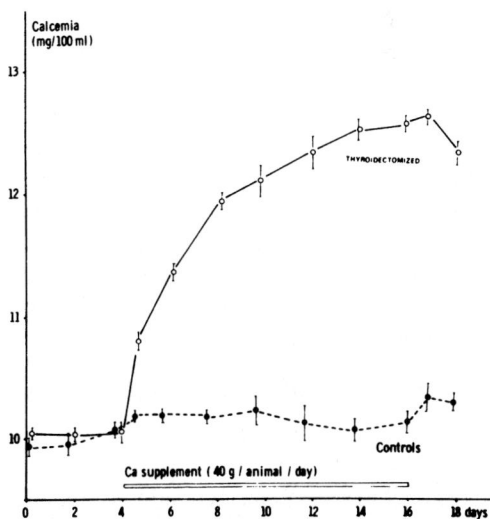

Fig. 4-35. Responses of cows without an endogenous source of calcitonin (thyroidectomized) and control cows with intact thyroid glands to an oral calcium load. (From: J. P. Barlet,[12] 1972).

Table 4-1   Evidence That Vitamin D Acts as a Hormone

1. Chemical structure resembles that of steroid hormones.

2. Very small quantities (ng) of active form required for full biologic activity.

3. Synthesized by one organ (skin) from precursor molecules (provitamins) by photoactivation; lesser amounts from dietary sources.

4. Transported by blood in bound form to target cells located primarily in intestine and bone.

5. Enhances rate of reactions in target cells to elicit a physiologic response.

6. Mechanism of action:
   —similar to steroid hormones, enters cell and binds to cytosolic receptor
   —hormone-receptor (HR) complex is transported to nucleus
   —HR complex binds to specific nuclear receptors
   —facilitates transcription of mRNA from DNA
   —increases protein synthesis in target cells, e.g., Calcium Binding Protein (CaBP).

7. Toxic in large amounts.

amounts in the diet and can be synthesized in the epidermis from precursor molecules (Fig. 4-36). This reaction is catalyzed by ultraviolet irradiation from the sun. A high-affinity vitamin D-binding protein in the serum transports cholecalciferol from its site of synthesis in the skin to the liver. In response to prolonged exposure to sunlight, previtamin D_3 is converted to lumisterol and tachysterol (Fig. 4-37). Because the vitamin D-binding protein has no affinity for lumisterol and minimal affinity for tachysterol, the translocation of these photoisomers into the circulation is negligible and they are sloughed with the natural turnover of the skin.

Cholecalciferol is absorbed from dietary sources by facilitated diffusion or synthesized from 7-dehydrocholesterol in the skin by a photochemical reaction caused by ultraviolet irradiation (Fig. 4-38). The cholecalciferol obtained from dietary resources or produced endogenously binds to an $alpha_2$-globulin in the blood for transport to the liver.

Metabolic Activation of Vitamin D_3

Vitamin D_3 must be metabolically activated into a physiologically active compound. The first step in the metabolic activation of vitamin D is the conversion of cholecalciferol to 25-hydroxycholecalciferol (25-OH-CC) in the liver[126] under the enzymatic control of a hepatic microsomal enzyme referred to as calciferol-25-

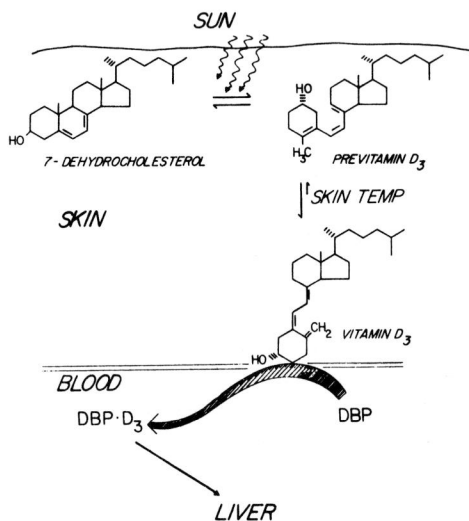

Fig. 4-36. Photochemical conversion of **7-dehydro-cholesterol** to **previtamin D_3** in the epidermis following exposure to ultraviolet radiation from sunlight. Previtamin D_3 subsequently undergoes thermal conversion to **vitamin D_3** (cholecalciferol), which enters dermal capillaries and binds to a specific binding protein (**DBP**) for vitamin D_3. Protein-bound vitamin D_3 is transported to the liver for the initial step of metabolic activation. (From: M. F. Holick,[135] 1981).

hydroxylase. Although 25-OH-CC may exert biologic effects when substantial amounts are present, it primarily serves as a precursor for the formation of the more active metabolites of vitamin D. High circulating levels of 25-OH-CC serve as a reservoir of vitamin D for the synthe-

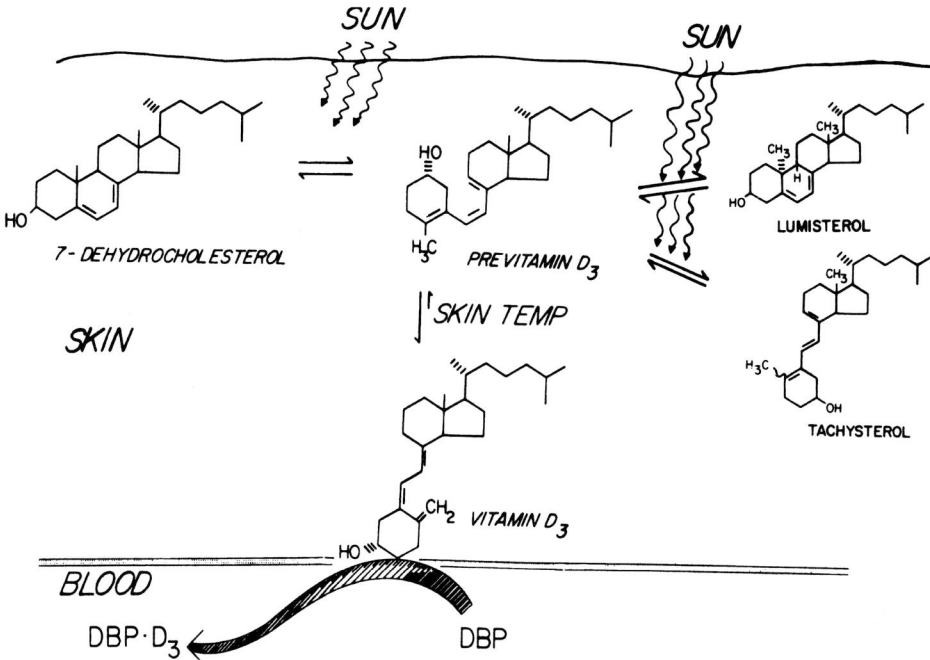

Fig. 4-37. Prolonged exposure to sunlight results in the photochemical conversion of excess **previtamin D$_3$** to **lumisterol** and **tachysterol**. These photoisomers remain in the epidermis and are lost with the natural turnover of the skin. The binding protein for vitamin D$_3$ has a low affinity for these isomers. (From: M. F. Holick,[135] 1981).

sis of the active forms of vitamin D by the kidney.

The 25-hydroxycholecalciferol synthesized in the liver is metabolized in the kidney (Figs. 4-16, 4-38, and 4-39) to 1,25-dihydroxy-cholecalciferol or 1,25-(OH)$_2$-CC. The rate of formation of 1,25-(OH)$_2$-CC in mitochondria of renal epithelial cells of the proximal convoluted tubules is catalyzed by 25-hydroxy-cholecalciferol-1α-hydroxylase. The conversion of 25-OH-CC to 1,25-(OH)$_2$-CC is the rate-limiting step in vitamin D metabolism and is the primary reason for the time elapsed between the administration of vitamin D and the expression of biologic effects.

The control of this final step in the metabolic activation of vitamin D is complex and appears to be regulated by the concentration of calcium in the plasma, which influences the rate of secretion of PTH and possibly calcitonin (Fig. 4-40). Parathyroid hormone increases the conversion of 25-OH-CC to 1,25-(OH)$_2$-CC (see Fig. 4-16), whereas calcitonin is inhibitory under certain conditions. A low concentration of phosphorus in the blood increases the rate of formation of 1,25-(OH)$_2$-CC (Fig. 4-40), whereas a high phosphorus concentration suppresses the formation of active hormone. Dihydroxyvitamin D$_3$ (1,25-(OH)$_2$-CC) is the major biologically active metabolite of cholecalciferol that interacts with target cells in the intestine and bone to enhance the rates of existing reactions and increase calcium mobilization under physiologic conditions (Fig. 4-21).[87] Hence, the onset of action is more rapid and the degree of potency is much greater than with either cholecalciferol or 25-OH-CC. A similar two-step process of metabolic activation also occurs with the irradiation of ergosterol to form vitamin D$_2$.

Hormones, such as prolactin, estradiol, placental lactogen, and possibly growth hormone enhance the activity of renal 1α-hydroxylase and the formation of 1,25-(OH)$_2$-CC. Participation of these hormones appears to be adaptive to meet the major calcium demands of the body and for the survival of the animal.

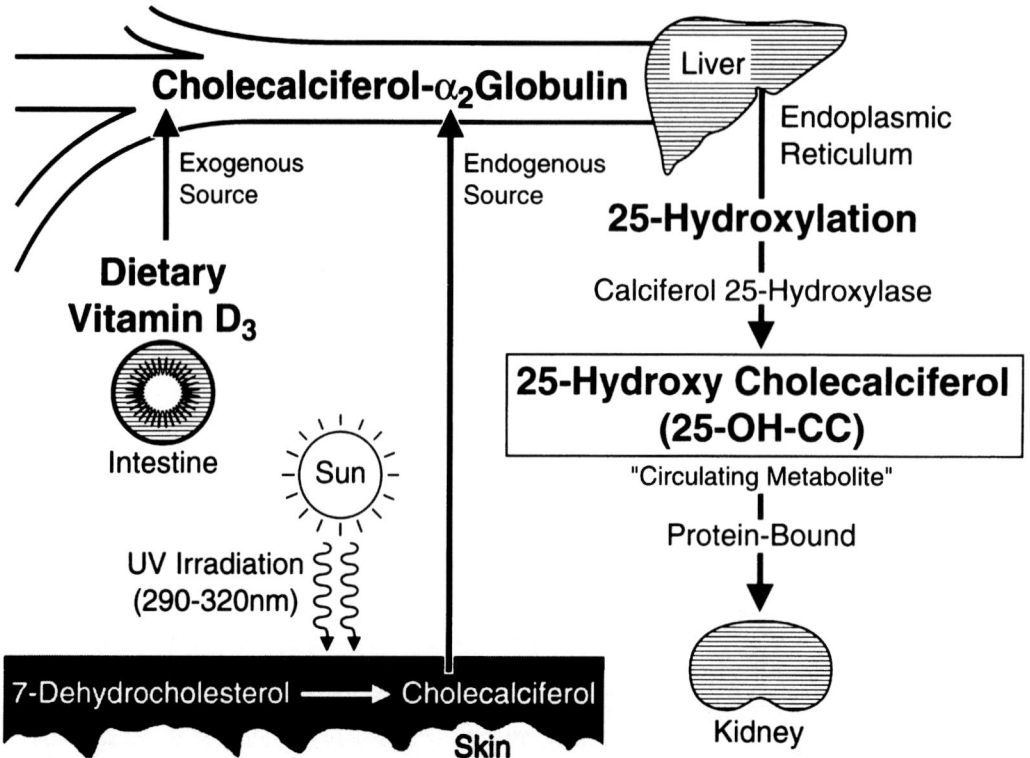

Fig. 4-38. Metabolism of vitamin D. The initial step in the metabolic activation of **vitamin D$_3$** from endogenous and dietary sources to form 25-hydroxycholecalciferol (**25-OH-CC**) occurs in the liver (**UV** = ultraviolet).

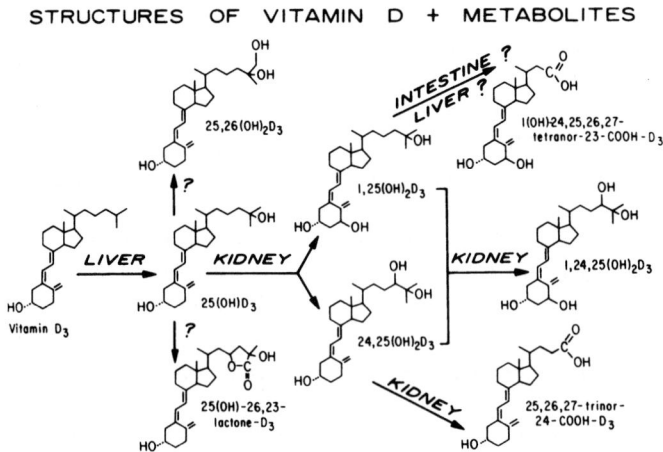

STRUCTURES OF VITAMIN D + METABOLITES

Fig. 4-39. The metabolic activation of cholecalciferol (**vitamin D$_3$**) begins in the liver with the formation of 25-hydroxycholecalciferol (**25(OH)D$_3$**) and is completed in the kidney. The (25(OH)D$_3$ molecule is converted to 1,25-dihydroxycholecalciferol (the principal biologically active metabolite) and several other less active metabolites by the epithelial cells lining the convoluted tubules of the kidney. (From: A. W. Norman and H. L. Henry,[203] 1979).

Multifactorial Control of Renal 1α-Hydroxylase

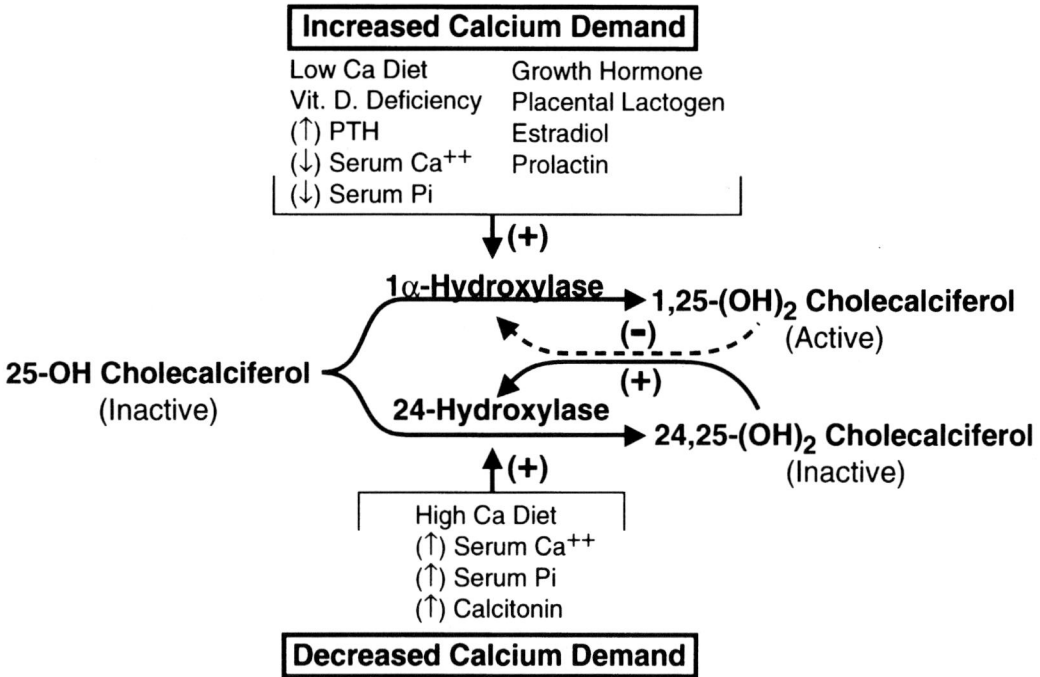

Increased Calcium Demand

Low Ca Diet   Growth Hormone
Vit. D. Deficiency   Placental Lactogen
($\uparrow$) PTH   Estradiol
($\downarrow$) Serum Ca^{++} Prolactin
($\downarrow$) Serum Pi

$\downarrow$**(+)**

1α-Hydroxylase → **1,25-(OH)$_2$ Cholecalciferol**
(−) (Active)

25-OH Cholecalciferol
(Inactive)

(+)

24-Hydroxylase

24,25-(OH)$_2$ Cholecalciferol
(Inactive)

$\uparrow$**(+)**

High Ca Diet
($\uparrow$) Serum Ca^{++}
($\uparrow$) Serum Pi
($\uparrow$) Calcitonin

Decreased Calcium Demand

Fig. 4-40. Multifactorial control of the final step of metabolic activation of vitamin D in the kidney. Conditions associated with increased calcium demand result in the stimulation of the production of **1,25-(OH)$_2$ cholecalciferol** from **25-OH cholecalciferol** by increasing the activity of **1α-hydroxylase** in the mitochondria of renal cells. Under conditions of decreased calcium demand the production of 1,25-(OH)$_2$ cholecalciferol is diminished and **24,25-(OH)$_2$ cholecalciferol** (an inactive metabolite) is formed by the enzymatic action of a **24-hydroxylase**.

Chemistry of Vitamin D and Metabolites

The chemical structure of vitamin D$_3$ resembles that of other steroid hormones (see Chapter 6; Fig. 6-3). During metabolic activation of cholecalciferol, hydroxyl groups are successively attached at positions 1 and 25 of the steroid nucleus by specific hydroxylases in the liver and kidney to form the hormonal or biologically active forms of vitamin D (Figs. 4-39 and 4-40).

There are a number of sterols closely related to cholecalciferol such as vitamin D$_2$ which is formed by the irradiation of the plant sterol referred to as ergosterol to form irradiated ergosterol. When irradiated ergosterol is ingested by the animal and absorbed from the intestine, it undergoes a series of steps of metabolic activation similar to those described for cholecalciferol (vitamin D$_3$). The more active metabolites of ergosterol are 25-hydroxyergosterol and 1,25-dihydroxyergosterol, synthesized by the liver and kidney, respectively.

Biologic Effects and Mechanism of Action of Vitamin D Metabolites

Vitamin D and its active metabolites function to increase the absorption of calcium and phosphorus from the intestine, thereby maintaining adequate levels of these electrolytes in the extracellular fluids in order to permit the appropriate mineralization of bone matrix (Fig. 4-19). From a functional point of view, vitamin D can be thought to act in such a way as to cause the retention of sufficient mineral ions to ensure that the mineralization of bone matrix is adequate, whereas PTH with the "permissive effect" of vitamin D maintains the proper ratio of calcium to phosphate in the extracellular fluids.

The major target for 1,25-dihydroxycholecalciferol is the absorptive cells of the mucosa of the small intestine (Fig. 4-41). In the proximal part of the small intestine 1,25-$(OH)_2$-CC increases the active transcellular transport of calcium and in the distal intestine, the transport of phosphorus. Following synthesis in the kidney, 1,25-$(OH)_2$-CC is bound to a protein and transported to specific target cells in the intestine (Fig. 4-41) and bone (Fig. 4-21). Circulating levels of the protein-bound 1,25-$(OH)_2$-CC are extremely low. Free 1,25-$(OH)_2$-CC penetrates the plasma membrane of target cells and initially binds to a cytoplasmic receptor in cells of the intestine (Fig. 4-41). Subsequently, the hormone-receptor

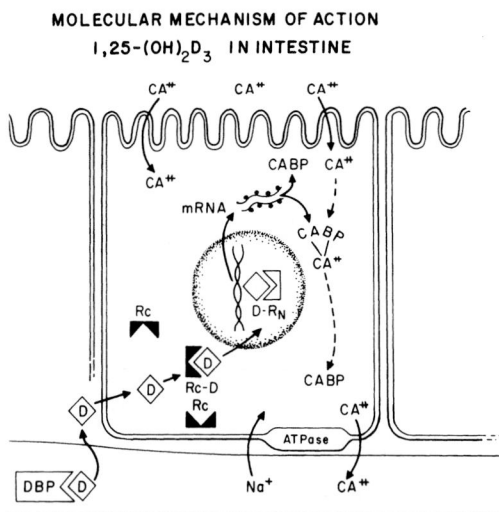

MOLECULAR MECHANISM OF ACTION
1,25-$(OH)_2D_3$ IN INTESTINE

Fig. 4-41. Molecular mechanisms for the action of 1,-25-dihydroxycholecalciferol (**1,25-$(OH_2)D_3$** in the intestine. The active hormone (**D**) is transported from the kidney to the intestine by a vitamin D-binding protein (**DBP**). The hydrophilic steroid penetrates the plasma membrane, binds to a cytoplasmic receptor in the target cell and is transported to the nucleus where it interacts with the nuclear chromatin to increase the formation of **mRNA**. The mRNA, associated with ribosomes on the endoplasmic reticulum, directs the synthesis of new proteins such as calcium-binding protein (**CABP**). The CABP is involved in the transcellular transport of calcium from the intestinal lumen to the basilar aspects of the intestinal absorptive cell where calcium enters the extracellular fluid compartment in exchange for sodium (R_c = cytoplasmic receptor; R_N = nuclear receptor).

complex is transferred to the nucleus and 1,25-$(OH)_2$-CC binds to specific receptors in the nuclear chromatin and stimulates gene expression leading to the increased synthesis of vitamin D-dependent proteins such as the calcium-binding protein (CaBP) produced by intestinal cells.

The luminal surface (brush border) of the intestinal absorptive cell is highly specialized and has numerous microvilli which further increase the surface area of the intestine (Figs. 4-42, 4-43, and 4-44).

In response to 1,25-dihydroxycholecalciferol, the absorptive cells of the intestine synthesize and secrete a specific calcium-binding protein. This protein (CaBP) has been isolated from several tissues including the small intestine, kidney, parathyroid gland, bone, mammary gland, and the shell gland of laying hens. A vitamin D-dependent calcium-binding protein also has been demonstrated in bone, particularly in the spongiosa and cartilaginous growth plate.[71]

The absorptive capacity of the intestine for calcium is a direct function of the amount of calcium-binding protein that is present. The administration of vitamin D or feeding low calcium and low phosphorus diets to animals has been shown to stimulate the synthesis of calcium-binding protein, which contributes to the increased absorption of calcium by intestine. The physiologic functions of this binding protein are related to the transcellular transport of calcium from the luminal to basilar border of intestinal absorptive cells and in the regulation intracellular calcium concentration. Calcium is exchanged for sodium at the basilar aspect of intestinal absorptive cells, and enters the extracellular fluid. Vitamin D may also exert an effect on the mitochondrial membrane and increase the accumulation of calcium granules within the mitochondria of intestinal cells.

The active metabolites of cholecalciferol also act on bone. In young animals, vitamin D is required for the orderly growth of bone and mineralization of cartilage in the growth plate (Fig. 4-45). Young animals fed diets deficient in vitamin D and housed indoors without exposure to ultraviolet irradiation develop rickets. Mineralization of the cartilaginous matrix fails to occur in affected animals and the formation of woven

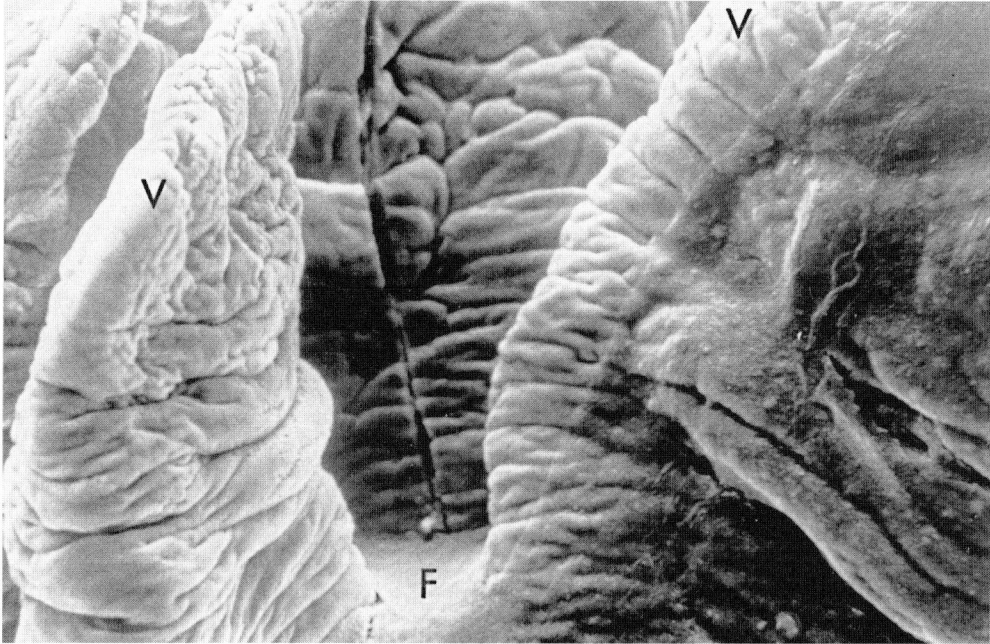

Fig. 4-42. Scanning electron micrograph illustrating the structure of the small intestine where absorption of dietary calcium occurs. Villi (**V**) project from the floor (**F**) of the intestine into the lumen and greatly increase the surface area. The surface of the intestinal villi appear relatively smooth at low magnification (300 ×).

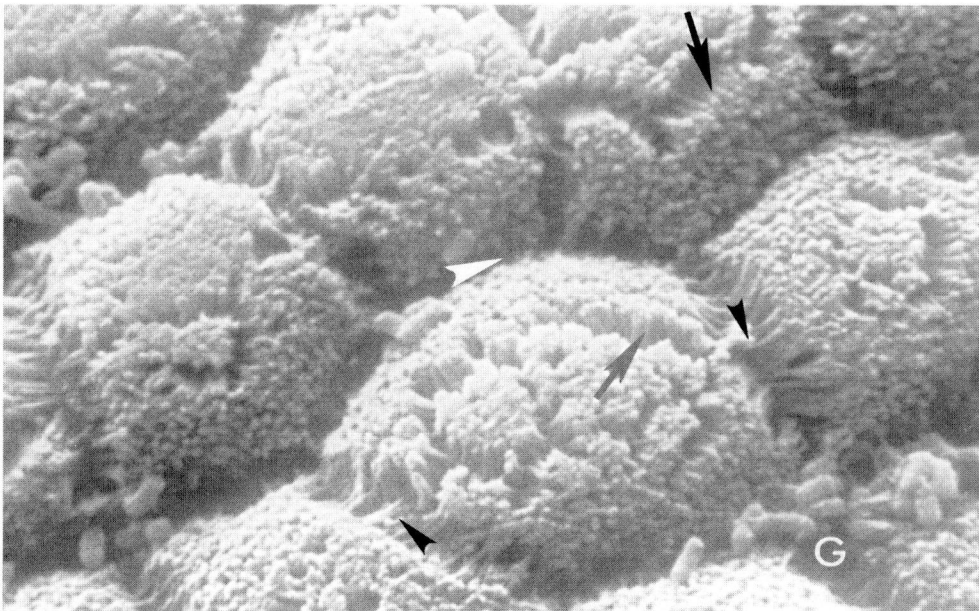

Fig. 4-43. Surface architecture of the intestinal villi illustrated in Figure 4-42 at higher magnification (3,000 x). Junctions can be visualized between absorptive cells (**arrow heads ➤**) and orifices of goblet cells (**G**). The area of the luminal surface of the intestinal cells is greatly increased by the presence of numerous microvilli (**arrows ➞**) which greatly increase the absorptive capacity of the cell.

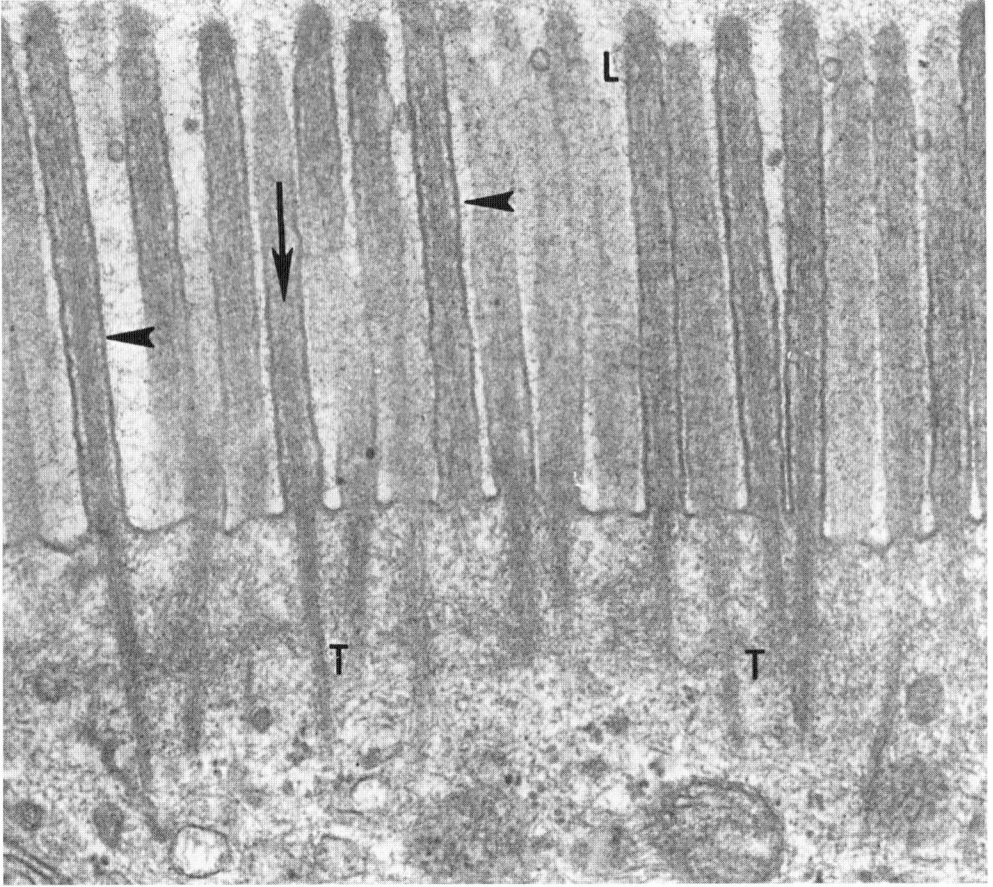

Fig. 4-44. Microvilli extending into the intestinal lumen (**L**). The trilaminar membrane of microvilli (**arrow heads ➤**) contain the vitamin D-dependent enzymes thought to be concerned with the translocation of calcium into the intestinal cell. Fine filaments in the cores of microvilli (**arrow ➝**) extend into the terminal web (**T**) of the absorptive cells. Magnification 21,750 ×.

bone on spicules of cartilage and subsequent remodeling to lamellar bone are blocked in this disease. The epiphyseal plate is irregularly thickened as progressively more primordial cartilaginous matrix accumulates and fails to mineralize. The administration of either cholecalciferol, 25-OH-CC or 1,25-(OH)$_2$-CC to animals leads to the reestablishment of a normal calcification front in the osteoid on bone surfaces and at the growth plate. Phosphorus deficiency will also result in rickets because of the failure to maintain an adequate ion product of serum calcium and phosphorous at the zones of mineralization in bone. However, phosphorus deficiency does not result in hypocalcemia and serum levels of 1,25-dihydroxyvitamin D are normal or increased. Rickets

seldom occurs in suckling animals unless the dam provides too little milk.

In addition to an effect on mineralization of bone matrix, vitamin D is necessary for osteoclastic resorption and calcium mobilization from bone. Small amounts of vitamin D or its active metabolite are necessary to permit osteolytic cells to respond to PTH ('permissive effect') under physiologic conditions. Cholecalciferol, 25-OH-CC, and 1,25-(OH)$_2$-CC in pharmacologic doses will stimulate osteoclastic proliferation and the resorption of bone *in vitro* and *in vivo*. Compared to 25-OH-CC, 1,25-dihydroxycholecalciferol is about 100 times more potent on a weight basis in stimulating the resorption of bone *in vitro*.

METAPHYSEAL GROWTH PLATE

EPIPHYSEAL VESSELS

EPIPHYSEAL BONE PLATE

PERICHONDRIAL RING

	germinal	
	proliferating	Zone of Growth
	palisading	
	hypertrophy	Zone of Cartilage Transformation
	calcification	
	degeneration	
	vascular entry	Zone of Ossification
	osteogenesis	
	remodelling	Metaphysis

metaphyseal vessels

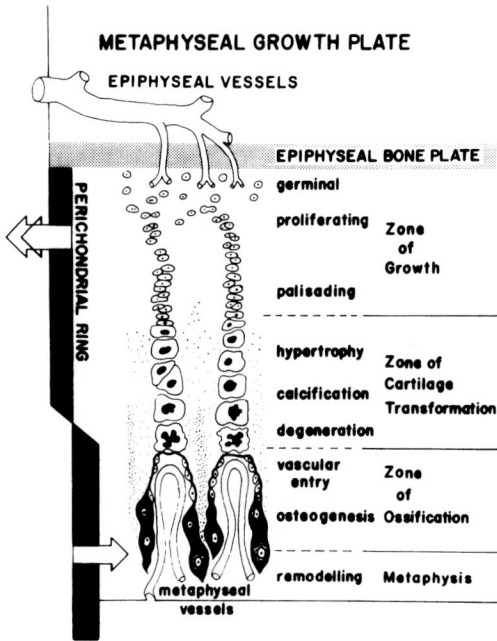

Fig. 4-45. Diagrammatic representation of the metaphyseal growth plate from a long bone. Vitamin D provides adequate concentrations of calcium and phosphorus in extracellular fluids to permit the mineralization of cartilaginous matrix that results in an orderly degeneration of chondrocytes and the eventual ingrowth of osteoblasts into the scaffold provided by the degenerating cartilage cells with formation of osteoid.

Deficiency of vitamin D also results from inadequate levels of renal 1α-hydroxylase, the enzyme that is essential for metabolic activation of precursor molecules (Fig. 4-39). Vitamin D-dependent rickets in both pigs and humans is a familiar disease inherited by an autosomal recessive gene. Newborn pigs appear healthy and have normal concentrations of calcium and phosphorus in the blood. Then, at 4 to 6 weeks of age, blood levels of calcium and phosphorus decrease while alkaline phosphatase activity increases (Fig. 4-46). Clinically detectable rickets develops during the following 3 to 4 weeks and affected pigs develop deformities of bone in the axial and abaxial skeleton and evidence severe pain, classical signs of rickets.

In response to the hypocalcemia caused by a deficiency in vitamin D, plasma levels of immunoreactive parathyroid hormone are elevated in pigs with vitamin D-dependent rickets (Fig. 4-47). Serum levels of 25-hydroxycholecalciferol (25-OH-CC) levels are strikingly elevated in pigs with clinical rickets, whereas the serum level of $1,25\text{-(OH)}_2\text{-CC}$ is markedly depressed.

Recent evidence suggests that the active metabolites of vitamin D also have a direct effect on the parathyroid gland, in addition to their well-characterized actions on intestine and bone. The parathyroid glands selectively localize $1,25\text{-(OH)}_2\text{-CC}$ and contain specific cytoplasmic and nuclear receptors for the active metabolites of vitamin D. Either alone or in combination, vitamin D metabolites directly interact with parathyroid cells to diminish the secretion of PTH, which in turn diminishes the formation of $1,25\text{-(OH)}_2\text{-CC}$ (Figs. 4-16 and 4-40). The active metabolites of vitamin D, in particular 1,25-dihydroxycholecalciferol, have many roles in health and disease beyond the regulation of calcium metabolism.[267] Vitamin D functions to regulate cell growth and differentiation and the vitamin D receptor is widespread in tissues, including: hematopoietic, muscle, skin, and lung cells, cells of endocrine glands, the gastrointestinal and urinary tracts, and the reproductive and nervous systems.

Assays for Metabolites of Vitamin D

Radioimmunoassays based on [125]iodine (^{125}I) are used to detect blood levels of 25-hydroxyvitamin D and 1,25-dihydroxyvitamin D.[144] Because the structure of the common vitamin D metabolites do not vary between species, the assays can be used to measure serum metabolites among species.[195] Measurement of serum levels of 25-hydroxyvitamin D is useful to evaluate the potential for a dietary deficiency of vitamin D or the excess intake of vitamin D.

Vitamin D Intoxication

The ingestion of small amounts of dried leaves from a plant (*Solanum malacoxylon*) indigenous to Argentina, Brazil, Chile, and probably other South American countries greatly increases the rate of intestinal calcium and phosphorus absorption and produces hyper-

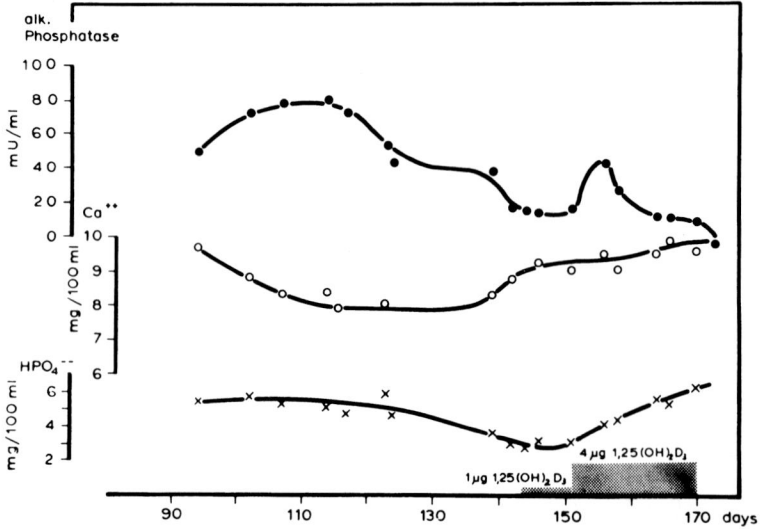

Fig. 4-46. Relationship between the serum levels of calcium (**Ca++**), phosphorus (**HPO$_4$$^{2-}$**), and alkaline (alk.) phosphatase in pigs with vitamin D-dependent rickets and following administration of 1 and 4 g 1,25-dihydroxy-cholecalciferol [**1,25(OH$_2$)D$_3$**]. (Courtesy of Dr. R. Wilke and Acta Endocrinologica *92*:295, 1979).

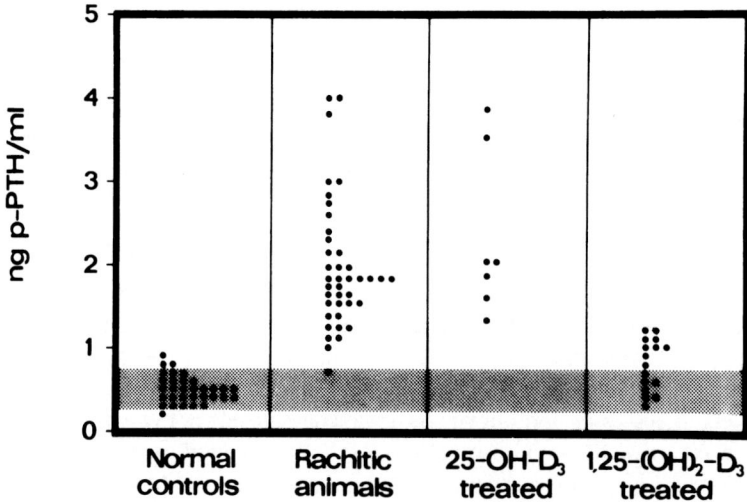

Fig. 4-47. Elevated plasma levels of immunoreactive parathyroid hormone (**PTH**) in pigs with vitamin D-dependent rickets compared with control pigs. Parathyroid hormone levels returned to the normal range following administration of active hormone, 1,25-dihydroxycholecalciferol (**1, 25-[OH]$_2$-D$_3$**) but not when treated with the precursor (**25-OH-D$_3$**). (Courtesy of Dr. R. Wilke and Acta Endocrinologica *92*:295, 1979).

calcemia and hyperphosphatemia in cattle (Fig. 4-48) and results in osteosclerosis, parathyroid atrophy, and hyperplasia of C-cells of the thyroid gland. Extracts of the leaves of *S. malacoxylon* contain an extremely potent, water-soluble, 1, 25-(OH)$_2$-D$_3$ which stimulates the calcium transport system of the intestine and causes the widespread mineralization of the cardiovascular system, lungs, kidneys, and other soft tissues. These lesions are similar

**EFFECT OF SOLANUM MALACOXYLON
ON SERUM CALCIUM AND PHOSPHORUS**

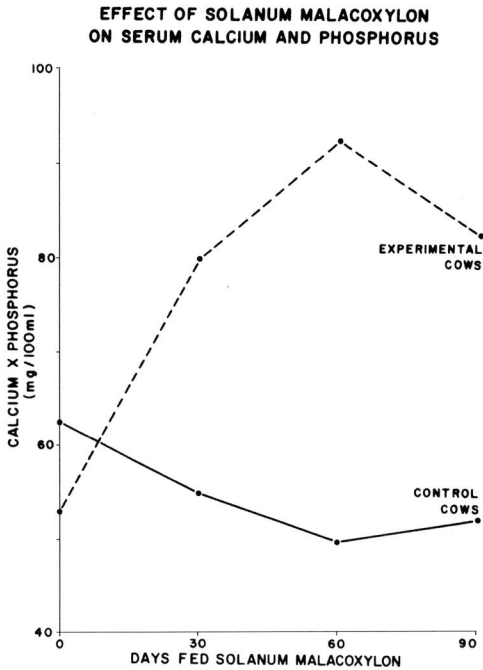

Fig. 4-48. Elevation of calcium x phosphorus ion product following ingestion of *Solanum malacoxylon*. The leaves of this calcinogenic plant contain large quantities 1,25 dihydroxycholecalciferol, the active metabolite of vitamin D. The chronic debilitating disease of cattle that is associated with the ingestion of calcinogenic plants causes major economic losses in several regions of the world.

to those produced by treatment of animals with high doses of vitamin D. The active principle has been shown to be 1,25-$(OH)_2$-CC that is conjugated to a glycoside. *Cestrum diurnum* ("day-blooming jessamine") is a plant that contains substantial amounts of 1,25-$(OH)_2$-CC and has caused a similar debilitating disease in cattle and horses in the southeastern part of the United States.

DISORDERS OF PARATHYROID FUNCTION

Hyperparathyroidism

Hyperparathyroidism is a metabolic disorder in which excessive amounts of PTH secreted by pathologic parathyroid glands cause disturbances of mineral and/or skeletal homeostasis. The predominant clinical features are the result of disturbances of serum levels of calcium and affects the metabolism of bone due to the prolonged hypersecretion of PTH. The skeletal lesion of generalized fibrous osteodystrophy (osteitis fibrosa) is characterized by increased bone resorption, decreased radiographic density, and incomplete fractures.[54] Two forms of the disorder are distinguished: Primary and secondary hyperparathyroidism.

Primary Hyperparathyroidism

Parathyroid hormone is produced in excess of normal in the primary type of hyperparathyroidism. This disease is encountered more frequently in older dogs but is less common than secondary hyperparathyroidism of either renal or nutrional origin. Hormone secretion is autonomous and the parathyroid gland produces excessive amounts of hormone in spite of the sustained increase in blood levels of calcium. Cells of the renal tubules are particularly sensitive to the amount of circulating PTH and the renal cells promote the excretion of phosphorus and the retention of calcium (Fig. 4-49).

Adenomas of chief cells are usually single and result in considerable enlargement of the parathyroid gland (Fig. 4-50). Radiographic evaluation reveals areas of subperiosteal cortical resorption, loss of lamina dura around the teeth (Fig. 4-51), soft tissue mineralization, bone cysts (Fig. 4-52), and a generalized decrease in bone density with multiple fractures. Mineralization of renal tubules (Fig. 4-53) and formation of multiple calculi (Fig. 4-54) may occur in advanced cases of primary hyperparathyroidism in the dog and are associated with substantial elevations of blood calcium. Hypercalcemia due to excessive PTH results in anorexia, vomiting, constipation, depression, and generalized muscular weakness due to a decrease in neuromuscular excitability.

Secondary Hyperparathyroidism

RENAL HYPERPARATHYROIDISM. This form of hyperparathyroidism (secondary renal hyperparathyroidism) is a metabolic disease characterized by an excessive, but not autonomous, rate of PTH secretion caused by chronic renal failure. This disorder is encountered most frequently in dogs but also occurs in cats and other

Primary Hyperparathyroidism

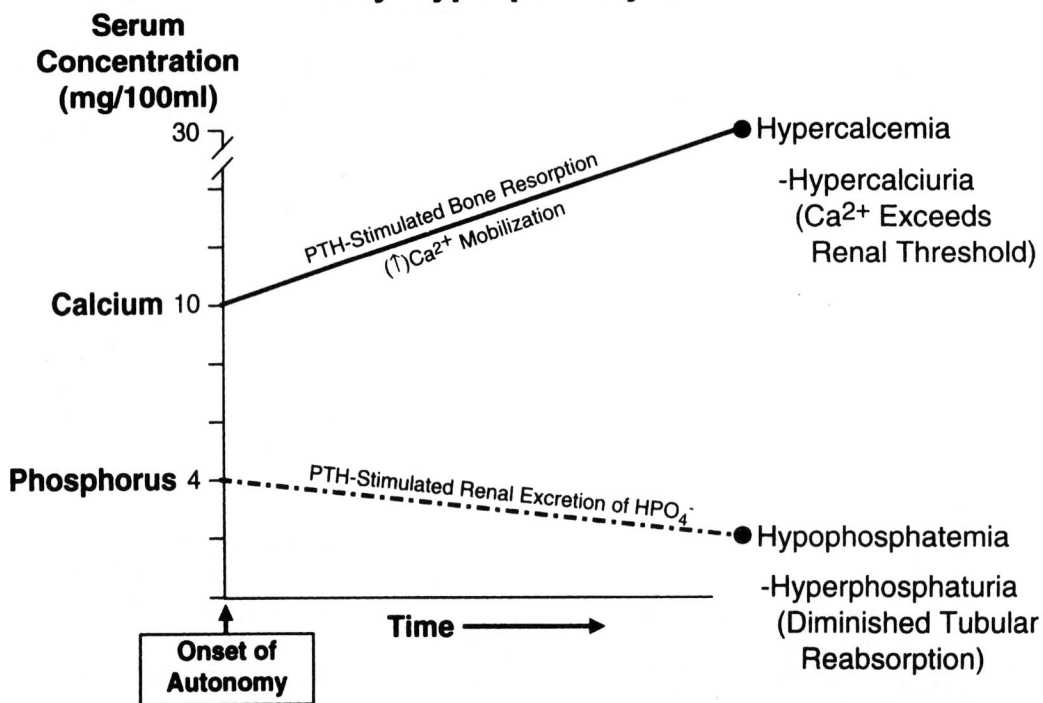

Fig. 4-49. Changes in the concentrations of calcium (**Ca^{2+}**) and phosphorus (**HPO_4^-**) in serum in response to the autonomous secretion of parathyroid hormone (primary hyperparathyroidism).

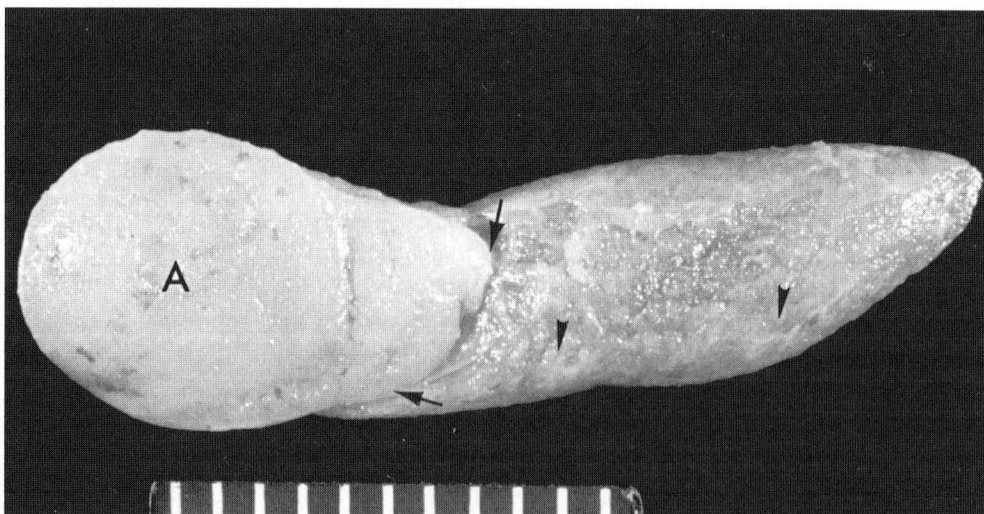

Fig. 4-50. Parathyroid adenoma (**A**) in the external parathyroid gland from a dog with primary hyperparathyroidism. The neoplasm is sharply demarcated (**arrow** ➤) from the adjacent thyroid parenchyma. The focal light areas in the thyroid gland represent areas of C-cell hyperplasia (**arrow heads** ➤) stimulated by the chronic hypercalcemia. The 1 cm scale is divided in mm.

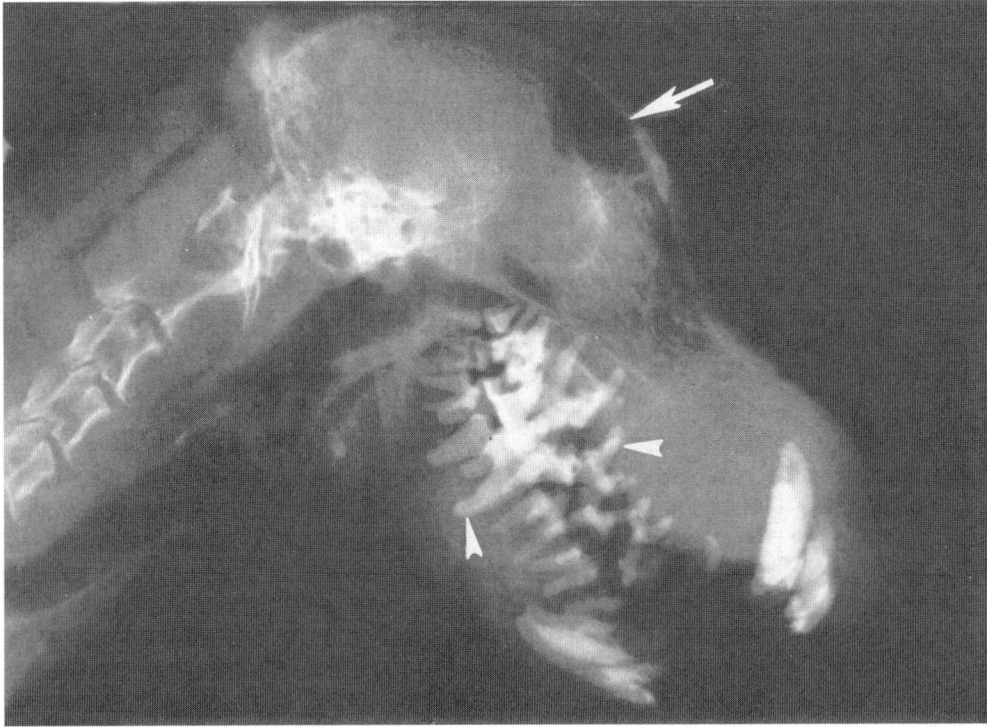

Fig. 4-51. Radiograph of the skull of a dog with primary hyperparathyroidism. As a result of the chronic hypersecretion of PTH, the cancellous bone of the maxilla, mandible, and skull has nearly resorbed to completion and has been replaced by an extensive proliferation of fibrous connective tissue, unmineralized osteoid, and neocapillaries. The *lamina dura dentes* and alveolar socket bone are extensively resorbed (**arrow ➤**) and the teeth are loosely embedded in connective tissue (**arrow heads ➤**).

animal species. The secretion of parathyroid hormone by the hyperplastic glands of animals affected with this disorder usually remains responsive to fluctuations in blood calcium.

Chronic renal insufficiency in older dogs from interstitial nephritis, glomerulonephritis, nephrosclerosis, or amyloidosis and congenital anomalies such as cortical hypoplasia, polycystic kidneys, and bilateral hydronephrosis in young dogs may result in a significant reduction in glomerular filtration rate leading to the retention of phosphorus and the development of progressive hyperphosphatemia (Fig. 4-55). The pathogenesis of secondary renal hyperparathyroidism is complex (Figs. 4-56 and 4-57).

Parathyroid stimulation in patients with chronic renal disease can be directly attributed to the hypocalcemia that develops due to the decreased release of 1,25 $(OH)_2$-CC by the diseased kidney. As the phosphorus concentration increases, blood calcium decreases reciprocally. All four parathyroid glands are enlarged (Fig. 4-58), initially this is due to organellar hypertrophy and later, cellular hyperplasia results in response to compensatory mechanisms to increase hormonal synthesis and secretion in response to hypocalcemia.

Although skeletal involvement is generalized with hyperparathyroidism, it does not affect all parts uniformly. Bone lesions include resorption of alveolar socket bone and loss of *lamina dura dentes* which occur early in the course of the disease. This results in loose teeth which may be dislodged easily and interfere with mastication. Cancellous bones of the maxilla and mandible also are sites of predilection in hyperparathyroidism. Due to the accelerated rate of resorption, bones become softened and are readily pliable (i.e. "rubber-jaw disease") and the jaws fail to close properly (Figs. 4-59 and 4-60). Long bones of the abaxial skeleton are less dramatically affected. Lameness, stiff gait, and fractures after relatively minor trauma may result from the increased resorption of bone. Areas of

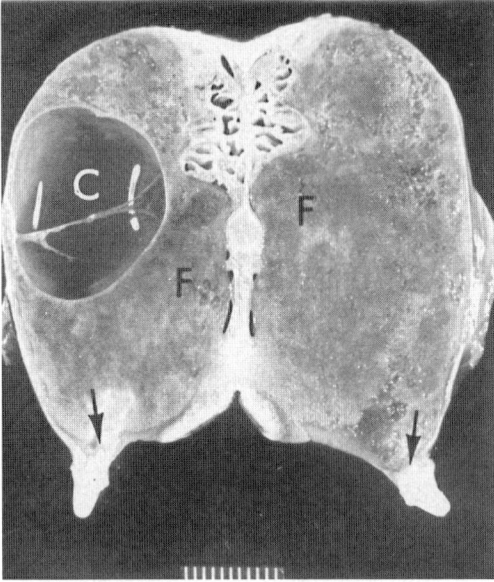

Fig. 4-52. Cross section of the maxilla of a dog with primary hyperparathyroidism illustrating severe hyperostotic fibrous osteodystrophy. Extensive proliferation of woven bone consisting of fibroblasts and osteoblasts with deposition of unmineralized osteoid (**F**) partially occlude the nasal cavity. A cystic area containing blood and fibrin strands (**C**) with extensive bone resorption is present in one side of the maxilla. The teeth are embedded in connective tissue and are freely movable in the sockets (arrows). Scale represents 1 cm.

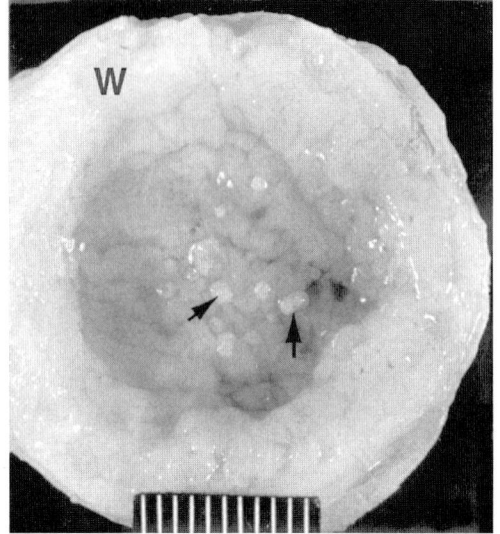

Fig. 4-54. Multiple small calculi (**arrows** ➤) in lumen of the urinary bladder from a dog with primary hyperparathyroidism. The wall of the urinary bladder (**W**) is thickened in response to the chronic irritation of the mucosa by the cystic calculi. The 1 cm scale is divided in mm.

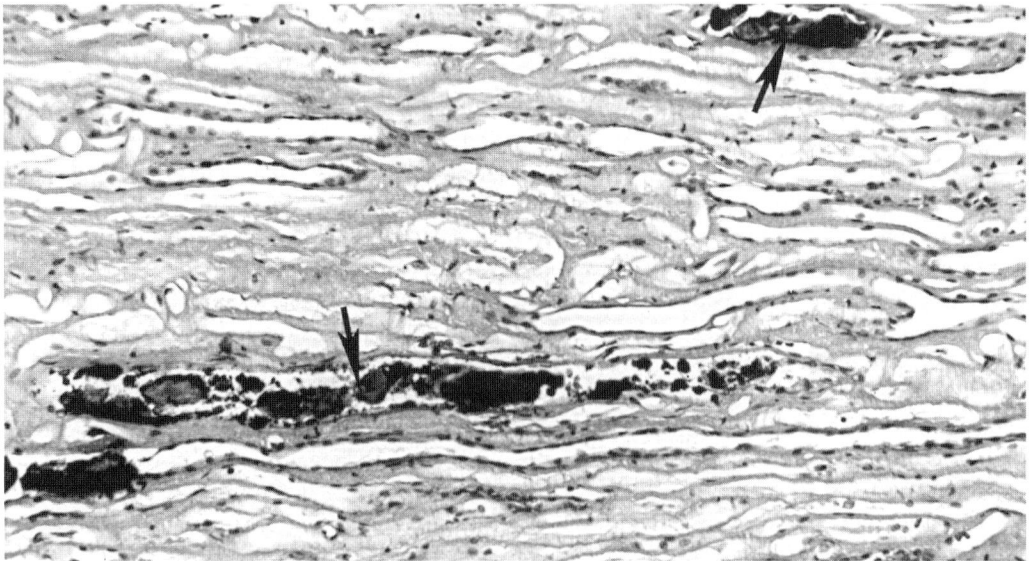

Fig. 4-53. Mineralization of the collecting tubules (**arrows** ➤) in the kidney of a dog due to the long-term hypercalcemia associated with primary hyperparathyroidism. Hematoxylin and eosin staining, magnification 62 ×.

Renal Secondary Hyperparathyroidism

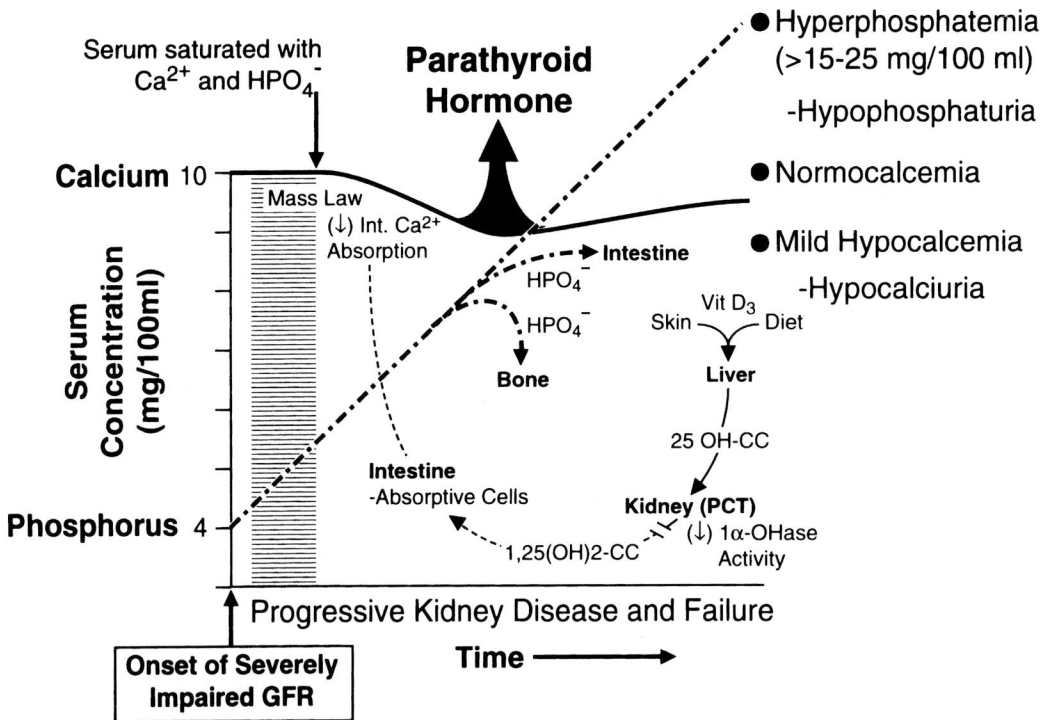

Fig. 4-55. Alterations in serum calcium (Ca^{2+}) and phosphorus (HPO_4^-) associated with progressive renal failure and events related to the pathogenesis of secondary hyperparathyroidism.

subperiosteal resorption by the numerous osteoclasts (see Fig. 4-22) may disrupt the osseous attachment of tendons, leading to elevation and stretching of the periosteum, bone pain, and inability to support the body's weight.

NUTRITIONAL HYPERPARATHYROIDISM. Nutritional hyperparathyroidism (secondary nutritional hyperparathyroidism) is characterized by the increased secretion of parathyroid hormone which develops as a compensatory mechanism to the disturbance of mineral homeostasis caused by nutritional imbalances. The disease is common in cats, dogs, certain non-human primates, and laboratory and farm animal species.

Dietary mineral imbalances of etiologic importance in the pathogenesis of nutritional hyperparathyroidism are: (a) a low content of calcium; (b) excessive phosphorus with normal or low levels of calcium; and (c) inadequate amounts of vitamin D_3. The end result is hypocalcemia which results in the stimulation of the parathyroid glands.

A diet low in calcium fails to supply the daily requirement and hypocalcemia develops even though a greater proportion of ingested calcium is absorbed (Fig. 4-61). Ingestion of excessive phosphorus results in the increased intestinal absorption and elevation of blood levels of phosphorus. Hyperphosphatemia does not stimulate the parathyroid gland directly but does so indirectly, by virtue of the ability to lower blood calcium when the serum becomes saturated with respect to these two ions. Diets containing inadequate amounts of vitamin D_3, even with normal levels of vitamin D_2, cause the diminished absorption of calcium by intestinal cells and results in hypocalcemia in certain New World monkeys.

In response to nutritionally-induced hypocalcemia, the parathyroid glands undergo cellular

Hyperparathyroidism and Chronic Renal Failure

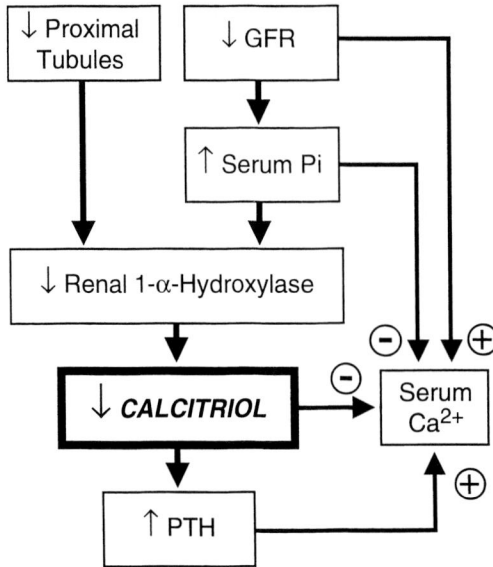

Fig. 4-56. Events associated with hyperparathyroidism and chronic renal failure. **Calcitriol** (1,25- dihydroxyvitamin D) plays a key role in the pathogenesis of renal secondary hyperparathyroidism (Ca^{2+} = ionized calcium; **GFR** = glomerular filtration rate, P_i = phosphorus, **PTH** = serum level of parathyroid hormone). (From: T. J. Rosol et al.,[234] 1995).

hypertrophy and hyperplasia. Active chief cells stimulated by this diet-induced hypocalcemia become larger and more tightly arranged together (Fig. 4-62A) compared to chief cells of normal animals (Fig. 4-62B). Because kidney function is normal, the increased levels of PTH result in the diminished rate of renal reabsorption of phosphorus, the increased renal reabsorption of calcium, and blood levels return toward normal (Fig. 4-61). The continued ingestion of an imbalanced diet sustains the state of compensatory hyperparathyroidism, which eventually leads to the progressive development of metabolic bone disease.

Nutritional hyperparathyroidism develops in young cats and dogs fed a nonsupplemented meat diet. Clinical signs are dominated by disturbances in locomotion manifested by a reluctance of animals to move, incoordinated gait, and posterior lameness (Fig. 4-63). Vertebral fractures with compression of spinal cord and

paralysis are common complications in kittens (Fig. 4-64) but are infrequent in adult cats.

Secondary hyperparathyroidism of nutritional origin also occurs in domestic and captive birds and primates (Figs. 4-65 and 4-66), caged lions and tigers, green iguanas, crocodiles in zoological parks, and laboratory animals used for research.

In horses, the most frequent nutritional imbalance involves the ingestion of excessive amounts of phosphorus. Horses that develop the disease usually have been fed high-grain diets with below-average quality roughage. Evidence of high phosphorus intake may be difficult to establish in horses, inasmuch as the excess phosphorus may be fed in the form of a bran supplement added to a grain diet in order to improve the health of the horse. The diet usually is palatable and nutritious except for the unbalanced and excessive phosphorus and the marginal or deficient calcium content. Occasionally, horses develop nutritional hyperparathyroidism after pasturing on grasses with a high oxalate content. This results in the intestinal malabsorption of calcium. The ingested oxalates appear to form insoluble complexes with calcium in the intestine resulting in an elevated fecal calcium:phosphorus ratio. The interference in intestinal absorption of calcium results in the progressive development of hypocalcemia that leads to the stimulation of the release of PTH and metabolic bone disease.

Hypoparathyroidism

Hypoparathyroidism results from the secretion of subnormal amounts of parathyroid hormone by pathologic parathyroid glands or the hormone that is secreted is unable to interact normally with target cells. Hypoparathyroidism has occasionally been recognized in dogs, particularly in the smaller breeds such as Schnauzers and Terriers. However, the incidence of hypoparathyroidism in dogs and cats is much less than that of hyperparathyroidism.

Inadequate secretion of parathyroid hormone may be caused by several mechanisms. The parathyroid glands may be damaged or inadvertently removed during the course of an operation on the thyroid gland. Agenesis of both pairs

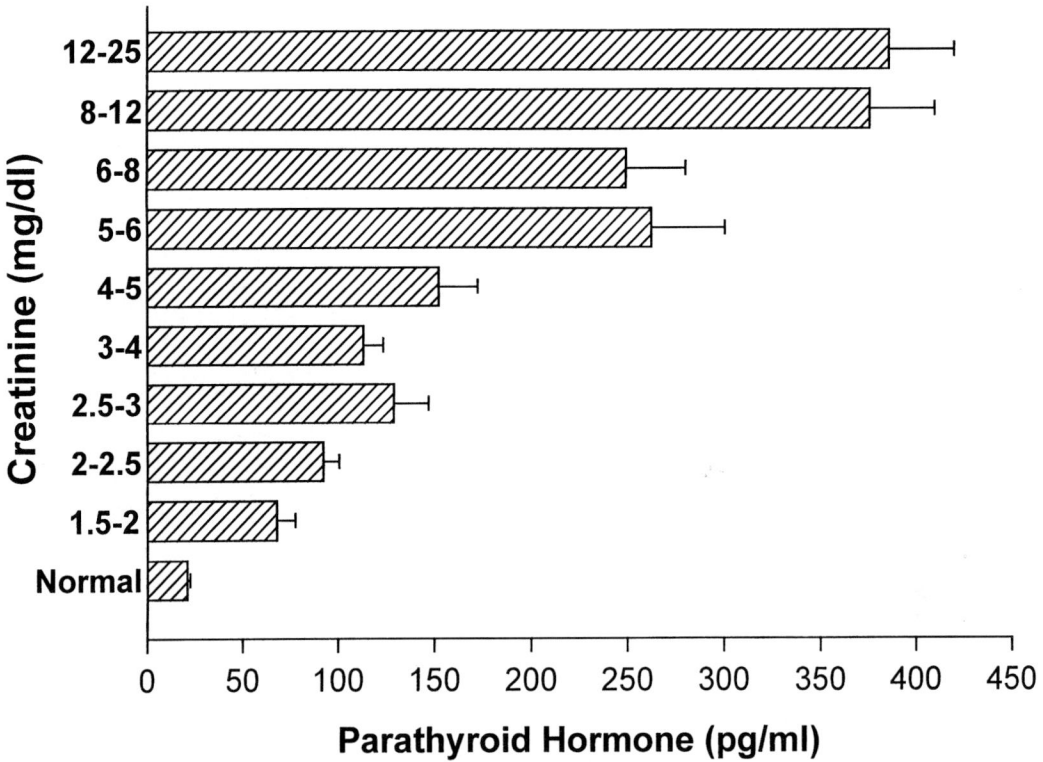

Fig. 4-57. Relationship between the concentration of serum N-terminal parathyroid hormone and creatinine levels in the serum from 35 normal dogs and 333 canine patients with clinical signs of uremia (Data are presented as the mean ± SEM). (From: L. A. Nagode and D. J. Chew,[196] 1992).

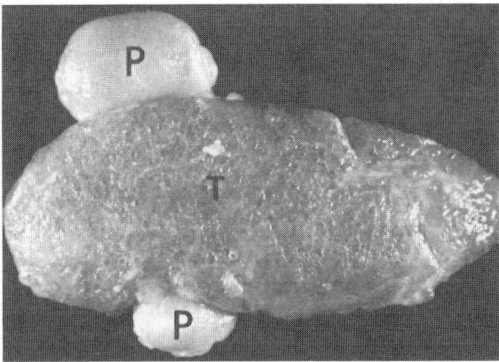

Fig. 4-58. Enlargement of the external and internal parathyroid glands (**P**) in a dog due to hypertrophy and hyperplasia of chief cells caused by renal secondary hyperparathyroidism. The adjacent tissue of the thyroid gland (**T**) appears normal.

of parathyroid glands is a rare cause of congenital hypoparathyroidism in pups. In adult dogs, idiopathic hypoparathyroidism is usually associated with diffuse lymphocytic parathyroiditis resulting in extensive degeneration of chief cells and partial replacement by fibrous connective tissue (Fig. 4-67). Invasion and destruction of the parathyroid glands by primary or metastatic neoplasms in the anterior cervical area may also cause hypoparathyroidism.

The functional disturbances and clinical manifestations of hypoparathyroidism are the result of increased neuromuscular excitability and tetany. Bone resorption is decreased and blood calcium levels progressively diminish (Fig. 4-68).

Other Related Abnormalities

Hypercalcemia is also associated with cancer in animals and humans. Elevated levels of calcium are due to the excessive production of PTHrP causes an imbalance between the rates of calcium release from bones, calcium absorption

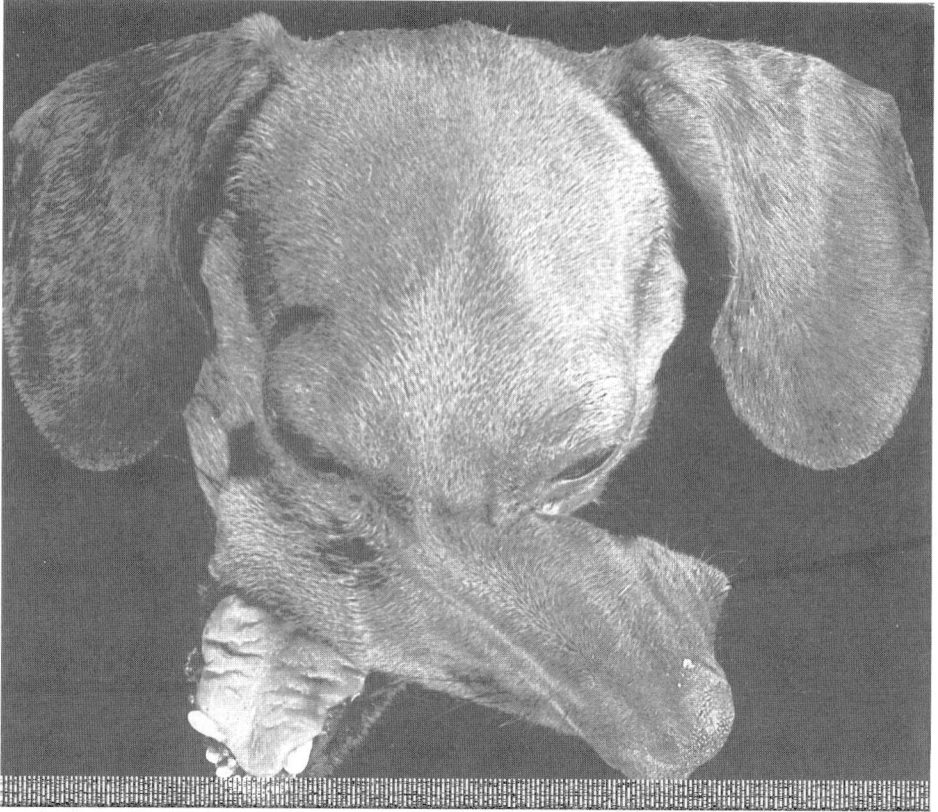

Fig. 4-59. Postmortem photograph of a 5-year-old Dachshund with extensive resorption of cancellous bone. The maxilla and mandible were extremely pliable and could be displaced with minimal pressure (see photo) due to the consequences of renal secondary hyperparathyroidism.

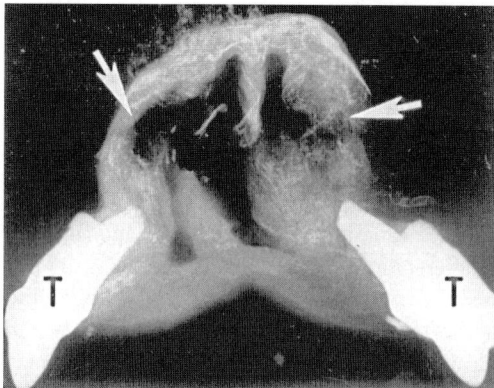

Fig. 4-60. Roentgenogram of a cross-section of the maxilla from the dog illustrated in Fig. 4-58. Under the influence of the chronic excess secretion of PTH, the cancellous bone of the maxilla is nearly completely resorbed and partially replaced by immature fibrous connective tissue, neocapillaries, and spicules of poorly mineralized osteoid (**arrows** ➤). The alveolar socket bone has been resorbed and the teeth (**T**) are loose.

by the intestine, and calcium excretion by the kidneys. Malignancies commonly associated with hypercalcemia include adenocarcinoma of the anal glands in dogs (Fig. 4-69), T-cell lymphomas, and miscellaneous carcinomas in cats and horses.

Compared to disorders of the parathyroid gland, abnormalities related to the secretion of calcitonin by the thyroid gland are rare. Abnormalities and syndromes that have been identified are attributed to the hypersecretion of calcitonin. Calcitonin-secreting C-cell neoplasms occur in bulls (Fig. 4-70), dogs, and horses.

Further description of the responses of animals to calcium imbalances and the pathology of diseased animals is beyond the scope of this textbook. The reader is encouraged to refer to articles included in the reference section for this chapter for additional information.

HYPOCALCEMIC SYNDROMES IN ANIMALS

A number of metabolic disorders have been characterized by the development of hypocalcemia and associated manifestations and these occur in several animal species (Table 4-2). Many of these syndromes develop near the time of the increased calcium demand associated with parturition and probably are a reflection of the temporary failure of calcium homeostatic mechanisms. Parturient hypocalcemia in dairy cows and puerperal tetany of bitches are examples of hypocalcemic syndromes of major economic and veterinary significance.

Parturient Hypocalcemia in Dairy Cows

Parturient hypocalcemia is a metabolic disease of high-producing dairy cows characterized by the development of severe hypocalcemia and hypophosphatemia (Fig. 4-71) result-

ing from the mineralization of fetal bones and the initiation of lactation, and is associated with paresis near the time of parturition (Fig. 4-72). The pathogenic mechanisms responsible for the rapid and precipitous decrease in calcium and phosphorus levels in the blood are complex and involve several interrelated factors.[45] Total and ionized calcium levels decrease progressively beginning several days before parturition (Fig. 4-71). Serum magnesium may increase reciprocally as calcium levels decline. The concentration of glucose in the blood is often increased in response to hypocalcemia (Fig. 4-71) due to interference with the secretion of insulin from the beta cells of the pancreas (see Chapter 5, Figs. 5-1 and 5-3). An adequate level of ionized calcium in the extracellular fluid is required for insulin secretion in response to glucose and other secretagogues for insulin (Fig. 4-73). However, the capability of

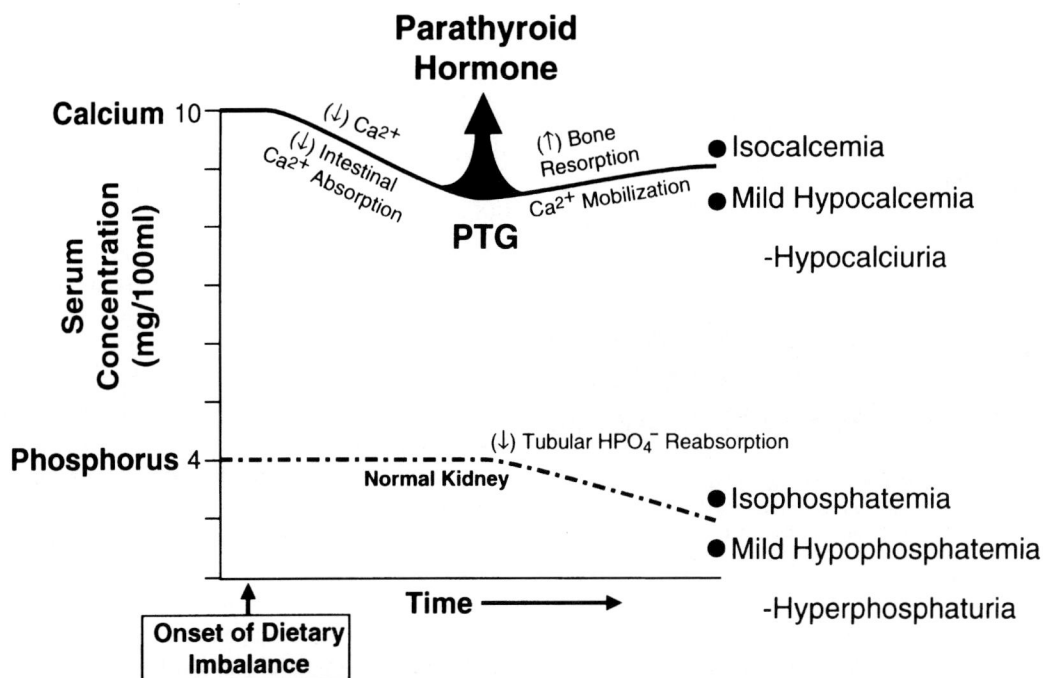

Fig. 4-61. Alterations in the levels of serum calcium (**Ca^{2+}**) and phosphorus (**HPO$_4^-$**) associated with the pathogenesis of secondary hyperparathyroidism caused by a diet low in calcium or deficient in cholecalciferol but with normal amounts of phosphorus. Compare these responses attributed to nutritional secondary hyperparathyroidism with to those indicated in Fig. 4-55 for animals affected by the renal disease.

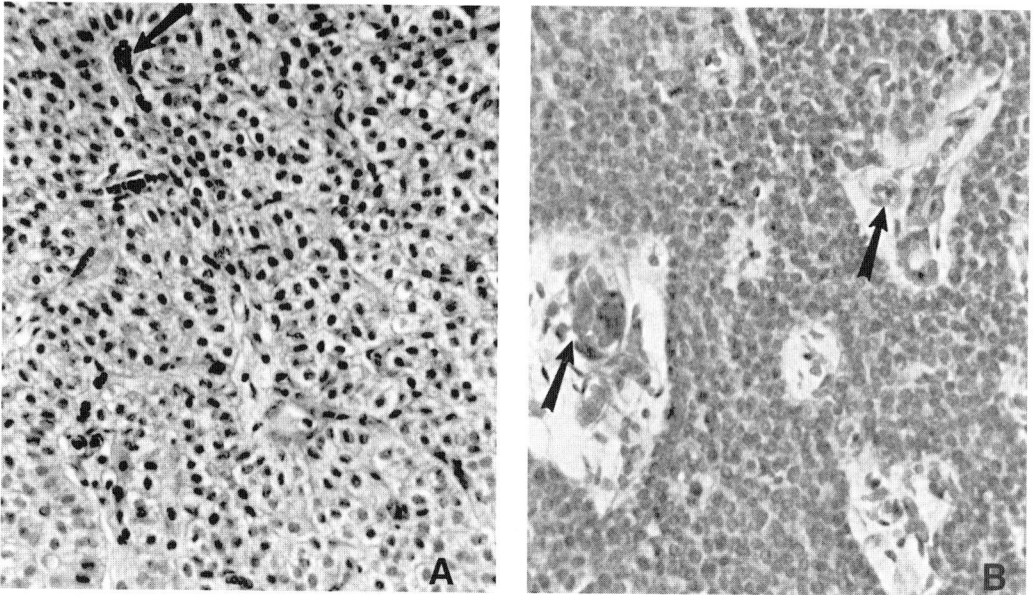

Fig. 4-62 A, (Left) Chief cell hyperplasia in the parathyroid gland of a cat with nutritional hyperparathyroidism. The hyperactive chief cells are enlarged, lightly eosinophilic, and closely packed together with narrow perivascular spaces (**arrow** ——➤). **B. (Right)** Chief cells in the parathyroid gland of a cat fed a balanced control diet. Compare with cells at same magnification for the cat with nutritional hyperparathyroidism (Fig. 4-62A). Note that the chief cells in the control cats are smaller (less cytoplasmic area), more loosely arranged, and the perivascular spaces (**arrows**) are more prominent. Hematoxylin and eosin staining, magnification 315 ×.

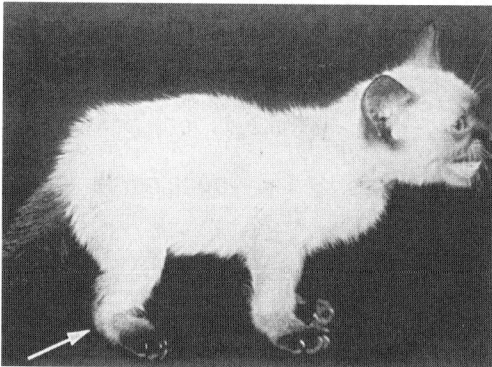

Fig. 4-63. Kitten with secondary hyperparathyroidism of nutritional (low calcium diet) origin. This kitten was reluctant to move due to bone pain and there was lateral deviation of the paws (**arrow** ——➤).

the parathyroid glands to respond to the challenge for the mobilization of additional calcium by the increased synthesis and secretion of parathyroid hormone (Fig. 4-74) does not appear to be defective in those cows that develop parturient hypocalcemia. Calcitonin release dur-

ing the prepartum period, especially in cows fed high calcium diets (Fig. 4-75), may be a factor that contributes to the inability of the increased levels of parathyroid hormone to mobilize calcium from skeletal reserves and maintain blood calcium levels within the normal range during the critical period near parturition. Administration of calcium to increase the levels of calcium in the extracellular fluids of affected animals will restore the responsiveness of the animal to PTH, trigger bone resorption, and correct the periparturient hypocalcemia.

Administration of vitamin D_2 or D_3 to dairy cows prepartum is an effective method for the prevention of parturient hypocalcemia and paresis. Feeding high levels of the parent vitamin D compound are known to increase the rate and quantity of calcium and phosphorus absorbed from the intestinal tract of cattle, to progressively elevate the blood levels of calcium and phosphorus levels within 3 to 5 days, and to increase the net deposition and retention of calcium in areas of new bone growth.

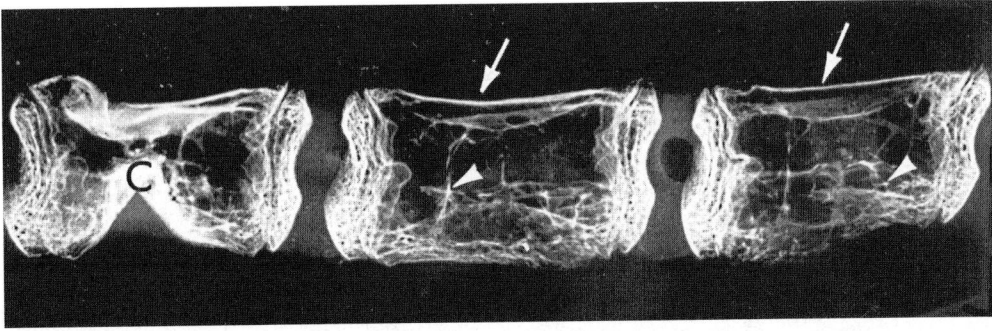

Fig. 4-64. Radiogram of the lumbar vertebrae from a kitten with nutritional hyperparathyroidism. Note the loss of trabecular bone (**arrow heads** ➤), thinning of the cortex (**arrows** ⟶), and cavitation (**C**) of the body of the vertebra on the left side of the figure.

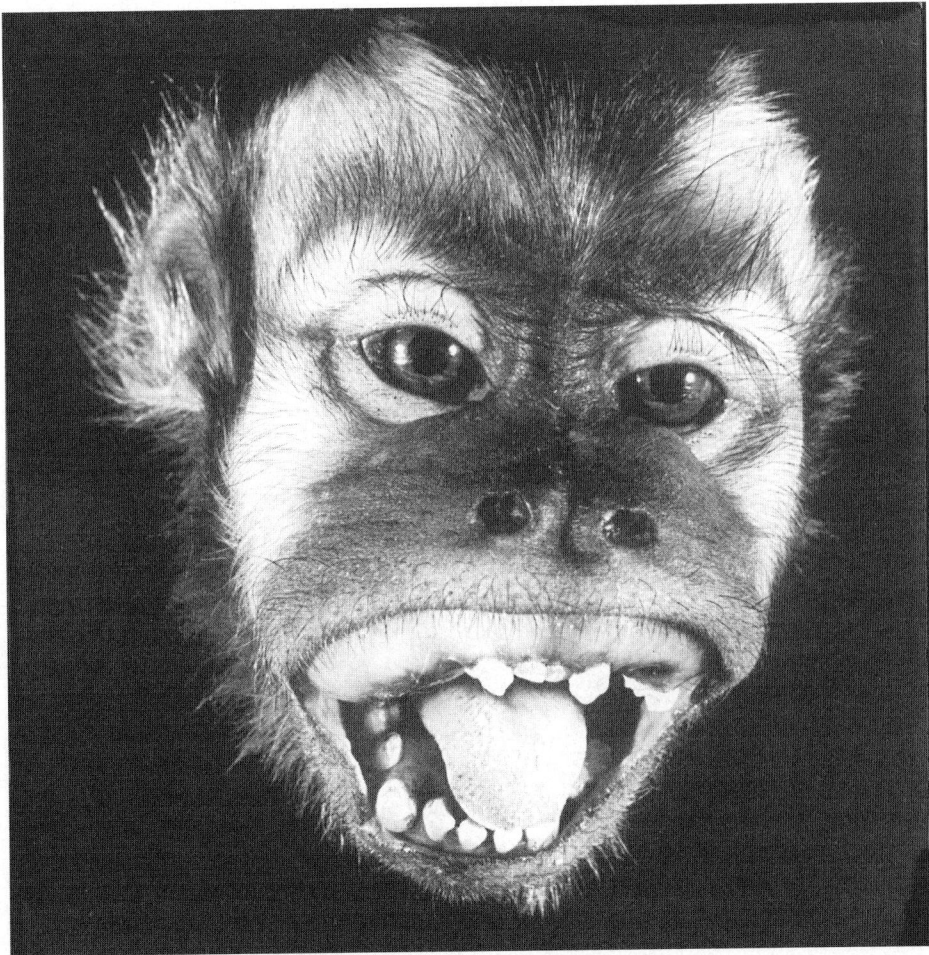

Fig. 4-65. Nutritional secondary hyperparathyroidism in a pet monkey causing difficulty with the mastication of food. The severe maxillary hyperostosis has caused distortion of the face and partial displacement of the teeth. The mouth could not be closed completely because of the proliferation of fibrous tissue and the deposition of poorly mineralized osteoid (i.e., woven bone).

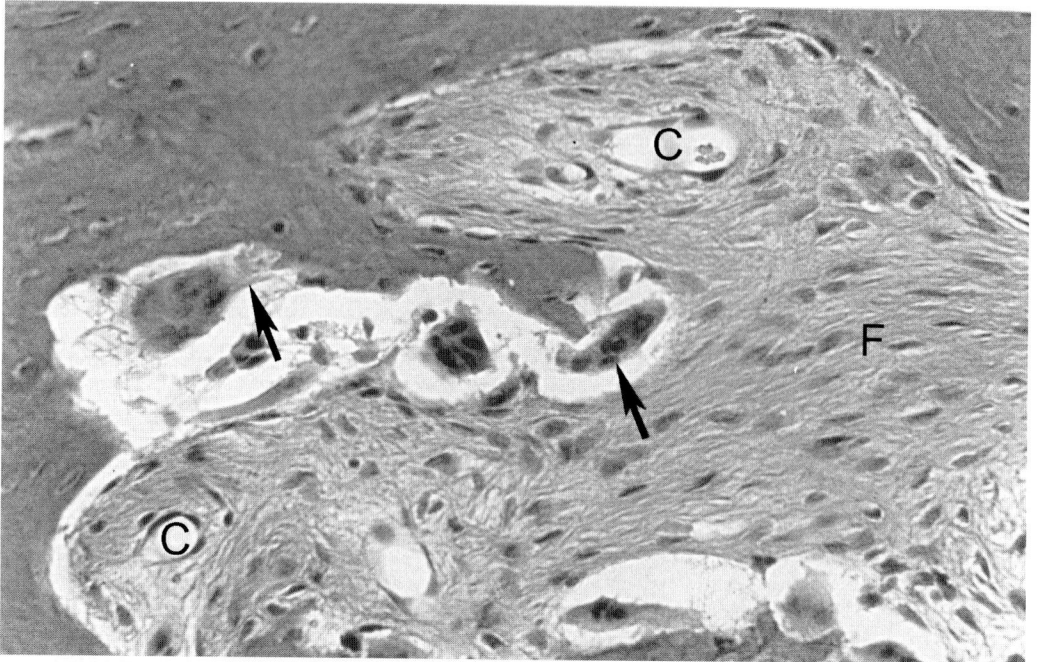

Fig. 4-66. Sites of osteoclastic resorption (**arrows** ➞) of trabecular bone in the rib of a New World primate with nutritional hyperparathyroidism. The long-term excess of PTH has increased the number of active osteoclasts and caused the breakdown of bone which is subsequently replaced by the proliferation of immature fibrous connective tissue (**F**) and neocapillaries (**C**). Hematoxylin and eosin staining, magnification 62 ×.

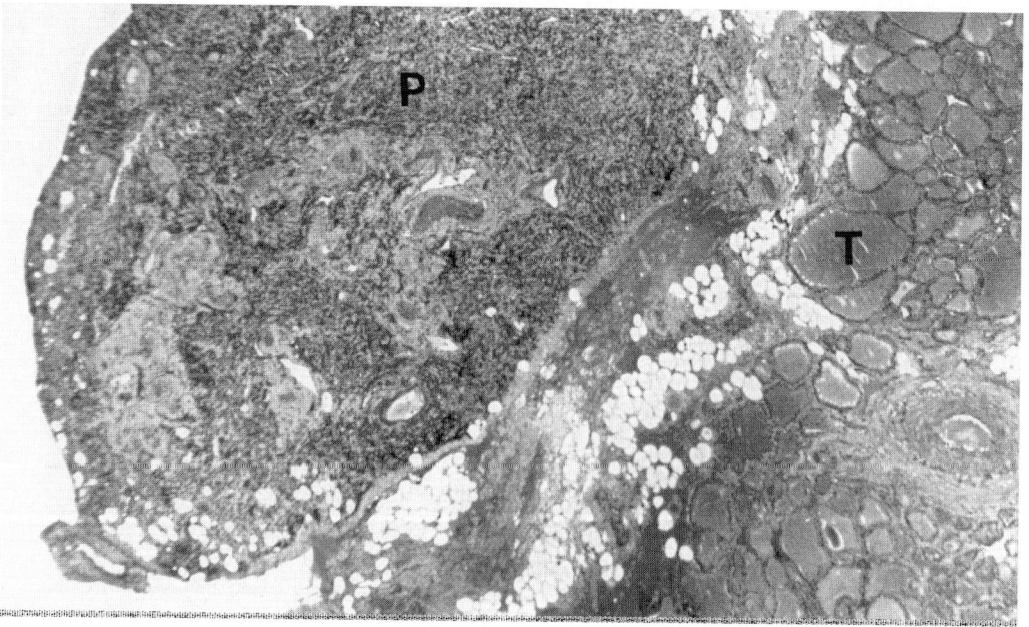

Fig. 4-67. Diffuse lymphocytic parathyroiditis (**P**) in a dog with hypoparathyroidism and hypocalcemia. The external parathyroid gland has been completely replaced by lymphocytes, plasma cells, fibroblasts, and neocapillaries (**T** = thyroid gland). Hematoxylin and eosin staining, magnification 32 ×.

Hypoparathyroidism

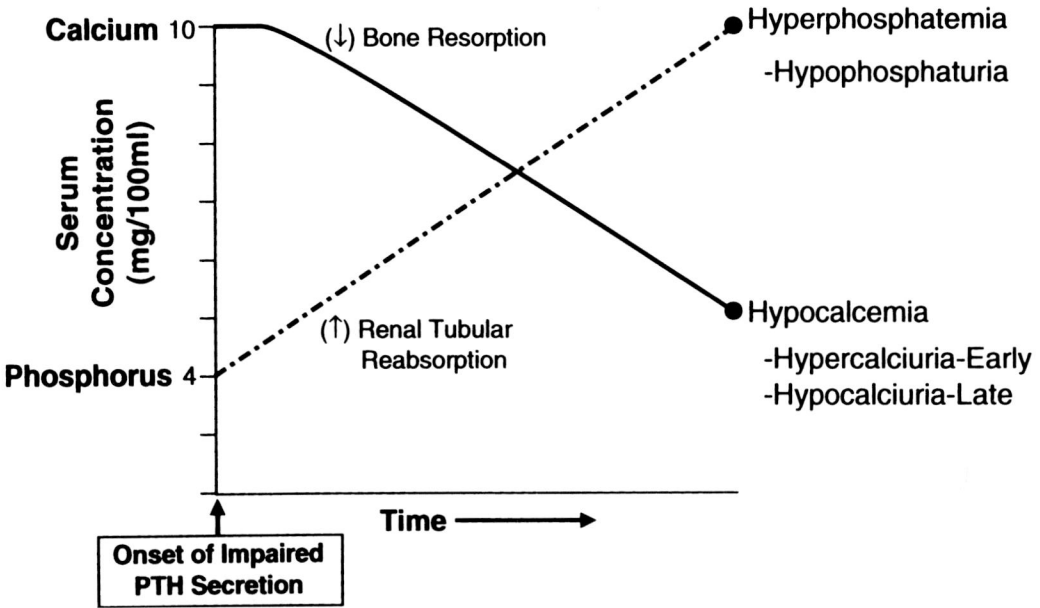

Fig. 4-68. Alterations in serum levels of calcium and phosphorus in response to the inadequate secretion of parathyroid hormone. There is a progressive increase in serum phosphorus and a marked decline in serum calcium that eventually results in neuromuscular tetany and death if untreated.

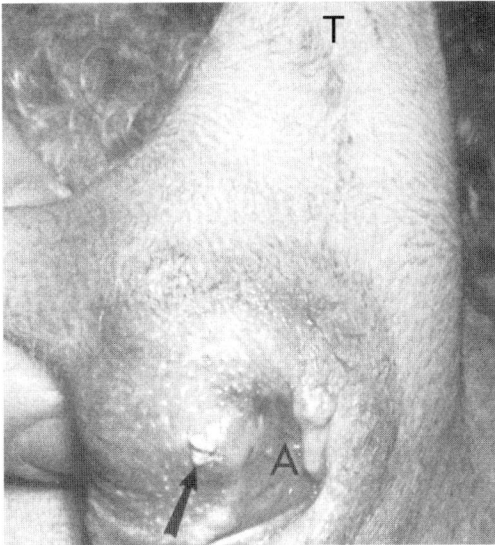

Fig. 4-69. Cancer-associated hypercalcemia. Perirectal region of a dog with hypercalcemia and a small adenocarcinoma (**arrow** ➤) derived from apocrine glands of the anal sac. (**A** = anus; **T** = tail).

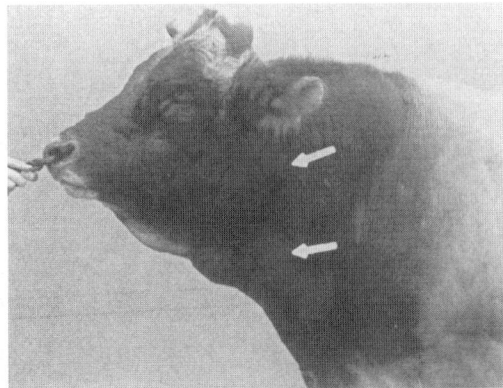

Fig. 4-70. An adult bull with a calcitonin-secreting C-cell (ultimobranchial) neoplasm. The thyroid tumor has resulted in a prominent enlargement of the anterior cervical region (**arrows** ➤) and had metastasized to several of the anterior cervical lymph nodes.

Puerperal Tetany in the Bitch

Little is known about the development of hypocalcemic syndromes in animal species other than the cow. Puerperal tetany resulting from hypocalcemia is frequently encountered in the small, hyperexcitable breeds of dogs. The clinical course is rapid and the bitch may proceed from premonitory signs including restlessness, panting, and nervousness to ataxia, trem-

Table 4-2 Hypocalcemic Syndromes in Animals

Species	Diseases
Cow	Parturient hypocalcemia ("milk fever")
Ewe	Pre- and postparturient paresis ("moss ill or staggers"; "lambing sickness")
Nanny goat	Hypocalcemia
Mare	Parturient eclampsia, postpartum tetany
Sow	Eclampsia
Bitch	Puerperal tetany, eclampsia
Queen	Puerperal tetany, eclampsia
Chinchilla	Hypocalcemia

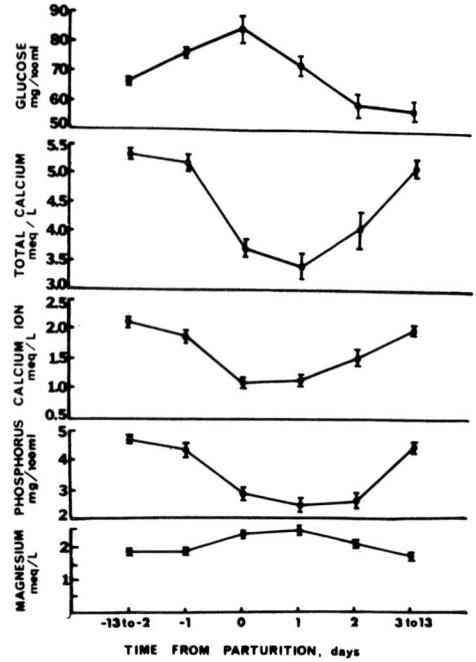

Fig. 4-71. Mean plasma concentrations of total and ionized calcium and inorganic phosphorus decrease rapidly near parturition in cows, however magnesium and glucose levels increase prior to parturition and during the development of the hypocalcemic state. (From: J. W. Blum et al.,[26] 1972).

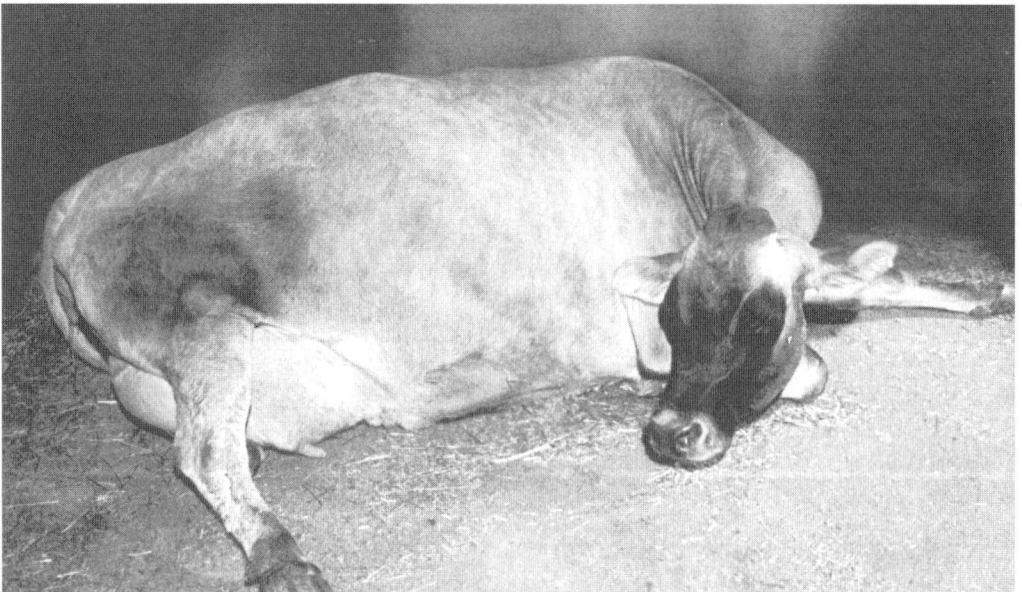

Fig. 4-72. Paresis in a Jersey cow with parturient hypocalcemia owing to a blockage in neuromuscular transmission.

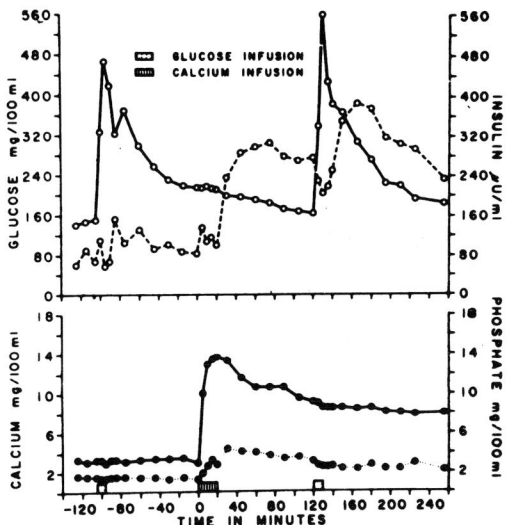

Fig. 4-73. Failure of insulin release in response to glucose infusion in cows with severe hypocalcemia. The ability to release insulin can be restored if calcium is injected to elevate blood calcium levels 2 hours before the second glucose infusion. (From: E. T. Littledike, S. C. Whipp, and L. Schroeder, Studies on parturient paresis. J. Am. Vet. Med. Assoc. *155*:1955, 1969).

bling, and muscular tetany (Fig. 4-76), and result in convulsive seizures within 8 to 12 hours. In the majority of bitches, administration of intravenous calcium counteracts the muscular tetany and when combined with a temporary decrease in the lactational drain of calcium by removing the pups, corrects the disruption of calcium homeostasis. In those bitches affected by puerperal tetany, dietary supplementation with calcium and vitamin D have proven useful to prevent relapses.

Hypocalcemia in Other Species

Metabolic disorders characterized by the development of hypocalcemia and associated manifestations occur in several animal species including queens, ewes, goats, mares, sows, and chinchillas. Many of these hypocalcemic syndromes develop near the period of increased calcium demand associated with parturition and probably are due to the temporary failure of calcium homeostatic mechanisms. A comparable hypocalcemic syndrome does not occur in hu-

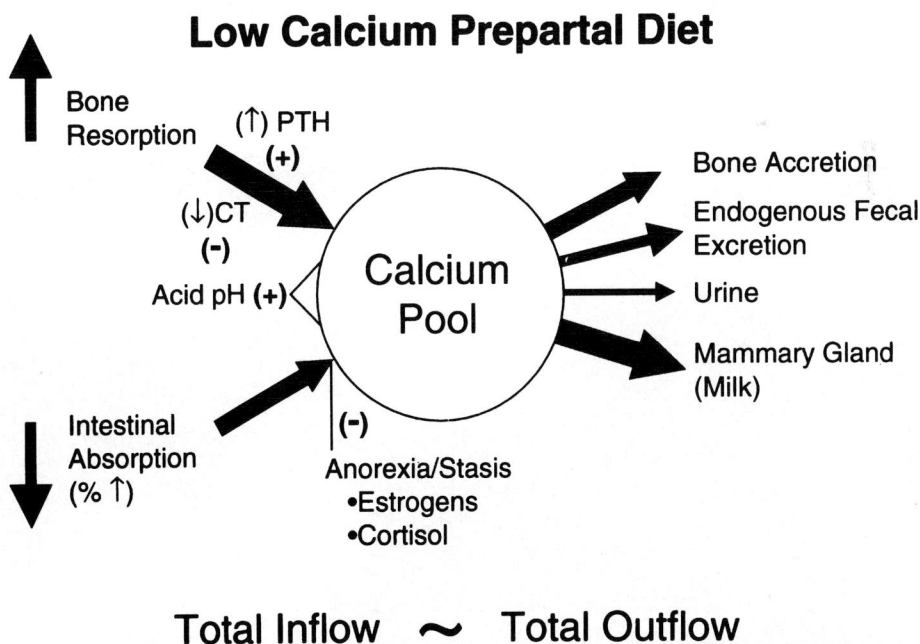

Fig. 4-74. Bone resorption and intestinal absorption contribute substantially to the availability of calcium in extracellular fluids. The anorexia and gastrointestinal stasis that often occur near parturition may temporarily interrupt calcium uptake from the intestine. Cows fed a low calcium prepartal diet maintain a pool of active bone-resorbing cells capable of responding to the increased secretion of **PTH**. These animals are less susceptible to the development of the progressive hypocalcemia associated with parturition. (Adapted from: G. P. Mayer,[176] 1971).

High Calcium Prepartal Diet

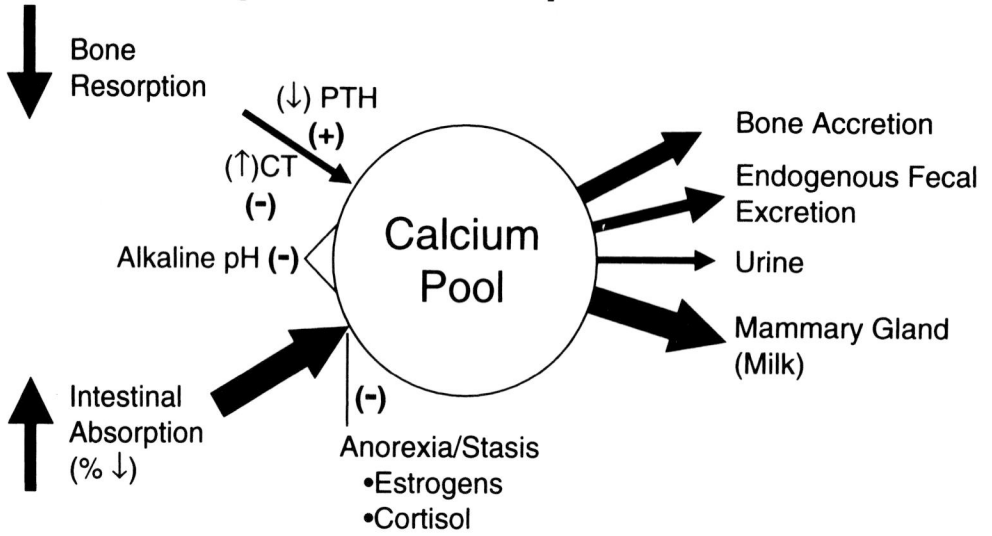

Bone Resorption

(↓) PTH (+)

(↑)CT (-)

Alkaline pH (-)

Calcium Pool

Bone Accretion

Endogenous Fecal Excretion

Urine

Mammary Gland (Milk)

Intestinal Absorption (% ↓)

(-)

Anorexia/Stasis
• Estrogens
• Cortisol

Total Inflow   <   Total Outflow

Fig. 4-75. Calcium homeostasis in cows fed a high calcium prepartal diet is primarily dependent on the regulation of the rate of calcium absorption by the intestine. The rate of bone resorption is low and the parathyroid glands are inactive. Anorexia and gastrointestinal stasis that often occur near the time of parturition interrupt the inflow of calcium into the extracellular fluid. Outflow of calcium with the onset of lactation exceeds the rate of inflow into the calcium pool and affected cows develop a progressive hypocalcemia and paresis. (Adapted from: G. P. Mayer,[176] 1971).

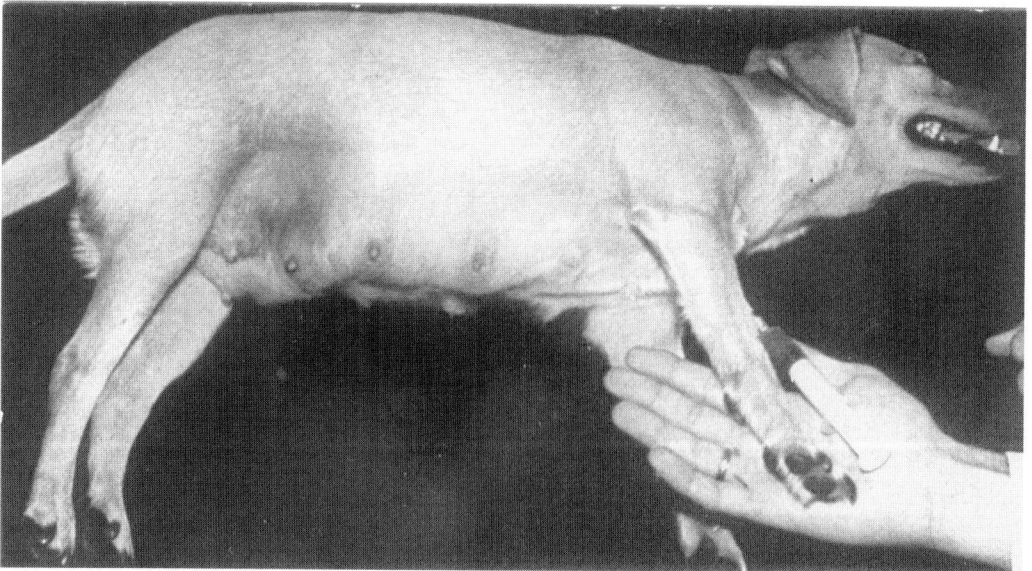

Fig. 4-76. Puerperal tetany in a bitch with hypocalcemia. Increased neuromuscular excitability occurs with hypocalcemia, because excitation-secretion coupling is maintained at the motor endplate.

mans. The eclampsia that develops in women is related to a toxemia of pregnancy and is associated with degenerative changes in the liver, kidney, and placenta, rather than disturbances in mineral homeostasis.

REFERENCES

1. Abou-Samra A.-B., Jüppner H., Force T., et al. (1992): Expression cloning of a common receptor for parathyroid hormone and parathyroid hormone-related peptide from rat osteoblast-like cells: A single receptor stimulates intracellular accumulation of both cAMP and inositol triphosphates and increases intracellular calcium. Proc. Nat. Acad. Sci., USA *89*:2732.
2. Altenähr, E. and Seifert, G. (1971): Ultrastruktureller Vergleich menschlicher Epithelkörperchen bei sekundärem Hyperparathyreodismus und primärem Adenom. Virchows Arch. Pathol. Anat. Physiol. Klin. Med. *353*:60.
3. Anderson, M. P. and Capen, C. C. (1976): Ultrastructural evaluation of parathyroid and ultimobranchial glands in iguanas with experimental nutritional osteodystrophy. Gen. Comp. Endocrinol. *30*:209.
4. Anderson, M. P. and Capen, C. C. (1976): Nutritional osteodystrophy in captive green iguanas (*Iguana iguana*). Virchows Arch. B Cell Pathol. *21*:229.
5. Argenzio, R. A., Lowe, J. E., Hintz, H. F., et al. (1974): Calcium and phosphorus homeostasis in horses. J. Nutr. *104*:18.
6. Arnaud, C. D. (1973): Parathyroid hormone: Coming of age in clinical medicine. Am. J. Med. *55*:577.
7. Arnaud, C. D. and Pun, K.-K. (1992): Metabolism and assay of parathyroid hormone. *In:* Disorders of Bone and Mineral Metabolism, edited by F. L. Coe and M. J. Favus. New York, NY, Raven Press, Ltd., p. 107.
8. Arnaud, C. D., Sizemore, G. W., Oldham, S. B., et al. (1971): Human parathyroid hormone: Glandular and secreted molecular species. Am. J. Med. *50*:630.
9. Arnold, B. M., Kovacs, K., Horvath, E., et al. (1974): Functioning oxyphil cell adenoma of the parathyroid gland: Evidence for parathyroid secretory activity of oxyphil cells. J. Clin. Endocrinol. Metab. *38*:458.
10. Avioli, L. V. and Haddad, J. G. (1973): Vitamin D: Current concepts. Metabolism *22*:507.
11. Barber, P. J., Elliott, J., and Torrance, A. G. (1993): Measurement of feline intact parathyroid hormone: Assay validation and sample handling studies. J. Small Anim. Pract. *34*:614.
12. Barlet, J. P. (1972): Calcium homeostasis in the normal and thyroidectomized bovine. Hormone Metab. Res. *4*:300.
13. Barlet, J. P., Abbas, S. K., Care, A. D., et al. (1993): Parathyroid hormone-related peptide and milking-induced phosphaturia in dairy cows. Acta Endocrinol. *129*:332.
14. Barlet, J. P., Champredon, C., Coxam, V., et al. (1992): Parathyroid hormone-related peptide might stimulate calcium secretion into the milk of goats. J. Endocrinol. *132*:353.
15. Barlet, J. P., Davicco, M. J., and Coxam, V. (1995): Physiologie de l'absorption intestinale du phosphore chez l'animal. Reprod. Nutr. Develop. *35*:475.
16. Bhattacharyya, M. H. and DeLuca, H. F. (1974): Subcellular location of rat liver calciferol-25-hydroxylase. Arch. Biochem. Biophys. *160*:58.
17. Biber J., Custer M., Magagnin S., et al. (1996): Renal Na/Pi-cotransporters. Kidney Int. *49*:981.
18. Bikle, D. D. (1992): Clinical counterpoint: Vitamin D: New actions, new analogs, new therapeutic potential. Endocrine Rev. *13*:765.
19. Bilezikian, J. P. (1992): Clinical utility of assays for parathyroid hormone-related protein. Clin. Chem. *38*:179.
20. Bindels, R. J. M. (1993): Calcium handling by the mammalian kidney. J. Exp. Biol. *184*:89.
21. Birkenhäger, J. C., Seldenrath, H. J., Hackeng, W. H. L., et al. (1973): Calcium and phosphorus metabolism, parathyroid hormone, calcitonin and bone histology in pseudohypoparathyroidism. Europ. J. Clin. Invest. *3*:27.
22. Black, H. E.,and Capen, C. C. (1971): Urinary and plasma hydroxyproline during pregnancy, parturition and lactation in cows with parturient hypocalcemia. Metabolism *20*:337.
23. Black, H. E., Capen, C. C., and Arnaud, C. D. (1973): Ultrastructure of parathyroid glands and plasma immunoreactive parathyroid hormone in pregnant cows fed normal and high calcium diets. Lab. Invest. *29*:173.
24. Black, H. E., Capen, C. C., Yarrington, J. T., et al. (1973): Effect of a high calcium prepartal diet on calcium homeostatic mechanisms in thyroid glands, bone, and intestine of cows. Lab. Invest. *29*:437.
25. Black, K. S. and Mundy, G. R. (1994): Other causes of hypercalcemia: Local and ectopic secretion syndromes. *In:* The Parathyroids, edited by J. P. Bilezikian, R. Marcus, and M. A. Levine. New York, NY, Raven Press, Ltd., p. 341.
26. Blum, J. W., Ramberg, C. F., Jr., Johnson, K. G., et al. (1972): Calcium (ionized and total), magnesium, phosphorus, and glucose in plasma from parturient cows. Am. J. Vet. Res. *33*:51.
27. Bouhtiauy, I., Lajeunesse, D., Christakos, S., et al. (1994): Two vitamin D_3-dependent calcium binding proteins increase calcium reabsorption by different mechanisms. I. Effect of CaBP 28K. Kidney Int. *45*:461.
28. Bouhtiauy, I., Lajeunesse, D., Christakos, S., et al. (1994): Two vitamin D_3-dependent calcium binding proteins increase calcium absorption by different mechanisms. II. Effect of CaBP 9K. Kidney Int. *45*:469.
29. Bowden, S. J., Hughes, S. V., and Ratcliffe, W. A. (1993): Molecular forms of parathyroid hormone-related protein in tumours and biological fluids. Clin. Endocrinol. *38*:287.
30. Boyle, I. T., Omdahl, J. L., Gray, R. W., et al. (1973): The biological activity and metabolism of 24,25-dihydroxyvitamin D_3. J. Biol. Chem. *248*:4174.
31. Brewer, H. B., Fairwell, T., Rittel, W., et al. (1974): Recent studies on the chemistry of human, bovine and porcine parathyroid hormone. Am. J. Med. *56*:759.
32. Brickman, A. S., Coburn, J. W., Massry, S. G., et al. (1974): 1,25 dihydroxy-vitamin D_3 in normal man and patients with renal failure. Ann. Intern. Med. *80*:161.

33. Bronner, F. (1989): Renal calcium transport: mechanisms and regulation - an overview. Am. J. Physiol. *257*:F707.

34. Brown, E. M. (1994): Homeostatic mechanisms regulating extracellular and intracellular calcium metabolism. *In:* The Parathyroids, edited by J. P. Bilezikian, R. Marcus, and M. A. Levine. New York, NY, Raven Press, Ltd., p. 15.

35. Brown, E. M., Gamba, G., Riccardi, D., et al. (1993): Cloning and characterization of an extracellular Ca^{2+}-sensing receptor from bovine parathyroid. Nature, London, England *366*:575.

36. Brown, E. M. and Hebert, S. C. (1996): A cloned extracellular Ca^{2+}-sensing receptor: Molecular mediator of the actions of extracellular Ca^{2+} on parathyroid and kidney cells? Kidney Int. *49*:1042.

37. Brown, E. M., Pollak, M., Seidman, C. E., et al. (1995): Calcium-ion-sensing cell-surface receptors. N. Engl. J. Med. *333*:234.

38. Brumbaugh, P. F. and Haussler, M. R. (1973): Nuclear and cytoplasmic receptors for 1,25-dihydroxycholecalciferol in intestinal mucosa. Biochem. Biophys. Res. Commun. *51*:74.

39. Brunette, M. G., Chan, M., Ferriere, C., et al. (1978): Site of 1,25 $(OH)_2$ vitamin D_3 synthesis in the kidney. Nature, London, England *276*:287.

40. Burtis, W. J. (1992): Parathyroid hormone-related protein: Structure, function, and measurement. Clin. Chem. *38*:2171.

41. Burtis, W. J., Brady, T. G., Orloff, J. J., et al. (1990): Immunochemical characterization of circulating parathyroid hormone-related protein in patients with humoral hypercalcemia of malignancy. N. Engl. J. Med. *322*:1106.

42. Burtis, W. J., Dann, P., Gaich, G. A., et al. (1994): A high abundance midregion species of parathyroid hormone-related protein: Immunological and chromatographic characterization in plasma. J. Clin. Endocrinol. Metab. *78*:317.

43. Campos, R. V., Asa, S. L., and Drucker, D. J. (1991): Immunocytochemical localization of parathyroid hormone-like peptide in the rat fetus. Cancer Res. *51*:6351.

44. Capen, C. C. (1971): Fine structural changes of parathyroid glands in response to experimental and spontaneous alterations of extracellular fluid calcium. Am. J. Med. *50*:598.

45. Capen, C. C. (1972): Endocrine control of calcium metabolism and parturient hypocalcemia in dairy cattle. *In:* Proc. 4th Annu. Conv. Am. Assoc. Bovine Pract., edited by E. I. Williams. Stillwater, OK, Heritage Press, p. 189.

46. Capen, C. C. (1975): Functional and fine structural relationships of parathyroid glands. *In:* Advances in Veterinary Sciences and Comparative Medicine. New York, NY, Academic Press Inc., p. 249.

47. Capen, C. C. (1982): Nutritional secondary hyperparathyroidism in horses. *In:* Current Therapy in Equine Medicine, edited by N. E. Robinson. Philadelphia, PA, W. B. Saunders Co., p. 160.

48. Capen, C. C. (1985): The endocrine glands. Chapter 3. *In:* Pathology of Domestic Animals. Third Edition, Volume III, edited by K. V. F. Jubb, P. C. Kennedy, and N. Palmer. New York, NY, Academic Press, Inc., p. 237.

49. Capen, C. C. (1985): Calcium-regulating hormones and metabolic bone disease. Chapter 59. *In:* Textbook of Small Animal Orthopaedics, edited by C. D. Newton and D. M. Nunamaker. Philadelphia, PA, J. B. Lippincott Co., p. 673.

50. Capen, C. C. (1988): Endocrine system. Chapter 9. *In:* Special Veterinary Pathology, edited by R. G. Thomson. Philadelphia, PA, B. C. Decker, Inc., p. 369.

51. Capen, C. C. (1989): The calcium regulating hormones: Parathyroid hormone, calcitonin, and cholecalciferol. *In:* Veterinary Endocrinology and Reproduction, 4th ed., edited by L. E. McDonald and M. H. Pineda. Philadelphia, PA, Lea & Febiger, p. 92.

52. Capen, C. C. and Black, H. E. (1974): Calcitonin-secreting ultimobranchial neoplasms of the thyroid gland in bulls: An animal model for medullary thyroid carcinoma in man (Sipple's syndrome). Am. J. Pathol. *74*:377.

53. Capen, C. C. and Black, H. E. (1975): Fine-structural evaluation of parathyroid glands of cows fed high-, normal-, and low-calcium diets. *In:* Electron Microscopic Concepts of Secretion: Ultrastructure of Endocrine and Reproductive Organs, edited by M. Hess. New York, NY, John Wiley & Sons, p. 379.

54. Capen, C. C., Black, H. E., and Arnaud, C. D. (1973): Fine structural evaluation of parathyroid glands from cows fed low and high calcium diets. *In:* 31st Annu. Proc. Electron Microscopy Soc. Amer., edited by C. J. Arceneaux. Baton Rouge, LA, Claitor's Publishing, p. 678.

55. Capen, C. C. and Martin, S. L. (1974): Hyperparathyroidism in animals. *In:* Current Veterinary Therapy, V, edited by R. W. Kirk. Philadelphia, PA, W. B. Saunders Co., p. 797.

56. Capen, C. C. and Martin, S. L. (1977): Calcium metabolism and disorders of parathyroid glands. Vet. Clin. North Am. *7*:513.

57. Capen, C. C. and Martin, S. L. (1982): Calcium regulating hormones and diseases of the parathyroid glands, Chapter 66. *In:* Textbook of Veterinary Internal Medicine, 2nd ed., edited by S. J. Ettinger. Philadelphia, PA, W. B. Saunders Co., p. 1550.

58. Capen, C. C. and Rosol, T. J. (1993): Hormonal control of mineral metabolism. *In:* Disease Mechanisms in Small Animal Surgery, 2nd ed., edited by M. J. Bojrab. Philadelphia, PA, Lea & Febiger, p. 841.

59. Capen, C. C. and Rosol, T. J. (1993): Pathobiology of parathyroid hormone and parathyroid hormone-related protein: Introduction and evolving concepts. *In:* Pathobiology of the Parathyroid and Thyroid Glands, edited by V. D. LiVolsi and R. A. DeLellis. Baltimore, MD, Williams & Wilkins, p. 1.

60. Capen, C. C. and Roth, S. I. (1973): Ultrastructural and functional relationships of normal and pathologic parathyroid cells. *In:* Pathobiology Annual, edited by H. L. Ioachim. New York, NY, Appleton-Century-Crofts, p. 129.

61. Care, A. D. (1991): Placental transfer of calcium. J. Develop. Physiol. *15*:253.

62. Care, A. D. (1994): The absorption of phosphate from the digestive tract of ruminant animals. Br. Vet. J. *150*:197.

63. Carothers, M. A., Chew, D. J., and Nagode, L. A. (1994): 25-OH-Cholecalciferol intoxication in dogs. Proc. Am. Coll. Vet. Int. Med. Forum *12*:822.

64. Chambers, T. J. (1980): The cellular basis of bone resorption. Clin. Orthop. Related Res. *151*:283.

65. Chambers, T. J. and Fuller, K. (1985): Bone cells predispose bone surfaces to resorption by exposure of mineral to osteoclastic contact. J. Cell Sci. *76*:155.

66. Chambers, T. J. and Mangus, C. J. (1982): Calcitonin alters behavior of isolated osteoclasts. J. Pathol. *136*:27.

67. Chambers, T. J. and Moore, A. (1983): The sensitivity of isolated osteoclasts to morphological transformation by calcitonin. J. Clin. Endocrinol. Metab. *57*:819.

68. Chambers, T. J., Revell, P. A., Fuller, K., et al. (1984): Resorption of bone by isolated rabbit osteoclasts. J. Cell. Sci. *66*:383.

69. Chattopadhyay, N., Mithal, A., and Brown, E. M. (1996): The calcium-sensing receptor: A window into the physiology and pathophysiology of mineral ion metabolism. Endocrine Rev. *17*:289.

70. Chew, D. J., Nagode, L. A., and Carothers, M. (1992): Disorders of calcium: Hypercalcemia and hypocalcemia. In: Fluid Therapy in Small Animal Practice, edited by S. P. DiBartola. Philadelphia, PA, W.B. Saunders, p. 116.

71. Christakos, S. and Norman, A. W. (1978): Vitamin D₃-induced calcium binding protein in bone tissue. Science *202*:70.

72. Chu, L. L. H., MacGregor, R. R., Anast, C. S., et al. (1973): Studies on the biosynthesis of rat parathyroid hormone and proparathyroid hormone: Adaptation of the parathyroid gland to dietary restriction of calcium. Endocrinology *93*:915.

73. Civitelli, R. and Avioli, L. V. (1994): Calcium, phosphate, and magnesium absorption. In: Physiology of the Gastrointestinal Tract, edited by L. R. Johnson. New York, NY, Raven Press, Ltd., p. 2173.

74. Cloutier, M., Rousseau, L., Gascon-Barré, M., et al. (1993): Immunological evidences for posttranslational control of the parathyroid function by ionized calcium in dogs. Bone Miner. *22*:197.

75. Cohn, D. V., Fasciotto, B. H., Zhang, J.-X., et al. (1994): Chemistry and Biology of chromogranin A (Secretory Protein I) of the parathyroid and other endocrine glands. In: The Parathyroids, edited by J. P. Bilezikian, M. A. Levine, and R. Marcus. New York, NY, Raven Press, Ltd., p. 107.

76. Cohn, D. V. and MacGregor, R. R. (1981): The biosynthesis, intracellular processing, and secretion of parathormone. Endocrine Rev. *2*:1.

77. Cohn, D. V., MacGregor, R. R., Chu, L. L. H., et al. (1974): Biosynthesis of proparathyroid hormone and parathyroid hormone. Chemistry, physiology and role of calcium in regulation. Am. J. Med. *56*:767.

78. Coleman, D. T., Fitzpatrick, L. A., and Bilezikian, J. P. (1994): Biochemical mechanisms of parathyroid hormone action. In: The Parathyroids, edited by J. P. Bilezikian, R. Marcus, and M. A. Levine. New York, NY, Raven Press, Ltd., p. 239.

79. Collins, W. T., Jr., Capen, C. C., Dobereiner, J., et al. (1977): Ultrastructural evaluation of parathyroid glands and thyroid C cells of cattle fed *Solanum malacoxylon*. Am. J. Pathol. *87*:603.

80. Cooper, C. W., Schwesinger, W. H., Ontjes, D. A., et al. (1972): Stimulation of secretion of pig thyrocalcitonin by gastrin and related hormonal peptides. Endocrinology *91*:1079.

81. Deftos, L. (1991): Chromogranin A: Its role in endocrine function and as an endocrine and neuroendocrine tumor marker. Endocrine Rev. *12*:181.

82. Deftos, L. J., Murray, T.M., Powell, D., et al. (1972): Radioimmunoassays for parathyroid hormone and calcitonins. In: Calcium, Parathyroid Hormone, and the Calcitonins, edited by R. V. Talmage and P. L. Munson. Amsterdam, The Netherlands, Excerpta Medica, p. 140.

83. DeGrandi, P. B., Kraehenbuhl, J. P., and Campiche, M. A. (1971): Ultrastructural localization of calcitonin in the parafollicular cells of the pig thyroid gland with cytochrome c-labeled antibody fragments. J. Cell Biol. *50*:446.

84. DeLuca, H. F. (1973): The kidney as an endocrine organ for the production of 1,25-dihydroxyvitamin D₃, a calcium-mobilizing hormone. N. Engl. J. Med. *289*:359.

85. DeLuca, H. F. (1974): Vitamin D—1973. Am. J. Med. *56*:871.

86. DeLuca, H. F. (1977): Vitamin D as a prohormone. Biochem. Pharmacol. *26*:563.

87. DeLuca, H. F. (1978): Vitamin D and calcium transport. Ann. N.Y. Acad. Sci. *307*:356.

88. DeLuca, H. F. and Schnoes, H. K. (1983): Vitamin D: Recent advances. Annu. Rev. Biochem. *52*:411.

89. Dennis, V. W. (1996): Phosphate metabolism: Contribution of different cellular compartments. Kidney Int. *49*:938.

90. DiBartola, S. P., Chew, D. J., and Jacobs, G. (1980): Quantitative urinalysis including 24-hour protein excretion in the dog. J. Am. Anim. Hosp. Assoc. *16*:537.

91. Dominguez, J. H. and Juhaszova, M. (1992): The renal sodium-calcium exchanger. J. Lab. Clin. Med. *1028*:2298

92. Done, S. H., Dobereiner, J., and Tokarnia, C. H. (1976): Systemic connective tissue calcification in cattle poisoned by *Solanum malacoxylon*: A histologic study. Br. Vet. J. *132*:28.

93. Dougherty, S. A., Center, S. A., and Dzanis, D. A. (1990): Salmon calcitonin as adjunct treatment for vitamin D toxicosis in a dog. J. Am. Vet. Med. Assoc. *196*:1269.

94. Ebashi, S. (1985): Ca²⁺ in biological systems. Experientia *41*:978.

95. Everhart-Caye, M., Inzucchi, S. E., Guinness-Henry, J., et al. (1996): Parathyroid hormone (PTH)-related protein (1-36) is equipotent to PTH(1-34) in humans. J. Clin. Endocrinol. Metab. *81*:199.

96. Favus, M. J. (1992): Intestinal absorption of calcium, magnesium, and phosphorus. In: Disorders of Bone and Mineral Metabolism, edited by F. L. Coe and M. J. Favus. New York, NY, Raven Press, Ltd., p. 57.

97. Felsenfeld, A. J. and Llach, F. (1993): Parathyroid gland function in chronic renal failure. Kidney Int. *43*:771.

98. Fenton, A. J., Kemp, B. E., Hammonds, R. G., Jr., et al. (1991): A potent inhibitor of osteoclastic bone resorption within a highly conserved pentapeptide region of parathyroid hormone-related protein; PTHrP[107-111]. Endocrinology *129*:3424.

99. Fenton, A. J., Kemp, B. E., Kent, G. N., et al. (1991): A carboxy-terminal peptide from the parathyroid hormone-related protein inhibits bone resorption by osteoclasts. Endocrinology *129*:1762.

100. Finco, D. R., Brown, S. A., Cooper, T., et al. (1994): Effects of parathyroid hormone depletion in dogs with induced renal failure. Am. J. Vet. Res. *55*:867.

101. Flanders, J. A. and Reimers, T. J. (1991): Radioimmunoassay for parathyroid hormone in cats. Am. J. Vet. Res. *52*:422.

102. Foster, G. V., Byfield, P. G. H., and Gudmundsson, T. V. (1972): Calcitonin. *In:* Clinics in Endocrinology and Metabolism, Vol. I, edited by I. MacIntyre. Philadelphia, PA, W. B. Saunders Co., p. 93.

103. Fraser, D., Jones, G., Kooh, S. W., et al. (1987): Calcium and phosphate metabolism. *In:* Fundamentals of Clinical Chemistry, 3rd ed., edited by N. W. Tietz. Philadelphia, PA, W.B. Saunders Co. p. 705.

104. Fraser, D. R. (1983): The physiological economy of vitamin D. Lancet, London, England *833*:969.

105. Fraser, D. R. and Kodicek, E. (1973): Regulation of 25-hydroxycholecalciferol-1α-hydroxylase activity in kidney by parathyroid hormone. Nature, London, England *241*:163.

106. Freitag, J., Martin, K. J., Hruska, D. A., et al. (1978): Impaired parathyroid hormone metabolism in patients with chronic renal failure. N. Engl. J. Med. *298*:29.

107. Fujii, H. and Isono, H. (1972): Ultrastructural observations on the parathyroid glands of the hen (*Gallus domesticus*). Arch. Histol. Jpn. *34*:155.

108. Gacad, M. A. and Adams, D. A. (1993): Identification of a competitive binding component in vitamin-D resistant new world primate cells with a low affinity but high capacity fo 1,25-dihydroxyvitamin D_3. J. Bone Miner. Res. *8*:27.

109. Garabedian, M., Holick, M. F., DeLuca, H. F., et al. (1972): Control of 25-hydroxycholecalciferol metabolism by parathyroid glands. Proc. Nat. Acad. Sci., USA *69*:1673.

110. Garrett, I. R. (1993): Bone destruction in cancer. Semin. Oncol. *20*:4.

111. Gerloff, B. J. and Swenson, E. P. (1996): Acute recumbency and marginal phosphorus deficiency in dairy cattle. J. Am. Vet. Med. Assoc. *208*:716.

112. Gilka, F. and Sugden, E. A. (1984): Ectopic mineralization and nutritional hyperparathyroidism in boars. Can. J. Comp. Med. *48*:102.

113. Goltzman, D., Bennett, H. P. J., Koutsilieris, M., et al. (1986): Studies of the multiple molecular forms of bioactive parathyroid hormone and parathyroid hormone-like substances. Recent Prog. Hormone Res. *42*:665.

114. Grau, H. and Dellmann, H. D. (1958): Über Tierärztliche Unterschiede der Epithelkörperchen unserer Haussäugetiere. Z. Zellforsch. Mikrosk. Anat. *64*:192.

115. Gray, R. W., Omdahl, J. L., Ghazarian, J. G., et al. (1972): 25-hydroxycholecalciferol-1α-hydroxylase: Subcellular location and properties. J. Biol. Chem. *247*:7528.

116. Gray, T. K. and Ontjes, D. A., (1975): Clinical aspects of thyrocalcitonin. Clin. Orthop. Related Res. *111*:238.

117. Gröne, A., Werkmeister, J. R., Steinmeyer, C. L., et al. (1994): Parathyroid hormone-related protein in normal and neoplastic tissues: Immunohistochemical localization and biochemical extraction. Vet. Pathol. *31*:308.

118. Grover, A. K. and Khan, I. (1992): Calcium pump isoforms: Diversity, selectivity and plasticity. Cell Calcium *13*:9.

119. Habener, J. F., Chang, H. T., and Potts, J. T., Jr. (1977): Enzymatic processing of proparathyroid hormone by cell-free extracts of parathyroid glands. Biochemistry *16*:3910.

120. Habener, J. F. and Potts, J. T., Jr. (1976): Chemistry, biosynthesis, secretion and metabolism of parathyroid hormone. Chapter 13. *In:* Handbook of Physiology, Section 7, Endocrinology Vol. II, Parathyroid Gland, edited by R. O. Greep and E. B. Astwood. Washington, D. C., American Physiological Society, p. 313.

121. Habener, J. F. and Potts, J. T., Jr. (1978): Biosynthesis of parathyroid hormone. N. Engl. J. Med. 299:580.

122. Habener, J. F., Powell, D., Murray, T. M., et al. (1971): Parathyroid hormone: Secretion and metabolism *in vitro*. Proc. Nat. Acad. Sci., USA *68*:2986.

123. Habener, J. F., Singer, F. R., Neer, R. M., et al. (1972): Metabolism of salmon and porcine calcitonin: An explanation for the increased potency of salmon calcitonin. *In:* Calcium, Parathyroid Hormone and the Calcitonins, edited by R. V. Talmage and P. L. Munson. Amsterdam, The Netherlands, Excerpta Medica, p. 152.

124. Hanafin, N. M., Chen, T. C., Heinrich, G., et al. (1995): Cultured human fibroblasts and not cultured human keratinocytes express a PTH/PTHrP receptor mRNA. J. Invest. Dermatol. *105*:133.

125. Harris, D. C. H., Gabow, P. A., Linas, S. L., et al. (1986): Prevention of hypercalcemia-induced renal concentrating defect and tissue calcium accumulation. Am. J. Physiol. *251*:F642.

126. Haussler, M. R., Boyce, D. W., Littledike, E. T., et al. (1971): A rapidly acting metabolite of vitamin D_3. Proc. Nat. Acad. Sci., USA *68*:177.

127. Haussler, M. R. and McCain, T. A. (1977): Basic and clinical concepts related to vitamin D metabolism and action. N. Engl. J. Med. *297*:974 (Part 1), 1041 (part 2).

128. Havinga, E. (1973): Vitamin D, example and challenge. Experientia *29*:1181.

129. Hazewinkel, H. A. W. (1991): Dietary influences on calcium homeostasis and the skeleton. *In:* Proc. 1st Purina Int. Nutr. Symp. Orlando, FL, Eastern States Vet. Conf., p. 51.

130. Henderson, J. E., Amizuka, N., Warshawsky, H., et al. (1995): Nucleolar localization of parathyroid hormone-related peptide enhances survival of chondrocytes under conditions that promote apoptotic cell death. Mol. Cell. Biol. *15*:4064.

131. Henry, H. L. and Norman, A. W. (1978): Vitamin D: Two dihydroxylated metabolites are required for normal chicken egg hatchability. Science *201*:835.

132. High, W. B., Black, H. E., and Capen, C. C. (1981): Histomorphometric evaluation of the effects of low dose parathyroid hormone administration on cortical bone remodeling in adult dogs. Lab. Invest. *44*:449.

133. High, W. B., Capen, C. C., and Black, H. E. (1981): Histomorphometric evaluation of the effects of inter-

mittent 1,25-dihydroxycholecalciferol administration on cortical bone remodeling in adult dogs. Am. J. Pathol. *104*:41.

134. Hoffsis, G. F., Capen, C. C., and Norman, A. W. (1978): The use of 1,25-dihydroxycholecalciferol in the prevention of parturient hypocalcemia in dairy cows. Bovine Pract. *13*:88.

135. Holick, M. F. (1981): The cutaneous photosynthesis of previtamin D_3: A unique photoendocrine system. J. Invest. Dermatol. *77*:51.

136. Holick, M. F. and Clark, M. B. (1978): The photobiogenesis and metabolism of vitamin D. Fed. Proc. *37*:2567.

137. Holick, M. F., Frommer, J. E., McNeill, S. C., et al. (1977): Photometabolism of 7-dehydrocholesterol to previtamin D_3 in skin. Biochem. Biophys. Res. Commun. *76*:107.

138. Holick, M. F., Ray, S., Chen, T. C., et al. (1994): A parathyroid hormone antagonist stimulates epidermal proliferation and hair growth in mice. Proc. Nat. Acad. Sci., USA *91*:8014.

139. Hruska, K. A., Kopelman, R., Rutherford, W. E., et al. (1975): Metabolism of immunoreactive parathyroid hormone in the dog. The role of the kidney and the effects of chronic renal disease. J. Clin. Invest. *56*:39.

140. Hruska, K. A., Martin, K., Mennes, P., et al. (1977): Degradation of parathyroid hormone and fragment production by the isolated perfused dog kidney. The effect of glomerular filtration rate and perfusate Ca^{++} concentrations. J. Clin. Invest. *60*:501.

141. Hughes, M. R. and Haussler, M. R. (1978): 1,25-dihydroxyvitamin D_3 receptors in parathyroid glands. J. Biol. Chem. *253*:1065.

142. Imamura, H., Sato, K., Shizume, K., et al. (1991): Urinary excretion of parathyroid hormone-related protein fragments in patients with humoral hypercalcemia of malignancy and hypercalcemia tumor-bearing nude mice. J. Bone Miner. Res. *6*:77.

143. Ingersoll, R. J., and Wasserman, R. H. (1971): Vitamin D_3-induced calcium-binding protein. J. Biol. Chem. *246*:2808.

144. Iqbal, S. J. (1994): Vitamin D metabolism and the clinical aspects of measuring metabolites. Ann. Clin. Biochem. *31*:109.

145. Isono, H., Sakurai, S., Fujii, H., et al. (1971): Ultrastructural change in the parathyroid gland of the phosphate treated newt, *Triturus pyrrhogaster* (Boié). Arch. Histol. Jpn. *33*:357.

146. Jacobs, J. W. (1985): Calcitonin gene expression. J. Bone Miner. Res. *3*:151.

147. Jorch, U. M., Anderson, C., Delaquerriere-Richardson, L. F. O., et al. (1982): Concentrations of plasma C-terminal immunoreactive parathyroid hormone in the standardized research Beagle. Am. J. Vet. Res. *43*:350.

148. Joyce, J. R., Pierce, K. R., Romane, W. M., et al.: (1971): Clinical study of nutritional secondary hyperparathyroidism in horses. J. Am. Vet. Med. Assoc. *158*:2033.

149. Kalina, M. and Pearse, A. G. E. (1971): Ultrastructural localization of calcitonin in C-cells of dog thyroid: An immunocytochemical study. Histochemie *26*:1.

150. Karaplis, A. C., Luz, A., Glowacki, J., et al. (1994): Lethal skeletal dysplasia from targeted disruption of the parathyroid hormone-related peptide gene. Genes Develop. *8*:277.

151. Karbach U. and Feldmeier H. (1993): The cecum is the site with the highest calcium absorption in rat intestine. Digest. Dis. Sci. *38*:1815.

152. Kasahara, H., Tsuchiya, M., Adachi, R., et al. (1992): Development of a C-terminal-region-specific radioimmunoassay of parathyroid hormone-related protein. Biomed. Res. *13*:155.

153. Kemper, B., Habener, J. F., Potts, J. T., Jr., et al. (1972): Parathyroid hormone: Identification of a biosynthetic precursor to parathyroid hormone. Proc. Nat. Acad. Sci., USA *69*:643.

154. Kempson, S. A. (1996): Peptide hormone action on renal phosphate handling. Kidney Int. *49*:1005.

155. Kodicek, E. (1974): The story of vitamin D from vitamin to hormone. Lancet, London, England *2*:325.

156. Kronenberg, H. M., Bringhurst, F. R., Segre, G. V., et al. (1994): Parathyroid hormone biosynthesis and metabolism. *In:* The Parathyroids, edited by J. P. Bilezikian, R. Marcus, and M. A. Levine. New York, NY, Raven Press, Ltd., p. 125.

157. Krook, L., Lutwak, L., Henrickson, P. A., et al.: (1971): Reversibility of nutritional osteoporosis: Physicochemical data on bones from an experimental study in dogs. J. Nutr. *101*:233.

158. Krook, L., Lutwak, L., and McEntee, K. (1969): Dietary calcium, ultimobranchial tumors and osteopetrosis in the bull. A syndrome of calcitonin excess? Am. J. Clin. Nutr. *22*:115.

159. Krook, L., Lutwak, L., McEntee, K., et al. (1971): Nutritional hypercalcitoninism in bulls. Cornell Vet. *61*:625.

160. Kruger, J. M., Osborne, C. A., Nachreiner, R. F., et al. (1996): Hypercalcemia and renal failure: Etiology, pathophysiology, diagnosis, and treatment. Vet. Clin. North Am., Small Anim. Pract. *26*:1417.

161. Lehner, N. D. M., Bullock, B. C., Clarkson, T. B., et al.: (1976): Biological activities of vitamin D_2 and D_3 for growing squirrel monkeys. Lab. Anim. Care *17*:483.

162. Long, P., Choi, G., and Rehmel, R. (1983): Oxyphil cells in a Red-tailed hawk (*Buteo jamaicensis*) with nutritional secondary hyperparathyroidism. Avian Dis. *27*:839.

163. Lötscher, M., Wilson, P., Nguyen, S., et al. (1996): New aspects of adaptation of rat renal Na-Pi contransporter to alterations in dietary phosphate. Kidney Int. *49*:1012.

164. MacGregor, R. R., Chu, L. L. H., Hamilton, J. W., et al. (1973): Studies on the subcellular localization of proparathyroid hormone and parathyroid hormone in the bovine parathyroid gland: Separation of newly synthesized from mature forms. Endocrinology *93*:1387.

165. MacGregor, R. R., Hamilton, J. W., and Cohn, D. V. (1978): The mode of conversion of proparathormone to parathormone by a particulate converting enzymic activity of the parathyroid gland. J. Biol. Chem. *253*:2012.

166. MacIntyre, I., Colston, K. W., Szelke, M., et al.: (1978): A survey of the hormonal factors that control calcium metabolism. Ann. N. Y. Acad. Sci. *307*:345.

167. MacIsaac, R. J., Caple, I. W., Danks, J. A., et al. (1991): Ontogeny of parathyroid hormone-related protein in the ovine parathyroid gland. Endocrinology *129*:757.

168. MacIsaac, R. J., Heath, J. A., Rodda, C. P., et al. (1991): Role of the fetal parathyroid glands and parathyroid hormone-related protein in the regulation of placental transport of calcium, magnesium, and inorganic phosphate. Reprod. Fertil. Develop. *3*:447.

169. Mallette, L. E. (1994): Parathyroid hormone and parathyroid hormone-related protein as polyhormones. *In:* The Parathyroids, edited by J. P. Bilezikian, R. Marcus, and M. A. Levine. New York, NY, Raven Press, Ltd., p. 171.

170. Mallette, L. E. and Tuma, S. N. (1984): A new radioimmunoassay for the midregion of canine parathyroid hormone. Miner. Electrolyte Metab. *10*:43.

171. Mangin, M., Ikeda, K., and Broadus, A. E. (1990): Structure of the mouse gene encoding parathyroid hormone-related protein. Gene *95*:195.

172. Martig, J. and Mayer, G. P. (1973): Diminished hypercalcemic response to parathyroid extract in prepartum cows. J. Dairy Sci. *56*:1042.

173. Martin, S. L. and Capen, C. C. (1980): Puerperal tetany. *In:* Current Veterinary Therapy VII, edited by R. W. Kirk. Philadelphia, PA, W. B. Saunders Co., p. 1027.

174. Martin, T. J. and Grill, V. (1992): Hypercalcemia and cancer. J. Steroid Biochem. Mol. Biol. *43*:123.

175. Mawer, E., B., Backhouse, J., Taylor, C. M., et al. (1973): Failure of formation of 1,25-dihydroxycholecalciferol in chronic renal insufficiency. Lancet, London, England 2:613.

176. Mayer, G. P. (1971): A rational basis for the prevention of parturient paresis. Bovine Pract. *6*:2.

177. Mayer, G. P., Habener, J. F., and Potts, J. T., Jr. (1973): Significance of plasma immunoreactive parathyroid hormone in hypocalcemic cows. *In:* Production Diseases in Farm Animals, edited by J. M. Payne, K. G. Hibbitt, and B. F. Sansom. London, England, Bailliere Tindall, p. 217.

178. Mayer, G. P. and Hurst, J. G. (1978): Comparison of the effects of calcium and magnesium on parathyroid hormone secretion rate in calves. Endocrinology *102*:1803.

179. Mayer, G. P., Ramberg, C. F., Jr., and Kronfeld, D. S. (1969): Calcium homeostasis in the cow. Clin. Orthop. Related Res. *62*:79.

180. McCauley, L. K., Rosol, T. J., Stromberg, P. C., et al. (1991): *In vivo* and *in vitro* effects of interleukin-1 and cyclosporin A on bone and lymphoid tissues in mice. Toxicol. Pathol. *19*:1.

181. McDowell, L. R. (1992): Calcium and phosphorus. *In:* Minerals in Animal and Human Nutrition, San Diego, CA, Academic Press, Inc., p. 26.

182. Melton, M. E., D'Anza, J. J., Wimbicus, S. A., et al. (1990): Parathyroid hormone-related protein and calcium homeostasis in lactating mice. Am. J. Physiol. *259*:E792.

183. Meuten, D. J., Cooper, B. J., Capen, C. C., et al. (1981): Hypercalcemia associated with an adenocarcinoma derived from the apocrine glands of the anal sac. Vet. Pathol. *18*:454.

184. Meuten, D. J., Kociba, G. J., Capen, C. C., et al. (1983): Hypercalcemia in dogs with lymphosarcoma.

Biochemical, ultrastructural, and histomorphometric investigations. Lab. Invest. *49*:553.

185. Meuten, D. J., Segre, G. V., Capen, C. C., et al. (1983): Hypercalcemia in dogs with adenocarcinoma derived from apocrine glands of the anal sac. Biochemical and histomorphometric investigations. Lab. Invest. *48*:428.

186. Midgett, R. J., Spielvogel, A. M., Coburn, J. W., et al. (1973): Studies on calciferol metabolism. VI. The renal production of the biologically active form of vitamin D, 1,25-dihydroxycholecalciferol; species, tissue and subcellular distribution. J. Clin. Endocrinol. Metab. *36*:1153.

187. Miller, R. J. (1992): Voltage sensitive Ca^{2+} channels. J. Biol. Chem. *267*:1403.

188. Mol, J. A., Kwant, M. M., Arnold, I. C. J., et al. (1991): Elucidation of the sequence of canine (pro)-calcitonin. A molecular biological and protein chemical approach. Regul. Pept. *35*:189.

189. Morris, M. L., Teeter, S. M., and Collins, D. R., (1971): The effects of the exclusive feeding of an all-meat dog food. J. Am. Vet. Med. Assoc. *158*:477.

190. Moseley, J. M. and Gillespie, M. T. (1995): Parathyroid hormone-related protein. Crit. Rev. Clin. Lab. Sci. *32*:299.

191. Moseley, J. M., Hayman, J. A., Danks, J. A., et al. (1991): Immunohistochemical detection of parathyroid hormone-related protein in human fetal epithelia. J. Clin. Endocrinol. Metab. *73*:478.

192. Muir, L. A., Hibbs, J. W., Conrad, H. R., et al. (1972): Effect of estrogen and progesterone on feed intake and hydroxyproline excretion following induced hypocalcemia in dairy cows. J. Dairy Sci. *55*:1613.

193. Murer H., Lötscher M., Kaissling B., et al. (1996): Renal brush border membrane Na/Pi- cotransport: Molecular aspects in PTH-dependent and dietary regulation. Kidney Int. *49*:1769.

194. Murray, T. M., Rao, L. G., and Rizzoli, R. E. (1994): Interactions of parathyroid hormone, parathyroid hormone-related protein, and their fragments with conventional and nonconventional receptor sites. *In:* The Parathyroids, edited by J. P. Bilezikian, M. A. Levine, and R. Marcus. New York, NY, Raven Press, Ltd., p. 185.

195. Nagode, L. A. and Chew, D. J. (1991): The use of calcitriol in treatment of renal disease of the dog and cat. *In:* Proc. 1st Purina Int. Nutr. Symp., Orlando, FL, Eastern States Vet. Conf., p. 39.

196. Nagode, L. A. and Chew, D. J. (1992): Nephrocalcinosis caused by hyperparathyroidism in progression of renal failure: Treatment with calcitriol. Seminar Vet. Med. Surg., Small Anim. *7*:202.

197. Nagode, L. A., Chew, D. J., and Podell, M. (1996): Benefits of calcitriol therapy and serum phosphorus control in dogs and cats with chronic renal failure. Vet. Clin. North Am., Small Anim. Pract. *26*:1293.

198. Nakagami, K., Warshawsky, H., and LeBlond, C. P. (1971): The elaboration of protein and carbohydrate by rat parathyroid cells as revealed by electron microscope radioautography. J. Cell Biol. *51*:596.

199. Nemere, I. and Norman, A. W. (1986): Parathyroid hormone stimulates calcium transport in perfused duodena from normal chicks: Comparison with the rapid (transcaltachic) effect of 1,25-dihydroxyvitamin D_3. Endocrinology *119*:1406.

200. Norman, A. W. (1980): 1,25-$(OH)_2$-D_3 as a steroid hormone. *In:* Vitamin D: Molecular Biology and Clinical Nutrition, edited by A. W. Norman. New York, NY, Marcel Dekker, Inc., p. 197.
201. Norman, A. W. and Henry, H. (1974): 1,25-Dihydroxycholecalciferol—a hormonally active form of vitamin D_3. Recent Prog. Hormone Res. *30*:43.
202. Norman, A. W. and Henry, H. (1974): The role of the kidney and vitamin D metabolism in health and disease. Clin. Orthop. Related Res. *98*:258.
203. Norman, A. W. and Henry, H. L. (1979): Vitamin D to 1,25-dihydroxycholecalciferol: Evolution of a steroid hormone. Trends Biochem. Sci. January: 14.
204. Nussbaum, S. R. and Potts, J. T., Jr. (1994): Advances in immunoassays for parathyroid hormone. *In:* The Parathyroids, edited by J. P. Bilezikian, R. Marcus, and M. A. Levine. New York, NY, Raven Press, Ltd., p. 157.
205. Olson, E. B., Jr., DeLuca, H. F., and Potts, J. T., Jr. (1972): The effect of calcitonin and parathyroid hormone on calcium transport of isolated intestine. *In:* Calcium, Parathyroid Hormone and the Calcitonins, edited by R. V. Talmage and P. L. Munson. Amsterdam, The Netherlands, Excerpta Medica, p. 240.
206. Omdall, J. L. and DeLuca, H. F. (1973): Regulation of vitamin D metabolism and function. Physiol. Rev. *53*:327.
207. Orloff, J. J., Ganz, M. B., Ribaudo, A. E., et al. (1992): Analysis of PTHRP binding and signal transduction mechanisms in benign and malignant squamous cells. Am. J. Physiol. *262*:E599.
208. Orloff, J. J., Reddy, D., dePapp, A. E., et al. (1994): Parathyroid hormone-related protein as a prohormone: Posttranslational processing and receptor interactions. Endocrine Rev. *15*:40.
209. Ornoy, A., Goodwin, D., Noff, D., et al. (1978): 24,-25-Dihydroxyvitamin D is a metabolite of vitamin D essential for bone formation. Nature, London, England *276*:517.
210. Osborne, C. A. and Stevens, J. B. (1973): Pseudohyperparathyroidism in the dog. J. Am. Vet. Med. Assoc. *162*:125.
211. Pandian, M. R., Morgan, C. H., Carlton, E., et al. (1992): Modified immunoradiometric assay of parathyroid hormone-related protein: Clinical application in the differential diagnosis of hypercalcemia. Clin. Chem. *38*:282.
212. Parfitt, A. M. (1977): The cellular basis of bone turnover and bone loss. Clin. Orthop. Related Res. *127*:236.
213. Parfitt, A. M. (1987): Bone and plasma calcium homeostasis. Bone *8* (Suppl. 1):S1.
214. Parsons, J. A. and Robinson, C. J. (1971): Calcium shift into bone causing transient hypocalcemia after injection of parathyroid hormone. Nature, London, England *230*:581.
215. Philbrick, W. M., Wysolmerski, J. J., Galbrath, S., et al. (1996): Defining the roles of parathyroid hormone-related protein in normal physiology. Physiol. Rev. *76*:127.
216. Pliam, N. B., Nyiredy, K. O., and Arnaud, C. D. (1982): Parathyroid hormone receptors in avian bone cells. Proc. Nat. Acad. Sci., USA *79*:2061.
217. Pollak, M. R., Brown, E. M., Chou, Y.-H. W., et al. (1993): Mutations in the human Ca^{2+}- sensing receptor gene cause familial hypocalciuric hypercalcemia and neonatal severe hypercalcemia. Cell *75*:1297.
218. Potts, J. T., Jr. (1976): Chemistry and physiology of parathyroid hormone. Clin. Endocrinol. *5* (Suppl.):307.
219. Powell, G. J., Southby, J., Danks, J. A., et al. (1991): Localization of parathyroid hormone-related protein in breast cancer metastases: Increased incidence in bone compared to other sites. Cancer Res. *51*:3059.
220. Prager, D., Rosenblatt, J. D., and Ejima, E. (1994): Hypercalcemia, parathyroid hormone-related protein expression and human T-cell leukemia virus infection. Leuk. Lymphoma *14*:395.
221. Raisz, L. G. and Kream, B. E. (1983): Regulation of bone formation. N. Engl. J. Med. *309*:29.
222. Raisz, L. G., Trummel, C. L., Holick, M. F., et al. (1972): 1,25-dihydroxycholecalciferol: A potent stimulator of bone resorption in tissue culture. Science *175*:768.
223. Rasmussen, H., Wong, M., Bikle, D., et al. (1972): Hormonal control of the renal conversion of 25-hydroxcholecalciferol to 1,25-dihydroxycholecalciferol. J. Clin. Invest. *51*:2502.
224. Ratcliffe, W. A. (1992): Role of parathyroid hormone-related protein in lactation. Clin. Endocrinol. *37*:402.
225. Reaven, E. P. and Reaven, G. M. (1974): A quantitative ultrastructural study of microtubule assembly and granule accumulation in parathyroid glands of control, phosphate, and colchicine treated rats. *In:* 56th Annu. Meeting of The Endocrine Society (p. A_182, Abstract).
226. Resnick, S. (1972): Hypocalcemia and tetany in the dog. Vet. Med./Small Anim. Clin. *67*:637.
227. Reynolds, J. J., Holick, M. F., and DeLuca, H. F. (1973): The role of vitamin D metabolites in bone resorption. Calcif. Tissue Res. *12*:295.
228. Rice, B. F., Roth, L. M., Cole, F. E. et al. (1975): Hypercalcemia and neoplasia. Biologic, biochemical and ultrastructural studies of a hypercalcemia-producing Leydig cell tumor of the rat. Lab. Invest. *33*:426.
229. Riond, J.-L., Kocabagli, N., Cloux, F., et al. (1996): Parathyroid hormone-related protein in the colostrum of paretic post parturient dairy cows. Vet. Rec. *138*:333.
230. Riond J.-L., Kocabagli N., Forrer R., et al. (1995): Repeated daytime measurements of the concentrations of PTHrP and other components of bovine milk. J. Anim. Physiol. Anim. Nutr. *74*:194.
231. Rodan, G. A. and Martin, T. J. (1981): The role of osteoblasts in hormonal control of bone resorption—A hypothesis. Calcif. Tissue Int. *33*:349.
232. Rosol, T. J. and Capen, C. C. (1988): Pathogenesis of humoral hypercalcemia of malignancy. Domestic Anim. Endocrinol. *5*:1.
233. Rosol, T. J. and Capen, C. C. (1992): Biology of disease: Mechanisms of cancer-induced hypercalcemia. Lab. Invest. *67*:680.
234. Rosol, T. J., Chew, D. J., Nagode, L. A., et al. (1995): Pathophysiology of calcium metabolism. Vet. Clin. Pathol. *24*:49.
235. Rosol, T. J., Nagode, L. A., Couto, C. G., et al. (1992): Parathyroid hormone (PTH)-related protein, PTH, and

1,25-dihydroxyvitamin D in dogs with cancer-associated hypercalcemia. Endocrinology *131*:1157.

236. Rosol, T. J., Nagode, L. A., Robertson, J. T., et al. (1994): Humoral hypercalcemia of malignancy associated with ameloblastoma in a horse. J. Am. Vet. Med. Assoc. *204*:1930.

237. Rosol, T. J., Steinmeyer, C. L., McCauley, L. K., et al. (1995): Sequences of the cDNAs encoding canine parathyroid hormone-related protein and parathyroid hormone. Gene *160*:241.

238. Roth, S. I. and Capen, C. C. (1974): Ultrastructural and functional correlations of the parathyroid glands. *In:* International Review of Experimental Pathology, Vol. 13, edited by G. W. Richter and M. A. Epstein. New York, NY, Academic Press, Inc., p. 162.

239. Rouse, D. and Suki, W. N. (1990): Renal control of extracellular calcium. Kidney Int. *38*:700.

240. Rowland, G. N., Capen, C. C., Young, D. M., et al. (1972): Microradiographic evaluation of bone from cows with experimental hypervitaminosis D, diet-induced hypocalcemia, and naturally occurring parturient paresis. Calcif. Tissue Res. *9*:179.

241. Schipani, E., Langman, C. B., Parfitt, A. M., et al. (1996): Constitutively activated receptors for parathyroid hormone and parathyroid hormone-related peptide in Jansen's metaphyseal chondrodysplasia. N. Engl. J. Med. *335*:708.

242. Schröder, B., Käppner, H., Failing, K., et al. (1995): Mechanisms of intestinal phosphate transport in small ruminants. Br. J. Nutr. *74*:635.

243. Segre, G. V. (1994): Receptors for parathyroid hormone and parathyroid hormone-related protein. *In:* The Parathyroids, edited by J. P. Bilezikian, R. Marcus, and M. A. Levine. New York, NY, Raven Press, Ltd., p. 213.

244. Sejersted, O. M., Steen, P. A., and Kiil, F. (1984): Inhibition of transcellular NaCl reabsorption in dog kidneys during hypercalcemia. Acta Physiol. Scand. *120*:543.

245. Seymour, J. F. and Gagel, R. F. (1993): Calcitriol: The major humoral mediator of hypercalcemia in Hodgkin's and non-Hodgkin's lymphomas. Blood *82*:1383.

246. Shannon, W. A. and Roth, S. I. (1971): Acid phosphatase activity in mammalian parathyroid glands. *In:* Proc. of the 29th Annu. Elect. Microsc. Soc. Amer., edited by C. J. Arceneaux. Baton Rouge, LA, Claitor's Publishing, p. 516.

247. Sherding, R. G., Meuten, D. J., Chew, D. J., et al. (1980): Primary hypoparathyroidism in the dog. J. Am. Vet. Med. Assoc. *176*:439.

248. Shirazi-Beechey, S. P., Penny, J. I., Dyer, J., et al. (1996): Epithelial phosphate transport in ruminants, mechanisms and regulation. Kidney Int. *49*:992.

249. Siesjö, B. K. (1989): Calcium and cell death. Magnesium *8*:223.

250. Silve, C. M., Hradek, G. T., Jones, A. L. et al. (1982): Parathyroid hormone receptor in intact embryonic chicken bone: Characterization and cellular localization. J. Cell Biol. *94*:379.

251. Silver, J. (1992): Regulation of parathyroid hormone synthesis and secretion. *In:* Disorders of Bone and Mineral Metabolism, edited by F. L. Coe and M. J. Favus. New York, NY, Raven Press, Ltd., p. 83.

252. Silverstein, D., Barac-Nieto, M., and Spitzer, A. (1996): Mechanism of renal phosphate retention during growth. Kidney Int. *49*:1023.

253. Singer, F. R., Melvin, K. W., and Mills, B. G. (1976): Acute effects of calcitonin on osteoclasts in man. Clin. Endocrinol. *5* (Suppl.): 333.

254. Soares, J. H., Jr. (1995): Phosphorus bioavailability. *In:* Bioavailability of Nutrients for Animals: Amino Acids, Minerals, and Vitamins. San Diego, CA, Academic Press, Inc., p. 257.

255. Steenbergh, P. H., Hoppener, J. W. M., Zandberg, J., et al. (1984): Calcitonin gene related peptide coding sequence is conserved in the human genome and is expressed in medullary thyroid carcinoma. J. Clin. Endocrinol. Metab. *59*:358.

256. Sutton, R. A. L. and Dirks, J. H. (1978): Renal handling of calcium. Fed. Proc. *37*:2112.

257. Suva, L. J., Winslow, G. A., Wettenhall, R. E. H., et al. (1987): A parathyroid hormone-related protein implicated in malignant hypercalcemia: Cloning and expression. Science *237*:893.

258. Swaminathan, R., Bates, R. F. L., and Care, A. D. (1972): Fresh evidence for a physiological role of calcitonin in calcium homeostasis. J. Endocrinol. *54*:525.

259. Szenci, O., Chew, B. P., Bajcsy, A. C., et al. (1994): Total and ionized calcium in parturient dairy cows and their calves. J. Dairy Sci. *77*:1100.

260. Tanaka, T. and DeLuca, H. F. (1974): Stimulation of 24,25-dihydroxyvitamin D_3 production by 1,25-dihydroxyvitamin D_3. Science *183*:1198.

261. Thiede, M. A. (1994): Parathyroid hormone-related protein: A regulated calcium-mobilizing product of the mammary gland. J. Dairy Sci. *77*:1952.

262. Thiele, J. and Wermbter, G. (1974): Die Feinstruktur der Aktivierten Hauptzelle der menschlichen Parathyroidea. Eine Darstellung mit Hilfe de Gefrierärztztechnik. Virchows Arch. *15*:251.

263. Thompson, G. E. (1993): Parathyroid hormone-related protein and mammary blood flow in the sheep. Exp. Physiol. *78*:499.

264. Thompson, K. G., Jones, L. P., Smylie, W. A., et al. (1984). Primary hyperparathyroidism in German Shepherd dogs: A disorder of probable genetic origin. Vet. Pathol. *21*:370.

265. Van Pelt, R. W. and Caley, M. T. (1974): Nutritional secondary hyperparathyroidism in Alaskan Red Fox kits. J. Wildlife Dis. *10*:47.

266. Vortkamp, A., Lee, K., Lanske, B., et al. (1996): Regulation of rate of cartilage differentiation by Indian hedgehog and PTH-related protein. Science *273*:613.

267. Walters, M. R. (1992): Newly identified actions of the vitamin D endocrine system. Endocrine Rev. *13*:719.

268. Walthall, J. C. and McKenzie, R. A. (1976): Osteodystrophia fibrosa in horses at pasture in Queensland: Field and laboratory observations. Aust. Vet. J. *52*:11.

269. Wasserman, R. H., Corradino, R. A., and Krook, L. (1975): *Cestrum diurnum*. A domestic plant with 1,25-dihydroxycholecalciferol-like activity. Biochem. Biophys. Res. Commun. *62*:85.

270. Wasserman, R. H. and Fullmer, C. S. (1983): Calcium transport proteins, calcium absorption, and vitamin D. Annu. Rev. Physiol. *45*:375.

271. Wasserman, R. H. and Taylor, A. N. (1972): Metabolic roles of fat-soluble vitamins D, E, and K. Annu. Rev. Biochem. *41*:179.

272. Weaver, C. M. (1990): Assessing calcium status and metabolism. J. Nutr. *120*:1470.

273. Wecksler, W. R., Henry, H. L., and Norman, A. W. (1977): Studies on the mode of action of calciferol: Subcellular localization of 1,25-dihydroxyvitamin D_3 in chicken parathyroid glands. Arch. Biochem. Biophys. *183*:168.

274. Weir, E. C. (1992): Hypercalcemia and malignancy. Proc. 10th American College of Veterinary Internal Medicine Forum, San Diego, CA.

275. Weir, E. C., Burtis, W. J., Morris, C. A., et al. (1988): Isolation of 16,000-dalton parathyroid hormone-like proteins from two animal tumors causing humoral hypercalcemia of malignancy. Endocrinology *123*:2744.

276. Weir, E. C., Norrdin, R. W., Matus, R. E., et al. (1988): Humoral hypercalcemia of malignancy in canine lymphosarcoma. Endocrinology *122*:602.

277. Weisbrode, S. E. and Capen, C. C. (1974): Ultrastructural evaluation of the effects of calcitonin on bone in thyroparathyroidectomized rats administered vitamin D. Am. J. Pathol. *77*:395.

278. Weisbrode, S. E., Capen, C. C., and Nagode, L. N. (1973): Fine structural and enzymatic evaluation of bone in thyroparathyroidectomized rats receiving various levels of vitamin D. Lab. Invest. *28*:29.

279. Werkmeister, J. R., Rosol, T. J., McCauley, L. K., et al. (1993): Parathyroid hormone-related protein production by normal human keratinocytes *in vitro*. Exp. Cell Res. *208*:68.

280. Wilson, J. W., Harris, S. G., Moore, W. D., et al. (1974): Primary hyperparathyroidism in a dog. J. Am. Vet. Med. Assoc. *164*:942.

281. Winkler, H. and Fischer-Colbrie, R. (1992): Chromogranins A and B: The first 25 years and future perspectives. Neuroscience *49*:497.

282. Witzel, D. A. and Littledike, E. T. (1973): Suppression of insulin secretion during induced hypocalcemia. Endocrinology *93*:761.

283. Wolfe, H. J. (1982): Calcitonin: Perspectives and current concepts. J. Endocrinol. Invest. *5*:423.

284. Wong, G. L. (1986): Skeletal effects of parathyroid hormone. J. Bone Miner. Res. *4*:103.

285. Wysolmerski, J. J. and Broadus, A. E. (1994): Hypercalcemia of malignancy: The central role of parathyroid hormone-related protein. Annu. Rev. Med. *45*:189.

286. Wysolmerski, J. J., McCaughern-Carucci, J. F., Daifotis, A. G., et al. (1995): Overexpression of parathyroid hormone-related protein or parathyroid hormone in transgenic mice impairs branching morphogenesis during mammary gland development. Development *121*:3539.

287. Yamaguchi, A., Kohno, Y., Yamazaki, T., et al. (1986): Bone in the marmoset: A resemblance to vitamin D-dependent rickets, type II. Calcif. Tissue Int. *39*:22.

288. Yanagawa, N. and Lee, D. B. N. (1992): Renal handling of calcium and phosphorus. *In:* Disorders of Bone and Mineral Metabolism, edited by F. L. Coe and M. J. Favus. New York, NY, Raven Press, Ltd., p. 3.

289. Yang, K. H., dePapp, A. E., Soifer, N. E., et al. (1994): Parathyroid hormone-related protein: Evidence for isoform- and tissue-specific posttranslational processing. Biochemistry *33*:7460.

290. Yarrington, J. T., Capen, C. C., and Black, H. E., (1977): Inhibition of bone resorption: An important mechanism in the pathogenesis of parturient hypocalcemia. Bovine Pract. *12*:30.

291. Yarrington, J. T., Capen, C. C., Black, H. E. et al. (1977): Effects of low calcium prepartal diet on calcium homeostatic mechanisms in the cow: Morphologic and biochemical studies. J. Nutr. *107*:2244.

292. Yarrington, J. T., Capen, C. C., Black, H. E., et al. (1977): Effect of dichloromethane diphosphonate on calcium homeostatic mechanisms in pregnant cows. Am. J. Pathol. *87*:165.

293. Youshak, M. S. and Capen, C. C. (1970): Fine structural alterations in parathyroid glands of chickens with osteopetrosis. Am. J. Pathol. *60*:257.

294. Youshak, M. S. and Capen, C. C. (1971): Ultrastructural evaluation of ultimobranchial glands from normal and osteopetrotic chickens. Gen. Comp. Endocrinol. *16*:430.

295. Zarrin, K. (1977): Naturally occurring parafollicular cell carcinoma of the thyroids in dogs. A histological and ultrastructural study. Vet. Pathol. *14*:556.

References Added in Proof

296. American Society for Bone and Mineral Research, Special Committee on Nomenclature (2000): Proposed standard nomenclature for new tumor necrosis factor members involved in the regulation of bone resorption. Bone *27*:761.

297. Angeletti, R. H., D'Amico, T., and Russell, J. (2000): Regulation of parathyroid secretion. Chromogranins, chemokines, and calcium. Adv. Exp. Med. Biol. *482*:217.

298. Aubin, J. E. and Bonnelye, E. (2000): Osteoprotegerin and its ligand: A new paradigm for regulation of osteoclastogenesis and bone resorption. Osteoporosis Int. *11*:905.

299. Goff, J. P. (2000): Pathophysiology of calcium and phosphorus disorders. Vet. Clin. North Am., Food Anim. Pract. *16*:319.

300. Hofbauer, L. C. (1999): Osteoprotegerin ligand and osteoprotegerin: Novel implications for osteoclast biology and bone metabolism. Europ. J. Endocrinol. *141*:195.

301. Hofbauer, L. C., Khosla, S., Dunstan, C. R., et al. (2000): The roles of osteoprotegerin and osteoprotegerin ligand in the paracrine regulation of bone resorption. J. Bone Miner. Res. *15*:2.

302. Rodan, G. A., and Martin, T. J. (2000): Therapeutic approaches to bone diseases. Science *289*:1508.

303. Schoenmakers, I., Nap, R. C., Mol, J. A., et al. (1999): Calcium metabolism: An overview of its hormonal regulation and interrelation with skeletal integrity. Vet. Quart. *21*:147.

304. Suda, T., Takahashi, N., Udagawa, N., et al. (1999): Modulation of osteoclast differentiation and function

by the new members of the tumor necrosis factor receptor and ligand families. Endocrine Rev. *20*:345.

305. Takahashi, N., Udagawa, N., and Suda, T. (1999): A new member of tumor necrosis factor ligand family, ODF/OPGL/TRANCE/RANKL, regulates osteoclast differentiation and function. Biochem. Biophys. Res. Commun. *256*:449.

306. Teitelbaum, S. L. (2000): Bone resorption by osteoclasts. Science *289*:1504.

The Endocrine Pancreas

P. A. Martin and M. H. Crump

5

INTRODUCTION

The pancreas is a glandular organ which has exocrine and endocrine roles in the ultimate regulation of the nutrition of animal cells. The exocrine secretions of the pancreas are controlled by pancreatic and gastrointestinal hormones and by the autonomic nervous system. As an exocrine gland, the pancreas secretes pancreatic juice, which consists of digestive enzymes, electrolytes, and water. The enzymes released in pancreatic juice are required for the digestion of complex substrates in food so the breakdown products of carbohydrates, proteins, and fats may be absorbed across the absorptive brush border of epithelial cells of the mucosa of the small intestine. The pancreatic enzymes are adsorbed on the glycocalyx and act in concert with brush border enzymes to ensure that the final breakdown of substrate occurs close to the cell membrane of absorptive epithelial cells. The breakdown products then enter the systemic circulation via the portal vein and lymphatics. The electrolytes from the exocrine pancreas aid in the maintenance of an optimum pH in the small intestine for enzyme action and in the proper acid-base balance of the body.

ANATOMY

The pancreas is located in the upper right quadrant of the abdominal cavity in close association with the duodenum. The pancreas is composed primarily of parenchymal or functional tissue with very little stromal or connective tissue and is supplied with extensive neural and vascular networks. The endocrine cells of the pancreas constitute 2 to 3% of the total pancreatic mass and are located in clusters of cells called islets of Langerhans. The cells of the pancreatic islets are richly innervated by sympathetic and parasympathetic branches of the autonomic nervous system, which influence the release of pancreatic hormones.

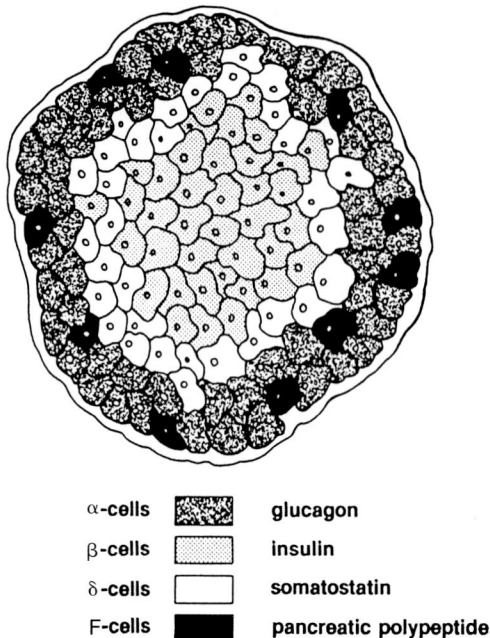

α-cells	(glucagon pattern)	glucagon
β-cells	(insulin pattern)	insulin
δ-cells	(somatostatin)	somatostatin
F-cells	(black)	pancreatic polypeptide

Fig. 5-1. Cell components of the pancreatic islet and their principal secretions.

Four functional cell types have been described in the islets of Langerhans: α, β, δ, and F (Fig. 5-1). These cell types are not randomly distributed within each islet. The β cells are located in the center of each islet and account for 60% of the total number of islet cells. The α cells are located in the periphery or outer part of the islet and comprise 30% of the islet cells. The δ cells are located between the α and β cells and account for approximately 10% of the islet cells. The F cells are not always found, but when present, they are few in number and are located in association with the α cells.

PANCREATIC HORMONES

As an endocrine gland, the pancreatic islets of Langerhans secrete insulin, glucagon, somatostatin, and pancreatic polypeptide. These hormones are secreted into the interstitial fluid, diffuse into capillaries, and are then carried by the portal vein to the liver and to all parts of the body. The major overall function of the pancreatic islets is the regulation of blood glucose through the action of pancreatic hormones. Insulin and glucagon are the major regulators of

blood glucose and, together, they maintain fairly stable concentrations of glucose and other nutrients in the blood. Insulin, which is synthesized and released from β cells, lowers blood glucose by facilitating the movement of glucose across cell membranes for energy or storage, thereby lowering the concentration of blood glucose. Conversely, glucagon, secreted by the α cells of islets, increases the concentration of glucose in the blood by stimulating hepatic glycogenolysis and gluconeogenesis. The endocrine regulation of glucose metabolism is of utmost importance in mammalian homeostasis because every cell requires an adequate supply of energy for survival. Insulin and glucagon are key hormones for the regulation of glucose metabolism.

Pancreatic somatostatin, a paracrine hormone secreted by δ cells, inhibits the release of insulin and glucagon. Paracrine hormones are synthesized and released by endocrine cells into the interstitial fluid and interact locally with membrane receptors of adjacent cells without entering the systemic circulation (see Chapter 1, Fig. 1-1C). The role of pancreatic polypeptide, secreted by F cells, has not been clearly established, but it appears to participate in the regulation of food intake by acting on the satiety center located in the hypothalamus. Thus, pancreatic polypeptide may indirectly contribute to the control of levels of glucose in the blood. In addition to these pancreatic hormones, other endocrine secretions, such as growth hormone, catecholamines, and glucocorticoids play important roles in the regulation of glucose metabolism by increasing glycogenolysis and gluconeogenesis.

The concentration of blood glucose varies among domestic animals (Table 5-1). Nonruminant animals, regardless of age, have concentrations of blood glucose which are in the range of 50 to 175 mg/dl. The concentration of glucose in the blood of ruminants varies with the age of the animal and development of the gastrointestinal tract. Adult ruminants have a well-developed, multicompartmental stomach which acts as a fermentation vat. Fermentation of carbohydrates takes place by bacteria and protozoa in the rumen, reticulum, and omasum

Table 5-1 *Levels of Glucose in the Blood in Normal, Pancreatectomized, and Alloxan-*
Induced Diabetic Animals[a]

Species	Blood Glucose in Normal Animals (mg/dl)		Treatment	Blood Glucose after Treatment (mg/dl)
Dog	90 ± 8[b]	65–118[c]	Pancreatectomized	475–510[c]
Cat	63 ± 7	50–75	Pancreatectomized	338–1050
Cattle	57 ± 7	45–75	Alloxan-induced	800–1400
Horse	95 ± 8	75–115	NA	— — —
Sheep	68 ± 6	50–80	Alloxan-induced	140–200
Goat	63 ± 7	50–75	Pancreatectomized	75–165
Llama	128 ± 2	103–160	NA	— — —
Pig	119 ± 2	85–150	NA	— — —
Monkey	107 ± 1	85–130	Pancreatectomized	200–400
Rabbit	73 ± 1	50–93	Alloxan-induced	476–581
			Pancreatectomized	400–500
Mouse	—[d]	62–175	Alloxan-induced	111–371
Rat	—[d]	50–135	Alloxan-induced	396–933
Duck	—[d]	97–133	Alloxan-induced	118–126

[a]For each species, normal and post-treatment values are from different groups of animals.
[b]Mean ± SD is shown for column data.
[c]Range is shown for column data.
[d]Mean was not provided and could not be calculated from data in the original publication.
NA = Not applicable. Studies not done or reported.
Adapted from: M. X. Zarrow, et al., *In:* Experimental Endocrinology. A Sourcebook of Basic Techniques, 1964, p. 390; J. J. Kaneko, et al., *In:* Clinical Biochemistry of Domestic Animals, 1997, p. 64; K. Hrapkiewiez, et al., *In:* Clinical Laboratory Animal Medicine, 1998, p. 261.

under anaerobic conditions, and the main by-products of incomplete oxidation are the short-chain fatty acids: Acetic, propionic, and butyric. Propionic acid is gluconeogenic, whereas acetic and butyric acids are ketogenic. These fatty acids are absorbed passively from the gastrointestinal tract and converted into glucose and fats. Glucose in the feed rarely ever reaches the small intestine because microbes in the forestomach compartments of the adult ruminant stomach metabolize all available carbohydrates. Thus, adult ruminants are in a constant state of gluconeogenesis and have blood glucose concentrations of only 45 to 80 mg/dl (Table 5-1). In contrast, neonatal ruminants have blood concentrations of glucose which resemble those of nonruminant animals. Blood glucose concentrations in young ruminants decline as the gastrointestinal tract becomes fully developed. Adult values for blood glucose concentrations in the bovine are attained by 6 months of age.

Diabetes mellitus is a metabolic dysfunction that results in hyperglycemia. This dysfunction is caused by insufficient production of insulin or by the development of resistance of tissues to respond to insulin. Cells and tissues of diabetic animals do not receive adequate nutrition because insulin is either not present in amounts sufficient to aid with the cellular uptake of glucose and amino acids or the cells of these animals are resistant to the actions of insulin. Hyperglycemia results in high levels of glucose in the glomerular filtrate which exceed the absorptive maximum of the kidney tubules. Excretion of glucose in the urine (**glucosuria**) along with water and electrolytes results in an osmotic diuresis, excessive loss of urine (**polyuria**), and increased thirst and ingestion of water (**polydipsia**). The clinical *sequelae* include faulty glucose, fatty acid, and amino acid metabolism, water and electrolyte loss, and eventually, metabolic acidosis. These metabolic disturbances will lead to coma and death unless insulin is administered therapeutically. Diabetic animals develop a voracious appetite (**polyphagia**) due to the lack of insulin to suppress the satiety center. Hence, polyphagia, glucosuria, polydipsia, and polyuria are considered the four cardinal signs of diabetes mellitus.

β CELL POLYPEPTIDES

Insulin

Structure of Insulin

Insulin is a polypeptide with a molecular weight of approximately 6,000 daltons. It consists of two chains, α and β, that are connected by two disulfide bonds. The amino acid sequence of canine and porcine insulin along with individual species differences are shown in Figure 5-2. The amino acid differences among species occur mainly at positions 8, 9, and 10 of the α chain. The administration of insulin from one species to another species will effectively lower the blood levels of glucose, but will eventually lead to the production of antibodies to the heterologous insulin. Differences in antigenicity of insulin from different species are directly related to variations in the amino acid sequence of the insulin molecule.

Biosynthesis of Insulin

The synthesis and secretion of insulin by β cells is stimulated by an increase in the blood concentration of glucose reaching the islets. The transcription of mRNA for the biosynthesis of insulin takes place in the nucleus and translation begins in the rough endoplasmic reticulum with the formation of preproinsulin on polysomes. This molecule (preproinsulin) consists of an N-terminal prepeptide, the β chain of insulin, a connecting peptide, and the α chain of insulin. Proinsulin is formed when the 23 amino acids of the N-terminal prepeptide are cleaved in the rough endoplasmic reticulum and the two disulfide bonds form between the α and β chains (see Chapter 1, Fig. 1-4). After the proinsulin molecule is transferred from the rough endoplasmic reticulum to the Golgi apparatus for packaging, the connecting peptide separates from the active moiety in the granules where insulin and the connecting peptide are stored. Insulin and connecting peptide are released from the cytosol of β cells in a ratio of 1:1.

Human insulin has been synthesized by genetically engineered *E. coli* bacteria. The α and β chains are produced separately and then combined to form the active molecule. The synthetic hormone is preferred for human patients because antibodies to insulin may develop in patients treated with heterologous, bovine or porcine insulin due to structural variations in insulin molecules originating from different species (Fig. 5-2). Synthetic, species-specific insulin for domestic animals is not commercially available.

Insulin: Dog, Pig, Sperm Whales and Fin Whales

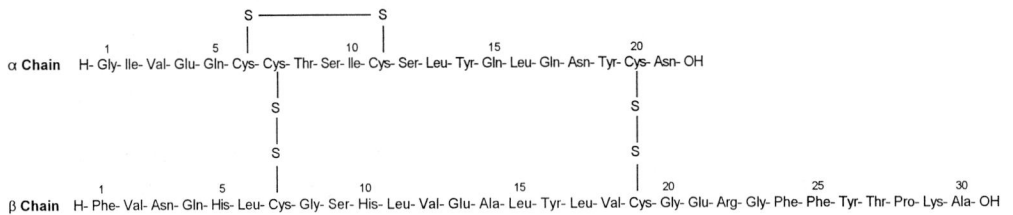

Species	α Chain Position					β Chain Position
	8	9	10	17	18	30
Human	--	--	--	--	--	Thr
Domestic Cat	Ala	--	Val	Glu	His	--
Cattle	Ala	--	Val	--	--	--
Sheep and Goat	Ala	Gly	Val	--	--	--
Horse	--	Gly	--	--	--	--
Elephant	--	Gly	Val	--	--	Thr
Rabbit	--	--	--	--	--	Ser

Fig. 5-2. The structure of insulin in various species. (Adapted from: D. F. Steiner,[112] 1976 and G. Hallden, et al.,[41] 1986).

Release of Insulin from Secretory Granules

Secretion of insulin takes place when the membrane-bound insulin granules translocate through the cytosol of the β cells and fuse with the cell membrane. The insulin and the connecting peptide are co-released from the β cell by exocytosis. The insulin and connecting peptide molecules then diffuse into capillaries and enter the portal system. Presently, it is not known if the connecting peptide has biological activity.

The effects of glucose on insulin release from β cells are believed to be mediated by the following secondary messengers: cAMP, inositol triphosphate, and diacylglycerol (Fig. 5-3). An increase in the level of glucose in β cells causes cAMP to form and phospholipase C to increase levels of diacylglycerol. These secondary messengers induce the activation of two different kinases, cAMP-dependent protein kinase A and diacylglycerol-dependent protein kinase C. These two kinases are believed to be responsible for the phosphorylation of proteins associated with exocytosis of the contents of secretory granules (Fig. 5-3). An increase in glu-

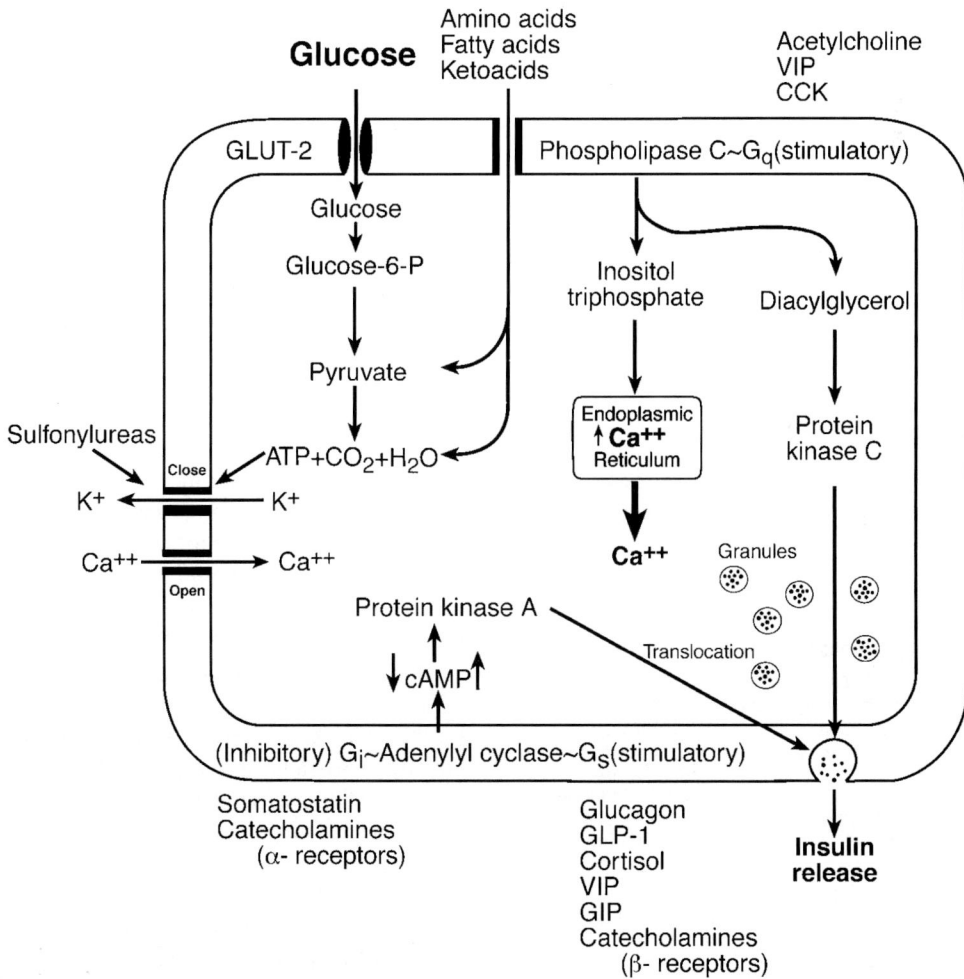

Fig. 5-3. Regulation of insulin secretion from β cells. Secondary messengers: **Inositol triphosphate, diacylglycerol**, and cyclic adenosine monophosphate (**cAMP**). Transporter proteins: **GLUT-2**, glucose transporter protein-2. Hormones: **VIP**, vasoactive intestinal peptide; **CCK**, cholecystokinin; **GLP-1**, glucagon-like polypeptide-1; **GIP**, gastric inhibitory polypeptide. (Adapted from: S. M. Genuth,[33] 1993, p. 857).

cose also causes an increase in inositol triphosphate which results in an immediate release of Ca^{2+} into the cytosol from sequestered sites in the endoplasmic reticulum. The increase of Ca^{2+} into the cytosol triggers the contraction of a network of microfilaments which moves secretory granules containing insulin from the cytosol to the cell membrane for release by exocytosis from the β cells (Fig. 5-3). This redistribution of intracellular Ca^{2+} is believed to be responsible for the surge of insulin into the circulation that results from the administration of glucose.

The sustained release of insulin results from the catabolism of glucose to pyruvate in β cells, which generates increased levels of ATP. This ATP is involved in the closure of ATP-sensitive K^+ channels and a decrease in the efflux of K^+, which leads to depolarization of the cell membrane. In turn, voltage-sensitive Ca^{2+} channels open and Ca^{2+} increases in the cytosol (Fig. 5-3). Hypercalcemia or the administration of calcium ionophores stimulates insulin release, whereas, hypocalcemia or the administration of calcium channel blockers decreases insulin release.

Regulation of Secretion of Insulin

Many factors influence the secretion of insulin (Table 5-2; Fig. 5-3). However, the concentration of energy substrates in the blood is by far the most important regulator of the secretion of insulin and of glucagon. Large amounts of insulin

are secreted during feeding and for several hours thereafter, when there is an abundance of energy substrates in the circulation. Concurrently, the secretion of glucagon is inhibited. This increase in the level of insulin lowers the concentration of energy substrates in the blood by promoting their uptake and storage in various tissues. When a deficit of energy substrates occurs between feedings, the secretion of glucagon is stimulated. Glucagon increases the concentration of energy substrates in the blood by promoting the release of energy stores, while simultaneously inhibiting some of the actions of insulin. Changes in the ratio of insulin and glucagon are largely controlled by the concentration of glucose in the circulation and, to a lesser extent, by the concentration of amino acids. The various actions of glucose have been investigated intensively, when compared to other energy substrates, due to the major role of glucose on the regulation of insulin secretion by β cells.

Following feedings that are high in protein and low in carbohydrate, large amounts of amino acids are absorbed from the gastrointestinal tract. Some amino acids are potent stimulators of insulin secretion. The essential amino acids, particularly arginine, lysine, and leucine, are secretagogues for insulin in humans, even in the absence of glucose. Arginine is also a secretagogue for domestic animals, but the role of lysine and leucine remains to be determined. In addition, some metabolites of amino acids stimulate the secretion of insulin, and most are effective in the absence of glucose. The mechanisms by which amino acids and their metabolites act on β cells to promote the secretion of insulin are unknown.

Fatty acids have very little effect on β cells and the secretion of insulin in humans. Short- and long-chain fatty acids are important secretagogues for the release of insulin in dogs, cats, and ruminants. Compared to glucose, little is known about the mechanisms by which fatty acids promote the secretion of insulin.

The relative importance of the direct effects of glucose, amino acids, and fatty acids on β cells depends, to a great extent, upon the natural diet for the species. In the United States, approximately half of human energy needs are met by carbohydrates. This is considerably more

Table 5-2 Factors Affecting Insulin Secretion

Stimulators	Inhibitors
Glucose	Somatostatin
Amino acids	Catecholamines
Fatty acids	Cortisol
GI hormones[a]	Growth hormone
Acetylcholine	Exercise
(muscarinic receptors)	Fasting
Glucagon	Hypokalemia
Ketoacids	Alloxan
Sulfonylureas	

Information compiled from various sources.

[a]GI hormones include gastric inhibitory peptide, cholecystokinin, glucagon-like peptide-1, gastrin, secretin, and glicentin.

than for many of the domestic species. For example, under normal circumstances, ruminants do not absorb glucose from the gastrointestinal tract. Ruminants obtain approximately 70% of their energy from short-chain fatty acids, the products of incomplete oxidation resulting from microbial fermentation under anaerobic conditions in the rumen, reticulum, and omasum. Butyrate and, to a lesser degree, propionate are potent stimulators of insulin release in ruminants. The lack of dietary glucose for intestinal absorption of glucose by ruminants precludes the portal vein from carrying high glucose loads to the liver and the stimulation of insulin secretion. As a result, ruminants evolved with very little hepatic glucokinase activity which converts glucose to glucose-6-phosphate. This conversion is essential before glucose can be used by hepatocytes. Thus, because dietary glucose is normally metabolized completely by the microflora, ruminants are in a continual state of gluconeogenesis.

Cats and other felines are strict carnivores whose natural diet contains very little carbohydrate. Their energy requirements are met almost entirely by dietary amino acids and fatty acids. As for ruminants, cats have very little hepatic glucokinase activity and they too are in a continual state of gluconeogenesis.

In contrast to cats, dogs and other canidae are not strict carnivores, and their natural diet can contain significant amounts of digestible carbohydrate. Dogs can utilize formulated diets that contain up to 65% carbohydrate. However, dogs can also be maintained on carbohydrate-free diets, even during late gestation and lactation when the demands for glucose are maximal.

In addition to nutrients absorbed from the gastrointestinal tract, there are other factors which stimulate the secretion of insulin. It has been known since the early 1900s that intravenous administration of a large amount of glucose to humans, dogs, and other animals is more effective for inducing glucosuria than the administration of glucose *per os*. This difference is due to the ability of oral glucose to evoke a greater release of insulin than that resulting from the parenteral administration of glucose. This suggests that oral glucose elicits some sort of anticipatory response signal or signals from

the gastrointestinal tract to stimulate additional secretion of insulin from pancreatic β cells. Thus, the gastrointestinal tract and the pancreas form an entero-pancreatic axis, not only for the digestion and absorption of nutrients, but also for controlling the utilization of glucose and other energy substrates within the body. The presence of glucose and other energy substrates in the gastrointestinal tract induce the biosynthesis and release of gastrointestinal hormones that act directly on β cells to augment insulin release (Fig. 5-3). The gastrointestinal hormones include gastric inhibitory polypeptide (GIP), also called glucose-dependent insulinotropic peptide, and a cohort of other hormones, including vasoactive intestinal peptide (VIP), secretin, cholecystokinin (CCK), glicentin (enteroglucagon), and glucagon-like peptide-1 and -2 (GLP-1 and GLP-2). These hormones share similarities in their chemical structure.

The first gastrointestinal hormone discovered which directly stimulated β cells was GIP. Secretion of GIP is stimulated by dietary glucose and fat. Cholecystokinin has a similar role in humans and animals, and its secretion is stimulated by dietary proteins and amino acids. High concentrations of GLP-1 are found in intestinal tissue and may be the most potent of the gastrointestinal hormones to stimulate the synthesis and release of insulin.

The endocrine pancreas has a role in the control of its own hormonal secretions. Insulin, glucagon, and pancreatic somatostatin modulate the secretion of each other through paracrine relationships (Fig. 5-4). The secretion of insulin is stimulated by the release of glucagon and related peptides and is inhibited by somatostatin. Hence, the paracrine interactions among islet cells form a key component of the entero-pancreatic axis that coordinates the digestion, absorption, and utilization of various energy substrates by the animal.

The autonomic nervous system also has a role on the synthesis and release of pancreatic hormones. Both sympathetic and parasympathetic branches of the autonomic system richly innervate the pancreatic islets and modulate their secretions. Autonomic input to the islets of Langerhans is largely regulated by the hypotha-

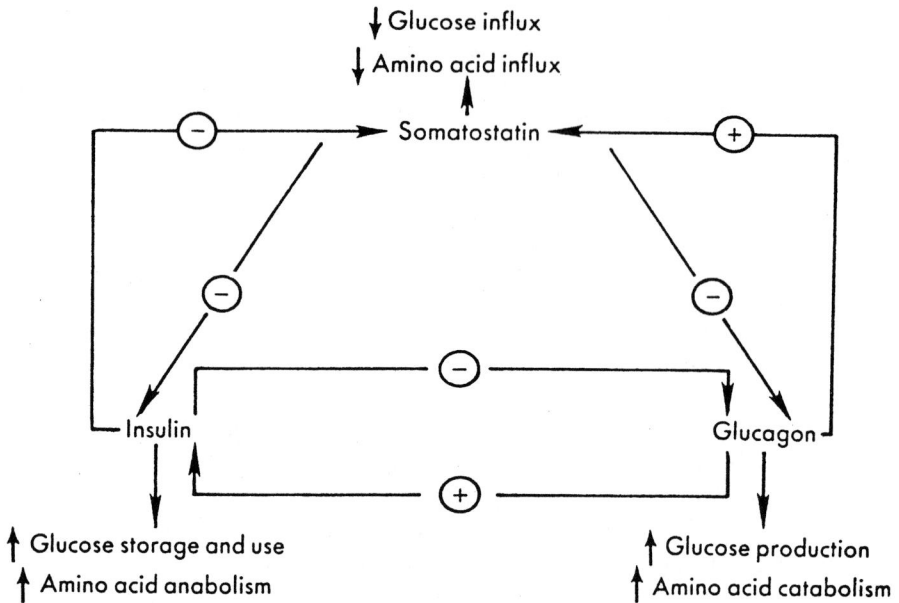

Fig. 5-4. Schematic representation of the interrelating and feedback effects of somatostatin, insulin, and glucagon on glucose and amino acid metabolism. (From: S. M. Genuth,[33] 1993, p. 872).

lamus. The hypothalamus also controls appetite and integrates feeding behavior through the appetite and satiety centers located in the ventrolateral and ventromedial hypothalamus, respectively. Some of the regulatory influences on these centers include gastrointestinal reflexes, the concentration of gastrointestinal hormones, and the concentration of energy substrates in the circulation.

During the prandial phase of digestion, the parasympathetic system stimulates the release of insulin. Stimulation of the vagus nerve or electrical stimulation of the ventrolateral hypothalamus leads to a rapid increase in the release of insulin by activating cholinergic (muscarinic) receptors on the β cells. Catecholamines resulting from the stimulation of the sympathetic nerves or electrical stimulation of the ventromedial hypothalamus inhibit the release of insulin and stimulate the release of glucagon. However, the predominant effect of catecholamines on the pancreas is mediated by α-adrenergic receptors and a subsequent decrease in cAMP to inhibit insulin release (Fig. 5-3). Exercise, hypoxia, hypothermia, burns, surgery, and other stressors can all lead to a suppression of insulin release by catecholamines acting on α2-adrenergic receptors. In the presence of drugs that block α2-adrenergic receptors, catecholamines can also activate β2-adrenergic receptors to increase insulin release. This latter action is also mediated by the adenyl cyclase system (Fig. 5-3), which, in this case, increases the cAMP levels of β cells. However, this is a pharmacological effect of catecholamines on the modulation of insulin release.

Mechanism of Action of Insulin

The hypoglycemic effects of insulin are essential to sustain life in humans and animals. Consequently, the effects of insulin on the metabolism and utilization of glucose are, by far, the most important effects of insulin. The major effect of insulin is to increase the permeability of cell membranes to glucose. Although the mechanisms are different, insulin also facilitates the cellular uptake of amino acids, potassium, phosphate, and magnesium. Metabolic responses are initiated when insulin binds to receptors on cell membranes. The receptor for insulin consists of two identical α and β subunits (Fig. 5-5). The two α subunits are located on the extracellular surface and bind the insulin

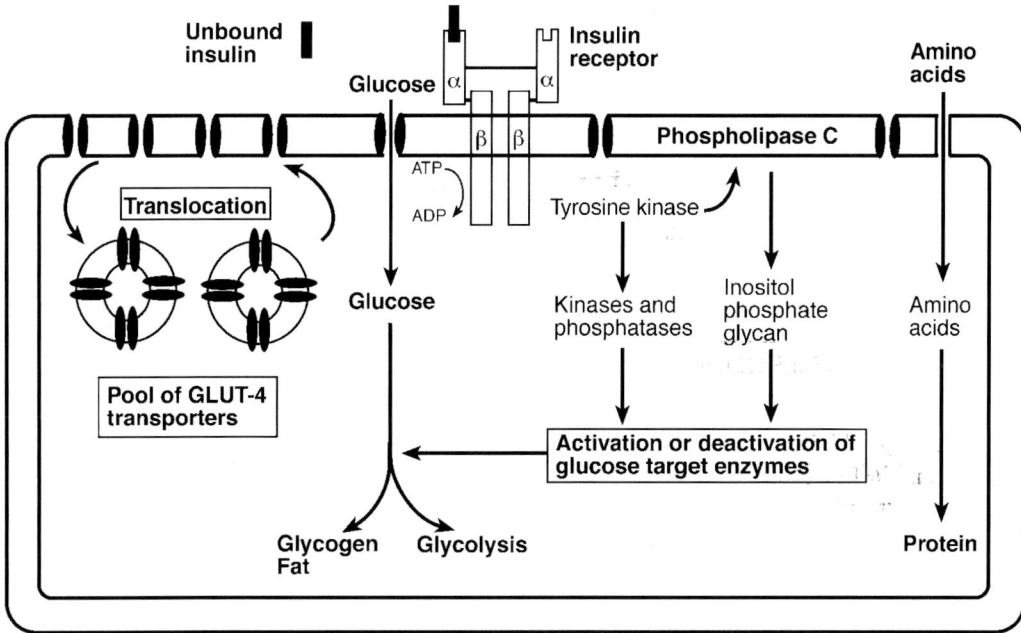

Fig. 5-5. The binding of insulin to membrane receptors of myocytes and adipocytes and effects of insulin on the cellular metabolic responses. (Adapted from: S. M. Genuth,[33] 1993, p. 861).

molecule. The two β subunits form the effector component of the protein-receptor complex. The β subunits span the cell membrane with one end of each subunit protruding into the cytoplasm. Although insulin binds preferentially to insulin receptors, insulin-like growth factors can also bind and activate insulin receptors.

When insulin binds to a receptor, autophosphorylation of the intracellular tyrosine kinase site of the β subunit occurs. The autophosphorylation of tyrosine kinase triggers a cascade of events which is essential for insulin to exert its biological effects. Within seconds of the binding of insulin to its receptor, the cell membrane becomes highly permeable to glucose, especially for muscle and fat cells in which glucose uptake may increase up to 20-fold. Five types of transporter proteins have been described for the facilitated transport of glucose into animal cells. More than one type of glucose transporter protein may be present in a cell. The type, location, and major function of glucose transporter proteins 1 through 5 are listed in Table 5-3. The molecular mechanisms responsible for the translocation of glucose transporter proteins

and changes in their cytosolic concentrations have not been determined. The rapid increase in glucose uptake by myocytes and adipocytes is made possible by the translocation of glucose transporter protein-4 (GLUT-4) from the cytosolic pool to the cell membrane (Fig. 5-5). The large increase in the number of GLUT-4 transporter proteins in the cell membrane results in a marked increase in the transport of glucose into cells. The GLUT-4 transporter proteins associated with the cell membrane are returned to the cytosolic pool as circulating levels of insulin decline. Molecular events responsible for the metabolism of glucose following the autophosphorylation of the tyrosine kinase site are poorly understood. However, it is known that activation of tyrosine kinase leads to the phosphorylation and dephosphorylation of numerous intracellular proteins, including kinases, phosphatases, and membrane-bound phospholipases and G-proteins, which direct the target cell's intracellular machinery to respond to insulin.

The overall effect of insulin is to stimulate enzyme systems that promote anabolism while

Table 5-3   *Function and Location of Glucose Transporter Proteins (GLUT) Responsible for Facilitated Diffusion of Glucose into Cells*

Transporter	Sites of Expression	Function
GLUT-1	Brain, red blood cells, kidneys, liver, and placenta	Basal glucose uptake
GLUT-2	β cells, liver, epithelium of small intestine, and kidneys	β cell glucose sensor; glucose transport in intestine and kidneys
GLUT-3	Brain, kidneys, and placenta	Basal glucose uptake
GLUT-4	Skeletal and cardiac muscle, and adipose tissue	Insulin-dependent glucose uptake
GLUT-5	Jejunum	Dietary absorption

Adapted from: G. I. Bell,[8] 1991, p. 417.

simultaneously inhibiting catabolic enzyme systems. The inhibitory effects of insulin on catabolic pathways may be mediated by intracellular levels of cAMP. It appears that insulin decreases cAMP levels largely by inactivation of the cAMP-dependent protein kinase and, to a lesser extent, by enhancing the breakdown of cAMP by increasing phosphodiesterase activity (see for reference Chapter 1, Fig. 1-10). For example, an insulin-induced decrease in cAMP in hepatocytes stimulates the synthesis of glycogen and triglycerides, while gluconeogenesis is inhibited. Conversely, catabolic hormones, such as glucagon and epinephrine increase intracellular levels of cAMP and inhibit and oppose the effects of insulin on hepatocytes.

Major Effects of Insulin

Major effects of insulin in animals are listed in Table 5-4. In addition to supplying energy to cells, large amounts of glucose are stored as glycogen in muscle, whereas, in adipose tissue large amounts of glucose are converted to glycerol-phosphate and ATP for synthesis and storage of triglycerides. Insulin also increases the entry of amino acids into cells while glucose supplies energy for the synthesis of these amino acids into protein.

Insulin also hyperpolarizes cell membranes by facilitating the influx of K^+. In clinical situations, hypoglycemia and hypokalemia may result from insulin therapy. Hypokalemia due to exogenously administered insulin may also result in cardiovascular disturbances.

Cells which do not require insulin for glucose transport include the liver, red and white blood cells, neural, renal, and intestinal epithelial cells (Fig. 5-6).

EFFECTS ON LIVER. One of the most important effects of insulin in the liver is the stimulation of glycogenesis in the hepatic cell (Fig. 5-7). The key enzymes that are activated and stimulated by insulin are glucokinase, which phosphorylates glucose to glucose-6-phosphate, and glycogen synthase, which is responsible for the polymerization of glucose-1-phosphate via uridine diphosphate glucose to form glycogen. Simultaneously, insulin inhibits enzymes responsible for glycogenolysis (glucose-6-phosphatase and phosphorylase). A small fraction of the excess glucose also enters the glycolytic pathway. Insulin stimulates glycolysis by stimulating phosphofructokinase and pyruvate kinase for oxidation of glucose-6-phosphate to pyruvate. Simultaneously, insulin decreases the hepatic uptake of amino acids and inhibits the gluconeogenic enzymes: Pyruvate carboxylase and phosphoenolpyruvate carboxykinase.

When the amount of glucose reaching the liver exceeds the metabolic needs for energy and storage of glycogen, insulin stimulates the conversion of excess glucose to fatty acids and triglycerides in hepatocytes. Simultaneously, insulin inhibits carnitine acyltransferase which is the key enzyme responsible for the conversion of fatty acid CoA to ketoacids (Fig. 5-7).

In summary, the overall effect of insulin on glucose metabolism by the liver is to stimulate

Table 5-4   Major Effects of Insulin

Liver

1. ↓ glucose output due to:
   a. ↑ glycogenesis
   b. ↓ gluconeogenesis
   c. ↑ glycolysis
2. ↑ lipogenesis
3. ↓ ketoacids
4. ↑ proteogenesis

Muscular Tissue

1. ↑ glucose uptake
2. ↑ glycolysis
3. ↑ glycogenesis
4. ↑ amino acid uptake
5. ↑ proteogenesis
6. ↑ ketoacid uptake
7. ↓ fatty acid uptake
8. ↑ K^+ uptake

Adipose Tissue

1. ↑ glucose uptake
2. ↑ glycolysis
3. ↑ synthesis of fatty acids
4. ↑ synthesis of glycerol-phosphate
5. ↑ lipogenesis
6. ↑ inhibition of hormone-sensitive lipase
7. ↑ K^+ uptake

Concentrations in the Blood

1. ↓ glucose
2. ↓ amino acids
3. ↓ fatty acids
4. ↓ ketoacids
5. ↓ K^+

Information compiled from various sources.

↑ = increase
↓ = decrease

hepatic, anabolic enzymes and pathways while at the same time, inhibiting hepatic enzymes and pathways that catabolize glycogen, amino acids, and fatty acids (Fig. 5-7).

EFFECTS ON MUSCLE. Quantitatively, the muscle mass is the largest target for insulin and the major depot for excess nutrients. Insulin stimulates the uptake of large quantities of circulating glucose by muscles and, to a lesser extent, amino acids. Much of the glucose entering myocytes is stored as muscle glycogen due to the action of insulin on glycogen synthase. The remainder of the glucose taken up by the muscle mass undergoes oxidation to produce ATP, creatine phosphate, carbon dioxide, metabolic water, and heat.

During periods of increased concentration of amino acids in the circulation, the myocytes become the major storage site for the sequestration of amino acids. Insulin stimulates the active transport of circulating amino acids and promotes protein synthesis in myocytes and other cells. Insulin is also a potent inhibitor of proteolysis. However, the mechanisms by which insulin promotes the storage of amino acids and proteins in muscle are poorly understood when compared to the mechanisms for the storage of carbohydrates and lipids in liver and fat cells, respectively.

The requirement of insulin for protein synthesis suggests that insulin is essential for the growth of animals. Indeed, insulin has effects on growth which are as important as those of growth

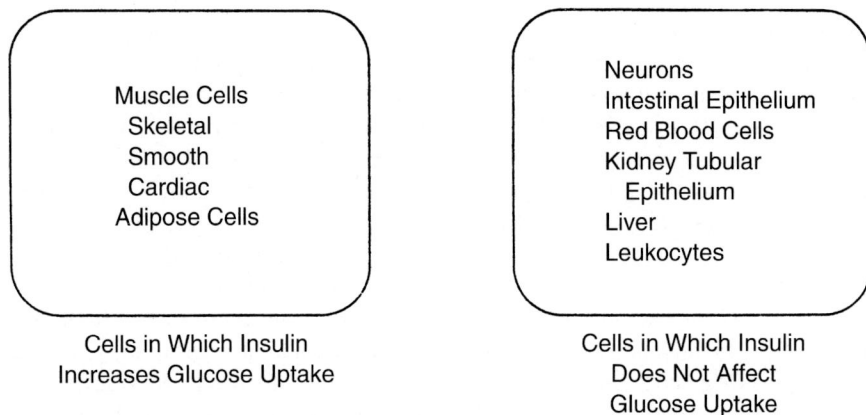

Muscle Cells
Skeletal
Smooth
Cardiac
Adipose Cells

Cells in Which Insulin
Increases Glucose Uptake

Neurons
Intestinal Epithelium
Red Blood Cells
Kidney Tubular
   Epithelium
Liver
Leukocytes

Cells in Which Insulin
Does Not Affect
Glucose Uptake

Fig. 5-6. The role of insulin on insulin-dependent and on insulin-independent cells.

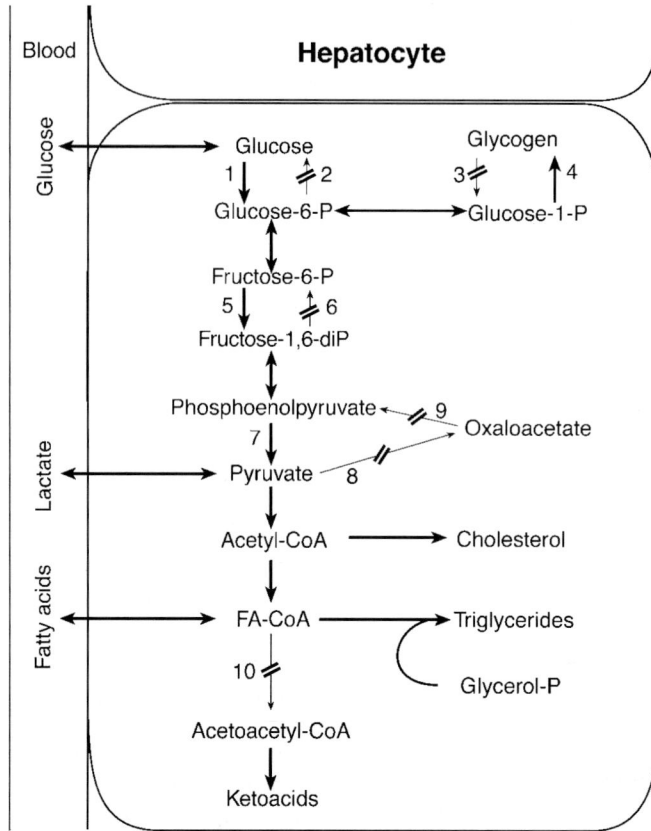

Fig. 5-7. Sites of action of insulin and glucagon on glucose and fatty acid metabolism in the liver. Key enzymes influenced by insulin and glucagon: **1**, glucokinase (hexokinase); **2**, glucose-6-phosphatase; **3**, phosphorylase; **4**, glycogen synthase; **5**, phosphofructokinase; **6**, fructose-1,6-diphosphatase; **7**, pyruvate kinase; **8**, pyruvate carboxylase; **9**, phosphoenolpyruvate carboxykinase; and **10**, carnitine acyltransferase. (Adapted from: S. M. Genuth,[33] 1993, p. 864). → = Increase in activity or concentration. ↛ = Decrease in activity or concentration.

hormone. When these two hormones are absent or secreted in very low amounts, young animals cease to grow. If only one of these two hormones is administered as a replacement therapy to affected animals, there will be very little effect on growth. However, if insulin and growth hormone are administered concurrently, growth resumes. Hence, insulin and growth hormone act synergistically to promote growth, with each hormone performing different functions.

EFFECTS ON ADIPOSE TISSUE. Another major target for insulin is the adipose cell. An increase in insulin promotes the storage of fat by stimulating the transport of glucose into adipocytes, where it is metabolized for energy and for the formation and storage of large amounts of glycerol-phosphate. The fatty acids combine with the glycerol-phosphate to form triglycerides, the major form of stored fats.

Perhaps of greater importance than the lipogenic effect of insulin on adipose tissue is the suppressive effect of insulin on hydrolysis of triglycerides to fatty acids and glycerol. Insulin is a potent inhibitor of hormone-sensitive lipase, the key enzyme for lipolysis in adipocytes. This effect of insulin on lipolysis is believed to be mediated by a decrease in cAMP and the inhibition of protein kinase A. As a result of insulin's effects on adipocytes, there is a marked reduction in circulating levels of fatty acids due to the effects of insulin on carnitine acyltransferase, as shown for the hepatocyte in Figure 5-7.

Adipose tissue produces the newly discovered[6] hormone, leptin. The major target for leptin is the hypothalamus where leptin appears to have specific effects on appetite, energy metabolism, and reproduction. Leptin inhibits feeding behavior by actions on the satiety center. In the presence of an abundant supply of stored energy, leptin stimulates the hypothalamic-growth hormone axis to promote protein synthesis and antagonizes the catabolic effects of glucocorticoids by inhibiting the hypothalamic-pituitary-adrenal axis. Leptin also appears to inhibit the secretion of insulin by direct action on β cells and attenuates the actions of insulin in muscle and adipose tissue.

Nutritional status plays a pivotal role in the timing of onset of puberty (see Chapter 12) and influences the resumption of estrous cycles following parturition or the period of seasonal anestrus. Leptin is believed[31] to be the hormonal signal that relays the nutritional status of the animal to the hypothalamic-pituitary-gonadal axis and influences reproductive activity by modulating the release of gonadotropin releasing hormone.

Islet Amyloid Polypeptide

Islet amyloid polypeptide (IAPP) is a polypeptide consisting of 37 amino acids in humans and animals. In the islets, IAPP is derived from a precursor molecule produced by β cells which is distinct from the precursor for insulin and connecting peptide. Interestingly, IAPP is stored and co-secreted with insulin. However, IAPP and insulin are not secreted in a 1:1 ratio, as is the case for insulin and connecting peptide. The ratio of insulin to IAPP varies from approximately 10:1 to 100:1. This suggests that IAPP may be regulated independently from insulin. Though it has not been determined in other animals, in fasted rats the ratio of insulin:IAPP is reduced in response to a glucose load, whereas rats made hyperglycemic have an increased ratio of insulin:IAPP. The structure of IAPP is related to calcitonin gene-related peptide; both consist of 37 amino acids. Islet amyloid polypeptide has been shown to displace calcitonin gene-related peptide from receptors in the brain, muscle, and liver.

The biological functions of IAPP remain to be elucidated. However, at pharmacological doses, IAPP inhibits basal and insulin-stimulated glycogenesis in muscle, impairs the suppressive effect of insulin on glucose output from the liver, and apparently reduces the uptake of glucose by peripheral tissues. In addition, IAPP is a potent vasodilator and hypocalcemic agent. Injection of IAPP into the hypothalamus of rats induces anorexia, which suggests that IAPP may also play a role in the control of food intake. Islet amyloid polypeptide has also been implicated in the pathogenesis of some forms of diabetes mellitus in cats, macaques, and humans in which amyloid is deposited in pancreatic islets.

INSULIN-LIKE GROWTH FACTORS

Insulin-like growth factors 1 and 2 (IGF-1 and IGF-2) are single-chain peptides. In several species, IGF-1 and IGF-2 consist of 70 and 67 amino acids, respectively. They are approximately 70% identical to each other. Insulin-like growth factors are also related to proinsulin and insulin. The α and β domains of IGFs are approximately 50% identical with the α and β chains of insulin, respectively. Though structurally related to insulin, most of the circulating IGFs originate from the liver and not from the pancreas. A minor part of the circulating IGFs are produced by other tissues where these IGFs are believed to act as paracrine or autocrine hormones.

The receptor for IGF-1 consists of two α and β subunits and a tyrosine kinase site. The structure of the IGF-1 receptor is very similar to that of the insulin receptor (Fig. 5-5). The IGF-1 receptor binds both IGF-1 and IGF-2 with high affinity and, to a lesser extent, insulin. The structure of the IGF-2 receptor is markedly different from IGF-1 and insulin receptors. The IGF-2 receptor consists of a single-chain glycosylated protein that has no tyrosine kinase activity. The IGF-2 receptor has high affinity for IGF-2, low affinity for IGF-1 and does not bind insulin.

The IGFs have a wide range of biological activity whose overall effects are anabolic. For instance, IGF-1 has potent insulin-like effects. As for insulin, administration of IGF-1 stimulates the uptake and utilization of glucose by muscle and adipose tissue, which results in a marked decrease in blood glucose. This hypoglycemic activity occurs even though IGF-1 inhibits the release of insulin. Although IGF-1 and insulin have similar effects on glucose metabolism in muscle and adipose tissue, there is an important difference in the actions of these two hormones in the liver. In contrast to insulin, IGF-1 has little, if any, ability to inhibit the release of hepatic glucose. This difference is attributed to the scarcity of hepatic IGF-1 receptors and, possibly, because IGF-1 does not inhibit glucagon release.

There are relatively few studies on the effects of IGF-2 on glucose metabolism. However, the actions of IGF-2 on glucose metabolism appear to be similar to those for IGF-1, though the potency of IGF-2 on glucose metabolism is lower than that for IGF-1. It is believed that most of the effects of IGF-2 on glucose metabolism are mediated by binding and activating the IGF-1 receptor rather than the IGF-2 receptor.

Except for steroid-producing glands, growth hormone is the major regulator of IGFs in most tissues. In steroid-producing glands, however, the stimulus is provided by the specific pituitary tropic hormone of the target gland to release the IGFs needed for the regulation and proliferation of steroid-producing cells. The action of IGFs on steroidogenic cells includes the potentiation of:

1. ACTH on cells of the adrenal cortex,
2. FSH on granulosa cells of ovarian follicles,
3. LH on thecal cells of ovarian follicles and luteal cells, and
4. LH on the Leydig cells of the testes.

α CELL POLYPEPTIDE

Glucagon

Shortly after the discovery of insulin, it became evident that the administration of crude pancreatic extracts to experimental animals was inconsistent in lowering the blood levels of glu-cose. By the contrary, in many cases, pancreatic extracts produced hyperglycemia. It was hypothesized that a hyperglycemic factor, which counteracted the insulin-induced hypoglycemia, was present in those extracts. This factor, named glucagon, was isolated and characterized in 1955, 30 years after the discovery of insulin.

Structure of Glucagon

Glucagon is a polypeptide which consists of a peptide chain of 29 amino acids (Fig. 5-8) and has a molecular weight of approximately 3,500 daltons. The amino acid sequence of glucagon appears to be identical for most mammalian species and glucagon's functions appear to be highly conserved.

Biosynthesis of Glucagon

The gene for glucagon belongs to a super-family of genes that also codes for other hormones, including glucagon-like polypeptide-1 and -2 (GLP-1 and GLP-2), gastric inhibitory polypeptide (GIP), secretin, growth hormone-releasing hormone (GHRH), and vasoactive intestinal polypeptide (VIP).

The processing of proglucagon differs markedly among different tissues (Fig. 5-9). In the α cells of the pancreatic islets, the primary cleavage products of proglucagon are glucagon and the amino- and carboxy-terminal peptides, which are, respectively, glicentin-related polypeptide (GRPP), also called enteroglucagon, and major proglucagon factor (MGF). The latter contains amino acid sequences for GLP-1 and GLP-2. In the L cells of the intestinal mucosa, proglucagon is processed to bioactive GLP-1, GLP-2, and glicentin. A portion of glicentin can also be cleaved to form GRPP and oxyntomodulin. Little is known about the functions of GLP-1 and GLP-2. However, GLP-1 has been shown to be a potent stimulator of insulin secretion and may be one of the factors largely responsible for the greater insulin response to oral glucose when compared to intravenous glucose administration.

NH₂ ... His·Ser·Glu·Gly·Thr·Phe·Thr·Ser·Asp·Tyr·Ser·Lys·Tyr·Leu·Asp·Ser·Arg·Arg·Ala·Glu·Asp·Phe·Val·Glu·Try·Leu·Met·Asp·Thr

Fig. 5-8. Amino acid sequence of glucagon.

Proglucagon

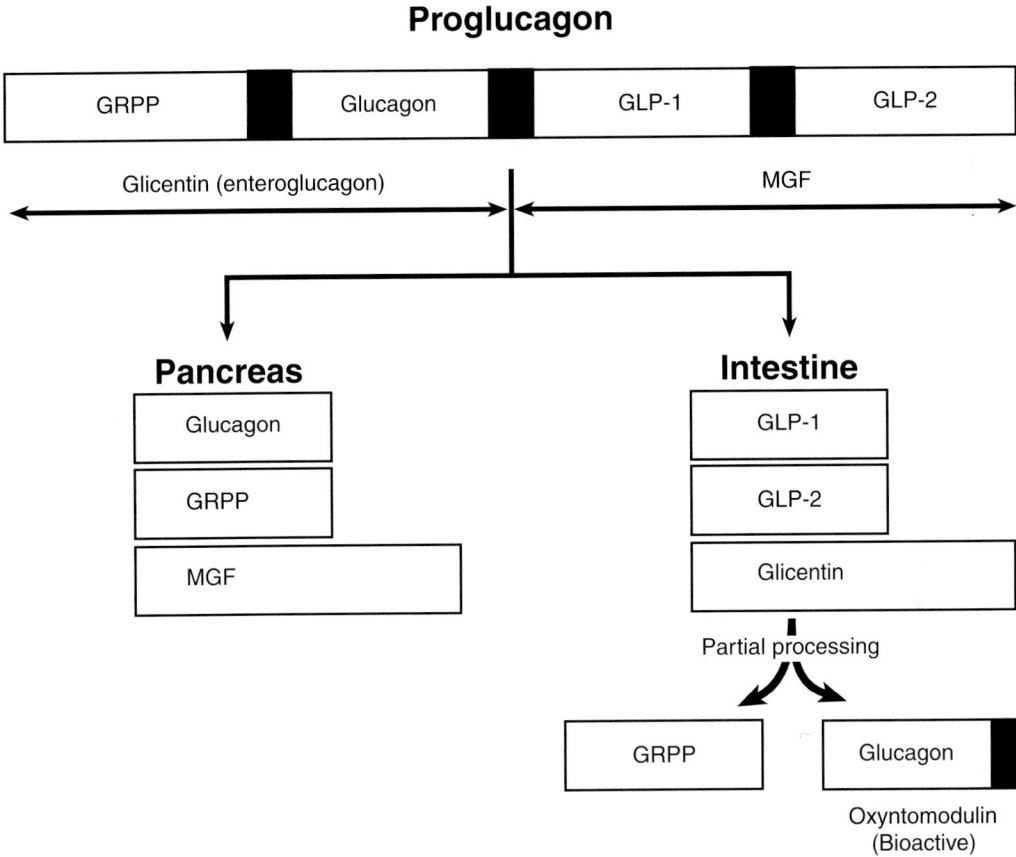

Fig. 5-9. Differential processing of proglucagon in the pancreas and intestine (**GRPP**, glicentin-related polypeptide; **GLP-1** and **GLP-2**, glucagon-like polypeptide-1 and -2, respectively; **MGF**, major proglucagon factor).

Table 5-5   Factors Affecting Glucagon Secretion

Stimulators	Inhibitors
Hypoglycemia	Hyperglycemia
Amino acids	Insulin
GI hormones[a]	Somatostatin
Catecholamines	Fatty acids
Acetylcholine	Ketoacids
Exercise	
Fasting	
Cortisol	
Growth hormone	

[a]GI hormones include cholecystokinin, vasoactive inhibitory polypeptide, and gastrin.

Regulation of Secretion of Glucagon

Some of the factors that influence the secretion of glucagon are summarized in Table 5-5.

By far, the most potent factor that regulates the secretion and release of glucagon from the α cells of the pancreatic islet is the concentration of glucose in the blood. Hypoglycemia results in a marked increase in glucagon secretion, whereas hyperglycemia is inhibitory. Thus, the effects of glucose in the blood on glucagon secretion and release from the islets are opposite to that of blood glucose on insulin secretion. These two hormones regulate the availability of glucose to the tissues.

Large amounts of amino acids are absorbed from the gastrointestinal tract following the feeding of protein. These amino acids act directly on α cells of the pancreatic islets to increase the biosynthesis and secretion of glucagon. In the absence of dietary carbohydrates, glucagon increases the hepatic output of glucose by stimulating gluconeogenesis. As indicated earlier, amino acids also act directly on β cells to increase the secretion of insulin required for the uptake and utilization of hepatic glucose and for the storage of amino acids as proteins. Although amino acids stimulate the release of both glucagon and insulin, the ratio of glucagon to insulin is such that normal levels of blood glucose are maintained.

Amino acids also have indirect effects on the secretion of glucagon. The absorption of amino acids from the intestine promotes the secretion of gastrointestinal hormones, such as gastrin, gastric inhibitory polypeptide, and cholecystokinin, which then stimulate the secretion of glucagon. Because of the effects of these gastrointestinal hormones, dietary amino acids are more effective than amino acids administered intravenously for stimulating the secretion of glucagon.

Glucagon secretion is also increased by activation of the sympathetic nervous system or administration of catecholamines. Exercise, starvation, and other forms of stress also stimulate the secretion of glucagon.

Effects of Glucagon on Liver and Other Tissues

The liver is the target of foremost importance for the metabolic activities controlled by glucagon. Glucagon's effect on the liver is to stimulate glycogenolysis. Glucagon also plays a major role in stimulating hepatic gluconeogenesis. The combined effects of glucagon on glycogenolysis and gluconeogenesis cause a marked increase in the output of glucose from the liver. Hepatic glucose is the body's major source of energy during the postabsorptive stage of digestion. Another hepatic effect of glucagon is to increase the synthesis and concentration of ketoacids in the circulation. In addition to its hyperglycemic effects, glucagon stimulates the synthesis and release of insulin from β cells. The increase in insulin potentiates the suppressive effect of hyperglycemia on glucagon release.

The initial effect of glucagon following binding to receptors on hepatic cell membranes is to increase the synthesis of cAMP (see Chapter 1, Fig. 1-10). The cAMP binds to and activates a cAMP-dependent protein kinase, which results in the phosphorylation and dephosphorylation of intracellular proteins that regulate nearly all of the known effects of glucagon in the liver. Glucagon stimulates glycogenolysis by activating phosphorylase and glucose-6-phosphatase while simultaneously inhibiting glycogen synthase and glucokinase (Fig. 5-7). Glucagon stimulates gluconeogenesis by activating pyruvate carboxylase, phosphoenolpyruvate carboxykinase, and fructose-1,6-diphosphatase while simultaneously inhibiting phosphofructose kinase and, possibly, pyruvate kinase (Fig. 5-7). Stimulation of gluconeogenesis by glucagon is accompanied by the simultaneous inhibition of glycolysis. The decrease in glycolysis leads to a decrease in the synthesis of fatty acids, triglycerides, and cholesterol and activation of carnitine acyltransferase, which is the key enzyme in the ketogenic pathway (Fig. 5-7).

Because glucagon inhibits the synthesis of fatty acids by the liver, fat depots become the primary source of fatty acid precursors for the formation of ketoacids. In addition to the liver, adipose tissue is an important target for glucagon. In adipocytes, glucagon is a potent lipolytic agent that acts by activating hormone-sensitive lipase to hydrolyze triglycerides to fatty acids and glycerol. The increase in the circulating levels of glycerol and fatty acids causes a marked increase in the uptake of these metabolites by the liver where, respectively, they become substrates for the formation of glucose and ketoacids. In the liver, glucagon directs fatty acids away from resynthesis to triglycerides and toward the formation of ketoacids. This glucagon-induced switch in the metabolism of fatty acids is accompanied by activation of a pivotal enzyme, carnitine acyltransferase, to form the fatty acid CoA precursors for synthesis of ketoacids (Fig. 5-7). Hence, the ketogenic effects of glucagon are the result of the combined effects of glucagon on the liver and adipose tissue.

The ketoacids produced by the liver are energy substrates utilized by most tissues, the liver being a notable exception. During periods of starvation, ketoacids become the major fuel for muscle cells. Hence, in normal animals, ketoacids are not harmful because even in the presence of low levels of insulin, ketoacids are metabolized by the body. In the diabetic animal there is no insulin to counteract the effects of glucagon. This leads to a marked increase in lipolysis, uptake of fatty acids by the liver, synthesis of ketoacids, and increased concentration of ketoacids in the blood. Furthermore, the lack of insulin decreases the utilization of ketoacids by peripheral tissues. The ensuing ketonemia can lead to ketoacidosis and death.

The effects of glucagon on lipolysis in adipose tissue and on the secretion of insulin and somatostatin from the pancreas have already been discussed. In the central nervous system, glucagon stimulates the secretion of growth hormone and may have a role in the control of the appetite center. Myocytes do not have receptors for glucagon, hence glucagon has little, if any, effects on muscle.

In summary, glucagon is a catabolic hormone whereas insulin is an anabolic hormone. Although other catabolic hormones also play a role in maintaining blood glucose, insulin and glucagon are paramount to glucose homeostasis. They function to maintain a fairly stable concentration of glucose in the blood to adequately meet the body's metabolic requirements. During the prandial and early postprandial periods, when there is a surplus of circulating energy substrates, insulin lowers blood glucose by facilitating the storage and utilization of glucose. When there is a decline in circulating energy substrate between feedings and during periods of high metabolic demand, glucagon acts to increase blood glucose through hepatic glycogenolysis and gluconeogenesis.

δ CELL POLYPEPTIDE

Somatostatin

Somatostatin was first isolated from the hypothalamus. Because the release of growth hormone was inhibited by somatostatin, at that time somatostatin was called somatotropin release-inhibiting factor (SRIF). Since the discovery of somatostatin in pituitary extracts, this peptide has been isolated from many other tissues, including the pancreas and gastrointestinal tract. In the pancreas, somatostatin is synthesized by the δ cells. In most species there are two major forms of somatostatin, distinguishable by the number of amino acids (14 or 28) in the molecule. The form with 14 amino acids predominates in the pancreas and hypothalamus, whereas the form with 28 amino acids predominates in the gastrointestinal tract. Both forms have similar biological activity in the inhibition of the release of somatotropin.

Pancreatic somatostatin inhibits the release of insulin, glucagon, and pancreatic juice. The 28-amino acid form of somatostatin is found throughout the gastrointestinal tract. It has been suggested that this hormone may act to coordinate the motility of the gut and gall bladder, their exocrine secretions, and the digestion and absorption of nutrients. Somatostatin also inhibits the endocrine secretions of the gastrointestinal tract such as GIP, CCK, VIP, GLP-1, GLP-2, and secretin.

The release of somatostatin from the pancreatic islets is stimulated by glucose, amino acids, fatty acids, gastrointestinal hormones, glucagon, and β-adrenergic and cholinergic neurotransmitters. The release of somatostatin is inhibited by insulin and α-adrenergic neurotransmitters. The low levels of somatostatin in the blood and its ubiquitous distribution in tissue have led many investigators to conclude that the known actions of somatostatin are primarily paracrine in nature. Gap junctions between cells in the islets of Langerhans facilitate intercellular communication due to displacement of fluid between cells.

F CELL POLYPEPTIDE

Pancreatic Polypeptide

Pancreatic polypeptide (PP) is a peptide hormone containing 36 amino acids which is synthesized by F cells in the islets. Pancreatic polypeptide is related to polypeptide YY, an intestinal peptide, and to neuropeptide Y, which is found in the brain and autonomic nervous system. All have 36 amino acids and are amidated at the C-terminal amino acid.

Secretion of PP is largely under vagal control and appears to be modulated by an entero-pancreatic reflex. Ingestion of protein stimulates the secretion of PP, as does fasting, exercise, and acute hypoglycemia. However, the parenteral injection of amino acids has no effect on PP secretion. Somatostatin and blood glucose inhibit the secretion of PP.

The functions of PP are not clear. The peptide does not appear to play a major role in the regulation of glucose metabolism. However, PP inhibits contractions of the gall bladder and the secretion of pancreatic juice and gastric acid. Therefore, the major functions of PP may be in dampening the flow of digestive juices following feedings. It has been postulated that PP may also inhibit food intake.

DYSFUNCTION OF THE ENDOCRINE PANCREAS

Diabetes Mellitus

Diabetes mellitus refers to an etiologically heterogeneous group of metabolic disorders characterized by hyperglycemia. It is an incurable disease which, if left untreated, leads to coma and death in humans and animals.

Diabetes mellitus is one of the most common endocrine diseases of dogs and cats and may occur at any age. The incidence of diabetes mellitus in dogs and cats varies from a ratio of 1:100 to 1:500. The incidence of diabetes mellitus is 2 to 3 times greater in female dogs than in male dogs. Diabetes mellitus in the female dog is frequently diagnosed during diestrus or pregnancy, when levels of progesterone are high and prolonged. The peak incidence of diabetes mellitus in dogs is at 7 to 9 years of age.

In cats, the majority of cases of diabetes mellitus are diagnosed after 6 years of age. The incidence may be approximately 1.5 times greater in male than in female cats. Neutered males appear to be more prone to diabetes than intact males.

Diabetes mellitus is seen occasionally in horses that are more than 7 years of age, with most cases (>80%) occurring in animals more than 15 years of age. Diabetes mellitus is rare in other domestic species.

Diabetes mellitus in domestic animals has been classified as insulin-dependent and non-insulin-dependent forms, which are clinical manifestations of the disease.

Insulin-dependent Diabetes Mellitus

Insulin-dependent diabetes mellitus (IDDM), frequently called Type 1 diabetes, is characterized by sudden onset and a marked decrease of insulin in the circulation. Histologically, there is a total or near total loss of β cells and a major decrease in the size of islets. In the severest cases, there may even be a marked reduction in the number of islets. Dogs and cats with IDDM are prone to ketoacidosis and require insulin therapy to sustain life.

Non-insulin-dependent Diabetes Mellitus

Non-insulin-dependent diabetes mellitus (NIDDM) occurs most frequently in domestic cats, macaques, and humans. In humans there is abundant evidence for a strong genetic component in the development of NIDDM. Obesity and sedentary lifestyles are important factors that contribute to increase the resistance of cells to insulin. A genetic predisposition for NIDDM in cats and other domestic animals has not been demonstrated. However, obesity appears to be a significant risk factor in increasing insulin resistance and the development of NIDDM. Amyloidosis of the pancreatic islets is the most striking pancreatic lesion in animals with NIDDM. Cats are especially prone to develop pancreatic amyloidosis, which begins well before the onset of symptoms of diabetes mellitus.

The liver and muscles are the major sites of insulin resistance. However, in contrast to muscle, the hepatic uptake of glucose is normal. Resistance occurs because insulin no longer inhibits critical enzymes in the gluconeogenic pathway. Thus, there is a marked overproduction of hepatic glucose via gluconeogenesis. In combination with hepatic insulin resistance, gluconeogenesis is stimulated by an increase in glucagon and a plentiful supply of amino acids. The elevated levels of fatty acids in these animals may also provide an important hepatic source of energy to drive gluconeogenesis.

Experimental Diabetes Mellitus

Much of the early work on insulin and the metabolic role of insulin was performed on pancreatectomized animals. These studies were confounded because of the difficulty in removing the entire pancreas and its endocrine islets. Today, it is possible to induce experimental diabetes with chemical agents without loss of the exocrine activities of the pancreas and complications of surgery. Alloxan and streptozotocin are two such drugs that selectively destroy β cells. These agents have also been used experimentally to treat animals with β-cell tumors. However, they are seldom used clinically be-

cause of their toxic effects on the liver, kidneys, and bone marrow.

Glucose Tolerance Test

When a large amount of glucose is given intravenously to fasted, glucose-tolerant animals, there is a moderate and short-lived elevation in blood glucose. This is referred to as a normal glucose tolerance curve or test. In glucose-intolerant or diabetic dogs and cats, the glucose tolerance curve is greatly exaggerated both in amplitude and duration (Fig. 5-10A and B). Non-diabetic, normoglycemic cats with impaired glucose tolerance have curves that are in-

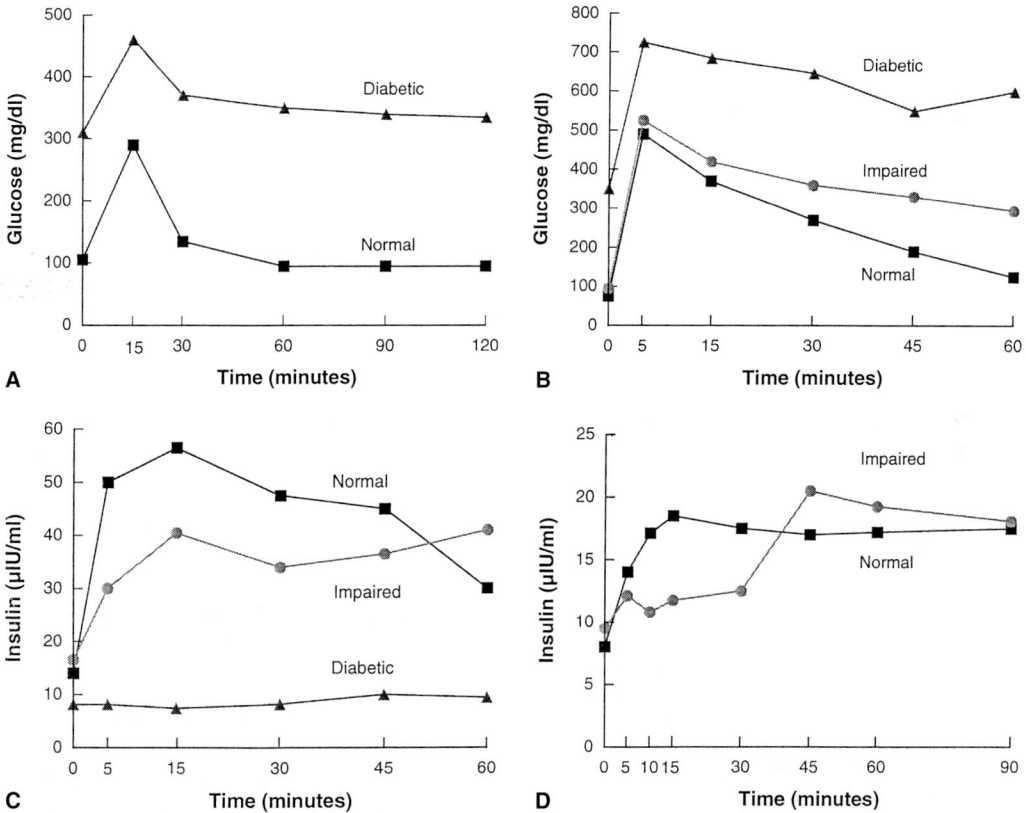

Fig. 5-10. Responses of dogs and cats to glucose tolerance test. **A.** Glucose tolerance test in normal (■–■) and in diabetic (▲–▲) dogs. Diabetes mellitus was induced with alloxan and streptozotocin. (Adapted from: S. L. Martin and C. C. Capen,[69] 1979, p. 1094). **B.** Glucose tolerance test in normal (■–■), normoglycemic, impaired glucose-tolerant (●–●), and in diabetic (▲–▲) cats. (Adapted from: T. D. O'Brien, et al,[85] 1985, pp. 254–256). **C.** Insulin levels in normal (■–■), normoglycemic, impaired glucose-tolerant (●–●), and in diabetic (▲–▲) cats during glucose tolerance tests. (Adapted from: T. D. O'Brien, et al.,[85] 1985, p. 256). **D.** Insulin levels in normal (■–■) and in normoglycemic, impaired glucose-tolerant (●–●) cats during glucose tolerance tests. (Adapted from: T. A. Lutz and J. S. Rand,[63] 1996, p. 31). Differences in the magnitude of blood levels shown in figure and among studies are attributable to assay conditions and to differential responses among test subjects.

termediate between normal and diabetic cats (Fig. 5-10B). Cats that are normoglycemic but have impaired glucose tolerance may exhibit one of two types of insulin release to the glucose challenge. Some cats have an attenuated insulin response to the test (Fig. 5-10C). Other cats may exhibit a marked delay in peak levels of insulin followed by an exaggerated release of insulin (Fig. 5-10D).

Hypoglycemia due to Hyperinsulinism

Hyperinsulinism is associated with improper care and management of dogs and cats with diabetes mellitus or caused by β-cell tumors that produce excessive amounts of insulin. These β-cell tumors are perhaps the sole cause of naturally occurring hypoglycemia and are uncommon in dogs and cats. The major effects of hypoglycemia caused by hyperinsulinism are common to various disorders that affect the central nervous system. Some of these signs are weakness, ataxia, strange behavior, lethargy, and seizures. The brain is particularly sensitive to acute hypoglycemia because, in contrast to other tissues, the brain's only energy substrate is glucose.

REFERENCES

1. Adashi, E. Y., Resnick, C. E., Hernandez, E. R., et al. (1988): Insulin-like growth factor 1 as an amplifier of follicle-stimulating hormone action: Studies on mechanism(s) and site(s) of action in cultured rat granulosa cells. Endocrinology *22:*1583.
2. Adashi, E. Y., Resnick, C. E., Svoboda, M. E., et al. (1986): Follicle-stimulating hormone enhances somatomedin C binding to cultured rat granulosa cells. Evidence for cAMP dependence. J. Biol. Chem. *261:*3923.
3. Ahren, B. (1999): Regulation of insulin secretion by nerves and neuropeptides. Ann. Acad. Med. *28:*99.
4. Asplin, C. M., Paquette, T. L., and Palmer, J. P. (1981): *In vivo* inhibition of glucagon secretion by paracrine ß cell activity in man. J. Clin. Invest. *68:*314.
5. Baker, J., Liu, J. P., Robertson, E. J., et al. (1993): Role of insulin-like growth factors in embryonic and postnatal growth. Cell *75:*73.
6. Barb, C. R. (1999): The brain-pituitary-adipocyte axis: Role of leptin in modulating neuroendocrine function. J. Anim. Sci. *77:*1249.
7. Behringer, R. R., Lewin, T. M., Quaife, C. J., et al. (1990): Expression of insulin-like growth factor I stimulates normal somatic growth in growth hormone-deficient transgenic mice. Endocrinology *127:*1033.
8. Bell, G. I. (1991): Molecular defects in diabetes mellitus. Diabetes *40:*413.
9. Black, H. E., Rosenblum, Y., and Capen, C. C. (1980): Chemically induced (streptozotocin-alloxan) diabetes mellitus in the dog. Biochemical and ultrastructural studies. Am. J. Pathol. *98:*295.
10. Blum, T. W., Wilson, R. B., and Kronfeld, D. S. (1973): Plasma insulin concentrations in parturient cows. J. Dairy Sci. *56:*459.
11. Bromer, W. W., Sinn, L. G., and Behrens, O. K. (1957): The amino acid sequence of glucagon. J. Am. Chem. Soc. *79:*2807.
12. Call, J. L., Mitchell, G. E., Jr., Ely, D. G., et al. (1972): Amino-acids, volatile fatty-acids, and glucose in plasma of insulin treated sheep. J. Anim. Sci. *34:*767.
13. Capen, C. C. and Martin, S. L. (1969): Hyperinsulinism in dogs with neoplasia of the pancreatic islets. A clinical, pathologic, and ultrastructural study. Pathol. Vet. *6:*309.
14. Caywood, D. D., Wilson, J. W., Hardy, R. M., et al. (1979): Pancreatic islet cell adenocarcinoma: Clinical and diagnostic features of six cases. J. Am. Vet. Med. Assoc. *174:*715.
15. Clark, A., Charge, S. B., Badman, M. K., et al. (1996): Islet amyloid in type 2 (non-insulin-dependent) diabetes. Acta Pathol. Microbiol. Immunol. Scand. *104:*12.
16. Considine, R. V. and Caro, J. F. (1997): Leptin and the regulation of body weight. Int. J. Biochem. Cell Biol. *29:*1255.
17. Cotton, R. B., Cornelius, L. M., and Theran, P. (1971): Diabetes mellitus in the dog: A clinicopathologic study. J. Am. Vet. Med. Assoc. *159:*863.
18. DeChiara, T. M., Efstratiadis, A., and Robertson, E. J. (1990): A growth-deficiency phenotype in heterozygous mice carrying an insulin-like growth factor II gene disrupted by targeting. Nature *345:*78.
19. DeChiara, T. M., Robertson, E. J., and Efstratiadis, A. (1991): Parental imprinting of the mouse insulin-like growth factor II gene. Cell *64:*849.
20. Dileepan, K. N. and Wagle, S. R. (1985): Somatostatin: A metabolic regulator. Life Sci. *37:*2335.
21. D'Mello, S. R., Galli, C., Ciotti, T., et al. (1993): Induction of apoptosis in cerebellar granule neurons by low potassium: Inhibition of death by insulin-like growth factor I and cAMP. Proc. Nat. Acad. Sci. USA *90:*10989.
22. Dobbins, R. L., Davis, S. N., Neal, D., et al. (1998): Rates of glucagon activation and deactivation of hepatic glucose production in conscious dogs. Metabolism *47:*135.
23. Dorrestijn, J., van Bussel, F. J., Maassen, J. A., et al. (1998): Early steps in insulin action. Arch. Physiol. Biochem. *106:*269.
24. Drago, J., Murphy, M., Carroll, S. M., et al. (1991): Fibroblast growth factor-mediated proliferation of central nervous system precursors depends on endogenous production of insulin-like growth factor I. Proc. Nat. Acad. Sci. USA *88:*2199.
25. Dupre, J., Ross, S. A., Watson, D., et al. (1973): Stimulation of insulin secretion by gastric inhibitory polypeptide in man. J. Clin. Endocrinol. Metab. *37:*826.
26. Dumonteil, E., Magnan, C., Ritz-Laser, B., et al. (2000): Glucose regulates proinsulin and prosomatostatin but not proglucagon messenger ribonucleic acid levels in rat pancreatic islets. Endocrinology *141:*174.

27. Eigenmann, J. E., Eigenmann, R. Y., Rijnberk, A., et al. (1983): Progesterone-controlled growth hormone overproduction and naturally occurring canine diabetes and acromegaly. Acta Endocrinol. *104:*167.

28. Elahi, D., Raizes, G. S., Andres, S., et al. (1982): Interaction of arginine and gastric inhibitory polypeptide on insulin release in man. Am. J. Physiol. *242:*E343.

29. Engler, D., Redei, E., and Kola, I. (1999): The corticotropin-release inhibitory factor hypothesis: A review of the evidence for the existence of inhibitory as well as stimulatory hypophysiotropic regulation of adrenocorticotropin secretion and biosynthesis. Endocrine Rev. 20:460.

30. Fehmann, H. C. and Habener, J. F. (1992): Insulinotropic hormone glucagon-like peptide-1(7–37) stimulation of proinsulin gene expression and proinsulin biosynthesis in insulinoma beta TC-1 cells. Endocrinology *130:*159.

31. Foster, D. L. and Nagatani, S. (1999): Physiological perspectives on leptin as a regulator of reproduction: Role in timing puberty. Biol. Reprod. *60:*205.

32. Frank, B. H. and Chance, R. E. (1983): Two routes for producing human insulin utilizing recombinant DNA technology. Münch. Med. Wochenschr. *125* (Suppl. 1):S14.

33. Genuth, S. M. (1993): Hormones of the pancreatic islets. *In:* Physiology, Section IX: The Endocrine System, 3rd ed., edited by R. M. Berne and M. N. Levy. St. Louis, MO, Mosby-Year Book, Inc., p. 851.

34. Gepts, W. and Toussaint, D. (1967): Spontaneous diabetes in dogs and cats. A pathological study. Diabetologia *3:*259.

35. Gerich, J. E. (1989): Oral hypoglycemic agents. N. Engl. J. Med. *321:*1231.

36. Gerich, J. E., Charles, M. A., and Grodsky, G. M. (1976): Regulation of pancreatic insulin and glucagon secretion. Annu. Rev. Physiol. *38:*353.

37. Gerich, J. E., Lorenzi, M., Bier, D. M., et al. (1975): Prevention of human diabetic ketoacidosis by somatostatin. Evidence for an essential role of glucagon. N. Engl. J. Med. *292:*985.

38. Gershwin, L. J. (1975): Familial canine diabetes mellitus. J. Am. Vet. Med. Assoc. *167:*479.

39. Gromada, J., Holst, J. J., and Rorsman, P. (1998): Cellular regulation of islet hormone secretion by the incretin hormone glucagon-like peptide 1. Pflugers Arch. *435:*583.

40. Guler, H. P., Zapf, J., Scheiwiller, E., et al. (1988): Recombinant human insulin-like growth factor I stimulates growth and has distinct effects on organ size in hypophysectomized rats. Proc. Nat. Acad. Sci., USA *85:*4889.

41. Hallden, G., Gafvelin, G., Mutt, V., et al. (1986): Characterization of cat insulin. Arch. Biochem. Biophys. *247:*20.

42. Hedeskov, C. J. (1980): Mechanism of glucose-induced insulin secretion. Physiol. Rev. *60:*442.

43. Hedo, J. A., Villanueva, M. L., and Marco, J. (1979): Influence of plasma free fatty acids on pancreatic polypeptide secretion in man. J. Clin. Endocrinol. Metab. *49:*73.

44. Heiman, M. L., Chen, Y., and Caro, J. F. (1998): Leptin participates in the regulation of glucocorticoid and growth hormone axes. J. Nutr. Biochem. *9:*553.

45. Hocquette, J. F. and Bauchart, D. (1999): Intestinal absorption, blood transport and hepatic and muscle metabolism of fatty acids in preruminant and ruminant animals. Reprod. Nutr. Develop. *39:*27.

46. Hoenig, M. (1995): Pathophysiology of canine diabetes. Vet. Clin. North Am., Small An. Pract. *25:*553.

47. Holz, G. G., IV, Kuhtreiber, W. M., and Habener, J. F. (1993): Pancreatic beta-cells are rendered glucose-competent by the insulinotropic hormone glucagon-like peptide-1(7–37). Nature *361:*362.

48. Hougen, T. J., Hopkins, B. E., and Smith, T. W. (1978): Insulin effects on monovalent cation transport on Na-K-ATPase activity. Am. J. Physiol. *234:*C59.

49. Houseknecht, K. L., Baile, C. A., Matteri, R. L., et al. (1998): The biology of leptin: A review. J. Anim. Sci. *76:*1405.

50. Janson, J., Ashley, R. H., Harrison, D., et al. (1999): The mechanism of islet amyloid polypeptide toxicity in membrane disruption by intermediate-sized toxic amyloid particles. Diabetes *48:*491.

51. Jeffrey, J. R. (1969): Diabetes mellitus secondary to chronic pancreatitis in a pony. J. Am. Vet. Med. Assoc. *153:*1168.

52. Johnson, R. K. (1977): Insulinoma in the dog. *In:* The Symposium on Endocrinology, edited by E. C. Feldman. Philadelphia, PA, W. B. Saunders, Co. Vet. Clin. North Am. *7:*629.

53. Jones, K. L., Bell, R. L., Oyler, J. M., et al. (1970): Hyperglycemic effects of sodium butyrate in normal and pancreatectomized sheep. Am. J. Vet. Res. *31:*81.

54. Karlsson, E. (1999): IAPP as a regulator of glucose homeostasis and pancreatic hormone secretion. Int. J. Mol. Med. *3:*577.

55. Kasson, B. G. and Hsueh, A. J. (1987): Insulin-like growth factor-I augments gonadotropin-stimulated androgen biosynthesis by cultured rat testicular cells. Mol. Cell Endocrinol. *52:*27.

56. Kieffer, T. J. and Habener, J. F. (2000): The adipoinsular axis: Effects of leptin in pancreatic B-cells. Am. J. Physiol. Endocrinol. Metab. *278:*E1.

57. Kirk, C. A., Feldman, E. C., and Nelson, R. W. (1993): Diagnosis of naturally acquired type I and type II diabetes mellitus in cats. Am. J. Vet. Res. *54:*463.

58. Larsson, L.I., Golterman, N., de Magistris, L., et al. (1979): Somatostatin cell processes as pathways for paracrine secretion. Science *205:*1393.

59. Lin, T., Blaisdell, J., and Haskell, J. F. (1987): Type I IGF receptors of Leydig cells are upregulated by human chorionic gonadotropin. Biochem. Biophys. Res. Commun. *149:*852.

60. Liu, J. P., Baker, J., Perkins, A. S., et al. (1993): Mice carrying null mutations of the genes encoding insulin-like growth factor I (Igf-1) and type 1 IGF receptor (Igf1r). Cell *75:*59.

61. Lutz, T. A. and Rand, J. S. (1993): A review of new developments in type 2 diabetes in human beings and cats. Br. Vet. J. *149:*527.

62. Lutz, T. A. and Rand, J. S. (1995): Pathogenesis of feline diabetes mellitus. Vet. Clin. North Am., Small Anim. Pract. *25:*527.

63. Lutz, T. A. and Rand, J. S. (1996): Plasma amylin and insulin concentrations in normoglycemic and hyperglycemic cats. Can. Vet. J. *37:*27.

64. Ma, Z., Westermark, G. T., Johnson, K. H., et al. (1998): Quantitative immunohistochemical analysis of

islet amyloid polypeptide (IAPP) in normal, impaired glucose tolerant, and diabetic cats. Amyloid *5:*255.

65. MacDonald, M. L., Rogers, Q. R., and Morris, J. G. (1984): Nutrition of the domestic cat, a mammalian carnivore. Annu. Rev. Nutr. *4:*521.

66. Magoffin, D. A., Kurtz, K. M., and Erickson, G. F. (1990): Insulin-like growth factor-I selectively stimulates cholesterol side-chain cleavage expression in ovarian theca-interstitial cells. Mol. Endocrinol. *4:*489.

67. Manns, J. G. and Boda, J. M. (1965): Control of insulin secretion in sheep: The effect of volatile fatty acids and glucose. Physiologist *8:*227.

68. Manns, J. G. and Martin, C. L. (1972): Plasma insulin, glucagon, and nonesterified fatty acid in dogs with diabetes mellitus. Am. J. Vet. Res. *33:*981.

69. Martin, S. L. and Capen, C. C. (1979): The endocrine system. *In:* Canine Medicine, Vol 4, edited by E. J. Catcott. Santa Barbara, CA, American Veterinary Publications, Inc., p. 1090.

70. Mattheeuws, D., Rottiers, R., Kaneko, J. J., et al. (1984): Diabetes mellitus in dogs: Relationship of obesity to glucose tolerance and insulin response. Am. J. Vet. Res. *45:*98.

71. McTigue, D. M. and Rogers, R. C. (1995): Pancreatic polypeptide stimulates gastric acid secretion through a vagal mechanism in rats. Am. J. Physiol. *269:*R983.

72. Meyer, D. J. (1977): Temporary remission of hypoglycemia in a dog with insulinoma after treatment with streptozotocin. Am. J. Vet. Res. *38:*1201.

73. Miller, R. E. (1981): Pancreatic neuroendocrinology: Peripheral neural mechanisms in the regulation of the islets of Langerhans. Endocrine Rev. *2:*471.

74. Morris, J. G. and Rogers, Q. R. (1983): Nutritional implications of some metabolic anomalies of the cat. Proc. Am. Anim. Hosp. Assoc., p. 325.

75. Moses, A. C., Nissley, S. P., Short, P. A., et al. (1980): Increased levels of multiplication-stimulating activity, an insulin-like growth factor, in fetal rat serum. Proc. Nat. Acad. Sci. USA *77:*649.

76. Nakaki, T., Nakadate, T., Ishii, K., et al. (1981): Postsynaptic alpha-2 adrenergic receptors in isolated rat islets of Langerhans: Inhibition of insulin release and cyclic 3',5'-adenosine monophosphate accumulation. J. Pharmacol. Exp. Ther. *216:*607.

77. Nelson, R. W. (1995): Diabetes mellitus. *In:* Textbook of Veterinary Internal Medicine. Diseases of the Dog and Cat, 4th ed., edited by S. J. Ettinger and E. C. Feldman. Philadelphia, PA, W. B. Saunders, Co., p. 1510.

78. Nelson, R. W. (1995): Insulin-secreting islet cell neoplasia. *In:* Textbook of Veterinary Internal Medicine. Diseases of the Dog and Cat, 4th ed., edited by S. J. Ettinger and E. C. Feldman. Philadelphia, PA, W. B. Saunders, Co., p. 1501.

79. Nelson, R. W., Feldman, E. C., Ford, S. L., et al. (1993): Effect of an orally administered sulfonylurea, glipizide, for treatment of diabetes mellitus in cats. J. Am. Vet. Med. Assoc. *203:*821.

80. Nelson, R. W., Himsel, C. A., Feldman, E. C., et al. (1990): Glucose tolerance and insulin response in normal-weight and obese cats. Am. J. Vet. Res. *51:*1357.

81. Niki, I. (1999): Ca2+ signaling and the insulin secretory cascade in the pancreatic beta-cell. Jpn. J. Pharmacol. *80:*191.

82. Nordlie, R. C., Foster, J. D., and Lange, A. J. (1999): Regulation of glucose production by the liver. Annu. Rev. Nutr. *19:*379.

83. Nussdorfer, G. G., Mazzocchi, G., and Malendowicz, L. K. (1998): The possible involvement of pancreatic polypeptide in the paracrine regulation of human and rat adrenal cortex. Endocrine Res. *24:*695.

84. O'Brien, T. D., Butler, P. C., Westermark, P., et al. (1993): Islet amyloid polypeptide: A review of its biology and potential roles in the pathogenesis of diabetes mellitus. Vet. Pathol. *30:*317.

85. O'Brien, T. D., Hayden, D. W., Johnson, K. H., et al. (1985): High dose intravenous glucose tolerance test and serum insulin and glucagon levels in diabetic and non-diabetic cats: Relationships to insular amyloidosis. Vet. Pathol. *22:*250.

86. O'Dell, S. D. and Day, I. N. (1998): Insulin-like growth factor II (IGF-II). Int. J. Biochem. Cell Biol. *30*:767.

87. Okita, M., Inui, A., Inoue, T., et al. (1998): Effects of corticotropin-releasing factor on feeding and pancreatic polypeptide response in the dog. J. Endocrinol. *156*:359.

88. Orci, L. (1982): Macro- and micro-domains in the endocrine pancreas. Diabetes *31:*538.

89. Panciera, D. L., Thomas, C. B., Eicker, S. W., et al. (1990): Epizootiologic patterns of diabetes mellitus in cats: 333 cases (1980–1986). J. Am. Vet. Med. Assoc. *197:*1504.

90. Penhoat, A., Jaillard, C., and Saez, J. M. (1989): Synergistic effects of corticotropin and insulin-like growth factor I on corticotropin receptors and corticotropin responsiveness in cultured bovine adrenocortical cells. Biochem. Biophys. Res. Commun. *165:*355.

91. Penhoat, A., Naville, D., Jaillard, C., et al. (1989): Hormonal regulation of insulin-like growth factor I secretion by bovine adrenal cells. J. Biol. Chem. *264:*6858.

92. Pipleers, D., Veld, P., Maes, E., et al. (1982): Glucose-induced insulin release depends on functional cooperation between islet cells. Proc. Nat. Acad. Sci. USA *79:*7322.

93. Pohlmann, R., Boeker, M. W. C., and Von Figura, K. (1995): The two mannose 6-phosphate receptors transport distinct complements of lysosomal proteins. J. Biol. Chem. *270:*27311.

94. Powell-Braxton, L., Hollingshead, P., Warburton, C., et al. (1993): IGF-I is required for normal embryonic growth in mice. Genes Develop. *7:*2609.

95. Prior, R. L. and Smith, S. B. (1983): Role of insulin in regulating animo acid metabolism in normal and alloxan-diabetic cattle. J. Nutr. *113:*1016.

96. Rinderknecht, E. and Humbel, R. E. (1978): The amino acid sequence of human insulin-like growth factor I and its structural homology with proinsulin. J. Biol. Chem. *253:*2769.

97. Rink, T. J., Beaumont, K., Koda, J., et al. (1993): Structure and biology of amylin. Trends Pharmacol. Sci. *14:*113.

98. Rogler, C. E., Yang, D., Rossetti, L., et al. (1994): Altered body composition and increased frequency of diverse malignancies in insulin-like growth factor-II transgenic mice. J. Biol. Chem. *269:*13779.

99. Romsos, D. R., Palmer, H. J., Muiruri, K. L., et al. (1981): Influence of a low carbohydrate diet on per-

formance of pregnant and lactating dogs. J. Nutr. *111:*678.

100. Salmon, W. D. and Daughaday, W. H. (1957): A hormonally controlled serum factor which stimulates sulfate incorporation by cartilage *in vitro.* J. Lab. Clin. Med. *49:*825.

101. Sanger, F. (1960): Chemistry of insulin. Br. Med. Bull. *16:*183.

102. Schaer, M. (1973): Diabetes mellitus in the cat. J. Am. Anim. Hosp. Assoc. *9:*548.

103. Schaer, M., Scott, R., Wilkins, R., et al. (1974): Hyperosmolar syndrome in the non-ketoacidotic diabetic dog. J. Am. Anim. Hosp. Assoc. *10:*357.

104. Schall, W. D. (1985): Pancreatic disorders. *In:* Handbook of Small Animal Therapeutics, edited by L. E. Davis. New York, NY, Churchill-Livingston, p. 485.

105. Schoenle, E., Zapf, J., Humbel, R. E., et al. (1982): Insulin-like growth factor I stimulates growth in hypophysectomized rats. Nature *296:*252.

106. Schoenle, E., Zapf, J., and Froesch, E. R. (1982): Insulin-like growth factors I and II stimulate growth of hypophysectomized rats. Diabetologia *23:*199.

107. Schwartz, M. W., Figlewicz, D. P., Baskin, D. G., et al. (1992): Insulin in the brain: A hormonal regulator of energy balance. Endocrine Rev. *13:*81.

108. Shetzline, M. A., Zipf, W. B., and Nishikawara, M. T. (1998): Pancreatic polypeptide: Identification of target tissues using an in vivo radioreceptor assay. Peptides *19:*279.

109. Shimazu, T. and Ishikawa, K. (1981): Modulation by the hypothalamus of glucagon and insulin secretion in rabbits: Studies with electrical and chemical stimulation. Endocrinology *108:*605.

110. Skottner, A., Clark, R. G., Fryklund, L., et al. (1989): Growth responses in a mutant dwarf rat to human growth factor I. Endocrinology *124:*2519.

111. Spencer, G. S., Hill, D. J., Garssen, G. J., et al. (1983): Somatomedin activity and growth hormone levels in body fluids of the fetal pig: Effect of chronic hyperinsulinemia. J. Endocrinol. *96:*107.

112. Steiner, D. F. (1976): Amino acid sequences of proteins - hormones (insulins). *In:* Handbook of Biochemistry and Molecular Biology, 3rd Edition, Proteins, Vol. III, edited by G. D. Fasman. Cleveland, OH, CRC Press, p. 378.

113. Stewart, C. E. H. and Rotwein, P. (1996): Growth, differentiation and survival: Multiple physiological functions for insulin-like growth factors. Physiol. Rev. *76:*1005.

114. Szecowka, J., Lins, P. E., and Efendic, S. (1982): Effects of cholecystokinin, gastric inhibitory peptide, and secretin on insulin and glucagon secretion in rats. Endocrinology *110:*1268.

115. Tannenbaum, G. S., Ling, N., and Brazeau, P. (1982): Somatostatin-28 is longer acting and more selective than Somatostatin-14 on pituitary and pancreatic hormone release. Endocrinology *111:*101.

116. Trenkle, A. (1978): Relation of hormonal variations to nutritional studies and metabolism of ruminants. J. Dairy Sci. *61:*281.

117. Unger, R. H. and Orci, L. (1981): Glucagon and the A cell. N. Engl. J. Med. *304:*1518.

118. Valverde, I., Vandermeers, A., Anjaneyulu, R., et al. (1979): Calmodulin activation of adenylate cyclase in pancreatic islets. Science *206:*225.

119. Van-Buul-Offers, S., Ueda, I., and Van-den-Brande, J. L. (1986): Biosynthetic somatomedin C (SM-C/IGF-I) increases the length and weight of Snell dwarf mice. Pediatr. Res. *20:*825.

120. Van Wyk, J. J., Underwood, L. E., Hintz, R. L., et al. (1974): The somatomedins: A family of insulin-like peptides under growth hormone control. Recent Prog. Horm. Res. *30:*259.

121. Washizu, T., Tanaka, A., Sako, T., et al. (1999): Comparison of the activities of enzymes related to glycolysis and gluconeogenesis in the liver of dogs and cats. Res. Vet. Sci. *67:*205.

122. Westermark, P., Wernstedt, C., Wilander, E., et al. (1987): Amyloid fibriles in human insulinoma and islets of Langerhans of the diabetic cat are derived from a neuro-peptide-like protein also present in normal islet cells. Pro. Nat. Acad. Sci., USA *84:*3881.

123. Witzel, D. A. and Littledike, E. T. (1973): Suppression of insulin secretion during induced hypocalcemia. Endocrinology *93:*761.

124. Wollheim, C. B. and Sharp, G. W. G. (1981): Regulation of insulin release by calcium. Physiol. Rev. *61:*914.

125. Zarrow, M. X., Yochim, J. M., McCarthy, J. L., et al. (1964): Experimental Endocrinology. A Sourcebook of Basic Techniques. New York, NY, Academic Press, Inc., p. 390.

The Adrenal Gland

P. A. Martin and M. H. Crump

6

INTRODUCTION

The adrenal glands are paired endocrine organs located within the abdominal cavity. Anatomically, each gland consists of two distinct parts, with different functions and embryonic origins. The outer part, or adrenal cortex, originates from mesodermal tissue located between the dorsal mesentery of the gut and the medial surface of the mesenteric kidney. The cortex synthesizes a wide range of steroid hormones which, collectively, are called corticosteroids. The inner part of the adrenal gland is the adrenal medulla which originates from neuroectodermal cells from the primitive ganglia of the celiac plexus. The adrenal medulla contains chromaffin cells which synthesize and release catecholamines, epinephrine and norepinephrine, in response to sympathetic stimulation. Thus, the adrenal medulla can be considered as an extension of the sympathetic nervous system.

Glucocorticoids and catecholamines secreted by the adrenal glands regulate a number of metabolic processes which enable animals to function in a constantly changing environment. The major effects of corticosteroids are on the regulation of metabolic processes for maintenance of the proper nutrition of cells, regulation of blood levels of Na^+ and K^+, and control of the volume of extracellular fluid. Catecholamines secreted by the adrenal glands influence the responsiveness of the animal to stressors, including the activation of the "fight or flight" response. Catecholamines also play a role in the regulation of metabolic processes by inhibiting the effects of insulin and increasing the levels of glucose in the blood. The corticosteroids and catecholamines are also involved in adaptive changes. In general, adaptive changes for corticosteroids occur over minutes, days, weeks, or even months, whereas, adaptive changes in response to catecholamines occur within seconds to minutes. Corticosteroids are critical for the animal's well being. Life cannot be maintained in the absence of functional adrenal cortices. In contrast, the catecholamines produced by adrenal medullae are not requisite for life.

The most common dysfunctions of the adrenal gland in clinical veterinary medicine are hypersecretion of the adrenal cortex or hyperadrenocorticism and hyposecretion of the adrenal cortex or hypoadrenocorticism. The most common clinical problem associated with the adrenal medulla is a tumor of the chromaffin cells called pheochromocytoma.

ANATOMY

The adrenal glands, literally "the glands next to the kidneys," are located retroperitoneally in close apposition to the anterior pole of the kidneys. All domestic animals have highly irrigated adrenal glands, receiving blood from several arterial sources. Only the thyroid gland may receive a greater flow of blood per gram of tissue. The arterial supply to the adrenal glands branches into an extensive network of arterioles located beneath the adrenal capsule. Most of the adrenal arterioles give rise to a dense network of sinusoidal capillaries which drain blood into medullary venules and, eventually, into the adrenal veins. Other arterioles traverse the adrenal cortex to supply blood directly to the medulla and this blood is also returned via the adrenal veins. The main nerve supply to the adrenal glands consists of sympathetic nerves that synapse with medullary cells. Only a few nerve fibers terminate in the adrenal cortex. The adrenal glands also receive a few parasympathetic fibers but little is known about their function.

Adrenal Cortex

The adrenal cortex constitutes approximately 80% to 90% of the mass of the adrenal gland. The parenchymal cells of the cortex, also called corticocytes, are the source of the various steroid hormones produced by the gland and corticocytes have unique characteristics that distinguish them from other cells. The cytoplasm of corticocytes have a large number of lipid-filled droplets. Most of the lipid is cholesterol which is the precursor for the steroid hormones produced by the adrenal glands. These cells also have an abundance of smooth endoplasmic reticulum, a paucity of rough endoplasmic reticulum, large Golgi complexes, and numerous mitochondria. Another distinguishing feature of corticocytes is their inability to store hormones in the cytoplasm as do cells that synthesize protein or peptide hormones. The large stores of cholesterol and the abundance of cytoplasmic organelles in corticocytes may be adaptations for the immediate response of these cells to their respective tropic hormones and to compensate for their inability to store hormone.

The adrenal cortex is characterized histologically by three distinct zones (Fig. 6–1). The *zona glomerulosa* is the thinnest and outermost zone. In ruminants and humans, it consists of clusters of small and darkly stained corticocytes arranged in whorls. In other domestic mammals, this zone is frequently called the *zona arcuata* because the corticocytes are grouped in the form of arcs. In dogs, cats, and other carnivores, however, the corticocytes of the *zona glomerulosa* are larger and lighter staining compared to those of other species. Depending on the species, the corticocytes in the *zona glomerulosa* appear to

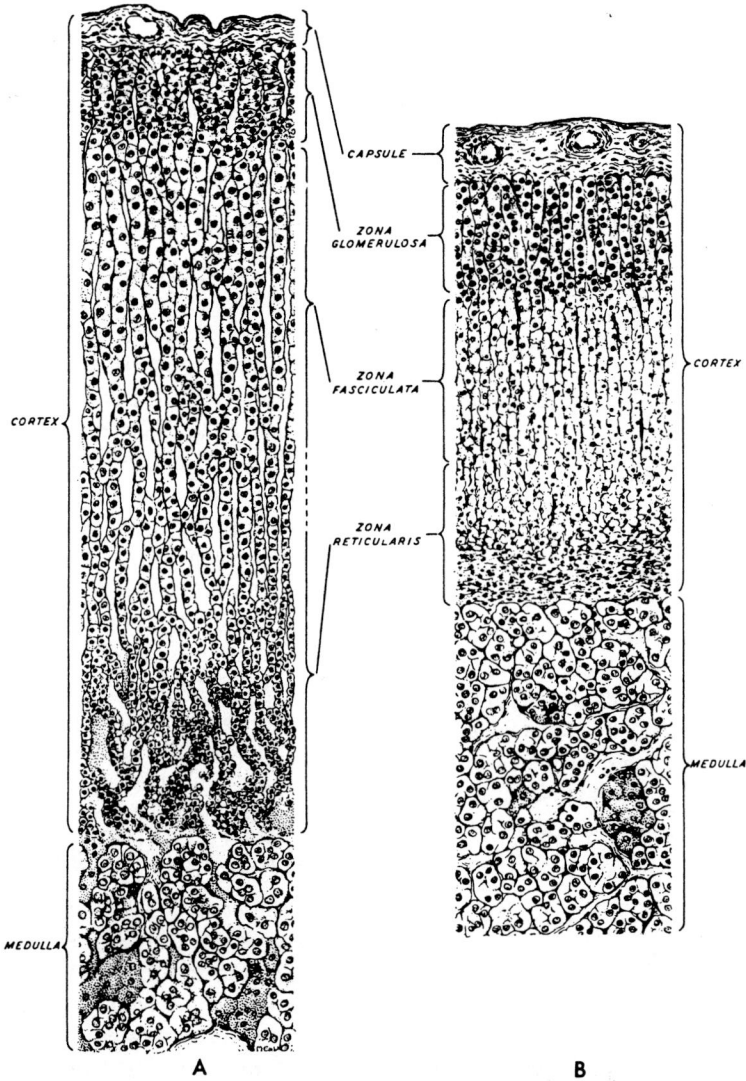

Fig. 6–1. Sections through the adrenal glands of normal (**A**) and hypophysectomized (**B**) rats. Because the functional capacity of the adrenal cortex is conditioned by the release of ACTH and other proopiomelanocortin-derived peptides, hypophysectomy results in a pronounced shrinkage of the *zona fasciculata* and *zona reticularis* of the cortex. The *zona glomerulosa* and the medulla are not influenced by hypophysectomy. Both sections are drawn to scale. (From: C. D. Turner,[188] et al., p. 293, 1976. Courtesy of W. B. Saunders Co., Philadelphia, PA).

be flattened or are polyhedral in outline. The *zona fasciculata* is the middle zone and is the thickest of the three zones. The cuboidal or polyhedral cells of the *zona fasciculata* form cords that are one cell wide and are perpendicular to the capsule of the gland. These cords are separated from each other by a rich network of sinusoidal capillaries. Cells in the cords are flanked by one to four of these sinusoidal capil-laries. The corticocytes of the *zona fasciculata* are large with large, vesicular nuclei and have an abundance of lipid and lipid droplets. As a consequence, their cytoplasm appears foamy and lightly-stained compared to the corticocytes found in the two adjoining zones. The *zona reticularis* is the innermost zone of the adrenal cortex and contains small corticocytes arranged in a network of anastomosing cords.

Adrenal Medulla

Chromaffin cells of the adrenal medulla of humans and animals are a part of the endocrine system and an important component of the sympathetic nervous system. These secretory cells contain enzymes for the synthesis of norepinephrine and many of the medullary cells contain the necessary enzymes and co-factors to form epinephrine. Chromaffin cells are innervated by cholinergic preganglionic nerve fibers which connect with the reticular formation of the medulla oblongata, pons, and hypothalamic centers. These preganglionic sympathetic fibers release acetylcholine which depolarizes the plasma membrane of medullary cells, thereby causing the release of norepinephrine and epinephrine to be distributed throughout the body by the circulatory system.

Norepinephrine and epinephrine secreting cells of the adrenal medulla may be distinguished histochemically and their relative number and distribution varies among species. In domestic ungulates, the adrenal medulla has two zones: An outer zone that contains mostly large, chromaffin cells that secrete epinephrine and an inner zone with mostly small cells that secrete norepinephrine.

MAINTENANCE AND GROWTH OF THE ADRENAL CORTEX

The maintenance and growth of the adrenal cortex is under the positive control of ACTH and other proopiomelanocortin-derived peptides secreted by the corticotropic cells of the adenohypophysis (see also, Chapter 2). After hypophysectomy, atrophy of the *zona glomerulosa* is limited but there is a marked decrease in the thickness of the *zona fasciculata* and *zona reticularis*. In contrast, hypersecretion of ACTH by pituitary corticotropes leads to a marked increase in the thickness of the *zona fasciculata* and *zona reticularis*.

Compared to other glands, the adrenal cortex has a high rate of turnover of cells. Every day large numbers of corticocytes die and are replaced by new cells. Therefore, maintenance of the adrenal cortex depends on an exquisite balance between mitosis and the genetically programmed cell death called apoptosis. Disturbances in this delicate balance due to over- or understimulation of the cortex lead, respectively, to an increase or decrease in the thickness and size of the adrenal cortex, particularly affecting the *zona fasciculata* and *zona reticularis*.

Adrenocorticotropic Hormone, ACTH

For many years, changes in the adrenal cortex were attributed solely to effects of ACTH on the corticocytes. Now, the role of ACTH is more controversial. Administration of high doses of ACTH or a synthetic analogue causes an increase in the size of the mitochondria, smooth endoplasmic reticulum, and the nucleus of corticocytes without a concurrent increase in cell numbers. This hypertrophy or increase in the size of corticocytes accounts for the increased mass of the adrenal cortex that is attributable to ACTH. Hypertrophy and ACTH-induced effects on adrenocortical steroidogenesis are mediated by insulin-like growth factors (IGFs).

It now appears that another factor, short N-terminal peptide, produced by corticotropic cells of the pituitary gland is responsible for the proliferation of corticocytes.

Short N-Terminal Peptide

The discovery that ACTH was not the only peptide secreted by adenohypophyseal corticotropes lead to the identification of additional peptides and elucidation of their physiological actions. Peptides produced by corticotropes originate from a large, precursor molecule called proopiomelanocortin (POMC, see also Chapter 1, Fig. 1–3) which is highly conserved among human, primate, and domestic animal species. Proopiomelanocortin is synthesized and processed by corticotropes of the *pars distalis* in all domestic animals. However, cells of the *pars intermedia* can also produce significant amounts of proopiomelanocortin, especially in dogs and horses. The regulation of the synthesis and the extent of post-translational processing of proopiomelanocortin differs among cells of the *pars distalis* and *pars intermedia* (Fig. 6–2). It appears that the primary peptides produced by corticotropes of the *pars distalis* are: Long N-terminal peptide, ACTH, and β-lipotropin. The long N-terminal peptide does not appear to be biologically active and must be processed to short N-terminal peptide (N-POMC). This peptide (N-POMC) induces a strong proliferative response in the atrophied adrenal cortex of hypophysectomized rats.

The major proopiomelanocortin-derived peptides produced and secreted from the cells of the *pars intermedia* are shown in Fig. 6–2. Whether or not proopiomelanocortin-derived peptides originate from cells of the *pars distalis* or *pars intermedia* can be of clinical significance[46] because corticotropes of the *pars distalis* are under the positive control of corticotropin-releasing hormone (CRH) whereas corticotropes of the *pars intermedia* are under the negative control of dopamine.[23,47]

Proopiomelanocortin is processed and the proopiomelanocortin-derived peptides are stored in the secretory granules of pituitary corticotropes. Hence, any stimulus that inhibits or stimulates the secretion of ACTH, also affects the secretion of other proopiomelanocortin-derived peptides. This would explain why hypo- or hypersecretion of corticotropes results in, respectively, atrophy of the adrenal cortex and low concentrations of circulating glucocorticoids or in an increase in the size of the adrenal cortex and high levels of glucocorticoids in the blood. Serum containing antibodies to N-POMC administered to normal, intact rats results in the inhibition of the proliferation of corticocytes without affecting glucocorticoid levels. In contrast, administration of an antiserum containing biologically active antibodies to ACTH does not inhibit the proliferation of corticocytes but results in a marked decrease in glucocorticoid levels. The secretion of fibroblast growth factors (FGFs) is stimulated by N-POMC, hence, FGFs may be the mediators of the mitogenic effect of N-POMC on adrenal corticocytes.

ADRENAL STEROIDS

The adrenal cortex produces steroid hormones and, without question, is the most versatile of the steroid-producing glands. The hormones produced are represented in each of the four major groups of steroid hormones: Glucocorticoids, mineralocorticoids, androgens, and estrogens. By far, the most important adrenocorticosteroids are the glucocorticoids, cortisol and corticosterone, and the mineralocorticoid, aldosterone (Fig. 6–3). The adrenal cortex also synthesizes small amounts of androgens, including dehydroepiandrosterone and androstenedione, as well as estrogens, including estradiol-

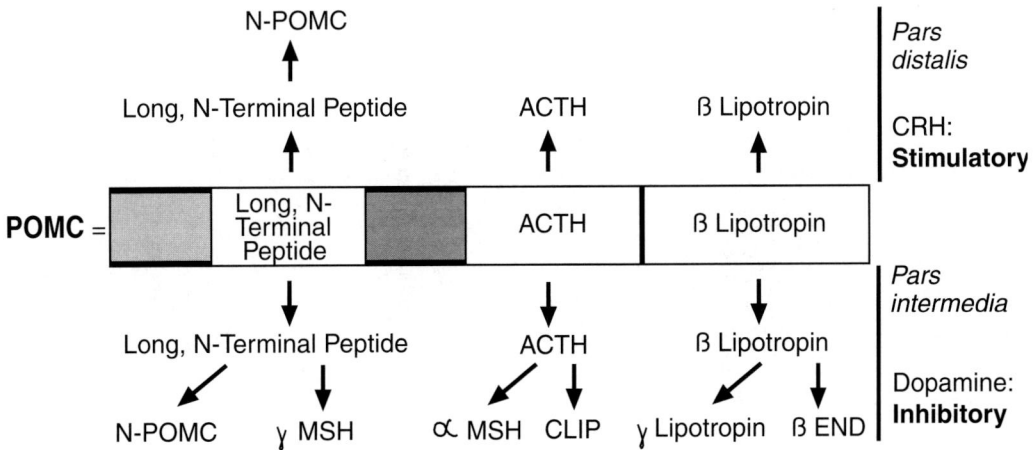

Fig. 6–2. Peptides derived from proopiomelanocortin (**POMC**) synthesized by corticotropes of the *pars distalis* and *pars intermedia* of the adenohypophysis (**ACTH** = adrenocorticotropic hormone; **CLIP** = corticotropin-like intermediate lobe peptide; **CRH** = corticotropin-releasing hormone; **END** = endorphin; **MSH** = melanocyte-stimulating hormone; **N-POMC** = Short N-terminal peptide). (Adapted from different sources, including: D. S. Bruyette,[23] et al., Vet. Clin. North Am., Small Anim. Pract. *27:*273, 1997; N. O. Dybdal,[47] et al., J. Am. Vet. Med. Assoc. *204:*627, 1994; N. Dybdal,[46] p. 499, 1997; and D. N. Orth and W. J. Kovaks,[142] p. 527, 1998).

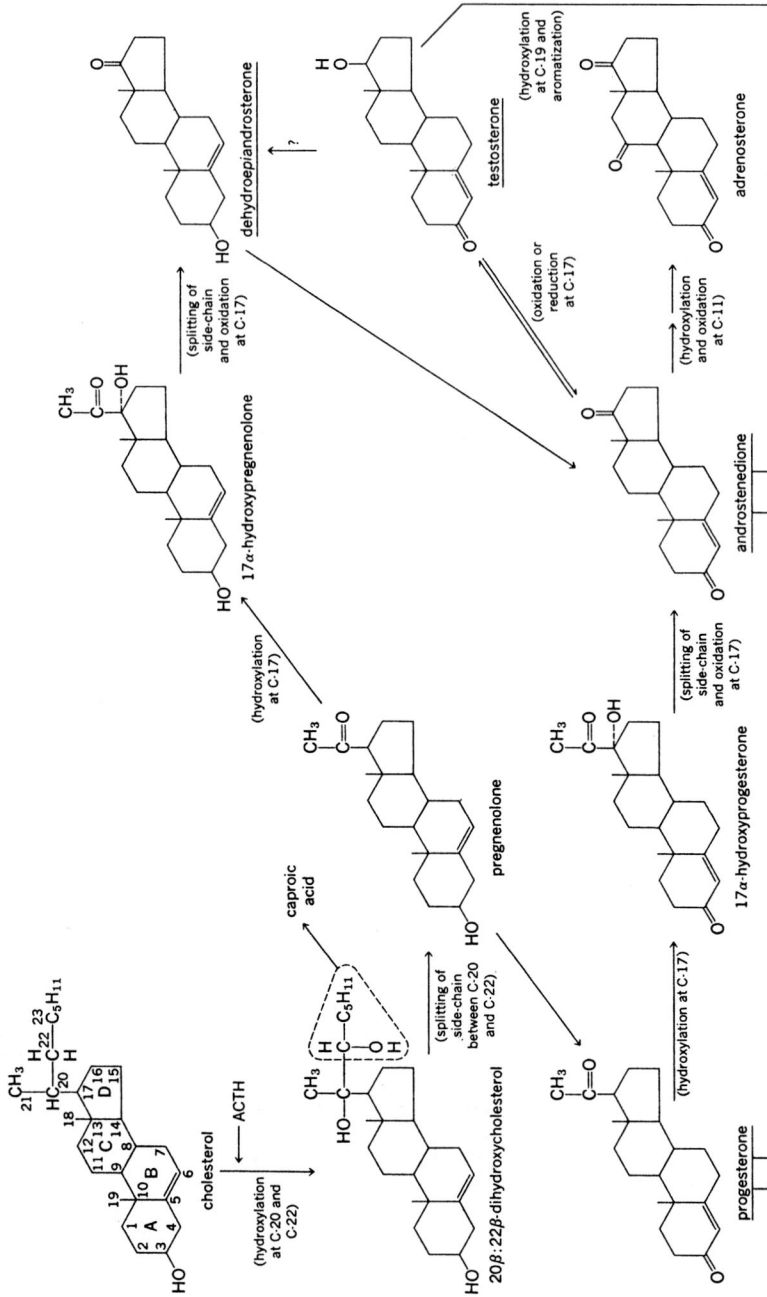

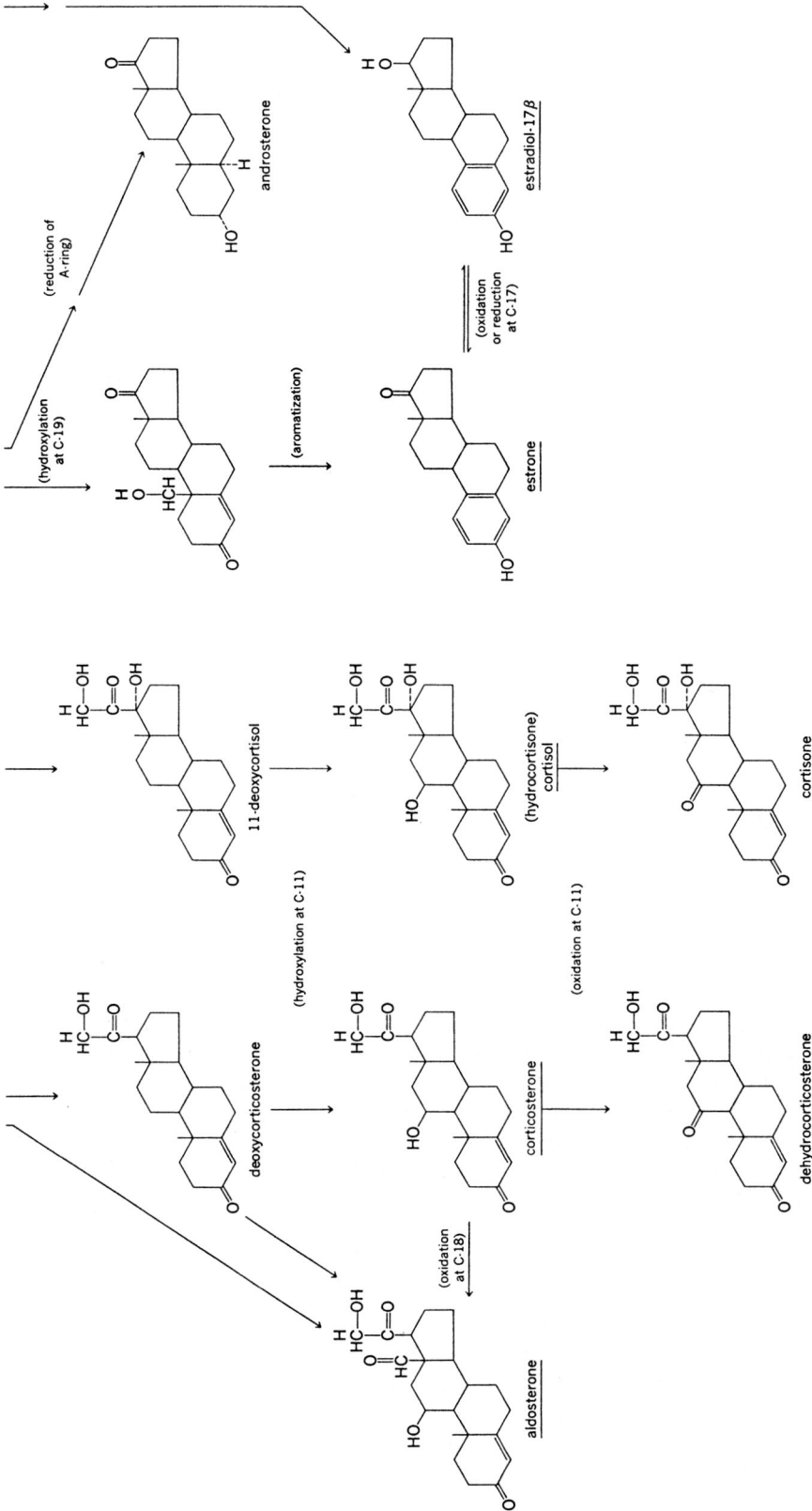

Fig. 6–3. Major metabolic pathways in biogenesis of steroid hormones. The principal secretory products of the steroidogenic organs are underlined. Specific enzymes have been characterized, and mitochondrial or microsomal participation has been determined for many of the steps shown. The 17- and 21-hydroxylations appear to require mitochondrial participation; the 11-hydroxylation, requires microsomal participation. Also, various co-factors have been specified for many of the steps. For example, reduced nicotinamide adenine dinucleotide phosphate (NADPH) and molecular O_2 are required for the various hydroxylations and for the side chain splitting (desmolase enzyme activity). In addition, certain ions are known to be required for the conversion of corticosterone to aldosterone by cells of the *zona glomerulosa*. The products of catabolism of the major steroid hormones are not shown. (From: A. Gorbman,[74] et al., p. 402, 1983. Courtesy of John Wiley and Sons, Inc., New York, NY).

17β (Fig. 6–3). The androgens and estrogens that are normally produced and released by the adrenal cortex in intact male and female animals constitute but a small portion of circulating androgens and estrogens. Thus, the androgens and estrogens produced by the adrenal cortex are insufficient to replace the loss of gonadal steroids in gonadectomized animals.

Structure and Biosynthesis

All steroid molecules and their precursor, cholesterol, contain the basic cyclopentanoperhydrophenanthrene ring structure which consists of three cyclohexane rings and one cyclopentane ring (Fig. 6–3). The molecules in this large family of steroids are closely related and very minor changes in molecular structure may result in a marked difference in biological activity, as exemplified by the similarities between cortisol (glucocorticoid) and aldosterone (mineralocorticoid), or estradiol-17β (estrogen) and testosterone (androgen).

The chemical nomenclature of steroid molecules follows internationally accepted conventions. The four rings and the number and location of the carbon atoms for cholesterol, the precursor for all steroids, are depicted in Figure 6–3. Double bonds in the structure are indicated by the Greek letter Δ, followed by a superscript number to indicate the specific carbon atom associated with the double bond. The carbon atom with the lower number is used to indicate the double bond (e.g., Δ^4 instead of Δ^5 for aldosterone and cortisol). Chemical groups attached to the steroid nucleus are designated according to their orientation relative to the horizontal plane of the steroid nucleus. Chemical groups projecting above the plane and toward the reader are β substituents (e.g., 11β-hydroxy) with their bonds designated by solid lines (—). Chemical groups below the plane and away from the reader are α substituents (e.g. 11α-hydroxy) with their bonds designated by dashed lines (– – –). Keto groups have double bonds and their location is identified by a number indicating the carbon atom to which they are attached (e.g., 3-keto). The chemical nomenclature for steroids is cumbersome and,

for that reason, trivial names are used for the more common steroids. For example, cortisol is seldom referred to by its chemical name, 4-pregnen-11β,17α,21-triol-3,20-dione. The total number of carbon atoms is 21 for glucocorticoids and progestagens, 19 carbons for mineralocorticoids and androgens, and 18 carbon atoms for estrogens. These steroidal groups are commonly referred to as C_{21}, C_{19}, and C_{18} steroids.

Biosynthesis of adrenocorticosteroids begins with cholesterol, the parent compound. Cholesterol can be absorbed directly from the gastrointestinal tract or synthesized *de novo* in the body from acetate. Corticosteroids are formed primarily from absorbed cholesterol. The remainder is formed from acetate in corticocytes. Because cholesterol is insoluble in water, it is transported to the adrenal cortical cells by low-density lipoproteins (LDLs, Fig. 6–4). After LDLs bind to the membrane of steroidogenic cells, the LDL-receptor complexes are internalized by receptor-mediated endocytosis. In the cell, the LDL-receptor complex dissociates and the receptor is reincorporated into the cell membrane, LDL is catabolized, and cholesterol is liberated. This intracellular cholesterol may be used directly for steroidogenesis or esterified and stored in lipid droplets (Fig. 6–4). Enzymes for steroidogenesis are located in the mitochondria and endoplasmic reticulum (Fig. 6–4). The final steroid products diffuse from the corticocyte into the circulation. Steroids are not stored in the cells of the adrenal cortex as are catecholamines in the medullary cells of the adrenal gland, or peptide and protein hormones produced by cells of other endocrine organs.

Transport, Metabolism, and Elimination

Steroids secreted by the adrenal glands enter the bloodstream as nonpolar molecules that are insoluble in water. Consequently, 60 to 95% of the adrenal steroids released into the circulation are reversibly bound to blood proteins. The major binding proteins for glucocorticoids, mineralocorticoids and progestagens, and for androgens and estrogens are respectively, transcortin, albumin, and sex hormone-

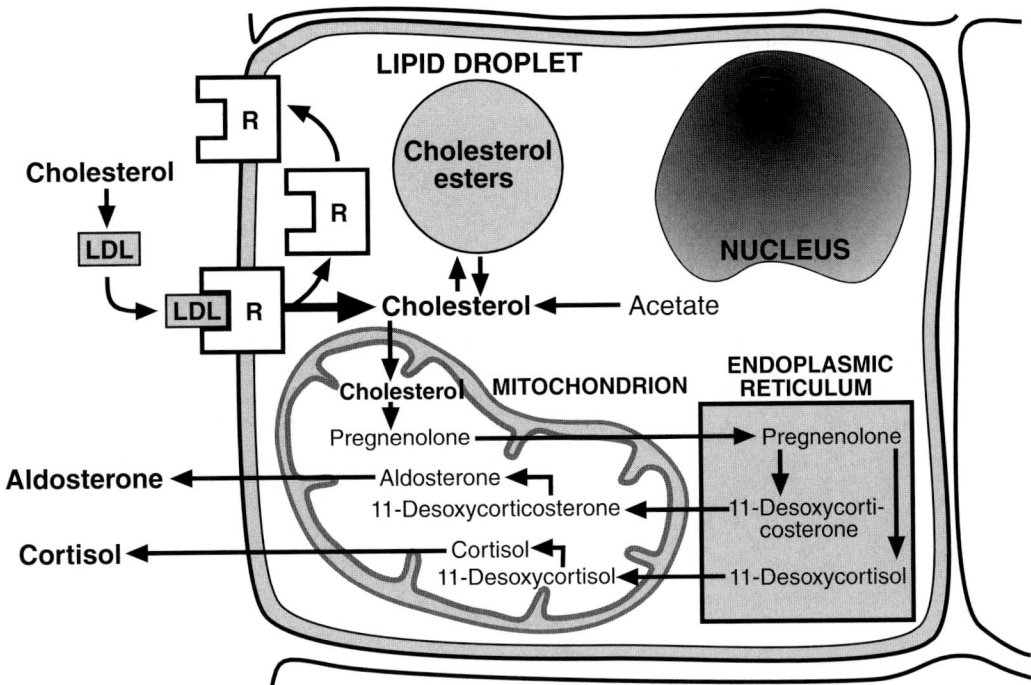

Fig. 6–4. Pathways and subcellular components involved in the biosynthesis of cortisol and aldosterone (**LDL** = low density lipoprotein; **R** = receptor).

binding globulin, all of which are produced by the liver. Because of the role blood proteins play in the binding of steroid hormones, diseases of the liver affecting protein synthesis or urinary losses of protein due to kidney disorders can alter blood levels of adrenal steroids in domestic animals.

Only free or unbound steroids passively diffuse through the lipid bilayer of the cell membrane of target cells to elicit biological effects. The half-life of cortisol is less than two hours but this is considerably longer than that of the catecholamines released from chromaffin cells of the adrenal medulla. The vast majority of steroids are degraded in the liver while the remainder is degraded in the kidneys. In the process of degradation, corticosteroids undergo various reductions, oxidations, and hydroxylations before conjugation with glucuronic acid or sulphates. These conjugated metabolites are water-soluble, which facilitates their excretion in urine (75%) and into the small intestine (25%) as a component of bile.

Mechanism of Action

Steroid hormones exert their effects by binding to and activating hormone-specific receptors in target cells. Steroid receptors for glucocorticoids, mineralocorticoids, androgens, estrogens, and progestagens belong to a superfamily of receptors that also include the non-steroidal receptors for thyroid hormones, vitamin D_3, retinoic acid, and a large number of 'orphan' receptors for which there are no known ligands. The molecular mechanism of the different steroid hormones is remarkably similar.

Glucocorticoids and mineralocorticoids enter cells by diffusion and bind to hormone-specific receptors in the cytoplasm of target cells to induce a conformational change in the receptor (Fig. 6–5). In the nucleus, dimers of the activated hormone-receptor complex bind with high affinity to specific DNA binding sites to direct gene transcription. After transcription and synthesis of biologically active mRNA (see also Chapter 1, Figures 1–7 and 1–8), hormone-induced proteins elicit the steroid-specific actions or functions in

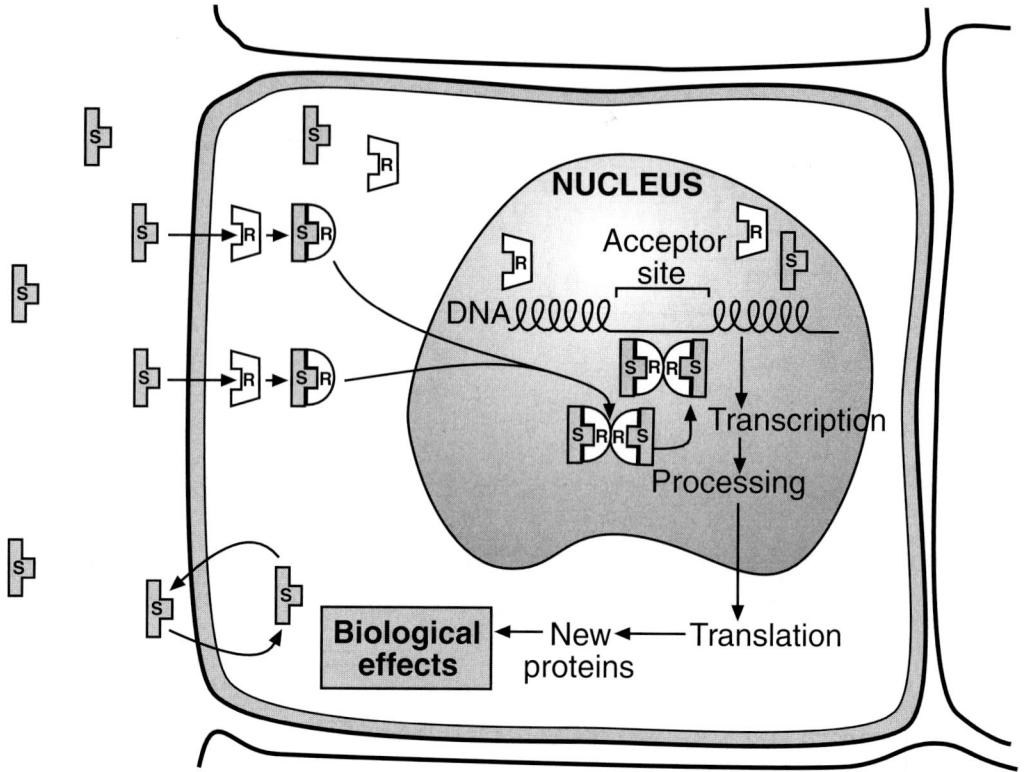

Fig. 6–5. Glucocorticoids and mineralocorticoids bind to cytoplasmic receptors and are translocated to the nucleus to form dimers which bind to **DNA.** The binding of the steroid-receptor complex to the acceptor site of nuclear chromatin initiates transcription and leads to the formation of new proteins which exert biological effects on the target cell (**S**=steroid hormone; **R**=receptor). (Adapted from: L. Chan,[29] et al., p. 698, 1978).

the target cell. Once the hormone-receptor complex has interacted with the gene, the receptor is recycled as inactive receptor and the steroid hormone passively diffuses from the cell.

GLUCOCORTICOIDS

Cortisol and corticosterone are the principal glucocorticoids produced and secreted by the adrenal cortex. Cortisol predominates in humans, horses, pigs, sheep, dogs, and cats, but corticosterone predominates in the rabbit, mouse, and rat. In newborn calves, cortisol is the major secretory product and corticosterone does not appear until 10 days after birth. Adult cattle secrete significant amounts of both glucocorticoids.

The approximate ratio of cortisol to corticosterone in adrenal venous blood of some mammals is as follows: Bovine, 0.05:1 to 1:1; sheep, 15:1 to 20:1; dogs, 2:1 to 5:1; humans and cats,

5:1 to 10:1; rats and rabbits, 0.05:1. The peripheral, circulating levels of cortisol in domestic animals are summarized in Table 6–1.

Regulation of Glucocorticoid Secretion

Basal levels of glucocorticoids are regulated by a negative feedback system that depends upon interactions between a functional hypothalamic-pituitary-adrenal axis and the associated hormones. The most important components of this feedback system are corticotropin-releasing hormone (CRH), ACTH, and cortisol (Fig. 6–6).

Effects of Corticotropin-releasing Hormone, Dopamine, and Vasopressin

Corticotropin-releasing hormone (CRH) is a peptide synthesized by parvocellular neurons in the paraventricular nucleus of the hypothalamus

Table 6-1   Levels of Cortisol* in the Plasma (ng/ml) of Adult Domestic Species

Species	Mean	Range	Reference Source
Cat	15	1 to 50	123, 153
Cattle			
Bull	19	16 to 21	162
Cow			
Dry	5	–**	197
Lactating, nonpregnant	8	–	197
Lactating, pregnant	8	–	169
Steer	11	–	175
Dog	21	6 to 48	9, 31
Goat			
Buck	21	–	61, 109
Doe, pregnant	18	–	135
Horse			
Gelding	42	15 to 97	104
Racing	72	–	151
Stallion	–**	36 to 46	181
Llama			
Pregnant	14	3 to 52	107
Pig			
Boar	25	2 to 134	115
Gilt, nonpregnant	14	–	7
Sow, pregnant	13	–	194
Sheep			
Ewe, anestrous	23	–	135
Ram	20	–	72
Wether	22	–	91

*Estimates calculated from data, as reported in the original publication(s). The numbers in the column for source are as listed in the reference section.
**A hyphen in the mean and/or range columns indicates missing information that was not provided or could not be estimated from the original publication.

and is the most potent and important factor that stimulates the release of ACTH. These parvocellular neurons store CRH in secretory granules until an appropriate stimulus induces the release of the hormone into the portal, hypophyseal blood for transport to the adenohypophysis, where CRH binds to specific receptors on the cell membrane of adenohypophyseal corticotropes of the *pars distalis*. The CRH-receptor complex activates adenyl cyclase in corticotropes and within seconds there is an increase in cAMP, which stimulates the release of ACTH into the blood.

The secretion of ACTH by the *pars intermedia,* which is well-developed in animals, is primarily under the negative regulation of dopamine (see Fig. 6–2). Thus, a decrease in the hypothalamic secretion of dopamine causes an increase in the synthesis and release of ACTH and other proopiomelanocortin-derived peptides from corticotropes in the *pars intermedia.*

Early in the search for CRH, it became apparent that there were other secretagogues that induced the synthesis and release of ACTH. The most potent of these secretagogues is vasopressin, which is secreted by the magnocellular neurons of the supraoptic and paraventricular nuclei and by parvocellular neurons in the paraventricular nucleus of the hypothalamus. Vasopressin and CRH are found in the same secretory granules of parvocellular neurons and are be-

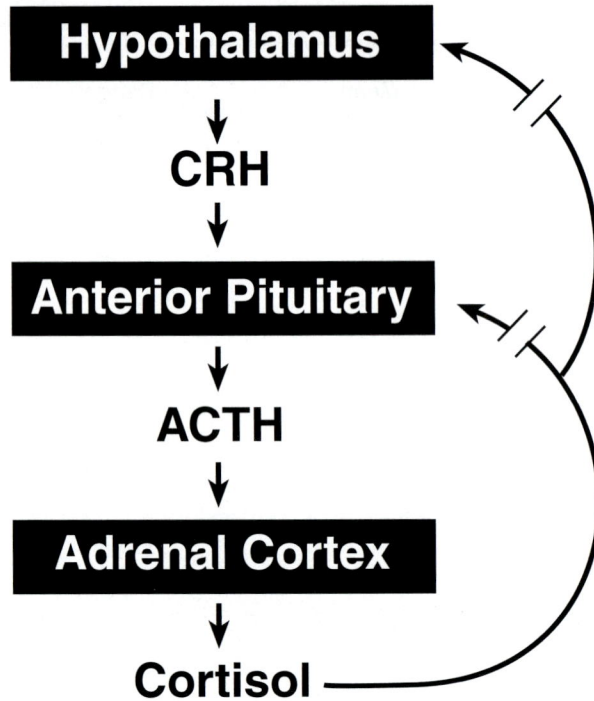

Fig. 6–6. Essential components of the hypothalamic-pituitary-adrenal axis and negative feedback control of the secretion of glucocorticoids.

⟶ = stimulation

⊣⟶ = inhibition

lieved to be co-secreted into the portal, hypophyseal blood. Compared to CRH, the intrinsic ACTH-releasing ability of vasopressin is weak. However, in the presence of CRH, vasopressin has strong synergistic actions on the secretion of ACTH. Vasopressin binds to specific cell membrane receptors and the vasopressin-receptor complex acts on corticotropes by greatly potentiating the CRH-induced increase in cAMP. This effect of vasopressin is mediated by activation of phospholipase C rather than by the activation of adenyl cyclase, as is the case for CRH. Various internal and external stimuli such as stress, depression, or adrenalectomy alter the percentage of parvocellular neurons in the paraventricular nucleus that synthesize and co-secrete CRH and vasopressin. Other secretagogues that act synergistically with CRH to stimulate the secretion of ACTH include catecholamines, angiotensins, serotonin, and several gastrointestinal hormones.

Elevated concentrations of glucocorticoids in the circulation have potent, direct inhibitory actions on the parvocellular neurons of the hypothalamus and corticotropes of the pituitary, which together, cause a decrease in the secretion of glucocorticoids. Thus, the concentration of circulating glucocorticoids is regulated by a negative feedback system (Fig. 6–6). Low concentrations of circulating glucocorticoids result in the increased release of CRH and ACTH to restore glucocorticoid levels.

Effects of ACTH

The secretion of steroids by all three zones of the adrenal cortex is influenced by ACTH, which is the tropic hormone that controls the basal secretion of glucocorticoids (Fig. 6–6). However, ACTH exerts only minor control over the secretion of mineralocorticoids. The immediate effect of ACTH on the adrenal gland of several species, including dogs, sheep, and cattle, is a marked increase in blood flow to the adrenal cortex. The increase in blood flow occurs within seconds and precedes the ACTH-mediated increase in glucocorticoids. This ACTH-induced increase in blood flow may be necessary for the efficient delivery of oxygen, nutrients, and hormones to the adrenal cortex and for the dispersion of adrenal hormones and the removal of waste products.

Steroidogenesis is initiated in the corticocyte by the binding of ACTH to receptors on the cell membrane and activation of adenyl cyclase and protein kinases (Fig. 6–7). Protein kinases promote the uptake of circulating cholesterol by up-regulating the number of low-density lipoprotein receptors on steroidogenic cells, increasing the storage of cholesterol in lipid droplets, and activating enzymes necessary for the conversion of cholesterol to steroid hormones (see also Fig. 6–4).

The actions of ACTH on the adrenal cortex can be divided into rapid, short-term, and long-term effects (Fig. 6–7). Rapid effects occur in a matter of seconds to minutes. For example, within seconds following the injection of ACTH in dogs, blood flow to the adrenals increases markedly and the secretion of cortisol begins. Measurable increases of cortisol in the peripheral circulation occur within two minutes. Short-term effects, such as increases in low-density lipoprotein receptors and steroidogenic enzymes, occur over a period of hours to days, whereas long-term effects such as cellular hypertrophy take weeks to months.

Chronic, high levels of circulating ACTH cause the long-term effects associated with high

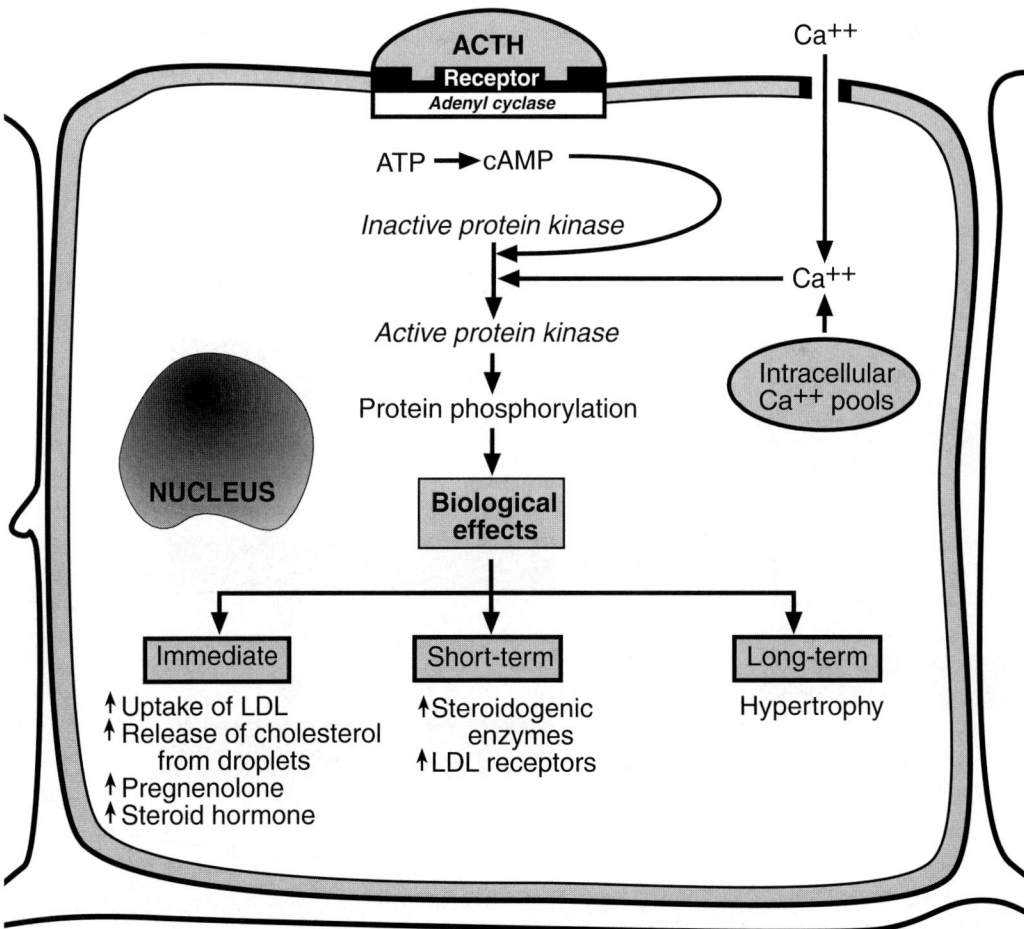

Fig. 6–7. Effects of adrenocorticotropic hormone (**ACTH**) on corticocytes (**ATP** = adenosine triphosphate; **cAMP** = cyclic adenosine monophosphate; **LDL** = low-density lipoprotein).

levels of glucocorticoids. Cellular changes include an increase in the size of the nucleus, the size and number of cell organelles, and an increase in the concentration of cellular enzymes and other proteins. These tropic effects appear to be mediated by the ACTH-induced secretion of local IGFs which influence the differentiation of adrenocortical cells and promote steroidogenesis in corticocytes.

Environmental Effects: Daily Rhythms and Stress

The intrinsic basal secretions of the hypothalamic-pituitary-adrenal axis can be affected by the central nervous system or by other hormonal factors (Fig. 6–8). Dogs and cats do not have a daily rhythm in the secretions of the hypothalamic-pituitary-adrenal axis. However, many species exhibit a circadian rhythm in the secretion of CRH, ACTH, and glucocorticoids. This rhythmic secretion of CRH is regulated by various inputs from the central nervous system to a "biological clock" located in the suprachiasmic nucleus of the hypothalamus. The suprachiasmic nucleus controls the secretion of CRH by afferent neural pathways to the paraventricular nucleus in the hypothalamus, such that the timing of the daily rhythm of CRH is synchronized with the sleep-wake cycle. Animals that are active during daylight, such as pigs, sheep, and horses, have a diurnal rhythm such that glucocorticoids levels may be several times greater during the early daylight hours than during the last hours of daylight. In contrast, animals that are active during the night, such as mice and rats, have a nocturnal rhythm. Nocturnal animals have higher levels of glucocorticoids during the early hours of darkness than during the waning hours of darkness. Endogenous hypersecretion of glucocorticoids or treatment with high doses of glucocorticoids can overwhelm the diurnal or nocturnal secretion of CRH, ACTH, and glucocorticoids.

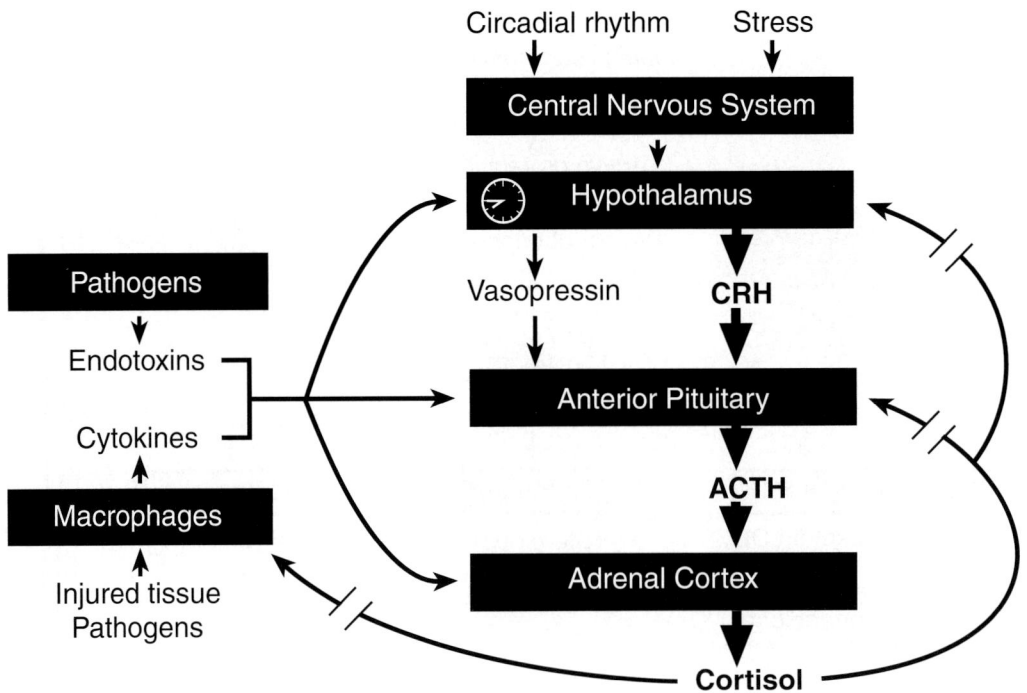

Fig. 6–8. Factors (circadial rhythms, stress, endotoxins, and cytokines) that affect the basal secretion of glucocorticoids from the adrenal cortex (**ACTH** = adrenocorticotropic hormone; **CRH** =corticotropin-releasing hormone).

⟶ = stimulation
⊣⟶ = inhibition

Corticotropin-releasing hormone is the primary hormone that regulates the response of animals to stress. All forms of stress, whether due to physical, chemical, thermal, microbial, or other factors, elicit profound stimulatory effects on the hypothalamic secretion of CRH (Fig. 6–8). These effects are mediated by neural and humoral factors, including catecholamines, serotonin, and neuropeptide Y. In addition, inflammatory cytokines, pyrogens, and bacterial endotoxins are humoral factors that can also stimulate the secretion of CRH (Fig. 6–8). Stress-induced secretion of CRH may cause up to a 20-fold increase in the levels of glucocorticoids. This marked increase in CRH and glucocorticoids can completely override the basal negative feedback of glucocorticoids on the hypothalamus and pituitary gland (see Fig. 6–8) and disrupt the diurnal or nocturnal rhythm in glucocorticoid levels.

Physiological Effects of Glucocorticoids

Glucocorticoids are major "permissive" hormones that appear to influence physiological processes of most cells and tissues. 'Permissive' hormones influence the full expression of certain activities or actions rather than the initiation of events. For example, in the absence of glucocorticoids, glucagon and epinephrine are essentially ineffective in stimulating gluconeogenesis. Glucocorticoids also decrease the rate of protein synthesis and enzyme production in cells. For cells of the hematopoietic and immune systems this can result in the decreased capacity of phagocytic cells to eliminate microorganisms and a reduction in antibody production, thereby increasing the vulnerability of the animal to disease.

Carbohydrate Metabolism

Some of the more important effects of glucocorticoids are those related to the metabolism of energy substrates. Glucocorticoids protect the body from hypoglycemia during the postabsorptive phase of digestion and during periods of stress. In this regard, glucocorticoids promote the output of hepatic glucose by: (a) stimulating gluconeogenesis; (b) enhancing the effects of glucagon and epinephrine on glu-

cose availability; and (c) inhibiting the effects of insulin on energy metabolism (see Chapter 5). Glucocorticoids stimulate hepatic glycogenolysis by activating glycogen phosphorylase, and stimulate gluconeogenesis by increasing the activity of gluconeogenic enzymes, while simultaneously inhibiting insulin-dependent hepatic enzymes. Levels of blood glucose can also be increased by glucocorticoid inhibition of the translocation of cytosolic glucose transporter protein-4 (GLUT-4) to the cell membrane, thereby decreasing the uptake and utilization of glucose by muscle and adipose tissue (see Chapter 5, Fig. 5–5).

At normal, basal concentrations, glucocorticoids enhance the effects of insulin on glucose utilization, glycogenesis, and lipogenesis.

Protein Metabolism

Glucocorticoids stimulate the catabolism of proteins, particularly when present at high concentrations in the blood. This leads to a negative nitrogen balance and to an increase in the urinary elimination of nitrogen as urea. Simultaneously, glucocorticoids inhibit the cellular uptake of amino acids, increase the concentration of amino acids in the circulation, and increase proteolysis in all tissues except the liver, where glucocorticoids stimulate the hepatic uptake of amino acids and protein synthesis. The increased availability of amino acids also stimulates gluconeogenesis, thereby increasing the levels of blood glucose (see Chapter 5, Fig. 5–7). The proteolytic effects of glucocorticoids are especially pronounced on myocytes. Glucocorticoids also have proteolytic effects on skin, connective tissue, and bone. In growing animals, an excess secretion of glucocorticoids stunts growth by inhibiting the secretion and release of growth hormone which is essential for muscle development and the proliferation, differentiation, and function of chondrocytes.

Fat Metabolism

Glucocorticoids are weak lipolytic agents that mobilize fatty acids from adipocytes and inhibit the uptake of fatty acids and the synthesis of fat in a manner that is analogous to the mobilization of amino acids from myocytes. Glucocorticoids permissively enhance the actions of glucagon, epinephrine, and growth hormone on the mobilization of fatty acids.

Neutral fat makes up the largest pool of energy in the body and is of utmost importance during periods of starvation and other forms of prolonged stress. Under these conditions, glucocorticoids shift the metabolism of cells from the utilization of glucose to the utilization of fatty acids for energy. In addition, glucocorticoids promote food intake by stimulating the appetite center in the hypothalamus. Thus, animals exposed to high concentrations of glucocorticoids develop a voracious appetite.

Endocrine System

Glucocorticoids interact with hormones that participate in the control of intermediary metabolism. In many respects, glucocorticoids antagonize the effects of insulin on muscle, adipose tissue, and the liver (see Chapter 5). Glucocorticoids also enhance the effects of glucagon and epinephrine on intermediary metabolism. These combined effects of glucocorticoids can induce hyperglycemia and hyperinsulinemia, which if prolonged, can lead to diabetes mellitus, especially in dogs.

Musculoskeletal System

In addition to their interactions with insulin, glucocorticoids also interact with hormones that affect the musculo-skeletal system. Hypersecretion of glucocorticoids stunts growth in young animals and causes wasting or atrophy of muscle tissue in adult animals, due to the catabolic effects of glucocorticoids on muscle protein. Muscle wastage in dogs can lead to muscle weakness causing difficulty or inability to ascend stairs even though these dogs descend stairs with ease. Bone mass can also be lost (**osteopenia**) by hypersecretion of glucocorticoids which depress the activity of osteoblasts and inhibit the synthesis of collagen, an essential component of bone. Glucocorticoids also antagonize the actions of vitamin D on the absorption of calcium from the intestine. Reduced levels of blood calcium cause an increase in the secretion of parathyroid hormone that leads to the demineralization of bone (**osteoporosis**).

Skin and Connective Tissue

Glucocorticoids modulate the proliferation and differentiation of fibroblasts which are responsible for maintenance of skin and connective tissue. Chronic excess of glucocorticoids results in the thinning of the skin and subcutis due to decreased proliferation of fibroblasts and decreased synthesis of collagen and mucopolysaccharides by connective tissue cells. As a consequence, subcutaneous vessels may be seen with ease in animals with light-colored skin. Animals with thinning of the skin and subcutis are also prone to bruising and wound healing is impaired. Frequently, hypersecretion of glucocorticoids leads to hyperpigmentation, pyoderma, and seborrhea. On occasion, deposits of calcium form in the dermis and subcutis (**calcinosis cutis**). Any of the latter skin conditions may lead to **pruritus** (itching). Another common disturbance of hypersecretion of glucocorticoids is atrophy of hair follicles and loss of hair (**alopecia**). This alopecia is bilaterally symmetrical and, typically, affects the trunk rather than the head and extremities of the animal (see Chapter 2, Fig. 2–9).

Cardiovascular System

The most important effects of glucocorticoids on the cardiovascular system are their contribution to the maintenance of normal vascular tone and blood pressure by enhancing the vascular response to vasoactive agents, such as catecholamines, angiotensins, and vasopressin. Glucocorticoids also enhance the activity of Na^+-K^+–ATPases in cardiocytes. This action may be responsible for the glucocorticoid-induced **positive inotropic** (increased force of contraction) and **positive chronotropic** (increased rate of contraction) effects on cardiac output.

Renal System

Glucocorticoids are required for normal renal function and water metabolism and cortisol and corticosterone have some inherent mineralocorticoid activity due to their binding to mineralocorticoid receptors. Hyposecretion of glucocorticoids impairs the ability of the kidneys to excrete a water load. The retention of water is caused by a decrease in the rate of glomerular filtration and by an increase in the secretion of vasopressin. High glucocorticoid levels increase the absorption of Na^+ and excretion of K^+ by the kidney by direct action on renal tubules and, indirectly, by the glucocorticoid-induced secretion of atrial natriuretic peptide from the heart.

Compared to aldosterone, which is the primary mineralocorticoid, the mineralocorticoid activity of glucocorticoids is weak (Table 6–2). Although the concentration of glucocorticoids in the circulation may be 200 to 1,000 times greater than that for mineralocorticoids, this is of little consequence to normal animals because the glucocorticoids that diffuse into renal cells that are targets for mineralocorticoids are inactivated by 11β-hydroxysteroid dehydrogenase. However, hypersecretion of glucocorticoids or treatments that overwhelm the activity of 11β-hydroxysteroid dehydrogenase in cells of the renal tubules, leads to the retention of salt and hypertension.

High levels of glucocorticoids cause blood flow to the kidneys to increase, possibly due to direct vasodilatory effects on renal vessels. Elevated glucocorticoid levels in the blood feedback to the hypothalamus to inhibit the release of CRH and vasopressin. The decrease in vasopressin leads to an increased clearance of water from the kidney causing the excretion of large volumes of urine. Thus, in addition to the development of a voracious appetite, polyuria and polydipsia are also clinical signs associated with hypersecretion of glucocorticoids in animals.

Hemopoietic and Immune Systems

Glucocorticoids are among the most widely used therapeutic agents in veterinary medicine due to their anti-inflammatory and immunosuppressive properties. Glucocorticoids decrease the number of circulating eosinophils, basophils, monocytes, and lymphocytes but increase the number of neutrophils, red blood cells, and platelets in the circulation. The neutrophilia induced by glucocorticoids results from an increase in the number of neutrophils entering the bloodstream from bone marrow, a diminished rate of removal from the circulation,

and inhibition of leukocyte migration to the site of inflammation. The administration of a single, pharmacological dose of glucocorticoids can cause eosinopenia, basopenia, monocytopenia, and lymphocytopenia within hours, and the condition may last for 12 to 48 hours.

Glucocorticoid-treated animals are more susceptible to infections than untreated animals and treatment of diseased animals with glucocorticoids may result in the rapid spread of microorganisms and septicemia. Hence, when infections are present and treatment with glucocorticoids is necessary, they should be administered in combination with antibiotics or antiviral agents.

Glucocorticoids powerfully inhibit immune processes, including: (a) secretion of cytokines produced by macrophages, helper T cells, and other cells of the immune system; (b) proliferation of immune cells; (c) synthesis of antibodies; and (d) cell-mediated and humoral immune responses. Persistent hypersecretion or prolonged therapy with glucocorticoids induces involution of the lymph nodes, thymus, and spleen by inhibiting the mitosis of lymphocytes. The thymus-derived lymphocytes decrease proportionally more than the lymphocytes derived from bone marrow.

Cattle and horses shipped for long distances are often stressed by exposure to extreme temperatures, fatigue, lack of food and water, and fright. These stressors cause massive release of glucocorticoids. As a result, the defense mechanisms of these animals are depressed and animals are more susceptible to infection, which frequently leads to a disease condition known as "shipping fever" or "transit fever".

Allergic reactions result from the binding of antigen to immunoglobulin (IgE) bound to mast cells. In affected animals, antigen binding triggers the immediate release of large amounts of histamine from mast cells. Glucocorticoids ameliorate and relieve the signs of asthma and allergic reactions by inhibiting the synthesis and release of histamine by mast cells. However, glucocorticoids have no effect on the binding of antigen to immunoglobulin or on the response of tissues to histamine that has been released from mast cells.

MINERALOCORTICOIDS

Mineralocorticoids, including aldosterone, deoxycorticosterone, and corticosterone, regulate the concentrations of sodium and potassium in the extracellular fluid by increasing the renal uptake of sodium and stimulating the excretion of potassium in the urine. The most important stimuli for the secretion of mineralocorticoids are changes in electrolyte levels and water balance.

Aldosterone is the most potent mineralocorticoid synthesized and released from the corticocytes of the *zona glomerulosa* of the adrenal cortex (see Table 6–2 and Fig. 6–1). The affinity of aldosterone for blood proteins is relatively low. Of the total amount of aldosterone in the blood, approximately 50% is loosely bound to albumin, 40% is unbound, and 10% is bound to transcortin. Mineralocorticoids, like glucocorticoids, diffuse passively across cell membranes and bind to specific receptors in the cytosol of target cells (see Chapter 1, Fig. 1–7 and Fig. 6–5). The responses of target cells to the action of aldosterone are not evident until 15 to 30 minutes after administration, due to the time required for protein synthesis. The half-life of aldosterone is approximately 15 minutes.

The major targets for mineralocorticoids are the epithelial cells of the collecting tubules of the kidney where mineralocorticoids increase the activity of the Na^+-K^+ATPases or Na^+-K^+ pumps located on the luminal membrane of the renal tubule. Activation of these Na^+-K^+ pumps causes reabsorption of Na^+ from the fluid in the renal tubules. Sodium reabsorption is coupled with the excretion of K^+ and H^+ into the urine. Mineralocorticoids also increase the activity of Na^+-K^+ATPases in the epithelial cells of sweat glands, stomach, colon, and ducts of the salivary glands, resulting in the reabsorption of Na^+ and excretion of K^+ and H^+.

Regulation of Mineralocorticoid Secretion

The basal secretion of mineralocorticoids is altered by circadian rhythms which are synchronized with the sleep-wake cycle, as was noted for the regulation of glucocorticoid secretion. Many animals that are active during daylight hours, such as pigs, sheep, horses, and humans, exhibit a diurnal rhythm in mineralocorticoid levels. Concentrations of mineralocorticoids in the blood of diurnal animals are higher in the morning than in the evening hours. In contrast, nocturnal animals have higher levels of mineralocorticoids during the early hours of darkness than during the waning hours of darkness. Dogs are an exception, they do not exhibit a daily rhythm in the secretion of mineralocorticoids.

The two most important factors that regulate the synthesis and secretion of aldosterone from corticocytes of the *zona glomerulosa* of the

Table 6-2   *Relative Potencies of Some Natural and Synthetic Corticosteroids*

	Relative Potency*	
Corticosteroid	**Glucocorticoid Activity**	**Mineralocorticoid Activity**
Natural		
Cortisol	1.0	1.0
Cortisone	0.8	0.8
Corticosterone	0.3	15
Deoxycorticosterone	0	100
Aldosterone	0.3	3000
Synthetic		
Dexamethasone	30	2
Prednisone	4	0.8
Flurocortisol	10	500

*Values are relative to the glucocorticoid and mineralocorticoid activity of cortisol.

adrenal cortex are the renin-angiotensin system and changes in the concentrations of Na^+ and K^+ in the extracellular fluid.

Effects of the Renin-angiotensin System and Potassium

The juxtaglomerular apparatus of the kidney nephron consists of: (a) the macula densa, a specialized tubular epithelium in contact with the glomerular arterioles; (b) extraglomerular mesangial cells which underlie the macula densa and provide structural support in the glomerulus; and (c) renin-producing granular (juxtaglomerular) cells. Cells of the macula densa monitor the concentration of NaCl in the tubular fluid of the thick ascending limb of the loop of Henle. The anatomical arrangement of the components of the juxtaglomerular apparatus provides for the interaction of the chemoreceptive cells of the macula densa with:

1. Smooth muscle surrounding the afferent arteriole; and
2. juxtaglomerular cells which synthesize and secrete renin.

Renin is a proteolytic enzyme synthesized and stored by the juxtaglomerular cells which surround the arterioles of renal glomeruli. The concentration of renin in the blood is the primary regulator of the production and release of mineralocorticoids.

The substrate for renin is angiotensinogen, an inactive plasma protein produced by the liver. Renin cleaves circulating angiotensinogen to angiotensin I, a decapeptide that does not appear to be biologically active. Angiotensin-converting enzyme, produced principally in the lungs, converts angiotensin I to angiotensin II, an octapeptide. Angiotensin II interacts with receptors on cells of the *zona glomerulosa* to induce the synthesis and secretion of mineralocorticoids by stimulating the enzymes that convert cholesterol to pregnenolone and corticosterone to aldosterone. In addition, angiotensin II: (a) feeds back to the juxtaglomerular cells to inhibit the secretion of renin; (b) is a potent vasoconstrictor, approximately 40 times more powerful than norepinephrine; (c) acts on the central nervous system to stimulate the thirst center; and (d) stimulates the release of vasopressin and ACTH.

Another member of the angiotensin family is angiotensin III which is a heptapeptide. This peptide can be formed by the cleavage of either angiotensin I or II. Angiotensin III has properties similar to angiotensin II and is known to stimulate the secretion of aldosterone in dogs, cats, sheep, humans, and rodents. As for angiotensin II, angiotensin III also inhibits the secretion of renin.

The half-life of angiotensin I, II, or III is approximately one to two minutes in most species. Angiotensinases that circulate in the blood inactivate these peptides.

The major factors that influence the secretion of renin are levels of Na^+, blood volume, blood pressure, and sympathetic nerve activity (Fig. 6–9). The concentration of Na^+ in the blood is monitored by the epithelial cells of the macula densa. Low levels of Na^+ cause the release of renin which leads to the synthesis and release of mineralocorticoids from the adrenal cortex, to increase the reabsorption of Na^+ and water by epithelial cells of the kidney tubules, thereby expanding the extracellular blood volume and increasing blood pressure. If the osmolarity of body fluids increases, vasopressin is released to stimulate the osmotic reabsorption of water by the kidney.

Blood pressure is also monitored by cells of the juxtaglomerular apparatus which function as miniature pressure transducers. A slight decrease in blood pressure in the afferent arterioles of renal glomeruli elicits an increase in the secretion of renin.

Secretion of renin is inhibited by an increase in Na^+ levels and blood pressure, and by angiotensins and vasopressin. As indicated earlier, ACTH plays a permissive role in the secretion of mineralocorticoids but it is not an important regulator of mineralocorticoid secretion.

An increase in the concentration of the ionic form of potassium in the extracellular fluid is a secondary stimulus to the renin-angiotensin system and causes the synthesis and release of aldosterone from corticocytes of the *zona glomerulosa*. Aldosterone stimulates the renal excretion of K^+ and also causes an increase in the reabsorption of Na^+ and water from the kidney tubules to increase blood volume. A decrease in the level of blood K^+ inhibits the secretion of aldosterone.

Effect of Atrial Natriuretic Peptide

Atrial natriuretic peptide (ANP) is a peptide hormone synthesized and released by myocytes of the right atrium. This peptide, secreted in response to increasing atrial stretch and pressure as a result of increased blood volume, is a powerful natriuretic agent that lowers blood volume and pressure in animals by increasing the urinary excretion of Na^+. The major physiological action of ANP on corticocytes is to inhibit the synthesis and release of mineralocorticoids. Indirect effects of ANP on electrolyte and water balance include the inhibition of the secretion of renin and the effects of angiotensin II and III on corticocytes, the secretion of vasopressin, and sympathetic nerve actions on the juxtaglomerular apparatus. Thus, ANP has potent natriuretic and diuretic actions.

The effects of the renin-angiotensin system, potassium, and ANP on the control of the balance of electrolytes and water are summarized in Figure 6–9.

DYSFUNCTIONS OF THE ADRENAL CORTEX

Hyperadrenocorticism

Primary and secondary hyperadrenocorticism are forms of a disease characterized by the hypersecretion of glucocorticoids (see also Chapter 1). The hypersecretion of glucocorticoids occurs spontaneously in humans and animals and is one of the most common endocrine diseases of the dog. This disease is seen occasionally in cats but is rare in horses and other domestic species. Affected dogs, humans, and certain other species often develop a peculiar redistribution of body fat and have a potbellied appearance (see Chapter 2, Fig. 2–9). Long-term treatment of animals with potent, synthetic glucocorticoids can have similar effects on animals and this condition is referred to as iatrogenic hyperadrenocorticism.

The adrenal cortex of animals with naturally occurring hyperadrenocorticism may also secrete excessive amounts of androgens and estrogens. However, overproduction of mineralocorticoids does not seem to occur in domestic animals with hyperadrenocorticism.

Primary Hyperadrenocorticism

Primary hyperadrenocorticism accounts for approximately 15% of all cases of naturally occurring hyperadrenocorticism in dogs; nearly all of which are caused by adenomas or carcinomas of the adrenal cortex. Primary hyperadrenocorticism due to neoplasms of the adrenal cortex occurs in 20% of cases in cats but rarely occurs in horses. The parvocellular neurons and pituitary corticotropes of animals with primary hyperadrenocorticism are atrophied due to the inhibitory effects of excess glucocorticoids.

Secondary Hyperadrenocorticism

Secondary hyperadrenocorticism accounts for 85% of the cases of naturally occurring hyperadrenocorticism in dogs and 90% of these are due to ACTH-producing neoplasms of the *pars distalis* or the *pars intermedia,* with the remaining cases (10%) due to hyperplasia and hypertrophy of ACTH-producing cells of the *pars distalis* or *pars intermedia.* In affected cats (80% of cases), the disease is primarily due to neoplasms of the *pars distalis* or *pars intermedia.* Secondary hyperadrenocorticism in horses is usually caused by hyperplasia or neoplasms of the *pars intermedia.*

Iatrogenic Hyperadrenocorticism

Iatrogenic or pharmacological hyperadrenocorticism is a syndrome that frequently occurs in dogs because of the widespread use of synthetic, long-acting glucocorticoids. Synthetic glucocorticoids are potent drugs and great care must be taken when administering them because even one large dose of a potent, long-acting glucocorticoid can lead to iatrogenic hyperadrenocorticism, followed by hypoadrenocorticism. The adrenal cortices, parvocellular neurons, and pituitary corticotropes are atrophied in animals affected by the prolonged treatment with natural or synthetic glucocorticoids. Hence, the abrupt discontinuation of glucocorticoid treatment frequently leads to iatrogenic hypoadrenocorticism.

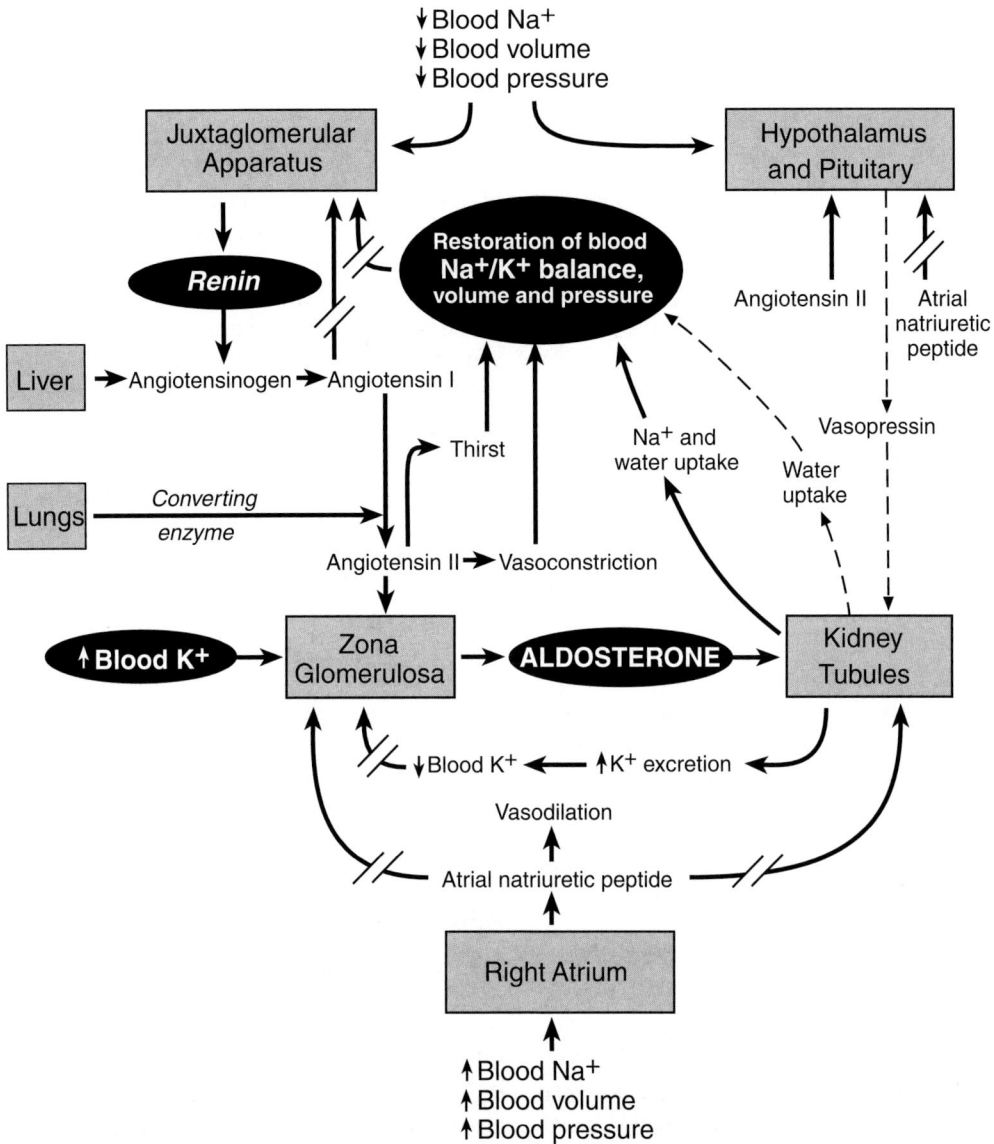

Fig. 6–9. Integration of mechanisms for the control of electrolytes and water in blood. (Adapted from: G. A. Vinson,[192] et al., p. 79, 1992).

⟶   = stimulation
⊣/⟶   = inhibition

Compared to dogs, cats are more resistant to the development of iatrogenic hyperadrenocorticism.

Hypoadrenocorticism

Hypoadrenocorticism occurs rarely in dogs, cats, and other species. Primary and secondary hypoadrenocorticism can be distinguished.

Primary Hypoadrenocorticism

Primary hypoadrenocorticism is the most common form of natural hypoadrenocorticism, accounting for nearly all cases of the disease. Primary hypoadrenocorticism is characterized by a deficiency in the secretion of both glucocorticoids and mineralocorticoids and is commonly associated with atrophy or destruction of the *zona fasciculata* and *zona reticularis* and less frequently with atrophy or degeneration of all three zones of the adrenal cortex.

Secondary Hypoadrenocorticism

Naturally occurring secondary hypoadreno-corticism is rare in domestic species. The natural disease is caused by hyposecretion of ACTH from the pituitary which, in turn, causes atrophy of the *zona fasciculata* and *zona reticularis* and results in glucocorticoid deficiency.

Iatrogenic Hypoadrenocorticism

In dogs, iatrogenic, hypoadrenocorticism is more frequent than the natural form of the disease and manifests itself after the abrupt withdrawal of treatment with glucocorticoids. Consequently, when glucocorticoid therapy is suddenly terminated, the hypothalamic-pituitary-adrenal axis is unable to respond to the sudden deficiency of glucocorticoids. The length of time needed for the normalization of the levels of glucocorticoids in the blood depends on the degree of atrophy of the anatomical components of the hypothalamic-pituitary-adrenal axis. Animals that have been treated for several months with high doses of glucocorticoids may take from six to nine months before normal adrenal function is restored.

Therapeutic Uses of Glucocorticoids and Mineralocorticoids

Glucocorticoids are among the most widely used therapeutic hormones used in veterinary medicine due to their: (a) anti-inflammatory and anti-allergic effects, their most common use; (b) replacement hormonal therapy for hypoadrenocorticism; (c) as an immunosuppressant factor for autoimmune disorders; and (d) as a palliative therapy for arthritis, arthrosis, and some other arthropathies.

Although infrequent, mineralocorticoid therapy is required for animals with adrenocortical insufficiency which leads to a life-threatening sodium and potassium imbalance. Emergency measures include: (a) intravenous fluid therapy to restore electrolyte levels; and (b) injections of corticosteroids and mineralocorticoids. In most cases, glucocorticoid and mineralocorticoid

therapy must be continued for the life of the animal.

ADRENAL MEDULLA

The chromaffin cells of the adrenal medulla can be distinguished histologically on the basis of the catecholamine (epinephrine or norepinephrine) synthesized and stored within secretory granules. Epinephrine and norepinephrine secreted by adrenomedullary cells bind to receptors on adipose, cardiovascular, hepatic, muscular, and pancreatic tissues to regulate metabolic processes and to receptors on nerve cells to influence neurogenic responses. The responses of cells and tissues to these two catecholamines are related to the nature of the adrenergic receptor (e.g., α, β) and the specific receptor sub-type (e.g., α_1, β_2) in the target tissue.

Catecholamines are referred to as the so-called emergency hormones that are released by activation of the "fight or flight" mechanism and factors such as cold, apnea, and hypoglycemia. Release of massive amounts of norepinephrine and epinephrine constitutes the principal regulatory mechanism to elicit the sympathetic responses that allow the animal to meet physical demands and respond to life-threatening challenges.

Biosynthesis of Catecholamines

Catecholamines include norepinephrine, epinephrine, and dopamine, a precursor for the synthesis of norepinephrine and epinephrine (Fig. 6–10). These compounds contain the catechol nucleus formed by a benzene ring with adjacent hydroxyl groups and an amine group. Catecholamines are synthesized from tyrosine by the chromaffin cells of the adrenal medulla and by adrenergic and dopaminergic neurons (Fig. 6–10). Most of the tyrosine utilized in the synthesis of catecholamines is of dietary origin, but tyrosine is also synthesized from phenylalanine in liver and other tissues. Tyrosine is absorbed directly from the blood into the cytosol of the chromaffin cells of the adrenal medulla and hydrolyzed to 3,4-dihydroxyphenylalanine (dopa), the rate limiting step for the synthesis of norepinephrine and epinephrine. Dopa is then decarboxylated in the cytosol to form dopamine.

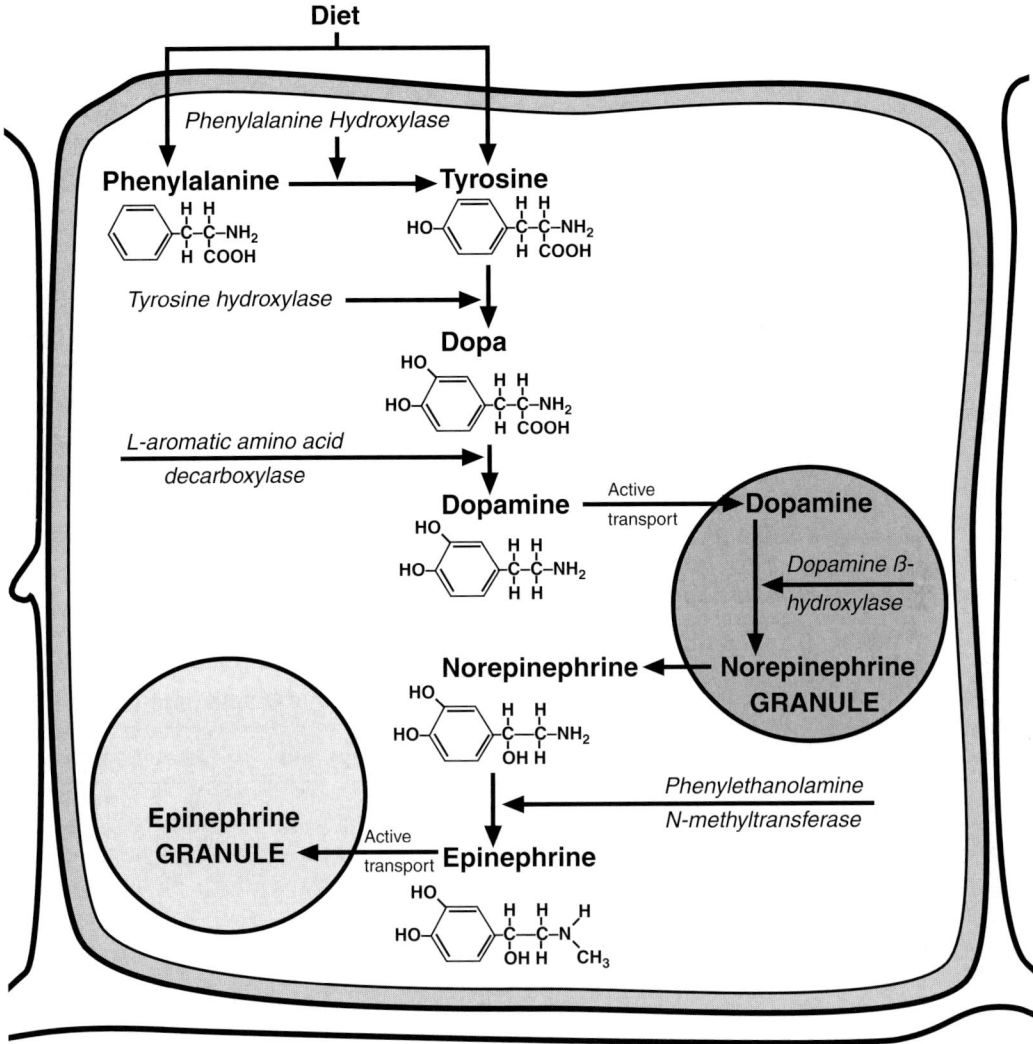

Fig. 6–10. Pathways for the biosynthesis of **norepinephrine** or **epinephrine** in chromaffin cells of the adrenal medulla.

After transport into the granules of chromaffin cells by an active process, dopamine is converted to norepinephrine by dopamine β-hydroxylase. In chromaffin cells devoid of phenylethanolamine N-methyltransferase, norepinephrine is stored in granules until it is secreted from the cell. The adrenal medullae of mammals also contain cells that have phenylethanolamine N-methyltransferase in the cytosol. In these cells, norepinephrine is released into the cytosol where a co-factor, S-adenosylmethionine, serves as the methyl donor for the synthesis of the epinephrine that is then stored in secretory granules for release into the circulation (Fig. 6–10).

Catecholamines are stored in secretory granules in adrenomedullary cells and in dopaminergic and adrenergic neurons throughout the body. The adrenal medulla is the primary source of epinephrine in animals, whereas norepinephrine is synthesized by the chromaffin cells of the adrenal medulla and by adrenergic neurons distributed throughout the body. The epinephrine content of the adrenal gland varies among species (Table 6–3). Depending on the cell type, each chromaffin cell has thousands of secretory granules which contain either epinephrine or norepinephrine. The primary catecholamine in the adrenomedullary cells of fetal animals is norepinephrine and, for several species studied (cat, cattle, dog, guinea pig, rabbit, and man), it appears that the capability of medullary cells to synthesize epinephrine and the relative amounts of epinephrine released in response to stimuli increases with age, until adulthood.

Release and Fate of Catecholamines

Calcium and energy in the form of ATP are required for the release of catecholamines from chromaffin cells. Acetylcholine released from preganglionic nerve fibers stimulates chromaffin cells of the adrenal medulla and postganglionic sympathetic nerve endings causing depolarization of the plasma membrane and a concomitant influx of Ca^{2+} into cells. In the adrenal medulla, membranes of the catecholamine-containing granules fuse with the plasma membrane of the chromaffin cell and the contents of the granule are expelled by exocytosis.

The ratio of epinephrine to norepinephrine released into the adrenal vein varies among species (Table 6–3). The adrenal glands of dogs, cattle, pigs, and man release mainly epinephrine, whereas the adrenal medullae of cats release mainly norepinephrine. The ratio of norepinephrine and epinephrine released from the adrenal medullae of adult animals is not con-

Table 6-3   Estimates* of the Epinephrine Ratio in Catecholamine Extracts of Adrenal Tissue and Basal Secretion Rates of Epinephrine and Norepinephrine from the Adrenal Gland of Adult Mammals

Animal Species	Epinephrine (%)		Adrenal Output (ng/Kg/min)	
	Mean	Range	Epinephrine	Norepinephrine
Cat	57	33–60	30	70
Cattle	69	–[a]	130[b]	40[b]
Dog	71	60–86	183	34
Goat	61	–	–	–
Horse	78	–	–	–
Man	81	78–88	9	–
Pig	49	–	11	–
Rabbit	96	86–98	–	–
Sheep	65	–	5	3
Whale	15	15–40	–	–
Carnivores	–	33–71	–	–
Primates	–	78–98	–	–
Rodents	–	48–96	–	–
Ungulates	–	48–83	–	–

*Estimate of the proportion of epinephrine in adrenal extracts is based on the formula: [100 - (percent norepinephrine + 2 percent for dopamine and other amine precursors)].

[a]Hyphen indicates that data were not available or that a range was not provided.
[b]Values obtained for calves ranging from 8 to 30 weeks of age.

(Adapted from various sources including: G. B. West,[199] p. 116; A. Gorbman and A. Bern,[73] p. 343; U. S. von Euler,[195] p. 269; and B. A. Callingham,[26] p. 427).

stant. For example, anxiety and hypoxia are followed by the release of more norepinephrine than epinephrine, whereas hypoglycemia and activation of the 'fight or flight' mechanism cause the release of more epinephrine than norepinephrine.

The half-life of catecholamines in the blood of animals is approximately two minutes. The degradation of circulating catecholamines occurs largely in the kidneys and liver by the combined actions of catechol-ortho-methyl transferase in the cytosol and the mitochondrial enzyme, monoamine oxidase. Catabolism of catecholamines begins either by ortho-methylation followed by deamination of intermediate metabolites, or by deamination followed by ortho-methylation of intermediate metabolites. Most of the conjugated metabolites of catecholamines are excreted in the urine and bile. Large amounts of these metabolites in the urine of animals are suggestive of chromaffin tumors.

The nerve endings of the sympathetic nervous system have an amine transport system which actively takes up approximately 50 percent of the norepinephrine discharged into the synaptic cleft. This norepinephrine is incorporated into the storage granules of the adrenergic neuron and recycled (Fig. 6–11).

Classification of Catecholamine Receptors

The concept of different categories of receptors for catecholamines was proposed in an effort to explain the pharmacological actions of catecholamines on various tissues; particularly due to the sensitivity of catecholamine receptors to certain drugs. Two major groups, adrenergic and dopaminergic receptors, are now recognized. The adrenergic receptors received their name because of their binding to epinephrine and norepinephrine, which in the European nomenclature are called adrenaline and noradrenaline, respectively. Epinephrine is the major hormone secreted by the cells of the adrenal medulla in man and was the first hormone[196] to be isolated (1898) and synthesized (1904). Dopaminergic receptors are activated by dopamine and dopamine agonists.

Adrenergic Receptors

Based on the results of pharmacologic studies, two major types, α- and β-adrenergic recep-

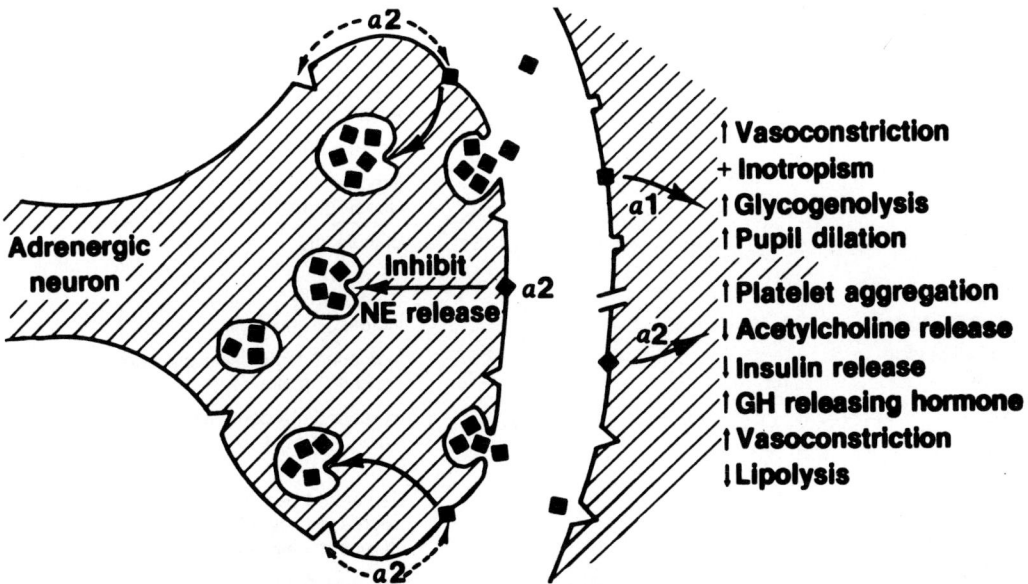

Fig. 6–11. Schematic representation of the synapse of a sympathetic (**adrenergic**) nerve ending showing the anatomical location of presynaptic and postsynaptic α-receptors and some of the effects mediated by them (**GH** = growth hormone; **NE** = norepinephrine).

tors, were first distinguished. It was determined that α receptors mediated the stimulatory effects of epinephrine and norepinephrine on smooth muscle, whereas β receptors mediated the inhibitory effects of these catecholamines. In cardiac muscle, β receptors mediated an increase in force (inotropic effect) and rate (chronotropic effect) of myocardial contraction. Adrenergic receptors also affected the release of certain hormones, including insulin and vasopressin. In this regard, α receptors generally mediated the inhibitory effects of catecholamines on insulin release, whereas, β receptors generally mediated the stimulatory effects of norepinephrine and epinephrine.

Adrenergic receptors were further classified as α_1, α_2, β_1, and β_2 (see Table 6–4) based on the physiological responses they mediate in animals and the identification of chemical antagonists. At this writing, several subtypes of α (α_{1A}, α_{1B}, α_{1C} and α_{2A}, α_{2B}, α_{2C}, α_{2D}) and β (β_1, β_2, and β_3) adrenergic receptors are recognized.

Table 6-4   Responses of Effector Organs to Norepinephrine and Epinephrine

Effector Organ	Type of Adrenergic Receptor	Responses
Eye		
Radial muscle, iris	α_1	Contraction
Ciliary muscle	β_2	Relaxation
Heart		
A-V and S-A nodes, atria, and ventricles	β_1; β_2	Increased activity
Blood Vessels		
Arterioles	α_1; β_2	Constriction; dilation
Veins (systemic)	α_1, α_2; β_2	Constriction; dilation
Lung		
Bronchial muscles	β_2	Relaxation
Bronchial glands	α_1; β_2	Decreased secretion; increased secretion
Gastrointestinal Tract		
Motility	α_1, α_2; β_2	Decrease
Sphincters	α_1	Contraction
Secretion	α_2	Inhibition
Kidney (Renin)	α_1; β_1	Decreased secretion; increased secretion
Uterus	α_1; β_2	Pregnant: contraction (α_1); relaxation (β_2) Nonpregnant: relaxation (β_2)
Sex Organs, Male	α_1	Ejaculation
Skin		
Pilomotor muscles	α_1	Contraction
Sweat glands	α_1	Increased secretion
Skeletal Muscle	β_2	Increased contractility, glycogenolysis, and K$^+$ uptake
Liver	α_1; β_2	Increased glycogenolysis and gluconeogenesis
Pancreas		
Acini	α	Decreased secretion
Islets (β cells)	α_2	Decreased secretion
	β_2	Increased secretion
Fat Cells	α_2; β_1	Decreased lipolysis; increased lipolysis
Posterior Pituitary (Vasopressin)	α_2; β_1	Decreased secretion; increased secretion

(Adapted from: R. J. Lefkowitz,[106] et al., pp. 110-111).

These receptor sub-types have been identified in humans and some animal species based on physiological responses to adrenergic hormones, effects of pharmacological agonists and antagonists, or by using molecular approaches to determine the amino acid sequences of receptor proteins.

Alternative classification schemes for responses mediated by receptors can also be used to explain the various physiological and pharmacological responses to adrenergic agonists and antagonists. These include the grouping of receptors based on the: (a) type of regulatory protein (e.g., G_s, G_i, G_o, G_p, or G_q); (b) catalytic unit (e.g., adenyl cyclase, phospholipase C) which is coupled with the cell membrane receptor; or (c) intracellular effectors (e.g., cAMP, IP_3, DAG, Ca^{2+}) that are integral to the signal transduction events governing the response of the target cell to the hormone or agonist.

Alpha$_1$ receptors are located on the postsynaptic nerve ending, whereas α_2 receptors are found in both pre- and postsynaptic sites (Fig. 6–11). The α_2 receptors of the presynaptic neuron regulate the secretion of norepinephrine into the synaptic cleft. High concentrations of norepinephrine activate presynaptic α_2 receptors resulting in the inhibition of norepinephrine release and stimulation of catecholamine uptake (Fig. 6–11).

Beta$_1$ receptors are located at postsynaptic sites and mediate effects such as the force and rate of myocardial contraction, intestinal relaxation, and lipolysis. Beta$_2$ receptors are also located pre- and postsynaptically. Activation of presynaptic β_2 receptors increases the release of norepinephrine into the synaptic cleft when the concentration of norepinephrine is low.

Agonists (activators) and antagonists (blockers) for α_1, α_2, β_1, and β_2 adrenergic receptors are listed in Table 6–5.

Table 6-5 *Representative* Agonists and Antagonists for Subclasses of Adrenergic and Dopaminergic Receptors*

α-Adrenergic Agonists
1. $\alpha_1 + \alpha_2$: Norepinephrine, epinephrine
2. α_1: Phenylephrine, methoxamine
3. α_2: Clonidine, xylazine

α-Adrenergic Antagonists
1. $\alpha_1 + \alpha_2$: Phentolamine, tolazoline
2. α_1: Phenoxybenzamine, prazosin
3. α_2: Yohimbine, idazoxan

β-Adrenergic Agonists
1. $\beta_1 + \beta_2$: Isoproterenol, epinephrine
2. β_1 : Norepinephrine, dopamine, dobutamine
3. β_2: Metaproterenol, albuterol

β-Adrenergic Antagonists
1. $\beta_1 + \beta_2$: Propranolol, nadolol
2. β_1: Metoprolol, atenolol
3. β_2: Butoxamine, ICI 118551[1]

Dopaminergic Agonists
1. $D_1 + D_2$: Dopamine
2. D_1: SK & F (SKF) 38393[2]
3. D_2: Apomorphine

Dopaminergic Antagonists
1. $D_1 + D_2$: Butaclamol
2. D_1: SCH 23390[3]
3. D_2: Haloperidol, domperidone

---

*Selected agonists and antagonists for α_1, α_2, β_1, or β_2 adrenergic and D_1 and D_2 dopaminergic receptors.

[1]ICI = Imperial Chemical Industries, Ltd.
[2]SKF = Smithkline Beecham Pharmaceuticals
[3]SCH = Schering-Plough Corporation

Dopaminergic Receptors

Dopaminergic receptors bind to dopamine or dopamine analogs to mediate the activity of vascular smooth muscle, endocrine glands, and responses of the central and peripheral nervous systems. Based on their interaction with adenyl cyclase, dopaminergic receptors have been classified into subtypes (e.g., D_1 and D_2) and at this writing, three other dopamine receptor subtypes have been identified. Activated D_1 receptors mediate the dilation of the vascular bed of the heart, kidneys, mesentery, and cerebrum. Activation of D_1 receptors also mediates the release of parathyroid hormone in cattle and possibly in other domestic animals. However, dopamine has no effect on the secretion of parathyroid hormone in humans. Activation of D_2 receptors inhibits the secretion of aldosterone, prolactin, and renin, and may cause emesis or vomiting in humans and animals. Presynaptic D_2 receptors located on sympathetic nerve endings also have a role in the inhibition of the release of norepinephrine into the synaptic cleft. In addition, activation of both D_1 and D_2 receptors seems to be necessary for normal neuromuscular control.

Specific agonists and antagonists for dopamine receptors are listed in Table 6–5.

Regulation of Catecholamine Receptors

Adrenergic and dopaminergic receptors are dynamic and undergo constant changes. Various mechanisms exist to regulate hormone receptors on target cells and the intracellular signals that are generated by hormone binding. These include: (a) hormone binding properties of receptors; (b) receptor concentration; (c) receptor signaling; and (d) post-receptor alterations. Together, they regulate the responsiveness of the target cell to catecholamines.

Changes which affect the response of the target cells or tissues due to the effects of the hormone itself are termed homologous regulation, whereas changes in the receptor-mediated responses of target cells due to other hormones or drugs are referred to as heterologous regulation. Alterations in the cellular response to hormone that can be attributed to the number of receptors on cells or tissues are classified as down-regulation (decreased concentration) or up-regulation (increased concentration) of receptors.

Prolonged exposure to high concentrations of epinephrine causes a decrease in the number of receptors and in the affinity of the receptors on the target cell for epinephrine (desensitization of the target cell). This can be referred to as "homologous down-regulation". The net effect is the decreased sensitivity of the target cell or tissue to the effects of epinephrine. Conversely, a decrease in the concentration of epinephrine in the circulation that results in an increase in the number of receptors on the target cell is called "up-regulation", and is associated with a concomitant increase in the affinity of the receptors for epinephrine and the responsiveness of the target cell to the hormone.

Adrenergic and dopaminergic receptors can also be affected by other factors in a process called heterologous regulation. For example, thyroid hormones increase the number of β_1-adrenergic receptors on cells in the myocardium. Therefore, thyroid hormones enhance the stimulatory effects of catecholamines on the heart. Steroid hormones also heterologously regulate receptors for catecholamines. For example, estrogens down-regulate the number of D_2 receptors in cells of the anterior pituitary of rats.

Mechanisms of Action

Although the mechanisms of action of catecholamines are not fully understood, certain cellular events have been elucidated. Activation of α_1 and α_2 receptors on target cells leads to an increase in the concentration of cytosolic Ca^{2+}. However, the sources of Ca^{2+} released by activation of α_1 and α_2 receptors appear to be different. Activation of α_1 receptors increases the release of Ca^{2+} from intracellular storage sites whereas activation of α_2 receptors increases the influx of Ca^{2+} from the extracellular fluid. In addition, α_2-adrenergic activity is associated with the inhibition of adenyl cyclase in some cells, such as β cells of the pancreas, adipocytes, and adrenergic nerve endings. An increase in adenyl cyclase activity is associated with activation of β_1 and β_2 receptors.

Dopamine binding to D_1 receptors activates adenyl cyclase and increases cAMP levels, whereas binding to D_2 receptors inhibits adenyl cyclase.

Effects of Epinephrine and Norepinephrine

Epinephrine and norepinephrine are found throughout the central nervous system and their effects range from depression to excitation. It appears that α_1 receptors mediate excitation whereas α_2 receptors mediate depression.

Catecholamines also have profound effects on the cardiovascular and respiratory systems, smooth muscle, and metabolism. Actions of norepinephrine and epinephrine on selected organs and tissues that have been deduced from pharmacological and *in vitro* studies are summarized in Table 6–4 or are described below.

Effects on the Cardiovascular System

Activation of the "fight or flight" response in animals due to the release of catecholamines causes vasoconstriction in the viscera and skin, dilation of coronary arteries and vessels in skeletal muscle, increases the force and rate of contraction of the heart, thereby increasing cardiac output, while having little effect on blood flow to the central nervous system. The net effect of these actions that are critical to the survival of the animal is to shunt the flow of blood and energy substrates to the heart and muscles and increase the efficiency of the heart. Epinephrine and norepinephrine increase the force of contraction of cardiac muscle by activation of α_1, β_1, and β_2 receptors, whereas heart rate is increased by activation of β_1 and β_2 receptors. The increase in blood flow to the more active heart is mediated by activation of β_2 receptors in the smooth muscle of the coronary arteries.

Additionally, catecholamines can stimulate contraction of pilomotor muscles causing the erection of hair that is part of the "fight or flight" response in many species. This effect is also mediated by α_1 receptors.

Effects on the Respiratory System

The intravenous administration of epinephrine to animals initially causes a brief period of apnea or temporary cessation of breathing. This apnea is probably due to a reflex inhibition of the respiratory center in the medulla oblongata via the pressor effects exerted on baroreceptors. Apnea may also be due to a direct inhibitory effect of epinephrine on the respiratory center.

Effects on Smooth Muscles

In general, constriction of smooth muscle by epinephrine and norepinephrine is mediated by α receptors, whereas muscle relaxation is usually attributed to activation of β receptors. In the urinary bladder, the smooth muscle of the body and neck or sphincter are regulated by β_2 and α_1 receptors, respectively. Epinephrine relaxes the body of the urinary bladder whereas epinephrine and norepinephrine cause contraction of the neck of the bladder. The overall effect is to retain urine.

Catecholamines can relax or inhibit the contraction of gastrointestinal smooth muscle via two mechanisms: (a) direct inhibition of contraction which is mediated by β_1-receptors on smooth muscle; and (b) indirectly by inhibiting acetylcholine release in Auerbach's (myenteric) plexus, mediated by the α_2 receptors of preganglionic parasympathetic fibers (Fig. 6–12).

Effects on Metabolism

Glycogenolysis in the liver and muscle of dogs and other animals is stimulated by norepinephrine and epinephrine and these actions are mediated mainly by β_2 receptors and to a lesser degree by α_1 receptors. In hepatic cells, binding of epinephrine to β_2 receptors leads to an increase in intracellular cAMP that stimulates protein kinases to activate phosphorylase which, in turn, metabolizes glycogen to glucose-6-phosphate (see for reference, Chapter 1, Fig. 1–10 and Chapter 5, Fig. 5–7). Hepatic stimulation of α_1-adrenergic receptors by epinephrine and norepinephrine also increases cytosolic Ca^{2+} by mobilizing this ion from intracellular storage sites.

Norepinephrine and epinephrine activate β_2-adrenergic receptors of the pancreatic islets to increase the release of insulin and glucagon, whereas activation of α_2-adrenergic receptors

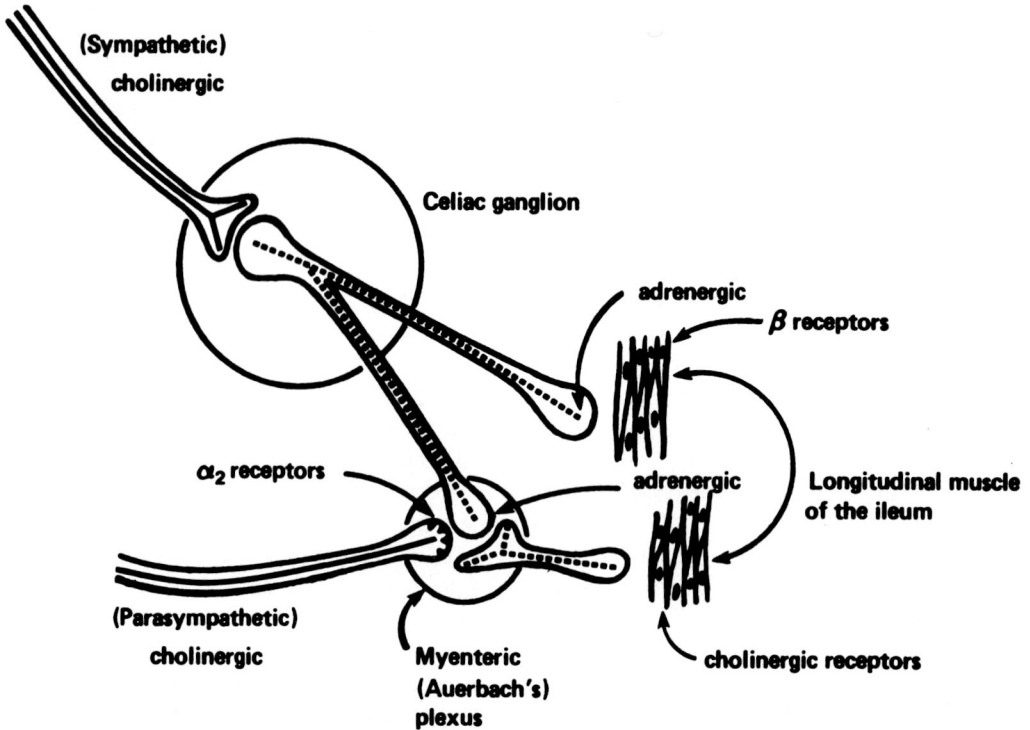

Fig. 6–12. Schematic representation of the autonomic control of longitudinal smooth muscle contraction in the ileum. Acetylcholine released from the preganglionic fibers stimulates the release of acetylcholine and norepinephrine from the postganglionic fibers of the respective parasympathetic and sympathetic nervous systems. Acetylcholine released from the postganglionic fibers stimulates the contraction of longitudinal smooth muscle by binding to cholinergic receptors. Norepinephrine released by post-ganglionic neurons inhibits longitudinal smooth muscle contraction via two mechanisms: (a) direct inhibition of muscle contraction by catecholamines released from postganglionic sympathetic neurons, an effect mediated through the β-receptors of myocytes; and (b) inhibition of acetylcholine release from Auerbach's plexus; mediated by the binding of catecholamines to the α_2-adrenergic receptors of preganglionic parasympathetic neurons.

decreases insulin release (see Chapter 5, Fig. 5–3).

HYPERFUNCTION OF THE ADRENAL MEDULLA (PHEOCHROMOCYTOMAS)

Pheochromocytomas are red-brown tumors that arise from chromaffin cells of the sympatho-adrenomedullary system. The catecholamines produced by pheochromocytomas may be secreted constantly or episodically. The reasons for this dichotomy in secretory patterns are not known. Pheochromocytomas may also produce various peptide hormones including ACTH, calcitonin, and somatostatin.[117]

The occurrence of pheochromocytomas has been reported for only a few of the domestic species. These tumors, though rare, have been observed in dogs, cats, and horses and most pheochromocytomas are thought to be benign. However, these tumors can secrete large quantities of catecholamines. The clinical diagnosis of pheochromocytoma in animals is difficult and approximately half of the pheochromocytomas in dogs and cats are detected after death and during routine necropsies.

REFERENCES

1. Adams, H. R. (1984): New perspectives in cardiopulmonary therapeutics: Receptor selective adrenergic drugs. J. Am. Vet. Med. Assoc. *185*:966.
2. Aguilera, G. and Rabadan-Diel, C. (2000): Vasopressinergic regulation of the hypothalamic-pituitary-adrenal axis: Implications for stress adaptation. Regul. Pept. *96*:23.

3. Ariens, E. J. and Simonis, A. M. (1983): Physiological and pharmacological aspects of adrenergic receptor classification. Biochem. Pharmacol. *32*:1539.
4. Ask, J. A. and Stene-Larsen, G. (1984): Functional alpha$_1$-adrenoceptors in the rat heart during beta-receptor blockade. Acta Physiol. Scand. *120*:7.
5. Balfour, W. E., Comline, R. S., and Short, R. V. (1959): Changes in the secretion of 20 alpha-hydroxypregn-4-en-3-one by the adrenal gland of young calves. Nature *183*:467.
6. Balow, J. E. and Rosenthal, A. S. (1973): Glucocorticoid suppression of macrophage migration inhibitory factor. J. Exp. Med. *137*:1031.
7. Barb, C. R., Kraeling, R. R., Rampacek, G. B., et al. (1986): Influence of stage of the estrous cycle on endogenous opioid modulation of luteinizing hormone, prolactin, and cortisol secretion in the gilt. Biol. Reprod. *35*:1162.
8. Baylink, D. J. (1983): Glucocorticoid-induced osteoporosis. N. Engl. J. Med. *309*:306.
9. Becker, M. J., Helland, D., and Becker, D. N. (1976): Serum cortisol (hydrocortisone) values in normal dogs as determined by radioimmunoassay. Am. J. Vet. Res. *37*:1101.
10. Berthelsen, S. and Pettinger, W. A. (1977): A functional basis for classification of alpha-adrenergic receptors. Life Sci. *21*:595.
11. Besedovsky, H. O. and del Rey, A. (1996): Immune-neuro-endocrine interactions: Facts and hypotheses. Endocrine Rev. *17*:64.
12. Besedovsky, H. O., del Rey, A., Klusman, I., et al. (1991): Cytokines as modulators of the hypothalamus-pituitary-adrenal axis. J. Steroid Biochem. Mol. Biol. *40*:613.
13. Bishop, C. R., Athens, J. W., Boggs, D. R., et al. (1968): Leukokinetic studies. XIII. A nonsteady-state kinetic evaluation of the mechanism of cortisone-induced granulocytosis. J. Clin. Invest. *47*:249.
14. Blair-West, J. R., Coghlan, J. P., Denton, D. A., et al. (1980): A dose-response comparison of the actions of angiotensin II and angiotensin III in sheep. J. Endocrinol. *87*:409.
15. Blaschko, H. (1959): Development of current concepts of catecholamine formation. Pharmacol. Rev. *11*:307.
16. Blatteis, C. M. (1990): Neuromodulative actions of cytokines. Yale J. Biol. Med. *63*:133.
17. Bonneau, N. and Reed, J. H. (1971): Adrenocortical insufficiency in a dog. Can. Vet. J. *12*:100.
18. Bornstein, S.R. and Chrousos, G.P. (1999): Clinical review 104. Adrenocorticotropin (ACTH)- and non-ACTH-mediated regulation of the adrenal cortex: Neural and immune inputs. J. Clin. Endocrinol. Metab. *84*:1729.
19. Bottoms, G. D., Roesel, O. F., Rausch, F. D., et al. (1972): Circadian variation in plasma cortisol and corticosterone in pigs and mares. Am. J. Vet. Res. *33*:785.
20. Boumpas, D. T., Paliogianni, F., Anastassiou, E. D., et al. (1991): Glucocorticoid action on the immune system: Molecular and cellular aspects. Clin. Exp. Rheumatol. *9*:413.
21. Braun, R. K., Bergman, E. N., and Albert, T. F. (1970): Effects of various synthetic glucocorticoids on milk production and blood glucose and ketone body concentrations in normal and ketotic cows. J. Am. Vet. Med. Assoc. *157*:941.
22. Brodde, O. E. (1986): Molecular pharmacology of beta-adrenoceptors. J. Cardiovasc. Pharmacol. *8*:S16.
23. Bruyette, D. S., Ruehl, W. W., Entriken, T., et al. (1997): Management of canine pituitary-dependent hyperadrenalcorticism with 1-deprenyl (Anipryl). Vet. Clin. North Am., Small Anim. Pract. *27*:273.
24. Buckingham, J. C. (1985): Two distinct corticotrophin releasing activities of vasopressin. Br. J. Pharmacol. *84*:213.
25. Burton, R. M. and Westphal, U. (1972): Steroid hormone binding proteins in blood plasma. Metabolism *21*:253.
26. Callingham, B. A. (1975): Catecholamines in blood. *In*: Handbook of Physiology, Section 7, Endocrinology, Vol. VI, Adrenal Gland, edited by R. O. Greep and E. B. Astwood. Washington, DC, American Physiological Society, p. 427.
27. Campbell, J. R. and Watts, C. (1973): Assessment of adrenal function in dogs. Br. Vet. J. *129*:134.
28. Canny, B. J., Funder, J. W., and Clarke, I. J. (1989): Glucocorticoids regulate ovine hypophysial portal levels of corticotropin-releasing factor and arginine vasopressin in a stress-specific manner. Endocrinology *125*:2532.
29. Chan, L. and O'Malley, B. W. (1978): Steroid hormone action: Recent advances. Ann. Intern. Med. *89*:694.
30. Chatterton, R. T. (1990): The role of stress in female reproduction: Animal and human considerations. Int. J. Fertil. *35*:8.
31. Chen, C. L., Kumar, S. A., Williard, M. D., et al. (1978): Serum hydrocortisone (cortisol) values in normal and adrenopathic dogs as determined by radioimmunoassay. Am. J. Vet. Res. *39*:179.
32. Cochnet, M., Chang, A. C. Y., and Cohen, S. N. (1982): Characterization of the structural gene and putative 5'-regulatory sequences for human pro-opiomelanocortin. Nature *297*:335.
33. Critchley, J. A., Ellis, P., and Ungar, A. (1980): The reflex release of adrenaline and noradrenaline from the adrenal glands of cats and dogs. J. Physiol. *298*:71.
34. Cupps, T. R. and Fauci, A. S. (1982): Corticosteroid-mediated immunoregulation in man. Immunol. Rev. *65*:133.
35. Dallman, M. F. (1984–85): Control of adrenocortical growth in vivo. Endocrine Res. *10*:213.
36. Davis, J. O. and Freeman, R. H. (1976): Mechanism regulating renin release. Physiol. Rev. *56*:1.
37. Daynes, R. A., Araneo, B. A., Hennebold, J., et al. (1995): Steroids as regulators of the mammalian immune system. J. Invest. Dermatol. *105* (Suppl 1):145.
38. DeBold, C. R., Sheldon, W. R., DeCherney, G. S., et al. (1984): Arginine vasopressin potentiates adrenocorticotropin release induced by ovine corticotropin-releasing factor. J. Clin. Invest. *73*:533.
39. De Goeij, D. C. E., Jezova, D., and Tilders, F. J. H. (1992): Repeated stress enhances vasopressin synthesis in corticotropin releasing factor neurons in the paraventricular nucleus. Brain Res. *577*:165.
40. De Goeij, D. C. E., Kvetnansky, R., Whitnall, M. H., et al. (1991): Repeated stress-induced activation of corticotropin-releasing factor neurons enhances vaso-

pressin stores and colocalization with corticotropin-releasing factor in the median eminence of rats. Neuroendocrinology *53*:150.

41. Delmage, D. A. (1972): Three cases of alopecia in the dog related to adrenocortical dysfunction. J. Small Anim. Pract. *13*:265.

42. Denault, D. L., Fejes-Toth, G., and Naray-Fejes-Toth, A. (1996): Aldosterone regulation of sodium channel gamma-subunit mRNA in cortical collecting duct cells. Am. J. Physiol. *271*:C423.

43. Dowling, P. M., Williams, M. A., and Clark, T. P. (1993): Adrenal insufficiency associated with long-term anabolic steroid administration in a horse. J. Am. Vet. Med. Assoc. *203*:1166.

44. Dunlop, D. G. and Shanks, R. G. (1968): Selective blockade of adrenoceptive beta-receptors in the heart. Br. J. Pharmacol. *32*:201.

45. Durant, S., Duval, D., and Homo-Delarche, F. (1986): Factors involved in the control of fibroblast proliferation by glucocorticoids: A review. Endocrine Rev. *7*:254.

46. Dybdal, N. (1997): Pituitary *pars intermedia* dysfunction (Equine Cushing's-like Disease) *In*: Current Therapy in Equine Medicine, edited by N. Dybdal. Volume 4. Philadelphia, PA, W. B. Saunders Co., p. 499.

47. Dybdal, N. O., Hargreaves, K. M., Madigan, J. E., et al. (1994): Diagnostic testing for pituitary pars intermedia dysfunction in horses. J. Am. Vet. Med. Assoc. *204*:627.

48. Eberhart, R. J. and Patt, J. A., Jr. (1971): Plasma cortisol concentrations in newborn calves. Am. J. Vet. Res. *32*:1291.

49. Edelman, I. S. and Marver, D. (1980): Mediating events in the action of aldosterone. J. Steroid Chem. *12*:219.

50. Eiler, H., Goble, D., and Oliver, J. (1979): Adrenal gland function in the horse: Effects of cosyntropine (synthetic) and corticotropin (natural) stimulation. Am. J. Vet. Res. *40*:724.

51. Enright, J. B., Goggin, J. E., Frye, F. L., et al. (1970): Effects of corticosteroids on rabies virus infections in various animal species. J. Am. Vet. Med. Assoc. *156*:765.

52. Estivariz, F. E., Lowry, P. J., and Jackson, S. (1992): Control of adrenal growth. *In*: The Adrenal Gland, 2nd ed., edited by V. H. T. James. New York, NY, Raven Press, Ltd., p. 43.

53. Farr, M. J. and Olsen, R. G. (1978): Suppression of the cell-mediated immune system of the horse by systemic corticosteroid administration. J. Equine Med. Surg. *2*:129.

54. Fauci, A. S., Dale, D. C., and Balow, J. E. (1976): Glucocorticosteroid therapy: Mechanisms of action and clinical considerations. Ann. Intern. Med. *84*:304.

55. Feige, J. J. and Baird, A. (1991): Growth factor regulation of adrenal cortex growth and function. Prog. Growth Factor Res. *3*:103.

56. Feldman, E. C. (1995): Hypoadrenocorticism. *In*: Textbook of Veterinary Medicine. Diseases of the Dog and Cat, 4th ed., Vol. 2, edited by S. J. Ettinger and E. C. Feldman. Philadelphia, PA, W. B. Saunders Co., p. 1538.

57. Fenske, M. (1997): Role of cortisol in the ACTH-induced suppression of testicular steroidogenesis in guinea pigs. J. Endocrinol. *154*:407.

58. Ferguson, J. L., Roesel, O. F., and Bottoms, G. D. (1978): Dexamethasone treatment during hemorrhagic shock: Blood pressure, tissue perfusion, and plasma enzymes. Am. J. Vet. Res. *39*:817.

59. Flower, R. J. (1986): The mediators of steroid action. Nature *320*:20.

60. Foster, L.J. and Klip, A. (2000): Mechanism and regulation of GLUT-4 vesicle fusion in muscle and fat cells. Am. J. Physiol. - Cell Physiol. *279*:C877.

61. Frandsen, J. C. (1987): Parasites and stressors: Plasma cortisol responses of goats infected with the stomach worm *Haemonchus contortus* to exogenous corticotropin (ACTH). Vet. Parasit. *23*:43.

62. Franklin, R. T. (1984): The use of glucocorticoids in treating cerebral edema. Comp. Cont. Educ. Pract. Vet. *6*:442.

63. Fuller, R. W. (1973): Control of epinephrine synthesis and secretion. Fed. Proc. *32*:177.

64. Fuller, P.J., Lim-Tio, S.S., and Brennan, F.E. (2000): Specificity in mineralocorticoid versus glucocorticoid action. Kidney Int. *57*:1256.

65. Gallo-Payet, N., Cote, M., Chorvatova, A., et al. (1999): Cyclic AMP-independent effects of ACTH on glomerulosa cells of the rat adrenal cortex. J. Steroid Biochem. Mol. Biol. *69*:335.

66. Ganjam, V. K. and Estergreen, V. L., Jr. (1970): Cortisol and corticosterone in bovine plasma and the effect of ACTH. J. Dairy Sci. *53*:480.

67. Gann, D. S., Dallman, M. F., and Engleland, W. C. (1981): Reflex control and modulation of ACTH and corticosteroids. Int. Rev. Physiol. *24*:157.

68. Garcia, M. C. and Beech, J. (1986): Endocrinologic, hematologic, and heart rate changes in swimming horses. Am. J. Vet. Res. *47*:2004.

69. Gensse, M., Vitale, N., Chasserot-Golaz, S., et al. (2000): Regulation of exocytosis in chromaffin cells by phosducin-like protein, a protein interacting with G protein betagamma subunits. FEBS Lett. *480*:184.

70. Giacchetti, G., Opocher, G., Sarzani, R., et al. (1996): Angiotensin II and the adrenal. Clin. Exp. Pharmacol. Physiol. *23* (Suppl. 3):S119.

71. Giguere, D. M. and Labrie, F. (1982): Vasopressin potentiates cyclic AMP accumulation and ACTH release induced by corticotropin-releasing factor (CRF) in rat anterior pituitary cells in culture. Endocrinology *111*:1752.

72. Gonzalez, R., Orgeur, P., and Signoret, J. P. (1988): Luteinizing hormone, testosterone and cortisol responses in rams upon presentation of estrus females in the nonbreeding season. Theriogenology *30*:1075.

73. Gorbman, A. and Bern, A. (1962): *In*: A Textbook of Comparative Endocrinology. New York, NY, John Wiley and Sons, Inc. p. 343.

74. Gorbman, A., Dickhoff, W. W., Vigna, S. R., et al. (1983): Steroid hormones and steroidogenesis. *In*: Comparative Endocrinology. New York, NY, John Wiley and Sons, Inc. p. 402.

75. Granelli-Piperano, A., Vassali, J. D., and Reich, E. (1977): Secretion of plasminogen activator by human polymorphonuclear leukocytes. Modulation of glucocorticoids and other effects. J. Exp. Med. *146*:1693.

76. Gwazdavkas, F. C., Thatcher, W. W., and Wilcox, C. J. (1972): Adrenocorticotropin alteration of bovine peripheral plasma concentrations of cortisol, corticosterone and progesterone. J. Dairy Sci. *55*:1165.

77. Hache, R.J., Tse, R., Reich, T., et al. (1999): Nucleo-cytoplasmic trafficking of steroid-free glucocorticoid receptor. J. Biol. Chem. *274*:1432.

78. Haidan, A., Bornstein, S. R., Glasow, A., et al. (1998): Basal steroidogenic activity of adrenocortical cells is increased 10-fold by coculture with chromaffin cells. Endocrinology *139*:772.

79. Harbuz, M. S. and Lightman, S. L. (1992): Stress and the hypothalamic-pituitary- adrenal axis: Acute, chronic and immunological activation. J. Endocrinol. *134*:327.

80. Hardee, G. E., Lai, J. W., Semrad, S. D., et al. (1983): Catecholamines in equine and bovine plasmas. J. Vet. Pharmacol. Therap. *5*:279.

81. Hate, T., Takimoto, E., Murakami, K., et al. (1994): Comparative studies on species-specific reactivity between renin and angiotensinogen. Mol. Cell. Biochem. *131*:43.

82. Hinshaw, L. B., Beller, B. K., Archer, L. T., et al. (1979): Recovery from lethal *E. coli* shock in dogs. Surg. Gynecol. Obstet. *149*:545.

83. Hirata, F., Schiffmann, E., Venkatasubramanian, K., et al. (1980): A phospholipase A2 inhibitory protein in rabbit neutrophils induced by glucocorticoids. Proc. Nat. Acad. Sci.; USA *77*:2533.

84. Hoffman, B. B. and Lefkowitz, R. J. (1980): Alpha-adrenergic receptor subtypes. N. Engl. J. Med. *302*:1391.

85. Hoffsis, G. F., Murdick, P. W., Tharp, V. L., et al. (1970): Plasma concentrations of cortisol and corticosterone in the normal horse. Am. J. Vet. Res. *31*:1379.

86. Hornsby, P. J. (1984–85): Regulation of adrenocortical cell proliferation in culture. Endocrine Res. *10*:259.

87. Horton, R. (1973): Aldosterone: Review of its physiology and diagnostic aspects of primary aldosteronism. Metabolism *22*:1525.

88. Imura, H., Fukata, J., and Mori, T. (1991): Cytokines and endocrine function: An interaction between the immune and neuroendocrine systems. Clin. Endocrinol. *35*:107.

89. Insel, P. A. (1984): Identification and regulation of adrenergic receptors in target cells. Am. J. Physiol. *247*:E53.

90. Jackson, S., Hodgkinson, S., Estivariz, F. E., et al. (1991): IGF 1 and 2 in two models of growth. J. Steroid Biochem. Mol. Biol. *40*:399.

91. Jephcott, E. H. and McMillen, I. C. (1986): Effect of electroimmobilization on ovine plasma concentrations of β-endorphin/β-lipotropin, cortisol and prolactin. Res. Vet. Sci. *41*:371.

92. Johnston, S. D. and Mather, E. C. (1978): Canine plasma cortisol measured by RIA. Am. J. Vet. Res. *39*:1766.

93. Johnston, S. D. and Mather, E. C. (1979): Feline plasma cortisol (hydrocortisone) measured by radioimmunoassay. Am. J. Vet. Res. *40*:190.

94. Judd, A.M., Call, G.B., Barney, M., et al. (2000): Possible function of IL-6 and TNF as intraadrenal factors in the regulation of adrenal steroid secretion. Ann. N. Y. Acad. Sci. *917*:628.

95. Kaiser, C. and Jain, T. (1985): Dopamine receptors: Functions, subtypes and emerging concepts. Med. Res. Quart. *5*:145.

96. Keller-Wood, M. E. and Dallman, M. F. (1984): Corticosteroid inhibition of ACTH secretion. Endocrine Rev. *5*:1.

97. Kelly, D. F., Siegel, E. T., and Berg, P. (1971): The adrenal gland in dogs with hyperadrenocorticalism. A pathologic study. Vet. Pathol. *8*:385.

98. Kooistra, H. S., Greven, S. H., Mol, J. A., et al. (1997): Pulsatile secretion of α-MSH and the differential effects of dexamethasone and haloperidol on the secretion of α -MSH and ACTH in dogs. J. Endocrinol. *152*:113.

99. Kristiansen, S. B., Endoh, A., Casson, P. R., et al. (1997): Induction of steroidogenic enzyme genes by insulin and IGF-I in cultured adult human adrenocortical cells. Steroids *62*:258.

100. L'Allemand, D., Penhoat, A., Lebrethon, M. C., et al. (1996): Insulin-like growth factors enhance steroidogenic enzyme and corticotropin receptor messenger ribonucleic acid levels and corticotropin steroidogenic responsiveness in cultured human adrenocortical cells. J. Clin. Endocrinol. Metab. *81*:3892.

101. Lands, A. M., Arnold, A., McAuliff, J. P., et al. (1967): Differentiation of receptor systems activated by sympathomimetic amines. Nature *214*:597.

102. Lang, R. E., Tholken, H., Ganten, D., et al. (1985): Atrial natriuretic factor—a circulating hormone stimulated by volume loading. Nature *314*:264.

103. Langer, S. Z. (1974): Presynaptic regulation of catecholamine release. Biochem. Pharmacol. *23*:1793.

104. Larsson, M., Edqvist, L. E., Ekman, L., et al. (1979): Plasma cortisol in the horse, diurnal rhythm and effects of exogenous ACTH. Acta. Vet. Scand. *20*:16.

105. Lavelle, R. B. (1976): The treatment of Cushing's disease in the dog. Vet. Rec. *98*:406.

106. Lefkowitz, R. J., Hoffman, B. B., and Taylor, P. (1996): Neurotransmission. The autonomic and somatic motor nervous systems. *In*: Goodman & Gilman's: The Pharmacological Basis of Therapeutics, edited by J. G. Hardman and L. E. Limbird. New York, NY, McGraw Hill, p. 110.

107. Leon, J. B., Smith B. B., Timm, K. I., et al. (1990): Endocrine changes during pregnancy, parturition and the early post-partum period in the llama (*Lama glama*). J. Reprod. Fert. *88*:503.

108. Lindner, H. R. (1959): Blood cortisol in the sheep: Normal concentration and changes in ketosis of pregnancy. Nature *184*:1645.

109. Lindner, H. R. (1964): Comparative aspects of cortisol transport: Lack of firm binding to plasma proteins in domestic ruminants. J. Endocrinol. *28*:301.

110. Ling, G. V., Stabenfeldt, G. H., Comer, K. M., et al. (1979): Canine hyperadrenocorticism: Pretreatment clinical and laboratory evaluation of 117 cases. J. Am. Vet. Med. Assoc. *174*:1211.

111. Liu, J. and DeFranco, D.B. (1999): Chromatin recycling of glucocorticoid receptors: Implications for multiple roles of heat shock protein 90. Mol. Endocrinol. *13*:355.

112. Livesey, J.H., Evans, M.J., Mulligan, R., et al. (2000): The interactions of CRH, AVP, and cortisol in the secretion of ACTH from perifused equine anterior pituitary cells: "Permissive" roles for cortisol and CRH. Endocrine Rev. *26:*445.

113. Love, S. (1993): Equine Cushing's disease. Br. Vet. J. *149:*139.

114. Lubberink, A. A. M. E., Rijnberk, A., der Kinderen, P. J., et al. (1971): Hyperfunction of the adrenal cortex: A review. Aust. Vet. J. *47:*504.

115. Lundström, K., Bosu, W. T. K., and Gahne, B. (1975): Peripheral plasma levels of corticosteroids in Swedish Landrace and Yorkshire boars. Swedish J. Agric. Res. *5:*81.

116. Macadam, W. R. and Eberhart, R. J. (1972): Diurnal variation in plasma corticosteroid concentration in dairy cattle. J. Dairy Sci. *55:*1792.

117. Maher, E. R., Jr. and McNeil, E. A., (1997): Pheochromcytoma in dogs and cats. Vet. Clin. North Am., Small Anim. Pract. *27:*359.

118. Maier, F. and Staehelin, M. (1968): Adrenal hyperaemia caused by corticotrophin. Acta Endocrinol. *58:*613.

119. Malbon, C. C., Rapiejko, P. J., and Watkins, D. C. (1988): Permissive hormone regulation of hormone sensitive effector systems. Trends Pharmacol. Sci. *9:*33.

120. Malmejac, J. (1964): Activity of the adrenal medulla and its regulation. Physiol. Rev. *44:*186.

121. Marple, D. N., Judge, M. D., and Aberle, E. D. (1972): Pituitary and adrenocortical function of stress susceptible swine. J. Anim. Sci. *35:*995.

122. Marver, D. (1980): Aldosterone action in target epithelia. Vitam. Horm. *38:*57.

123. Medleau, L., Corvan, L. A., and Cornelius, L. M. (1987): Adrenal function testing in the cat: The effect of low dose intravenous dexamethasone administration. Res. Vet. Sci. *42:*260.

124. Meij, B. P., Mol, J. A., Bevers, M. M., et al. (1997): Alterations in anterior pituitary function of dogs with pituitary-dependent hyperadrenocorticism. J. Endocrinol. *154:*505.

125. Meijer, J. C., de Bruijne, J. J., Rijnberk, A., et al. (1978): Biochemical characterization of pituitary-dependent hyperadrenocorticism in the dog. J. Endocrinol. *77:*111.

126. Meijer, J. C., Mulder, G. H., Rijnberk, A., et al. (1978): Hypothalamic corticotrophin releasing factor activity in dogs with pituitary-dependent hyperadrenocorticism. J. Endocrinol. *79:*209.

127. Messer, N. T., Johnson, P. J., Refsal, K. R., et al. (1995): Effect of food deprivation on baseline iodothyronine and cortisol concentrations in healthy, adult horses. Am. J. Vet. Res. *56:*116.

128. Michelotti, G.A., Price, D.T., and Schwinn, D.A. (2000): Alpha 1-adrenergic receptor regulation: Basic science and clinical implications. Pharmacol. Therap. *88:*281.

129. Mizelle, H. L., Hildebrandt, D. A., Gaillard, C. A., et al. (1990): Atrial natriuretic peptide induces sustained natriuresis in conscious dogs. Am. J. Physiol. *258:*R1445.

130. Moore, J. N., Steiss, J., Nicholson, W. E., et al. (1979): A case of pituitary adrenocorticotropin-dependent Cushing's syndrome in the horse. Endocrinology *104:*576.

131. Morrison, S.F. and Cao, W.H. (2000): Different adrenal sympathetic preganglionic neurons regulate epinephrine and norepinephrine secretion. Am. J. Physiol. - Regul. Integr. Comp. Physiol. *279:*R1763.

132. Mouri, T., Itoi, K., Takahashi, K., et al. (1993): Colocalization of corticotropin-releasing factor and vasopressin in the paraventricular nucleus of the human hypothalamus. Neuroendocrinology *57:*34.

133. Mulrow, P.J. (1999): Angiotensin II and aldosterone regulation. Regul. Pept. *80:*27.

134. Munck, A., Guyre, A. P., and Holbrook, N. J. (1984): Physiological functions of glucocorticoids in stress and their relation to pharmacological actions. Endocrine Rev. *5:*25.

135. Muñoz, M. L., Ramírez, C. M. R., and Rodríguez, C. V. (1990): Ensayo, por competencia de unión a proteínas para cuantificar sin purificacíon previa cortisol o corticosterona en el suero de algauns especies animales. Vet Mex. Mexico City, Mexico *31:*115.

136. Nagayama, T., Matsumoto, T., Kuwakubo, F., et al. (1999): Role of calcium channels in catecholamine secretion in the rat adrenal gland. J. Physiol. *520* (Pt. 2):503.

137. Nakanishi, S., Inoue, A., Kita, T., et al. (1979): Nucleotide sequence of cloned cDNA for bovine corticotropin-beta-lipotropin precursor. Nature *278:*423.

138. Nankova, B.B. and Sabban, E.L. (1999): Multiple signaling pathways exist in the stress-triggered regulation of gene expression for catecholamine biosynthetic enzymes and several neuropeptides in the rat adrenal medulla. Acta Physiol. Scand. *167:*1.

139. Nara, P. L., Krahowka, S., and Powers, T. E. (1979): Effects of prednisolone on the development of immune responses to canine distemper virus in Beagle pups. Am. J. Vet. Res. *40:*1742.

140. O'Malley, B. (1974): Steroid hormone receptors. Session IX. Fifty-sixth Annual Meeting of the Endocrine Society. Atlanta, GA. Endocrinology *94:*21.

141. Orth, D. N., Holscher, M. A., Wilson, M. G., et al. (1982): Equine Cushing's disease: Plasma immunoreactive proopiolipomelanocortin peptide and cortisol levels basally and in response to diagnostic tests. Endocrinology *110:*1430.

142. Orth, D. N. and Kovaks, W. J. (1998) The adrenal cortex, Chapter 12. *In*: Williams Textbook of Endocrinology, 9th Edition, edited by J. D. Wilson, D. W. Foster, H. M. Kronenberg, and P. R. Larsen. Philadelphia, PA, W. B. Saunders, Inc., p. 517.

143. Osbaldiston, G. W. and Johnson, J. H. (1972): Effect of ACTH and selected glucocorticoids on circulating blood cells in horses. J. Am. Vet. Med. Assoc. *161:*53.

144. Paape, M. J., Desjardins, C., Schultze, W. D., et al. (1972): Corticosteroid concentrations in jugular and mammary vein blood plasma of cows after overmilking. Am. J. Vet. Res. *33:*1753.

145. Parrillo, J. E. and Fauci, A. S. (1979): Mechanism of glucocorticoid action on immune processes. Annu. Rev. Pharmacol. Toxicol. *19:*179.

146. Penhoat, A., Chatelain, P. G., Jaillard, C., et al. (1988): Characterization of insulin-like growth factor I and insulin receptors on cultured bovine adrenal fasciculata cells. Role of these peptides on adrenal cell function. Endocrinology *122:*2518.

147. Penhoat, A., Leduque, P., Jaillard, C., et al. (1991): ACTH and angiotensin II regulation of insulin-like growth factor-I and its binding proteins in cultured bovine adrenal cells. J. Mol. Endocrinol. 7:223.

148. Penhoat, A., Rainey, W. E., Viard, I., et al. (1994): Regulation of adrenal cell- differentiated functions by growth factors. Hormone Res. 42:39.

149. Perchellet, J. and Sharma, R. K. (1979): Mediating role of calcium and guanosine 3', 5'-monophosphate in adrenocorticotropin induced steroidogenesis by adrenal cells. Science 23:1259.

150. Perretti, M. and Ahluwalia, A. (2000): The microcirculation and inflammation: Site of action for glucocorticoids. Microcirculation 7:147.

151. Persson, S. G. B., Larsson, M., and Linholm, A. (1980): Effects of training on adreno-cortical function and red-cell volume in trotters. Zbl. Vet. Med. 27:261.

152. Peterson, M. E., Greco, D. S., and Orth, D. N. (1989): Primary hypoadrenocorticism in ten cats. J. Vet. Intern. Med. 3:55.

153. Peterson, M. E., Kemppainen, R. J., and Orth, D. N. (1994): Plasma concentrations of immunoreactive proopiomelanocortin peptides and cortisol in chronically normal cats. Am. J. Vet. Res. 55:295.

154. Peterson, M. E., Kintzer, P. P., and Kass, P. H. (1996): Pretreatment clinical and laboratory findings in dogs with hypoadrenocorticism: 225 cases (1979–1993). J. Am. Vet. Med. Assoc. 208:85.

155. Plotsky, P. M., Cunningham, E. T., Jr., and Widmaier, E. P. (1989): Catecholaminergic modulation of corticotropin-releasing factor and adrenocorticotropin secretion. Endocrine Rev. 10:437.

156. Quinn, S. J. and Williams, G. H. (1988): Regulation of aldosterone secretion. Annu. Rev. Physiol. 50:409.

157. Raadsheer, F. C., Hoogendijk, W. J. G., Stam, F. C., et al. (1994): Increased numbers of corticotropin-releasing hormone expressing neurons in the hypothalamic paraventricular nucleus of depressed patients. Neuroendocrinology 60:436.

158. Rao, A. J., Long, J. A., and Ramachandran, J. (1978): Effects of antiserum to adrenocorticotropin on adrenal growth and function. Endocrinology 102:371.

159. Rebuffe, S. M., Walsh, U. A., McEwen, B., et al. (1992): Effect of chronic stress and exogenous glucocorticoids on regional fat distribution and metabolism. Physiol. Behav. 52:583.

160. Reichlin, S. (1993): Neuroendocrine-immune interactions. N. Engl. J. Med. 329:1246.

161. Reid, I. A., Morris, B. J., and Ganong, W. F. (1978): The renin-angiotensin system. Annu. Rev. Physiol. 40:377.

162. Rhynes, W. E. and Ewing, L. L. (1973): Plasma corticosteroids in Hereford bulls exposed to high ambient temperature. J. Anim. Sci. 36:369.

163. Richkind, M. and Edqvist, L. E. (1973): Peripheral plasma levels of corticosteroids in normal Beagles and Greyhounds measured by a rapid competitive protein binding technique. Acta Vet. Scand. 14:745.

164. Rivier, C. and Vale, W. (1983): Interaction of corticotropin-releasing factor and arginine vasopressin on adrenocorticotropin secretion in vivo. Endocrinology 113:939.

165. Ross, J. N. (1979): Comprehensive patient management in shock. J. Am. Vet. Med. Assoc. 175:92.

166. Sansom, S. C. and O'Neil, R. G. (1985): Mineralocorticoid regulation of apical cell membrane Na^+ and K^+ transport of the cortical collecting duct. Am. J. Physiol. 248:F858.

167. Santen, R. J. (1980): Adrenal of male dog secretes androgens and estrogens. Am. J. Physiol. 239:E109.

168. Schechter, R. D., Stabenfeldt, G. H., Gribble, D. H., et al. (1973): Treatment of Cushing's syndrome in the dog with an adrenocorticolytic agent (o,p'-DDD). J. Am. Vet. Med. Assoc. 162:629.

169. Schwalm, J. W. and Tucker, H. A. (1978): Glucocorticoids in mammary secretions and blood serum during reproduction and lactation and distributions of glucocorticoids, progesterone, and estrogens in fractions of milk. J. Dairy Sci. 61:550.

170. Scott, D. W. and Greene, C. E. (1974): Iatrogenic secondary adrenocortical insufficiency in dogs. J. Am. Anim. Hosp. Assoc. 10:555.

171. Scott, D. W., Kirk, R. W., and Bentinck-Smith, J. (1979): Some effects of short-term methylpredisolone therapy in normal cats. Cornell Vet. 69:104.

172. Sebranek, J. G., Marple, D. N., Cassens, R. G., et al. (1973): Adrenal response to ACTH in the pig. J. Anim. Sci. 36:41.

173. Seren, E. (1973): ACTH and glucocorticoids in cattle. Folia Vet. Latina 3:584.

174. Sigala, S., Missale, C., Tognazzi, N., et al. (2000): Differential gene expression of dopamine D-2 receptor subtypes in rat chromaffin cells and sympathetic neurons in culture. Neuroreport 11:2467.

175. Slight, S., Ganjam, V. K., and Weber, K. T. (1994): Species diversity of 11- beta-hydroxysteroid dehydrogenase in the cardiovascular system. J. Lab. Clin. Med. 124:821.

176. Solomon, S. (1999): POMC-derived peptides and their biological action. Ann. N. Y. Acad. Sci. 885:22.

177. Sosa, R. E., Volpe, M., Marion, D. N., et al. (1986): Relationship between renal hemodynamic and natriuretic effects of atrial natriuretic factor. Am J. Physiol. 250:F520.

178. Stark, K. (1977): Regulation of noradrenaline release by presynaptic receptor systems. Rev. Physiol. Biochem. Pharmacol. 77:1.

179. Steinberg, D. (1966): Catecholamine stimulation of fat mobilization and its metabolic consequences. Pharmacol. Rev. 18:217.

180. Swift, G. A. and Brown, R. H. (1976): Surgical treatment of Cushing's syndrome in the cat. Vet. Rec. 99:374.

181. Tamanini, C., Giordano, N., Chiesa F., et al. (1983): Plasma cortisol variations induced in the stallion by mating. Acta Endocrinol. 102:447.

182. Temple, T. E. and Liddle, G. W. (1970): Inhibitors of adrenal steroid synthesis. Annu. Rev. Pharmacol. 10:199.

183. Thompson, E. B. and Lippman, M. E. (1974): Mechanism of action of glucocorticoids. Metabolism 23:159.

184. Thurley, D. C. (1972): Prenatal growth of the adrenal gland in sheep. N. Z. Vet. J. 20:177.

185. Tohei, A., Tomabechi, T., Mamada, M., et al. (1997): Effects of repeated ether stress on the hypothalamic-pituitary-testes axis in adult rats with special reference to inhibin secretion. J. Vet. Med. Sci. 59:329.

186. Tumisto, J. and Mannisto, P. (1985): Neurotransmitter regulations of anterior pituitary hormones. Pharmacol. Rev. *37*:249.

187. Turek, F. W. (1994): Circadian rhythmns. Recent Prog. Hormone Res. *49*:43.

188. Turner, C. D. and Bagnara, J. T. (1976): The adrenal medulla: Chromaffin tissue. Chapter 10. *In*: General Endocrinology. 6th ed., edited by C. D. Turner and J. T. Bagnara. Philadelphia, PA., W. B. Saunders Co., p. 291.

189. Twedt, D. C. and Wheeler, S. L. (1984): Pheochromocytoma in the dog. Vet. Clin. North Am., Small Anim. Pract. *14*:767.

190. Unger, A. and Phillps, J. H. (1983): Regulation of the adrenal medulla. Physiol. Rev. *63*:687.

191. Vendeira, P., Pignatelli, D., Neves, D., et al. (1999): Effects of prolonged infusion of basic fibroblast growth factor and IGF-I on adrenocortical differentiation in the autotransplanted adrenal: An immunohistochemical study. J. Endocrinol. *162*:21.

192. Vinson, G. A., Whitehouse, B., and Hinson, J. (1992): Physiological and cellular aspects of the control of adrenocortical hormone secretion. Chapter 3. *In*: The Adrenal Cortex, edited by G. P. Vinson, B. Whitehouse, and J. Hinson. Englewood Cliffs, NJ, Prentice-Hall Inc., p. 79.

193. Vittet, D., Ciais, D., Keramidas, M., et al. (2000): Paracrine control of the adult adrenal cortex vasculature endothelial growth factor. Endocrine Res. *26*:843.

194. Von Borell, E. and Hurnik, J. F. (1991): Stereotypic behavior, adrenocortical function, and open field behavior of individually confined gestating sows. Physiol. Behav. *49*:709.

195. Von Euler, U. S. (1963): Chromaffin cell hormones, Chapter 7. *In*: Comparative Endocrinology, Vol. 1, edited by U. S. von Euler and H. Heller. New York, Academic Press, p. 258.

196. Von Euler, U. S. (1966): Twenty years of noradrenaline. Pharmacol. Rev. *18*:29.

197. Wagner, W. C. and Oxenreider, S. L. (1972): Adrenal function in the cow. Diurnal changes and the effects of lactation and neurohypophyseal hormones. J. Anim. Sci. *34*:630.

198. Weber, M. M., Simmler, P., Fottner, C., et al. (1995): Insulin-like growth factor II (IGF-II) is more potent than IGF-I in stimulating cortisol secretion from cultured bovine adrenocortical cells: Interaction with the IGF-I receptor and IGF-binding proteins. Endocrinology *136*:3714.

199. West, G. B. (1955): The comparative pharmacology of the suprarenal medulla. Quart. Rev. Biol. *30*:116.

200. Westley, H. J. and Kelley, K. W. (1984): Physiological concentrations of cortisol suppress cell-mediated immune events in the domestic pig. Proc. Soc. Exp. Biol. Med. *177*:156.

201. Whipp, S. C., Wood, R. L., and Lyon, N. C. (1970): Diurnal variation in concentrations of hydrocortisone in plasma of swine. Am. J. Vet. Res. *31*:2105.

202. Whitnall, M. H., Mezey, E., and Gainer, H. (1985): Co-localization of corticotropin-releasing factor and vasopressin in median eminence neurosecretory vesicles. Nature *317*:248.

203. Whitworth, E. and Vinson, G.P. (2000): Zonal differentiation in the rat adrenal cortex. Endocrine Res. *26*:973.

204. Williams, G. H. and Dluhy, R. G. (1972): Aldosterone biosynthesis. Am. J. Med. *53*:595.

205. Windle, R. J., Wood, S. A., Shanks, N., et al. (1998): Ultradian rhythm of basal corticosterone release in the female rat: Dynamic interaction with the response to acute stress. Endocrinology *139*:443.

206. Wright, R. D. (1963): Blood flow through the adrenal gland. Endocrinology *72*:418.

207. Wurtman, R. J., Pohorecky, L. A., and Baliga, B. S. (1972): Adrenocortical control of the biosynthesis of epinephrine and proteins in the adrenal medulla. Pharmacol. Rev. *24*:411.

208. Young, D. B. (1988): Quantitative analysis of aldosterone's role in potassium regulation. Am. J. Physiol. *255*:F811.

209. Yovich, J. V., Horney, F. D., and Hardee, G. E. (1984): Pheochromocytoma in the horse and measurement of norepinephrine levels in horses. Can. Vet. J. *25*:21.

The Biology of Sex

M. H. PINEDA

7

"There is no such biological entity as sex. What exists in nature is a dimorphism within species into male and female individuals, which differ with respect to contrasting characters, for each of which in any given species we recognize a male form and a female form, whether these characters be classed as of the biological, or psychological, or social orders. Sex is not a force that produces these contrasts, it is merely a name for our total impression of the differences."

(From: F. R. Lillie, 1932, quoted by Ursula Mittwoch, in Sex determination and sex reversal: Genotype, phenotype, dogma and semantics. Human Genet. *89*: 467–479, 1992.)

INTRODUCTION

FOR the purposes of this chapter, sex is defined as the total morphologic, physiologic, and psychologic differences that distinguish a male from a female. Chromosomal and phenotypic sex are recognized.

SEXUALITY

Reproduction is essential to the continuity of the species in all living organisms. The lower forms of life are more or less fixed in their habitat, and reproduction by mitotic cellular division is advantageous, because seeking and recognizing a suitable mate is unnecessary. This form of reproduction is found in mammalian somatic cells and in the proliferative stages of gametogenesis, prior to the formation of male and female gametes. The principal disadvantage of mitosis is the uniformity of the genotype of daughter cells. Except for occasional mutants, every progeny originated during mitosis is identical to its progenitor.

Evolution of Sex

In mammals, reproduction depends upon the union of anisogametes produced by dimorphic individuals designated as male and female. The evolution of sexuality in multicellular organisms is an adaptation to specialized function. Division of genetic materials between male and female provides for specialization of social function as well as reproductive function. The most important evolutionary advantage gained by sexual reproduction is the increase in genetic variability afforded by meiotic division to form haploid gametes which, at fertilization, will reconstitute the diploid number. Variability in the offspring is produced by chiasma formation, random segregation, and recombination of chromosomal genes.

Although sexual reproduction is advantageous in terms of adaptation, the union of anisogametes from dimorphic parents is subject to temporal and spatial hazards. If gametes were released independently of coordinating activities by the two sexes, this type of reproduction would likely lead to extinction. Thus, even in the lowest bisexual species, there are stimuli that tend to synchronize male and female partners to release their gametes at nearly the same time and in close proximity. These adversities were further complicated as land-dwelling species evolved and the gametes could no longer be released directly into an aqueous environment. Fertilization became an internal process in the oviducts of the female, and uterine gestation evolved. A further hazard in sexual reproduction is that the progeny must pass through critical stages of development.

Chromosomal Sex

Chromosomal sex is determined by a single pair of sex chromosomes and results in the formation of either testes or ovaries. The sex having similar sex chromosomes is the homozygous sex. The heterozygous sex has dissimilar sex chromosomes. Among domestic animals, the female is the homogametic sex and is designated XX. The mammalian male is the heterogametic sex and is designated XY. In poultry, hens are heterogametic and are designated ZW. Roosters are homogametic and are designated ZZ.

Chromosomal sex can be ascertained by examining interphase nuclei of somatic cells. The nuclei of somatic cells containing two X chromosomes contain a characteristic chromatin mass, the Barr body. The Barr body represents a single inactive X chromosome of an XX individual, which forms a loop structure. Nuclei containing Barr bodies are chromatin-positive. The number of Barr bodies is one less than the total number of X chromosomes in diploid cells. Normal males are chromatin-negative.

Gene expression in one of the X chromosomes of the XX somatic cells of the female appears to be inactivated or repressed early during embryonic or fetal development in eutherian mammals. This results in a ratio of sex chromosome to autosomes similar to that of the XY cells of the male, compensating for the X sex chromosomal difference in the 2X females and 1X males. For a given individual female, the inactivation of the X chromosome from either progenitor, paternal X or maternal X, may be of random occurrence. Recent evidences suggest that the paternal X chromosome seems to be inactivated in the trophodermic cells of the developing embryo more frequently than the maternal X chromosome, as the embryonic cells differentiate from the totipotent lineage. The inactivation of the paternal X chromosome of the inner cell mass appears to be random and clonal. Once the inactivation has occurred, it remains fixed in the heredity of the somatic cells of that individual. During oogenesis, the inactivated X chromosome becomes active again while the oocyte undergoes meiosis so that each oocyte will contain an active X chromosome.

Anomalous sex chromosomal complements result from nondisjunction of the sex chromosomes during meiosis (Fig. 7-1). Best-documented among these are the XXY nuclei of individuals

			OOCYTE		
			Normal	Nondisjunctive	
			x	xx	o
SPERM	Normal	x	xx (=normal female)	xxx	xo
		y	xy (=normal male)	xxy	yo
	Nondisjunctive	xy	xxy		
		o	xo		

Fig. 7-1. Diagram showing how normal and abnormal sex-chromosome constitutions can arise at fertilization. An **O** spermatozoon or oocyte is one that carries neither an **X** nor a **Y** chromosome. Nondisjunctive gametes arise through faulty sharing out (nondisjunctive) of the sex chromosomes; **YO** individuals are probably not viable; human **XXX** individuals in man are sterile females.

affected with Klinefelter's syndrome (seminiferous tubule dysgenesis) and the XO nuclei of individuals affected with Turner's syndrome (ovarian agenesis) in man and animals. An XXY chromosomal constitution associated with testicular hypoplasia and azoospermia has been reported in bulls, horses, pigs, rams, and cats. An XO syndrome associated with inactive ovaries has also been reported in the mare. Patients with Klinefelter's disease are chromatin-positive, and those with Turner's syndrome are chromatin-negative.

Table 7-1 shows the diploid number of chromosomes of domestic species. Chromosome number plays an important role in maintaining genetic purity in nature. Interspecific mammalian hybrids, usually produced for commercial purposes, are possible. The mule and its reciprocal hybrid, the hinny, are examples. However, such hybrid progeny are usually sterile. The sterility of mules is due to chromosomal incompatibility. Mules of both sexes occasionally produce gametes, but most germ cells degenerate early in gametogenesis, probably because of a block in meiosis due to the unequal number of chromosomes between the paternal (donkey,

62) and maternal (horse, 64) chromosomes. The mule and the hinny both have 63 chromosomes with unevenly matched pairs. Lack of pairing of homologous chromosomes in the few gametes produced by mules would not allow normal development and fertilization by interaction of their own gametes. However, mules undergo estrous cycles and are capable of gestation to term of transferred equine embryos.

The South American camelids, such as alpacas, llamas, guanacos, and vicuñas, all have 37 pairs of chromosomes and can interbreed and produce fertile offspring.

Characteristic club-shaped nuclear appendages termed drumsticks occur in a small proportion of segmented neutrophils of XX genetic females. Drumsticks are equivalent to the sex chromatin mass of Barr bodies in the nuclei of other somatic cells.

Technical advances in chromosomal analysis have contributed to the value of determination of sex chromatin and the understanding of sexual abnormalities resulting from chromosomal aberrations. Cytogenetics, the science dealing with karyotype, has become a routine procedure in many pathology laboratories to aid in the diagnosis of developmental abnormalities.

Phenotypic Sex

Potentiality toward the development of both male or female exist in every embryo. Most individuals differentiate in accord with their chromosomal sex, but all degrees of expression of the genetic sex may occur. Furthermore, individuals may differentiate toward the sex contrary to their chromosomal sex, resulting in intersexuality. Complete sex reversals are known in some species. Genetic sex is unalterably fixed at fertilization, but phenotypic sex differentiation is influenced by a number of factors such as hormones, temperature extremes, and probably other agents.

Oocytes from normal females carry only an X chromosome, whereas 50% of spermatozoa carry an X chromosome, and 50% carry a Y chromosome. Theoretically, 50% of the embryos should be males, and 50% should be females (Fig. 7-2).

Sex ratio is expressed as the percentage of males or as **the number of males per 100**

Table 7-1   Numbers of Chromosomes

Animal	Diploid No.
Alpaca	74
Barbary sheep	58
Cat	38
Cattle, domestic	60
Cattle, Zebu	60
Chicken	
Rooster	78
Hen	77
Dog	78
Donkey	62
Goat	60
Goat, Rocky Mountain	42
Hinny	63
Horse	64
Llama	74
Mule	63
Pig	38
Sheep	54
Vicuña	74

Adapted from several sources, including: S. P. Pakes and R. A. Griesemer, J. Am. Vet. Med. Assoc. *146*:138, 1965; and S. Ohno, Annu. Rev. Genet. *3*:495, 1969.

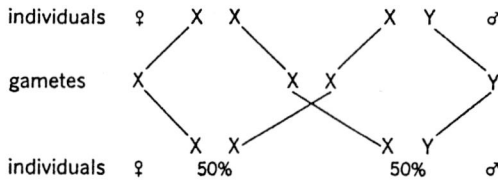

Fig. 7-2. Theoretic sex ratio at fertilization.

females. Primary sex ratio is the ratio at conception. This is a theoretic value, but sex ratio can be determined early in embryonal development by sex chromatin techniques. Secondary sex ratio is the proportion of males at birth, and tertiary sex ratio is the ratio at puberty. The secondary sex ratios of a number of species are displayed in Table 7-2.

The perfection of sex control on a practical scale by artificial insemination with sexed spermatozoa or transfer of sexed embryos would be a great asset to genetic progress in the livestock industry. Females could be ranked according to their genetic worth for highly heritable economic traits. A small percentage of the most desirable females could be bred to selectively produce male progeny for use as seminal donors. The next most valuable females could be bred to produce female replacements, and the remainder of females could produce males or females, depending on economic demand. Sex ratios have been reported to be modified by genetic selection, frequency of ejaculation, and parity of the dam. Separation of X and Y spermatozoa would be the simplest method to achieve this end. Successful attempts at separating male- and female-determining spermatozoa from domestic species have been reported, but these results are not yet repeatable for routine field applications.

Because the Y chromosome contains less material than the X chromosome, the Y-bearing spermatozoon has less mass. Centrifugation, sedimentation, electrophoresis, and flow cytometric sorting have been used to separate the two types of spermatozoa. Separation of spermatozoa on the basis of nuclear mass or membrane potential to obtain sufficient number of sexed spermatozoa for artificial insemination has not been reliably achieved on a practical scale. Another route of further investigation lies in the distinct antigenic properties of the X- and Y-bearing spermatozoa, which would allow sex control by immunologic technics. The use of immunologic methods to detect the H-Y antigen, a gene product of the Y chromosome, is also being investigated. Production of sexed offsprings from oocytes fertilized *in vitro* has been obtained in some species, and the *in vitro* fertilization of oocytes with either X- or Y-bearing spermatozoa would then allow for the generation of sexed embryos for transfer and obtainment of offsprings of predetermined sex.

Female monozygotic mice have been produced by microsurgical removal of the male pronucleus from a fertilized oocyte. Diploidy is achieved by inducing the haploid female pronucleus to replicate its chromosomes by culturing in a medium containing cytochalasin B. The re-

Table 7-2   *Secondary Sex Ratios Commonly Observed in Some Mammals and Domestic Chicken*

Species	Number Observed	Percentage of Males (High Ratio)	Number Observed	Percentage of Males (Low Ratio)
Cattle	4,900	51.8	982	48.6
Dog	1,400	55.4	6,878	52.4
Domestic chicken	20,037	48.6	2,501	46.8
Horse	25,560	49.9	135,826	49.1
Pig	2,357	52.8	16,233	48.8
Sheep	50,685	49.5	8,965	49.2

Data modified from various sources, especially from: P. S. Lawrence, Quart. Rev. Biol. *16:*35, 1941; and A. V. Nalbandov, Reproductive Physiology, 2nd ed. San Francisco, CA, W. H. Freeman and Co., 1964.

moval of the female pronucleus would generate lethal YY individuals.

None of these approaches have consistently produced reproducible results for field application to livestock species. Hybridization for DNA sequences specific to the Y or X chromosomes is also being investigated for application to separation of X- or Y-bearing spermatozoa.

DEVELOPMENT OF MALE AND FEMALE REPRODUCTIVE ORGANS

Sexual differentiation, like the differentiation of other systems, proceeds in consecutive steps (Fig. 7-3). Chromosomal sex is determined at fertilization; the establishment of gonadal sex is followed by the differentiation of the Müllerian

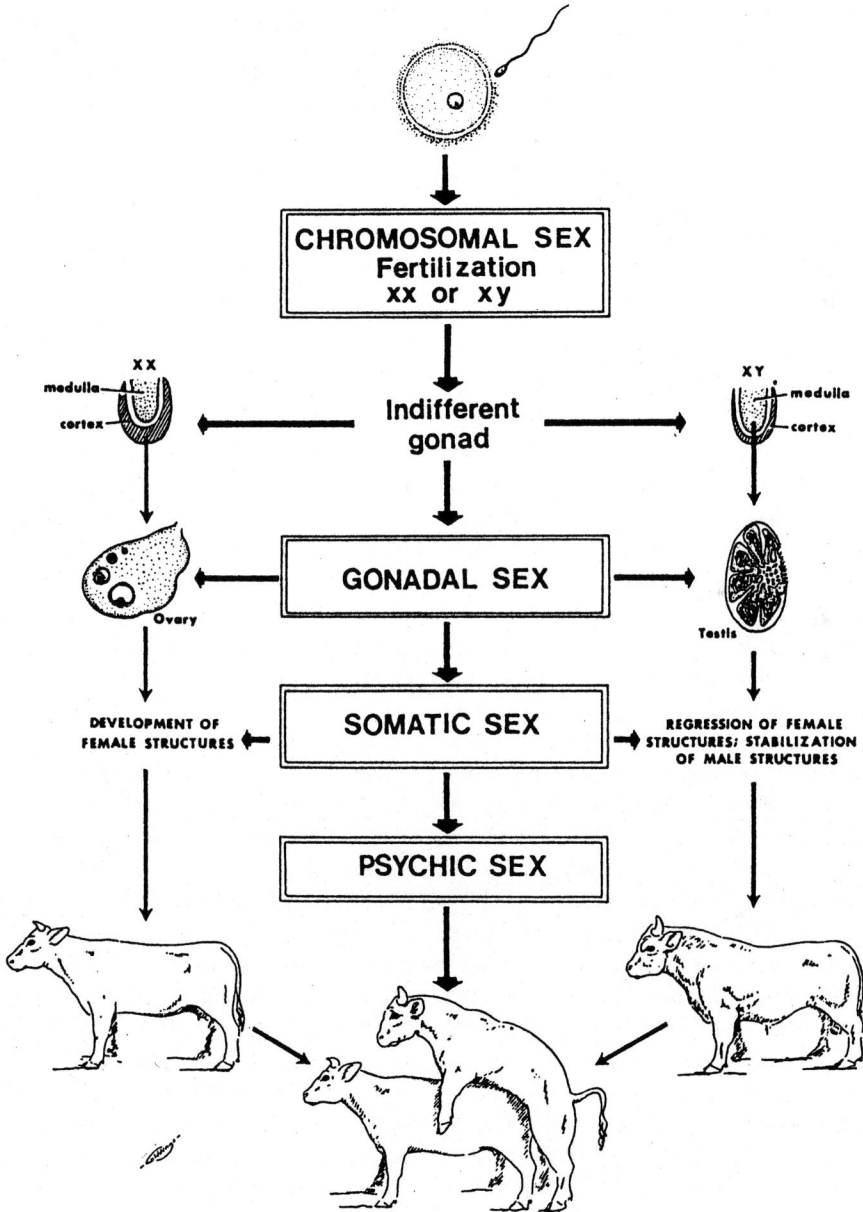

Fig. 7-3. Diagram representing four consecutive steps of sexual differentiation.

or Wolffian duct system into the female or male accessory genitalia, respectively. The final step is the establishment of the psychic sex with the characteristic male or female sexual behavior.

Gonadal Sex

Although the genetic sex of the conceptus is unalterably determined by its sex chromosome complement, each embryo is potentially capable of developing the genitalia of either sex because the primitive gonad has all of the cellular elements to give origin to a testicle or to an ovary. Each undifferentiated gonad consists of an inner medulla surrounded by an outer cortex (Fig. 7-3). In a normal XY sex chromosomal individual, each medulla will give origin to testes, whereas in a normal XX sex chromosomal individual, each cortex will give origin to ovaries. The differentiation of sexual characteristics depends upon the quantitative relationship between male- and female-determining genes and their interaction with the internal environment.

Genes associated with female characteristics are believed to be located on the X chromosome. Homologous (XX) chromosomes appear to be necessary for the differentiation of the normal ovary. In Turner's syndrome (XO), diagnosed in man, rats, cats, sows, ewes, and mares, the adult gonad is an elongated mass of connective tissue. Genes for male development are located on autosomes and on the Y chromosome. To develop as a normal male, genes for masculinity on the autosomes and on the Y chromosome must overcome and prevail over the dominant female-determining genes on the single X chromosome of an XY individual. The presence of a Y chromosome, irrespective of the number of X chromosomes, or some other form of chromosomal X-Y interaction is responsible for the differentiation of the testes. In man, individuals with 45,XO syndrome are females, whereas those with 46,XY; 47,XXY; 48,XXXY; and 49,XXXXY are all males. However, the dominant effect of the Y chromosome insofar as related to testicular development is diminished as the number of X chromosomes increases. Normally, the XX chromosomic constitution of a normal female embryo provides an abundance of female-determining genes, and the embryo

develops as a female. Evidences accumulated in the past few years indicate that maleness and testicular differentiation in mammals is dependent upon both the Y chromosome and other associated and interacting factors. The Y chromosome has in one of its short arms a maleness gene called sex-determining region Y-gene, or sry-gene for short, which was first identified in mice and later in other species, including man. This gene has also been named SRY-gene and TDF-gene, an acronym that stands for testis-determining factor. The sry-gene triggers the genital ridges of each developing gonad of a normal XY embryo to develop as testicles.

The sry-gene encodes a number of transcription factors, among these a protein that contains a 79-amino acid motif called high-mobility-group (HMG) box protein, which appears to be conserved and is homologous among species. Outside of the HMG box, however, the amino acid sequence of the sry-gene is dissimilar among species. Sex determination is generally believed to involve a cascade of gene expression that induces conformational changes in its target DNA. This leads the undifferentiated gonad to develop as testis when the sry-gene is present and functioning normally or as ovary if the sry-gene is absent or not functional. As of the writing of this chapter, the sry-gene has been identified as a testes-determining factor in the boar, bull, stallion, tiger, mouse, and human, and it has been cloned in the pig and mouse. Given the universality of the sex-determining activity of genes in the Y chromosome, it is reasonable to expect the presence of a sry-gene regulating maleness in all species with biparenteral reproduction.

Gonadogenesis begins with the formation of the genital ridges in close association with the mesonephros, also called Wolffian body (Fig. 7-4). Primordial germ cells migrate from the yolk sac endoderm to the genital ridges. The gonads at this stage are still sexually bipotent and consist of an inner medulla and an outer cortex. As stated earlier, the mammalian embryo has an inherent tendency to develop as a female; castration of male feti at early stages of development consistently results in their development as females. Primordial germ cells invade the medulla

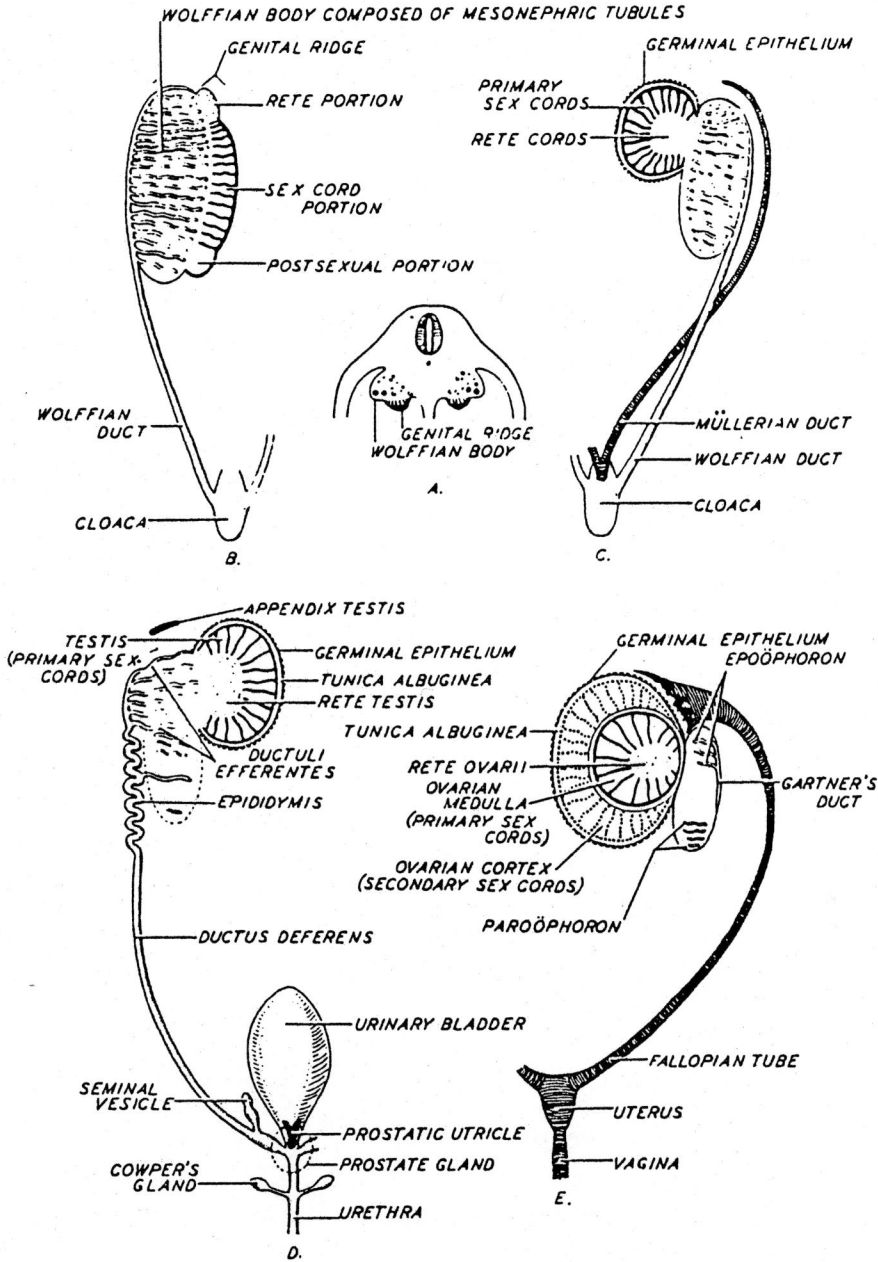

Fig. 7-4. Embryogenesis of the genital system in amniotes. **A.** Section through the dorsal region of an early embryo, showing the Wolffian bodies (mesonephric kidneys) and the genital ridges on their mediolateral surfaces. **B.** The Wolffian body and genital ridge in sagittal section. With respect to the fate of its parts, the genital ridge is divisible into three general regions. The Wolffian (mesonephric) ducts drain the kidneys, but genital ducts as such are not present. **C.** The indifferent (ambisexual) stage. The rete cords have become enclosed by the primary sex cords. The Müllerian ducts appear and temporarily coexist with the Wolffian ducts in both genetic males and females. **D.** Differentiation of the male genitalia. **E.** Differentiation of the female genitalia.

The primary sex cords are shown in solid black, whereas the secondary sex cords are represented by large stipples. The Müllerian ducts and their derivatives are heavily cross-hatched; the Wolffian ducts are relatively unshaded. (By permission from: C. D. Turner, General Endocrinology, 3rd ed., edited by C. D. Turner. Philadelphia, PA, W. B. Saunders Co., 1960).

to form the primary sex cords. At this time, gonadal differentiation occurs, and bipotentiality no longer exists. When genes for masculinity of an XY individual prevail, the medulla persists, cortical development is inhibited, and a testis develops. When genes for femaleness predominate in the XX embryo, the medulla is inhibited, and the cortex develops. In this case, the persisting primordial germ cells in the epithelium invade the cortex as the secondary sex cords, and an ovary develops. Thus, spermatozoa are derived from progenitors in the primary sex cords, and cells in the secondary sex cords are the ancestors of oocytes.

During the indifferent or bisexual stage, the gonad is potentially capable of either testis or ovary formation. Furthermore, discrete primordia for development of complete accessory sex structures of either sex are present. Table 7-3 shows the homologous structures that differentiate from the indifferent rudiments.

Following gonadal differentiation, the accessory genitalia develop under the influence of the gonad. When a testis has formed, the female (Müllerian) duct system regresses to vestigial rudiments, and the male (Wolffian) elements develop under the influence of morphogenic agents secreted by the newly formed testes: Androgens and Müllerian-inhibiting hormone (MIH), which is also known as anti-Müllerian hormone. The androgens, mainly testosterone, secreted by the fetal testes or their metabolites, mainly 5α-dihydrotestosterone (5α-DHT), masculinize the embryo and stimulate the growth and development

Table 7-3   *Homologies of Male and Female Reproductive Systems*

Indifferent	Male	Female
INTERNAL GENITALIA		
Gonad	Testis Rete testis	Ovary Rete ovarii[a]
Mesonephric tubules	Vas efferens Paradidymis[a] Vas aberrans[a]	Epoophoron[a] Paroophoron[a]
Mesonephric duct	Epididymis Vas deferens Ejaculatory duct Seminal vesicle Appendix of the epididymis[a]	Duct part of epoophoron[a] (Gartner's duct)
Müllerian duct	Appendage of the testis[a]	Appendage of the ovary[a] (hydatid) Fimbria of oviduct Oviduct
	Prostatic utricle[a] (uterus masculinus)	Uterus Vagina [all or part?]
Urogenital sinus	Prostatic, membranous, and cavernous urethra	Urethra Vestibule Vagina [in part?]
	Bulbourethral glands (Cowper's glands)	Vestibular glands (Bartholin's glands)
	PROSTATE	**PARAURETHRAL GLANDS**
EXTERNAL GENITALIA		
Genital tubercle	Glans penis Corpus penis	Glans clitoris Corpus clitoridis
Urethral folds	Raphe of scrotum and penis	Labia minora
Labioscrotal swellings	Scrotum	Labia majora

[a]Rudimentary.
From: A. V. Nalbandov, Reproductive Physiology, 2nd ed. San Francisco, CA, W. H. Freeman and Co., 1964.

of the Wolffian system and the male external genitalia of the fetus. The onset of testosterone synthesis by the fetal testes corresponds closely with the differentiation of the fetal Leydig cells. The Müllerian-inhibiting hormone blocks the development of the Müllerian system. Müllerian-inhibiting hormone is a macromolecular, glycoproteic hormone containing 575 amino acids in the bovine. The bovine MIH gene was cloned in 1986. Müllerian-inhibiting hormone is produced by the Sertoli cells of the fetal testis and by the granulosa cells of the postnatal ovary. The physiologic role of MIH in the postnatal female has not been determined (see Chapter 9). The inhibitory activity of MIH on the Müllerian system of the male fetus is limited to a short, sensitive period early in fetal development. In the calf, this sensitive period for the activity of MIH extends to day 62 of gestation. In pig feti, this period extends up to day 35 of gestation. Notwithstanding, it now appears that a discrete secretion of MIH continues after testicular differentiation until the initiation of puberty, suggesting that the expression of MIH is not totally repressed in the postnatal testis.

When an ovary has formed, the absence of the testicular morphogenic agents permits the Müllerian system to develop, and the Wolffian ducts and tubules regress to vestigial rudiments. Ablation of the fetal male gonad prior to differentiation of the Wolffian system causes differentiation of the Müllerian system in individuals with XY constitution. The urogenital sinus, genital tubercle, and genital folds normally differentiate in accord with the Wolffian or Müllerian duct system (Table 7-3). In addition to the sry-gene, the full expression of maleness and testicular differentiation is also dependent on the production of a discrete peptide factor called the H-Y (histocompatibility-Y) antigen. This antigen appears encoded by a gene termed SMCY for "selected mouse cDNA on Y" located on the Y chromosome. The H-Y antigen has been detected on preimplantation embryos and is thought to be a major sex determiner. The presence of the H-Y antigen and its interaction with cells of the undifferentiated, developing gonad would signal for the formation of the testis. Thus, the undifferentiated gonad becomes a tes-

tis when the sry-gene is present and active on the Y chromosome of the heterogametic XY male and the H-Y antigen is fully expressed. When the Y chromosome is absent or if the Y chromosome is present, but the sry-gene and the H-Y antigen are not fully expressed, the undifferentiated gonad will become an ovary. The endogenous H-Y antigen is not recognized as foreign by the immune system of mammals. In the avian species, however, the H-Y (H-W) antigen is present in the female, which is the heterogametic sex. It appears that antibodies against the H-Y antigen are generated by the immune system of the female bird, which would neutralize the H-Y antigen, preventing its male-determining activity.

Despite the male-determining role of the Y chromosome in mammals, a gene on the X chromosome appears to be necessary for testosterone secretion. Moreover, hermaphroditic development has been observed in Cocker Spaniel dogs, gilts, goats, mares, mice, and men with the XX karyotype. The cause of sex reversal in XX males has not been determined. In the species mentioned, XX males were positive for H-Y antigen. The finding of mares with an XY karyotype has also been reported. These mares were infertile and had underdeveloped gonads and uteri, resembling those of females with an XO karyotype. The case of a fertile mare with an XY constitution and low blood levels of H-Y antigen has also been reported.

Many of these developmental abnormalities can now be explained with the identification of the sry-gene and discovery of its role in the establishment of maleness. XY individuals develop as females if they lose the sry-gene during embryogenesis, or XX individuals may develop as males owing to the inheritance of a fragment of the short arm of the Y chromosome containing the sry-gene. Failure to express the H-Y antigen on the cells of the undifferentiated gonads results in degeneration of the Wolffian ducts and development of Müllerian structures, conducive to establishing a female phenotype. A similar situation occurs if XY-male feti are experimentally castrated at the critical period, before the testes begin to secrete testosterone. Castrated XY feti develop phenotypically as females.

However, from the evolutionary point of view, it seems that the Y chromosome is losing its preeminence as a result of the lack of gene recombination with those of the X chromosome. In some vertebrate species, the male-determining genes are concentrated in a single locus. In others, like certain species of fish, the Y chromosome has simply disappeared, and sex is more simply determined by a pair of XX chromosomes for the female or by an XO sex chromosomic constitution with a single X chromosome for the male.

Genes inherited from the mother are more methylated than those from the male and are less likely to be expressed owing to a phenomenon called genomic imprinting. Genes contributed by the male are usually expressed without interference. Experimentally, embryos manipulated to contain either two maternal or two paternal genomes die before or shortly after implantation, whereas embryos manipulated to contain both a maternal and a paternal genome survive after implantation. These studies emphasize the fact that the biparenteral genome is essential for normal implantation, gestation, and birth of offspring. Furthermore, though there is no doubt that the sry-gene determines maleness and testes development in XY individuals, Y-chromosomal genes, other than the sry-gene, and genes in the X chromosome are needed in mammals in general and in the domestic species in particular for the full expression of maleness and for the development of a functional and fertile male.

A series of major developmental changes begin to occur in the testes during the fetal period. These changes continue after birth in the late postnatal period until puberty is reached and the full expression of the male reproductive function has been established. During the early fetal period, the germinal cells of the developing testes undergo mitotic proliferation and differentiate into Sertoli and fetal Leydig cells. The fetal Leydig cells secrete androgens, which influence the differentiation of the male reproductive system. In the late fetal and early postnatal periods, the germinal cells cease to divide and the Leydig cells undergo regressive changes while the Sertoli cells proliferate. As puberty approaches, the Leydig cells resume their secre-

tory activity and differentiate into the adult type. The Sertoli cells also undergo further differentiation and morphogenic changes that lead to the establishment of a blood-testis barrier. In the prepubertal period, the germinal cells resume their mitotic activity and differentiate into spermatogonia as spermatogenesis progresses.

The testes are in the abdominal cavity during the embryonal and fetal stages. However, in most mammals, the testes descend to the scrotum at variable periods prior to or after birth. The extra-abdominal location of the testes in domestic mammals is indispensable for normal spermatogenesis. In other species, the testes are in the scrotum only during periods of sexual activity and ascend into the inguinal canal during sexual quiescence. In birds and a few mammals, the testes are permanently intra-abdominal.

Development of the reproductive system is a complex series of events involving a number of developmental actions and interactions subject to error at the following stages.

1. The distribution of sex chromosomes during meiotic or mitotic divisions may result in sex chromosome aneuploidy in gametes. Moreover, fragments of sex chromosomes or of autosomes bearing sex-influencing genes may be abnormally distributed as a result of partial or complete deletion or translocation during chiasma formation.

2. Gonadal morphogenesis may be disturbed because of abnormal corticomedullary relationships.

3. Secondary and accessory genital structures may develop abnormally under the influence of an irregular endocrine environment, or

4. They may develop as a result of teratogenic factors.

The classic example of intersexuality in veterinary medicine is the freemartin heifer. The freemartin is a genetic XX female that has been modified in the male direction by masculinizing factors such as sry-genes, fetal testicular androgens, H-Y antigen, and MIH from a heterozygous male twin. These factors from the male twin enter the vascular system of the female co-twin when anastomosis of placental blood vessels has occurred. Placental fusion with vascular anastomosis is said to occur in about 92% of bovine twin pregnancies. Because the testicular morphogenic agents from the male twin exert their influence before the development of the ovary and Müllerian system in the female twin, the sexual apparatus of the freemartin is stimulated to develop male structures. All degrees of masculinization are observed, presumably owing to variable amounts of a male morphogenic substance, likely MIH, reaching the reproductive system of the female co-twin. The female gonads resemble testes to some degree, the Müllerian duct system is inhibited, and Wolffian ducts remain and are differentiated in varying degrees. The secretion of estrogens by the fetal ovary is impaired in the freemartin heifer, probably because of inhibition of 17β-hydroxysteroid dehydrogenase followed later by inhibition of aromatase. Postnatal treatment of freemartin heifers with estrogens induces mammary growth, whereas postnatal treatment with androgens stimulates clitoral development with little effect on the other reproductive organs. The finding that many freemartins are chimeric (XY/XX) gave impetus to the cellular theory of freemartinism. XY cells from the male co-twin concurrently with the H-Y antigen and fetal MIH instruct the developing female system to masculinize. Singleton freemartins with 60 XX/60 XY chimeric karyotype have been reported. These probably result from the early death and absorption of the male twin fetus. Similar intersexes in XX individuals have been reported in dogs, goats, pigs, and sheep.

A large percentage of the bulls born co-twin with freemartin heifers have impaired testicular steroidogenesis and reduced reproductive capability, including low spermatozoal output or even azoospermia and a high incidence of abnormal spermatozoa in their ejaculates. The finding of XX spermatogonia and primary spermatocytes in the testes of some bulls born co-twin with freemartin heifers suggests that XX germinal cells from the female co-twin have altered spermatogenesis in these chimeric bulls.

Female pseudohermaphrodites have essentially normal internal genitalia but intermediate external genitalia. The external genitals may vary from a nearly normal vulva with an enlarged clitoris to a nearly normal penis, usually with hypospadias. The male pseudohermaphrodite, with abdominal or subcutaneous testes and intermediate external genitalia, is more common among domestic species than the female pseudohermaphrodite.

SEXUAL BEHAVIOR

Sexual behavior includes mating behavior, maternal behavior, and social mannerisms. This discussion is limited to mating behavior and social mannerisms related to mating behavior.

Mating behavior has two components. The first is sex drive, or libido. The second includes all phases of copulation, such as postural adjustments, intromission, ejaculation, orgasm, and postcopulatory behavior.

Internal Factors

There is a generally close relationship between ovarian function and sexual behavior in female mammals. Sexual receptivity is largely limited to periods of maximal development of ovarian follicles and the secretion of estrogens. Sexual receptivity is the ultimate criterion of estrus. However, receptive behavior sometimes occurs at other stages in the ovarian cycle and occasionally during pregnancy. Prepubertal gonadectomy usually prevents the development of mating behavior. Ovariectomy of sexually mature females immediately abolishes mating behavior, in contrast to the gradual loss of mating behavior that follows orchiectomy.

Adequate doses of estrogen administered to ovariectomized adult females restore manifestations of estrus, including mating behavior in most domestic species. In several species, and particularly in the bitch, treatment with estrogens followed by progesterone is needed to induce estrous behavior in ovariectomized animals. The first pubertal cycle of ewes and heifers and the first ovulatory cycle of the breeding season of ewes are "silent" and usually not accompanied by normal mating behavior, presumably because progesterone from a corpus luteum of a preceding cycle is absent.

Exogenous gonadotropins may initiate mating behavior in pubertal or adult females by stimulating the secretion of ovarian steroids. In some species, estrogens alone restore mating behavior in hypophysectomized females, confirming that estrogens are the primary regulators of female mating behavior for most of the domestic species.

The consequences of gonadectomy in the male are generally less dramatic than in the female, especially when castration is performed in sexually experienced adult males. Prepubertal orchiectomy prevents normal mating patterns. Adult castration is followed by a gradual diminution of copulatory responses and sex drive, in that order. In castrated males, behavioral response to erogenous stimuli and copulatory responses, in that order, are restored by treatment with androgens.

The role of androgens in male sexual behavior is twofold. During fetal life of males, or within a few days after birth, androgens organize neural centers that will mediate male mating behavior. In pubertal males, androgens activate these centers.

Experimental masculinization of the developing female brain has been achieved in several species, including dogs, by the administration of androgens during the critical fetal period of development. Masculinized females are incapable of displaying female sexual behavior, even in response to the administration of ovarian hormones. On the other hand, orchiectomy or the administration of antiandrogens during the critical fetal period renders males to act psychologically as females. These feminized males display lordosis in response to mounting.

In contrast to the ability of androgens to organize neural centers for the mediation of male mating behavior, injections of estrogen in females during the period when the neural centers are organized inhibit adult female behavior. Thus, the absence of androgen rather than the presence of estrogen during the period of differentiation induces female mating patterns.

The neural centers mediating estrous behavior are located in the mammillary bodies or in other areas of the hypothalamus. Centers for male sexual behavior are less defined, but certain cortical and hypothalamic lesions cause decreased sexual activity. Lesions in the region of the amygdala of male cats apparently destroy a sex-inhibiting center, resulting in hypersexuality. Castration abolishes this hypersexuality, and testosterone restores it in the castrate.

Mating behavior is dependent upon functional levels of other hormonal factors as well. The thyroidal secretion influences behavioral response to sexual steroids. Thyroidal activity also modifies the rate of secretion of gonadal steroids. The adrenal glands are capable of secreting androgens and estrogens, and their activity must be considered when evaluating the effects of gonadectomy.

Mating behavior varies with genotype. Sex drive, like many other measures of reproductive function, is subject to heterosis, or hybrid vigor. Homozygous twin bulls showed great similarities of the sexual pattern within pairs of twins and great differences between pairs. Beef bulls generally exhibit much less sex drive and require more sexual preparation than dairy bulls. These factors all indicate a genetic basis for male sexual behavior.

External Factors

The effects of season and nutrition are the most profound of the environmental factors that influence mating behavior. Seasonal effects are discussed in Chapter 11, Patterns of Reproduction. Light and temperature influence mating behavior through neural pathways that modify the function of the pituitary and by altering the sensitivity of the somatic substrate to endocrine stimulation.

Mating activity almost invariably occurs at that portion of the year that assures an adequate supply of feed at the time the offspring are born. Nutritional deficiencies, especially inadequate caloric intake, delay the onset of puberty in both males and females. Conversely, high-energy diets hasten puberty. After puberty, females are more sensitive to dietary insufficiencies than males because of the increased demands imposed in the reproductively active female by pregnancy and lactation.

Species differ in their response to confinement and domestication. Reproduction fails in several wild species when confined in zoos, whereas domestication with attendant provision of shelter and food has nearly obliterated seasonal reproductive activity in cattle and swine. The history of domesticated species is thus a record of the species' ability to adapt physiologically to a life of confinement.

Social interactions in groups of prepubertal companions are a necessary learning experience in the formation of sexual behavior. In several species and notably among certain subhuman primates, behavioral deficiencies develop in males reared in isolation. Males reared in isolation display arousal to the same degree as normal males, but copulatory responses are uncoordinated, and intromission is rarely achieved. These behavioral deficiencies are not corrected by injections of testosterone. Deficiencies in copulatory behavior have been observed in boars, bulls, dogs, and stallions. However, deficient males can be taught the proper copulatory patterns through patient training. The effect of rearing females in isolation is less pronounced, and puberty is hastened in gilts having contact with a boar.

When groups of rams are joined with ewes, mature rams dominate the yearling rams. Dominance also occurs within both yearling and mature groups of rams. Rams joined with ewes prior to the first (silent) ovulation of the breeding season hasten the onset of estrus. Vasectomized teasers are less effective, possibly owing to a loss of libido as a function of time following surgery; postsurgical loss of libido has also been observed in vasectomized dogs and men.

Pheromones

Chemical communication between animals is well documented, especially among the lower phyla, and is implicated as the prime mode of communication. Sex communicants are among the compounds known as pheromones. Pheromones affect behavioral centers and may alter the function of the anterior pituitary by influencing the release of hypothalamic-releasing or hypothalamic-inhibiting hormones. Pheromones, acting through olfaction and taste, influence patterns of sexual behavior in most species of domestic animals. Sociosexual interaction influences reproduction, facilitating the encounter of males with females in estrus and influencing the female responses so that mating and fertilization can be successfully completed. Pheromones from the ram's fleece induce changes in the pulsatile rhythm of the secretion of LH, which is ultimately conducive to the surge and release of LH and ovulation in the ewe. The presence of ewes in estrus can stimulate LH release and increased testosterone secretion in rams. Male goats, their pheromones, and social interactions exert profound influences on the female goat, inducing short estrous cycles, due to short-lived corpora lutea (see Chapter 14). Surprisingly, however, pheromones from the male goat can also influence the reproductive activity of the ewe, suggesting that the species barrier, in relation to pheromone activity, could be overcome between sheep and goats. Pheromones activate the vomeronasal organ, located within the septum of the nose, which contains bipolar, sensory neurons. These neurons send axons to the olfactory bulb, which projects to a vomeronasal nucleus in the amygdala and then to the hypothalamus, from where neuroendocrine responses are elicited. Pheromones activate the vomeronasal organ to elicit reproductive and social behaviors and provide information about gender, dominance, and reproductive status. Genes likely to encode mammalian pheromone receptors have been recently isolated. Quantitative screening of genomic libraries and hybridizations to the genomic DNA have allowed the characterization of six subfamilies of about 30 receptor genes.[94]

Sex pheromones elicit one or both of two responses: Attraction and mating behavior. Anosmic rams display normal sex drive and copulatory behavior, but their ability to discriminate between estrous ewes and ewes not in estrus is impaired. Anosmic but experienced rams approach ewes at random and must rely on the precopulatory behavior of estrous ewes to discern receptive females. Rams with unimpaired olfactory capacity are capable of rapidly detecting those ewes that are more apt to accept their precopulatory advances.

Estrous bitches attract males over a considerable distance. The anal glands, vaginal secretion, and urine have been postulated as sources of sex pheromones. Saliva, urine, and preputial washings of the boar attract sows in estrus, and boars exert an estrous-synchronizing effect on gilts. Steroidal compounds comprising 5α-androsterone, 3α-androstenol and other 16-androstenes have been isolated from the saliva, urine, and spermatic venous blood of boars and implicated as pheromones for the sow. These compounds are part of the boar-taint and produce the unpleasant odor of cooked pork meat. Valeric acid in the urine of the female cat may play an important role in facilitating mating behavior in the male cat.

In addition to olfactory and gustatory stimuli, visual, tactile, and auditory stimuli arouse mating behavior. Animals with one of these senses impaired compensate by increased reliance on the remaining senses.

The homosexual behavior of heifers and cows helps range bulls to identify estrous females. Allowing bulls to observe seminal collection procedures stimulates their ejaculatory responsiveness at artificial insemination centers (see Chapter 10). Similarly, boars, bulls, dogs, and stallions become excited when they observe other males mating.

The males of most species use tactile stimuli to identify estrous females. Licking and rubbing of the female external genitalia are almost universal among domestic species. Stallions often nibble the mare's neck or withers to test receptivity, and the auditory response from the mare may in turn stimulate the horse. Rams test receptivity in ewes by thumping the ewe's chest with the foreleg. Bulls and rams are often seen to rest the head and chin on the female's rump prior to mounting.

Mating experience is an important factor in sexual behavior. Experienced males usually achieve copulation in less time than inexperienced males. Males trained to serve the artificial vagina learn to rely heavily on tactile stimuli. Temperature and tactile receptors on the penis are important to intromission. Learning of copulatory patterns decreases the dependence of neural sex centers for endocrine stimuli. For instance, sexually experienced stallions may maintain sex drive for more than 500 days following castration.

GAMETOGENESIS

Gametogenesis refers to the formation of the male and female gametes, the spermatozoon and the oocyte, respectively. Gametogenesis is a highly regulated event of specialized cellular proliferation that involves mitosis, meiosis, and cellular differentiation, which are conducive to the formation of the male and female gametes. The genetic control of these processes is of a superbly fine-tuned and evolutionarily conserved nature. The male and female primordial germinal cells populate the genital ridges of the developing gonads of the genetically male or female embryo, respectively. In the fetal male, the primordial germinal cells continue to proliferate mitotically and become surrounded by developing seminiferous cords. During this period, the male germinal cells cease to divide and grow, instead becoming gonocytes, which remain arrested, for most species until the time of birth. At this time the gonocytes of the male resume mitosis and differentiate into spermatogonia, entering in the process of spermatogenesis. In the fetal female, however, after entering the developing gonad, the gonocytes, which are the product of mitotic proliferating of the primordial germinal cells, become oogonia and continue mitotic divisions for most of the domestic species until prior to birth, when they become oocytes. At this point, the oocytes enter into meiosis and progress up to the diplotene stage of prophase of meiosis I, which is also called the dictyate stage. The oocytes remain arrested at the dictyate stage, each within an ovarian follicle surrounded by a layer of granulosa cells until puberty.

The identification of genes that regulate the mitotic and meiotic proliferation of germinal cells is an area of intense research, and a series of "cyclin-genes" and cyclin-dependent kinases are under study to determine their activity and function during the male and female germinal cell cycle and on factors controlling the replicative DNA synthesis during mitosis of oogonia and spermatogonia.

Apoptosis of Germinal Cells

The process of apoptosis, programmed cell death or suicide, as it has also been called, is a physiologic process of normal occurrence in all tissues. Contrary to the unprogrammed cell death or necrosis caused by acute injury, apoptosis is an active, orderly, and genetically governed process of selective cell elimination. Apoptosis is characterized by chromatin condensation, phagocytosis, and cell disintegration without tissue inflammation. Apoptotic cells do not burst but shrink and condense and are rapidly phagocytized, whereas the cells that undergo necrosis rupture and empty their contents, inflaming neighboring tissue.

Apoptotic cell death begins during early embryonic cleavage and development and continues during the life of an individual as a regulator of growth of tissues and organs. It should not be surprising, then, that the apoptotic rate is high in rapidly dividing cells with short cell cycles.

Apoptosis plays a vital role as regulator of cell division and proliferation of the germinal cells in the seminiferous tubules during spermatogenesis. As will be discussed later, spermatogenesis, once initiated, is a continued process extending from fetal life until senescence. Apoptosis serves the purpose to maintain a fine-tuned balance between germinal cell divisions and cell death to prevent uncontrolled tissue proliferation and growth. Apoptosis affects more frequently the spermatogonia in the prepubertal animal than the spermatocytes and spermatids. The process is reversed in the adult animal in which the spermatocytes are more often affected. Characteristic changes in the increased production of spermatozoa at the beginning of the breeding season in males of seasonally breeding species is negatively correlated with the rate of testicular apoptosis. As a result, the testicular and epididymal weight and daily sperm production and output are greater during the rutting period, when they are needed the most.

Contrary to the continued nature of the spermatogenic process in the male, the oocytes of the female remain arrested at the diplotene stage of the prophase of meiosis I, as dictyate oocytes. Then, the female gamete is induced to resume meiosis beyond the dictyate stage by stimulation with gonadotropic hormones, which induce the maturation and final growth of follicles and subsequently, ovulation. Hence, the major rate of apoptotic death in the female apparently occurs first in the granulosa cells of those follicles that do not enter the ovulatory process. These follicles and oocytes undergo atresia and degenerative changes and thus are eliminated from the pool of ovarian follicles available for growth, maturation, and ovulation.

Interestingly, spermatogenesis proceeds with the germinal cells undergoing meiotic divisions within the microenvironment of the adluminal compartment. This compartment is formed by tight junctions of the nongerminal Sertoli cells. The oocyte also needs the microenvironment provided by the nongerminal granulosa cells of the follicular wall, cumulus oophorus, and corona radiata for nourishment while at the dictyate stage of meiosis and for maturational growth when the follicle that contains the oocyte is recruited and gonadotropically stimulated to ovulate (see Chapter 9).

Spermatogenesis

Spermatogenesis refers to the complex process of cell division and differentiation conducive to the formation of spermatozoa. Spermatozoa are formed in the seminiferous tubules by a series of cell divisions, followed by a metamorphosis that results in a highly differentiated and potentially motile cell, the spermatozoon. The seminiferous tubules form a complex system that constitutes about 90% of the testicular mass in the adult. Spermatogenesis can be divided into two phases: Spermatocytogenesis and spermiogenesis. **Spermatocytogenesis** is the proliferative phase in which spermatogonial cells multiply by a series of mitotic divisions followed by the meiotic divisions which produce the haploid state. In most of the domestic species, spermatocytogenesis begins shortly after birth. **Spermiogenesis** is the differentiative phase in which the nucleus and cytoplasm undergo morphologic changes to form the spermatozoon. The phase of spermiogenesis is completed at puberty.

Spermatocytogenesis begins with the mitotic division of spermatogonia in close proximity to the basement membrane (Fig. 7-5) and proceeds toward the lumen. Spermatogonia are activated to form active, type A spermatogonia. There

Basement Membrane of
Seminiferous Tubule

Spermatogonium

Type A Spermatogonia
(may be several generations)

Resting Spermatogonium

Intermediate
Spermatogonia

MITOSIS
(2n)

Type B
Spermatogonia

Primary
Spermatocyte

─── ─ · ─ ─ ─ ─ ─ ─ ─➤ 1st MEIOTIC DIVISION
(n)

Secondary Spermatocytes

─── ─ · ─ · ─ ─ ─ ─ ─➤ 2nd MEIOTIC DIVISION
(n)

Spermatids

Spermatozoa

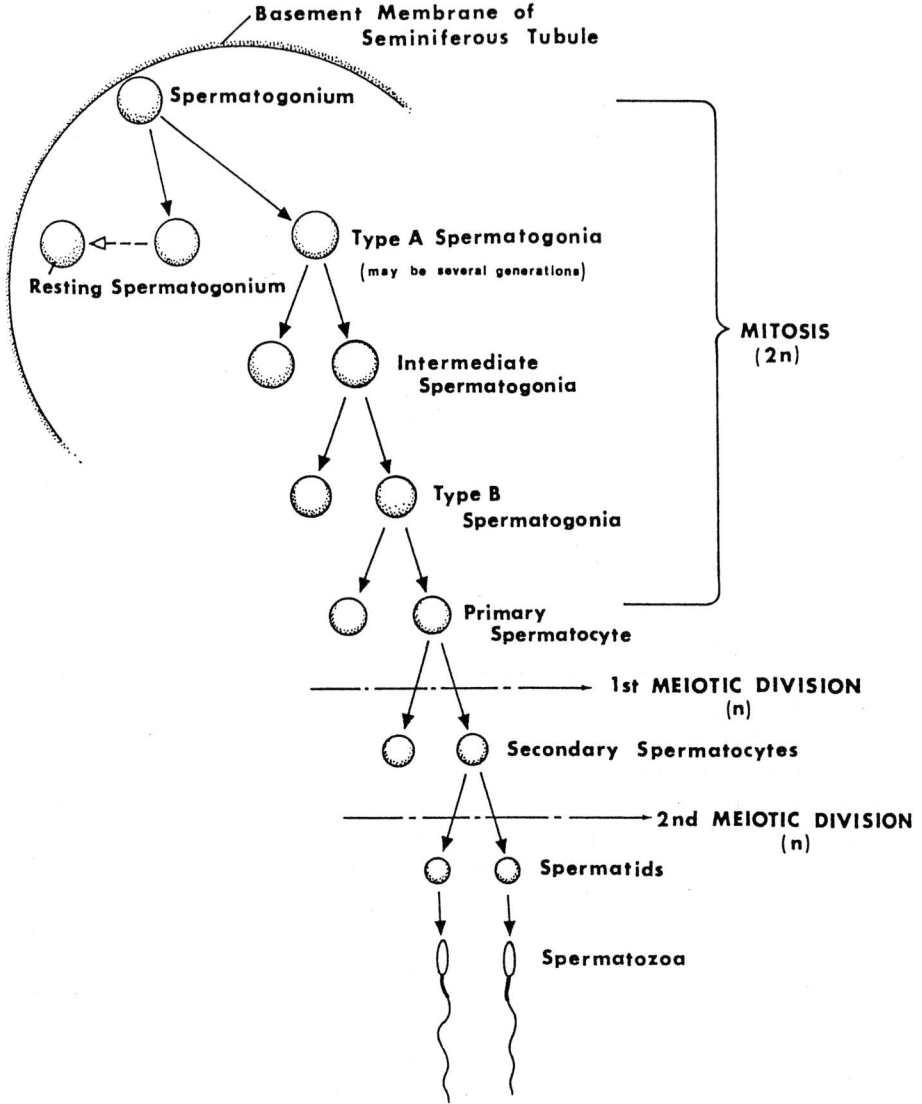

Fig. 7-5. Diagrammatic representation of spermatogenesis.

may be several generations of type A spermatogonia, depending on the species. Most of the type A spermatogonia divide to form intermediate spermatogonia; certain type A cells are retained as resting-type A spermatogonia. In this way, the type A cells provide daughter cells for the formation of spermatozoa but are not normally depleted in the process. Intermediate spermatogonia divide to form type B spermatogonia, which undergo the last of the mitotic divisions to form primary spermatocytes. Primary spermatocytes undergo final synthesis of DNA prior to the first reductional meiotic division to produce secondary spermatocytes and divide by meiosis to produce round spermatids. Spermatocytogenesis is concluded by the meiotic divisions, which produce secondary spermatocytes, then spermatids (Fig. 7-5). Round spermatids, cells that have completed meiosis, can, under appropriate experimental conditions, be micromanipulated and injected to fertilize an oocyte. In fact, intracytoplasmic injection of a round spermatid into an oocyte resulted in fertilization and then in the gestation and birth of mouse and rabbit offspring when the embryos so generated were transferred to recipients. These results suggest that the nuclei of the spermatids are genomically imprinted.

The formation of spermatids marks the end of spermatocytogenesis and the beginning of spermiogenesis. **Spermiogenesis,** or **spermateliosis** as it is also called, begins in the seminiferous tubules and is completed in the epididymis as the animal approaches puberty. Spermiogenesis has been intensively studied because normal or abnormal morphologic forms develop during this phase. A series of complex structural reorganizations occurs during spermiogenesis (Fig. 7-6).

Although reproductive behavior and spermatogenesis of most domestic males are relatively independent of cyclic variations, very definite cyclic activity is seen in the seminiferous tubules. In the postpubertal male, the cells of the germinal epithelium are organized in cellular associations that are about the same stage of development. They evolve synchronously from the basement membrane of the seminiferous tubule to its lumen. These cellular associations succeed one another at a point in the seminiferous tubule over time and are called stages in the cycle of the seminiferous epithelium (Fig. 7-7). One cycle of the seminiferous epithelium, then, includes the series of changes in the cells at a specific location in the tubule between two successive appearances of the same cellular association. Each successive cell layer in a given stage, or cellular association, is derived from a cell that has completed the changes of one cycle of the seminiferous epithelium. Thus, each cycle of the seminiferous epithelium constitutes a generation interval.

The spermatogenic cycle consists of several cycles of the seminiferous epithelium and includes all events from activation of the resting spermatogonium to the release of spermatozoa generated from it. In Figure 7-7, the spermatogenic cycle of the bull is depicted as consisting of $4^1/_2$ cycles of the seminiferous epithelium. The linear movement of cells is confined to progression between the basement membrane and lumen of the tubule during the spermatogenic cycle and does not occur along the long axis of the tubule.

Various investigators have classified the cellular associations in the cycle of the seminiferous epithelium into more or less distinct stages. Because the criteria for classification are arbitrary and the starting points in the cycle have not been uniform in these studies, the number of stages and their relation to the classifications of other authors are variable.

The duration of the cycle of the seminiferous epithelium and the duration of the spermatogenic cycle are variable among species, but they are constant for a given species (Table 7-4). The durations of the cycle of the seminiferous epithelium have been accurately determined. For practical purposes, the duration of spermatogenesis can be calculated by multiplying the duration of the cycle of the seminiferous epithelium by 4, because spermatogenesis extends over approximately four consecutive cycles (3.9 to 4.7 cycles, according to criteria for classification and species).

Although the Sertoli cells are the only nongerminal cells in the seminiferous epithelium, they are fundamental to normal spermatogenesis. The Sertoli cells, also called supporting or sustentacular cells, extend from the basement membrane to the lumen of the seminiferous tubules. Cytoplasmic processes from the Sertoli cells surround clusters of germinal epithelial cells. This arrangement allows the Sertoli cells to receive and convey signals and metabolic products from the extratubular environment through the basement membrane to the meiotically dividing germinal cells. Plasma membranes form tight junctions between adjacent Sertoli cells that divide the seminiferous epithelium into basal and adluminal compartments. These compartments constitute part of a blood-testis barrier and serve to provide a special testosterone-enriched microenvironment necessary for meiosis and spermiogenesis (Fig. 7-8). The number of junctional strands in Sertoli cell tight junctions, as determined for the guinea pig and mink, surpasses 100. The clusters of actively dividing germinal cells migrate from the

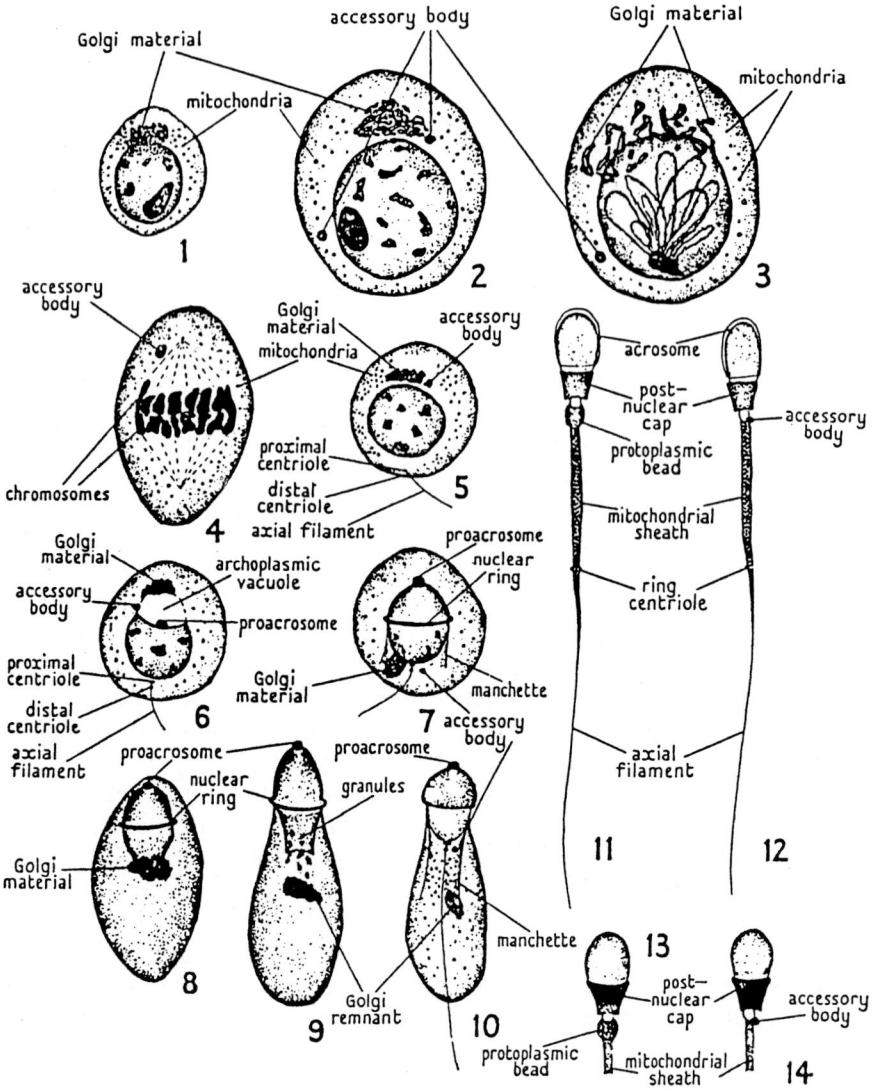

Fig. 7-6. Formation of a spermatozoon. Note the process of spermiogenesis and the responsible cellular inclusions. **1.** Spermatogonium. **2.** Primary spermatocyte. **3.** Primary spermatocyte–early prophase. **4.** Primary spermatocyte–early anaphase. **5.** Young spermatid. **6–8.** Spermatids. **9, 10.** Late spermatids. **11.** Spermatozoon. **12.** Spermatozoon, showing accessory body; the protoplasmic bead is not shown. **13.** Spermatozoon. **14.** Spermatozoon, showing accessory body; the protoplasmic bead is not shown. (By permission from: R. A. R. Gresson and I. Zlotnik, Quart. J. Microbiol. Sci. *89*:219, 1948).

basal to the adluminal compartment of the seminiferous epithelium by coordinated breakdown and reconstitution of the tight junctions between Sertoli cells. The morphological transformation of spermatids during spermiogenesis occurs while the spermatids are embedded within cytoplasmic pockets of individual Sertoli cells. The Sertoli cells support the spermatogenic epithelium, have endocrine activity, and participate in spermiogenesis by phagocytosis of the residual bodies shed by the maturing spermatids. The release of spermatozoa from the cytoplasmic

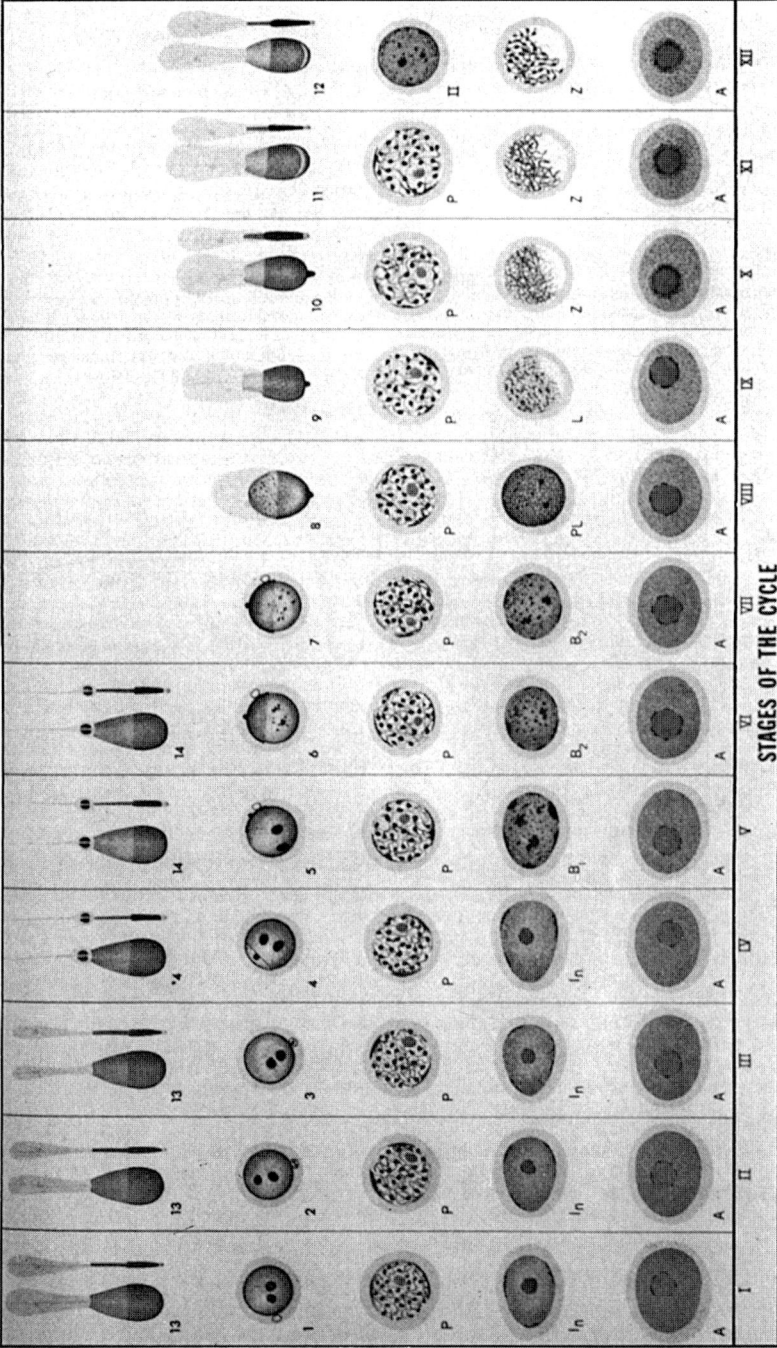

Fig. 7-7. Stages of the cycle of the seminiferous epithelium in the bovine testis. Columns, represented by Roman numerals **I–XII**, depict cellular associations at each of the 12 stages. Fourteen steps of spermiogenesis were identified and illustrated by spermatids (numbered **1–14**) in the upper two rows with the lateral profile of the elongated spermatids (steps **10–14** of spermiogenesis) included. The types of germ cells observed in sequence are: **A**, type A spermatogonia; **I_n**, intermediate spermatogonia; **B_1**, type B_1 spermatogonia; **B_2**, type B_2 spermatogonia; **PL**, prelep-totene primary spermatocytes; **L**, leptotene primary spermatocytes; **Z**, zygotene primary spermatocytes; **P**, pachytene primary spermatocytes; and **II**, secondary spermatocytes. (By permission from: W. E. Berndtson and C. Desjardins, Am. J. Anat. *140*:167, 1974).

Table 7-4 Duration of the Cycle of the Seminiferous Epithelium and of Spermatogenesis in Some Mammals

Species	Duration in Days	
	Cycle	Spermatogenesis
Boar	8.6	34.4
Bull	13.5	54[a]
Coyote	13.6	54.4[a]
Dog	13.6	54.4[a]
Man	16	64
Monkey (*Macaca fasicularis*)	9.3	37.2[a]
Monkey (*Macaca mulatta*)	10.5	42[a]
Rabbit	10.3, 10.7, 10.9	51.8, 42–47, 48
Ram	10.4	49
Rat (Sprague-Dawley)	12.9	51.6
Rat (Wistar)	13	52
Stallion	12.2	48.8[a]

[a]Duration of spermatogenesis calculated by multiplying duration of the cycle by 4. Adapted from: Y. Clermont, Physiol. Rev. *52*:198, 1972. Data for the dog and coyote from: R. H. Foote, et al., Anat. Rec. *173*:341, 1972; and J. J. Kennelly, J. Reprod. Fertil. *31*:163, 1972. Data for the stallion from: E. E. Swierstra et al., J. Reprod. Fertil. *40*:113, 1974.

pockets of the Sertoli cell, called **spermiation**, involves marked swelling of the Sertoli cell.

The vascular supply to the germinal epithelium is outside the basement membrane of the seminiferous tubule. Sertoli cells serve to convey nutrients and metabolites between the spermatogenic cells and the peritubular capillaries. In line with their role in sustaining the maturing germinal elements during spermatogenesis, Sertoli cells undergo a cyclic transformation that is coextensive with those of the germinal epithelial cells undergoing a cycle of the seminiferous epithelium. The Sertoli cell cycle may, in fact, be the most important coordinating factor in the spermatogenic cycle. The long-held view that the number of Sertoli cells is established before or during puberty and remains stable in the adult male may no longer be tenable. Evidences accumulated in the last few years indicate that there are seasonal variations in the number and volume of Sertoli cells in the stallion and man. Sertoli cell numbers increase during the breeding season and decrease during the winter months of the year. However, the junctional membrane design and compartmentalization of the seminiferous epithelium remain in the testes during the nonbreeding season in seasonal breeder species. Age-related changes in the numbers of Sertoli cells have been observed in human testes, and similar changes may occur in other species, as well.

Oogenesis

Oogenesis refers to the formation, development, and maturation of the female gamete, called oocyte, which results from the divisions of oogonia (Fig. 7-9). Oogonia are produced by mitotic proliferation of primordial germ cells. It is not clear for all species whether all oogonia are the direct descendants of germinal cells in the secondary sex cords, or whether some of them arise by transition of peritoneal cells covering the ovary (referred to as "germinal epithelium").

Oogonia multiply by mitosis until the final generation of oogonia enter the prophase of the first meiotic division, at which point they are primary oocytes. The primary oocyte consists of the ooplasm, or vitellus, and a large spherical nucleus, sometimes called the germinal vesicle. During the first meiotic prophase, primary oocytes are surrounded by a flattened layer of follicular epithelium to form primary or primordial follicles. In domestic mammals, with the exception of the bitch and the female cat, the queen, oogonia develop into primary oocytes before or shortly after birth (Fig. 7-9). In the bitch and queen, oogenesis extends after birth. In the female

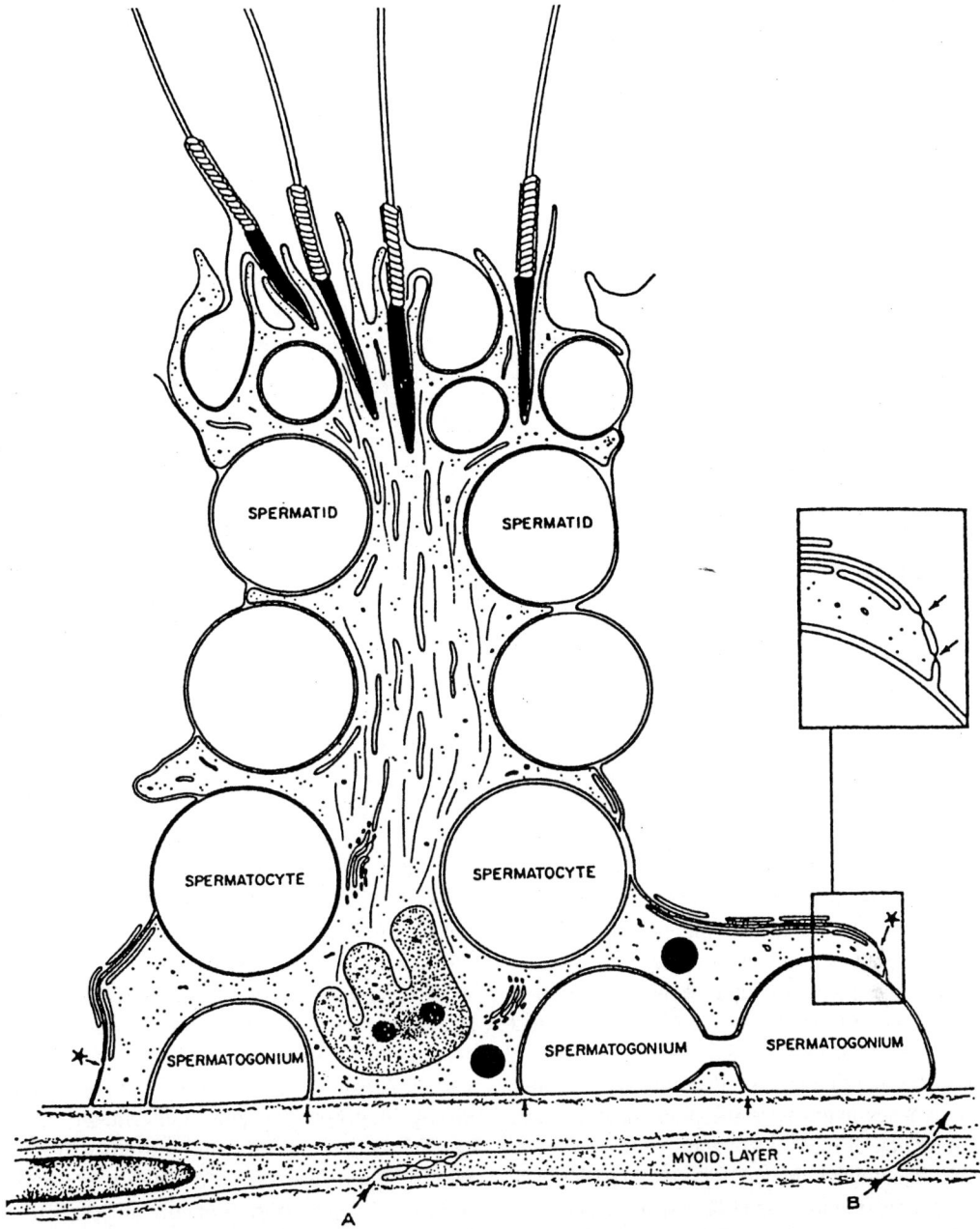

Fig. 7-8. Diagram depicting localization of the blood-testis barrier and compartmentalization of the germinal epithelium by tight junctions between adjacent Sertoli cells. Note the germ cells and their relationship to a columnar Sertoli cell. The primary barrier to substances penetrating from the interstitium is the myoid layer. The majority of cell junctions in this layer are closed by a tight apposition of membranes (**A**). Over a small fraction of the tubule surface, the myoid junctions exhibit a 200 Å-wide interspace and are therefore open (**B**). Material gaining access to the base of the epithelium by passing through open junctions in the myoid layer is free to enter the intercellular gap between spermatogonia and Sertoli cells. Deeper penetration is prevented by occluding junctions (**stars**) on the Sertoli-Sertoli boundaries. These tight junctions constitute a second and more-effective component of the blood-testis barrier. In effect, Sertoli cells and their tight junctions delimit a **basal** compartment in the germinal epithelium, containing the spermatogonia and early preleptotene spermatocytes, and an **adluminal** compartment, containing the spermatocytes and spermatids. Substances traversing open junctions in the myoid cell layer have direct access to cells in the basal compartment, but to reach the cells in the adluminal compartment, substances must pass through the Sertoli cells. (By permission from: M. Dym and D. W. Fawcett, Biol. Reprod. 3:308, 1970).

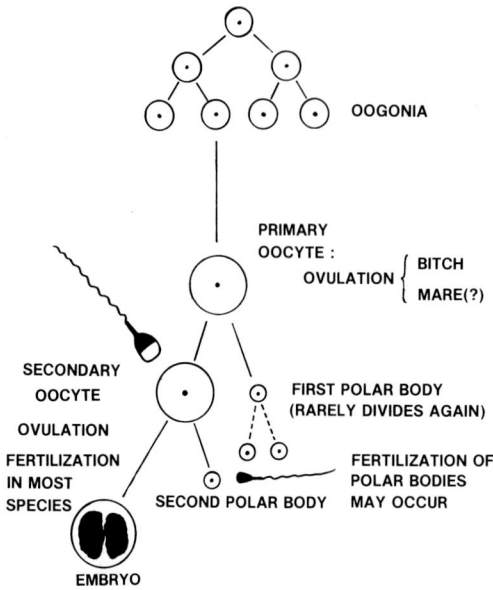

Fig. 7-9. Diagrammatic representation of oogenesis in domestic species.

pup, primary oocytes are present in the ovarian follicles by approximately 50 to 60 days of age.

The nucleus of the primary oocyte enters the dictyate, or resting, stage of the first meiotic prophase. The dictyate stage is specific to meiotic prophase in the female, as there is not a corresponding stage in spermatocytogenesis. The nucleus of the primary oocyte remains in the dictyate stage during growth of the oocyte and follicle, and for most of the domestic species it completes the first meiotic division when the follicle reaches maturity at the preovulatory stage. Resumption of meiosis beyond the dictyate stage in the mammalian oocyte depends upon the ovulatory surge of luteinizing hormone (LH). At each estrous cycle, a number of follicles from the pool of available follicles are recruited to respond to gonadotropic stimulation to grow, mature, and ovulate. However, the great majority of primordial follicles with their contained oocytes remain unresponsive and impervious to endogenous gonadotropic stimulation. In women, primary oocytes may remain viable within the follicle up to 50 years of age. If one accepts that oogenesis for most species stops at the dictyate stage of meiosis at the time of birth and that there are no further cell divisions that would replace these oocytes, one would have no choice but to recognize that the oocyte has got to be one of the longest-lasting viable cells.

The granulosa cells form a diffusion barrier between the blood and the oocyte so that the ovarian follicle provides the oocyte with an appropriate microenvironment for oocyte nourishment and maturation. This includes the maintenance of an intrafollicular temperature, particularly at the preovulatory stage, which is about $2°$ to $3°C$ lower than the systemic temperature in the female rabbit and woman, species for which this lower intrafollicular temperature has been reported. The primordial follicle consists of a primary oocyte surrounded by a single layer of follicular cells, which will proliferate and develop into the membrana granulosa. Follicles containing more than one oocyte occur rarely in adult domestic animals. However, follicles with multiple oocytes are seen in the fetal ovaries and in ovaries of newborn and adult queens and bitches. At first, the follicular cells of primordial follicles are in intimate contact with the vitelline membrane, or cellular membrane of the oocyte. As the follicle grows, a complex glycoproteic layer, which will later form the zona pellucida, is deposited in isolated patches between the vitelline membrane and the inner layer of granulosa cells, or *corona radiata*. These patches of zona material gradually coalesce to form a continuous structure around the oocyte. As the follicle matures, the zona thickens by incorporating zona material produced by the follicular cells and possibly by the oocyte. There are species differences in the process of zona formation, but in general, it follows the general pattern indicated above. Cellular processes from the corona cells and oocyte plasma membrane maintain contact between the granulosa cells and the oocyte. These cellular extensions probably serve to nourish the oocyte. Contact between the oocyte and the granulosa cells prevents maturation of the oocyte beyond the dictyate stage. A small peptide factor called Oocyte Maturation Inhibitor (OMI), produced by the granulosa cells of the follicle (Fig. 7-10), maintains the oocyte

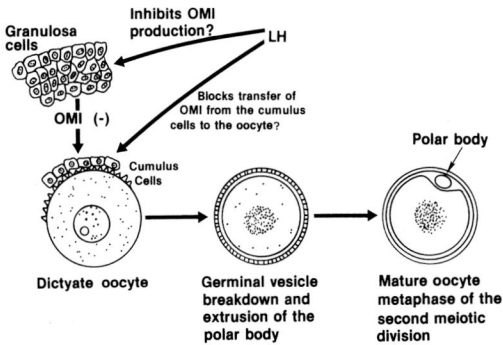

Fig. 7-10. Postulated control of meiotic maturation of mammalian oocytes. (Adapted from: A. Tsafriri, et al., *J. Reprod. Fertil. 64*:541, 1982).

at the dictyate stage of meiosis. Oocyte Maturation Inhibitor is present in the developing follicles, and its concentration in the follicular fluid declines as the follicles mature. It is now known that OMI is absent in the follicular fluid of follicles approaching ovulation. The ovulatory surge of LH presumably blocks the transfer of OMI from the cumulus cells to the oocyte, allowing meiosis to resume at the time of ovulation (Fig. 7-10). Oocytes isolated from preovulatory follicles resume meiosis spontaneously *in vitro*. Oocytes in developing follicles remain at the dictyate stage when cultured *in vitro* unless they have been exposed to gonadotropins *in vivo* or when cultured in a medium containing gonadotropins.

As the follicle grows, lacunae are formed between the follicular cells. These lacunae coalesce to form an antrum or cavity, which fills with the *liquor folliculi*. At this stage the primary oocyte is surrounded by the *cumulus oophorus,* a mass of granulosa cells that projects into the antrum. Many of the follicular cells in this mass are expelled with the oocyte at ovulation. During follicular growth, cells of the surrounding connective tissue differentiate as theca interna and theca externa cells.

At the termination of follicular growth, the oocyte resumes the meiotic or maturation divisions. During the first division, the oocyte nucleus migrates toward the plasma membrane, the nuclear membrane and nucleoli disappear, and the chromosomes dispersed in the cyto-

plasm undergo the first meiotic division. Half of the chromatin and a small amount of cytoplasm are extruded as the **first polar body**.

In most domestic species, the first meiotic division is completed a few hours before ovulation, and the cell is then a secondary oocyte (Fig. 7-9). However, in the bitch, Silver and Blue foxes, and possibly other canidae, the first maturation division and abstriction of the first polar body occur after ovulation (Fig. 7-9). Abstriction of the first polar body may be delayed for a few days following ovulation, and this delay probably accounts for the prolonged period of viability of tubal oocytes, up to 7 days in these species.

The mare is a special case; in some mares the oocyte is ovulated at the dictyate stage, as in the bitch, and the abstriction of the first polar body occurs in the oviduct. In other mares, the first meiotic division is completed shortly before ovulation, and the oocyte is ovulated as a secondary oocyte. The causes for the dichotomous release of oocytes at ovulation as primary or secondary oocytes in mares are not known.

Except for the bitch and some mares, the secondary oocyte of the other domestic species enters the second meiotic division and is usually in metaphase II at the time of ovulation. The tubal oocyte normally completes the second maturation division when a spermatozoon penetrates the oocyte envelopes to 'activate' the oocyte (Fig. 7-11). When the oocyte is activated, the second maturation division is completed with the formation of the **second polar body**. At this time, the germinal cell is momentarily a cytula until the first embryonic cleavage occurs and the 2-cell embryo is formed. The first polar body occasionally undergoes division to form two polar bodies.

The fate of ovulated but unfertilized oocytes has been studied in several species. In most laboratory and domesticated animals, fertilized and unfertilized oocytes reach the uterus 3 to 6 days after ovulation. The unfertilized oocytes of most species undergo degeneration and fragmentation in the uterus. In the mare, however, only fertilized oocytes pass through the oviduct and enter the uterus, whereas unfertilized oocytes are retained in the oviducts. Thus, for the mare and possibly

CORONA RADIATA

ZONA PELLUCIDA

VITELLUS

CUMULUS OOPHORUS

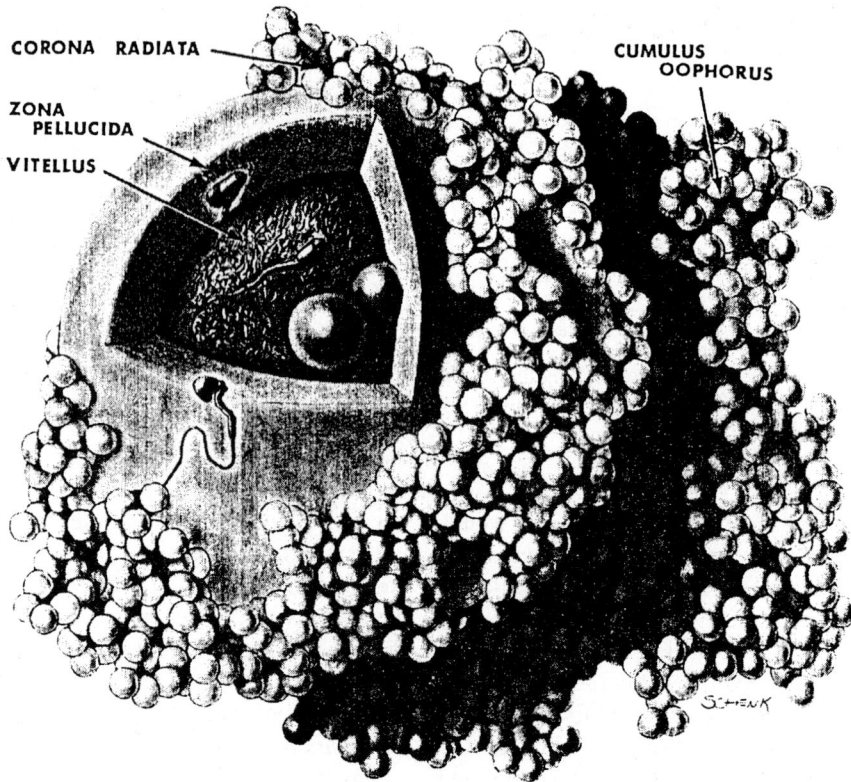

Fig. 7-11. Drawing of the layers surrounding the rabbit oocyte. (By permission from: K. G. Gould, Fed. Proc. *32*:2071, 1973).

for other equidae, degeneration and fragmentation of the unfertilized oocyte occur in the oviduct.

FERTILIZATION

Fertilization can be defined as a multiple-step phenomenon initiated by the interaction, binding, and subsequent association of the male and female pronuclei. This process culminates in the formation of a single cell of a new individual, conventionally called the zygote, which has biparental nuclear heredity. The term zygote, as applied to mammalian embryos, is an homology from terminology applicable to the product of fertilization of invertebrate oocytes. **Cytula** is a more appropriate term for the ephemeral 1-cell embryo of mammals. From the embryologic and genetic points of view, the essential aspect of fertilization is the association of the maternal (from the oocyte) and the paternal (from the spermatozoon) genomes.

Gametic Encounter

Spermatozoa encounter and unite with the oocytes in the *ampulla* of the oviduct where fertilization occurs in domestic species. Testicular spermatozoa of most species are immotile, and movement into the epididymis is entirely passive. The forces involved include the pressure of spermatozoa and fluids in the seminiferous tubules, ciliary movements in the efferent ductuli, epididymal contractions, and absorption of seminal fluid. In the epididymis, spermatozoa are moved passively toward the epididymal tail. Ejaculated spermatozoa become motile after exposure to accessory sex gland secretions.

Ejaculation is the result of a series of muscular contractions along the male excurrent tract. The neural impulse for ejaculation is initiated by thermal and pressure receptors, which are located primarily in the glans penis. The afferent pathway is via the internal pudic nerve to the lumbosacral section of the cord. The efferent impulse is via the *erigens* nerves to the hypogastric plexus.

During mating or artificial insemination, the estrogen-sensitized uterus responds with muscular contractions owing to the reflexogenic release of oxytocin in response to genital stimulation. At least for a short time after natural insemination through mating or after artificial insemination, uterine contractions are far more important than spermatozoal motility in spermatozoal transport within the female genitals. However, spermatozoal motility does enhance the probability of a spermatozoon-oocyte collision and facilitates the penetration of the oocyte envelopes. The progressive motility of the spermatozoa depends on the intrinsic flagellar motor activity, including the participation of the mitochondrial system of enzymes and influx of Ca^{2+}, as well as on factors from the female genitalia.

Ovulated oocytes normally are captured by and enter the fimbria of the ipsilateral oviduct, which is in close contact with the ovary during estrus. The proper transport of fertilized oocytes in the oviducts is essential to assure their arrival in the uterus at the proper time. Premature or delayed arrival results in embryonal death. Transport within the oviducts depends upon ciliary movements, segmental and peristaltic contractions of the oviduct, and probably the flow of oviductal secretions.

Oocytes are capable of fertilization and development for 12 to 24 hours following ovulation in most species. In the bitch, the oocyte may be viable and fertilizable for several days after ovulation. Fertilizability of oocytes is highest in the *ampulla*, decreases significantly in the isthmus, and is lost in the uterus.

Capacitation

Ejaculated spermatozoa of several mammalian species must be exposed to secretions of the female reproductive tract for a variable period of time before they attain the capacity to fertilize oocytes. This process of enabling a spermatozoon for the *in vivo* fertilization is termed capacitation. The secretions of the uterus and oviducts participate in the capacitation process,

and the follicular fluid released at ovulation may also contribute to capacitation.

A need for the capacitation of ejaculated spermatozoa has been demonstrated for the bull, boar, cat, and several species of laboratory rodents. The evidence for the necessity of capacitation in the ram, stallion, dog, and man, although generally accepted, is still equivocal (Table 7-5). It is generally believed that capacitation involves release or activation of enzymes, possibly associated with loosening or detachment of the acrosome, which enhances spermatozoal penetration of the cumulus and zona pellucida.

Capacitation can be reversed in previously capacitated spermatozoa by incubating them in seminal plasma. Thus, **capacitation** would involve the destruction or removal of a macromolecular decapacitation factor in the seminal plasma. Spermatozoa collected from the proximal part of the *vas deferens* in cats or from the epididymal tail in rabbits can fertilize oocytes *in vitro* without a period of *in vivo* capacitation. Even though spermatozoal viability may not always be optimal when spermatozoa are deposited in a foreign female tract, *in vivo* interspecies spermatozoal capacitation is possible. Furthermore, seminal plasma from the bull, boar, ram, stallion, dog, and tomcat contain decapacitating activity for rabbit spermatozoa, suggesting that the decapacitation factor is not species-specific. Thus, the presence or absence of decapacitation factor in the seminal plasma of a given species may indicate the requirement for capacitation to occur in that species (Table 7-5). Ejaculated spermatozoa from several species have been

Table 7-5 Need for Capacitation of Ejaculated Spermatozoa

Species	Capacitation Required	Decapacitation Factor in Semen
Boar	Yes	Yes
Bull	Yes	Yes
Cat	Yes	Yes
Dog	Probably	Yes
Man	Probably	Yes
Ram	Probably	Yes
Stallion	Probably	Yes

"capacitated" *in vitro* by incubation with enzymes or by inactivation of the decapacitation factor by incubation in chemically defined media. *In vivo*, capacitation may represent a selective process to prevent fertilization by weak or abnormal spermatozoa, because these cells must survive several hours in the female tract. Capacitation is more effective during the estrous phase of the ovarian cycle than during the progestational phase, and the efficiency of capacitation seems to be related to optimal levels of estrogens and gonadotropins because it may be modified by exogenous hormones.

Phases of Fertilization

Encounters between spermatozoa and oocytes in the oviduct depend upon the number of oocytes released, the concentration and motility of spermatozoa, and of factors that participate in the displacement of the oocytes. Thus, the transport of a population of spermatozoa from the site of seminal deposition in the female genitals at ejaculation to the ampullary region of the oviducts is essential for successful fertilization. The process of fertilization can be divided into three phases: (a) gametic encounter and binding of the spermatozoon to the oocyte; (b) initiation and completion of the acrosome reaction, which is an exocytotic process conducive to the release of enzymes; and (c) the actual penetration of the spermatozoon through the zona pellucida and plasma membrane into the oocyte cytoplasm, with the concurrent male and female pronuclear formation and association. Gametic encounter and binding of the spermatozoon to the oocyte is a receptor-mediated process, in which a glycoprotein from the zona pellucida called ZP3 functions as a receptor. Tubal oocytes of some mammals are surrounded for several hours by granulosa cells (*corona radiata* and *cumulus oophorous*). Enzymes in the spermatozoal head are released, exposed, or activated to attack and penetrate successive oocyte investments. The *cumulus* of most domestic species disintegrates within a few hours after ovulation. Hyaluronidase from spermatozoa may in some species enhance penetration of the cumulus (Figs. 7-12A, B and 7-13A, B). Acrosomal enzymes exposed during the acrosomal reaction disperse the *cumulus* and *corona radiata* (Fig. 7-12B). After reaching the zona pellucida, the spermatozoon binds to the ZP3 receptor in the zona, triggering the acrosome reaction in the spermatozoal head. The ZP3 glycoprotein receptor specificity seems to be a factor on the selective intraspecies binding of the spermatozoon to the zona pellucida and may be a major factor in preventing the binding, penetration, and ultimately the fertilization of the oocyte by spermatozoa from a different species. Proteolytic activity is essential to penetration of the zona pellucida, which appears to be the most difficult of the oocyte envelopes for the spermatozoa to penetrate. Active dispersal factors, such as neuraminidase and hyaluronidase, and trypsin-like enzymes, such as acrosin, are present in the acrosome. During passage through the zona pellucida, the spermatozoon undergoes the acrosome reaction and gradually loses its outer acrosomal membrane (Fig. 7-13C to E). Spermatozoa reaching the vitelline membrane are divested of the acrosome (Fig. 7-12C). Upon entrance of the spermatozoon into the perivitelline space, microvilli from the oocyte plasma membrane fuse with the plasma membrane at the equatorial segment of the spermatozoon (Fig. 7-13F, G). Cytoplasmic materials from the oocyte mix with that of the spermatozoon (Fig. 7-13H). The interaction of spermatozoal components with the oocyte cytoplasm is essential for the formation of the male pronucleus (Fig. 7-13I).

Oocytes of higher mammals normally undergo monospermic fertilization. The zona pellucida of most mammals allows a single spermatozoon to reach the plasma membrane of the oocyte and to fuse with the plasma membrane of the oocyte, which causes a rapid depolarization of the oocyte plasma membrane to inhibit the fusion of additional spermatozoa. The depolarization reaction is associated with the release of calcium ions from calmodulin in the plasma membrane into the cytoplasm of the oocyte, increasing the intracytoplasmic calcium, which induces the activation of the oocyte. The enzymatic digestion of the zona pellucida allows for the *in vitro* interspecies fertilization. In the normal oocyte, however, the zona pellucida is an effective barrier to prevent the fertilization of an

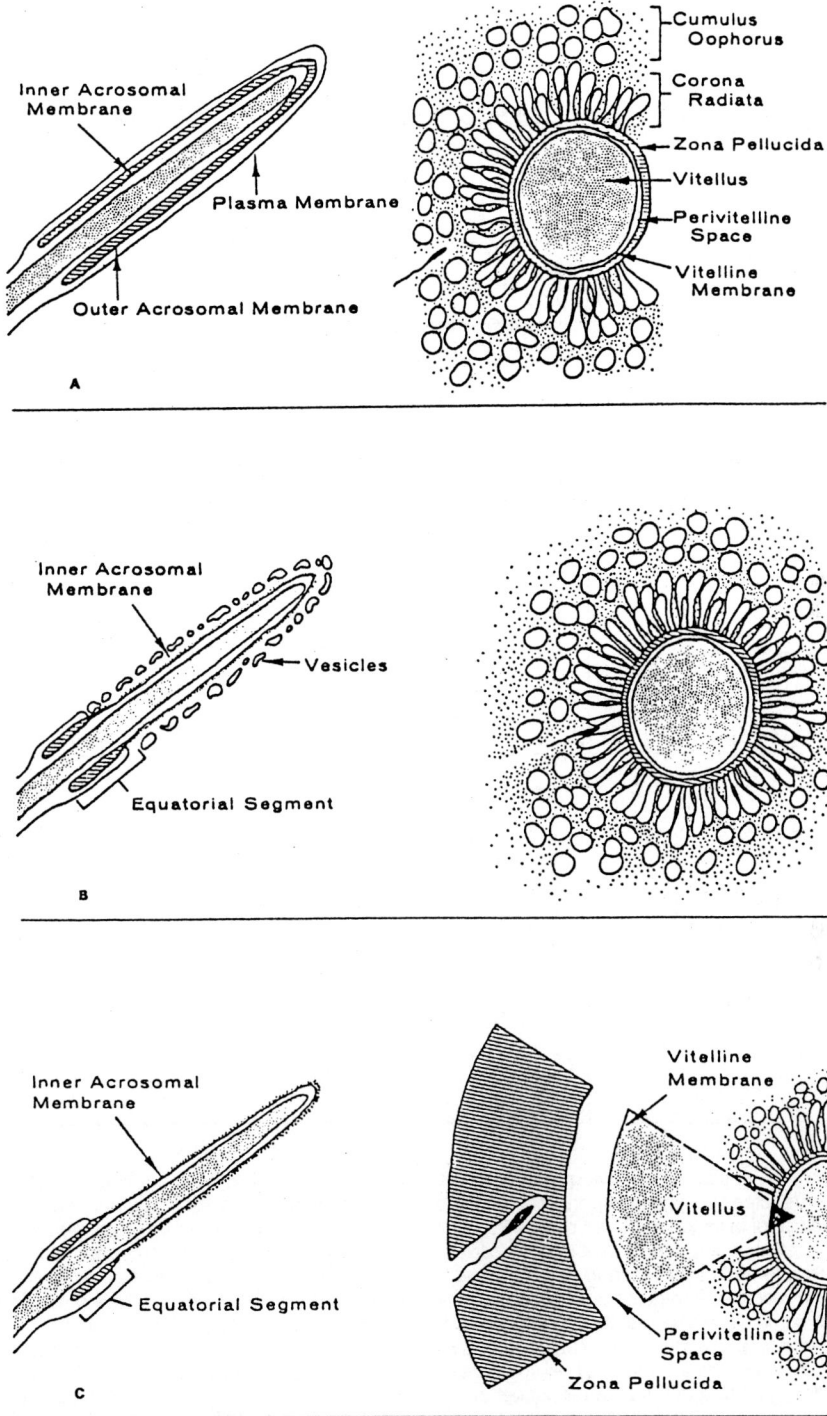

Fig. 7-12. Penetration of spermatozoa. **A**. Status of a capacitated spermatozoon (**left**) as it penetrates *cumulus oophorus* (**right**). **B**. Acrosome reaction of a spermatozoon (**left**) as it penetrates the *corona radiata* (**right**). **C**. Status of a reacted spermatozoon (**left**) as it penetrates the zona pellucida (**right**). (Reprinted with permission from: R. A. McRorie and W. L. Williams, Ann. Rev. Biochem. *43:*778, 779, 1974).

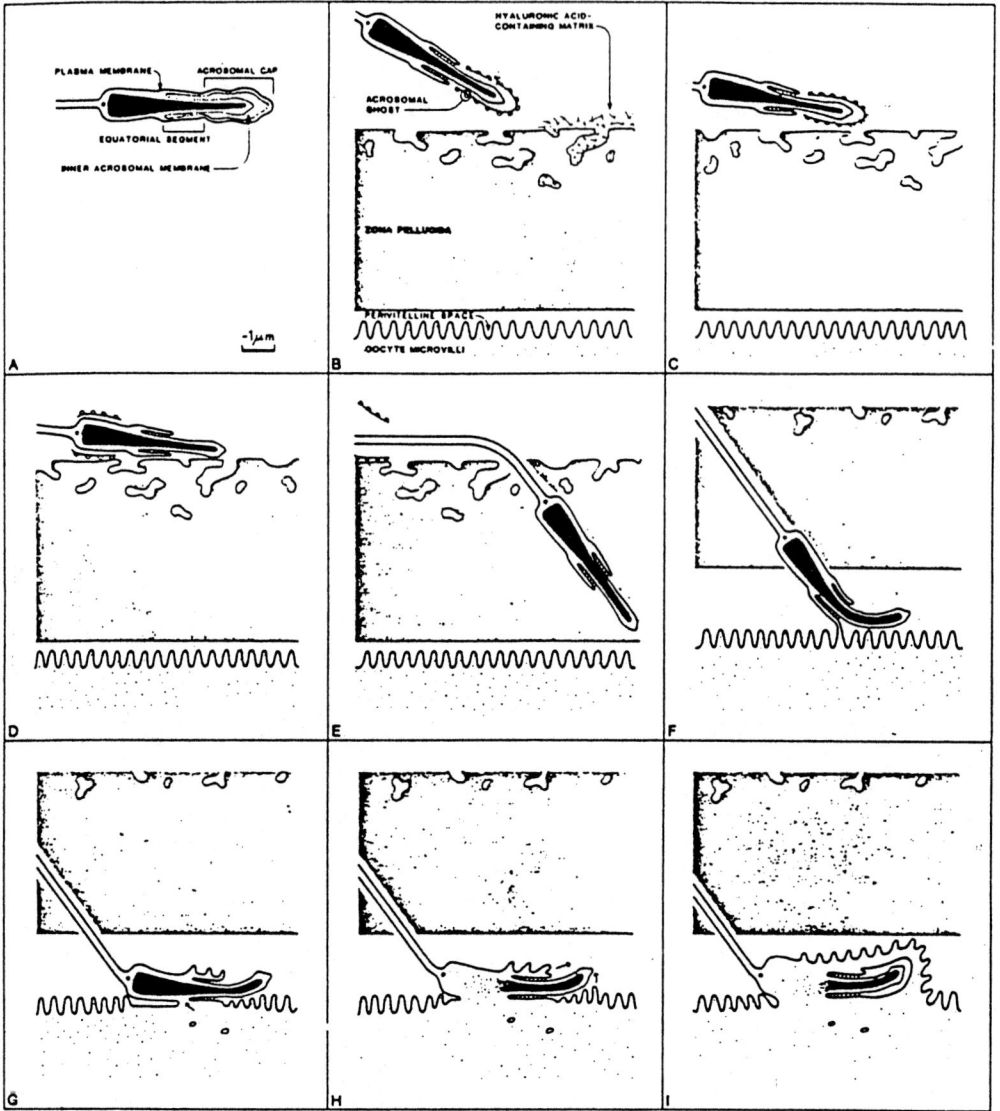

Fig. 7-13. Schematic diagram showing ultrastructural aspects of the fertilization sequence in eutherian mammals. **A**. An unreacted mammalian spermatozoal head is shown; the acrosome consists of a cap and equatorial segment. The site of initiation of the acrosome reaction is not known, but it is probably at the *cumulus/corona radiata* or zona pellucida surface. **B**. A spermatozoon that has started a normal acrosome reaction is shown; the plasma membrane and outer acrosomal membrane have vesiculated, and the soluble acrosomal vesicle contents (AVC) can escape. The acrosomal ghost is formed. A granule/filament matrix containing hyaluronic acid is present in the *cumulus/corona radiata* and outer region of the zona pellucida (only a small portion of this matrix is shown). In some species, this matrix is also abundant in the perivitelline space. **C**. The spermatozoon has attached to the zona pellucida surface by its acrosomal ghost (vesicle plus insoluble AVC). **D**. The spermatozoon then swims through a split in the anterior aspect of the ghost. **E**. The spermatozoon enters the zona pellucida at an angle; the equatorial segment remains intact, and the ghost is left on the zona surface. A narrow slit forms in the zona. **F, G**. The spermatozoon enters the perivitelline space, where the oocyte microvilli fuse with the plasma membrane overlying the equatorial segment. **H**. Ooplasm flows into the sperm, and the posterior aspect of the nucleus begins decondensing. **I**. The perforatorium enters the oocyte last, probably in a phagocytic vesicle. In stages **G** and **H**, the spermatozoon head bends. The equatorial segment is drawn into the oocyte while the anterior and posterior regions deflect upward toward the zona pellucida. These diagrams are approximately to scale. (Reprinted with permission from: P. Talbot, Am. J. Anat. *174*:331–346, 1985).

oocyte by spermatozoa from a different species, in agreement with the concept that views species as reproductively isolated populations. According to this concept, individuals from the same species are interfertile, whereas individuals from a different species do not naturally mate and if they do, given the chance because of changes in the habitat or by direct human intervention, the offspring resulting from the interfertilization of their oocytes is sterile. This emphasizes hybrid sterility as a major factor for the maintenance and protection of species as separate reproductive units. The zona pellucida of the mare's oocyte is penetrated by the donkey's spermatozoon, or the donkey's oocyte is penetrated by the stallion's spermatozoon, resulting in the birth of a mule or a hinny, respectively. Both are sterile hybrids. Similarly, intermatings of sheep and goats results in the fertilization of oocytes and restricted development of the hybrid embryos, which are aborted early in pregnancy. On the other hand, South American camelids, such as llamas, alpacas, and guanacos (also correctly spelled as huanacos) naturally interbreed and produce fertile hybrids. It is not clear, although possible, that llamas, alpacas, guanacos, and even vicuñas are varieties of the same species that had evolved phyletically and not by speciation.

In the rabbit and a few other mammals, several spermatozoa (supplementary spermatozoa) penetrate the zona to reach the perivitelline space, but only a single spermatozoon normally penetrates the vitellus. Thus, monospermic fertilization safeguards the constancy of the DNA content for the species. Among domestic animals, the primary block to polyspermy is a reaction in the zona pellucida. The reaction is secondary to changes in the vitelline cortex and the release of agents that alter the zona pellucida. Aging of mammalian eggs decreases the efficiency of the block to polyspermy.

In summary, fertilization is associated with three major events: (a) the continuation of meiosis and maturation of the oocyte; (b) spermatozoal penetration and the development of the parental pronuclei; and (c) the early stages of embryonic mitotic cleavage and development (Figs. 7-14 and 7-15). A detailed description of the events of fertilization is beyond the scope of this chapter. The reader is urged to refer to the pertinent references listed at the end of this chapter.

Mitochondrial DNA

Experimental evidences accumulated over the past few years clearly indicate that the cytoplasmic inheritance of mitochondrial DNA is an important component of eukaryotic inheritance. Mitochondria in all metazoan animals so far studied possess double-stranded DNA, which is distinguishable from nuclear DNA. The mitochondrial DNA is greatly amplified during oogenesis, and mammalian oocytes are rich in mitochondria and mitochondrial DNA. It is estimated that an oocyte contains approximately 92,000 mitochondria. However, the number of mitochondria in the midpiece is low in the mammalian spermatozoon, about 72 mitochondria in the bull spermatozoon. Mitochondrial DNA is maternally inherited—that is, the offspring, regardless of their homo- or heterozygosity, including reciprocal crosses of horses and donkeys, will have the mitochondrial DNA of the mother. The maternal inheritance of mitochondrial DNA has been explained on the basis of the small number of mitochondria contributed to the oocyte by the fertilizing spermatozoon. The midpiece containing spermatozoal mitochondria enters the oocyte at fertilization in several mammalian species. Hence, it is not possible to rule out a role for the paternal mitochondrion on maternal mitochondrial replication during embryonic development. Maternal inheritance of the mitochondrial DNA may simply be the result of an overwhelming preponderance of maternal mitochondria in the oocyte.

Unequal amplification and segmentation of mitochondrial DNA during oogenesis and possibly polymorphism resulting from maternal and paternal mitochondrial interactions at fertilization, and subsequently during embryonic development, may influence the survivability of the embryo to term. A further understanding of cytoplasmic inheritance might allow for the improvement of production traits in livestock animals and resistance to diseases of importance to the veterinary profession.

Oocyte Maturation Following the Ovulatory Surge of LH

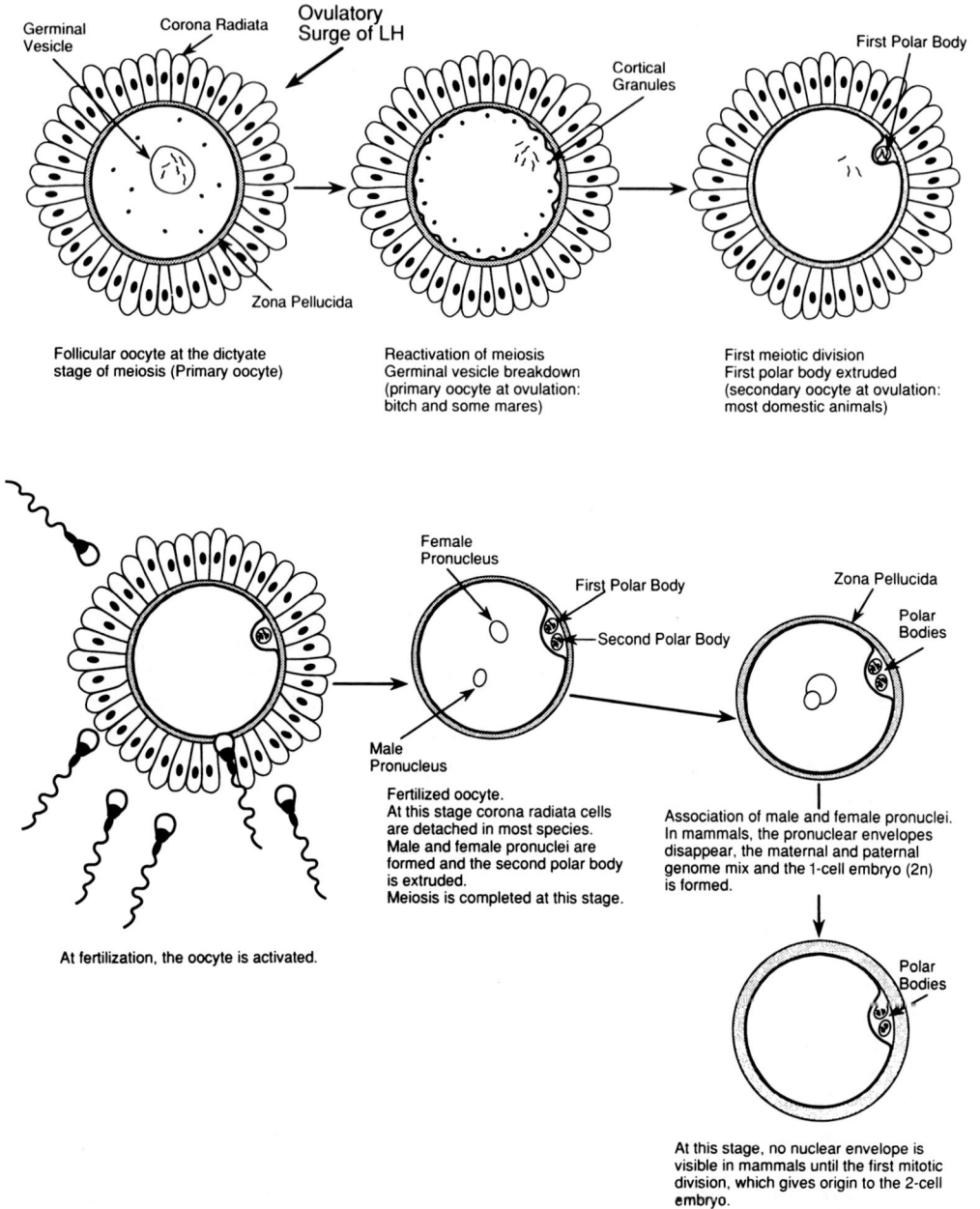

Germinal Vesicle

Corona Radiata

Ovulatory Surge of LH

Zona Pellucida

Cortical Granules

First Polar Body

Follicular oocyte at the dictyate stage of meiosis (Primary oocyte)

Reactivation of meiosis
Germinal vesicle breakdown
(primary oocyte at ovulation:
bitch and some mares)

First meiotic division
First polar body extruded
(secondary oocyte at ovulation:
most domestic animals)

Female Pronucleus

First Polar Body

Second Polar Body

Male Pronucleus

Zona Pellucida

Polar Bodies

At fertilization, the oocyte is activated.

Fertilized oocyte.
At this stage corona radiata cells are detached in most species. Male and female pronuclei are formed and the second polar body is extruded.
Meiosis is completed at this stage.

Association of male and female pronuclei. In mammals, the pronuclear envelopes disappear, the maternal and paternal genome mix and the 1-cell embryo (2n) is formed.

Polar Bodies

At this stage, no nuclear envelope is visible in mammals until the first mitotic division, which gives origin to the 2-cell embryo.

Fig. 7-14. Process of oocyte maturational changes induced by the ovulatory surge of luteinizing hormone (LH) and the activation of the oocyte by the fertilizing spermatozoon.

Embryonic Cleavage

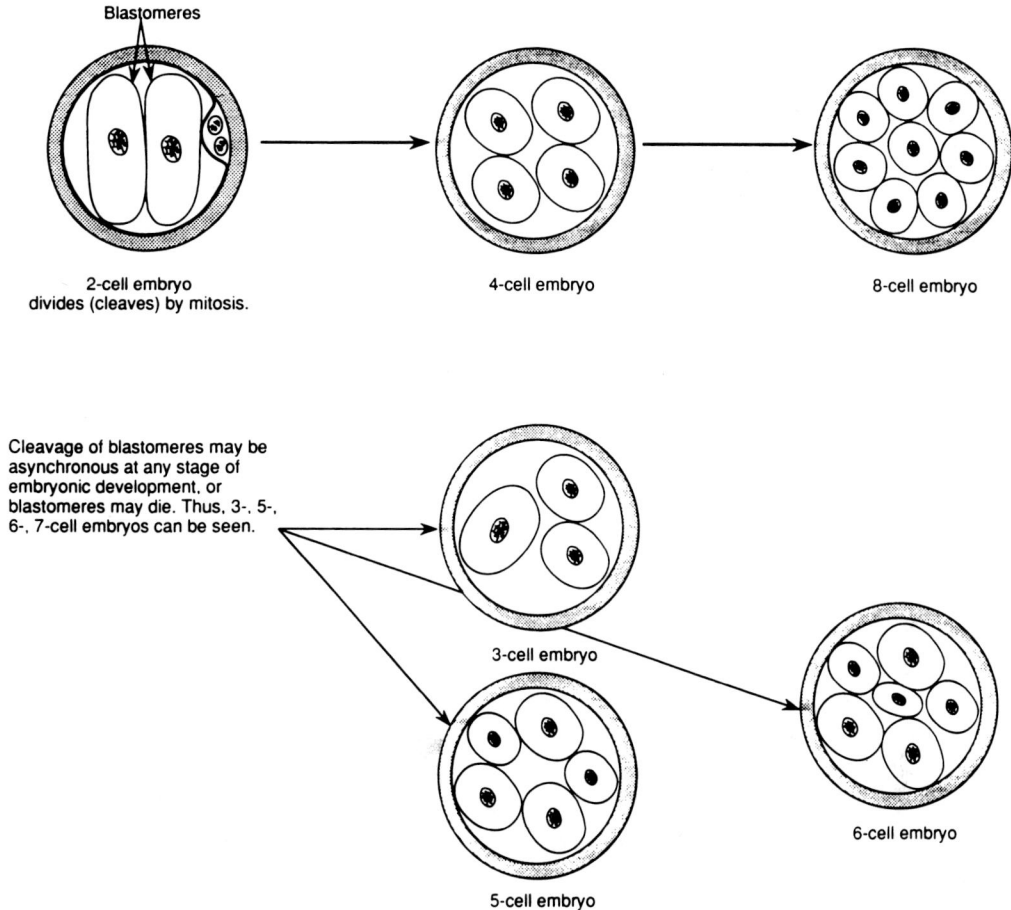

2-cell embryo divides (cleaves) by mitosis.

4-cell embryo

8-cell embryo

Cleavage of blastomeres may be asynchronous at any stage of embryonic development, or blastomeres may die. Thus, 3-, 5-, 6-, 7-cell embryos can be seen.

3-cell embryo

5-cell embryo

6-cell embryo

Fig. 7-15. Synchronous and asynchronous cleavage of blastomeres from the 2-cell embryo.

Extraordinary Fertilization

Polyspermy, a condition that develops when more than one spermatozoon enters the ooplasm to form multiple male pronuclei, is pathologic in mammals. Multiple pronuclei may also result from monospermic fertilization of binucleate oocytes. Two female pronuclei may develop from binucleate primary oocytes or as a result of failure to abstrict the polar body at one of the maturation divisions. These multinucleate oocytes, like polyspermic oocytes, are destined to developmental failure, because the pronuclei fuse and polyploidy results. Few polyploid embryos survive to birth.

A single nucleus undergoes cleavage without syngamy in parthenogenesis, gynogenesis, or androgenesis. The process by which the oocyte nucleus is activated in the absence of fertilization is called **parthenogenesis**. In **gynogenesis**, the oocyte is activated by a spermatozoon, which takes no further part in the development of the embryo. In **androgenesis**, the oocyte nucleus fails to participate. These resulting embryos, like polyploid embryos, generally fail to develop to birth.

Development of the embryo is further discussed in Chapter 19.

REFERENCES

Sexuality

1. Bianchi, N. O. (1991): Sex determination in mammals. How many genes are involved? Biol. Reprod. *44*:393.
2. Blottner, S., Pitra, C., and Berger, U. (1992): Y-chromosome-specific fluorescence (F-body) of poorly decondensed bovine spermatozoa. Andrology *24*:255.
3. Bruere, A. N., Marshall, R. B., and Ward, D. P. J. (1969): Testicular hypoplasia and XXY sex chromosome complement in two rams: The ovine counterpart of Klinefelter's syndrome in man. J. Reprod. Fertil. *19*:103.
4. Buoen, L. C., Eilts, B. E., Rushmer, A., et al. (1983): Sterility associated with an XO karyotype in a Belgian mare. J. Am. Vet. Med. Assoc. *182*:1120.
5. Centerwall, W. R. and Benirschke, K. (1975): An animal model for the XXY Klinefelter's syndrome in man: Tortoiseshell and Calico male cats. Am. J. Vet. Res. *36*:1275.
6. Cran, D. B., Johnson, L. A., Miller, N. G. A., et al. (1993): Production of bovine calves following separation of X- and Y-chromosome bearing sperm and *in vitro* fertilization. Vet. Rec. *132*:40.
7. Dunn, H. O., Lein, D. H., and McEntee, K. (1980): Testicular hypoplasia in a Hereford bull with 61, XXY karyotype: The bovine counterpart of human Klinefelter's syndrome. Cornell Vet. *70*:137.
8. Epstein, C. J. (1983): Sex chromosome expression in embryonic development. Differentiation *23* (Suppl.): S31.
9. Garner, D. L., Gledhill, B. L., Pinkel, D., et al. (1983): Quantification of the X- and Y-chromosome-bearing spermatozoa of domestic animals by flow cytometry. Biol. Reprod. *28*:312.
10. Gartler, S. M. and Riggs, A. D. (1983): Mammalian X-chromosome inactivation. Annu. Rev. Genet. *17*:155.
11. Gledhill, B. L. (1988): Selection and separation of X- and Y-chromosome-bearing mammalian sperm. Gamete Res. *20*:377.
12. Grant, S. G. and Chapman, V. M. (1988): Mechanisms of X-chromosome regulation. Annu. Rev. Genet. *22*:199.
13. Hare, W. C. D. and Betteridge, K. J. (1978): Relationship of embryo sexing to other methods of prenatal sex determination in farm animals: A review. Theriogenology *9*:27.
14. Hernández-Jauregui, P. and Márquez, H. (1977): Fine structure of mule testes: Light and electron microscopy study. Am. J. Vet. Res. *38*:443.
15. Hunter, R. H. F., Baker, T. G., and Cook, B. (1982): Morphology, histology and steroid hormones of the gonads in intersex pigs. J. Reprod. Fertil. *64*:217.
16. Jamieson, R. V., Tam, P. P. L., and Gardiner-Garden, M. (1996): X-chromosome activity: Impact of imprinting and chromatin structure. Int. J. Develop. Biol., *40*:1065.
17. Johnson, L. A., Flook, J. P., and Hawk, H. W. (1989): Sex preselection in rabbits: Live births from X and Y sperm separated by DNA and cell sorting. Biol. Reprod. *41*:199.
18. Johnson, L. A., Cran, D. G., and Polge, C. (1994): Recent advances in sex preselection of cattle: Flow cytometric sorting of X- and Y-chromosome-bearing sperm based on DNA to produce progeny. Theriogenology *41*:51.
19. Johnson, L. A. (1992): Gender preselection in domestic animals using flow cytometrically sorted sperm. J. Anim. Sci. *70*:8.
20. Jost, A. and Magre, S. (1984): Testicular development phases and dual hormonal control of sexual organogenesis. *In:* Sexual Differentiation: Basic and Clinical Aspects, edited by M. Serio, et al. New York, NY, Raven Press, p. 1.
21. Kay, G. F., Barton, S. C., Surani, M. A., et al. (1994): Imprinting and X chromosome counting mechanisms determine *Xist* expression in early mouse development. Cell *77*:639.
22. Koopman, P. (1995): The molecular biology of SRY and its role in sex determination in mammals. Reprod. Fertil. Develop. *7*:713.
23. Koopman, P., Gubbay, J., Vivian, N., et al. (1991): Male development of chromosomally female mice transgenic for SRY. Nature *351*:117.
24. McFeely, R. A. (1975): A review of cytogenetics in equine reproduction. J. Reprod. Fertil. (Suppl. 23):371.
25. Merchant-Larios, H. and Taketo, T. (1991): Testicular differentiation in mammals under normal and experimental conditions. J. Elect. Microsc. Tech. *19*:158.
26. Moruzzi, J. F. (1979): Selecting a mammalian species for the separation of X- and Y-chromosome-bearing spermatozoa. J. Reprod. Fertil. *57*:319.
27. Nagai, Y. (1992): Primary sex determination in mammals. Zool. Sci. *9*:475.
28. Nalbandov, A. V. (1964): The biology of sex. *In:* Reproductive Physiology, 2nd ed., edited by A. V. Nalbandov. San Francisco, CA, W. H. Freeman & Co., p. 3.
29. Ohno, S. (1969): Evolution of sex chromosomes in mammals. Annu. Rev. Genet. *3*:495.
30. Pääbo, S. (1995): The Y chromosome and the origin of all of us (men). Science *268*:1141.
31. Picard, J.-Y. and Josso, N. (1984): Purification of testicular anti-Müllerian hormone allowing direct visualization of the pure glycoprotein and determination of yield and purification factor. Mol. Cell. Endocrinol. *34*:23.
32. Selden, J. R., Wachtel, S. S., Koo, G. C., et al. (1978): Genetic basis of XX male syndrome and XX true hermaphroditism: Evidence in the dog. Science *201*:644.
33. Simoni, M. (1994): Transgenic animals in male reproduction research. Exp. Clin. Endocrinol. *102*:419.
34. Trujillo, J. M., Ohno, S., Jardine, F. H., et al. (1969): Spermatogenesis in a male hinny: Histological and cytological studies. J. Hered. *60*:79.
35. Vendeberg, J. L. (1983): Developmental aspects of X chromosome inactivation in eutherian and metatherian mammals. J. Exp. Zool. *228*:271.
36. Van Vliet, R. A., Verrinder, A. M., and Walton, J. S. (1989): Livestock embryo sexing: A review of current methods, with emphasis on Y-specific DNA probes. Theriogenology *32*:421.
37. Wachtel, S. S. (1984): H-Y antigen in the study of sex determination and control of sex ratio. Theriogenology *21*:18.

38. Walker, C. L., Cargile, C. B., Floy, K. M., et al. (1991): The Barr body is a looped X chromosome formed by telomere association. Proc. Nat. Acad. Sci., USA 88:6191.

39. Windsor, D. P., Evans, G., and White, I. G. (1993): Sex predetermination by separation of X and Y chromosome-bearing sperm: A review. Reprod. Fertil. Develop. 5:155.

40. Winter, H. and Pfeffer, A. (1977): Pathogenic classification of intersex. Vet. Rec. 100:307.

Development of Male and Female Reproductive Organs

41. Basrur, P. K. and Kanagawa, H. (1971): Sex anomalies in pigs. J. Reprod. Fertil. 26:369.

42. Behringer, R. R., Finegold, M. J., and Cate, R. L. (1994): Müllerian-inhibiting substance function during mammalian sexual development. Cell 79:415.

43. Daneau, I., Ethier, J.-F., Lussier, J. G., et al. (1996): Porcine SRY gene locus and genital ridge expression. Biol. Reprod. 55:47.

44. Daneau, I., Houde, A., Ethier, J.-F., et al. (1994): SRY gene in bull and boar show greater similarity to human than to mouse gene. Biol. Reprod. 50 (Suppl. 1):412 Abstract.

45. Daneau, I., Houde, A., Ethier, J.-F., et al. (1995): Bovine SRY gene locus: Cloning and testicular expression. Biol. Reprod. 52:591.

46. Dominguez, M. M., Liptrap, B. A., Croy, B. A., et al. (1990): Hormonal correlates of ovarian alterations in bovine freemartin fetuses. Anim. Reprod. Sci. 22:181.

47. Donahoe, P. K., Ito, Y., Price, J. M., et al. (1977): Müllerian-inhibiting substance activity in bovine fetal, newborn and prepubertal testes. Biol. Reprod. 16:238.

48. Dunn, H. O., McEntee, K., Hall, C. E., et al. (1979): Cytogenetic and reproductive studies of bulls born co-twin with freemartins. J. Reprod. Fertil. 57:21.

49. Gladue, B. A., Green, R., and Hellman, R. E. (1984): Neuroendocrine response to estrogen and sexual orientation. Science 225:1496.

50. Goodfellow, P. N. and Lovell-Badge, R. (1993): SRY and sex determination in mammals. Annu. Rev. Genet. 27:71.

51. Greene, W. A., Mogil, L. G., Lein, D. H., et al. (1979): Growth and reproductive development in freemartins hormonally treated from 1 to 79 weeks of age. Cornell Vet. 69:248.

52. Guerrier, D., Boussin, L., Mader, S., et al. (1990): Expression of the gene for anti-Müllerian hormone. J. Reprod. Fertil. 88:695.

53. Haqq, C. M., King, C. Y., Ukiyama, E., et al. (1994): Molecular basis of mammalian sexual determination: Activation of Müllerian-inhibiting substance gene expression by SRY. Science 266:1494.

54. Hughes, J. P. and Trommershausen-Smith, A. (1977): Infertility in the horse associated with chromosomal abnormalities. Aust. Vet. J. 53:253.

55. Huhtaniemi, I. and Pelliniemi, L. J. (1992): Fetal Leydig cells: Cellular origin, morphology, life span, and special functional features. Proc. Soc. Exp. Biol. Med. 201:125.

56. Huhtaniemi, I. T. and Warren, D. W. (1990): Ontogeny of pituitary-gonadal interactions. Current advances and controversies. Trends Endocrinol. Metab. 1:356.

57. Inomata, T., Inoue, S., Sugawara, H., et al. (1993): Developmental changes in paramesonephric and mesonephric ducts and the external genitalia in swine fetuses during sexual differentiation. J. Vet. Med. Sci. 55:371.

58. Josso, J. (1973): In vitro synthesis of Müllerian-inhibiting hormone by seminiferous tubules isolated from the calf fetal testis. Endocrinology 93:829.

59. Josso, N. (1986): Antimüllerian hormone: New perspectives for a sexist molecule. Endocrine Rev. 7:421.

60. Josso, N., Forest, M. G., and Picard, J-Y. (1975): Müllerian-inhibiting activity of calf fetal testes: Relationship to testosterone and protein synthesis. Biol. Reprod. 13:163.

61. Jost, A., Vigier, B., and Prepin, J. (1972): Freemartins in cattle: The first steps of sexual organogenesis. J. Reprod. Fertil. 29:349.

62. Kent, M. G., Schneller, H. E., Hegsted, R. L., et al. (1988): Concentration of serum testosterone in XY sex reversed horses. J. Endocrinol. Invest. 11:609.

63. Long, S. E. (1988): Chromosome anomalies and infertility in the mare. Equine Vet. J. 20:89.

64. Maekawa, M., Kamimura, K., and Nagano, T. (1996): Peritubular myoid cells in the testis: Their structure and function. Arch. Histol. Cytol. 59:1.

65. Meck, J. M. (1984): The genetics of the H-Y antigen system and its role in sex determination. Perspect. Biol. Med. 27:561.

66. Merchant-Larios, H. and Taketo, T. (1991): Testicular differentiation in mammals under normal and experimental conditions. J. Elect. Microsc. Tech. 19:158.

67. Meyers-Wallen, V. N., Donahoe, P. K., Manganaro, T., et al. (1987): Müllerian-inhibiting substance on sex-reversed dogs. Biol. Reprod. 37:1015.

68. Meyers-Wallen, V. N., MacLaughlin, D., Palmer, V., et al. (1994): Müllerian-inhibiting substance secretion is delayed in XX sex-reversed dog embryos. Mol. Reprod. Develop. 39:1.

69. Meyers-Wallen, V. N. and Patterson, D. F. (1989): Sexual differentiation and inherited disorders of sexual development in the dog. J. Reprod. Fertil. (Suppl. 39):57.

70. Mittwoch, U. (1989): Sex differentiation in mammals and tempo of growth: Probabilities vs. switches. J. Theor. Biol. 137:445.

71. Mittwoch, U. (1992): Sex determination and sex reversal: Genotype, phenotype, dogma and semantics. Human Genet. 89:467.

72. Mittwoch, U., Delhanty, D. A., and Beck, F. (1969): Growth of differentiating testes and ovaries. Nature 224:1323.

73. Nalbandov, A. V. (1964): Reproductive Physiology, 2nd ed., edited by A. V. Nalbandov. San Francisco, CA, W. H. Freeman & Co., p. 5.

74. Ohno, S., Nagai, Y., Ciccarese, S., et al. (1979): Testis-organizing H-Y antigen and the primary sex-determining mechanism of mammals. Recent Prog. Hormone Res. 35:449.

75. Pailhoux, E., Popescu, P. C., Parma, P., et al. (1994): Genetic analysis of 38XX males with genital ambiguities and true hermaphrodites in pigs. Anim. Genet. 25:299.

76. Saba, N., Cunningham, N. F., and Millar, P. G. (1975): Plasma progesterone, androstenedione and testosterone concentrations in freemartin heifers. J. Reprod. Fertil. 45:37.

77. Sharp, A. J., Wachtel, S. S., and Benirschke, K. (1980): H-Y antigen in a fertile XY female horse. J. Reprod. Fertil. *58*:157.

78. Shore, L. S., Shemesh, M., and Mileguir, F. (1984): Foetal testicular steroidogenesis and responsiveness to LH in freemartins and their male co-twins. Int. J. Androl. *7*:87.

79. Solter, D. (1988): Differential imprinting and expression of maternal and paternal genomes. Annu. Rev. Genet. *22*:127.

80. Turner, C. D. (1960): The biology of sex and reproduction, Ch. 8. *In:* General Endocrinology, 3rd ed., edited by C. D. Turner. Philadelphia, PA, W. B. Saunders Co., p. 272.

81. Van Vorstenbosch, C. J. A. H. V., Spek, E., Colenbrander, B., et al. (1987): The ultrastructure of normal fetal and neonatal pig testis germ cells and the influence of fetal decapitation on the germ cell development. Development *99*:553.

82. Vigier, B., Tran, D., Legeai, L., et al. (1984): Origin of anti-Müllerian hormone in bovine freemartin fetuses. J. Reprod. Fertil. *70*:473.

83. Vigier, B., Watrin, F., Magre, S., et al. (1988): Anti-Müllerian hormone and freemartinism: Inhibition of germ cell development and induction of seminiferous cord-like structures in rat fetal ovaries exposed *in vitro* to purified bovine AMH. Reprod. Nutr. Develop. *28*:1113.

84. Wachtel, S. S., Hall, J. L., and Cahill, L. T. (1981): H-Y antigen in primary sex determination. *In:* Bioregulators of Reproduction, 1st ed., edited by G. Jagiello and H. J. Vogel. New York, NY, Academic Press, Inc., p. 9.

85. Wai-Sum, O. and Baker, T. G. (1978): Germinal and somatic cell interrelationships in gonadal sex differentiation. Ann. Biol. Anim. Biochim. Biophys. *18*:351.

86. White, K. L., Anderson, G. B., and Bondurant, R. H. (1987): Expression of a male-specific factor on various stages of preimplantation bovine embryos. Biol. Reprod. *37*:867.

87. Wijeratne, W. V. S., Munro, I. B., and Wilkes, P. R. (1977): Heifer sterility associated with single-birth freemartinism. Vet. Rec. *100*:333.

88. Wartenberg, H. (1983): Morphological aspects of gonadal differentiation. Structural aspects of gonadal differentiation in mammals and birds. Differentiation *23* (Suppl.):S64.

Sexual Behavior

89. Aronson, L. R. and Cooper, M. L. (1974): Olfactory deprivation and mating behavior in sexually experienced male cats. Behav. Biol. *11*:459.

90. Bland, K. P. (1979): Tom-cat odour and other pheromones in feline reproduction. Vet. Sci. Comm. *3*:125.

91. Brooks, P. H. and Cole, D. J. A. (1970): The effect of the presence of a boar on the attainment of puberty in gilts. J. Reprod. Fertil. *23*:435.

92. Bruce, H. M. (1960): A block of pregnancy in the mouse caused by proximity of strange males. J. Reprod. Fertil. *1*:96.

93. Doty, R. L. and Mare, C. J. (1974): Color, odor, consistency and secretion rate of anal sac secretions from male, female, and early androgenized female Beagles. Am. J. Vet. Res. *35*:669.

94. Dulac, C. and Axel, R. (1995): A novel family of genes encoding putative pheromone receptors in mammals. Cell *83*:195.

95. Edgar, D. G. and Bilkey, D. A. (1964): The influence of rams on the onset of the breeding season in ewes. Proc. N. Z. Soc. Anim. Prod. *23*:79.

96. Gower, D. B. (1972): 16-unsaturated C_{19} steroids. A review of their chemistry, biochemistry and possible physiological role. J. Steroid Biochem. *3*:45.

97. Gower, D. B. and Ruparelia, B. A. (1993): Olfaction in humans with special reference to odorous 16-androstenes: Their occurrence, perception and possible social, psychological and sexual impact. J. Endocrinol. *137*:167.

98. Levine, S. (1966): Sex differences in the brain. Sci. Am. *214*:84.

99. Lichtenwalner, A. B., Woods, G. L., and Weber, J. A. (1996): Ejaculatory pattern of llamas during copulation. Theriogenology *46*:285.

100. Lichtenwalner, A. B., Woods, G. L., and Weber, J. A. (1996): Seminal collection, seminal characteristics and pattern of ejaculation in llamas. Theriogenology *46*:293.

101. Heindel, J. J. and Treinen, K. A. (1989): Physiology of the male reproductive system: Endocrine, paracrine and autocrine regulation. Toxicol. Pathol. *17*:411.

102. Meyers-Wallen, V. N., Donahoe, P. K., Ueno, S., et al. (1989): Müllerian-inhibiting substance is present in testes of dogs with persistent Müllerian duct syndrome. Biol. Reprod. *41*:881.

103. Signoret, J. P. (1974): Rôle des différentes informations sensorielles dans l'attraction de la femelle en oestrus par le mâle chez les porcins. Ann. Biol. Anim. Biochim. Biophys. *14*:747.

104. Signoret, J. P. (1991): Sexual pheromones in the domestic sheep: Importance and limits in the regulation of reproductive physiology. J. Steroid. Biochem. Mol. Biol. *39*:639.

105. Tischner, M., Kosiniak, K., and Bielanski, W. (1974): Analysis of the pattern of ejaculation in stallions. J. Reprod. Fertil. *41*:329.

106. Wheeler, J. W. (1976): Insect and mammalian pheromones. Lloydia *39*:53.

107. Whitten, W. K., Bronson, F. H., and Greenstein, J. A. (1968): Estrus-inducing pheromone of male mice: Transport by movement of air. Science *161*:584.

Gametogenesis

108. Allan, D. J., Harman, B. V., and Roberts, S. A. (1992): Spermatogonial apoptosis has three morphologically recognizable phases and shows no circadian rhythm during normal spermatogenesis in the rat. Cell Prolif. *25*:241.

109. Amann, R. P. and Schanbacher, B. D. (1983): Physiology of male reproduction. J. Anim. Sci. *57* (Suppl. 2):380.

110. Andersen, A. C. and Simpson, M. E. (1973): The Ovary and Reproductive Cycle of the Dog (Beagle). Los Altos, CA, Geron-X, Inc., p. 48.

111. Berndtson, W. E. and Desjardins, C. (1974): The cycle of the seminiferous epithelium and spermatogenesis in the bovine testes. Am. J. Anat. *140*:167.

112. Billig, H., Furuta, I., and Hsueh, A. J. W. (1994): Gonadotropin-releasing hormone (GnRH) directly in-

duces apoptotic cell death in the rat ovary: Biochemical and *in situ* detection of DNA fragmentation in granulosa cells. Endocrinology *134*:245.

113. Billig, H., Furuta, I., Revier, C., et al. (1995): Apoptosis in testis germ cells: Developmental changes in gonadotropin dependence and localization to selective tubule stages. Endocrinology *136*:5.

114. Buccione, R., Schroeder, A. C., and Eppig. J. J. (1990): Interactions between somatic cells and germ cells throughout mammalian oogenesis. Biol. Reprod. *43*:543.

115. Burgoyne, P. S. (1978): The role of sex chromosomes in mammalian germ cell differentiation. Ann. Biol. Anim. Biochim. Biophys. *18*:317.

116. Carreau, S., Foucault, P., and Drosdowsky, M. A. (1994): La cellule de Sertoli: Aspects fonctionnels comparés chez le rat, le porc et l'homme. Ann. Endocrinol. Paris, France *55*:203.

117. Clarke, P. G. H. and Clarke, S. (1996): Nineteenth century research on naturally occurring cell death and related phenomena. Anat. Embryol. *193*:81.

118. Crisp, T. M. (1992): Organization of the ovarian follicle and events in its biology: Oogenesis, ovulation or atresia. Mutation Res. *296*:89.

119. Clermont, Y. (1972): Kinetics of spermatogenesis in mammals: Seminiferous epithelium cycle and spermatogonial renewal. Physiol. Rev. *52*:198.

120. De Rooij, D. G. (1988): Regulation of the proliferation of spermatogonial stem cells. J. Cell Sci. (Suppl. 10):181.

121. Dym, M. and Cavicchia, J. C. (1978): Functional morphology of the testis. Biol. Reprod. *18*:1.

122. Fawcett, D. W. (1975): The mammalian spermatozoan. Develop. Biol. *44*:394.

123. Foote, R. H., Swiestra, E. E., and Hunt, W. L. (1972): Spermatogenesis in the dog. Anat. Rec. *173*:341.

124. Grinsted, J., Kjer, J. J., Blendstrup, K., et al. (1985): Is low temperature of the follicular fluid prior to ovulation necessary for normal oocyte development? Fertil. Steril. *43*:34.

125. Hecht, N. B. (1995): The making of a spermatozoon: A molecular perspective. Develop. Genet. *16*:95.

126. Heindel, J. J. and Treinen, K. A. (1989): Physiology of the male reproductive system: Endocrine, paracrine and autocrine regulation. Toxicol. Pathol. *17*:411.

127. Hingst, O., Blottner, S., and Meyer, H. H. D. (1996): Role of apoptosis in seasonal involution and recrudescence of testis. Z. Saügertierkunde *61*:59.

128. Hochereau de Reviers, M. T. and Courot, M. (1978): Sertoli cells and development of seminiferous epithelium. Ann. Biol. Anim. Biochim. Biophys. *18*:573.

129. Hunter, R. H. F. (1989): Differential transport of fertilised and unfertilised [sic] eggs in equine fallopian tubes: A straightforward explanation. Vet. Rec. *125*:304.

130. Hyttel, P., Callesen, H., and Greve, T. (1986): Ultrastructural features of preovulatory oocyte maturation in superovulated cattle. J. Reprod. Fertil. *76*:645.

131. Hyttel, P., Farstad, W., Mondain-Monval, M., et al. (1990): Structural aspects of oocyte maturation in the blue fox (*Alopex lagopus*). Anat. Embryol. *181*:325.

132. Ibach, B., Weissbadi, L., and Hilscher, B. (1976): Stages of the cycle of the seminiferous epithelium in the dog. Andrologia *8*:297.

133. Jégou, B. (1992): The Sertoli cell. Bailliere's Clin. Endocrinol. Metab. *6*:273.

134. Johnson, L. and Thompson, D. L., Jr. (1983): Age-related and seasonal variation in the Sertoli cell population, daily sperm production and serum concentrations of follicle-stimulating hormone, luteinizing hormone and testosterone in stallions. Biol. Reprod. *29*:777.

135. Kennelly, J. J. (1972): Coyote reproduction. I. The duration of the spermatogenic cycle and epididymal sperm transport. J. Reprod. Fertil. *31*:163.

136. Kruip, T. A. M., Cran, D. G., Van Beneden, T. H., et al. (1983): Structural changes in bovine oocytes during final maturation *in vivo*. Gamete Res. *8*:29.

137. Mather, J. P., Gunsalus, G. L., Musto, N. A., et al. (1983): The hormonal and cellular control of Sertoli cell secretion. J. Steroid Biochem. *19*:41.

138. Matsuda, Y., Seki, N., Utsugi-Takeushi, T., et al. (1989): Changes in x-ray sensitivity of mouse eggs from fertilization to the early pronuclear stage, and their repair capacity. Int. J. Rad. Biol. *55*:233.

139. Mauléon, P. (1967): Cinétique de l'ovogenèse chez les mammiféres. Arch. d'Anat. Microsc. Morphol. Exp. *56*:125.

140. Norton, J. N. and Skinner, M. K. (1989): Regulation of Sertoli cell function and differentiation through the actions of a testicular paracrine factor P-Mod-S. Endocrinology *124*:2711.

141. Oakberg, E. F. (1978): Differential spermatogonial stem-cell survival and mutation frequency. Mutation Res. *50*:327.

142. Ogura, A. and Yanagimachi, R. (1993): Round spermatid nuclei injected into hamster oocytes form pronuclei and participate in syngamy. Biol. Reprod. *48*:219.

143. Ogura, A. and Yanagimachi, R. (1995): Spermatids as male gametes. Reprod. Fertil. Develop. *7*:155.

144. Ohuma, H. and Ohnamiu, Y. (1975): Retention of tubal eggs in mares. J. Reprod. Fertil. (Suppl. 23):507.

145. Osman, D. I. and Plöen, L. (1979): Fine structure of the modified Sertoli cells in the terminal segment of the seminiferous tubules of the bull, ram and goat. Anim. Reprod. Sci. *2*:343.

146. Park, Y. S., Abe, M., Takehana, K., et al. (1993): Three-dimensional structure of dog Sertoli cells: A computer-aided reconstruction from serial semi-thin sections. Arch. Histol. Cytol. *56*:65.

147. Pelletier, R.-M. (1988): Cyclic modulation of Sertoli cell junctional complexes in a seasonal breeder: The mink (*Mustela vison*). Am. J. Anat. *183*:68.

148. Pelletier, R.-M. and Byers, S. W. (1992): The blood-testis barrier and Sertoli cells junctions: Structural considerations. Microsc. Res. Tech. *20*:3.

149. Phillips, D. M. and Dekel, N. (1991): Maturation of the rat cumulus-oocyte complex: Structure and function. Mol. Reprod. Develop. *28*:297.

150. Ross, M. H. (1976): The Sertoli cell junctional specialization during spermiogenesis and at spermiation. Anat. Rec. *186*:79.

151. Ross, G. T. and Lipsett, M. B. (1978): Homologies of structure and function in mammalian testes and ovaries. Int. J. Androl. (Suppl. 2):39.

152. Sakai, Y. and Yamashina, S. (1990): Spermiation in the mouse: Contribution of the invading Sertoli cell

process to adluminal displacement of the spermatid head. Develop. Growth Differ. *39*:389.

153. Schwartz, L. M. and Osborne, B. A. (1993): Programmed cell death, apoptosis and killer genes. Immunol. Today *14*:582.

154. Seidl, K. and Holstein, A.-F. (1990): Organ culture of human seminiferous tubules: A useful tool to study the role of nerve growth factor in the testis. Cell Tissue Res. *261*:539.

155. Seidl, K. and Holstein, A.-F. (1990): Evidence for the presence of nerve growth factor (NGF) and NGF receptors in human testis. Cell Tissue Res. *261*:549.

156. Setchell, B. P. and Waites, G. M. H. (1975): The blood-testis barrier. *In:* Handbook of Physiology, Section 7: Endocrinology, Vol. V, Male Reproductive System, edited by D. W. Hamilton and R. O. Greep. Washington, DC, American Physiological Society, p. 143.

157. Sharpe, R. M., Maddocks, S., and Kerr, J. B. (1990): Cell-cell interactions in the control of spermatogenesis as studied using Leydig cell destruction and testosterone replacement. Am. J. Anat. *188*:3.

158. Shehata, R. (1974): Polyovular graafian follicles in a newborn kitten with a study of polyovuly in the cat. Acta Anat. *89*:21.

159. Skinner, M. K. (1991): Cell-cell interactions in the testes. Endocrine Rev. *12*:45.

160. Sofikitis, N. V., Miyagawa, I., Agapitos, E., et al. (1994): Reproductive capacity of the nucleus of the male gamete after completion of meiosis. J. Assist. Reprod. Genet. *11*:335.

161. Spano, M. and Evenson, D. P. (1993): Flow cytometric analysis for reproductive biology. Biol. Cell *78*:53.

162. Sprando, R. L. and Russell, L. D. (1987): Germ cell-somatic cell relationships. A comparative study of intercellular junctions during spermatogenesis in selected non-mammalian vertebrates. Scanning Microsc. *1*:1249.

163. Steffenhagen, W. P., Pineda, M. H., and Ginther, O. J. (1972): Retention of unfertilized ova in uterine tubes of mares. Am. J. Vet. Res. *33*:2391.

164. Steinberger, A. (1979): Inhibin production by Sertoli cells in culture. J. Reprod. Fertil. *26*:31.

165. Steinberger, A., Heindel, J. J., Lindsay, J. N., et al. (1975): Isolation and culture of FSH responsive Sertoli cells. Endocrine Res. Commun. *2*:261.

166. Steller, H. (1995): Mechanisms and genes of cellular suicide. Science *267*:1445.

167. Swierstra, E. E. (1968): Cytology and duration of the cycle of the seminiferous epithelium of the boar; duration of the spermatozoan transit through the epididymis. Anat. Rec. *161*:171.

168. Swierstra, E. E., Gebauer, M. R., and Pickett, B. W. (1974): Reproductive physiology of the stallion. I. Spermatogenesis and testis composition. J. Reprod. Fertil. *40*:113.

169. Tapanainen, J. S., Tilly, J. L., Vihko, K. K., et al. (1993): Hormonal control of apoptotic cell death in the testis: Gonadotropins and androgens as testicular cell survival factors. Mol. Endocrinol. *7*:643.

170. Tesoriero, J. V. (1984): Comparative cytochemistry of the developing ovarian follicles of the dog, rabbit, and mouse: Origin of the zona pellucida. Gamete Res. *10*:301.

171. Tiba, T., Matsuzaki, S., and Kojima, Y. (1994): Examination of spermatogonial multiplication in the bull using whole-mount seminiferous tubules. Reprod. Domestic Anim. *29*:458.

172. Tsafriri, A., Debel, N., and Bar-Ami, S. (1982): The role of oocyte maturation inhibitor in follicular regulation of oocyte maturation. J. Reprod. Fertil. *64*:541.

173. Vanha-Pertula, T. (1978): Spermatogenesis and hydrolytic enzymes. A review. Ann. Biol. Anim. Biochim. Biophys. *18*:633.

174. Van den Wiel, D. F. M., Bar-Ami, S., Tsafriri, A., et al. (1983): Oocyte maturation inhibitor, inhibin and steroid concentrations in porcine follicular fluid at various stages of the oestrous cycle. J. Reprod. Fertil. *68*:247.

175. Van Niekerk, C. H. and Gerneke, W. H. (1966): Persistence and parthenogenic cleavage of tubal ova in the mare. Onderstepoort J. Vet. Res. *31*:195.

176. Vaux, D. L. and Strasser, A. (1996): The molecular biology of apoptosis. Proc. Nat. Acad. Sci., USA. *93*:2239.

177. Vaux, D. L., Haecker, G., and Strasser, A. (1994): An evolutionary perspective on apoptosis. Cell *76*:1.

178. Wolgemuth, D. J., Rhee, K., Wu, S., et al. (1995): Genetic control of mitosis, meiosis and cellular differentiation during mammalian spermatogenesis. Reprod. Fertil. Develop. *7*:669.

179. Zamboni, L. (1970): Ultrastructure of mammalian oocytes and ova. Biol. Reprod. *2*:44.

180. Zamboni, L. (1974): Fine morphology of the follicle wall and follicle cell-oocyte association. Biol. Reprod. *10*:125.

Fertilization

181. Alcivar, A. A., Dooley, M. P., and Pineda, M. H. (1995): Effect of mitochondrial DNA (mtDNA) type on pregnancy rate after embryo transfer in rats. Theriogenology *44*:773.

182. Bedford, J. M. (1983): Significance of the need for sperm capacitation before fertilization in eutherian mammals. Biol. Reprod. *28*:108.

183. Bell, B. R., McDaniel, B. T., and Robinson, O. W. (1985): Effects of cytoplasmic inheritance on production traits of dairy cattle. J. Dairy Sci. *68*:2038.

184. Berruti, G. (1981): Multiple forms of bovine acrosin: Purification and characterization. Comp. Biochem. Physiol. *69B*:323.

185. Bowen, R. (1977): Fertilization *in vitro* of feline ova by spermatozoa from the ductus deferens. Biol. Reprod. *17*:144.

186. Corselli, J. and Talbot, P. (1986): An *in vitro* technique to study penetration of hamster oocyte-cumulus complexes by using physiological numbers of sperm. Gamete Res. *13*:293.

187. Crozet, N., Théron, M. C., and Chemineau, P. (1987): Ultrastructure of *in vivo* fertilization in the goat. Gamete Res. *18*:191.

188. Dale, B. and Monroy, A. (1981): How is polyspermy prevented? Gamete Res. *4*:151.

189. Dietl, J. A. and Rauth, G. (1989): Molecular aspects of mammalian fertilization. Human Reprod. *4*:869.

190. Epel, D. (1990): The initiation of development at fertilization. Cell Differ. Develop. *29*:1.

191. Francisco, J. F., Brown, G. G., and Simpson, M. V. (1979): Further studies in types A and B rat mtDNAs: Cleavage maps and evidence for cytoplasmic inheritance in mammals. Plasmid *2*:426.

192. Gould, K. G. (1973): Application of *in vitro* fertilization. Fed. Proc. *32*:2069.

193. Grant, V. (1994): Evolution of the species concept. Biol. Zent. bl. *113*:401.

194. Grivell, L. A. (1983): Mitochondrial DNA. Sci. Am. *248*:78.

195. Gustafson, R. A., Anderson, G. B., BonDurant, R. H., et al. (1993): Failure of sheep-goat hybrid conceptuses to develop to term in sheep-goat chimaeras. J. Reprod. Fertil. *99*:267.

196. Hamner, C. E., Jennings, L. L., and Sojka, N. J. (1970): Cat (*Felis catus L.*) spermatozoa require capacitation. J. Reprod. Fertil. *23*:477.

197. Hawk, H. W. (1987): Transport and fate of spermatozoa after insemination of cattle. J. Dairy Sci. *70*:1487.

198. Herz, Z., Northey, D., Lawyer, M., et al. (1985): Acrosome reaction of bovine spermatozoa *in vivo:* Sites and effects of stages of the estrous cycle. Biol. Reprod. *32*:1163.

199. Holst, P. A. and Phemister, R. D. (1974): Onset of diestrus in Beagle bitch: Definition and significance. Am. J. Vet. Res. *35*:401.

200. Hunter, R. H. F. (1977): Physiological factors influencing ovulation, fertilization, early embryonic development and establishment of pregnancy in pigs. Br. Vet. J. *133*:461.

201. Hunter, R. H. F. and Hall, J. P. (1974): Capacitation of boar spermatozoa: Synergism between uterine and tubal environments. J. Exp. Zool. *188*:203.

202. Hunter, R. H. F. and Nichol, R. (1988): Capacitation potential of the Fallopian tube: A study involving surgical insemination and the subsequent incidence of polyspermy. Gamete Res. *21*:255.

203. Hutchinson, C. A., III, Nebold, J. E., Potter, S. S., et al. (1974): Maternal inheritance of mammalian mitochondrial DNA. Nature *251*:536.

204. Iritani, A. and Niwa, K. (1977): Capacitation of bull spermatozoa and fertilization *in vitro* of cattle follicular oocytes matured in culture. J. Reprod. Fertil. *50*:119.

205. Kopf, G. S. and Wilde, M. W. (1990): Signal transduction processes leading to acrosomal exocytosis in mammalian spermatozoa. Trends Endocrinol. Metab. *1*:362.

206. Leman, A. D. and Dziuk, P. J. (1971): Fertilization and development of pig follicular oocytes. J. Reprod. Fertil. *26*:387.

207. Lindemann, C. B. and Kanous, K. S. (1989): Regulation of mammalian sperm motility. Arch. Androl. *23*:1.

208. Longo, F. J. (1973): Fertilization: A comparative ultrastructural review. Biol. Reprod. *9*:149.

209. MacLaren, L. A., Anderson, B. G., BonDurant, R. H., et al. (1993): Reproductive cycles and pregnancy in interspecific sheep-goat chimaeras. Reprod. Fertil. Develop. *5*:261.

210. Mahi, C. A. and Yanagimachi, R. (1978): Capacitation, acrosome reaction, and egg penetration by canine spermatozoa in a simple defined medium. Gamete Res. *1*:101.

211. Mahi, C. A. and Yanagimachi, R. (1976): Maturation and sperm penetration of canine ovarian oocytes *in vitro*. J. Exp. Zool. *196*:189.

212. Mattner, P. E. (1963): Capacitation of ram sperm and penetration of the ovine egg. Nature *199*:772.

213. McLaren, A. (1974): Fertilization, implantation and cleavage. *In:* Reproduction in Farm Animals, 3rd ed., edited by E. S. E. Hafez. Philadelphia, PA, Lea & Febiger, p. 143.

214. McRorie, R. A. and Williams, W. L. (1974): Biochemistry of mammalian fertilization. Annu. Rev. Biochem. *43*:777.

215. Metz, C. B. (1972): Effects of antibodies on gametes and fertilization. Biol. Reprod. *6*:358.

216. Michaels, G. S., Hauswirth, W. W., and Laipis, P. J. (1982): Mitochondrial DNA copy number in bovine oocytes and somatic cells. Develop. Biol. *94*:246.

217. Miller, D. J. and Ax, R. L. (1990): Carbohydrates and fertilization in animals. Mol. Reprod. Develop. *26*:184.

218. Moore, H. D. M. and Bedford, J. M. (1978): Ultrastructure of the equatorial segment of hamster spermatozoa during penetration of oocytes. J. Ultrastruct. Res. *62*:110.

219. Morton, D. B. (1975): Acrosomal enzymes: Immunochemical localization of acrosin and hyaluronidase in ram spermatozoa. J. Reprod. Fertil. *45*:375.

220. Phillips, D. M. (1977): Surface of the equatorial segment of the mammalian acrosome. Biol. Reprod. *16*:128.

221. Plöen, L. (1971): A scheme of rabbit spermateleosis [sic] based upon electron microscopical observations. Z. Zellforsch. *115*:553.

222. Pollard, J. W., Martino, A., Rumph, N. D., et al. (1996): Effect of ambient temperature during oocyte recovery on *in vitro* production of bovine embryos. Theriogenology *46*:849.

223. Rogers, B. J. (1978): Mammalian sperm capacitation and fertilization *in vitro:* A critique of methodology. Gamete Res. *1*:165.

224. Saling, P. M. and Bedford, J. M. (1981): Absence of species specificity for mammalian sperm capacitation *in vivo*. J. Reprod. Fertil. *63*:119.

225. Singhas, C. A. and Oliphant, G. (1978): Ultrastructural observations of the time sequence of induction of acrosomal membrane alterations by ovarian follicular fluid. Fertil. Steril. *29*:194.

226. Snell, W. J. and White, J. M. (1996): The molecules of mammalian fertilization. Cell *85*:629.

227. Steger, K. and Wrobel, K.-H. (1996): Postnatal development of ovine seminiferous tubules: An electron microscopical and morphometric study. Ann. Anat. *178*:201.

228. Sun, F. Z., Bradshaw, J. P., Galli, C., et al. (1994): Changes in intracellular calcium concentration in bovine oocytes following penetration by spermatozoa. J. Reprod. Fertil. *101*:713.

229. Talbot, P. (1985): Sperm penetration through oocyte investments in mammals. Am. J. Anat. *174*:331.

230. Thompson, R. S. and Zamboni, L. (1975): Anomalous patterns of mammalian oocyte maturation and fertilization. Am. J. Anat. *142*:233.

231. Umansky, S. R. (1996): Apoptosis: Molecular and cellular mechanisms (a review). Mol. Biol. *30*:285.

232. Vander Vliet, W. L. and Hafez, E. S. E. (1974): Survival and aging of spermatozoa: A review. Am. J. Obstet. Gynecol. *118*:1006.

233. Wagner, R. P. (1972): The role of maternal effects in animal breeding: II. Mitochondria and animal inheritance. J. Anim. Sci. *35*:1280.

234. Wassarman, P. M. (1983): Oogenesis: Synthetic events in the developing mammalian egg. *In:* Mechanism and Control of Animal Fertilization, edited by J. F. Hartmann. New York, NY, Academic Press, Inc., p. 1.

235. Williams, W. L., Abney, T. O., Chernoff, H. N., et al. (1967): Biochemistry and physiology of decapacitation factor. J. Reprod. Fertil. (Suppl. 2):11.

236. Whitaker, M. (1996): Control of meiotic arrest. Rev. Reprod. *1*:127.

237. Wolgemuth, D. J., Rhee, K., Wu, S., et al. (1995): Genetic control of mitosis, meiosis and cellular differentiation during mammalian spermatogenesis. Reprod. Fertil. Develop. *7*:669.

References Added in Proof

238. Evans, J. P. (2000): Getting sperm and egg together:Things conserved and things diverged. Biol. Reprod. *63*:355.

239. Evans, J. P. and Kopf, G. S. (1998): Molecular mechanisms of sperm-egg interactions and egg activation. Andrologia *4-5*:297.

240. Graves, J. A. (1998): Evolution of the mammalian Y chromosome and sex-determining genes. J. Exp. Zool. *281*:472.

241. Koopman, P. (1999): Sry and Sox 9:Mammalian testis-determining genes. Cell. Mol. Life Sci. *55*:839.

242. Lau, Y. F. and Zhang, J. (1998): Sry interactive proteins: Implication for the mechanisms of sex determination. Cytogenet. Cell Genet. *80*:128.

243. Longo, F. J., Cook, S., McCulloh, D. H. et al. (1994): Stages leading to and following fusion of sperm and egg plasma membranes. Zygote *2*:317.

244. Mather, J. P., Moore, A., and Li, R-H. (1997): Activins, inhibins, and follistatins: Further thoughts on a growing family of regulators. Proc. Soc. Exp. Biol. Med. *215*:209.

245. Mori, T., Guo, M. W., Sato, E., et al. (2000): Molecular and immunological approaches to mammalian fertilization. J. Reproductive Immunol. *47*:139.

246. Pevny, L. H. and Lovell-Badge, R. (1997): Sox genes find their feet. Curr. Opinion Genetics Develop. *7*:338.

247. Wakayama, T. and Yanagimachi, R. (1998): The first polar body can be used for the production of normal offspring in mice. Biol. Reprod. *59*:100.

Male Reproductive System

M. H. PINEDA

8

INTRODUCTION

The male gonads or testes are the primary organs of reproduction in the male. The gonads of male and female fulfill two essential functions: Gametogenesis and steroidogenesis. In the postpubertal animal, both male and female gonads share compartmentalization homologies provided by nongerminal, somatic cells. The Sertoli cells in the seminiferous tubules of the testes and the granulosa cells in the ovarian follicles form diffusion barriers between the germinal cells and the blood. These compartmentalizations provide a microenvironment for meiosis and normal gametogenesis.

REGULATION OF GONADAL ACTIVITIES

Both gametogenic and steroidogenic testicular functions are regulated by gonadotropins, which are secreted in and released from the adenohypophyseal cells in a pulsatile fashion. Most of our knowledge of pituitary regulation of gonadal function is based upon the effects of hypophysectomy and replacement therapy. Unfortunately, hypophysectomy removes not only gonadotropins but also other tropic hormones from the anterior pituitary and nontropic hormones from the posterior pituitary. Hypophysectomy is a difficult surgical procedure, and our knowledge of the effects of hypophysectomy is based upon data from a limited number of species. Moreover, it has not been possible to prepare pure gonadotropins, free of contaminating activities from other pituitary hormones, for use in replacement studies. Added to these problems is the inadequate knowledge of the secretion, biologic life, and metabolic clearance rates of a hormone from a given species when given to individuals from the same or a different species. All of these factors influence the physiologic levels in the blood and in target tissues. In addition, little is known regarding the activity of hormonal metabolites and species specificity of gonadotropins. Selective depletion of a single pituitary hormone without disturbing the independent activities of other pituitary hormones may be achieved by monospecific, active, or passive immunization. Hormone-specific antibodies

239

have also been used to study the sites of pituitary hormone production, circulating levels of pituitary hormones, and the binding of hormones to receptors in target tissues.

Control of Spermatogenesis

In general, the seminiferous tubules do not respond to gonadotropins in juvenile male mammals as they do in adult males, indicating an effect of somatic age independent of gonadotropins. Other factors, as yet unknown, must act upon the germinal cells to make them sensitive to gonadotropin stimulation.

There is no question, however, that the pituitary gland is essential to the function of seminiferous tubules. Normal spermatogenesis requires the synergistic activities of luteinizing hormone (LH, also known for the male as Interstitial Cell Stimulating Hormone, ICSH), follicle-stimulating hormone (FSH), prolactin, androgens, and probably other hormones (Fig. 8-1). The respective roles for these hormones in the spermatogenic process are not fully established, and the precise mechanisms and hormonal requirements for quantitative maintenance of normal spermatogenesis are unknown for most domestic animals. The unavailability of pure LH and FSH complicates the separation of their roles in spermatogenesis. Experimental evidence suggests that LH stimulates both steroidogenic and gametogenic testicular functions. The stimulatory activity of LH on spermatogenesis appears to be indirect and exerted through the action of testosterone secreted by the Leydig cells. FSH is involved in spermiogenesis by its activity on the Sertoli cells. The secretory, functional activity of the Sertoli cells shows cyclic variation in accordance to the complex requirements of spermatogenesis. Furthermore, the secretion of insulin-like growth factor 1 (IGF-1) is emerging as another important product of the Sertoli cells. The IGF-1 produced by the liver cannot cross the blood testis barrier. However, the IGF-1 produced locally by the Sertoli cells is made available, in a paracrine fashion, to the spermatocytes undergoing meiosis in the adluminal compartment of the seminiferous epithelium. Sertoli and germinal cells contain receptors for

IGF-1 and for insulin-like growth factor 2 (IGF-2), although IGF-2 has not been found expressed in the Sertoli cells.

Unilateral castration in males of several species results in increased blood levels of LH and FSH, which stimulate a compensatory hypertrophy of the remaining testis.

It is evident that the activity of gonadotropic hormones on the testicular, gametogenic, and steroidogenic cells is under the paracrine interactive control of intratesticular factors, including growth factors. This is discussed in corresponding sections of this chapter.

Noxious Agents

In general, the sensitivity of germinal cells of the seminiferous epithelium to harmful agents increases as differentiation proceeds to the spermatid stage. One of the earliest changes induced by harmful agents that cause degeneration of the seminiferous epithelium is the appearance in the semen of spermatids and multinucleated cells from the luminal layers of the spermatogenic epithelium. The harmful effect of testicular irradiation is an exception to this rule, because irradiation produces its greatest destructive effect on dividing cells, and spermatogonia are more sensitive than spermatocytes. On the other hand, the most serious effects of irradiation may be on the genetic apparatus. These effects would include mutations, translocations, and deletions. Spermatids are sensitive to the mutagenic effects of X-irradiation, spermatozoa are somewhat less sensitive, and spermatogonia are the least sensitive.

The interval between testicular damage and the appearance of abnormal cells in semen and changes in seminal quality depends on the nature of the insult, the cell types affected, spermatogonia versus spermatids, the duration of spermatogenesis, and epididymal migration time in that species. Table 8-1 shows the total epididymal migration time for some domestic and nondomestic species. The transit time from the head or caput to the body or corpus of the epididymis varies from 2 to 5 days for most of the species. This suggests that the time available for spermatozoal maturation in these two active areas of the epididymis is less than 5 days. If ep-

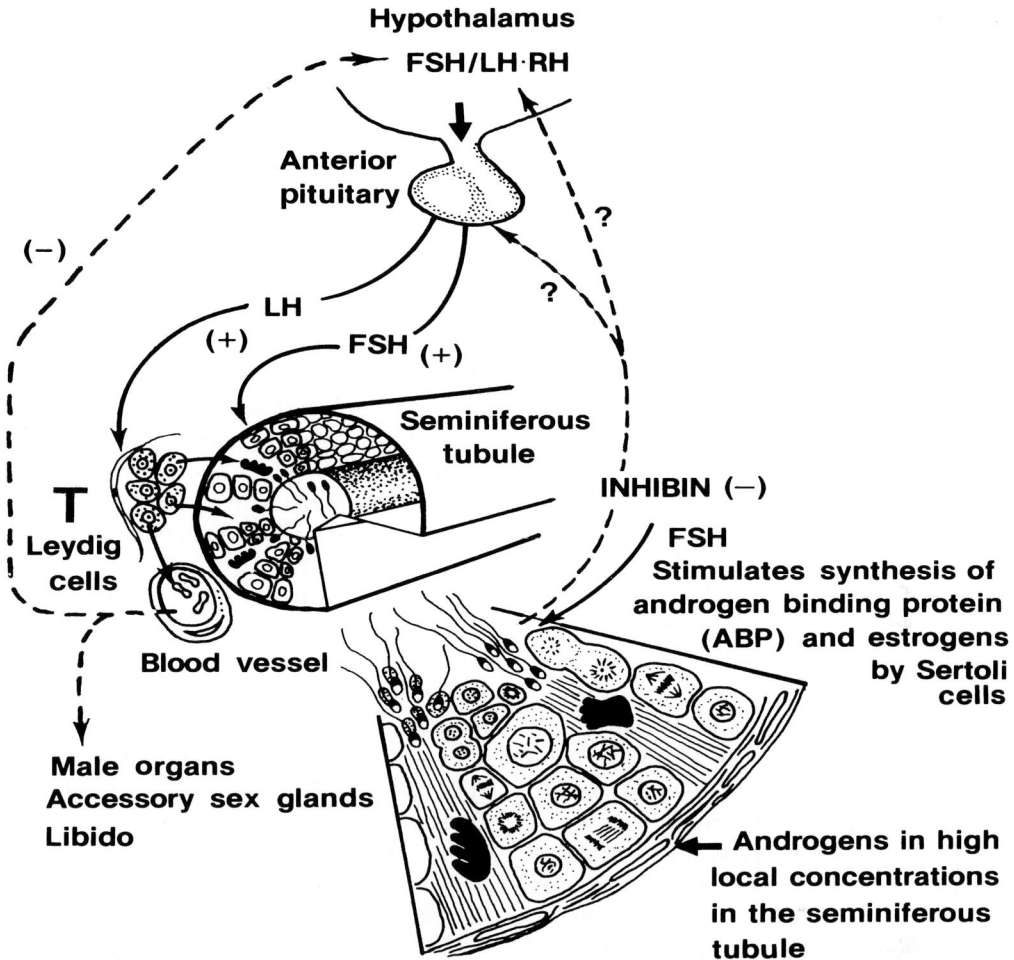

Fig. 8-1. Interrelationships in the hormonal control of testicular function. Luteinizing hormone (LH) stimulates (+) the secretion of testosterone by the Leydig cells, while FSH stimulates (+) cell divisions of the germinal epithelium, particularly in the prepubertal male. Follicle-stimulating hormone (FSH) also stimulates the Sertoli cells to uptake androgens to metabolize them to estrogens. Testosterone (T) produced by the Leydig cells enters the systemic circulation to reach and stimulate the androgen-dependent organs of the male and feedback negatively (−) on the hypothalamus, decreasing the release of GnRH (**FSH/LH-RH**). High local concentrations of testosterone directly stimulate the germinal epithelium. FSH stimulates the synthesis of androgen-binding protein (**ABP**). Inhibin secreted by the Sertoli cells suppresses plasma levels of FSH.

Table 8-1 *Epididymal Migration Time*

Species	Migration Time (days)
Boar	9 to 14
Bull	8 to 11
Coyote	14
Dog	7 to 10
Rabbit	10
Ram	13
Stallion	3 to 7

Compiled from different sources.

ididymal spermatozoa are damaged, the semen is affected soon after application of the noxious agent. If the effect is on spermatogonia, the damage will not be apparent in the semen for several weeks after the damage is done.

In addition, the type of change in seminal quality is related to the type of damage produced, i.e., death of germinal cells causes decreased numbers of spermatozoa; abnormal spermateliosis results in morphologic defects; and damage to the spermatozoal genetic apparatus results in embryonal and fetal death or teratogeny.

Sertoli cells are resistant to nearly all factors that harm germinal cells and often are the only tubular cells remaining after prolonged testicular insult. It remains possible, however, that damage to the Sertoli cells is responsible for at least some of the apparent damage to germinal cells. For example, the sloughing of spermatids and formation of multinucleated cells may actually result from functional damage to Sertoli cells, even though their morphologic integrity is undisturbed. Whereas the Leydig cells respond relatively fast to hypophysectomy with morphologic changes, the response of the Sertoli cells is delayed and will require a prolonged posthypophysectomy period to display reduction in nuclear volume and retrogressive changes.

Seasonal Variations

Females of domestic mammals show reproductive periodicity (see Chapter 9), but males of these species show a less pronounced seasonal variation in testicular function. In general, the quality and fertility of ejaculates for males of seasonal breeder species are optimal during the reproductive season. Similarly, seasonal changes in the concentrations of LH, FSH, and testosterone are influenced by the photoperiod. In addition, testicular weight and male sexual behavior are influenced by the season and photoperiod. Interestingly, male rats, as they gain sexual experience, "learn" to discharge pituitary gonadotropins in anticipation of copulation. Similar situations occur in males from other species, such as bulls in artificial insemination centers, that are trained and conditioned to regular and frequent ejaculations. The presence of the female does not seem to be a requirement to evoke this response. For some species, seminal quality and male fertility tend to decline during the hot summer months, but it is not clear whether this is attributable to the effects of season on hypothalamo-hypophyseal pathways or to a direct effect of temperature on the testis and epididymis.

Scrotal Position

In many species, the testes are normally located extrascrotally, in either the abdominal cavity or the inguinal canal. For these species, spermatogenesis proceeds normally at the higher body or systemic temperature. However, normal adult males of domestic mammals have scrotal testes, and the scrotal position with the associated lower intratesticular temperature is essential to normal gametogenic function. Males with bilateral cryptorchidism are sterile. Unilaterally cryptorchid males have lower testicular and epididymal weight in the undescended testis and display impaired spermatogenesis. The descent of the testes to the scrotum may be an evolutionary trait to maintain an intratesticular temperature 2° to 4°C lower than the abdominal temperature, resulting from the storage of spermatozoa in the tail of the epididymides, which is even cooler than in the testes. Different theories have been proposed; the reader is addressed to a review by Freeman,[19] for further discussion.

Experimentally, spermatogenesis is impaired when heat is applied to the scrotum or when the scrotum is insulated against heat loss. The extent of spermatozoal degeneration is proportional to the degree and duration of temperature elevation.

Intrascrotal deposits of fat are also detrimental to spermatogenesis, probably because the fat acts as an insulator. For some species and breeds, there may be a genetic predisposition for the deposition of fat in the scrotum.

The scrotum, the cremaster muscles, and the spermatic vasculature constitute an efficient thermoregulatory mechanism (Fig. 8-2). The tunica dartos and cremaster muscles regulate scrotal surface area and the position of the testes with respect to the abdominal wall, and the spermatic artery and pampiniform plexus provide a heat-exchange mechanism.

Both scrotal surface area and the position of the testes regulate heat loss. In hot weather, the tunica dartos and cremaster muscles are fully relaxed, and the testes are separated from the abdominal wall to allow maximum heat loss. In cold weather, these muscles contract to reduce

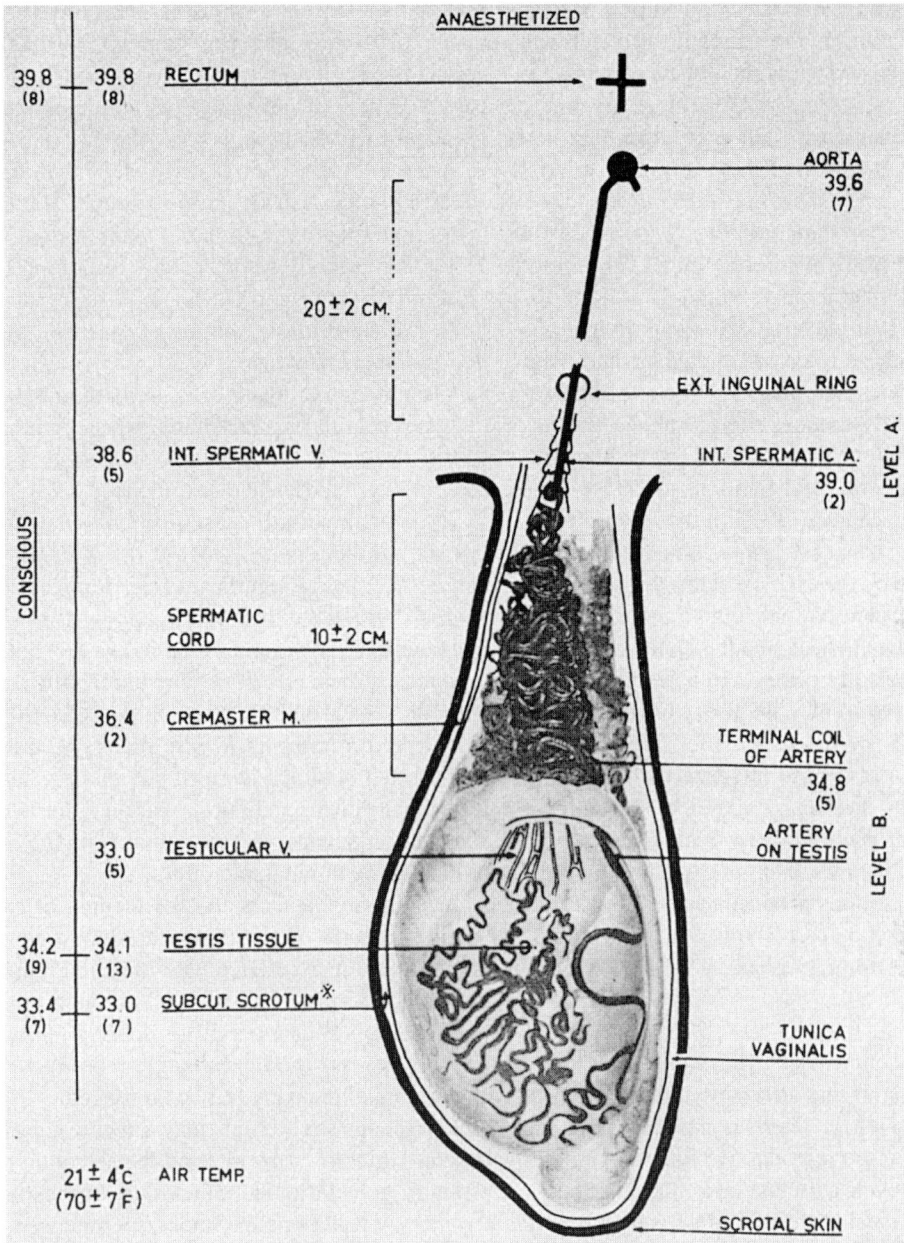

Fig. 8-2. Sites of measurements and comparisons of the temperatures recorded from conscious and anesthetized rams. Lateral aspect. The internal spermatic artery has been filled with neoprene, and the cast has been exposed by removal of the pampiniform plexus and the tunica albuginea over the artery on the testis. Figures in parentheses give the number of measurements from which the average was obtained. *Subcutaneous scrotal measurements were made beneath the posterior skin and not the anterior as shown here for the purposes of illustration only. (Reprinted with permission from: G. M. H. Waites and E. R. Moule, J. Reprod. Fertil. *2*:217, 1961).

heat loss. Arterial blood is cooled as it passes among the vessels of the pampiniform plexus and courses on the surface of the testicle before passing into the testis. Venous return blood is warmed by heat exchange with the artery, resulting in a decreased temperature of the testicular arterial blood.

Normal spermatogenesis also depends on general homeothermy. Febrile states causing increased testicular temperature may result in disturbed spermatogenesis. Testicular hypoxia probably plays a role in heat damage and other spermatogenic disturbances. The Sertoli cells of experimentally-induced cryptorchidia in rats produce a mitogenic factor that, while stimulating Leydig cell proliferation, decreases the number of receptors to LH in the Leydig cells. This results in a net decrease in the secretion of testosterone by the cryptorchid testes.

Spermatogenesis seems to be more resistant to cooling than to heat, and the tunica dartos and cremaster muscles contract to protect the testes from the effects of cold. Low environmental temperatures ($-15°$ to $-20°C$) during winter months do not seem to interfere with testicular development, sperm production, or semen quality in boars. Within a herd, bulls that suffered scrotal frostbite as a result of exposure to severe blizzard conditions produced semen of inferior quality as compared to bulls that were not affected with scrotal necrosis.

Nutrition

Specific deficiencies in the intake and utilization of nutrients can adversely influence reproductive efficiency. There is no doubt that the fulfillment of the reproductive function, including estrous cycles, pregnancy, milk production, and nourishment of the offspring, is by far more energy demanding for the female than the fulfillment of the reproductive function for the male of the species. However, premating interactions, search for females in estrus, love fights with other males, and repeated copulations are also energy consuming for the male. Energy costs of mating could be considerable, particularly during the breeding season for males of wild species, as reflected by a decline in feeding and heavy weight loss. Malnutrition constitutes

a greater stress to spermatogenesis in prepuberal males than in postpubertal males. A markedly deficient caloric intake in prepubertal males causes hypoplasia of the testes and accessory sex glands and delays puberty.

There is evidence that energy-deficient diets adversely affect gonadotropin secretion. Mature males underfed to the point of inanition (loss of 25 to 35% of body weight) show decline in libido, suffer damage to the seminiferous epithelium, and have a low volume of ejaculate and poor seminal quality.

Germinal and Leydig cells are both affected by hypovitaminosis A, resulting in poor seminal quality, testicular atrophy, hypoplasia of the accessory sex glands, and delayed puberty.

Hypovitaminosis E causes testicular damage in rats, but there is no evidence that vitamin E deficiency plays a significant role in infertility among domestic animals. Prolonged vitamin E deficiency in the ration of dairy cows and bulls produced some cases of cardiac failure but was without a measurable effect on reproduction. Very young ruminants require dietary sources of the water-soluble vitamins, but animals with functional rumens and normal ruminal flora get adequate amounts of these vitamins from the activities of the ruminal microflora.

Mineral deficiencies and the feeding of excessive amounts of phytoestrogens, goitrogens, and nitrates are associated with impaired reproductive performance in males. Although optimal nutrition after a period of deprivation appears to reverse the degenerative reproductive changes, total recovery can be prolonged.

Exogenous sex steroids may affect testicular function directly or by altering the secretion of pituitary gonadotropins. Small doses of testosterone may feed back and impair spermatogenesis by suppressing gonadotropin secretion from the pituitary. Prolonged treatment with large doses while suppressing the pituitary can maintain the seminiferous epithelium, allowing spermatogenesis to proceed. In some species, steroidal suppression of the gametogenic function of the testis has been followed by a "rebound phenomenon" after withdrawal of the steroid. Testicular rebound is presumably due to released gonadotropin secretion following withdrawal of the exogenous steroid. Testosterone injected into intact bulls severely depressed semen quality by 11 weeks (approximately the time required for spermatogenesis and epididymal migration) after the injections were stopped, suggesting that the greatest effect was on spermatogonia. Seminal quality returned to pretreatment levels between 12 and 37 weeks after testosterone withdrawal.

Estrogens administered to 2- to 3-month-old calves retard development of the seminiferous tubules and inhibit development of accessory glands. Progestins are also potent inhibitors of spermatogenesis by blocking the release of LH from the pituitary. The pituitary-suppressing activities of sex steroids make them useful as contraceptives.

Steroidogenic Function

The fetal testes synthesize androstenedione and testosterone before and during differentiation of the accessory reproductive organs and regression of the Müllerian system. The male tubular genitalia, accessory sex glands, and secondary sexual characters develop and function under the influence of testicular androgens.

Secondary sexual characters can be classified as special or general and are not directly related with the reproductive process, although they may be important to identification and mating behavior. Special sex characters are organs or appendages that serve for adornment, attraction, or combat, and these characters often differ qualitatively between sexes. Sex plumage of birds is an outstanding example of a special secondary sex character. In some species, including deer and elk, antlers are limited to males. General sex characters, unlike special sex characters, differ quantitatively between the sexes. Muscular and skeletal development are the most notable examples of general sexual characters (Fig. 8-3).

The extratesticular role of androgens in maintaining male secondary sex characteristics is well established. Androgens also support spermatogenesis. The germinal epithelium has a higher testosterone requirement for normal function than other androgen-dependent tissues. In fact, the close association of the Leydig cells

with the seminiferous tubules (Figs. 8-1 and 8-4) provides high local concentrations of testosterone to the tubules. Intratesticular changes in testosterone concentration may act as a regulatory mechanism on capillary permeability and flow, altering the secretion of testosterone by the Leydig cells. This regulatory mechanism may be exerted directly on the Leydig cells or indirectly on the Sertoli cells. A small peptide, a GnRH-like factor called gonadocrinin, is produced by the Sertoli cell. Gonadocrinin appears to act locally at the interstitial-tubular system to serve as an intratesticular regulator of testosterone secretion (Fig. 8-4). This GnRH-like factor increases the Ca^{2+} permeability of the Leydig cells. The Sertoli cells also produce an androgen-binding protein (ABP), which serves as a protein carrier for testosterone. This ABP protein apparently maintains a high concentration of testosterone within the tubular compartments of the mammalian testis. The concentration of testosterone in the testicular artery leaving the pampiniform plexus is consistently higher than the concentration of testosterone in the systemic blood in the monkey, rat, ram, and bull. This suggests a transfer of steroids from testicular venous blood to the testicular artery in the pampiniform plexus. The venous-arterial transfer of steroids may function to enrich the supply of testosterone and other steroids to the testes and epididymides.

The interstitial Leydig cells of the testis produce androgens, including testosterone, in response to LH (ICSH) stimulus and in synergy with FSH and probably with prolactin. Prolactin regulates secretion of testosterone by the Leydig cells by increasing the number and affinity of receptors for LH on the Leydig cells. The interaction of LH with receptors in the Leydig cells activates the adenyl cyclase system, including protein kinase activation and RNA synthesis, resulting in an increased production of pregnenolone from cholesterol by the mitochondria in the Leydig cell (Fig. 8-5). Intracellular enzymatic side-chain cleavage of pregnenolone occurs in the mitochondrion and leads to the production and finally release of testosterone by the Leydig cells (Fig. 8-5). The Leydig cell appears to be the only testicular cell that can synthesize

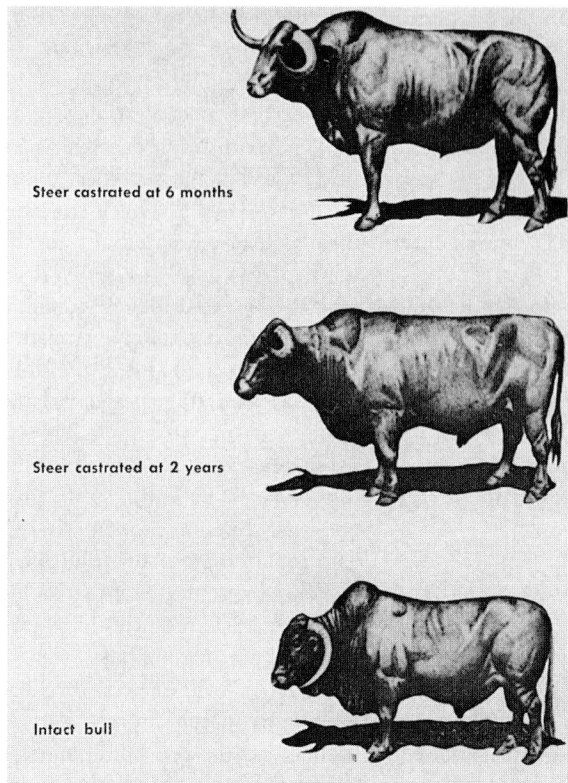

Fig. 8-3. Influence of sex hormones on hair, muscular development, and skeletal growth. All three animals are 12 years old. (Source: J. C. Bonsma, Wortham Lectures in Animal Science. College Station, TX, Texas A & M University Press, 1965).

testosterone from cholesterol. For some species, there are evidences indicating that testosterone produced by the Leydig cells is uptaken in a paracrine fashion by the Sertoli cell, which, under the influence of FSH, converts it to estradiol (Fig. 8-6). The estradiol produced by the Sertoli cells may in turn have a regulatory activity in the production of testosterone by the Leydig cells, because specific receptors for estradiol have been demonstrated in the Leydig cells of some species. Thus, normal spermatogenesis in the adult testes represents the result of a complex interaction between the cells of the germinal epithelium, the Leydig cells and the secretion of testosterone, the Sertoli cells and the secretion of estrogens, and gonadotropins from the pituitary gland. Growth factors such as IGF-1 and -2 and other local regulators, perhaps acting in an autocrine fashion, may also participate in the control of Leydig and Sertoli cell secretions. The adrenal cortex also secretes androgens, but the amounts normally secreted must be small.

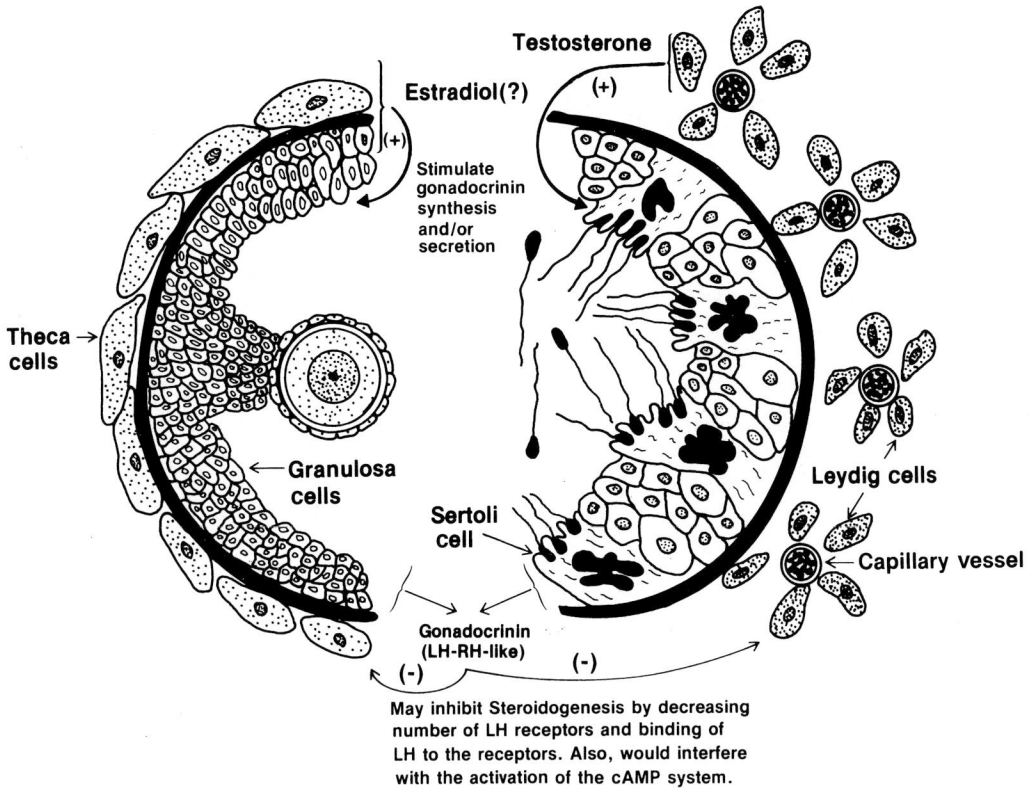

Fig. 8-4. Postulated physiologic function of gonadocrinin on the Sertoli, Leydig, and granulosa cells. (Adapted from different sources, including: R. M. Sharp, J. Reprod. Fertil. *64*:517, 1982).

Orchiectomy in animals with intact adrenals undergo profound atrophy of accessory sex organs and secondary sex characters. In dogs, bilateral orchiectomy is followed by a rapid decline in blood levels of testosterone associated with an increase in blood levels of LH and FSH.

Puberty, the onset of reproductive capacity, is the result of complex interactions of the hypothalamus, the anterior pituitary gland, the gonads, conditioning of the target organs or "aging" of the somatic substrate, and environmental factors such as nutrition. An animal that has reached puberty becomes puberal or pubertal. These terms are synonymous. Pubertal, postpubertal, and adult types of Leydig cells can be observed in the stallion and other species, reflecting the maturational and physiologic changes for the transitional period from prepu-

berty to puberty and adult Leydig cell steroid secretion. Function of the Leydig cells precedes the formation of spermatozoa, suggesting that androgens condition the seminiferous tubules to respond to gonadotropic stimulation and spermatogenesis.

Sexual maturity is the state of full reproductive capacity. The interval between puberty and sexual maturity is adolescence. Several seminal characteristics have been shown to change quantitatively during adolescence. As the animal approaches puberty, changes in the androstenedione/testosterone ratios with advancing age and an increased concentration of 17β-hydroxysteroid dehydrogenase activity in the testes of bulls, rams, rats, stallions, Rhesus monkeys, and men are indicative of the establishment of the adult pattern of testicular secretion.

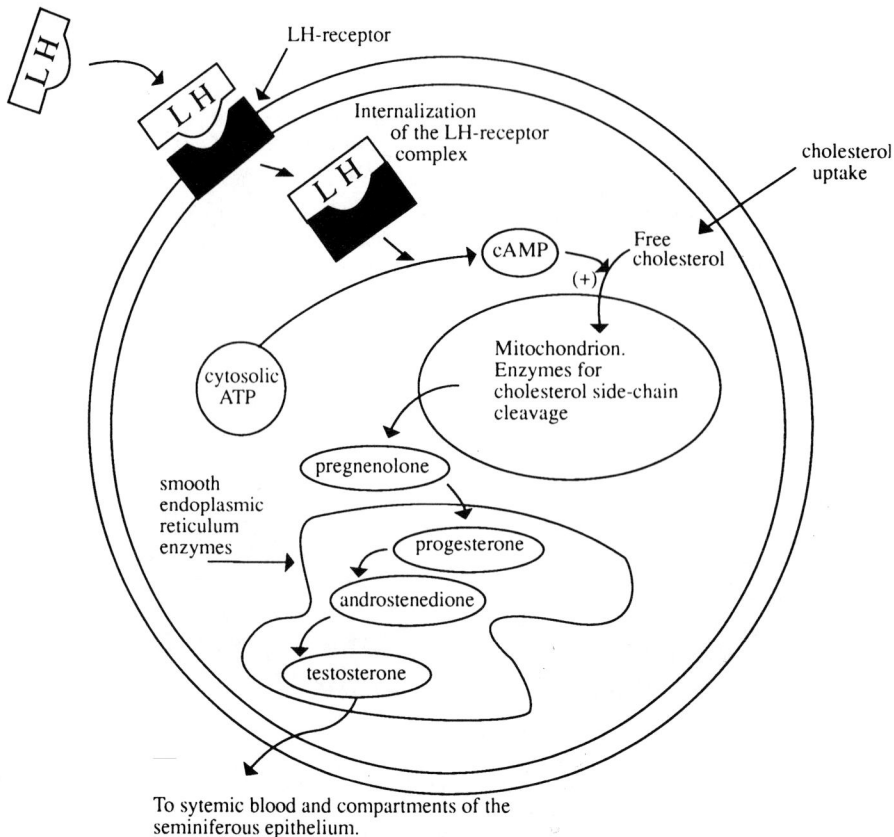

Fig. 8-5. Synthesis and production of testosterone by the Leydig cell. (Adapted from: A. H. Payne and G. L. Youngblood, Biol. Reprod. *52*:217, 1995).

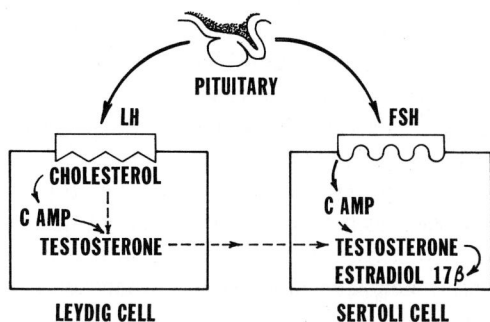

Fig. 8-6. Paracrine interactions between Leydig and Sertoli cells.

Table 8-2   Levels of Testosterone (ng/ml) in the Systemic Blood

Species	Testosterone (mean ± standard error of the mean)
Alpaca	0.20 − 1.50[a]
Boar	4.00 ± 0.50
Bull	6.70 ± 0.20
Cat	6.33 ± 0.35
Dog	2.20 ± 0.70
Goat	6.22 ± 0.70
Llama	0.30 − 0.65[a]
Ram	5.22 ± 0.66
Stallion	2.10 ± 0.10

Adapted from: Ø. Andresen, J. Reprod. Fertil. *48*:51, 1976; L. V. Swanson, et al. J. Anim. Sci. *33*:823, 1971; V. K. Ganjam and R. M. Kenney, J. Reprod. Fertil. *52*:67, 1975; B. D. Schanbacher and J. J. Ford, Endocrinology *99*:752, 1976; G. Zlotnik, J. Reprod. Fertil. *32*:287, 1973; L. De Palatis, et al., J. Reprod. Fertil. *52*:201, 1978; M. B. Taha and D. E. Noakes, J. Small Anim. Pract. *23*:351, 1982; and I. P. Johnstone, et al., Anim. Reprod. Sci. *7*:363, 1984.

[a]Values shown for the llama and alpaca are ranges. (From: P. W. Bravo, Vet. Clin. N. A., *10*:259, 1994).

Blood levels of testosterone are shown in Table 8-2. The concentration of steroids and other hormones per unit volume of blood is highly variable among individuals and over time in the same individuals, particularly for those that are seasonal breeders. Hormonal levels in the blood are dependent upon not only secretion, release, and metabolic clearance rates but also the age of the animal, season of the year, time of day, and circadian rhythms. The frequency of sampling, conditions of sampling (sexually stimulated versus nonstimulated; conscious versus anesthetized), and the sensitivity and specificity of the immunoassay system also affect the values obtained.

The classic methods of studying the effects of testicular hormones are castration or bilateral orchiectomy and replacement therapy. Interpretation of the results of these methods must include several important considerations. The changes occurring after bilateral orchiectomy may reflect the residual effects of extragonadal influences, which are synergized or antagonized by testicular steroids. The effects of replacement therapy may be primary or secondary to effects on other systems. Testicular steroids may exert permissive effects on target organs that allow the effects of a second factor to be expressed.

Male sex steroids have both androgenic and anabolic activities at the target cell level (Fig. 8-7). The androgenic activity stimulates growth and function of accessory reproductive organs and the development of special sex characters, which constitutes the basis for bioassay of these hormones. The anabolic activity stimulates constructive metabolism and the development of general sex characters (Fig. 8-7).

Body Size and Shape

Larger body size with more massive development of component parts in males is nearly

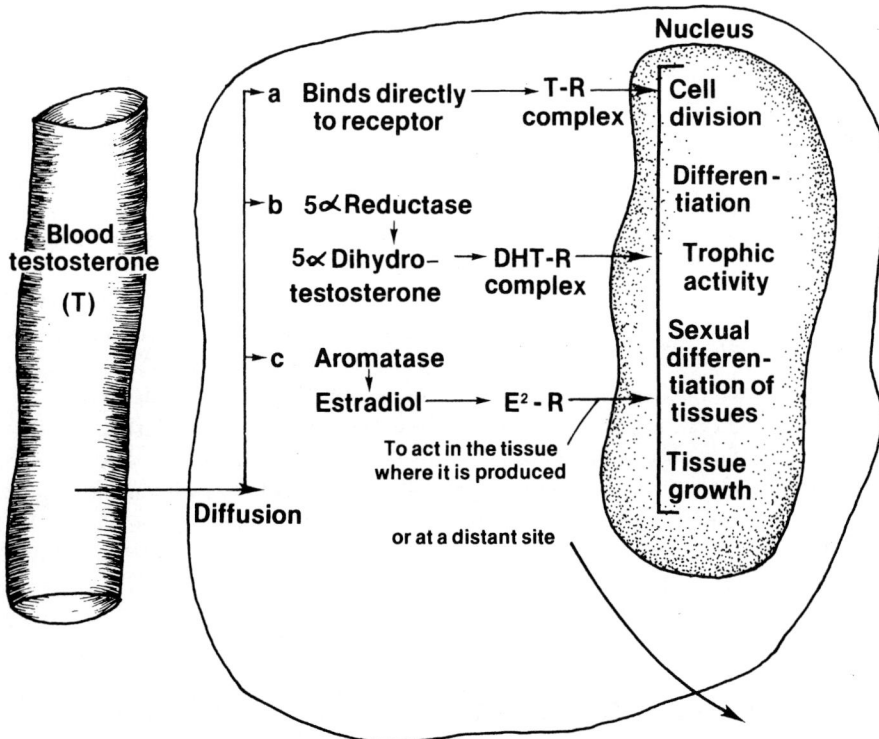

Fig. 8-7. Major pathways of metabolism of testosterone in target cells. (Adapted from: C. W. Bardin and J. F. Catterall, Science *211*:1285, 1981).

universal among animals. Bulls, in which mature body weight is frequently double the weight of mature females of the same breed, are extraordinary examples. Gonadal steroids influence ossification of the epiphyses in both sexes.

Steroids with androgenic activity have myotropic activity. Massive muscular development in the male can be related to copulatory postural requirements and aggressive social mannerisms related to mating behavior.

Complex interrelationships exist between fat compartments and sexual function. Excessive fat deposition has been related to lowered reproductive function in both sexes. Excessive fat deposits in the neck of the scrotum appear to lower seminal quality, probably by insulating against normal heat loss. Effects of fat deposits on the steroidogenic function are unknown. Fat deposits may cause reproductive impairment by sequestering the fat-soluble steroid hormones.

Other Characteristics

Greater longevity of the females than of the males of several species is known, but it is not always clear whether the difference is a direct effect of gonadal steroids. Male sex steroids influence hair pigmentation and growth in mammals and feather pigmentation and growth in poultry. The hair coat of highly masculine males tends to be darker, especially in certain body regions, than the coat of castrates or females. Hair fibers of males are coarser than those of females or castrates.

Testis-Pituitary Relationships

The pituitary gland has several sexual dichotomies. The female generally has a larger gland than the male. Sex differences in the relative percentages of acidophils, basophils, and chromophobes, as well as differences in the staining qualities of the chromophilic granules, have been reported. Sex differences in total gonadotropic potency and the relative activities of FSH and LH are common, but considerable species variation exists as to which sex has the greater potencies. The preoptic area of the female hypothalamus contains a center that regulates the ovulatory surge of LH. This center is not functional in males.

Leydig cell function declines as the male ages. The mechanisms acting to induce a hypofunctional activity of the Leydig cells in the aged animal remain undetermined. In some species, such as in rodents, total gonadotropic output declines with age, whereas it increases in other species, such as in humans. Age-related intracellular changes in the Leydig cells may influence the response of these cells to local intratesticular factors and to pituitary control of their secretory activity.

Following castration, the male hypophysis enlarges more than the female gland, abolishing the sex difference in size. Vacuolated "signet ring" basophils form in the pituitary glands of both sexes in some species following castration, and the percentage of basophils and gonadotropic activity increase. Estrogens are generally more effective than androgens in preventing castrational changes in the pituitary of either sex.

Testosterone inhibits the secretion of pituitary gonadotropins by a negative feedback mechanism (Fig. 8-1). The relative pituitary-depressing and androgenic activities, like the relative anabolic and androgenic activities, vary among the androgenic steroids. Thus, some androgens suppress pituitary gonadotropin secretion to a greater extent than they stimulate spermatogenesis, development of accessory sex organs, and expression of secondary sex characters.

The existence of inhibin, a nonsteroidal pituitary inhibitor of gonadal origin, was first postulated by McCullagh in 1932.[109] Inhibin is produced by the Sertoli cells and is present in testicular fluid, seminal plasma, and the ovarian follicular fluid. Inhibin selectively suppresses plasma levels of FSH without altering LH levels in castrated animals. In intact animals, inhibin appears to participate in the control of FSH secretion by the pituitary gland through a negative feedback control. Main products secreted by the Sertoli cells are presented in Table 8-3.

Testis-Adrenal Relationships

Adrenal cortices normally produce androgens, and adrenal androgen secretion may be greatly increased in a variety of pathological

Table 8-3 Secretory Products of the Sertoli Cells

Product	Function
ABP, androgen binding protein	Androgen transport to the male reproductive organs.
Estrogens, estradiol-17β	Control secretion of FSH and in a paracrine fashion, inhibit androgen secretion by the Leydig cells.
Essential nutritional components, including enzymes and amino acids, that cannot cross the blood testis barrier	Needed for the metabolism and survival of germinal cells, mainly those undergoing meiosis in the adluminal compartment of the seminiferous epithelium.
Gonadocrinin	Regulates LH secretion by decreasing the number of receptors to LH and the binding of LH to the receptors on the Leydig cells.
Inhibin	Control of FSH secretion.
IGF-1, Insulin-like growth factor 1	Growth and differentiation of germinal cells, possibly interacting with Leydig cells for steroid production.
IGF-2, Insulin-like growth factor 2	Presence in the Sertoli cells postulated.
MIH, Müllerian Inhibiting Hormone, produced by the Sertoli cells of the fetal testis	Prevents development of Müllerian organs in the fetal male.

Compiled from different sources, including: M. K. Skinner, Endocrine Rev. *12:*45, 1991; and B. P. Bullaney and M. K. Skinner, Bailliére's Clin. Endocrinol. Metab. *5:*771, 1991.

conditions, including adrenal hyperplasia or neoplasia, nymphomania in cattle, and adrenal virilism in women.

Special Sex Characters

In some species and in certain breeds within species, some body characters are qualitatively different according to sex and, thus are special sex characters. These include dichromism of the pelage (hair coat), horns in ungulates, vocalization, and behavior at urination.

The production of pheromones (See Chapter 7) is, in some cases, a secondary sex character because some pheromones are sex-specific and dependent on gonadal steroids. The Bruce and Whitten factors refer to pheromones produced by male rodents, which affect the reproductive cycle in females. Androgenic (C_{19}–Δ^{16}) steroids synthesized by the testes of the boar are released into the systemic circulation during sexual excitement. These steroids are metabolized to 5α-androsterone type of steroids in the salivary glands and are released in the saliva of the boar, bound to pheromaxein, a pheromone-binding protein. The ligands for pheromaxein are androstenol and other Δ^{16}-androstene-related androgens. These steroids induce a pheromonal response in the female pig in estrus, which results in the mating stance. These C_{19}–Δ^{16} steroids are also stored in the fat of the male and are responsible for the boar taint, the unpleasant, urine-like odor of cooked pork meat. In postpubertal boars, orchiectomy abolishes the androgenic activities of these substances. Fat content of 5α-androstenone is reduced in boars immunized against LHRH. Other chemical communicants are concerned with sexual behavior and identification of appropriate sex partners, and gonadectomy alters these activities. Moreover, castration has been reported to alter the development of olfactory perception.

Testis-Accessory Sexual Organ Relationships

The male accessory sex organs include the efferent ducts, epididymides, vasa deferentia and their ampullae, vesicular glands, prostate, bulbourethral glands, urethra, urethral glands, prepuce, preputial glands, penis, and scrotum. The effects of castration on these organs vary with the age and stage of development at which orchiectomy is performed. In general, prepuberal castration prevents normal development of accessory sex organs, whereas postpubertal castration leads to atrophy. In adults, function is a more accurate index of androgenic activity than size of the sexual accessory organs. The accessory sexual organs of males castrated as adults may retain their precastration size because the stroma is maintained while function is severely impaired.

In addition to stimulating growth of the penis, androgens stimulate cleavage of the preputial lamellae to form the preputial cavity. Preputial adhesions in prepuberal bulls may be mistaken for a pathologic process when electroejaculation is used to stimulate protrusion of the penis. The development of the penile spines in the cat is directly related to androgen levels, and the spines undergo atrophy after bilateral orchiectomy.

Hypertrophic or hyperplastic enlargement of the prostate is a common ailment in intact, aged male dogs. Castration often corrects the condition.

Seminal fructose levels decline rapidly following castration, and injections of testosterone restore the function of the vesicular glands. There appears to be a progressive loss of sensitivity of the vesicular glands to androgen stimulation following orchiectomy, and estrogens may synergize with testosterone or act to sensitize the vesicular glands to the stimulatory effect of testosterone.

Factors Affecting Leydig Cell Function

As would be expected, the steroidogenic function of the testis parallels the gametogenic activity in seasonal and continuous breeder animals. As a result, the accessory glands and special sex characters undergo corresponding changes in these species.

In contrast to the severe damaging effect of the intra-abdominal or other ectopic position of the testes on the germinal epithelium and spermatogenesis, the Leydig cells of artificially induced cryptorchid testes are functional for a time, as evidenced by the size of accessory sex glands, male aggressiveness, and libido. However, in time, cryptorchid testes weigh less, are less capable than scrotal testes to respond to gonadotropic stimulation, and may not secrete androgens normally. The endocrine activity of the Sertoli cells is also affected by cryptorchidism. In some species, high blood levels of FSH have been associated with cryptorchidism, suggesting that inhibin secretion is impaired.

Restriction of dietary intake, resulting in energy deficiency, causes atrophy and functional depression of the accessory sex glands. Energy restriction in rams reduces the testicular blood flow and uptake of oxygen and glucose as well as the daily output of testosterone. Exposure to severe cold ($-5°C$) causes atrophy of the accessory sex glands similar to that resulting from restriction of dietary energy. Low temperatures may reduce the flow of blood to the testis and thus cause a depression in androgen secretion.

The results of experiments to evaluate the effects of exogenous testosterone on Leydig cell function must be evaluated considering that doses equal to or greater than physiologic levels may suppress Leydig cell function, yet still maintain functional androgen-dependent organs.

Testicular Estrogens

Estrogens have been isolated from the testes of stallions, bulls, boars, dogs, and men. Estrogens may play a role in the pathogenesis of prostatic hyperplasia common in aged dogs, and estrogen receptors are present in the prostatic urethra and prostatic glands of dogs. The level of estrogenic activity in testicular venous blood from stallions is 20 times greater than the level in peripheral blood. Levels of estrogens in the blood of the spermatic vein draining the testis are higher than those in the peripheral blood of several species, including the canine. Estrogens, like androgens, are transferred from the testicular vein to the testicular artery. In several species, levels of estrogens in the blood of the testicular artery are consistently higher than the levels of estrogens in systemic blood. In bulls, about 12% of the estrogens in testicular venous blood are transferred to the testicular artery. The mechanisms involved in the transfer of steroids from the testicular vein to the artery in the pampiniform plexus and its physiologic role remains to be determined.

The ability of the testes to synthesize estrogens implies the presence of enzymes necessary for aromatization of the A ring and removal of the C-19 methyl group of the steroid molecule. Sertoli cells, under the control of FSH, contain the necessary enzymes for the conversion of testosterone to estrogens in general and estradiol-17β in particular.

The urine of stallions and male mules is one of the richest sources of estrogens, and the daily output of urinary estrogen in the stallion exceeds that of the nongravid mare by a factor of 100 to 200. In spite of this, the stallion is one of the most impressively masculine of all males of domestic species. Estrone is the major urinary estrogen in the stallion; there are relatively small levels of estradiol and no detectable levels of estriol. Estrone is also the major estrogen in the urine of male mules. The testes of the stallion have a low 17β-(testosterone) dehydrogenase activity and very high 19-(androstenedione) hydroxylase and aromatizing activities, compared to other species. As a consequence, most of the androstenedione, which serves as a precursor for both testosterone and estrone, is converted to estrone.

The ejaculate of the bull, stallion, and particularly the boar contains relatively high concentrations of estrogens. It has not been conclusively established whether the estrogens in the semen are contributed by the testes, the accessory sex glands, or both. Spermatozoa released from the Sertoli cells at spermiation may act as estrogen carriers.

Sertoli cells are the source of testicular estrogens and generally, Sertoli cell tumors in dogs are feminizing and contain high levels of estrogenic activity (see Chapter 16). Canine Sertoli cell tumors produce estrone and estradiol-17β. Unexpectedly, however, peripheral levels of inhibin are high in dogs with Sertoli cell tumors, and the peripheral levels of LH and testosterone are lower than in normal dogs. The blood levels of estradiol were not suppressed in spite of lower levels of FSH, suggesting that tumorous Sertoli cells respond differently than normal Sertoli cells to FSH stimulation. Because estrogens are more potent than androgens in inhibiting pituitary gonadotropin secretion, estrogens in the male may play an important role in regulating the pituitary-gonadal axis. Furthermore, in several species estrogens inhibit Leydig cell secretion of testosterone. In addition, β-endorphins produced by the fetal Leydig cells may, in a paracrine fashion, control Sertoli cell function during the fetal and the prepubertal and postpubertal period, including modulation of testicular tubular function during the adult life.

EXCURRENT TRACT

The excurrent tract includes the rete testis, efferent ducts, epididymis, vas deferens, and urethra. Semen is composed of spermatozoa and other cellular elements, as well as fluids contributed by a number of organs, including the accessory sex glands (Fig. 8-8). The relative contribution of the organs participating in the formation of semen varies between species and even between ejaculates from the same animal. The rete testis is a network of straight tubules connecting the convoluted seminiferous tubules with the efferent ducts. The convoluted seminiferous tubules are the sperm-producing tubules; the straight tubules do not have germinal epithelium but a simple, cuboidal epithelium. The rete testis tubules are mostly intratesticular, but they become extratesticular after penetrating the tunica albuginea to join the efferent ducts. The union of the rete tubules with the efferent ducts is extratesticular in the stallion and ram and probably also in other domestic species. The number of efferent ducts (ductuli efferentes) for the domestic species is shown in Table 8-4.

The simple cuboidal epithelium of the rete tubules becomes columnar, containing both ciliated and nonciliated cells at the union with the efferent ducts. The efferent ducts lie under the head of the epididymis and converge to form the epididymal tubule. The epididymal tubule is a single, highly convoluted tubule that may be as long as 50 meters in the bull and 70 meters in the stallion. Anatomically, the epididymis is divided into the head (caput), body (corpus), and tail (caudum) components. However, this anatomic division of the epididymis does not correspond with its histologic and functional characteristics.

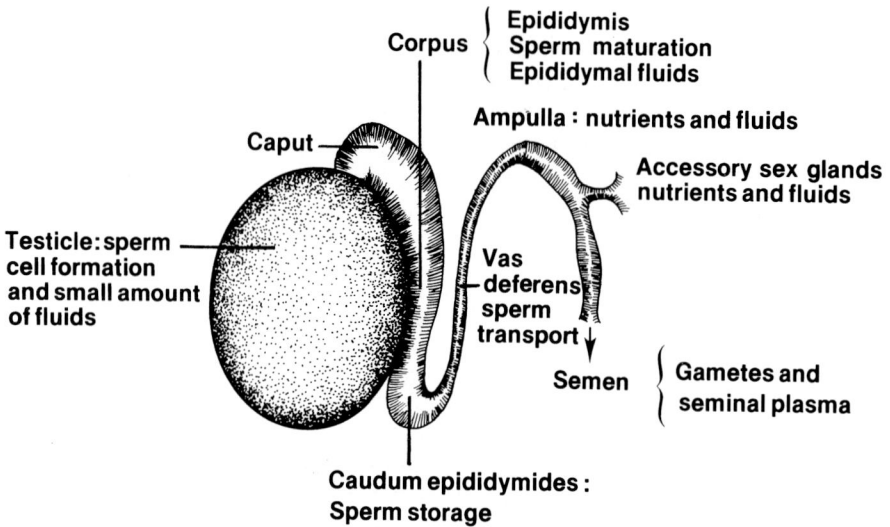

Fig. 8-8. Organs participating in the formation of semen.

Table 8-4   Number of Ductuli Efferentes in Domestic Species

Species	Range	Relative Frequency[a] of Blind-ending Ductuli
Boar	14–16	–
Bull	13–16	Common
Cat	14–17	–
Dog	13–15	–
Goat	18–19	Common
Ram	17–20	Common
Stallion	14–17	Common

[a]Spermiostasis in the head of the epididymis is common in the goat, ram, and bull, and may be associated with the number of blind-ending ductuli.
Adapted from: N. A. Hemeida, et al., Am. J. Vet. Res. *39:*1892, 1978; and H. O. Gayal and C. S. Williams, Anat. Rec. *220:*58, 1988.

The term **spermateliosis**, or **spermiogenesis**, is usually applied only to that phase of spermatogenesis in which spermatids are transformed into spermatozoa before spermiation, which is the release of spermatozoa from the Sertoli cells into the lumen of the seminiferous tubules. Spermatozoa do, however, undergo additional physicochemical changes between the rete testis and the *cauda epididymis.* These changes are described as maturational and are necessary for the spermatozoon to acquire fertilizing capability.

The nonmotile spermatozoa released into the seminiferous tubules are propelled through the rete testis into the epididymis by the contracting activity of myoid elements in the testicular capsule and the periphery of the seminiferous tubules and by the flow of testicular fluids (Fig. 8-9). During migration through the epididymis, spermatozoa develop the capacity for motility and fertility, whereas their resistance to thermal stress is decreased. Spermatozoa acquire the progressive, forward motility typical of mature sperm as they pass through the epididymides. The metabolic pattern of testicular spermatozoa differs from epididymal and ejaculated cells, indicating enzymatic changes within the cells, a change in metabolic substrate, or both.

Testicular fluid is absorbed in the efferent ducts and *caput epididymis,* causing sperm concentration to fluctuate throughout the epididymis. The absorptive capacity of the epididymis may be related to the fact that it develops from the mesonephros. The specific gravity of spermatozoa in the caudum or tail is greater than that of spermatozoa in the caput or head of the

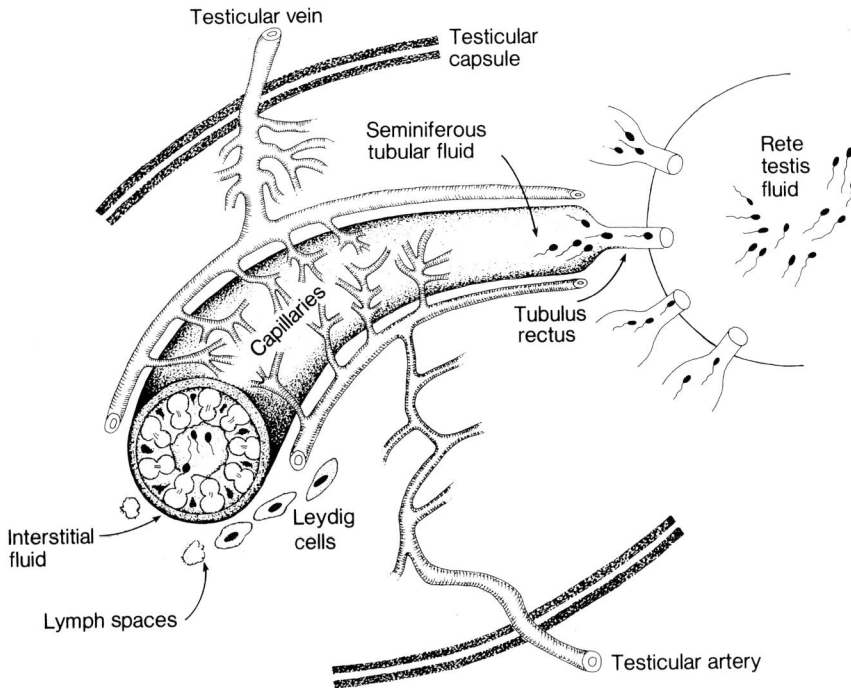

Fig. 8-9. Fluid compartments of the testis.

epididymis. Changes in the fluid environment of spermatozoa in the epididymis include changes in the concentration of electrolytes, especially sodium, potassium, and chloride, and of amino acids and proteins, phospholipids, and enzymes.

Sodium and potassium are reciprocally related in the spermatozoa and seminal plasma of several species. Potassium is concentrated in the cells, whereas the sodium concentration is high in seminal plasma.

Testicular and ejaculated spermatozoa from the boar, bull, and ram show qualitative and quantitative changes in phospholipid and fatty acids during epididymal passage and ejaculation. Epididymal spermatozoa of these species contain more total lipid than ejaculated cells. These changes in cellular lipids suggest that certain lipids are implicated in spermatozoal maturation, perhaps by serving as metabolic substrates for spermatozoa during their passage through the epididymis.

Testicular spermatozoa are more resistant to cold shock than epididymal spermatozoa, and resistance to thermal stress decreases from the head to the tail of the epididymis. Ejaculated spermatozoa have even less thermal resistance, and spermatozoa from second ejaculates survive freezing or cold shock better than those from the first ejaculate. Changes in cellular lipids may be associated with the degree of susceptibility of the cells to thermal shock, probably as a result of changes in membrane permeability.

As spermatids differentiate into spermatozoa, most of the cytoplasm enters into the formation of the midpiece and tail. Some of this cytoplasm persists at the base of the head (proximal droplet), moves down to the end of the midpiece (distal droplet), and is eventually lost from most spermatozoa during epididymal passage; the residual bead of cytoplasm is called the cytoplasmic or kinoplasmic droplet.

No physiological role has been defined for the cytoplasmic droplet, although the rods and granules in the droplet have been postulated to constitute an endogenous source of energy for spermatozoa in the proximal epididymis. These droplets are rich in hydrolase enzymes, and their disappearance from spermatozoa in the distal epididymis and ejaculate may thus be related to observed differences in metabolism of cells from various segments of the excurrent ducts. Large numbers of spermatozoa with droplets, particularly proximal droplet, in ejaculated spermatozoa indicate a disturbance in maturation or suggest frequent ejaculations.

In summary, the epididymis participates in three major functions, including spermatozoal transport, maturation, and protection of spermatozoa during storage, mainly in the tail of the epididymides. For most species, the bulk of ejaculated spermatozoa originates from the spermatozoa stored in the tail of the epididymides, with minor contribution from spermatozoa stored in the *vasa deferentia* and *ampullae.*

Spermatogenesis proceeds throughout the year in most domestic males, even though females may be out of season. This fact raises the question of the disposition of unejaculated spermatozoa during periods of sexual rest. In some rodents, spermiophages from the basal layer of cells lining the epididymis phagocytize spermatozoa in cases of obstructive azoospermia. However, in vasectomized animals or animals with obstruction of the vas deferens, spermatozoa accumulate in the epididymis, to the point of causing dilation and rupture of the epididymal tubule. Furthermore, there is a constant flow of semen from bulls and rams with fistulated *vas deferens,* suggesting the unejaculated spermatozoa are constantly eliminated through the vas deferens into the urethra. It is generally believed that the daily produced but unejaculated spermatozoa are released into the urethra and washed out during micturition because variable but considerable numbers of spermatozoa are found in the urine of sexually rested animals and men. However, spermatozoa have been found before ejaculation in the urine withdrawn with a catheter from the urinary bladder of rams or by cystocentesis from the bladder of dogs and cats, indicating that spermatozoa had flowed into the bladder during sexual rest. A series of old, but largely ignored, and new evidence clearly indicates that the pathway of least resistance in

nonejaculatory situations is for the flow of fluid and spermatozoa into the bladder, probably because of a relative higher resistance to the outflow presented by the penile urethra. Thus, retrograde flow of spermatozoa into the bladder during periods of sexual rest may provide a mechanism for the disposal of the daily produced but unejaculated spermatozoa. Furthermore, recent studies (Table 8-5) have demonstrated that there is retrograde flow of spermatozoa into the urinary bladder during electroejaculation in the cat, boar, bull, ram, lion-tailed macaques (*Macaca silenus*), Lowland gorilla, and men and, as a consequence, considerable losses of spermatozoa in the urine. Retrograde flow of spermatozoa into the bladder is not limited to ejaculation induced by electrical stimulation, because cats, dogs, and rams in which semen was collected with an artificial vagina had significant numbers of spermatozoa in the bladder (Table 8-5). Similarly, retrograde flow of spermatozoa into the bladder also occurs during mating in cats. The percentage of retrograde flow, estimated by dividing the total number of spermatozoa in the urine by the total number of spermatozoa displaced during ejaculation (the total number of spermatozoa in the urine plus the total number of spermatozoa in the ejaculate) varies considerably among species, between and within animals, and with seminal collections. The retrograde displacement of spermatozoa into the urinary bladder can be induced or prevented pharmacologically.[144,154,168] The percentage of retrograde flow may reach values as high as 50% or even exceed 90%. A retrograde flow of 100% of the spermatozoa displaced should be termed retrograde ejaculation because the anterograde or antegrade ejaculate would be devoid of spermatozoa. Retrograde ejaculation is a pathologic condition that appears to be more frequent in men than in domestic animals. However, the retrograde flow of spermatozoa into the bladder, defined as the displacement of part of an ejaculate into the urinary bladder, appears to be a component of the ejaculatory process when semen is collected by artificial means and probably occurs at the beginning of the seminal emission (Fig. 8-10).

Table 8-5 *Summary of Studies on Retrograde Flow of Spermatozoa into the Urinary Bladder of Domestic Animals*

Animals	Method to Collect Semen	Method to Collect Urine	Percentage of Retrograde Flow[a] Mean	SD	Range	Reference[b]
Boar	DM	Catheterized bladder	0.15[c]	0.78	0–2.10	1
	DM	Catheterized bladder	0.03[c]	0.16	0–0.25	1
	EE(A)	Catheterized bladder	7.51[c]	17.80	0–32.69	2
Bull	EE(C)	Micturition	21.00[d]	17.00	1.00–50.00	3
Cat	EE(A)	Cystocentesis	68.33[d]	21.14	39.00–94.00	4
	EE(A)	Cystocentesis	69.05[c]	25.90	14.28–92.95	5
	AV	Cystocentesis	46.82[d]	31.67	14.56–90.32	5
Dog	DM	Cystocentesis	24.67[c]	33.98	0–99.75	6
Ram	EE(C)	Micturition	28.30[c]	30.00	0.30–100	7
	EE(C)	Catheterized bladder	20.10[c]	20.80	0.10–79.00	7
	EE(C)	Micturition	15.28[c]	29.89	0.03–94.60	8
	AV	Micturition	2.70[c]	4.78	0.21–19.38	8

[a]Percentage of retrograde flow: Total number of spermatozoa in the urine/total number of spermatozoa in the ejaculate or electroejaculate plus the total number of spermatozoa in the urine.

[b]Adapted from:
1. P. A. Martin, et al., Theriogenology *39:*945, 1993.
2. P. A. Martin, et al., Theriogenology *41:*869, 1994.
3. M. P. Dooley, et al., Theriogenology *26:*101, 1986.
4. M. P. Dooley, et al., Proc. 10th Int. Congr. Anim. Reprod. and A. I., Univ. Illinois, Champaign/Urbana, 1984, Vol. III, Brief Comm. No. 363.
5. M. P. Dooley, et al., Am. J. Vet. Res. *52:*687, 1991.
6. M. P. Dooley, et al., Am. J. Vet. Res. *51:*1574, 1990.
7. M. H. Pineda, Am. J. Vet. Res. *48:*562, 1987.
8. M. H. Pineda, Am. J. Vet. Res. *52:*307, 1991.

[c]Mean adjusted percentage of retrograde flow was obtained by subtracting for each animal the concentration of spermatozoa in the pre-ejaculation or pre-electroejaculation urine from the concentration of spermatozoa in the postejaculation or postelectroejaculation urine.

[d]Mean unadjusted percentage of retrograde flow.

Abbreviations: DM, digital manipulation, using the glove-hand method for the boar or the cone method for the dog; EE(C), electroejaculation, conscious; EE(A), electroejaculation, anesthetized; AV, artificial vagina.

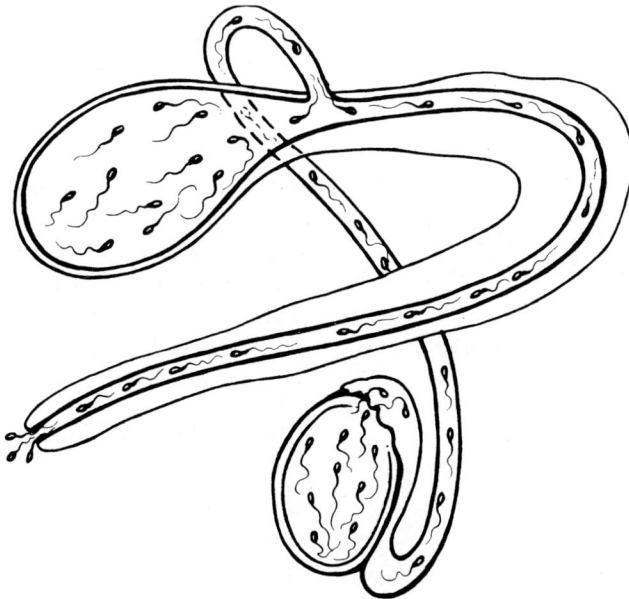

Fig. 8-10. Pathways of spermatozoal displacement during ejaculation.

In addition to its roles in sperm transport and maturation, the epididymis functions to store viable spermatozoa. Spermatozoa accumulate in the tail of the epididymis, which acts as a reservoir. Ejaculated spermatozoa in man, cat, dog, stallion, and probably in other species originate mainly from their site of storage in the *cauda epididymides* and to a lesser degree from the *vasa deferentia*. A large reservoir of mature spermatozoa in the tail of the epididymis is important for species, such as the ram, that copulate frequently or for species that produce ejaculates of large volume such as the boar and stallion. The location of the tail of the epididymis in the most distal, cooler part of the scrotum may be related to the storage function. While stored in the tail of the epididymis, spermatozoa from several species are immotile and do not acquire motility until exposed to the accessory sex gland secretions during ejaculation. Epididymal spermatozoa, however, can be rendered motile experimentally by incubation in their own epididymal fluid (Table 8-6) or in appropriate, chemically defined solutions. The existence of "immobilin", a high-molecular-weight epididymal glycoprotein, has been postulated. Immobilin would inhibit spermatozoal motility by creating a viscoelastic epididymal environment for the spermatozoa stored in the tail of the epididymis.

Epididymal dysfunction has been related to altered seminal quality, including increased spermatozoal morphologic defects and akinesia. Spermatozoal morphologic defects have also been related to degeneration of the epididymal epithelium. Bulls, rams, and dogs with microscopic and focal interstitial epididymitis frequently have lowered seminal quality, including an abnormally high percentage of spermatozoa displaying morphologic defects.

Epididymal function depends on androgen stimulation. In some species, such as rodents and monkeys, the need for androgens to maintain the structural and functional integrity of the epididymis is higher than that of other accessory sex glands. This is apparently true for other species as well.

During emission, spermatozoa and testicular and epididymal fluids are conveyed into the pelvic urethra by peristaltic contractions of the muscular walls of the excurrent ducts. Near the pelvic urethra of some species, an increase in the glandular elements of the deferent ducts forms the *ampullae* of the vasa. The glands of the ampullae are similar to those of the vesicular glands (which also are embryologic tributaries of the Wolffian duct), and their secretion provides the first notable carbohydrate substrate to semen. No distinct *ampulla* is formed in the boar or the tomcat.

The urethra receives ducts of a number of glandular tributaries, of which the accessory glands are prominent. Urethral or Littre's glands have not been extensively studied in domestic mammals, but urethral glands are not found in the bull or the dog.

Emission of contributions from the excurrent ducts and various accessory glands occurs in sequential fashion in the stallion, boar, and dog. In the bull and ram, emission is nearly instantaneous, with a mixing of contributions from various portions of the tract. However, presperm, sperm-rich, and postsperm fractions of bull ejaculates have been collected with an electro-ejaculator and on occasions during collection with an artificial vagina.

ACCESSORY SEX GLANDS

The accessory glands include the vesicular glands, the prostate, and the bulbourethral (Cowper's) glands. The occurrence and development of these structures vary widely among species (Fig. 8-11). Unlike mammals, birds,

Table 8-6   Motility of Spermatozoa Incubated in Their Own Epididymal Fluid

Source of Spermatozoa	Species		
	Boar	Bull	Ram
Testis	–	–	–
Epididymis			
caput	–	–	–
corpus	–	+	+
cauda	–	++	+++

Adapted from: J. L. Dacheux and M. Paquignon, Reprod. Nutr. Develop. *20:*1085, 1980.

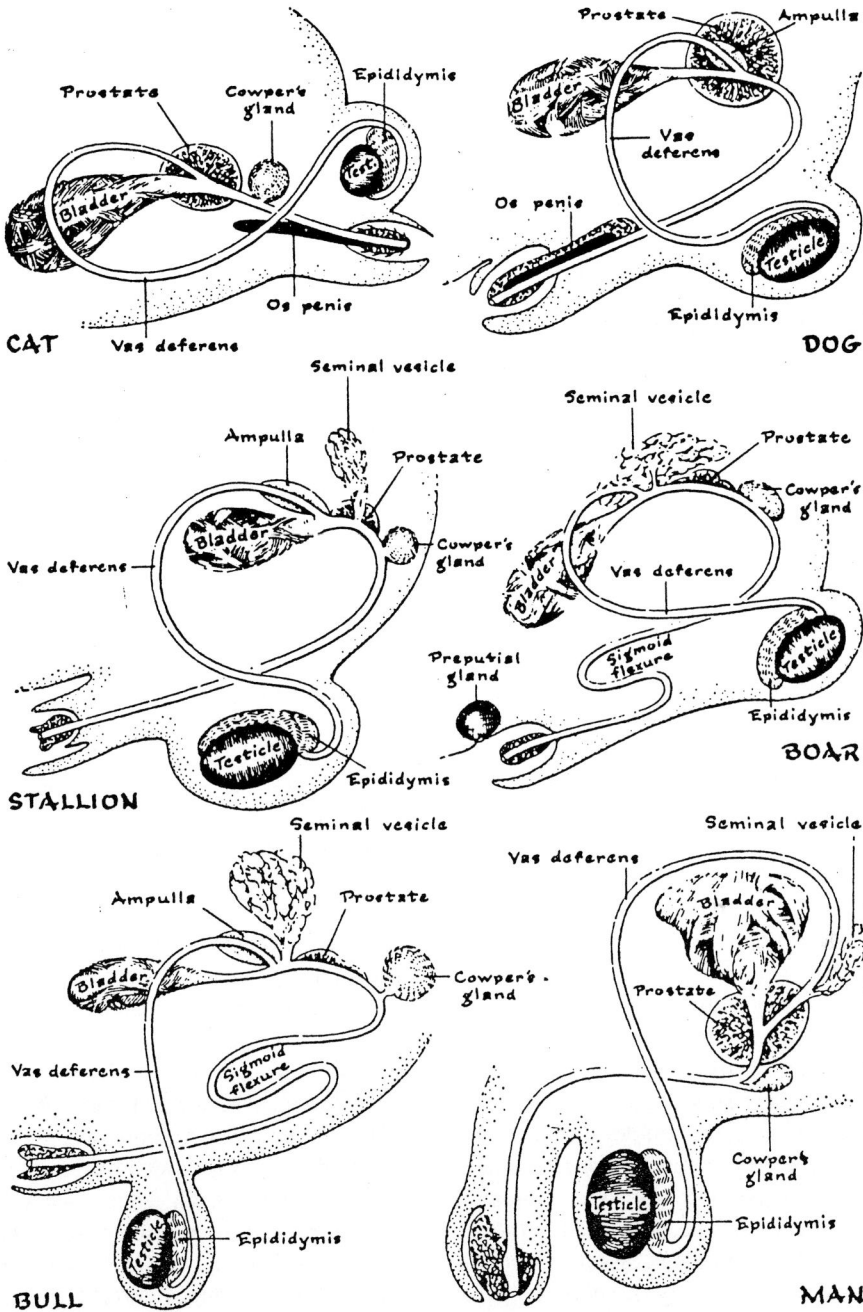

Fig. 8-11. Reproductive systems of the male cat, the dog, the stallion, the boar, the bull, and man. Compare the relative sizes of the various accessory glands and note that all these species have the prostate gland; that the dog and the cat have no seminal vesicles; that the dog has no Cowper's gland; that the cat, the boar, and man have no ampullar swelling; that the bull and the boar have the sigmoid flexure of the penis; that the dog and the cat have the os penis; that only the boar has the preputial pouch. (Reprinted with permission from: A. V. Nalbandov, Reproductive Physiology, 2nd ed. San Francisco, CA, W. H. Freeman and Co., 1964).

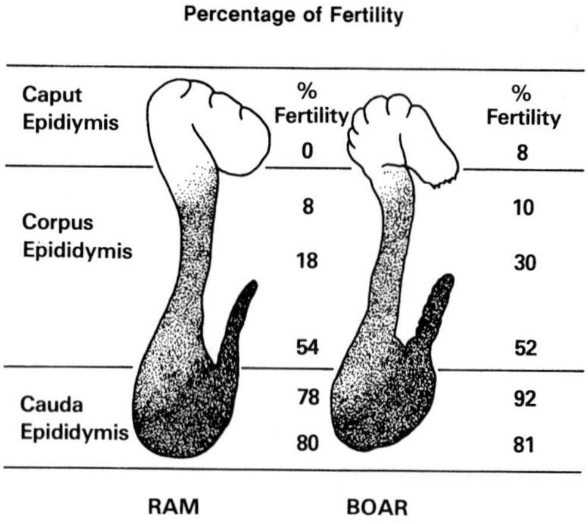

Percentage of Fertility

Caput Epididymis	% Fertility 0		% Fertility 8
	8		10
Corpus Epididymis	18		30
	54		52
	78		92
Cauda Epididymis	80		81

RAM   BOAR

Fig. 8-12. Fertility of spermatozoa from different regions of the epididymis in the ram and boar. (Adapted from: J. L. Dacheux and M. Paquignon, Reprod. Nutr. Develop. *20*:1085, 1980).

Table 8-7 Accessory Glands in Domestic Species and Camelids

Species	Vesicular Glands	Prostate	Cowper's
Bovine	+	+	+
Canine	−	+	−
Equine	+	+	+
Feline	−	+	+
Llamas and alpacas	−	+	+
Ovine	+	+	+
Porcine	+	+	+

such as the chicken and turkey, do not have accessory sex glands, but rather secretory cells in the epithelium of the excurrent ducts that add products to the semen.

Normal development and function of the accessory sex glands are controlled by testosterone, and the synergistic action of estrogens may also be required. In some species, testosterone must be converted to dihydrotestosterone to be physiologically active on the accessory glands.

The accessory glands contribute most of the volume to the ejaculate. Motility and metabolic activity of sperm are stimulated as the accessory gland secretions are added to the contributions from the testes and epididymides during ejaculation. Sperm-coating antigens are also secretory products of the accessory sex glands. A great deal of study has been devoted to the effects of constituents in the accessory glandular secretion on the physiology of sperm *in vitro,* but remarkably little is known about the role of normal or abnormal accessory glandular secretions in the function of spermatozoa while in the female tract.

Artificial insemination of caput and corpus epididymal and even testicular spermatozoa results in fertilized oocytes, but the fertility of

these cells is less than that of mature spermatozoa (Fig. 8-12).

Epididymal rabbit spermatozoa and spermatozoa from the vas deferens in cats are capable of fertilizing oocytes *in vitro,* without previous capacitation in the female tract. Ejaculated spermatozoa, however, require capacitation in most species.

The vesicular and prostate glands have been removed from boars and rats without impairing fertility, and the breeding efficiency of bulls in natural service has been acceptable following seminal vesiculectomy. The seminal vesicles are not, as their name implies, places of sperm storage. Vesicular glands is a preferable designation and more accurately describes the function of these glands. Sixty to ninety percent of the volume of fluid in normal ejaculates originates from the accessory glands, and the vesicular glands when present contribute a major portion. Vesicular glands are absent in the dog, llama, alpaca, and tomcat (Table 8-7).

The bovine and porcine prostate glands are composed of a body, which overlies the origin of the pelvic urethra, and a disseminate prostate, which surrounds the pelvic urethra. The ram's prostate consists of two lateral lobes that are connected by an isthmus dorsal to the origin of the pelvic urethra. The prostate gland of the dog, being the only accessory gland present, is well developed, contributes a large volume of fluid to the ejaculate, and is mostly delivered as part of the postsperm fraction of the ejaculate.

The bulbourethral (Cowper's) glands of most species of domestic mammals are relatively small, compact, round bodies located above the urethra near the pelvic outlet. The bulbourethral glands of the boar are large and cylindrical.

PENIS AND PREPUCE

With the exception of the dog, vaginal intromission of the penis requires full erection. The penis of the dog contains a bone, the os penis, which facilitates vaginal entry without full erection. In fact, the fully erected dog's penis cannot enter the bitch's vagina. Erection is accomplished by synergy of two mechanisms. The cavernous bodies of the penis become engorged through expansion of the arterioles, while the corresponding venules, which have strategically placed valves, contract. Secondly, the ischiocavernosus and bulbospongiosus muscles contract to compress the dorsal vein of the penis against the ischial arch. Structural abnormalities in the blood vessels of the penis may cause impotency in bulls, boars, and males of other species because of a deficient penile erection or the inability to sustain an erection until ejaculation has occurred. A pressure, greatly exceeding the systemic arterial pressure, develops in the corpus cavernosum penis during erection, reaching a peak pressure at ejaculation. For the bull, the pressure in the corpus cavernosum reaches a mean of more than 14,000 mm of Hg during ejaculation. Pressures of this magnitude help to explain the development and frequency of hematomas of the penis, a common clinical entity in bulls.

The extent to which the cavernous bodies expand to enlarge the penis during erection depends upon the development and composition of the tunic of connective tissue that surround and send trabeculae into the spongy tissues. Ruminants and boars have fibroelastic penes that enlarge slightly during erection, and protrusion of the penis is primarily achieved by straightening of the sigmoid flexure as a result of relaxation of the retractor penis muscle. The body of the dog's penis has considerable fibrous tissue, whereas the connective tissues of the glans are weakly developed and consist of a large proportion of elastic fibers and smooth muscle. Erection involves primarily the glans penis. In the

dog, enlargement of the *bulbus glandis* and contraction of vestibular muscles after intromission 'lock' the penis in the bitch's vagina. The stallion has no sigmoid flexure, and protrusion results by enlargement of the highly vascular penis, which is invested with elastic fibers and smooth muscle. The pressure in the corpus cavernosum of the stallion seldom reaches pressures higher than 1,500 mm of Hg during ejaculation.

The glans penis of the cat has cornified spines that function to stimulate the ovulatory response of the queen, the female cat, in this reflexogenously ovulating species. The canine glans penis has a long collum glandis and a prominent *bulbus glandis*. A distinct corona glandis appears just behind the urethral process in the erect canine penis.

The bull's penis is surrounded by lamellae important in the support and protrusion of the penis, which appears to be peculiarly susceptible to deviations during erection and protrusion. Spiral deviation of the bull's penis commonly occurs within the vagina during normal ejaculation. The architecture of the lamellae suggests that the penis is structurally adapted to perform this spiral deviation. In the clinical condition known as 'corkscrew penis', mating is prevented because spiraling occurs before intromission.

Except for the cat, the penes of most domestic animals are suspended by the prepuce from the ventral abdomen. The dog's prepuce is loose, allowing the glans penis to deflect posteriorly when the *bulbus glandis* engages the vulva and is anchored in the vestibule when the dog, while still ejaculating, dismounts the bitch. The penis of the cat is directed backward and downward from the ischial arch.

The penis is not free in the preputial cavity at the time of birth in most domestic animals. At birth, the epithelial surfaces of the penis and sheath are adhered as the balanopreputial fold. The fold is split into parietal and visceral layers by a cytolytic process that forms vesicles that coalesce to form the preputial cavity. Separation of the parietal and visceral layers is influenced by androgens.

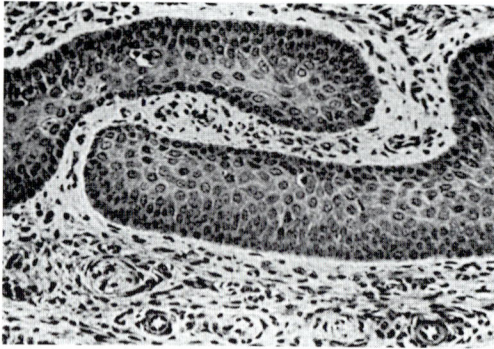

Fig. 8-13. Glans from a pup, showing an "S"-shaped mesodermal **primordium** of the **frenulum** interrupting the balanopreputial fold ventral to the urethra. Trichrome stain; ×350. (Reprinted with permission from: M. B. Bharadwaj and M. L. Calhoun, Am. J. Vet. Res. *22*:767, 1961).

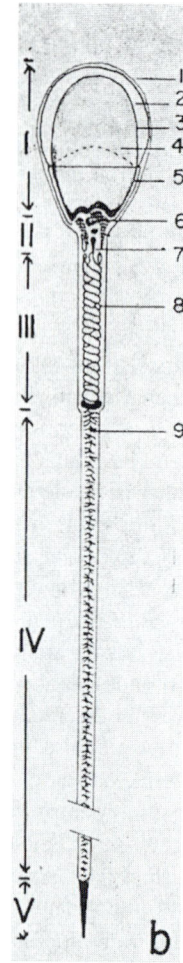

Fig. 8-14. Diagrammatic representation of a bovine spermatozoon. Parts are labeled with terms largely according to those suggested by Fawcett. **I**, head. **II,** neck. **III**, middle piece. **IV**, principal piece. **V**, end piece. **1**, cytoplasmic membrane. **2**, acrosome. **3**, nuclear membrane. **4**, nucleus. **5**, postnuclear cap. **6**, proximal centriole. **7**, axial filament. **8**, mitochondrial helix; and **9**, fibrous sheath. (Reprinted with permission from: S. H. Wu and J. D. Newstead, J. Anim. Sci. *25*:1186, 1966).

The balanopreputial fold is continuous in the boar. In dogs and bulls, the fold is discontinuous ventral to the urethra, leaving a band of fibrous tissue between the ends of the solid primary fold (Fig. 8-13). This band forms the frenulum in the dog and may persist in the bull to cause severe deviation of the penis or to prevent complete protrusion.

BIOLOGY OF SPERMATOZOA

The spermatozoon is a highly specialized cell that has evolved to perform the sole function of fertilizing an oocyte. The head is specialized to penetrate the oocyte to deliver its genetic payload. The tail contains the metabolic machinery to produce energy and provides the propelling mechanism for motility. Figure 8-14 is a diagrammatic representation of a bovine spermatozoon.

The head, which is usually flattened, is primarily a nucleus covered anteriorly by the acrosome (*galea capitis*, or head cap) composed of an outer and inner acrosomal membrane, connected by bridges, which apparently maintain the spacing and parallel arrangement of the acrosomal membranes. The nucleus is covered posteriorly by the postnuclear membrane. Between the nucleus and the acrosome lies the perinuclear substance. The perforatium or apical body is part of the perinuclear substance and

may play a role in fertilization (see Chapter 7). The ultrastructural features of the head of a bull's spermatozoon are illustrated in Figure 8-15. The shape of the head varies greatly among species. During spermateliosis, the spermatid nucleus gradually takes the shape characteristic of the species as the chromatin condenses.

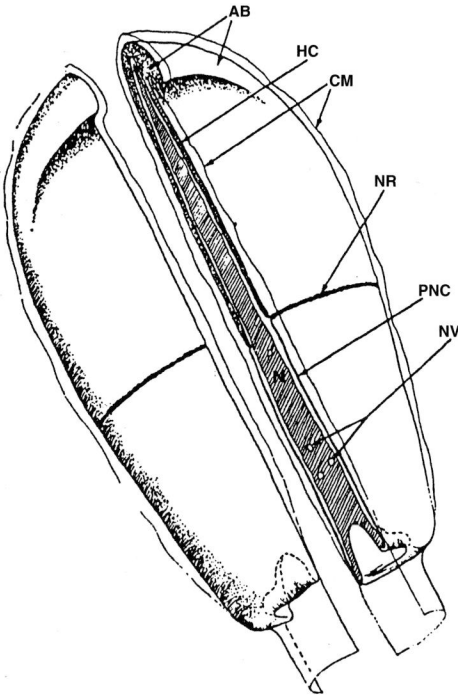

Fig. 8-15. Ultrastructural features of the bovine sperm head. Apical body (**AB**); head cap (**HC**); cell membrane (**CM**); nuclear ring (**NR**); nucleus (**N**); postnuclear cap (**PNC**); nuclear vacuoles (**NV**). (Reprinted with permission from: R. G. Saacke and J. O. Almquist, Am. J. Anat. *115*:144, 1964).

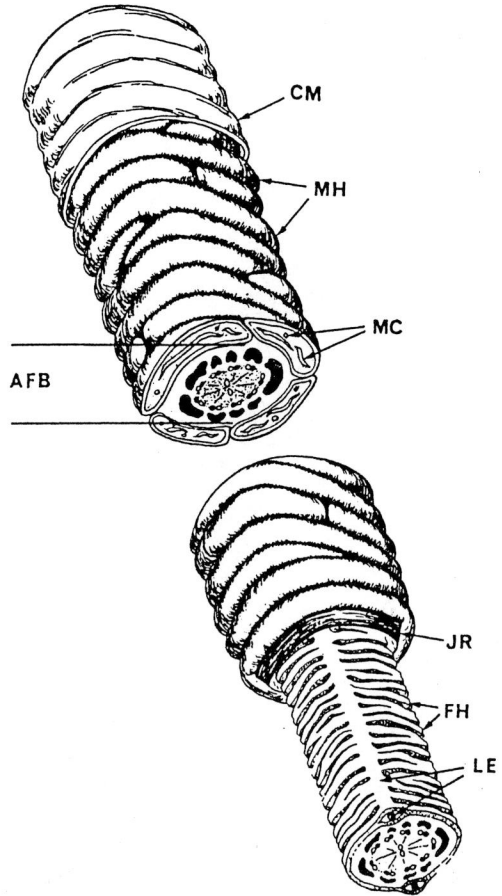

Fig. 8-16. Ultrastructural features of the middle piece and anterior portion of the principal piece of the tail of the spermatozoon. The cell membrane has been partially removed and the flagellum cut to show the internal structure. Cell membrane (**CM**); mitochondrial helix (**MH**); mitochondrial cristae (**MC**); Jensen's ring (**JR**); fibrous helix (**FH**); longitudinal element (**LE**); axial fiber bundle (**AFB**), consisting of the nine outer coarse fibers, the nine inner fibers or doublets, and the central pair of fibers. (Reprinted with permission from: R. G. Saacke and J. O. Almquist, Am. J. Anat. *115*:165, 1964).

The tail consists of the middle piece, principal piece, and terminal piece. A delicate neck joins the middle piece and head. The metabolic apparatus, a sheath of mitochondria, surrounds the flagellar filament in the middle piece. When compared to the mammalian oocyte, the number of mitochondria in the middle piece is small, around 80 to 100 mitochondria. Spermatozoal mitochondria, as the oocyte mitochondria, contain DNA, but the contribution of spermatozoal mitochondrial DNA to the oocyte during fertilization appears to be negligible, because the mitochondrial DNA is maternally inherited in the offspring (see Chapter 7). The flagellar fibrils extend the length of the tail. Figures 8-16 and 8-17 illustrate the ultrastructure of the spermatozoal tail.

Our meager knowledge of the physiology of spermatozoa after deposition in the female genital tract limits the usefulness of measurements of seminal characteristics *in vitro*. This is particularly true of measures of metabolic activity. One of the first decisive discoveries of the influence of the female environment on spermatozoal function was the phenomenon of spermatozoal capacitation (see Chapter 7).

Substantial concentrations of glycerylphosphorylcholine, primarily an epididymal contri-

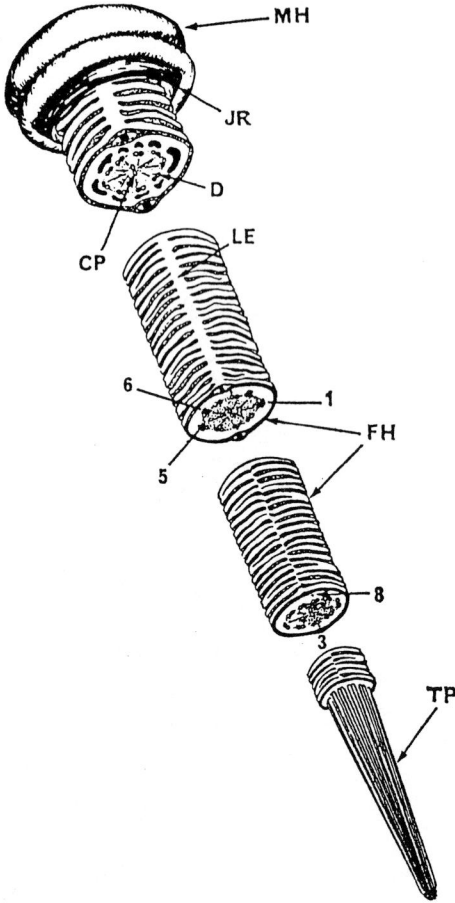

Fig. 8-17. Graphic illustration of the principal piece and terminal piece of tail of the spermatozoon. The cell membrane has been removed and the principal piece has been cut at various locations to show the internal structure. Mitochondrial helix (**MH**); Jensen's ring (**JR**); central pair of fibers (**CP**); doublet (**D**); longitudinal element (**LE**); fibrous helix (**FH**); terminal piece (**TP**). (Reprinted with permission from: R. G. Saacke and J. O. Almquist, Am. J. Anat. *115*:169, 1964).

erol and phosphoglycerol, could serve as energy sources by entering the glycolytic pathway. Secretions of the female reproductive tract stimulate the metabolic activity of boar, bull, rabbit, dog, ram, and rooster spermatozoa.

An overwhelming abundance of spermatozoa are deposited in the female tract during each natural service, and the apparent requirement for a minimum number of motile sperm in the artificial insemination dose ensures the presence of large numbers of motile cells in the female tract following insemination. Among domestic mammals, the survival of sperm in the female genital tract is usually limited to a few days at or near the time of ovulation. The dog is a notable exception, as motile and fertile spermatozoa are present in large numbers for at least 6 days after copulation and motile spermatozoa are present as long as 11 days after mating. Removal of ejaculated spermatozoa from the female tract after mating is accomplished by mechanical evacuation through the vulva, leukocytic phagocytosis, and cytolysis.

SEMEN

The efficient production of meat, milk, and other animal products depends first and foremost upon successful reproduction. The maximal utilization of superior genetic material in the gametes of companion, sporting, and work animals is of primary concern to the breeders of these animals. At the present stage of technology in animal reproduction, the greatest selection pressure is exerted against the male's gametes. The male is immensely more capable of yielding a harvest of germinal cells than is the female, and spermatozoa from single sires are used to fertilize oocytes in as many dams as possible. From this point of view, submaximal fertility in individual males is of greater consequence than submaximal fertility in individual females. However, the development and use of superovulation and embryo recovery and transfer techniques facilitates the utilization of superior genes in females. Thus, the role of the female's fertility is important to increase reproductive rates in species such as the bovine and equine, which have characteristically low reproductive rates.

bution, are found in the semen of rams, bulls, stallions, goats, rabbits, and men. Spermatozoa are incapable of metabolizing this abundant seminal substrate *in vitro,* but glycerylphosphorylcholine diesterase activity has been found in the uterine washings of the ewe, cow, sow, rat, and mouse. Uterine glycerylphosphorylcholine diesterase activity is regulated by ovarian steroids and is greatest when estrogen levels are high. The products of uterine hydrolysis, glyc-

Evaluation of Seminal Quality

Lagerlöf[234] reviewed the history of the evaluation of seminal quality and histologic investigations of the testes associated with infertility. An evaluation of seminal quality is an important consideration in assessing fertility levels and for diagnosing male reproductive disorders. Histologic examinations of tissues from the male reproductive tract are essential to the understanding of seminal physiology and pathology, but they are of distinctly limited value in clinical veterinary medicine. Often the biopsy of testicular tissue *per se* causes permanent damage to the testes. These techniques should be used sparingly until biopsy techniques for obtaining meaningful samples of tissue are perfected.

There are some distinct limitations to relating seminal quality to fertility that must be appreciated. The ejaculate is a composite of contributions from the testes, excurrent ducts, and accessory sex glands. The seminal sample reflects the function of each contributing portion of the reproductive tract and its interactions with all other portions. Because the secretion of accessory glandular fluid is reasonably concurrent with ejaculation, the accessory gland contributions are a fairly accurate reflection of current functional status. The epididymal and testicular contributions, on the other hand, reflect past events in these portions of the tract.

Physical and Chemical Properties of Semen

The composition of semen varies among species, individuals of the same species, and ejaculates from the same individual. Seminal quality may be modified by disease, frequency of ejaculation (including masturbation), nutrition, and other management factors, such as season, age, amount of sexual preparation, method of collection, and magnitude of retrograde flow of semen into the urinary bladder. Also, procedures of handling the ejaculate during and after collection, analytic techniques and variation among technicians, pharmacologic agents, and normal physiologic variation are all sources of variation that affect seminal quality. Each potential source of variation should be recognized

and accounted for in the interpretation of analyses of seminal quality. Many of these sources of variation can be controlled. Collection, handling, and analytic techniques for semen evaluation should be standardized, and the analytic procedures should be as objective, repeatable, and reliable as possible.

No single measurement of seminal quality has been found to be a reliable criterion for predicting fertility of a given male. Correlations of fertility with measures of quality in semen used for artificial insemination have the distinct advantage that individual ejaculates are used to inseminate relatively large numbers of females. Correlation coefficients based on the results of artificial insemination are usually biased, however, by the large number of normal, motile spermatozoa inseminated and by the use of semen that has been selected for high quality. Seminal characteristics are better correlated to fertility when the samples are drawn from an unselected population. Many biologic correlations are not linear for the range of all possible values for the independent variable (Fig. 8-18). Hence, correlation between a seminal characteristic and fertility will depend upon the range of values of the characteristic in the seminal samples used to determine the relationship.

In addition to the possibility of bias in the samples of semen used in computing relationships between seminal quality and fertility, there is the possibility of bias in the female population. Seminal quality must be characterized

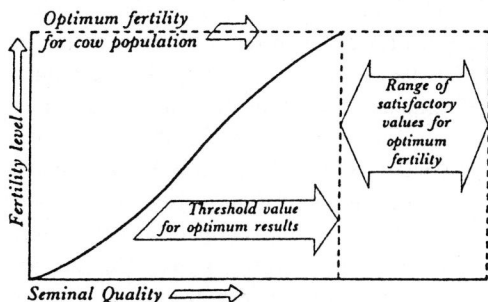

Fig. 8-18. Fertility increases with increasing quality of bull semen until the threshold for optimum fertility is reached. (Reprinted with permission from: G. W. Salisbury and N. L. VanDemark, Physiology of Reproduction and Artificial Insemination of Cattle. San Francisco, CA; W. H. Freeman & Co., 1961).

before or after the breeding period, and the number of females exposed per unit time is restrictive. The more females that are inseminated by single ejaculates, the less will be the bias in this direction. A further advantage of computing the relationship of seminal quality to fertility in artificial insemination programs is that male mating behavior is eliminated as a variable. Moreover, the inseminating dose, within the limits of processing and technician errors, is the same for all inseminations.

It is nearly impossible to obtain reliable coefficients of correlation that apply to natural mating. Single females are naturally inseminated during mating by a single ejaculate containing large yet variable numbers of spermatozoa. Furthermore, there is no way to separate the contributing secretions from the female's tract to accurately measure the seminal characteristics of that ejaculate.

The evaluation of seminal quality should incorporate as many useful measurements of seminal characteristics as possible within the limits of practicality. The procedures used should be based on the purpose of the evaluation. Routine seminal analyses at artificial insemination centers usually include volume, spermatozoal concentration, total number of spermatozoa per ejaculate, and percentage and rate of motility as minimal procedures. Examinations of seminal quality for research purposes usually include these plus a variety of additional measures of physical, chemical, and metabolic characteristics. In evaluating sires for potential breeding soundness, the results of the seminal analysis must always be interpreted in terms of the intended use of the sire and after a thorough physical examination. Valuable sires, especially those destined for service in artificial insemination centers, should be examined for venereal diseases or other infectious diseases that may be transmitted through insemination. Attempts to diagnose specific infertility may include hormone assays, microscopic examination of tissues obtained by testicular biopsy, chemical analysis of semen to assess testicular and accessory sex glandular function, special studies of spermatozoal morphology and ultrastructure, *in vitro* fertilization of zona free, homologous and heterologous oocytes, and heterospermic inseminations.

A thorough discussion of the properties of semen and evaluation of seminal quality is beyond the scope of this chapter. Table 8-8 summarizes published values of seminal characteristics; in addition, the reader should address reviews and original papers listed in the reference section under the headings of Biology of Spermatozoa, Evaluation of Seminal Quality, and Physical and Chemical Properties of Semen.

MATING

Copulatory behavior is composed of several elements that vary among species and individuals, but the pattern is remarkably similar among species. The male mounts the female from the rear and **clasps** his forelegs about her laterolumbar region (Fig. 8-19A). Rapid movement of the forelegs along the female's sides is termed **palpation**. Palpation is frequently accompanied by rapid, piston-like movements of the pelvis, called **pelvic thrusts** (Fig. 8-19B). If intromission is not achieved and the male dismounts, the mount is termed an **attempt** or **incomplete copulation**. When intromission is achieved, with or without ejaculation, the mount is called a **complete copulation** (Figs. 8-19C and D). Copulatory behavior of the male goat is depicted in Figure 8-20. Copulation with ejaculation is followed by a **refractory period**, during which mating behavior in the male is not aroused by any sexual stimuli. The refractory period may be shortened by intensifying the sexual stimulus. When the refractory period is excessively prolonged, the male is said to be **satiated**. Satiation is followed by a **recovery period**.

Frequency of copulation varies with the species, among the domestic species, and with a number of factors such as breed, health, ratio of males to females, and dimensions of the breeding area. Rams and tom cats may copulate several times in an hour. Some rams have been observed to copulate over 50 times in 24 hours. Bulls are also frequent copulators, especially after a period of sexual rest. Stallions and boars may copulate 3 to 4 times in a day but are satiated after fewer ejaculations than the ram or bull. Dogs, probably because of the prolonged

Table 8-8 Composition of Semen as Collected with an Artificial Vagina or by Digital Manipulation of the Penis in Boars and Dogs (values are mg/100 ml unless otherwise indicated)

Constituent or Property	Bull	Ram	Goat	Stallion	Boar	Dog	Cat	Llama
1. Volume of ejaculate, ml	4.0(2.0–10.0)	1.0(0.7–2.0)	0.80–0.98	70(30–300)	250(150–500)	6.0(2.0–16.0)	0.06(0.03–0.09)	1.7(0.4–4.3)
2. Spermatozoa, millions/ml	1,000(300–2,000)	3,000(2,000–5,000)	2,940–3,330	120(30–800)	100(25–300)	65(10–300)	---	0.35–0.60
3. Total number of spermatozoa in ejaculate (millions)	4,000 (2,000–12,000)	3,000 (2,000–11,000)	2,352–3,263	8,400 (3,600–13,000)	25,000 (15,000–50,000)	390(60–3,000)	61(22–117)	0.60–1.02
4. Spermatozoa, size,[a] μm	65; 9 × 4 × 1; 13; 44	---	8 × 4	58; 7 × 4 × 2; 10; 42	57; 8 × 4 × 1; 11; 38	60; 7 × 4 × 1; 10; 34	---	---
5. Specific gravity	1.034(1.015–1.053)	---	---	---	---	1.011	---	---
6. Freezing point depression, –°C	0.61(0.54–0.73)	0.64(0.55–0.70)	---	0.60(0.58–0.62)	0.62(0.59–0.63)	0.58–0.60	---	---
7. Conductivity, mho × 10^{-4}	105(90–115)	63(50–80)	---	123(110–130)	129(125–134)	129–138	---	---
8. pH	6.9(6.4–7.8)	6.9(5.9–7.3)	7.0–7.2	7.4(7.2–7.8)	7.5(6.8–7.9)	6.4(6.1–7.0)	8.3(8.1–8.6)	---
9. Water, g/dl	90(87–95)	85	---	98	95(94–98)	98	---	---
10. Carbon dioxide, ml/dl	16	16	---	24	50	---	---	---
11. Sodium	230(140–280)	190(120–250)	103(60–183)	70–275	650(290–850)	89(56–124)[b]	---	---
12. Potassium	140(80–210)	90(50–140)	158(76–255)	60–103	240(80–380)	8.2(8–8.3)[b]	---	---
13. Calcium	44(35–60)	11.6(10–15)	11.3(5–15)	26	5(2–6)	0.7(0.4–0.9)[b]	---	---
14. Magnesium	9(7–12)	8(2–13)	3(1–4)	3–9	11(5–15)	0.5(0.3–1.00)[b]	---	---
15. Chloride	180(110–290)	142	125(82–215)	270(90–450)	330(260–430)	151	---	---
16. Phosphorus, total	82	132	---	19	357	13	---	---
17. Acid-soluble P	35	12	---	14	171	---	---	---
18. Inorganic P	9	9	---	17	6	---	---	---
19. Lipid P	9	3	---	---	2.2	---	---	---
20. Zinc	2.8(2.6–3.7)	0.28	---	---	6	7.1–8.7	---	---
21. Nitrogen, total	897(441–1,169)	875	---	310	615(335–765)	361(299–406)	---	---
22. Nitrogen, nonprotein	48	57	---	55	22(15–31)	25	---	---
23. Ammonia	2	2	---	1	1	---	---	---
24. Urea	4	44	---	3	5	---	---	---
25. Uric acid	3	4–23	---	---	3	---	---	---
26. Creatine	3	21	---	3	---	---	---	---
27. Creatinine	12	---	---	12	0.3	---	---	---
28. Ergothioneine	0–trace	0–trace	---	7.6	15	---	---	---
29. Spermine	0	---	---	0	0	---	---	---
30. Phosphorylcholine	Trace	0	---	0	0	---	---	---
31. Glucose	300	0	Trace	82	0	116	---	---
32. Glycerylphosphorylcholine	350(100–500)	1,650(1,100–2,100)	809	40–100	110–240	180(110–240)	---	---
33. Fructose	530(150–900)	250–372	875	2(0–6)	13(3–50)	Trace	---	---
34. Citric acid	720(340–1,150)	140(110–260)	---	26(8–53)	130(30–330)	0–30	---	---
35. Lactic acid	30(15–40)	---	73	15(9–15)	30	44(22–77)	---	---
36. Inositol	35(25–46)	12(7–41)	---	30(11–47)	530(380–630)	---	---	---
37. Ascorbic acid	6(3–9)	5(2–8)	---	---	3.5(2–5)	---	---	---
38. Phosphatase, acid[c] U/dl	170(50–340)	High	---	---	---	---	---	---
39. Phosphatase, alk.[c] U/dl	400(100–3,500)	---	---	---	---	---	---	---
40. Amylase	---	---	---	---	+	---	---	---
41. Arysulfatase activity (μmol/hr/mg protein)	0.08 spermatozoa; 0.21 seminal plasma	---	---	0.28 spermatozoa; 0.11 seminal plasma	0.40 spermatozoa; 0.55 seminal plasma	0.75 spermatozoa; 1.01 seminal plasma	---	---
42. Cholinesterase	+	++	---	---	---	---	---	---
43. Cytochrome	++	+	---	+	+	+	---	---
44. β-glucuronidase	+++	++	---	+	0	---	---	---
45. Hyaluronidase	+++	---	---	---	++	+	---	---
46. 5-Nucleotidase	+++	+	---	---	+	---	---	---

[a] Values are, respectively: total length; length × width × thickness of head; length of mid-piece; length of tail.

[b] m Eq/L

[c] U = units, one unit indicating activity necessary for liberation of 1 mg, phenol from monophenylphosphate in one hour at 37°C.

Single values represent means and ranges are not given unless information was provided in the original publication. Only ranges are given when not enough data is available to establish a representative mean.

Adapted from different sources, including: I. G. White, Anim. Breed. Abst. 26:110, 1958; J. H. Boucher, et al., Cornell Vet. 48:67, 1958; K. L. Polakoski and M. Kopta. In: Biochemistry of Mammalian Reproduction, 1982, p. 97; T. T. Olar, et al., Biol. Reprod. 29:1114, 1983; M. P. Dooley and M. H. Pineda, Am. J. Vet. Res. 47:286, 1986; B. M. Gadella et al., Biol. Reprod. N. A. 10:259; G. Mendoza et al., Theriogenology 32:455, 1989; C. G. Gravance et al., Theriogenology 44:989, 1995.

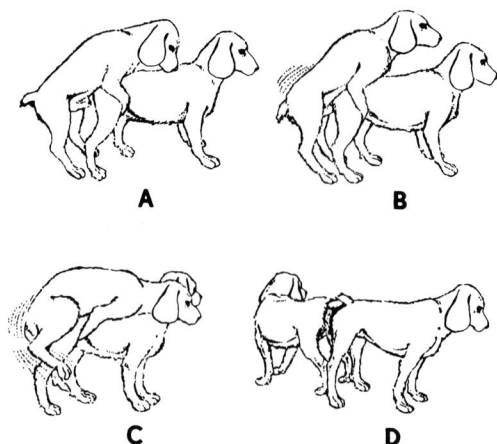

Fig. 8-19. Different stages in mating behavior of the male dog (drawn from motion picture prints): **A,** mounting and clasping. **B,** pelvic thrusting. **C,** intense ejaculatory reaction. **D,** copulatory lock. (Reprinted with permission from: B. J. Hart, J. Comp. Physiol. Psychol. *64*:390, 1967).

ejaculation with vaginal locking, and boars, because of the prolonged ejaculation and large volume of ejaculate, are capable of only a few ejaculations in a 24-hour period.

Sexual experience is an important factor in sexual behavior. Sexual behavior persists for variable periods after castration. Postcastration sexual behavior depends upon the species, age, and sexual experience of the male.

Ejaculation depends on the normal integrity and function of the autonomic nervous system, which coordinates seminal emission, closure of the urinary bladder sphincters, and ejaculatory displacement of seminal components through the penile urethra. The contractile activity of the urethral musculature seems to be under the control of catecholamines, and adrenergic receptors in the urethra of horses and dogs have been reported.

Copulatory patterns are influenced by the anatomy of the penis and the contributions of the accessory glands to seminal volume (Table 8-9). The duration of copulation is roughly proportional to the duration of ejaculation. Copulation is rapid in the bull, billy goat, and ram, which have fibroelastic penes and ejaculate relatively small volumes of semen. The refractory period

is relatively short in these species. The boar also has a fibroelastic penis, but the volume of the ejaculate is remarkably large, and copulation is prolonged. The male llama also has a fibroblastic type of penis and ejaculates a small volume of ejaculate, but the copulation is prolonged. The stallion has a vascular penis and ejaculates a large volume of semen; copulation is accordingly prolonged. The dog's penis is uniquely adapted to the prolonged emission of the prostatic fluid, while the *bulbus glandis* is engaged in the vulva. The "belling" of the glans of the stallion's penis probably plays a similar role. Copulation may be characterized by repeated intromissions in species, such as the cat and rabbit, in which LH, the ovulatory hormone, is released from the pituitary of the female by a neuroendocrine reflex elicited by the penial stimulation of the vagina.

Optimal copulation frequency varies considerably among unselected males. Thus, it is difficult to make general recommendations. Each male should be used according to his own capabilities within the limits of the conditions under which he is used. Among the factors to be considered are:

1. **Physical Condition**. Males with acquired physical impairments must be used in limited service. Excessively fat or thin males are considered debilitated for breeding purposes.

2. **Seminal Quality and Sperm Reserves**. Males with semen of high quality and a high daily output of spermatozoa should be used heavily. Males with inferior seminal quality or low daily spermatozoal output should not be used or used only in limited service and only when of superior genetic value. **Daily spermatozoal production** (DSP) refers to the number of spermatozoa produced daily by the testes and can be expressed as the number of spermatozoa produced per gram of testis or as the total number of spermatozoa produced. DSP is estimated by quantitative histologic analysis of testicular tissue. **Daily spermatozoal output** (DSO) refers to the number of spermatozoa ejaculated and collected with an artificial vagina or by electroejaculation after a period of frequent collections to deplete the spermatozoal reserves.

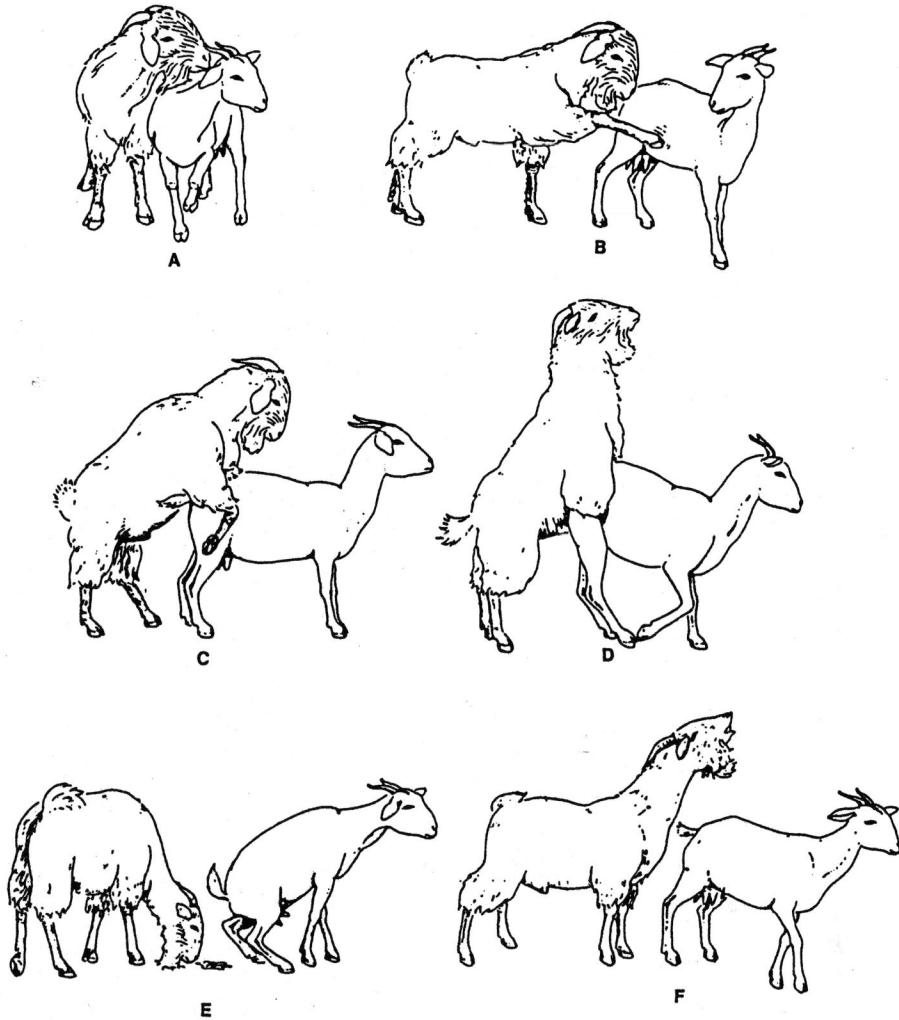

Fig. 8-20. Sexual responses of the male goat. **A**. Nudging the female. **B**. Flexing the foreleg against the female in short, choppy kicking motions. **C**. Mounting without intromission. **D**. Mounting with intromission and ejaculation as characterized by a deep penile thrust and backward retraction of the forelegs. The upward head bounce, shown here, evidently occurs at the moment of ejaculation. **E**. Olfactory investigation of female urine. **F**. Characteristic posture of the Flehmen response that occurs just after sniffing urine of an estrous or anestrous female. (Adapted from: B. L. Hart and T. O. A. C. Jones, Hormones and Behav. *6*:251, 252, 1975).

The DSP and DSO, as expected, are lower for postpubertal males, but increase as the animal approaches sexual maturity. The DSP and DSO for sexually mature animals are presented in Table 8-10.

For all of the domestic species studied to date, the DSP is higher than the DSO (Table 8-10). Several factors, including spermatozoal losses in the collection equipment, phagocytosis and epididymal absorption of spermatozoa, or overestimation of the DSP, have been considered to explain the difference between the DSP and DSO. Lino[162] and coworkers first proposed in 1967 that the DSP for the ram could be estimated by determining the number of spermatozoa voided daily in the urine during periods of sexual rest. Lino's observations were largely ignored or disputed on the assumption that the large number of spermatozoa in the urine of sexually rested rams was due to unnoticed mastur-

Table 8-9   Relationship Between Type of Penis, Volume of Ejaculate, Type of Copulation, and Site of Seminal Deposition

Species	Type of Penis	Volume of Ejaculate (ml)		Type of Copulation	Site of Deposition
		Mean	Range		
Billy goat	Fibroelastic	0.70	0.5–0.9	Rapid	Vagina
Boar	Fibroelastic	250.00	150–500	Prolonged	Uterus
Bull	Fibroelastic	4.00	1.7–10.0	Rapid	Vagina
Cat	Vascular (os penis) with spines	0.06	0.03–0.09	Rapid	Vagina
Dog	Vascular (os penis)	6.00	2.0–16.0	Prolonged	Vagina
Llama	Fibroelastic	1.70	0.4–4.3	Prolonged	Cervical/uterus
Ram	Fibroelastic	1.00	0.7–2.0	Rapid	Vagina
Stallion	Vascular	70.00	30–300	Prolonged	Uterus

Table 8-10   Daily Sperm Production and Daily Sperm Output in Six Domestic Species

Species	Daily Sperm (10^9)			
	Production		Output	
	Mean	Range	Mean	Range
Boar	16.5	---	16.3	---
Bull	5.3	3.2–6.7	2.7	1.7–4.0
Dog	0.48	---	0.37	---
Goat	---	4.0–6.4	---	---
Ram	10.5	7.8–13.9	2.9	5.5–8.6
Stallion	8.0	5.7–10.6	7.0	4.4–8.7

Adapted from: E. E. Swierstra, Biol. Reprod. *2:*23, 1970 (boar); E. E. Swierstra, Can. J. Anim. Sci. *46:*107, 1968 (bull); T. T. Olar et al., Biol. Reprod. *29:*1114, 1983 (dog); A. J. Ritar et al., J. Reprod. Fertil. *95:*97, 1992 (goat). Data for the ram estimated from: R. P. Amann (1970): Sperm Production Rates. *In:* The Testis, edited by A. D. Johnson, W. R. Gomes, and N. L. VanDemark, New York, NY, Academic Press, Inc. p. 433; R. Ortavant and C. Thibault, Compt. Rend. Soc. Biol. *150:*358, 1956; and A. W. N. Cameron, et al., Vol. II. Comm. 266, 10th Int. Congr. Anim. Reprod. A. I., 1984. M. B. Gebauer, et al., J. Anim. Sci. *39:*732, 1974 (stallion).

bation. The finding of a significant percentage of retrograde flow of spermatozoa into the bladder (Table 8-5) during electroejaculation of rams, bulls, and cats, during ejaculation within an artificial vagina in rams and cats, during natural matings in cats, or during ejaculation induced by digital manipulation of the penis in dogs strongly suggests that the determination of the total number of spermatozoa in the ejaculate and in the urine collected immediately after ejaculation would accurately estimate the total number of spermatozoa displaced during the ejaculatory process. In boars, the overall mean percentage of total urinary losses of spermatozoa during ejaculation, including retrograde flow into the bladder and urethral retention, is less than 0.5% (Table 8-5) of the total number of spermatozoa displaced during the ejaculatory process.[163] This is consistent with the fact that for boars, the DSO is nearly 100% of the DSP (Table 8-10). Thus, Lino's approach[162] could be adapted to noninvasively monitor the DSP of individual animals in a variety of experimental or field situations.

Testicular diameter is a simple clinical measurement that, in some but not all of the domestic species, correlates with spermatogenic activity. Spermatogenic deficiencies that are heritable should not be perpetuated, and males with such deficiencies should not be used as sires. Fortunately, some reproductive deficiencies are self-limiting. Unfortunately, sires with such deficiencies may be outstanding in other characteristics upon which selection is based, and a sound reproductive apparatus has been historically overlooked as a criterion for selection.

3. **Breeding Management.** The ultimate efficiency in the use of a male is obtained through artificial insemination. Males used in handbreeding programs, in which estrous females are presented to the male for single or limited multi-

ple services, may be used to inseminate more females than when pasture or random mating is practiced.

The size and topography of the breeding pastures limit the number of females that may be assigned to a male in pasture breeding programs. When several males are together in a breeding pasture, social dominance and fighting reduce the effectiveness of individual sires. Males in multi-sire pastures should be kept dispersed to reduce this problem to a minimum.

4. **Length of Breeding Season.** A male may be used to inseminate more females in a prolonged breeding season if the number of females is evenly distributed over the breeding period.

5. **Individual Mating Behavior.** Some easily measured criteria that correlate with mating behavior are sorely needed. For example, some bulls are known to inseminate cows with a single mating, then move on to seek other estrous cows; other bulls mate repeatedly with a single female before searching for other cows in heat. Some bulls travel over large pastures daily in search of estrous cows; other bulls wait for cows in heat to come to water or a salt lick; still other bulls prefer to group and fight. Unfortunately, the complex interactions between males and females may limit the usefulness of measures of mating behavior. For example, bulls are known to "fall in love" with certain females, and the bull will devote his undivided attention to a single cow throughout estrus, and sometimes proestrus as well, while other cows in heat are ignored and unable to attract his service.

Recommendations for service frequency are presented for each of the domestic species in the corresponding Chapters for Reproductive Patterns.

SPERMATOZOAL TRANSPORT

Efficient transport of a number of viable spermatozoa from the site of deposition during mating (Table 8-9) or insemination to the site of gametic encounter in the ampulla of the oviduct is essential to successful fertilization. In most mammals, the transport of spermatozoa is rapid; they reach the oviduct shortly after insemination.

The highest concentration of spermatozoa is found at the site of seminal deposition, and the number of spermatozoa decreases rapidly in the ovarian direction so that few spermatozoa reach the site of gametic encounter in the oviducts.

For a short time following mating or artificial insemination, uterine contractions are more important to the transport of spermatozoa in the female tract than is spermatozoal motility. The rate of transport through the tract is too rapid to be accounted for by the spermatozoa progressive motility. Moeller and VanDemark[323] estimated the maximum velocity of bull spermatozoa *in vitro* as 126 cm per hour. Because the bovine reproductive tract is about 65 cm in length, the fastest spermatozoon would require about 30 minutes to reach the ampulla of the oviduct. Notwithstanding, bull spermatozoa have been found in the ovarian portion of the oviduct within 2.5 minutes following intracervical deposition of motile cells and within 4.3 minutes following insemination of nonmotile cells. Although few spermatozoa are rapidly transported to the ampullary region of the oviducts, these may not participate in the fertilization of the oocyte. The establishment of a population of viable, fertile spermatozoa within the oviducts is a much slower process. In the sheep, significant numbers of viable spermatozoa enter the oviducts within 6 to 8 hours after mating and remain arrested in the caudal isthmus until the time of ovulation, when they are transported to the anterior oviduct. Similar rates in the transport of a population of spermatozoa have been observed for heifers, gilts, and laboratory rodents. It is possible that the retention of spermatozoa in the isthmus is related to a more efficient spermatozoal capacitation and may serve to protect the capacitated spermatozoa from the anterior oviductal environment, because spermatozoa that are capacitated are relatively fragile and short-lived. Contractility of the female genital tract appears to be the dominant force in transporting spermatozoa to the oviducts in other species, too. Spermatozoal motility, however, does influence transcervical migration and distribution of spermatozoa in the female tract and may be important in the penetration of the oocyte during fertilization.

The reflexogenous release of oxytocin in response to visual and tactile stimuli also plays a role in the transport of spermatozoa in cattle, in which natural mating and artificial insemination cause milk ejection and increased uterine contractions. Motile or nonmotile bull spermatozoa were transported from the cervix to the tubal infundibulum of excised cow tracts in 2.5 to 5 minutes when oxytocin was present in the perfusate. When oxytocin was absent from the perfusate, cells did not penetrate beyond the body of the uterus. Epinephrine inhibits the effect of oxytocin in stimulating both milk ejection and uterine motility in the cow. For this reason, cows should be handled as quietly as possible in preparation for milking or breeding. However, oxytocin secreted at the time of mating does not seem to have a significant effect on spermatozoal transport in ewes.

Spermatozoal transport into and through the cervix was inhibited in ewes that had grazed subterranean clover with estrogenic activity. Because ewes that graze pastures containing plants with high estrogenic activity also have a high incidence of maternal dystocia (difficult birth) due to uterine inertia, the impaired transport of spermatozoa may also be due to the inhibition of myometrial activity. Foreign devices such as an intrauterine plastic spiral in one horn of the uterus in ewes prevent spermatozoal transport in both horns, probably as a result of impairment of neurogenic stimuli for myometrial activity. Uterine contractions in the form of segmentation waves would tend to disperse semen throughout the uterus. Seminal plasma, identified by its characteristic components or by radioactive labeling of components, is distributed rapidly throughout the uterus. Relaxin, produced by the prostate gland, appears to stimulate spermatozoal motility when spermatozoa are exposed to the secretion of the accessory glands. Relaxin in the seminal plasma of several domestic species and humans may also contribute to spermatozoal penetration of the oocyte envelopes.

Although uterine contractions are unquestionably important for the rapid transport of spermatozoa in most species, other mechanisms of transport cannot be regarded as unimportant

to the reproductive process. Natural insemination through mating usually occurs several hours before ovulation, and the rate of transport may be less important to conception and fertilization rates than the number of capacitated spermatozoa at the fertilization site in the ampulla of the oviduct. Additional factors influencing spermatozoal transport include the negative intrauterine pressure, the movement of genital fluids, the propensity of spermatozoa for rheotaxis (counterflow orientation), ciliary movements in the oviduct, and the volume and concentration of spermatozoa in the inseminating dose.

The cervix, the uterotubal junction, and possibly the isthmus of the oviduct are especially critical barriers for spermatozoal transport, and only a fraction of the cells in the preceding segment of the tract pass through these areas (Figs. 8-21 and 8-22). The glans penis of the boar pen-

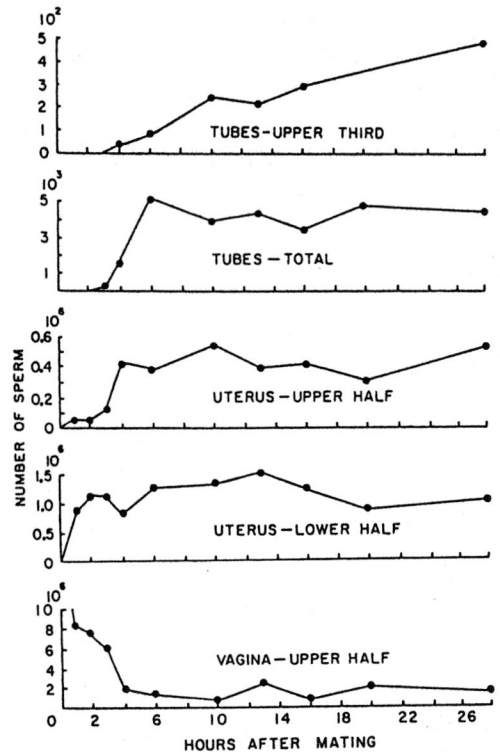

Fig. 8-21. Changes in spermatozoal number in various sections of the genital tract of the female rabbit after copulation. (A. W. H. Braden, Aust. J. Biol. Sci. 6:693, 1953).

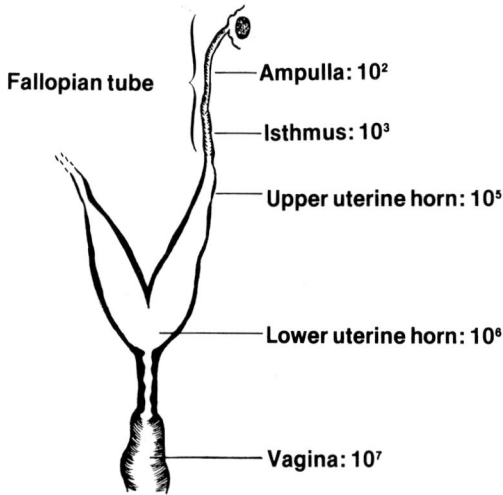

Fig. 8-22. Declining gradient in numbers of spermatozoa within the reproductive tract of the cow. (Compiled from different sources).

etrates the cervix of the sow, and the cervix is fully relaxed at the height of estrus in mares. Thus, the cervix is not a critical barrier for the spermatozoa of these two species. However, for the other species, transport through the cervix may be influenced by the flow of cervical mucus, which undergoes physical and chemical changes related to the ovarian cycle. Muscular contractions of the uterus and cervix, a negative uterine pressure owing to a pumping action of the abdomen, and spermatozoal motility can also influence the passage of spermatozoa through the cervix.

Segmenting and peristaltic contractions occur in the wall of the oviduct, but these peristaltic waves progress from the uterine to the ovarian end during the follicular phase of the cycle and from the ovarian toward the uterine end of the oviduct during the luteal phase of the cycle. Ciliary movements are also abovarian, but the flow of oviductal fluids may then orient the spermatozoa toward the ovary. There is controversy concerning the selectivity of the uterotubal barrier. Motile rat spermatozoa freely penetrate the uterotubal junction in estrous or diestrous rats, but dead rat spermatozoa and inert particles do not pass. On the other hand, foreign spermatozoa pass the uterotubal junction even in the presence of an intrauterine for-

eign body. Stallion spermatozoa are efficiently transported through the reproductive tract of the female donkey or jenney; the reciprocal effect is true for mares inseminated with jackass spermatozoa. The resulting product is a viable hybrid, the mule or the hinney, respectively. Goat spermatozoa are successfully transported through the reproductive tract of the ewe, and the reciprocal effect is also true, so goat oocytes can be fertilized by ram spermatozoa and ewe oocytes can be fertilized by the billy goat spermatozoa. However, intergeneric goat/sheep embryos do not develop to term because of chromosomal and placental incompatibility (see Chapter 14).

REFERENCES

Control of Spermatogenesis

1. Anderson, L. L. (1977): Development in calves and heifers after hypophysial stalk transection or hypophysectomy. Am. J. Physiol. *232*:E497.
2. Babol, J., Squires E. J., and Bonneau, M. (1996): Factors regulating the concentrations of 16-androstene steroids in submaxillary salivary glands of pigs. J. Anim. Sci. *74*:413.
3. Baumans, V., Dijkstra, G., and Wensing, C. J. G. (1981): Testicular descent in the dog. Zbl. Vet. Med. C. *10*:97.
4. Bellvé, A. R. and Feig, L. A. (1984): Cell proliferation in the mammalian testis: Biology of the seminiferous growth factor (SGF). Recent Prog. Hormone Res. *40*:531.
5. Berndtson, W. E. (1977): Methods for quantifying mammalian spermatogenesis: A review. J. Anim. Sci. *44*:818.
6. Bowler, K. (1972): The effect of repeated applications of heat on spermatogenesis in the rat: A histological study. J. Reprod. Fertil. *28*:325.
7. Brown, B. W. (1994): A review of nutritional influences on reproduction in boars, bulls and rams. Reprod. Nutr. Develop. *34*:89.
8. Bustos-Obregon, E., Courot, M., Flechon, J. E., et al. (1975): Morphological appraisal of gametogenesis. Spermatogenic process in mammals with particular reference to man. Andrologia *7*:141.
9. Clarke, P. G. H. and Clarke, S. (1996): Nineteenth century research on naturally occurring cell death and related phenomena. Anat. Embryol. *193*:81.
10. Clay, C. M., Squires, E. L., Amann, R. P., et al. (1987): Influences of season and artificial photoperiod on stallions: Testicular size, seminal characteristics, and sexual behavior. J. Anim. Sci. *64*:517.
11. Clay, C. M., Squires, E. L., Amann, R. P., et al. (1988): Influences of season and artificial photoperiod on stallions: Luteinizing hormone, follicle-stimulating hormone, and testosterone. J. Anim. Sci. *66*:1246.
12. Cook, R. B., Coulter, G. H., and Kastelic, J. P. (1994): The testicular vascular cone, scrotal thermoregulation, and their relationship to sperm production and seminal quality in beef bulls. Theriogenology *41*:653.

13. Coulter, G. H., Senger, P. L., and Bailey, D. R. C. (1988): Relationship of scrotal surface temperature measured by infrared thermography to subcutaneous and deep testicular temperature in the ram. J. Reprod. Fertil. *84*:417.

14. Courot, M., Hochereau-de-Reviers, M.-T., Monet-Kuntz, C., et al. (1979): Endocrinology of spermatogenesis in the hypophysectomized ram. J. Reprod. Fertil. (Suppl. 26):165.

15. Daneau, I., Ethier, J.-F., Lussier, J.G., et al. (1996): Porcine SRY gene locus and genital ridge expression. Biol. Reprod. *55*:47.

16. Dorrington, J. H., Roller, N. F., and Fritz, I. B. (1975): Effects of follicle-stimulating hormone on cultures of Sertoli cell preparations. Mol. Cell Endocrinol. *3*:57.

17. Fabbri, A., Knox, G., Buczko, E., et al. (1988): β-endorphin production by the fetal Leydig cell: Regulation and implications for paracrine control of Sertoli cell function. Endocrinology *122*:749.

18. Forest, M. G. (1983): Role of androgens in fetal and pubertal development. Hormone Res. *18*:69.

19. Freeman, S. (1990): The evolution of the scrotum: A new hypothesis. J. Theor. Biol. *145*:429.

20. Frey, H. L., Peng, S., and Rajfer, J. (1983): Synergy of abdominal pressure and androgens in testicular descent. Biol. Reprod. *29*:1233.

21. Fritz, I. B., Louis, B. G., Tung, P. S., et al. (1978): Action of hormones on Sertoli cells during maturation. Ann. Biol. Anim. Biochim. Biophys. *18*:555.

22. Gebauer, M. R., Pickett, B. W., and Swierstra, E. E. (1974): Reproductive physiology of the stallion. III. Extra-gonadal transit time and sperm reserves. J. Anim. Sci. *39*:737.

23. Ghosh, S., Bartke, A., Grasso, P., et al. (1992): Structural response of the hamster Sertoli cell to hypophysectomy: A correlative morphometric and endocrine study. Anat. Rec. *234*:513.

24. Glitteman, J. L. and Thompson, S. D. (1988): Energy allocation in mammalian reproduction. Am. Zool. *28*:863.

25. Glover, T. D. and Young, D. H. (1963): Temperature and the production of spermatozoa. Fertil. Steril. *14*:441.

26. Hart, B. L. and Ladewig, J. (1979): Serum testosterone of neonatal male and female dogs. Biol. Reprod. *21*:289.

27. Hees, H., Kohler, T., Leiser, R., et al. (1990): Gefäß-Morphologie des Rinderhodens. Licht-und Rasterelektronenmikroskopische Studien. Anat. Anz., Jena, Germany *170*:119.

28. Heindel, J. J. and Treinen, K. A. (1989): Physiology of the male reproductive system: Endocrine, paracrine and autocrine regulation. Toxicol. Pathol. *17*:411.

29. Heyns, C. F. and Hutson, J. M. (1995): Historical review of theories on testicular descent. J. Urol. *153*:754.

30. Hidiroglou, M. (1979): Trace elements deficiencies and fertility in ruminants: A review. J. Dairy Sci. *62*:1195.

31. Hoagland, T. A. and Bolt, D. J. (1986): Serum follicle-stimulating hormone, luteinizing hormone, and testosterone in sexually stimulated intact and unilaterally castrated rams. Theriogenology *26*:671.

32. Hoagland, T. A., Mannen, K. A., Dinger, J. E., et al. (1986): Effects of unilateral castration on serum luteinizing hormone, and testosterone concentrations in one-, two-, and three-year-old stallions. Theriogenology *26*:407.

33. Hoagland, T. A., Ott, K. M., Dinger, J. E., et al. (1986): Effects of unilateral castration on morphologic characteristics of the testis in one-, two-, and three-year-old stallions. Theriogenology *26*:407.

34. Howard, B., Jr. (1969): Fertility in the ram following exposure to elevated ambient temperature and humidity. J. Reprod. Fertil. *19*:179.

35. Jégou, B. (1992): The Sertoli cell. Baillière's Clin. Endocrinol. Metab. *6*:273.

36. Kennelly, J. J. (1972): Coyote reproduction. I. The duration of the spermatogenic cycle and epididymal sperm transport. J. Reprod. Fertil. *31*:163.

37. Kroes, R., Berkvens, J. M., Loendersloot, H. J., et al. (1971): Oestrogen-induced changes in the genital tract of the male calf. Zbl. Vet. Med. *18*:717.

38. Leung, P. C. K. and Steele, G. L. (1992): Intracellular signaling in the gonads. Endocrine Rev. *13*:476.

39. Maekawa, M., Kamimora, K., and Nagano, T. (1996): Peritubular myoid cells in the testis: Their structure and function. Arch. Histol. Cytol. *59*:1.

40. Mather, J. P., Gunsalus, G. L., Musto, N. A., et al. (1983): The hormonal and cellular control of Sertoli cell secretion. J. Steroid Biochem. *19*:41.

41. Moyle, W. R., Kuczek, T., and Bailey, C. A. (1985): Potential of a quantal response as a mechanism for oscillatory behavior: Implications of our concepts of hormonal control mechanisms. Biol. Reprod. *32*:43.

42. Mullaney, B. P. and Skinner, M. K. (1991): Growth factors as mediators of testicular cell-cell interactions. Baillière's Clin. Endocrinol. Metab. *5*:771.

43. Myrén, C. J. and Einer-Jensen, N. (1992): Microvascular transposition of the arterial supply to the testis of the boar. J. Exp. Anim. Sci. *35*:80.

44. Olar, T. T., Amann, R. P., and Pickett, B. W. (1983): Relationships among testicular size, daily production and output of spermatozoa, and extragonadal spermatozoal reserves of the dog. Biol. Reprod. 29:1114.

45. Price, C. A. (1991): The control of FSH secretion in the larger domestic species. J. Endocrinol. *131*:177.

46. Roser, J. F., McCue, P. M., and Hoye, E. (1994): Inhibin activity in the mare and stallion. Domestic Anim. Endocrinol. *11*:87.

47. Ross, G. T. and Lipsett, M. B. (1978): Homologies of structure and function in mammalian testes and ovaries. Int. J. Androl. *1* (Suppl. 2):39.

48. Sanborn, B. M., Tsai, Y. H., Steinberger, A., et al. (1978): Biochemical aspects of the interaction of androgens with Sertoli cells. Ann. Biol. Anim. Biochim. Biophys. *18*:615.

49. Schanbacher, B. D. and Ford, J. J. (1979): Photoperiodic regulation of ovine spermatogenesis: Relationship to serum hormones. Biol. Reprod. *20*:719.

50. Sharpe, R. M. (1984): Intratesticular factors controlling testicular function. Biol. Reprod. *30*:29.

51. Sharpe, R. M., Maddocks, S., and Kerr, J. B. (1990): Cell-cell interactions in the control of spermatogenesis as studied using Leydig cell destruction and testosterone replacement. Am. J. Anat. *188*:3.

52. Solari, A. J. and Fritz, I. B. (1978): The ultrastructure of immature Sertoli cells. Maturation-like changes

during culture and the maintenance of mitotic potentiality. Biol. Reprod. *18*:329.

53. Steinberger, E. (1971): Hormonal control of mammalian spermatogenesis. Physiol. Rev. *51*:1.

54. Stone, B. A. (1981/1982): Heat-induced infertility of boars: The inter-relationship between depressed sperm output and fertility and an estimation of the critical air temperature above which sperm output is impaired. Anim. Reprod. Sci. *4*:283.

55. Swierstra, E. E. (1968): Cytology and duration of the cycle of the seminiferous epithelium of the boar; duration of spermatozoa transit through the epididymis. Anat. Rec. *161*:171.

56. Swierstra, E. E. (1970): The effect of low ambient temperatures on sperm production, epididymal sperm reserves, and semen characteristics of boars. Biol. Reprod. *2*:23.

57. Terner, C. (1977): Progesterone and progestins in the male reproductive system. Ann. N. Y. Acad. Sci. *286*:313.

58. Van der Molen, H. J., Van Beurden, M. O., Blankenstein, M. A., et al. (1979): The testis: Biochemical actions of trophic hormones and steroids on steroid production and spermatogenesis. J. Steroid Biochem. *11*:13.

59. Voglmayr, J. K., Setchell, B. P., and White, I. G. (1971): The effects of heat on the metabolism and ultrastructure of ram testicular spermatozoa. J. Reprod. Fertil. *24*:71.

60. Wu, N. and Murono, E. P. (1996): Temperature and germ cell regulation of Leydig cell proliferation stimulated by Sertoli cell-secreted mitogenic factor: A possible role in cryptorchidism. Andrologia *28*:247.

Steroidogenic Function

61. Abdel-Raouf, M. (1960): The postnatal development of the reproductive organs in bulls with special reference to puberty. Acta Endocrinol. *34* (Suppl. 49):1.

62. Almahbobi, G., Papadopoulos, V., Carreau, S., et al. (1988): Age-related morphological and functional changes in the Leydig cells of the horse. Biol. Reprod. *38*:653.

63. Amann, R. P. and Ganjam, U. K. (1976): Steroid production by the bovine testis and steroid transfer across the pampiniform plexus. Biol. Reprod. *15*:695.

64. Andresen, Ø. (1976): Concentrations of fat and plasma 5α-androstenone and plasma testosterone in boars selected for rate of body weight gain and thickness of back fat during growth, sexual maturation, and after mating. J. Reprod. Fertil. *48*:51.

65. Aronson, L. R. and Cooper, M. L. (1967): Penile spines of the domestic cat. Anat. Rec. *157*:71.

66. Babol, J., Squires, E. J., and Bonneau, M. (1996): Factors regulating the concentrations of 16-androstene steroids in submaxillary salivary glands of pigs. J. Anim. Sci. *74*:413.

67. Bardin, C. W. and Catterall, J. F. (1981): Testosterone: A major determinant of extragenital sexual dimorphism. Science *211*:1285.

68. Barenton, B., Blanc, M. R., Caraty, A., et al. (1982): Effect of cryptorchidism in the ram: Changes in the concentrations of testosterone and estradiol and receptors for LH and FSH in the testis, and its histology. Mol. Cell Endocrinol. *28*:13.

69. Bartke, A., Hafiez, A. A., Bex, F. J., et al. (1978): Hormonal interactions in the regulation of androgen secretion. Biol. Reprod. *18*:44.

70. Benahmed, M., Bernier, M., Ducharme, J. R., et al. (1982): Steroidogenesis of cultured purified pig Leydig cells: Secretion and effects of estrogens. Mol. Cell. Endocrinol. *28*:705.

71. Bergh, A. (1983): Paracrine regulation of Leydig cells by the seminiferous tubules. Int. J. Androl. *6*:57.

72. Berndtson, W. E., Pickett, B. W., and Nett, T. M. (1974): Reproductive physiology of the stallion. IV. Seasonal changes in the testosterone concentration of peripheral plasma. J. Reprod. Fertil. *39*:115.

73. Booth, W. D. and White, C. A. (1988): The isolation, purification and some properties of pheromaxein, the pheromonal steroid-binding protein, in porcine submaxillary glands and saliva.J. Endocrinol. *118*:47.

74. Bravo, P. W. (1994): Reproductive physiology of the male camelid. Vet. Clin. North Am. *10*:259.

75. Brooks, R. I. and Pearson, A. M. (1986): Steroid hormone pathways in the pig, with special emphasis on boar odor: A review. J. Anim. Sci. *62*:632.

76. Bubenik, G. A., Brown, G. M., and Grota, L. J. (1975): Localization of immunoreactive androgen in testicular tissue. Endocrinology *96*:63.

77. Cahoreau, C., Blanc, M. R., Dacheux, J. L., et al. (1979): Inhibin activity in ram rete testis fluid: Depression of plasma FSH and LH in the castrated and cryptorchid ram. J. Reprod. Fertil. (Suppl. 26):97.

78. Caraty, A. and Bonneau, M. (1986): Immunisation active du porc mâle contre la gonadolibérine: Effects sur la sécrétion d'hormones gonadotropes et sur la teneur en 5α-androst-16-ène-3-one du tissu adipeux. Compt. Rend. Acad. Sci., Paris, France *303*:673.

79. Carroll, E. J., Aanes, W. A., and Ball, L. (1964): Persistent penile frenulum in bulls. J. Am. Vet. Med. Assoc. *144*:747.

80. Chari, S., Duraiswami, S., and Franchimont, P. (1978): Isolation and characterization of inhibin from bull seminal plasma. Acta Endocrinol. *87*:434.

81. Claus, R. and Hoffmann, B. (1980): Oestrogens, compared to other steroids of testicular origin, in blood plasma of boars. Acta Endocrinol. *94*:404.

82. Claus, R., Schopper, D., and Hoang-Vu, C. (1985): Contribution of individual compartments of the genital tract to oestrogen and testosterone concentrations in the ejaculates of the boar. Acta Endocrinol. *109*:281.

83. Comhaire, F., Mattheeuws, D., and Vermeulen, A. (1974): Testosterone and oestradiol in dogs with testicular tumors. Acta Endocrinol. *77*:408.

84. Davies, A. G. (1981): Role of FSH in the control of testicular function. Arch. Androl. *7*:97.

85. De Palatis, L., Moore, J., and Falvo, R. E. (1978): Plasma concentrations of testosterone and LH in the male dog. J. Reprod. Fertil. *52*:201.

86. Eik-Nes, K. B. (1975): Biosynthesis and secretion of testicular steroids. *In:* Handbook of Physiology, Section 7, Vol. V, Male Reproductive System, edited by D. W. Hamilton and R. O. Greep. American Physiological Society, Washington, DC, p. 95.

87. Ewing, L. L., Zirkin, B. R., Cochran, R. C., et al. (1979): Testosterone secretion by rat, rabbit, guinea

pig, dog, and hamster testes perfused *in vitro:* Correlation with Leydig cell mass. Endocrinology *105*:1135.

88. Flor-Cruz, S. V. and Lapwood, K. R. (1978): A longitudinal study of pubertal development in boars. Int. J. Androl. *1*:317.

89. Fonda, E. S., Diehl, J. R., Barb, C. R., et al. (1981): Serum luteinizing hormone, testosterone production and cortisol concentrations after PGF2α in the boar. Prostaglandins *21*:933.

90. Franchimont, P. (1982): Intragonadal regulation of reproduction. 2nd Int. Congr. Androl., Tel Aviv, Israel, June 28. Int. J. Androl. (Suppl. 5):157.

91. Ganjam, V. K. and Kenney, R. M. (1975): Androgens and oestrogens in normal and cryptorchid stallions. J. Reprod. Fertil. (Suppl. 23):67.

92. Gastal, M. O., Henry, M., Beker, A. R., et al. (1996): Sexual behavior of donkey jacks: Influence of ejaculatory frequency and season. Theriogenology *46*:593.

93. Ginther, O. J., Mapletoft, R. J., Zimmerman, N., et al. (1974): Local increase in testosterone concentration in the testicular artery in rams. J. Anim. Sci. *38*:835.

94. Godfrey, R. W., Randel, R. D., Forrest, D. W., et al. (1985): The concentration of estradiol-17β in bovine semen. J. Anim. Sci. *60*:760.

95. Gray, R. C., Day, B. N., Lasley, J. F., et al. (1971): Testosterone levels of boars at various ages. J. Anim. Sci. *33*:124.

96. Grootenhuis, A. J., Van Sluijs, F. J., Klaij, I. A., et al. (1990): Inhibin, gonadotrophins, and sex steroids in dogs with Sertoli cell tumours. J. Endocrinol. *127*:235.

97. Harris, J. M., Irvine, C. H. J., and Evans, M. J. (1983): Seasonal changes and serum levels of FSH, LH and testosterone and in semen parameters in stallions. Theriogenology *19*:311.

98. Hsueh, A. J. W. and Schaeffer, J. M. (1985): Gonadotropin-releasing hormone as a paracrine hormone and neurotransmitter in extra-pituitary sites. J. Steroid Biochem. *23*:757.

99. Huhtaniemi, I. and Pelliniemi, L. J. (1992): Fetal Leydig cells: Cellular origin, morphology, life span, and special functional features. Proc. Soc. Exp. Biol. Med. *201*:125.

100. Huhtaniemi, I. T. and Warren, D. W. (1990): Ontogeny of pituitary-gonadal interactions. Current advances and controversies. Trends Endocrinol. Metab. *1*:356.

101. Johnson, L. and Thompson, D. L., Jr. (1983): Age-related and seasonal variation in the Sertoli cell population, daily sperm production and serum concentrations of follicle-stimulating hormone, luteinizing hormone, and testosterone in stallions. Biol. Reprod. *29*:777.

102. Johnstone, I. P., Bancroft, B. J., and McFarlane, J. R. (1984): Testosterone and androstenedione profiles in the blood of domestic tom cats. Anim. Reprod. Sci. *7*:363.

103. Jost, A. (1965): Gonadal hormones in the sex differentiation of the mammalian fetus. *In:* Organogenesis, edited by R. L. DeHaan and H. Ursprung. New York, NY, Holt, Rinehart and Winston, p. 611.

104. Kawakami, E., Tsutsui, T., Yamada, Y., et al. (1987): Spermatogenesis and peripheral spermatic venous plasma androgen levels in the unilateral cryptorchid dogs. Jpn. J. Vet. Sci. *49*:349.

105. Lacroix, A. and Pelletier, J. (1979): LH and testosterone release in developing bulls following LH-RH

treatment. Effect of gonadectomy and chronic testosterone propionate pre-treatment. Acta Endocrinol. *91*:719.

106. Lieberman, S., Greenfield, N. J., and Wolfson, A. (1984): A heuristic proposal for understanding steroidogenic processes. Endocrinology *5*:128.

107. Lloyd, J. W., Thomas, J. A., and Mawhinney, M. G. (1975): Androgens and estrogens in the plasma and prostatic tissue of normal dogs and dogs with benign prostatic hypertrophy. Invest. Urol. *13*:220.

108. Lluarado, J. G. and Dominguez, O. V. (1963): Effect of cryptorchidism on testicular enzymes involved in androgen biosynthesis. Endocrinology *72*:292.

109. McCullagh, D. R. (1932): Dual endocrine activity of the testis. Science *76*:19.

110. Olson, P. N., Mulnix, J. A., and Nett, T. M. (1992): Concentrations of luteinizing hormone and follicle-stimulating hormone in the serum of sexually intact and neutered dogs. Am. J. Vet. Res. *53*:762.

111. Payne, A. H. and Youngblood, G. L. (1995): Regulation of expression of steroidogenic enzymes in Leydig cells. Biol. Reprod. *52*:217.

112. Peters, H. (1976): Intrauterine gonadal development. Fertil. Steril. *27*:493.

113. Peyrat, J.-P., Meusy-Desolle, N., and Garnier, J. (1981): Changes in Leydig cells and luteinizing hormone receptors in porcine testis during postnatal development. Endocrinology *108*:625.

114. Pierrepoint, C. G., Galley, J. McI., Griffiths, K., et al. (1967): Steroid metabolism of a Sertoli cell tumor of the testis of a dog with feminization and alopecia and of the normal canine testis.J. Endocrinol. *38*:61.

115. Rawlings, N. C., Hafs, H. D., and Swanson, L. V. (1972): Testicular and blood plasma androgens in Holstein bulls from birth through puberty. J. Anim. Sci. *34*:435.

116. Reiffsteck, A., Dehennin, L., and Scholler, R. (1982): Estrogens in seminal plasma of human and animal species: Identification and quantitative estimation by gas chromatography-mass spectrometry associated with stable isotope dilution. J. Steroid Biochem. *17*:567.

117. Ritar, A. J. (1991): Seasonal changes in LH, androgens and testes in the male Angora goat. Theriogenology *36*:959.

118. Ritar, A. J., Mendoza, G., Salamon, S., et al. (1992): Frequent semen collection and sperm reserves of the male Angora goat (*Capra hircus*). J. Reprod. Fertil. *95*:97.

119. Rowson, L. E. A. and Skinner, J. D. (1968): Some effects of orchiopexy on the testes of unilateral cryptorchid pubescent rams. Proc. 6th Int. Congr. Anim. Reprod. A. I., Paris, France, Vol. 1, p. 313.

120. Sanford, L. M., Simaraks, S., Palmer, W. M., et al. (1982): Circulating estrogen levels in the ram: influence of season and mating, and their relationship to testosterone levels and mating frequency. Can. J. Anim. Sci. *62*:85.

121. Sanford, L. M., Winter, J. S. D., Palmer, W. M., et al. (1974): The profile of LH and testosterone in the ram. Endocrinology *96*:627.

122. Schulze, H. and Barrack, E. R. (1987): Immunocytochemical localization of estrogen receptors in the normal male and female canine urinary tract and prostate. Endocrinology *121*:1773.

123. Setchell, B. P. and Main, S. J. (1975): The bloodtestis barrier and steroids. *In:* Hormonal Regulation of Spermatogenesis, edited by F. S. French, V. Hansson, E. M. Ritzen, and S. N. Neyfeh. New York, NY, Plenum Press, p. 513.

124. Setchell, B. P., Laurie, M. S., Flint, A. P. F., et al. (1983): Transport of free and conjugated steroids from the boar testis in lymph, venous blood and rete testis fluid. J. Endocrinol. *96*:127.

125. Setoguti, T., Esumi, H., and Shimizu, T. (1974): Electron microscopic studies on dog testicular interstitial cells. Arch. Histol. Jpn. *37*:97.

126. Sharpe, R. M. (1982): Cellular aspects of the inhibitory actions of LH-RH on the ovary and testis. J. Reprod. Fertil. *64*:517.

127. Sharpe, R. M. (1984): Intratesticular factors controlling testicular function. Biol. Reprod. *30*:29.

128. Shupnik, M. A. (1996): Gonadotropin gene modulation by steroids and gonadotropin-releasing-hormone. Biol. Reprod. *54*:279.

129. Singer, A. G. (1991): A chemistry of mammalian pheromones. J. Steroid Biochem. Mol. Biol. *39*:627.

130. Skinner, M. K. (1991): Cell-cell interactions in the testis. Endocrine Rev. *12*:45.

131. Steinberger, A. (1979): Inhibin production by Sertoli cells in culture. J. Reprod. Fertil. *26*:31.

132. Swierstra, E. E., Gebauer, M. R., and Pickett, B. W. (1974): Reproductive physiology of the stallion. I. Spermatogenesis and testis composition. J. Reprod. Fertil. *40*:113.

133. Taha, M. B. and Noakes, D. E. (1982): The effect of age and season of the year on testicular function in the dog, as determined by histological examination of the seminiferous tubules and the estimation of peripheral plasma testosterone concentrations. J. Small Anim. Pract. *23*:351.

134. Tilley, W. D., Marcelli, M., and McPhaul, M. J. (1990): Recent studies of the androgen receptor: New insights into old questions. Mol. Cell. Endocrinol. *68*:C7.

135. Vincent, D. L., Kepic, T. A., Lathrop, J. C., et al. (1979): Testosterone regulation of luteinizing hormone secretion in the male dog. Int. J. Androl. 2:241.

136. Wrobel, K.-H., Sinowatz, F., and Mademann, R. (1981): Intertubular topography in the bovine testis. Cell Tissue Res. *217*:289.

137. Zlotnik, G. (1973): Testosterone levels in intersex goats. J. Reprod. Fertil. *32*:287.

Excurrent Tract

138. Amann, R. P. (1970): Sperm production rates. *In:* The Testis, edited by A. D. Johnson, W. R. Gomes, and N. L. Vandemark. New York, NY, Academic Press, p. 433.

139. Amann, R. P., Johnson, L., and Pickett, B. W. (1977): Connection between the seminiferous tubules and the efferent ducts in the stallion. Am. J. Vet. Res. *38*:1571.

140. Brooks, D. E. (1983): Epididymal functions and their hormonal regulation. Aust. J. Biol. Sci. *36*:205.

141. Cameron, A. W. N., Fairnie, I. J., Curnow, D. H., et al. (1984): The output of spermatozoa of naturally mated rams. Proc. 10th Int. Congr. Anim. Reprod. A. I., Univ. Illinois, Champaign/Urbana, IL, Vol. II, Brief Comm. No. 266.

142. Dacheux, J. L. and Paquignon, M. (1980): Relations between the fertilizing ability, motility and metabolism of epididymal spermatozoa. Reprod. Nutr. Develop. *20*:1085.

143. Dooley, M. P., Pineda, M. H., Hopper, J. G., et al. (1984): Retrograde flow of semen caused by electroejaculation in the domestic cat. Proc. 10th Int. Congr. Anim. Reprod. A. I. Univ. Illinois, Champaign/Urbana, IL, Vol. III, Brief Comm. No. 363.

144. Dooley, M. P., Pineda, M. H., Hopper, J. G., et al. (1990): Retrograde flow of spermatozoa into the urinary bladder of dogs during ejaculation or after sedation with xylazine. Am. J. Vet. Res. *51*:1574.

145. Dooley, M. P., Pineda, M. H., Hopper, J. G., et al. (1991): Retrograde flow of spermatozoa into the urinary bladder of cats during electroejaculation, collection of semen with an artificial vagina, and mating. Am. J. Vet. Res. *52*:687.

146. Dooley, M. P., Pineda, M. H., Maurer, R. R., et al. (1986): Evidence for retrograde flow of spermatozoa into the urinary bladder of bulls during electroejaculation. Theriogenology *26*:101.

147. Dym, M. (1976): The mammalian rete testis a morphological examination. Anat. Rec. *186*:493.

148. Ellis, L. C., Groesbeck, M. D., Farr, C. H., et al. (1981): Contractility of seminiferous tubules as related to sperm transport in the male. Arch. Androl. *6*:283.

149. Essenhigh, D. M., Chir, M., Adran, G. M., et al. (1969): The vesical sphincters and ejaculation in the ram. Br. J. Urol. *41*:190.

150. Frenette, M. D., Dooley, M. P., and Pineda, M. H. (1986): Effect of flushing the vasa deferentia at the time of vasectomy on the rate of clearance of spermatozoa from the ejaculates of dogs and cats. Am. J. Vet. Res. *47*:463.

151. Garbers, D. L., Wakabayashi, T., and Reed, P. W. (1970): Enzyme profile of the cytoplasmatic droplet from bovine epididymal spermatozoa. Biol. Reprod. *3*:327.

152. Goyal, H. O. and Williams, C. S. (1988): The ductuli efferentes of the goat: A morphological study. Anat. Rec. *220*:58.

153. Hemeida, N. A., Sack, W. O., and McEntee, K. (1978): Ductuli efferentes in the epididymis of boar, goat, ram, bull, and stallion. Am. J. Vet. Res. *39*:1892.

154. Hernandez, F. I., Dooley, M. P., and Pineda, M. H. (1992): Effect of xylazine on retrograde flow of spermatozoa into the urinary bladder or rams. In: 1992 Beef and Sheep Research Report, Iowa State University, Ames, IA, p. 160.

155. Hinton, B. T., Palladino, M. A., Rudolph, D., et al. (1995): The epididymis as protector of maturing spermatozoa. Reprod. Fertil. Develop. 7:731.

156. Hirsch, I. H., Sedor, J., Jeyendran, R. S., et al. (1992): The relative distribution of viable sperm in the antegrade and retrograde portions of ejaculates obtained after electrostimulation. Fertil. Steril. *57*:399.

157. Hovell, G. J. R., Ardran, G. M., Essenhigh, D. M., et al. (1969): Radiological observations on electrically-induced ejaculation in the ram. J. Reprod. Fertil. *20*:383.

158. Johnson, A. L. and Pursel, V. G. (1975): Cannulation of ductus deferens of the boar: A surgical technique. Am. J. Vet. Res. *36*:315.

159. Johnson, L., Amann, R. P., and Pickett, B. W. (1980): Maturation of equine epididymal spermatozoa. Am. J. Vet. Res. *41*:1190.

160. Jones, R. (1978): Comparative biochemistry of mammalian epididymal plasma. Comp. Biochem. Physiol. *61B*:365.

161. Koefoed-Johnsen, H. H. (1964): "Sperm production in bulls. The excretion of sperm with the urine at each ejaculation frequences" (sic). In Danish, title from English summary. Ann. Report Royal Veterinary and Agricultural College, Copenhagen, Denmark, A/S Carl F. R. Mortensen, p. 23.

162. Lino, B. F., Braden, A. W. H., and Turnbull, K. E. (1967): Fate of unejaculated spermatozoa. Nature *213*:594.

163. Martin, P. A., Dooley, M. P., Hembrough, F. B., et al. (1993): Urinary losses of spermatozoa during ejaculation are negligible in boars. Theriogenology *39*:945.

164. Martin, P. A., Dooley, M. P., Hembrough, F. B., et al. (1994): Retrograde flow of spermatozoa into the urinary bladder of boars during collection of semen by electroejaculation. Theriogenology *41*:869.

165. Oslund, R. M. (1928): The physiology of the male reproductive system. J. Am. Med. Assoc. *40*:829.

166. Ortavant, R. and Thibault, C. (1956): Influence de la durée d'éclairment sur les productions spermatigues du belier. Compt. Rend. Soc. Biol., Paris, France *150*:358.

167. Pineda, M. H. and Dooley, M. P. (1991): Effect of method of seminal collection on the retrograde flow of spermatozoa into the urinary bladder of rams. Am. J. Vet. Res. *52*:307.

168. Pineda, M. H. and Dooley, M. P. (1994): Yohimbine prevents the retrograde flow of spermatozoa into the urinary bladder of dogs induced by xylazine. J. Vet. Pharmacol. Therap. *17*:169.

169. Pineda, M. H., Dooley, M. P., Hembrough, F. B., et al. (1987): Retrograde flow of spermatozoa into the urinary bladder of rams. Am. J. Vet. Res. *48*:562.

170. Pineda, M. H., Reimers, T. J., and Faulkner, L. C. (1976): Disappearance of spermatozoa from the ejaculates of vasectomized dogs. J. Am. Vet. Med. Assoc. *168*:502.

171. Quinn, P. J., White, I. G., and Wirrick, B. R. (1965): Studies of the distribution of the major cations in semen and male accessory secretions. J. Reprod. Fertil. *10*:379.

172. Robaire, B. and Viger, R. S. (1995): Regulation of epididymal epithelial cell functions. Biol. Reprod. *52*:226.

173. Rodríguez, H. and Bustos-Obregon, E. (1994): Seasonal and epididymal maturation of stallion spermatozoa. Andrologia *26*:161.

174. Schaffer, N. E., Cranfield, M., Fazleabas, A. T., et al. (1989): Viable spermatozoa in the bladder after electroejaculation of Lion-tailed macaques (*Macaca silenus*). J. Reprod. Fertil. *17*:459.

175. Schaffer, N., Jeyendran, R. S., and Bechler, B. (1991): Improved sperm collection from the Lowland gorilla: Recovery of sperm from bladder and urethra following electroejaculation. Am. J. Primatol. *24*:265.

176. Scott, T. W., Voglmayr, J. K., and Setchell, B. P. (1967): Lipid composition and metabolism in testicular and ejaculated ram spermatozoa. Biochem. J. 102:456.

177. Smith, C. L., Peter, A. T., and Pugh, D. G. (1994): Reproduction in llamas and alpacas: A review. Theriogenology *41*:573.

178. Tischner, M. (1971): Transport of unejaculated spermatozoa through the pelvic part of the urogenital tract in the ram.J. Reprod. Fertil. *24*:271.

179. Tischner, M. (1972): The role of the vasa deferentia and the urethra in the transport of semen in rams. Acta Agr. et Silv. *12*:77.

180. Usselman, M. C. and Cone, R. A. (1983): Rat sperm are mechanically immobilized in the caudal epididymis by "immobilin," a high-molecular-weight glycoprotein. Biol. Reprod. *29*:1241.

181. Voglmayr, J. K., Waites, G. M. H., and Setchell, B. P. (1966): Studies on spermatozoa and fluid collected directly from the testis of the conscious ram. Nature *210*:861.

Accessory Sex Glands

182. Barnes, G. W. (1972): The antigenic nature of male accessory glands of reproduction. Biol. Reprod. *6*:384.

183. Boesel, R. W., Klipper, R. W., and Shain, S. A. (1977): Identification of limited capacity androgen-binding components in nuclear and cytoplasmic fractions of canine prostate. Endocrine Res. Commun. *4*:71.

184. Bowen, R. A. (1977): Fertilization *in vitro* of feline ova by spermatozoa from the ductus deferens. Biol. Reprod. *17*:144.

185. Davies, D. C., Hall, G., Hibbitt, K. G., et al. (1975): The removal of the seminal vesicles from the boar and the effects on the semen characteristics. J. Reprod. Fertil. *43*:305.

186. MacMillan, K. L. and Hafs, H. D. (1969): Reproductive tract of Holstein bulls from birth through puberty. J. Anim. Sci. *28*:233.

187. Rodger, J. C. (1976): Comparative aspects of the accessory sex glands and seminal biochemistry of mammals. Comp. Biochem. Physiol. *55B*:1.

188. Wales, R. G. and White, I. G. (1965): Some observations on the chemistry of dog semen. J. Reprod. Fertil. *9*:69.

189. Wilson, J. D. and Gloyna, R. E. (1970): The intranuclear metabolism of testosterone in the accessory organs of reproduction. Recent Prog. Hormone Res. *26*:309.

Penis and Prepuce

190. Ashdown, R. R. (1962): Persistence of the penile frenulum in young bulls. Vet. Rec. *74*:1464.

191. Ashdown, R. R. and Gilanpour, H. (1974): Venous drainage of the corpus cavernosum penis in impotent and normal bulls.J. Anat. *117*:159.

192. Ashdown, R. R. and Pearson, H. (1973): Studies on "Corkscrew Penis" in the bull. Vet. Rec. *93*:30.

193. Ashdown, R. R., Barnett, S. W., and Ardalani, G. (1981): Impotence in the boar: Angioarchitecture and venous drainage of the penis in normal boars. Vet. Rec. *109*:375.

194. Ashdown, R. R., Barnett, S. W., and Ardalani, G. (1982): Venous drainage of the bovine corpus cavernosum penis. J. Anat. *134*:621.

195. Ashdown, R. R., David, J. S. E., and Gibbs, C. (1979): Impotence in the bull: (1) Abnormal venous drainage of the corpus cavernosum penis. Vet. Rec. *104*:423.

196. Ashdown, R. R., Gilanpour, H., David, J. S. E., et al. (1979): Impotence in the bull: (2) Occlusion of the longitudinal canals of the corpus cavernosum penis. Vet. Rec. *104*:598.

197. Ashdown, R. R., Ricketts, S. W., and Wardley, R. C. (1968): The fibrous architecture of the integumentary coverings of the bovine penis. J. Anat. *103*:567.

198. Beckett, S. D., Hudson, R. S., Walker, D. F., et al. (1973): Blood pressures and penile muscle activity in the stallion during coitus. Am. J. Physiol. *225*:1072.

199. Beckett, S. D., Walker, D. F., Hudson, R. S., et al. (1974): Corpus cavernosum penis pressure and penile muscle activity in the bull during coitus. Am. J. Vet. Res. *35*:761.

200. Beckett, S. D., Walker, D. F., Hudson, R. S., et al. (1975): Corpus spongiosum penis pressure and penile muscle activity in the stallion during coitus. Am. J. Vet. Res. *36*:431.

201. Grandage, J. (1972): The erect dog penis: A paradox of flexible rigidity. Vet. Rec. *91*:141.

202. Kainer, R. A., Faulkner, L. C., and Abdel-Raouf, M. (1969): Glands associated with the urethra of the bull. Am. J. Vet. Res. *30*:963.

203. Seidel, G. E. and Foote, R. H. (1967): Motion picture analysis of bovine ejaculation. J. Dairy Sci. *50*:970.

Biology of Spermatozoa

204. Atherton, R. W. (1979): A review of the spectrometric quantitation of spermatozoal motility. *In:* The Spermatozoon, edited by D. W. Fawcett and J. M. Bedford. Baltimore, MD, Urban and Schwarzenberg, p. 421.

205. Bahr, G. F. and Engler, W. F. (1970): Considerations of volume, mass, DNA, and arrangement of mitochondria in the midpiece of bull spermatozoa. Exp. Cell Res. *60*:338.

206. Bravo, P. W. (1994): Reproductive physiology of the male camelid. Vet. Clin. N.A. *10*:259.

207. Doak, R. L., Hall, A., and Dale, H. E. (1967): Longevity of spermatozoa in the reproductive tract in the bitch. J. Reprod. Fertil. *13*:51.

208. Dott, H. M. (1975): Morphology of stallion spermatozoa. J. Reprod. Fertil. *23*:41.

209. Fawcett, D. W. (1970): A comparative view of sperm ultrastructure. Biol. Reprod. 2(Suppl. 2):90.

210. Fawcett, D. W. (1975): The mammalian spermatozoon. Develop. Biol. *44*:394.

211. Fawcett, D. W. (1977): What makes cilia and sperm tails beat? N. Engl. J. Med. *297*:46.

212. Fawcett, D. W. Anderson, W. A., and Phillips, D. M. (1971): Morphogenic factors influencing the shape of the sperm head. Develop. Biol. *26*:220.

213. Garner, D. L., Gledhill, B. L., Pinkel, D., et al. (1983): Quantification of the X- and Y-chromosome-bearing spermatozoa of domestic animals by flow cytometry. Biol. Reprod. *28*:312.

214. Gledhill, B. L. (1970): Enigma of spermatozoal deoxyribonucleic acid and male infertility: A review. Am. J. Vet. Res. *31*:539.

215. Jones, R. C. (1973): The plasma membrane of ram, boar and bull spermatozoa. J. Reprod. Fertil. *33*:179.

216. Kozima, Y. (1966): Electron microscopic study of the bull spermatozoon. Jpn. J. Vet. Res. *14*:1.

217. Phillips, D. M. (1972): Comparative analysis of mammalian sperm motility. J. Cell Biol. *53*:561.

218. Plattner, H. (1971): Bull spermatozoa: A reinvestigation by freeze-etching using widely different cryofixation procedures.J. Submicr. Cytol. *3*:19.

219. Revell, S. G. and Wood, P. D. P. (1978): A photographic method for the measurement of motility of bull spermatozoa. J. Reprod. Fertil. *54*:123.

220. Russell, L., Peterson, R. N., and Freund, M. (1980): On the presence of bridges linking the inner and outer acrosomal membranes of boar spermatozoa. Anat. Rec. *198*:449.

221. Saacke, R. G. and Almquist, J. O. (1964): Ultrastructure of bovine spermatozoa. I. The head of normal, ejaculated sperm. Am. J. Anat. *115*:143.

222. Sharma, O. P. (1976): Scanning electron microscopy of equine spermatozoa. J. Reprod. Fertil. *48*:413.

223. Weiss, G. (1989): Relaxin in the male. Biol. Reprod. *40*:197.

224. Wu, S. H. and Newstead, J. D. (1966): Electron microscope study of bovine epididymal spermatozoa. J. Anim. Sci. *25*:1186.

Evaluation of Seminal Quality

225. Almquist, J. O. (1982): Effect of long-term ejaculation at high frequency on output of sperm, sexual behavior, and fertility of Holstein bulls; relation of reproductive capacity to high nutrient allowance. J. Dairy Sci. *65*:814.

226. Boucher, J. H., Foote, R. H., and Kirk, R. W. (1958): The evaluation of semen quality in the dog and the effects of frequency of ejaculation upon semen quality, libido, and depletion of sperm reserves. Cornell Vet. *48*:67.

227. Carroll, E. J., Ball, L., and Scott, J. A. (1963): Breeding soundness in bulls–a summary of 10,940 examinations. J. Am. Vet. Med. Assoc. *142*:1105.

228. Corselli, J. and Talbot, P. (1986): An *in vitro* technique to study penetration of hamster oocyte-cumulus complexes by using physiological numbers of sperm. Gamete Res. *13*:293.

229. Hackett, A. J. and Macpherson, J. W. (1965): Some staining procedures for spermatozoa, a review. Can. Vet. J. 6:55.

230. Hartman, C. G. (1965): Correlations among criteria of semen quality. Fertil. Steril. *16*:632.

231. Hemsworth, P. H. and Galloway, D. B. (1979): The effect of sexual stimulation on the sperm output of the domestic boar. Anim. Reprod. Sci. 2:387.

232. Hirao, K. (1975): A multiple regression analysis of six measurements of bovine semen characteristics for fertility. Int. J. Fertil. *20*:204.

233. Johnson, L. and Thompson, D. L., Jr. (1983): Age-related and seasonal variation in the Sertoli cell population, daily sperm production and serum concentrations of follicle-stimulating hormone, luteinizing hormone, and testosterone in stallions. Biol. Reprod. *29*:777.

234. Lagerlöf, N. (1966): The history of cytological and histological examination of sperm and testis. Proc. Int. Symp. on Physiol. Pathol. Spermatogenesis, Rijksuniversiteit, Gent, Belgium, p. 5.

235. Linford, E., Glover, F. A., Bishop, C., et al. (1976): The relationship between semen evaluation methods and fertility in the bull. J. Reprod. Fertil. *47*:283.

236. Mader, D. R. and Price, E. O. (1984): The effects of sexual stimulation on the sexual performance of Hereford bulls. J. Anim. Sci. *59*:294.

237. Nunes, J. F., Corteel, J.-M., Combarnous, Y., et al. (1982): Role du plasma seminal dans la survie in vitro des spermatozoides de bouc. Reprod. Nutr. Develop. *22*:611.

238. Olar, T. T., Amann, R. P., and Pickett, B. W. (1983): Relationships among testicular size, daily production and output of spermatozoa, and extragonadal spermatozoal reserves of the dog. Biol. Reprod. *29*:1114.

239. Quinn, P. J. and White, I. G. (1966): Variation in semen cations in relation to semen quality and methods of collection. Fertil. Steril. *17*:815.

240. Saacke, R. G. (1982): Components of seminal quality. J. Anim. Sci. *55*(Suppl. 2):1.

241. Seidel, G. E., Jr. and Foote, R. H. (1969): Influence of semen collection techniques on composition of bull seminal plasma. J. Dairy Sci. *52*:1080.

242. Seidel, G. E., Jr. and Foote, R. H. (1973): Variance components of semen criteria from bulls ejaculated frequently and their use in experimental design. J. Dairy Sci. *56*:399.

243. Weisgold, A. D. and Almquist, J. O. (1979): Reproductive capacity of beef bulls. VI. Daily spermatozoal production, spermatozoal reserves, and dimensions and weight of reproductive organs. J. Anim. Sci. *48*:351.

Physical and Chemical Properties of Semen

244. Bartlett, D. J. (1962): Studies on dog semen. I. Morphological characteristics. J. Reprod. Fertil. *3*:173.

245. Bartlett, D. J. (1962): Studies on dog semen. II. Biochemical characteristics. J. Reprod. Fertil. *3*:190.

246. Berger, T., Drobnis, E. Z., Foley, L., et al. (1994): Evaluation of relative fertility of cryopreserved goat sperm. Theriogenology *41*:711.

247. Bielanski, W. (1975): The evaluation of stallion semen in aspects of fertility control and its use for artificial insemination. J. Reprod. Fertil. (Suppl. 23):19.

248. Boucher, J. H., Foote, R. H., and Kirk, R. W. (1958): The evaluation of semen quality in the dog and the effects of frequency of ejaculation upon semen quality, libido, and depletion of sperm reserves. Cornell Vet. *48*:67.

249. Brotherton, J. (1975): The counting and sizing of spermatozoa from ten animal species using a Coulter counter. Andrologia *7*:169.

250. Brown-Woodman, P. D. C. and White, I. G. (1974): Amino acid composition of semen and secretions of the male reproductive tract. Aust. J. Biol. Sci. *27*:415.

251. Calvete, J. J., Nessau, S., Maun, K., et al. (1994): Isolation and biochemical characterization of stallion seminal-plasma proteins. Reprod. Domestic Anim. *29*:411.

252. Casillas, E. R., Elder, C. M., and Hoskins, D. D. (1978): Adenyl cyclase activity in maturing bovine spermatozoa. Activation by GTP and polyamines. Fed. Proc. *37*:1688.

253. Crabo, B., Gustafsson, B., Bane, A. P., et al. (1967): The concentration of sodium, potassium, calcium, inorganic phosphate, protein, and glycerylphosphorylcholine in the epididymal plasma of bull calves. J. Reprod. Fertil. *13*:589.

254. Crump, J., Jr. and Crump, J. (1989): Stallion ejaculation induced by manual stimulation of the penis. Theriogenology *31*:341.

255. Dacheux, J. L., O'Shea, T., and Paquignon, M. (1979): Effects of osmolality, bicarbonate and buffer on the metabolism and motility of testicular epididymal and ejaculated spermatozoa of boars. J. Reprod. Fertil. *55*:287.

256. Dooley, M. P. and Pineda, M. H. (1986): Effect of method of collection on seminal characteristics of the domestic cat. Am. J. Vet. Res. *47*:286.

257. Gadella, B. M., Colenbrander, B., and Lopes-Cardozo, M. (1991): Arylsulfatases are present in seminal plasma of several domestic mammals. Biol. Reprod. *45*:381.

258. Gebauer, M. R., Pickett, B. W., and Swierstra, E. E. (1974): Reproductive physiology of the stallion. II. Daily production and output of sperm. J. Anim. Sci. *39*:732.

259. Gravance, C. G., Lewis, K. M., and Casey, P. J. (1995): Computer automated sperm head morphometry analysis (ASMA) of goat spermatozoa. Theriogenology *44*:989.

260. Hood, R. D., Witters, W. L., Foley, W. C., et al. (1967): Free amino acids in porcine spermatozoa. J. Anim. Sci. *26*:1101.

261. Hudson, M. T., Wellerson, R., Jr., and Kupferberg, A. B. (1965): Sialic acid in semen, spermatozoa and serum of mammals. J. Reprod. Fertil. *9*:189.

262. James, R. W., Heywood, R., and Street, A. E. (1979): Biochemical observations on Beagle dog semen. Vet. Rec. *104*:480.

263. King, G. J. and Macpherson, J. W. (1966): Alkaline and acid phosphatase activity, pH and osmotic pressure of boar semen. Can. J. Comp. Med. Vet. Sci. *30*:304.

264. Komarek, R. J., Pickett, B. W., Gibson, E. W., et al. (1965): Lipid of porcine spermatozoa, seminal plasma and gel. J. Reprod. Fertil. *9*:131.

265. Komarek, R. J., Pickett, B. W., Gibson, E. W., et al. (1965): Composition of lipids in stallion semen. J. Reprod. Fertil. *10*:337.

266. MacMillan, K. L., Desjardins, C., Kirton, K. T., et al. (1967): Relationship of glycerylphosphorylcholine to other constituents of bull semen. J. Dairy Sci. *50*:1310.

267. Mann, T. (1964): The Biochemistry of Semen and of the Male Reproductive Tract, 2nd ed. New York, NY, John Wiley & Sons, Inc.

268. Mann, T. (1975): Biochemistry of stallion semen. J. Reprod. Fertil. (Suppl. 23):47.

269. Matousek, J. (1985): Biological and immunological roles of proteins in the sperm of domestic animals (review). Anim. Reprod. Sci. *8*:1.

270. Mendoza, G., White, I. G., and Chow, P. (1989): Studies of chemical components of Angora goat seminal plasma. Theriogenology *32*:455.

271. Pickett, B. W. and Back, D. G. (1973): Procedures for preparation, collection, evaluation, and insemination

of stallion semen. Colorado State University, Animal Reproduction Laboratory, Ft. Collins, CO, Information Series #2-1.

272. Pickett, B. W., Faulkner, L. C., and Sutherland, T. M. (1970): Effect of month and stallion on seminal characteristics and sexual behavior. J. Anim. Sci. *31*:713.

273. Pickett, B. W., Sullivan, J. J., and Seidel, G. E., Jr. (1975): Reproductive physiology of the stallion. V. Effect of frequency of ejaculation on seminal characteristics and spermatozoal output. J. Anim. Sci. *40*:917.

274. Pineda, M. H., Dooley, M. P., and Martin, P. A. (1984): Long-term study on the effect of electroejaculation on seminal characteristics of the domestic cat. Am. J. Vet. Res. *45*:1038.

275. Pineda, M. H. and Dooley, M. P. (1984): Effects of voltage and order of voltage application on seminal characteristics of electroejaculates of the domestic cat. Am. J. Vet. Res. *45*:1520.

276. Polakoski, K. L. and Kopta, M. (1982): Seminal plasma. Chapter 4. *In:* Biochemistry of Mammalian Reproduction, edited by L. J. D. Zaneveld and R. T. Chatterton. New York, NY, John Wiley and Sons, Inc., pp. 97, 99–101, 103, 112.

277. Quinn, P. J., White, I. G., and Wirrick, B. R. (1965): Studies of the distribution of the major cations in semen and male accessory secretions. J. Reprod. Fertil. *10*:379.

278. Saito, S., Zeitz, L., Bush, I. M., et al. (1967): Zinc content of spermatozoa from various levels of canine and rat reproductive tracts. Am. J. Physiol. *213*:749.

279. Scott, T. W., Voglmayr, J. K., and Setchell, B. P. (1967): Lipid composition and metabolism in testicular and ejaculated ram spermatozoa. Biochem. J. *102*:456.

280. Seidel, G. E., Jr. and Foote, R. H. (1970): Compartmental analysis of sources of the bovine ejaculate. Biol. Reprod. *2*:189.

281. Setchell, B. P. (1974): Secretions of the testis and epididymides. J. Reprod. Fertil. *37*:165.

282. Skalet, L. H., Rodriguez, H. D., and Goyal, H. O. (1988): Effects of age and season on the type and occurrence of sperm abnormalities in Nubian bucks. Am. J. Vet. Res. *49*:1284.

283. Strezežek, J., Torska, J., Borkowski, K., et al. (1995): The biochemical characteristics of boar seminal plasma during high ejaculation frequency. Reprod. Domestic Anim. *30*:77.

284. Strezežek, J., Kordan, W., Glogowski, J., et al. (1995): Influence of semen-collection frequency on sperm quality in boars, with special reference to biochemical markers. Reprod. Domestic Anim. *30*:85.

285. Wales, R. G., Wallace, J. C., and White, I. G. (1966): Composition of bull epididymal and testicular fluid. J. Reprod. Fertil. *12*:139.

286. Wales, R. G. and White, I. G. (1965): Some observations on the chemistry of dog semen. J. Reprod. Fertil. *9*:69.

287. White, I. G. (1958): Biochemical aspects of mammalian semen. Anim. Breed. Abst. *26*:109.

288. White, I. G. and Lincoln, G. J. (1960): The yellow pigmentation of bull semen and its content of riboflavin, niacin, thiamine and related compounds. Biochem. J. *76*:301.

Mating

289. Aron, C. (1979): Mechanisms of control of the reproductive function by olfactory stimuli in female mammals. Physiol. Rev. *59*:229.

290. Aronson, L. R. and Cooper, M. L. (1974): Olfactory deprivation and mating behavior in sexually experienced male cats. Behav. Biol. *11*:459.

291. Beach, F. A. (1970): Coital behavior in dogs. IX. Sequelae to "coitus interruptus" in males and females. Physiol. Behav. *5*:263.

292. Carter, C. S. and Davis, J. M. (1977): Biogenic amines, reproductive hormones and female sexual behavior: A review. Behav. Rev. *1*:213.

293. Garcia-Sacristan, A., Casanueva, C. R., Castilla, C., et al. (1984): Adrenergic receptors in the urethra and prostate of the horse. Res. Vet. Sci. *36*:57.

294. Gebauer, M. R., Pickett, B. W., and Swierstra, E. E. (1974): Reproductive physiology of the stallion. II. Daily production and output of sperm. J. Anim. Sci. *39*:732.

295. Hart, B. L. and Jones, T. O. A. C. (1975): Effects of castration on sexual behavior of tropical male goats. Hormones and Behav. *6*:247.

296. Hopkins, S. G., Schubert, T. A., and Hart, B. L. (1976): Castration of adult male dogs: Effects on roaming, aggression, urine marking, and mounting. J. Am. Vet. Med. Assoc. *168*:1108.

297. Jarman, P. (1983): Mating system and sexual dimorphism in large, terrestrial, mammalian herbivores. Biol. Rev. *58*:485.

298. Kedia, K. and Markland, C. (1975): The effect of pharmacological agents on ejaculation. J. Urol. *114*:569.

299. Kimura, Y. (1970): On peripheral nerves controlling ejaculation. Tohoku J. Exp. Med. *105*:177.

300. Kimura, Y., Miyamoto, A., Urano, S., et al. (1982): The spinal monoaminergic systems relating to ejaculation. I. Ejaculation and dopamine. Andrologia *14*:341.

301. Lande, R. and Arnold, S. J. (1985): Evolution of mating preference and sexual dimorphism. J. Theor. Biol. *117*:651.

302. Lino, B. F. (1972): The output of spermatozoa in rams. II. Relationship to scrotal circumference, testis weight and the number of spermatozoa in different parts of the urogential tract. Aust. J. Biol. Sci. *25*:359.

303. Lino, B. F., Braden, A. W. H., and Turnbull, K. E. (1967): Fate of unejaculated spermatozoa. Nature *213*:594.

304. MacLusky, N. J. and Naftolin, F. (1981): Sexual differentiation of the central nervous system. Science *211*:1294.

305. Naden, J., Amann, R. P., and Squires, E. L. (1990): Testicular growth, hormone concentrations, seminal characteristics and sexual behavior in stallions. J. Reprod. Fertil. *88*:167.

306. Olar, T. T., Amann, R. P., and Pickett, B. W. (1983): Relationships among testicular size, daily production and output of spermatozoa, and extragonadal spermatozoal reserves of the dog. Biol. Reprod. *29*:1114.

307. Swierstra, E. E. (1966): Structural composition of Shorthorn bull testes and daily spermatozoa production as determined by quantitative testicular histology. Can. J. Anim. Sci. *46*:107.

308. Swierstra, E. E. (1970): The effect of low ambient temperatures on sperm production, epididymal sperm reserves, and semen characteristics of boars. Biol. Reprod. 2:23.

309. Tischner, M., Kosiniak, K., and Bielanski, W. (1974): Analysis of the pattern of ejaculation in stallions. J. Reprod. Fertil. *41*:329.

Spermatozoal Transport

310. Austin, C. R. (1975): Sperm fertility, viability and persistence in the female tract. J. Reprod. Fertil. (Suppl. 22):75.

311. Baker, R. D. and Degen, A. A. (1972): Transport of live and dead boar spermatozoa within the reproductive tract of gilts. J. Reprod. Fertil. *28*:369.

312. Baker, R. D., Dziuk, P. J., and Norton, H. W. (1968): Effect of volume of semen, number of sperm and drugs on transport of sperm in artificially inseminated gilts. J. Anim. Sci. *27*:88.

313. Hunter, R. H. F. (1975): Physiological aspects of sperm transport in the domestic pig, *Sus scrofa.* I. Semen deposition and cell transport. Br. Vet. J. 131:565.

314. Hunter, R. H. F. (1975): Physiological aspects of sperm transport in the domestic pig, *Sus scrofa.* II. Regulation, survival and fate of cells. Br. Vet. J. 131:681.

315. Hunter, R. H. F. (1981): Sperm transport and reservoirs in the pig oviduct in relation to the time of ovulation. J. Reprod. Fertil. *63*:109.

316. Hunter, R. H. F. and Nichol, R. (1983): Transport of spermatozoa in the sheep oviduct: Preovulatory sequestering of cells in the caudal isthmus. J. Exp. Zool. *228*:121.

317. Hunter, R. H. F. and Wilmut, I. (1982/1983): The rate of functional sperm transport into the oviducts of mated cows. Anim. Reprod. Sci. *5*:167.

318. Hunter, R. H. F., Barwise, L., and King, R. (1982): Sperm transport, storage and release in the sheep oviduct in relation to the time of ovulation. Br. Vet. J. 138:225.

319. Larsson, B. and Larsson, K. (1985): Distribution of spermatozoa in the genital tract of artificially inseminated heifers. Acta Vet. Scand. *26*:385.

320. Lightfoot, R. J., Corker, K. P., and Neil, H. G. (1967): Failure of sperm transport in relation to ewe infertility following prolonged grazing on oestrogenic pastures. Aust. J. Agric. Res. *18*:755.

321. Lightfoot, R. J. and Restall, B. J. (1971): Effects of site of insemination, sperm motility, and genital tract contractions on transport of spermatozoa in the ewe. J. Reprod. Fertil. *26*:1.

322. Mattner, P. E. and Braden, A. W. H. (1963): Spermatozoa in the genital tract of the ewe. I. Rapidity of transport. Aust. J. Biol. Sci. *16*:473.

323. Moeller, A. N. and VanDemark, N. L. (1955): *In vitro* speeds of bovine spermatozoa. Fertil. Steril. *6*:506.

324. Parker, W. G., Sullivan, J. J., and First, N. L. (1975): Sperm transport and distribution in the mare. J. Reprod. Fertil. (Suppl. 23):63.

325. Phillips, D. M. (1972): Comparative analysis of mammalian sperm motility. J. Cell Biol. *53*:561.

326. VanDemark, N. L. and Moeller, A. N. (1951): Speed of spermatozoan transport in reproductive tract of estrous cow. Am. J. Physiol. *165*:674.

References Added In Proof

327. Carreau, S., Genissel, C., Bilinska, B., et al. (1999): Sources of oestrogen in the testis and reproductive tract of the male. Int. J. Androl. *22*:211.

328. De Kretser, D, M., Meinhardt, A., Meehan, T., et al. (2000): The roles of inhibin and related peptides in gonadal function. Mol. Cell. Endocrinol. *161*:43.

329. Guraya, S. S. (2000): Cellular and molecular biology of capacitation and acrosome reaction in spermatozoa. Int. Rev. Cytol. *199*:1.

330. Hess, R. A. (2000): Oestrogen in fluid transport in efferent ducts of the male reproductive tract. Rev. Reprod. 5:84.

331. Hull, K. L. And Harvey, S. (2000): Growth hormone: Roles in male reproduction. Endocrine *13*:243.

332. Jones, R. C. (1999): To store or mature spermatozoa? The primary role of the epididymis. Int. J. Androl. *22*:57.

333. McLachlan, R. I. (2000): The endocrine control of spermatogenesis. Baillières Clin. Endocrinol. Metab. *14*:334.

334. Mather, J. P., Moore, A., and Li, R-H. (1997): Activins, inhibins, and follistatins: Further thoughts on a growing family of regulators. Proc. Soc. Exp. Biol. Med. *215*:209.

335. Nagata, S-i, Tsunoda, N., Nagamine, N., et al. (1998): Testicular inhibin in the stallion: Cellular source and seasonal changes in its secretion. Biol. Reprod. *59*:62.

336. Resko, J. A., Perkins, A., Roselli, C. E., et al. (1999): Sexual behaviour of rams: Male orientation and its endocrine correlates. J. Reprod. Fertil. (Suppl. 54):259.

337. Risbridger, G. P. And Cancilla, B. (2000): Role of activins in the male reproductive tract. Rev. Reprod. 5:99.

Female Reproductive System

M. H. Pineda

9

"Classical physiologists, by tradition, have generally sought to ascertain principles governing the steady state. The most notable feature of the female reproductive system is the total absence of a steady state. By virtue of its ever-changing functional status, the female reproductive system is clearly the prime example of a dynamic system. Its changes may be subtle, but just as small daily lengthenings of sunlight yield a season, so do subtle changes in hormonal status yield a reproductive cycle. Some events in the cycle can be traced on a day-to-day basis, but others occur at such a pace that a reading must be made every 3 hr or even more often in order to obtain a true account of the shifting functional status. Even during long periods of gestation, the physiological indicators must show a constantly unfolding pattern, else the pregnancy cannot progress. Although the underlying morphological and biochemical processes that manifest these cyclic events and the neural and endocrine mechanisms that generate the cyclicity are only partially understood, a massive volume of information is at hand."

(From: R. O. Greep, Preface to Handbook of Physiology, Section 7, Am. Physiol. Soc., Washington, D.C., 1973).

INTRODUCTION

Like the male gonad of mammals, the female gonad also produces gametes and hormones that regulate and integrate the functional activity of the female reproductive system. However, the homology probably ends at this point because the participation of the female in the reproductive processes is more intense and demanding of bodily energetic expenditures than those of the male of the species. Spermatozoal production in the postpubertal animal is continuous for males of both monoestric and seasonally breeding species, and fertile ejaculates are possible in the nonbreeding season. The reproductive processes of the female are cyclic, and substantially fewer gametes are released at each ovulation as compared to the number of gametes released by the male at each ejaculation. The reproductive participation of the male ends with deposition of semen in the genitals of the female at the time of mating. At this time, the reproductive participation of the female is only beginning, because she must contribute to the gestation, development, and survival of the offspring. To be successful, the reproductive activities of females and males must be exquisitely coordinated. The female releases her gametes at ovulation in synchrony with behavioral changes which ensure the attraction of the male for mating and natural insemination. In addition, the female must provide synchronous and adequate oviductal and uterine environments for gametic encounter and fertilization and for embryonic development, attachment, gestation, and successful completion of pregnancy. On top of all of these biologically costly and debilitating demands, the pregnant female has to provide for the delivery, feeding, and protection of the newborn after parturition.

Reproduction, essential as it is for the survival of the species, is not necessary for the survival of the individual. If one considers the demands imposed by the reproductive processes upon the female of the species, it should not be surprising that the reproductive activities are often the first to be arrested when the female is confronted with debilitating nutritional deficiencies or with life-threatening diseases. In many ways, years of domestication and selection for specific traits, such as milk production, have imposed further burdens on the female and, as a consequence, nonpregnant cycles are increasingly common or even the norm. In the nondomesticated, wild species in which there has been no man-made selection for production traits, the nonpregnant cycle is an oddity.

The female reproductive system consists of the ovaries, oviducts (also called uterine tubes and, with less frequency, Fallopian tubes), uterus, cervix, vagina, and vulva. The ovary is the female gonad; the vulva and clitoris form the external genitalia, and the other organs are referred to as the internal genitalia. Students are encouraged to review, in appropriate textbooks, the macro- and microscopic anatomy of the female reproductive system. Figure 9-1 shows the genitalia of the mare.

ORIGIN AND DEVELOPMENT OF THE REPRODUCTIVE ORGANS

The embryologic development of the male and female reproductive organs is the same prior to sexual differentiation (see Chapter 7, Biology of Sex). Reference is made to Table 7-3 for the homologies of the male and female reproductive systems). Failure of differentiation of these systems in whole, or in part, can lead to some of the intersexes and sterility in domestic animals.

OVARIES

The ovaries, as the testes, are paired organs that serve both a gametogenic and an endocrine function. This dual role is complementary, interdependent, and necessary for successful reproduction.

Gross Anatomy

The ovaries of the normal XX embryo are formed under the influence of the X chromosomes (see Chapter 7). The differentiation of the ovary begins slightly later than that of the testis. The initiation of meiosis, the formation of follicles, and differentiation of steroidogenic cells are the three major events in the development of the ovary. The female gonad remains perma-

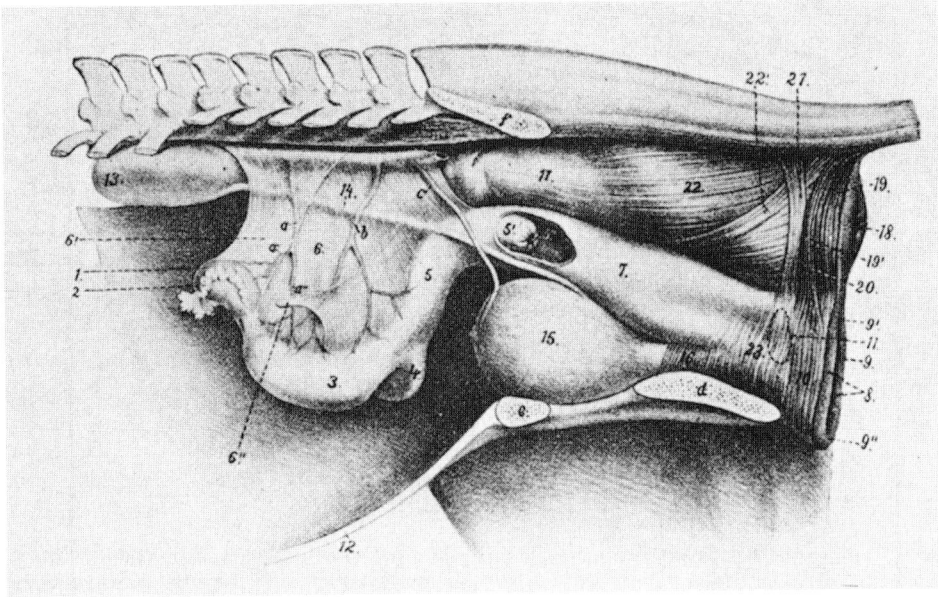

Fig. 9-1. Lateral view of genital organs and adjacent structures of the mare. Removal of the other abdominal viscera has allowed the ovaries and uterus to sink down; this has, however, the advantage of showing the broad ligaments of the uterus. **1,** left ovary; **2,** uterine or fallopian tube; **3,** left cornu uteri; **4,** right cornu uteri; **5,** corpus uteri; **5',** portio vaginalis uteri, and **5",** os uteri, seen through window cut in vagina; **6,** broad ligament of uterus; **6",** round ligament of uterus; **7,** vagina; **8,** labia vulvae; **9,** rima vulvae, **9',** dorsal commissure, and **9"** ventral commissure of vulva; **10,** constrictor vulvae; **11,** position of vestibular bulb; **12,** ventral wall of abdomen; **13,** left kidney; **14,** left ureter; **15,** urinary bladder; **16,** urethra; **17,** rectum; **18,** anus; **19, 19',** unpaired and paired parts of sphincter ani externus; **20,** retractor ani cut at disappearance under sphincter ani externus; **21,** suspensory ligament of anus; **22,** longitudinal muscular layer of rectum; **22',** rectococcygeus; **23,** constrictor vaginae; **a,** utero-ovarian artery, with ovarian (**a'**) and uterine (**a"**) branches; **b,** uterine artery; **c,** umbilical artery; **d,** ischium; **e,** pubis; **f,** ilium. (After Ellenberger, *In:* Leisering's Atlas; Sisson and Grossman: The Anatomy of the Domestic Animals. Courtesy of W. B. Saunders Co., Philadelphia, PA, 1975).

nently located in the abdominal cavity during development and completion of differentiation.

The shape of the ovary varies according to the species and stage of the estrous cycle, but there are some generalizations that can be made depending upon whether the female is a **polytocous** (litter-bearing; see Fig. 9-24) or a **monotocous** (single-bearing) species. The functional ovary of a polytocous animal (sow, bitch, or cat) has several follicles or has several corpora lutea which give the appearance of a cluster of grapes. The monotocous animal (cow, ewe, and mare) has an ovoid-shaped ovary unless a follicle or corpus luteum is present, then the ovary takes on a distorted shape depending on the size of the structure, whether an antral follicle or a fully developed corpus luteum. The mare has a kidney-shaped ovary because of the ovulation fossa, which is normally the site of all ovula-

tions. Table 9-1 gives some pertinent data for domestic animals.

Figure 9-2 shows the anatomic relationship between the ovary and the oviduct in the ewe. Figure 9-3 depicts an idealized section showing the sequence of events in a mammalian ovary, including follicular growth and maturation, ovulation and release of the oocyte, and corpus luteum formation and regression. The figure is composite and idealized because it shows all the ovarian events as occurring at the same time, without distinction to a prevailing follicular or luteal phase of the cycle.

The epithelium covering the mammalian ovary is a single layer of cuboidal or low columnar cells called the **germinal epithelium.** This layer covers the entire ovary except in the mare, where it is limited to the ovulation fossa. Beneath the germinal epithelium is the tunica al-

Table 9-1 **Comparative Anatomy of the Adult Ovary and Reproductive Tract of Domestic Animals**[a]

	Bitch	Cat	Cow	Ewe	Goat	Llama	Mare	Sow
Ovary								
Shape	Oval, slightly flattened, covered by a bursa with a slit	Oval, slightly flattened	Almond-shaped	Almond-shaped	Round or oval	Oval, covered by the bursa	Kidney-shaped; with ovulation fossa	Berry-shaped (cluster of grapes)
Weight of one ovary (g)	0.1–1.5 (in nonpregnant bitches)	0.1–0.3	10–20	3–4	1.8–3.5	2–2.5	40–80	3–10
Mature Graafian follicles								
Number	3–15	2–10	1–2	1–4	2–8	1–6	1–2	10–25
Diameter (mm)	2–14	1–2	12–19	5–10	up to 12	8–12	25–70	8–12
Ovary that is the more active	---	---	Right	Right	Right	---	Left	Left
Mature corpus luteum								
Shape	Spheroid	Spheroid	Spheroid or ovoid	Spheroid or ovoid	---	Spheroid to ovoid	Pear-shaped	Spheroid or ovoid
Diameter (mm)	2–5	1.5–3	20–25	9	---	10–15	10–25	10–15
Maximum size attained on (days from ovulation)	5–14	5–14	10	7–9	---	---	14	14
Regression starts (days from ovulation)	---	---	---	14–15	12–14	---	---	17
Oviduct								
Length (cm)	4–7	3–5	25	15–19	---	---	20–30	14–30
Uterus								
Type	Bicornuate	Bicornuate	Bipartite	Bipartite	Bipartite	Bicornuate	Bipartite	Bicornuate
Length of horn (cm)	10–14	6–10	35–40	10–12	---	---	15–25	40–110
Length of body (cm)	1.4–2	1.5–2	2–4	1–2	---	---	15–20	5
Surface lining of endometrium	Longitudinal folds	Longitudinal folds	70–120 caruncles	60–100 caruncles	115–120 caruncles	---	Conspicuous longitudinal folds	Slight longitudinal folds
Cervix								
Length (cm)	1.5–2	1–1.5	8–10	4–10	5–6	---	7–8	10–23
Outside diameter (cm)	0.5–1.5	0.4–0.6	3–4	2–3	---	---	3.5–4	2–3
Cervical lumen								
Shape	Irregular	Irregular	2–5 annular rings	Annular rings	Up to five annular rings	Spiral fold, gives the appearance of three rings	Conspicuous folds	Corkscrew-like
Os uteri								
Shape	Slightly protruding	---	Small & protruding	Small & protruding	Protruding	---	Clearly defined	Poorly defined
Anterior vagina								
Length (cm)	5–10	---	25–30	10–14	7.3	---	20–35	10–23
Hymen	Poorly defined	Poorly defined	Poorly defined	Well developed	---	---	Well developed	Poorly defined
Vestibule								
Length (cm)	2–5	0.5–1.5	10–12	2.5–3	3.6	---	10–12	6–8

[a]Data are estimates. Actual values vary with age, breed, and parity.
Adapted from different sources, including: E. S. E. Hafez, Reproduction in Farm Animals, 5th ed., Philadelphia, PA, Lea & Febiger, 1987; H. H. Cole and P. T. Cupps, Reproduction in Domestic Animals, 3rd ed. New York, NY, Academic Press, 1977; F. T. Cowan and J. W. MacPherson, Can. J. Comp. Med. Vet. Sci 30:107, 1966; A. C. Andersen and M. E. Simpson, The Ovary and Reproductive Cycle of the Dog (Beagle), 1st ed. Los Altos, CA, Geron-X, Inc., 1973; C. L. Smith, et al., Theriogenology 41:573, 1994; P. W. Bravo, Vet. Clin. North Am. 10:265, 1994; M. C. Smith Reproductive anatomy of the female goat. In: Current Therapy in Theriogenology 2, D. A. Morrow, ed. Philadelphia, PA, W. B. Saunders, 1986; J. H. Sokolowski, et al., Am. J. Vet. Res. 34:1001, 1973.

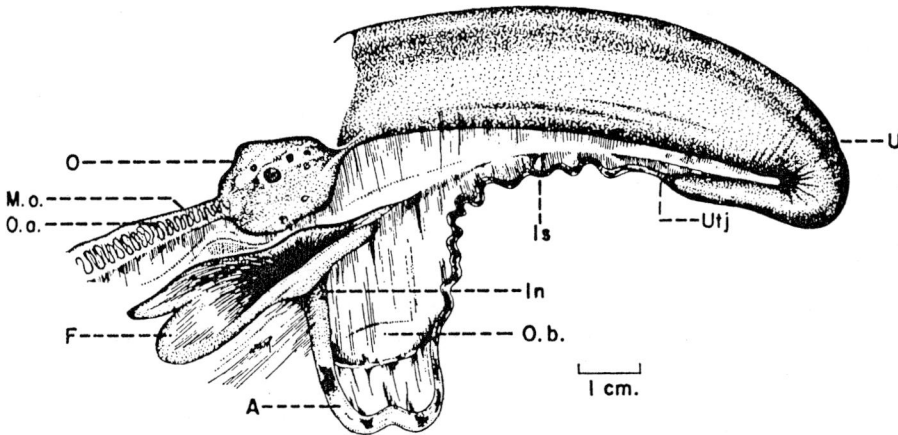

Fig. 9-2. Anatomical relationship between the ovary and the oviduct in the ewe. **A**, ampulla; **F**, fimbriae; **In**, infundibulum; **Is**, isthmus; **M.o.**, mesovarium; **O**, ovary; **O.a.**, ovarian artery; **O.b.**, ovarian bursa; **U**, uterus; **Utj**, uterotubal junction. Note the suspended loop to which the ovarian bursa is attached. The oviduct in the ewe is pigmented. (from Hafez, E. S. E., Reproduction in Farm Animals, 5th ed. Philadelphia, PA, Lea & Febiger, 1987).

buginea and then the ovarian cortex, where the large mass of follicles are located.

Transrectal ultrasonography has emerged as a valuable technique in veterinary medicine for the noninvasive visualization and evaluation of the functional status of female reproductive organs. The technique is particularly useful for the *in vivo*, day-to-day evaluation of the morphological and functional status of ovarian follicles and corpora lutea in the cycling animal.

Ovarian Follicles

The embryonic origin of the cells which eventually form the ovarian follicle is one of the most controversial and still unresolved problem in embryology. Recent studies indicate that the undifferentiated and the differentiated gonads are colonized by invasive mesonephric cells which become associated with the germinal cells of the ovarian surface. The ovigerous cords, which are transitory, are formed in close association with the mesonephric cells (Fig. 9-3). These mesonephric cells later participate in the organization and probably in the formation of definite ovarian structures such as follicles. The superficial epithelium of the ovary penetrates the albuginea of the ovary and forms cords and crypts in the ovarian cortex. These cords and crypts were formerly thought to contribute to

the oocyte population, and the name germinal epithelium is derived from this belief. Some invaginations of the superficial epithelium terminate in fragmented cords, forming nests of epithelial-like cells in close proximity to growing follicles. The close association of these nests of cells from the superficial epithelium to the follicle may provide a continuous source of granulosa cells to the growing follicles during postpubertal life.

From the morphologic point of view, the ovarian follicles may be classified (Fig. 9-4) in three major groups:

1. primordial or unilaminar follicles,
2. growing follicles, and
3. Graafian follicles.

It must be noted, however, that **folliculogenesis,** defined as the formation of a mature or Graafian follicle from a pool of primordial, nongrowing follicles, is a highly dynamic and rapid process that occurs during the follicular phase of the estrous cycle of the female.

PRIMORDIAL (PRIMARY) FOLLICLES consist of an oocyte surrounded by a single layer of epithelial, flattened granulosa cells with irregularly-shaped nuclei. Thecal cells are not present at this stage of folliculogenesis. Primordial,

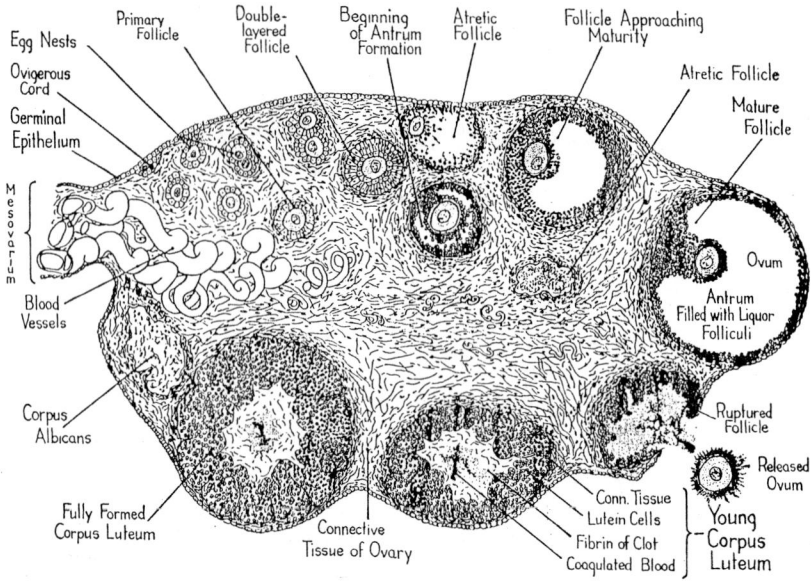

Fig. 9-3. Schematic diagram of an ovary, showing the sequence of events in origin, growth, and rupture of an ovarian (Graafian) follicle and formation and retrogression of the corpus luteum. Follow clockwise around ovary, starting at the mesovarium. (B. M. Patten, Human Embryology. Courtesy of Blakiston Division of McGraw-Hill Book Co., New York, NY, 1946).

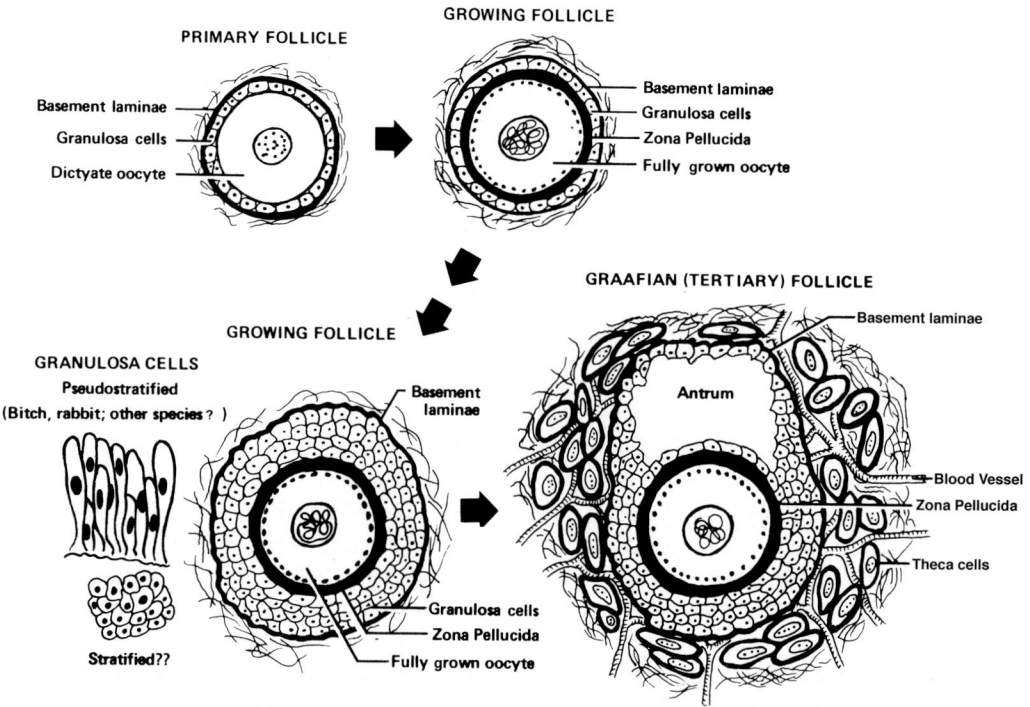

Fig. 9-4. Schematic representation of ovarian follicular growth. (Adapted from different sources, including G. F. Erickson, et al., Endocrine Rev., *6*:371, 1985).

unilaminar follicles lack a distinct vasculature. A discrete follicular capillary bed develops later in the growing follicles (Fig. 9-4). This unilaminar stage of development is reached at birth in the newborn heifer, and the ovary may contain as many as 150,000 of these follicles (Fig. 9-5). The number of primordial follicles decreases to as few as 1,000 in a cow by 15 to 20 years of age. A similar age-related decline in the number of primordial follicles present in the ovaries of newborn animals occurs in other species. The number of primordial follicles that undergo folliculogenesis to reach the mature, Graafian stage from puberty on is only a small fraction of the number of follicles available in the pool of primordial follicles. Most follicles will either un-

dergo a process of regression called **atresia** at some stage of folliculogenesis or remain as primordial follicles with no sign of growth. Primordial follicles containing more than one oocyte (polyovular) have been observed in several species (Fig. 9-6). Figures 9-6 through 9-9 show aspects of folliculogenesis in the heifer.

GROWING FOLLICLES are follicles that have left the resting stage as primordial follicles and have begun growth, but have not yet developed a thecal layer or antrum (cavity). In at least two species, the rabbit[115] and the bitch,[2] the granulosa cells form a pseudostratified epithelium, with each granulosa cell reaching the basal lamina of the follicular wall. The position of the nucleus and the height of the cell gives the appear-

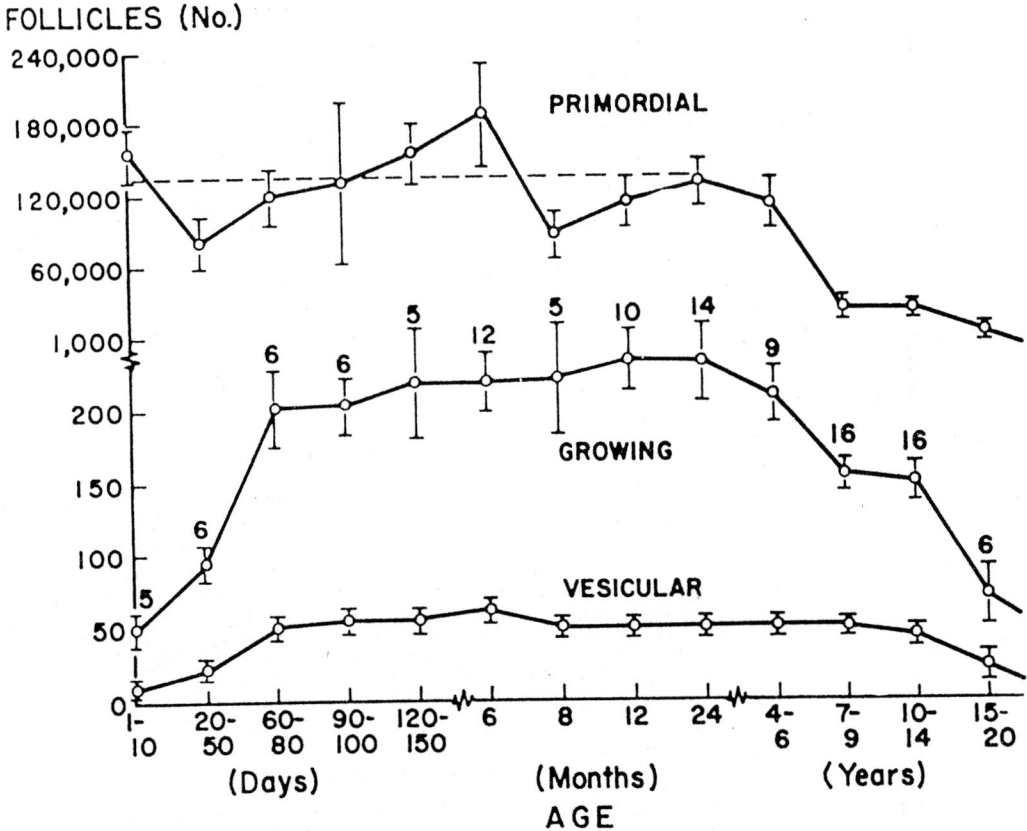

Fig. 9-5. Development and senescence of follicles of the postnatal bovine ovary. Quantitative analysis of the follicles of the postnatal bovine ovary. Primordial follicles encompassed by a single layer of follicle cells. Broken line represents average for animals aged 0 to 24 months. Growing follicles with two or more layers of follicle cells, but without a fully-formed vesicle. Vertical bars and numerals represent the standard error and number of ovarian pairs analyzed, respectively. (After: B. H. Erickson, J. Anim. Sci. *25*:800, 1966).

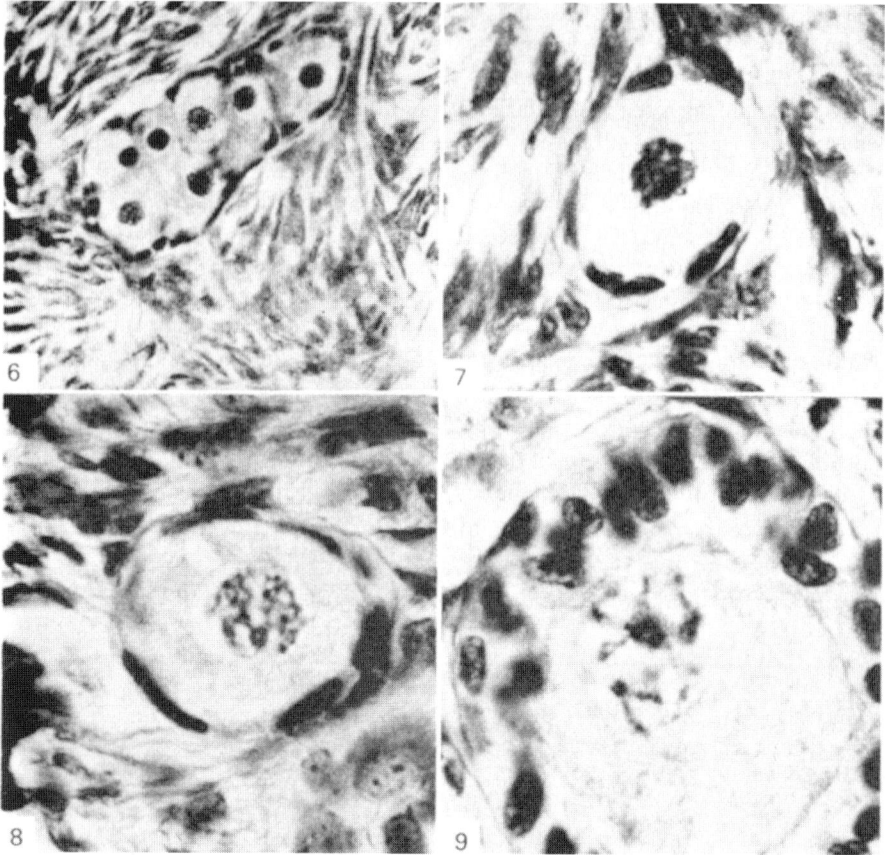

Fig. 9-6. Three primordial follicles from a cow ovary. The one on the left contains 5 oocytes. The two oocytes to the right form solitary primordial follicles. 395 × H. E. (From: E. Rajakoski, Acta Endocrinol. *34* (Suppl. 52):1, 1960).

Fig. 9-7. Primordial follicle from a cow ovary with oocyte and its nucleus. The chromosomes form a compact cluster which occupies only a portion of the nucleus. 990 × H. E. (From: E. Rajakoski, Acta Endocrinol. *34* (Suppl. 52):1, 1960).

Fig. 9-8. Eccentric section through an oocyte nucleus in a primordial follicle from a cow. The chromosomes are in the pachytene stage and the nucleolus is visible, although weakly stained. 990 × H. E. (From: E. Rajakoski, Acta Endocrinol. *34* (Suppl. 52):1, 1960).

Fig. 9-9. Growing follicle from a cow ovary with a 2-layered epithelium. Chromosomes are in the pachytene stage; the nucleolus is visible. 990 × H. E. (From: E. Rajakoski, Acta Endocrinol. *34* (Suppl. 52):1, 1960).

ance of stratification in cross sections of growing and mature follicles. Hence, it is not only possible, but also likely, that a similar arrangement and pseudostratification may be also the norm for growing and mature follicles of the other domestic species. This may be particularly true for those species that have large follicles and a thick follicular wall. Reaching the base-ment membrane would allow an equal and better distribution of nutrients to each and all of the granulosa cells. In this chapter, reference is made to the 'layer' of granulosa cells only to indicate the histologic appearance of the granulosa cells in thick, cross sections of the follicle, not necessarily to truly imply stratification of cells.

A growing follicle is characterized as developing two or more 'layers' of granulosa cells surrounding the oocyte (Figs. 9-4 and 9-9 through 9-11). With continued growth, additional 'layers' of granulosa cells appear to surround the oocyte. A zona pellucida surrounding the oocyte may be seen at this stage (see Chapter 7). The number of growing follicles in an ovary at a given time is relatively small in the domestic species and varies with the stage of the estrous cycle. By the onset of puberty, as many as 200 growing follicles may be present in the ovary of a heifer.

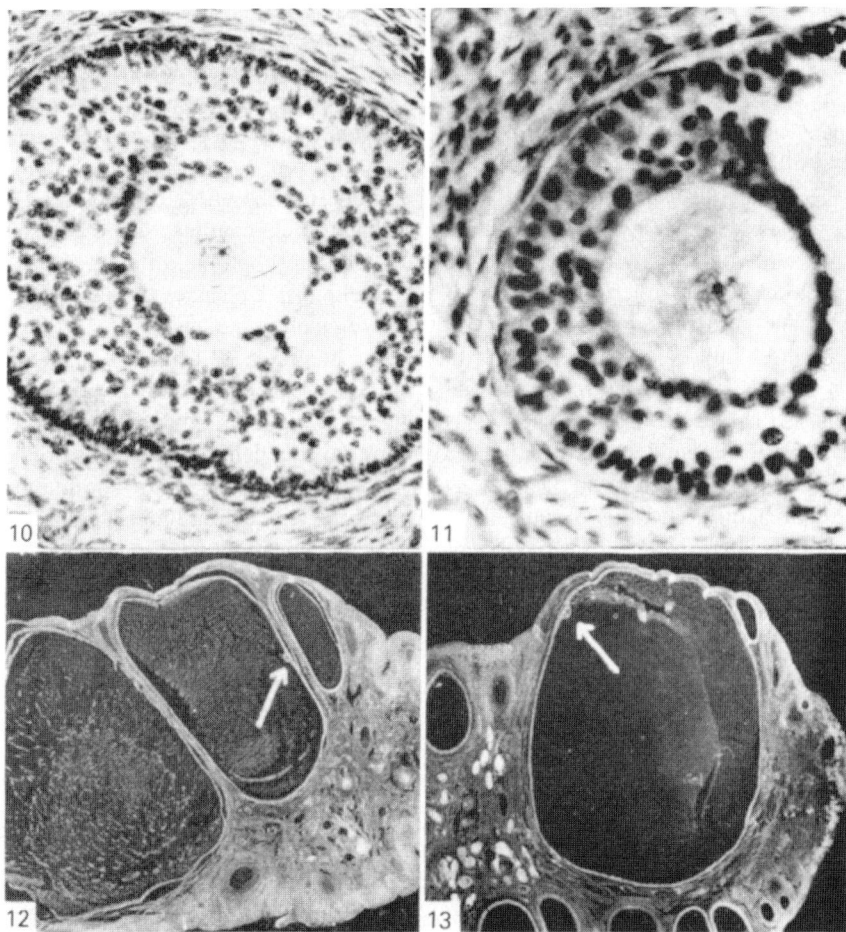

Fig. 9-10. Transitional phase between growing and Graafian follicles. Note the pools of liquor folliculi in the granulosa cells. 200 × H. E. (From: E. Rajakoski, Acta Endocrinol. *34* (Suppl. 52):1, 1960).

Fig. 9-11. Small Graafian follicle. Liquor folliculi fills the antrum, the granulosa is compact. 200 × H. E. (From: E. Rajakoski, Acta Endocrinol. *34* (Suppl. 52):1, 1960).

Fig. 9-12. Photograph of a serial section of the ovary taken from a heifer on the twentieth day of the cycle. Cumulus oophorus (**arrow**) in a normal follicle with a diameter of 8.3 mm. 4 ×. (From: E. Rajakoski, Acta Endocrinol. *34* (Suppl. 52):1, 1960).

Fig. 9-13. Photograph of a serial section of the ovary taken from a heifer on the twenty-first day of the cycle. Cumulus oophorus (**arrow**) in a normal follicle 12.5 mm in diameter. 4 ×. (From: E. Rajakoski, Acta Endocrinol. *34* (Suppl. 52):1, 1960).

GRAAFIAN FOLLICLES (vesicular follicles) are follicles in which an antrum is clearly visible (Figs. 9-4 and 9-10 through 9-13). The Graafian follicle protrudes from the surface of the ovary (Fig. 9-3 and Fig. 9-21) and as the antrum enlarges, the granulosa layer is evened out except at the *cumulus oophorus,* where the oocyte rests in a nest of granulosa cells. The diameter of the primary oocyte of the cow is 80 to 120 μm at this stage and is surrounded by the zona pellucida. Two layers of thecal cells, theca interna and theca externa, are now discernible; and, together with the granulosa cells, form the wall of the follicle (Fig. 9-14). The **theca externa,** formed by myoid-type (muscle) cells and fibrocytes, is the outermost layer of the follicular wall. These myoid cells have cytoplasmic features, such as parallel microfilaments containing actin and myosin, suggesting a role in follicular contractility. The **theca interna** (Fig. 9-14) is formed by ovarian fibrocytes and stromal cells as the follicle matures. These cells undergo dramatic differentiation into epithelioid cells, rich in granules and cytoplasmic organelles. Maximal differentiation of the cells of the theca interna occurs late in the process of

follicular maturation, in the large antral follicles present at the time of estrus. The innermost layer of the follicular wall is formed by granulosa cells (Figs. 9-11 and 9-14), which are separated from the thecal cells and ovarian stroma throughout folliculogenesis by a well-defined basal lamina or basement membrane. This membrane becomes discontinuous near the time of follicular rupture during ovulation. The granulosa cells maintain contact with the oocyte during folliculogenesis and in the preantral and antral stages they form the *cumulus oophorus.* The cumulus cells maintain contact with the oocyte, even as the follicular fluid fills the antrum and eccentrically displaces the oocyte. As the follicle matures, the granulosa cells also undergo morphologic differentiation, including epithelioid-like changes and increased cytoplasmic organelles, indicative of steroidogenic function. The granulosa cells, and to a lesser degree the cells of the theca interna, show adherens and gap types of intercellular junctions. Gap junctions are abundant between cells of the cumulus oophorus and the oocyte. The number of gap junctions between granulosa cells increases as folliculogenesis progresses toward the mature Graafian stage of the follicle. Gap junctions between granulosa cells play an important role in the movement of small molecules, ions, and nutrients from the basement membrane toward the antrum. In addition, intercellular gap junctions may serve as channels for hormonal communication between the peripheral cells of the follicle and the oocyte.

Primordial follicles lack an independent vasculature. The capillary bed, confined to the thecal layer, develops around the follicle as the thecal cells are formed. These thecal capillaries increase in size and concentrate in the theca interna in close proximity to the basement membrane. Blood flow through these capillaries also increases as the follicle matures.

The permeability of the follicular wall increases in the preovulatory period in several species. In general, the follicular wall appears to offer little resistance to the entry of blood constituents into the follicle, since the composition of the follicular fluid is similar to that of the blood plasma. However, either through metabolic or se-

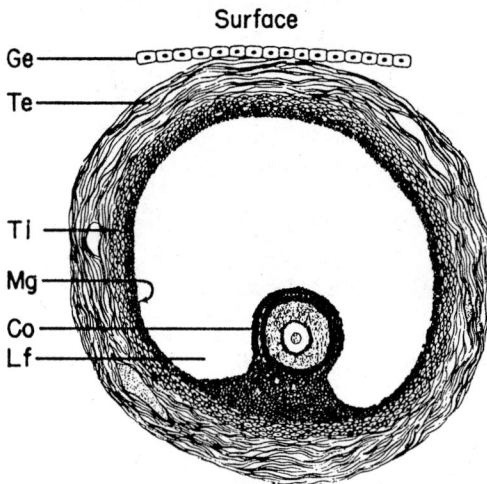

Surface

Ge

Te

Ti

Mg

Co

Lf

Fig. 9-14. Graafian follicle. **Co,** cumulus oophorus; **Ge,** germinal epithelium; **Lf,** liquor folliculi; **Mg,** membrana granulosa; **Te,** theca externa; **Ti,** theca interna. (From: E. S. E. Hafez, ed. *In:* Reproduction in Farm Animals, 5th ed. Philadelphia, PA, Lea & Febiger, 1987).

cretory activities of the follicular cells, the follicular fluid has a lower concentration of gonadotropins and a higher concentration of steroid hormones than that of the peripheral blood. Thus, the follicular fluid may serve the function of storing the steroid hormones produced by the follicular cells. In addition, the follicular fluid functions as a vehicle for the transport of the oocyte through the oviduct from the rupturing follicle in the ovaries to the uterus. The follicular and oviductal fluids concurrently provide factors for spermatozoal capacitation, fertilization of the oocyte, and initial embryonic development.

FOLLICULAR ATRESIA. Few of the follicles and oocytes that undergo growth and maturation at each cycle are destined to ovulate. In fact, in most species, the great majority of follicles present in the ovaries at birth will undergo degenerative changes and atresia as the animal ages. The atretic changes of the follicle may occur at any stage of follicular development. Cells from the granulosa membrane are most frequently affected by apoptosis, defined as programmed cell death[196, 200] (see Chapter 7), and by degenerative changes characteristic of atresia. Observation of the apoptotical cell death of granulosa cells was made by Wagener as early as 1879 and by Flemming in 1895 (cited by Clarke and Clarke[35]). Only recently, apoptosis of granulosa cells has been revisited and regained popularity among researchers. Interestingly, recent evidences indicate that in pigs, apoptosis occurs in the granulosa cells of antral follicles undergoing atresia but not in the cumulus cells, which surround the oocyte. Many theories have been proposed to explain this wastage of follicles and oocytes, including the participation of androgens secreted by the ovary, yet the factors and mechanisms causing it remain largely undetermined. The concurrent establishment of basal follicular endothelia, which are part of a rich capillary bed around the follicle, and the associated increase in blood blow, would provide nutrients needed for follicular cell survival, possibly retarding or "rescuing" follicular cells from a programmed apoptotic death in those follicles that mature and eventually ovulate. There appears to be a common apoptotical pathway for granulosa, thecal, and luteal cells, which would involve genes encoding for certain proteins that act as intracellular effectors.[196] Readers seeking further discussion of mechanisms regarding physiological, programmed cell death are referred to the excellent reviews by Clarke and Clarke[35] and Tilly.[196]

The Ovarian Follicle as a Functional Unit

The ovarian follicle (Tables 9-2 and 9-3) is a structural and functional unit which produces steroid hormones (androgens and estrogens), peptide hormones, including inhibin, oocyte maturation inhibition factors, insulin growth factor 1, oxytocin in some species, gonadocrinin, a GnRH-like hormone, and possibly other factors, such as activin and follistatin, which are under study to clarify their physiological role. Most of the peptide factors, likely in a paracrine form of communication, act as intraovarian coordinating factors for the activities of the follicular cells. The steroidogenic function of the ovarian follicle, its gonadotropic, and its local control will be discussed later in this chapter, under the heading of Ovarian Hormones.

The follicle provides a chemical and physical microenvironment, including lower temperature than the somatic temperature, for oocyte growth and maturation. As discussed in Chapter 7, the oocyte is in a quiescent stage of meiosis in the primordial follicle, arrested at the diplotene stage or dictyate stage (germinal vesicle). These oocytes are devoid of receptors to LH; however, during the preovulatory growth of the follicle, likely under the influence of LH mediated by the

Table 9-2 Progesterone Levels in Peripheral Plasma During the Follicular and Luteal Phases

Species[a]	Follicular Phase (ng/ml)	Luteal Phase (ng/ml)
Cow	0.4	6.6
Gilt	0.5	12.0
Ewe	0.25	3.7
Llama	< 1.0	1.0 –> 2.0[b]
Mare	0.4	7.7 to 9.5
Bitch	< 1.0	23.0
Queen	< 1.0	24.6 to 25.8

[a]Notice higher levels in the polytocous species.
[b]Varies during pregnancy.
Compiled from different sources.

Table 9-3   Secretory Products of Ovarian Follicular Cells

Product	Secretory Cell(s)	Function
Androgens (androsterone, testosterone)	Metabolic products of thecal cells steroidogenesis.	Accumulate in the follicular fluid. May participate in feedback control for LH.
Estrogens (Estradiol-17β)	Metabolization of androgens to estrogens by the granulosa cells.	Maintenance of the normal morphologic and functional status of female reproductive organs.
Gonadocrinin	GnRH-like decapeptide produced by the granulosa cells.	Regulates number of receptors for LH on thecal cells.
Inhibin	Glycoprotein produced by the granulosa cells. Heterodimer composed of α and β subunits.	Involved in the regulation of follicular development by controlling the secretion of FSH.
Insulin-like Growth Factor 1	Peptide produced by the granulosa cells.	Participates in the amplification of gonadotropin steroidogenic activity by granulosa and thecal cells.
Müllerian-inhibiting Hormone (MIH)	Granulosa cells of developing follicles.	Its role in the female is undetermined.
Oocyte Maturation Inhibitor (OMI)	Granulosa cells of primordial and developing follicles.	Maintains oocytes arrested at the dictyate stage of meiosis.
Oxytocin	Granulosa and luteal cells.	May exert a paracrine control of steroidogenesis.
Relaxin	Polypeptide produced by granulosa cells	Role of relaxin in the cycling animal has not been established.
Other potential factors under study include: Activin, the β-subunit of inhibin; β-endorphins; follistatin, interleukin-I system, and insulin-like growth factor-2.	Not clearly established.	Postulated roles are related to integrative modulation of gonadotropin activity.

Compiled from different sources.

follicular cells, the oocyte undergoes in most species the meiotic maturation and becomes a secondary oocyte (Fig. 9-15). This process takes place around 12 hours prior to ovulation in most of the domestic species. The oocyte maturation inhibiting factor (OMI; see Chapter 7, Fig. 7-10) plays an important role to maintain the oocyte in the arrested, dictyate stage of meiosis. The close association of the oocyte with the cells of the *cumulus oophorus* and *corona radiata* during follicular maturation and the presence of numerous gap junctions among the cells of the cumulus facilitate factors secreted by follicular cells and nutrients present in the follicular fluid to reach, stimulate, nourish, and control the growth and maturation of the oocyte.

The ovulating follicle emerges from a group of follicles that grow in response to gonadotropic stimulation. The number of follicles

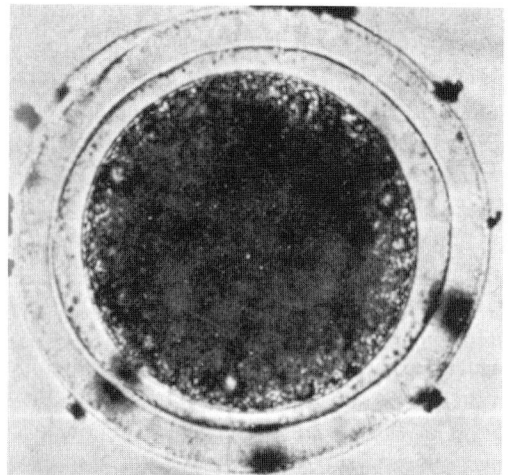

Fig. 9-15. Unfertilized oocyte of a cow (400 ×). (From: J. Hammond, *In:* Physiology of Farm Animals. London, England, Butterworths Scientific Publications, 1957). See Chapter 19 for pictures of fertilized oocytes.

that reach the stage of mature, Graafian follicles at each estrous cycle is set by the genetic make-up of the species, e.g., monotocous or single-bearing species grow, mature, and later ovulate a single follicle, whereas polytocous or litter-bearing species mature and ovulate several follicles at each follicular phase of the estrous cycle. The interaction of follicular estradiol with pituitary gonadotropins appears to play a major role in determining the number of follicles that ovulate. Possibly, a fine-tuned feedback mechanism[75] in which inhibin, estradiol-17β, number of receptors for FSH and LH in the follicular cells, and intraovarian factors, including growth factors, modulate the number of follicles that mature and ovulate at each cycle. The amount of gonadotropins, particularly FSH, undoubtedly has a significant role in the control of the number of follicles that reach the ovulatory stage. This is clearly exemplified by the magnitude of superovulatory responses obtainable from single-bearing species, such as the cow, when induced to superovulate with exogenous gonadotropins. It is not unusual to recover, after treatment with gonadotropins, as many as 40 oocytes or embryos from the oviducts of an animal that seldom matures more than one follicle and releases more than one oocyte from the ovaries at each estrous cycle (see Chapter 19).

Avian Ovaries

The avian ovary is an unusual organ. Domestic fowls have been selected to lay large numbers of eggs, far beyond the need for perpetuation of the species. Birds are oviparous and must provide for the nutrition of the embryo outside the body of the female. Consequently, a large amount of yolk must be provided for nutrition of the embryo in birds. In birds, only the left ovary is functional under normal conditions. The right ovary is rudimentary and ordinarily nonfunctional. This condition sets the stage for a phenomenon of sex-reversal sometimes reported in the popular press, whereby a hen is reported to have changed sex and become a rooster. If the left ovary ceases its function due to destruction by disease, accident, or surgical removal, then the rudimentary right ovary may become an ovotestis and secrete androgens. Under this con-

dition, the female develops secondary sex characteristics of the male including comb, plumage, spurs, and behavioral changes such as crowing and copulatory attempts. The Wolffian duct system does not develop, so there is no connection between the newly developed testes and the exterior.

Unequal Function of Ovaries

The two ovaries do not function equally in most domestic species, and through sequential estrous cycles, one of the ovaries is more active than the other. Ewes, cows, and goats ovulate more frequently from the right than from the left ovary. In the ewe and goat, 54 to 60% of the ovulations occur in the right ovary, and in the cow, 60 to 65% of the oocytes are released from the right ovary. The proximity of the left ovary to the rumen may be responsible for the unequal activity of the left ovary of ruminants, possibly due to extrinsic factors such as temperature fluctuations and mechanical effects caused by contractions of the rumen.

In the sow, the left ovary is the most functional, providing 55 to 60% of the oocytes. The mare ovulates approximately 60% of the oocytes from the left ovary, possibly because the right ovary is close to the cecum.

While unilateral orchiectomy is followed by a moderate hypertrophy of the contralateral testis, unilateral ovariectomy in adult cycling animals is always followed in time by a compensatory and functional hypertrophy of the remaining ovary. The number of follicles that ovulate from the remaining ovary increases after unilateral ovariectomy in litter-bearing species, and the number of offspring born after compensatory hypertrophy is established is not different from the number of offspring produced by the two ovaries of intact females. Lipschütz[116] postulated in 1928 the law of follicular constancy, stating that, for a given species, the number of follicles that ovulate at each cycle remains constant, suggesting again that the number of follicles that grow, mature, and ovulate is genetically preestablished for the species. Compensatory hypertrophy may result from more gonadotropins becoming available to the remaining ovary. Surprisingly, however, the side of ovariectomy (left versus right) does not seem to influence the compensatory response of the remaining ovary, which suggests again, a genetic control of the number of follicles that reach the mature ovulatory stage.

TUBULAR GENITAL TRACT

The tubular components of the female genital tract are the oviducts, uterus, and vagina. The tubular genital tract of the female serves as the transportation route for the spermatozoa to the *ampulla* of the oviduct, where fertilization occurs. In addition, the fimbriated end of the oviduct captures the oocytes at ovulation, and the oviducts serve as a route for the movement of the developing embryo to the uterus, where gestation occurs. Finally, at the end of gestation, the fetus is expelled through the cervix and vagina at parturition and is termed a **newborn.**

The cyclic physiological changes of the tubular genital tract (Table 9-4) will be considered in

Table 9-4   *Mucosal Changes in the Reproductive Tract of the Cow During the Estrous Cycle*

Area of Tract	Proestrus	Estrus	Postestrus
Vestibule and posterior vagina	Congestion; edema	Congestion; edema	2 days: mucus-secreting cells 9 days: cornification
		Leukocyte infiltration; extravasation of blood	8–11 days: leukocyte infiltration, extravasation of blood
Anterior vagina	Large, wide mucous cells; 2–3 layers of epithelial cells; stroma edematous	Tall, narrow, columnar mucous cells; 2–3 layers epithelial cells; stroma edematous; leukocytes abundant	2 days: several layers of epithelial cells 8–11 days: vacuolar and degenerate epithelium 9–16 days: cornified cells in smears rise rapidly; leukocytes present in all smears
Cervix	Mucus-secreting cells	Cells loaded with mucus, many emptying; edema and hyperemia	1–2 days: mucus-loaded cells disappear; regeneration of mucous membrane; less congestion 3 days on: cells filled with mucus, but low; few cells emptying mucus; stroma compact; little or no congestion
Uterus	Cells tallest; cell length to nucleus length 4:1; marked edema	Congested blood vessels; edema of stroma; cells tall 2:1, glands straight with large lumens	Cells vacuolize just after estrus 2 days: cells lowest, 1.5:1 cell to nucleus 2 days: glandular growth starts 1–8 days: increased glandular secretion 8–11 days: glandular hypertrophy 8–12 days: glandular cell height increases; greatest coiling of glands
Oviducts	Cilia present and active; edema; granules in epithelial cells; cells 33 μm high; cytoplasmic projections from cells	Cilia present and active; edema; granules in epithelial cells; cells 45 μm high	Cilia present and active 1–2 days: edema and granules in cells 1–5 days: epithelial height 44 μm 3–4 days: mucus-like material in oviducts 6–15 days: epithelial height 27 μm

Reprinted with permission from: G. W. Salisbury and N. L. VanDemark, Physiology of Reproduction and Artificial Insemination of Cattle. San Francisco, CA, W. H. Freeman and Co., 1961.

the section on the estrous cycle and in each of the chapters on patterns of reproduction. Table 9-1 describes and Figure 9-16 shows the comparative anatomy of the uterus of the various species. This varies from a duplex uterus with two separate, independent cervices in the rabbit to a rather simple uterus in primates. The pig has a bicornuate uterus with well-developed elongated uterine horns, so that litters may be accommodated adequately. The cat and dog (Fig. 9-16) utilize the bicornuate uterus for somewhat equal distribution of the embryos of the litter. The cow and some breeds of ewes, which are monotocous, utilize only one horn during pregnancy. However, there may be some utilization of the other horn by the fetal membranes for placentation. The mare's uterus approaches the form of the primate's uterus, which lacks distinct uterine horns.

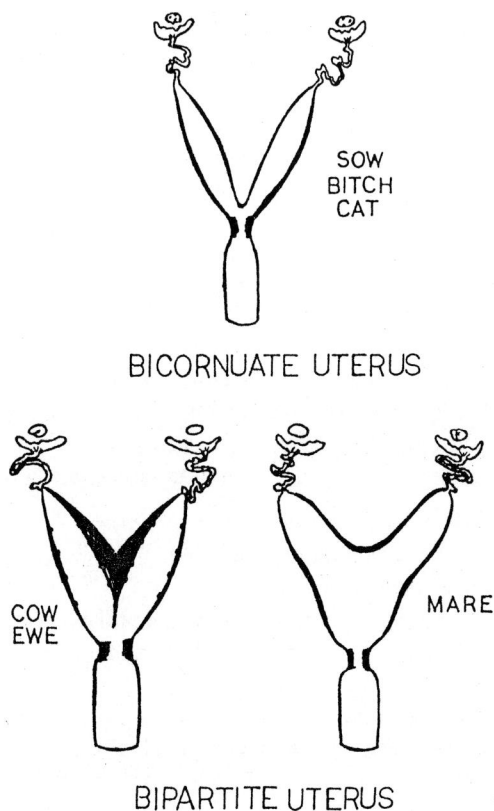

BICORNUATE UTERUS

SOW
BITCH
CAT

COW
EWE

MARE

BIPARTITE UTERUS

Fig. 9-16. Schematic gross anatomy of the uteri of several domestic species.

Oviducts (Uterine Tubes)

The oviducts, also called uterine tubes and less frequently Fallopian tubes, are paired convoluted tubes that extend from the ovaries to the uterus. The *rete ovarii* in the adult animal, considered to be the homologue of the *rete testis,* is a complex and open tubular system that communicates the ovary with the oviductal infundibulum. The physiological role of this structure has not been determined. The ovarian end of the oviduct is funnel-shaped and, depending on the species, embraces the ovary in varying degrees at ovulation. In the rat and the mouse, the ovarian end completely envelops the ovary to form a sac commonly referred to as the *bursa ovarica.* A small opening permits communication with the peritoneal cavity. In the bitch and mink, the bursa has a slit large enough to permit the ovary to move through it. The infundibulum of the sow almost completely envelops the ovary, particularly at the time of ovulation. The fingered or fimbriated ends of the oviducts do not enclose the ovary in other domestic animals. In the cow and the ewe, the ovarian bursa is only partially complete, whereas in the mare, the bursa encloses only the ovulation fossa.

The bursa consists of a thin peritoneal fold of the mesosalpinx. At the time of ovulation, the fimbriated end of the oviduct embraces the ovary and captures the oocytes. The efficiency of oocyte pickup seems to be as good in the nonbursal- as in the bursal-containing species.

The portion of the oviduct closer to the ovary is called the *ampulla,* and the portion next to the uterus is the isthmus. There does not seem to be a well-developed valve at the junction of the oviduct and uterus. However, there is good evidence for several species that the folds of the oviductal mucosa may serve as a deterrent to the movement of fluids from the oviduct into the uterus except at the luteal phase of the cycle. The degree of edema of the folds may control the patency of the uterotubal junction. This junction may prevent the movement of bacteria from the uterus into the oviduct and peritoneal cavity. Yet, it must allow semen ejaculated in the female genitals during copulation to pass into the oviduct. Also, the embryo (Fig. 9-17) moves through this junction into the uterus at

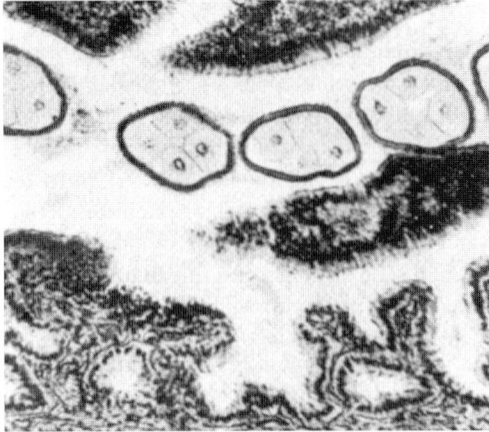

Fig. 9-17. Photograph of the four-cell stage of segmenting embryos in the oviduct of the dog. (Reproduced by permission from: H. M. Evans and H. H. Cole, The Oestrous Cycle in the Dog, Memoirs, Univ. of California Press, Berkley, CA, 9, no. 2).

the proper time. The embryo remains in the oviduct for 3 to 7 days in domestic animals. This delay is critical and necessary for further embryonic development and survival.

The oviduct is a tortuous organ of small diameter in all domestic species. The lumen of the oviduct is honeycombed in appearance, as seen in Figure 9-18A. The muscular wall of the oviduct is well developed and constricts in response to hormones. Estrogen priming enhances the response of the oviductal musculature to oxytocin. Oxytocin appears to cause the infundibular end of the oviduct to embrace the ovary. Estrogen dominance enhances the activity of cilia in the upper oviduct and facilitates the rapid transport of oocytes from the fimbria to the *ampulla* of the oviduct. Volume of fluid and protein composition of fluids in the oviduct change according to the phases of the estrous cycle, and the volume of fluid and total protein are higher during the period of estrus. The final stages of spermatozoal capacitation and fertilization occur here, and the embryos remain in this middle part of the oviduct, but near the ampulla-isthmus junction, for 2 to 3 days. Muscular contractions probably displace the embryos the remaining distance into the uterus in one more day, except in the bitch and mare, which require about 6 to 7 days for embryos to enter the uterus.

Timing of the displacement of the embryos into the uterus is important for continued development. A too-early or too-late uterine entry will result in death of the embryo due to asynchrony between the needs and stage of embryonic development and those of the endometrial and uterine development to provide for embryonic needs.

The epithelial lining of the lumen of the oviduct is simple columnar and ciliated. If both ends of the oviduct are ligated, fluid accumulates which is high in glucose, lactate, pyruvate, amino acids, sodium, and calcium ions. Therefore, the oviduct contributes ions and fluid for transporting spermatozoa, oocytes, or embryos and provides a microenvironment favorable for initial embryonic development.

Uterus

In domestic animals, the uterus consists of two horns (*cornua*) and a body. The development of long uterine horns is common to litter-bearing species, such as the sow, bitch, and queen (Fig. 9-16). The broad ligament supports the uterus and is subject to considerable stretching during pregnancy. In the nonpregnant female the uterus is held in the dorsal pelvic area. In the mare and cow, the uterus can be palpated through the rectal wall. For pregnancy diagnosis, restricted rectal palpation is possible in large ewes, goats, llamas, and sows by individuals with small hands and thin arms. The uterus is a remarkable organ in that it can enlarge and extend itself to accommodate the growth of concepti yet retain the capacity to involute following parturition, even approaching the original size and form.

The uterus is composed of three distinct layers:

1. the **serous membrane,** which is an extension of the peritoneum;

2. the **myometrium,** consisting of three muscle layers, which are subject to considerable hypertrophy; and

3. the **endometrium,** consisting of the epithelial lining of the lumen, the glands, and the connective tissue.

There is a rich blood supply to the uterus which varies according to the stage of the es-

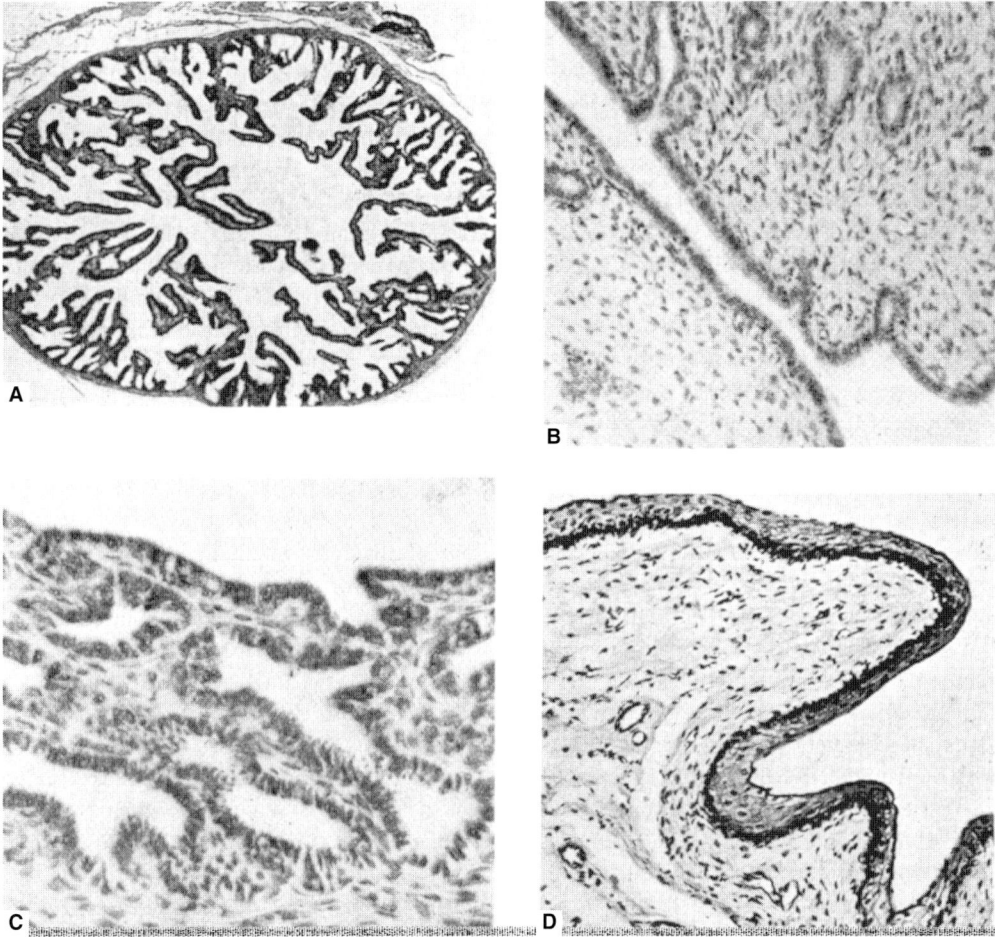

Fig. 9-18. Female duct system. **A,** oviduct. **B,** uterus of estrous rabbit. **C,** uterus of luteal phase rabbit. **D,** vagina. (From: L. E. McDonald, et al., Am. J. Vet. Res. *12:*419, 1952).

trous cycle and in the pregnant animal increases as gestation progresses, because the developing fetus and enlarged uterus require additional blood nutrients.

The highest concentration of estrogen and progesterone receptors is localized in the horns and uterine body. Myometrial and endometrial changes (Table 9-4) occur during every cycle under direct control of the ovarian hormones, estrogen and progesterone. These changes are similar to but less intense than those that occur during pregnancy. The myometrium is responsible for uterine contractions during estrus and copulation and for limited uterine activity throughout the estrous cycle. The uterine mus-

cular activity during early pregnancy enhances the spacing of fetuses in polytocous species. At the time of parturition and also during the follicular phase of the cycle, the myometrium is primed by estrogens and becomes at this time very sensitive to oxytocin.

The endometrial epithelium lining the uterus is simple columnar in most species. This epithelium extends into the uterine glands. Endometrial glandular development is cyclic, responding to rising levels of estrogen and progesterone during the estrous cycle and pregnancy. Figure 9-18B and C, shows the glandular development of the uterus. The uterine epithelium contacts the fetal membranes and is the site for exchange of nutrients and waste. The type of placental attachment varies greatly with the species (see Chapters 12-18). Ruminants have specialized sites of attachment called cotyledonary areas. These are highly specialized localized points of contact with the fetal membranes; consequently, glandular development does not occur at these points.

The uterus serves several functions other than to be an incubator for the embryo or fetus during gestation. The existence of a blood-uterine lumen barrier has been proposed. This barrier, whose main component would be the endometrial epithelium, would act as a limiting boundary between blood components and the lumen of the uterus, serving the physiological purpose to provide a favorable environment for the developing embryo. The uterine glands secrete "uterine milk", which serves as the nutrient medium for the free-living embryo for several weeks preceding implantation or attachment. In addition to the role of the uterus as a preselector and passageway to the oviduct for spermatozoa deposited in the vagina or cervix (see Chapter 8), the uterus and associated structures perform endocrine functions in both the cycling and pregnant animal. During implantation, in conjunction with developing placental structures, the uterus acts as a barrier to the maternal immunological rejection of the embryo or fetus. From this point of view, the spermatozoa and seminal components from the male's ejaculate, deposited in the female tract during mating, are the first foreign, antigenic challenges to the female immune system. The seminal plasma, however, appears to contain immunosuppressants that may protect the spermatozoa from local, uterine, and oviductal immune reactions. Once fertilization has occurred, the developing embryo, which, as a new entity is immunologically dissimilar to the female, is not rejected by the mother. On the contrary, the embryo attaches to the endometrium and normally develops to term. Several theories have been proposed to explain the lack of maternal immune rejection of the embryo or fetus. It is noteworthy to point out here, however, that during the period of implantation and for most of gestation, the female is under the influence of progesterone, which is a hormone with powerful immunosuppressive properties.

A nonimmunological embryonic reduction occurs in the uterus of the mare when more than one embryo have entered the uterus. The incidence of double ovulation is estimated to be about 16% for the mare, but the incidence of twin births is approximately 1%. The embryo that reaches the uterus first somehow prevents the development or interferes with the survival of the embryo reaching the uterus later. This phenomenon occurs between days 17 and 40 of pregnancy.

Cervix

The cervix is the doorway to the uterus, a physiological barrier separating the external environment from the internal environment of the animal. Outside the cervix lies the vagina, which is usually contaminated with microorganisms from the external environment.

The cervix is a thick-walled sphincter-like organ. It has a thick, muscular wall capable of contracting to close the passageway during gestation or of relaxing after mating at estrus to allow the passage of semen or for the passage of the fetus at parturition. The lumen of the cervix is tortuous and has folds that fit together. The cow, ewe, and sow have transverse ridges known as annular rings. In the sow, the rings display a corkscrew appearance. The spiral twisting of the tip of the boar's penis penetrates these rings in the sow. Ring development is less apparent in the mare, but the vaginal end of the cervix is well constricted to form the *os uteri*.

The cervix has a tall columnar epithelium interspersed with goblet cells, which have an important secretory function (Table 9-4). Goblet cell secretion is a mucus which varies in amount and viscosity depending on the gonadal hormone balance. Uterine fluids move through the cervix during the flushing process occurring at estrus. During estrus, the cervix is hyperemic, and at midcycle, or during pregnancy, the cervix is blanched and constricted. Under the influence of progesterone, the goblet cells secrete a thick, sticky, mucus which is so tenacious that it forms a definite barrier. Such mucus is sometimes referred to as the "cervical seal". The mucous seal of pregnancy should not be penetrated by an instrument such as an artificial insemination pipet. If the natural flora of the vagina are carried into the uterus, particularly during the luteal, progesterone-dominated phase of the cycle, it can become easily infected and the fetus may die. This is one of the hazards of intrauterine insemination in dairy cattle, because estrus sometimes occurs during pregnancy in the cow (3 to 5% of all cows).

Vagina

The vagina serves as a passageway inwardly for semen following copulation and outwardly for the fetus at parturition. In addition, the exterior limits of the vagina mark the confluence of the urinary tract with the reproductive tract.

The epithelial lining of the vagina (Fig. 9-18D) undergoes cyclic changes under the influence of the ovarian hormones (Table 9-4). Under the influence of estrogens in general and of estradiol-17β in particular, the epithelium becomes stratified and squamous, whereas during midcycle, under the influence of progesterone, the epithelium has low, cuboidal cells. The vaginal smear can be used to determine accurately the stage of the estrous cycle in the rat. Among domestic species, however, the bitch is the only one to have a distinct vaginal smear suitable to serve as an indicator of the stage of the estrous cycle. The mucous secretions in the vagina come mostly from the uterus through the cervix, because most of the vagina does not have glands.

The hymen is a transverse fold of the posterior portion of the vagina which is broken at the time of the first copulation. Occasionally, especially in the heifer, the hymen forms an unusually persistent band of connective tissue that must be relieved by a minor surgical procedure.

White Shorthorns are affected by a recessive hereditary condition called "white heifer disease". The condition is recognized by abnormal development of the reproductive tract. The most common manifestations are persistent hymen or absence of the cervix or of portions of the uterus.

EXTERNAL GENITALIA

The external genitalia consists of the *labia majora* and *minora* and the clitoris. The clitoris is the embryological homologue of the penis and consists of erectile tissue. The *labia* are the homologues of the scrotum. The *labia minora* are poorly developed in domestic animals, but the *labia majora* are well developed. The *labia majora* respond to the cyclic levels of estrogen and progesterone (Table 9-4). During proestrus and estrus, while estrogen dominates, the *labia* are swollen, congested, and edematous in domestic animals. These are useful signs for breeding management. Sebaceous glands surrounding the vulva and the glands of Bartholin within the vestibule secrete a lubricating mucus that facilitates the copulatory process.

PUBERTY

Puberty is defined as the age at which the female or the male gonad becomes capable of releasing gametes; oocytes or spermatozoa. In the female, this is associated with estrus and ovulation. For the female, however, puberty is customarily defined as the age at which she will display the first overt estrus or heat, because the signs of estrus are easily detectable. Animals that have reached puberty are called puberal or pubertal, terms that are synonymous. It must be noted that puberty in the female, as in the male (see Chapter 8), is not a sudden event, but the result of a gradual process of maturation of the endocrine and reproductive systems, conducive to the sexual maturity of the female and competence to reproduce successfully.

Many aspects of the endocrine events occurring during the transitional period leading to puberty remain unclear or undetermined. For instance, the pituitary gland of fetal and newborn animals responds to exogenous stimulation with GnRH by secreting and releasing gonadotropins, as a postpubertal animal would. Furthermore, the gonads of prepubertal animals are capable of superovulatory responses to stimulation with exogenous gonadotropins, even when given well in advance to the normal age of puberty. The quality of the superovulatory response, however, increases as the animal approaches the expected age of puberty for the species. This indicates the need for a certain degree of somatic development before spontaneous gonadotropin surges and puberty can occur. For most of the domestic species, the available evidence indicates that hypothalamic centers are sensitive, in a negative feedback fashion, to small amounts of steroid hormones secreted by the prepubertal gonads, mainly estradiol-17β for the female and androgens, mainly testosterone, for the male. As the animal matures, the hypothalamus becomes less sensitive to the negative feedback of gonadal steroids and begins to respond by secreting gonadotropin-releasing factors. The pituitary gland subsequently responds by secreting gonadotropins, which in turn stimulate the gonads. Thus, puberty could be considered as a series of hypophysial and gonadal endocrine events which are dependent on the release from the hypothalamic repression. This release occurs when a suitable stage of somatic development is attained.

The modulating activity of the brain, concurrent with the participation of other endocrine glands, such as the thyroid, pineal, and thymus, appears to be needed for the occurrence of puberty.

Some domestic species, such as the heifer and the ewe-lamb, undergo one or more 'silent or quiet' estruses and ovulations before they display full estrous behavior and establish the characteristic pattern of cyclic activity of the female. Progesterone secreted by a short-lived corpus luteum, concurrent with the shift from a high to low hypothalamic sensitivity to the negative feedback of gonadal steroids and changes in the patterns of LH secretion, have a major role in the establishment of the postpubertal, estrual cyclicity of the female.

Factors Affecting Puberty

Many factors, including interaction with the opposite sex, high levels of nutrition, favorable climate, and lack of a stressful environment, favor the onset of puberty. Other factors, such as confinement of females, probably because of pheromones, undernutrition, and adverse climate and environment, delay the onset of puberty. Particular characteristics for a species and breed differences in the onset of puberty are discussed in Chapters 12 to 18.

Breed and Genetic Influences

In general, smaller breeds experience puberty at an earlier age. Bitches of small breeds frequently experience first estrus several months earlier than bitches of large breeds. Jersey heifers have an average age of puberty of 8 months, Guernseys and Holsteins at 11 months, and Ayrshires 13 months. Perhaps the selection for genes controlling breed size was concurrent with the selection of other genetic traits such as age at puberty.

Climatic Effects

Puberty in man occurs earlier in the tropics than in the temperate zones. But good comparative data are not available in domestic animals. However, temperate climates, including the interaction of temperature, humidity, diurnal variation, and daylight, favor early puberty in all animals.

Seasonal Effects

An unusual situation exists in the seasonal-breeding sheep, because age at puberty can be overridden to some extent by the occurrence of the breeding season. If the hypothalamo-pituitary-ovarian axis is sufficiently developed in the ewe-lamb, then puberty can be initiated at an early date. For example, ewe-lambs born early in the Spring may show first estrus the following Fall when they are only 150 days of age. But ewe-lambs born late in the Spring or in the early Summer may not show first estrus until the next breeding season, in the Fall of the following year, when these females have reached 400 to 500 days of age.

Effect of Nutrition

A well-balanced diet and a high plane of nutrition favors an earlier puberty. Conversely, a low plane of nutrition delays puberty. This is particularly true for nonseasonal-breeding animals. Considerable work has been done in this area, especially in heifers, and a more complete discussion can be found in Chapter 12. Apparently there is an interaction of nutrition, body weight gain, and age, since animals maintained under good nutrition reach puberty at an earlier age. **But poor nutrition is not able to prevent the eventual onset of puberty,** although severe delays can be caused to the extent that the age of puberty can be doubled.

Effect of Sex

The generalization that females of all species reach puberty at an earlier age than males is traditionally found in textbooks dealing with animal reproduction. However, evidence to the contrary is abundant, and the statement may be incorrect. For instance, more bull calves, lambs, billy goats, dogs, and likely males from other species as well, produce ejaculates containing spermatozoa and therefore have reached puberty at an earlier age than the majority of females display the signs of the first overt estrus. Beagle dogs reach puberty as early as 6 months of age, whereas Beagle bitches seldom reach puberty before 10 months of age. Holstein bull calves produce ejaculates with significant numbers of spermatozoa by 8 to 9 months of age, whereas Holstein heifers usually come into estrus about 9 to 13 months of age. Comparative studies to determine age of puberty in males and females of the same species and genetic background, using animals reared and maintained under the same conditions of feeding and management, need to be performed. The behavioral signs of estrus are easily detected, as opposed to the difficulties of collecting ejaculates from untrained, pubescent males. This may have contributed to the misbelief that the age of puberty is earlier for the female than for the male of the species.

THE ESTROUS CYCLE

At puberty, the female develops a rhythmic pattern of physiologic events which induce detectable morphologic changes in the reproductive system and behavioral changes in the animal. These physiologic and behavioral changes are cyclic and repeated over time, unless normally interrupted by pregnancy or abnormally by a variety of pathologic conditions. Behavioral changes are easier to detect than the morphologic changes within the reproductive organs; and hence, it is customary to use the period of sexual receptivity of the female for mating, called estrus or heat, as the central pivot for the cyclic changes. During the period of estrus or heat, the females will stand and accept the advances of the male for mating. During any other part of the cycle, the female rejects the mating advances of the male. Because there is only one period of estrus in each cycle, conventionally the sequence of events that occur between two successive estruses is termed an estrous or estrual cycle. The interestrous interval is for most species the time in days elapsed from the beginning of an estrus to the beginning of the next estrus. This interestrous interval is then used as a conventional unit of measurement for the duration of the estrous cycle. The period of estrus or heat varies, according to the species, from a few hours to several days. There is also variation in the length of estrus between individuals of the same species. It is conventional to designate the day or days of estrus as Day 0 of the cycle, regardless if the length of estrus is less than or more than one day. When needed, and particularly for species that normally have several days of estrus, each day of estrus may be designated as E1, E2, and so forth.

Ovulation occurs during estrus in most of the domestic species or, like in the cow, shortly after estrus. The behavioral and physiologic changes associated with ovulation, development, and full attainment of functional activity of the corpus luteum, and the associated behavioral changes of the female, including rejection to mating, are used to describe the estrous cycle. The first day the female refuses to mate is referred to as the first day of diestrus or day 1 of the cycle. Pertinent endocrine events and associated changes in the reproductive organs will be discussed later in this chapter.

According to the periodicity of presentation of estrous cycles, the domestic species can be classified as monoestric or polyestric. Monoestric species, such as the bitch, have only one estrous cycle per breeding season, and bitches may have two breeding seasons per year. Monoestric species typically present a prolonged period of sexual inactivity called anestrus. Polyestric species are those that, in the absence of mating or when mated with a sterile male, have several estrous cycles during the year. These can be further classified as seasonally polyestrous or seasonal breeders and continuously polyestrous or nonseasonal breeders. Seasonal breeders such as the ewe, goat, and mare present several cycles, but only during a particular season of the year. Continuously polyestrous or nonseasonal breeders, such as the cow and the sow, cycle year around. This classification is somewhat arbitrary, because changes in the geographic location and climate and the provision of favorable environmental conditions may induce seasonally polyestrous species to become continuously polyestrous, or at the very least, extend the breeding season.

Based on ovarian changes, which can be categorized according to the role of copulation in ovulation, the activity or inactivity of the resulting corpus luteum, and the associated behavioral responses of the female, it is possible to classify species into three general types: 1, 2, and 3.

1. This type is exemplified by nonseasonal breeders, such as the cow and sow, or by the seasonal breeders, such as the mare and ewe during the breeding season. The infertile cycle in these species culminates in spontaneous ovulation of mature follicles. Corpora lutea automatically form and become functional for a definite period of time. However, in the absence of pregnancy, the corpus luteum regresses and a subsequent cycle ensues. The bitch fits this pattern insofar as ovulation and luteal function are concerned. However, the bitch differs from the other species in this category in that the corpora lutea of the bitch remain functional for approximately the same length of time whether pregnancy had occurred or not. In addition, a long period of anestrus follows the functional demise of the corpus luteum.

2. The rat and mouse provide an example of another type of estrous cycle in which ovulation is spontaneous but the corpora lutea which form are not functional unless mating occurs. These estrous cycles are short (4 to 5 days) when female rats are not mated and longer (12 days) if cervical stimulation takes place.

3. The third type of estrous cycle is one in which ovulation does not occur unless the male copulates with the female. The South American camelidae, rabbit, cat, and mink are examples of this type and are commonly referred to as reflex or induced ovulators. Spontaneous ovulations may occur in the camelidae, also termed

camelids or cameloids, but most ovulate within 30 hours after mating in females that have antral, mature follicles in the ovaries. Mating of female camelids that have large regressing follicles induces luteinization without ovulation. In llamas, the incidence of hemorrhagic follicles, detected ultrasonographically, is greater in nonmated than in mated llamas. The physiological significance has not been determined, but the hemorrhagic follicles may represent follicles that failed to ovulate. Some of these unovulated follicles may become luteinized. In the rabbit, successive groups of follicles mature and degenerate rhythmically, and at any time there are a number of follicles capable of being stimulated to ovulate if copulation occurs. The queen, another induced ovulator, has periods of anestrus during the year and seasonal periods of breeding in which ovarian follicles develop and secrete estrogens to induce behavioral responses and definite estrous stances that last for several days (see Chapter 17). If mating does not occur, these follicles regress, and subsequent periods of follicular growth and estrus recur several times during the breeding season. From this point of view, the queen could be classified as a seasonally pseudopolyestrous species. Copulation in these species stimulates afferent neural pathways via the hypothalamus, causing release of luteinizing hormone, which in turn promotes the ovulatory process.

Phases of the Estrous Cycle

The estrous cycle of domestic animals is traditionally classified into five somewhat arbitrary and sometimes difficult-to-distinguish sequential stages called phases of the estrous cycle. These phases are called **proestrus, estrus, metestrus, diestrus,** and **anestrus** (Fig. 9-19). All of these terms are nouns, and their corresponding adjectives are estrous, metestrous, diestrous, and anestrous.

Proestrus is the period of rapid follicular growth under gonadotropic stimulation and also the period in which the corpus luteum from the previous cycle completes regression in polyestrous species. At this stage, the animal is exposed and behaviorally responds to the progressively increasing levels of estrogens secreted by

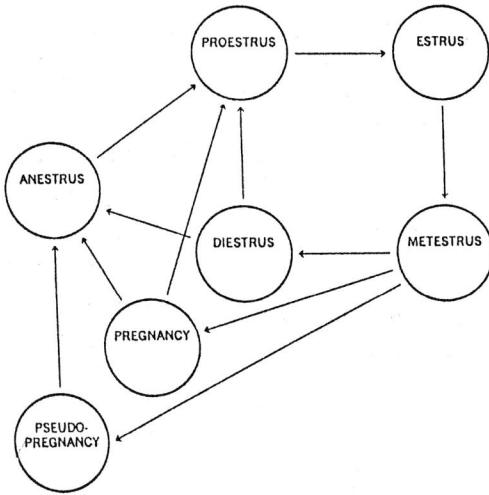

Fig. 9-19. The reproductive cycle of domestic animals.

the developing follicles. In most of the domestic species, proestrus is associated with progressively declining levels of progesterone due to the regression of the corpus luteum from the preceding cycle. In the bitch, proestrus lasts for 7 to 9 days and is clearly identifiable by well-defined changes in the external genitalia and behavioral signs due to increasing sexual excitement. Proestrus lasts only for 2 to 3 days in the other domestic species and it is not as clinically evident or distinguishable.

Estrus is defined as the period of **sexual receptivity,** during which mating and ovulation occur and the corpus (corpora) luteum (lutea) begins to form in most species.

The beginning of estrus is a gradual phenomenon, and thus the detection of the precise time of the onset of estrus is difficult. Duration of estrus is usually estimated by the duration of the period of acceptance of the male for mating and varies from 14 to 18 hours in the cow to 7 to 10 days in the mare and 2 to 15 days in the bitch. Breed, age, and environmental temperature may influence the duration of estrus. High environmental temperatures shorten the duration of estrus in gilts and sows. Copulation early in estrus will usually shorten the period of sexual receptivity. Split estrus is common in mares: Estrus usually lasts 7 to 10 days, but there may be 1 to 2 days in this period when the mare is not sexu-

ally receptive. **Proestrus and that portion of the period of estrus prior to ovulation form part of the follicular phase of the cycle.**

Metestrus is the transitional period between ovulation and the full development of the corpus luteum. During metestrus, the endocrine ovary switches from secretion of estrogens to progesterone secretion, and the reproductive system is then exposed to progesterone dominance. Because the location of metestrus in relation to the other phases of the cycle is variable among species, the phase of metestrus is only of academic significance. For most domestic species, such as the bitch, mare, sow, ewe, and goat that ovulate before the end of estrus, or for the reflex ovulator species (queen and camelids), the period of metestrus is either partially or totally included within the phase of estrus. For species that ovulate after the end of estrus (cow), the phase of metestrus forms part of the diestrual phase of the cycle.

Diestrus is the phase of the cycle during which the corpus luteum fully develops and the reproductive organs are under the dominant influence of progesterone. Metestrus and diestrus form part of the luteal phase of the cycle for those species that ovulate late in the cycle or that are induced ovulators.

The duration of diestrus depends primarily on the occurrence or nonoccurrence of conception and pregnancy. In the nonpregnant animal, diestrus is the longest phase of the cycle, lasting from 13 to 16 days for most of the domestic species, with the exception of the bitch and the queen. The duration of diestrus for the bitch is about 64 days, the same whether the bitch is pregnant or not (see Chapter 16). The queen will not undergo diestrus unless ovulation has been induced by mating or by other means, and the duration of diestrus will depend if the animal becomes pseudopregnant or pregnant (see Chapter 17). In the pregnant queen, diestrus becomes the period of gestation.

In the nonmated animal, in those mated with sterile males, or in those in which conception did not occur, the corpus luteum regresses at the end of diestrus, and diestrus is followed by either proestrus and a subsequent estrous cycle in the continuously polyestrous, and in the seasonally polyestrous species, during the breeding season. In monoestric species, diestrus is followed by a period of sexual inactivity, or anestrus.

Anestrus is a stage of sexual quiescence characterized by the lack of estrous behavior and is a normal stage of the reproductive function in the prepubertal and in the aged animals of all species. Anestrus is also normal for the pregnant animal of all species. In fact, pregnancy is the most common cause of anestrus in polyestrous species. After puberty, anestrus is normal in nonpregnant animals for the monoestric species, such as the bitch, for the seasonally polyestrous species during the nonbreeding season, and for the lactating female of some species.

The endocrine mechanisms involved in anestrus are not clearly defined. For some species, such as the bitch, endogenous gonadotropic stimulation of the ovaries is high during anestrus, as demonstrated by follicular development and estrogen secretion. However, the bitch does not express estrous behavior, possibly because corpora lutea are not formed and progesterone, which in the bitch is needed for the full expression of estrous behavior, is not secreted during anestrus. Silent ovulatory cycles without behavioral signs of estrus occur at the time of puberty in some species and at the beginning or end of the breeding season in seasonally polyestrous species.

In all domestic species, anestrus may occur as a pathological condition caused by a variety of factors, including nutritional deficiencies, environmental influences that cause endocrine imbalances, diseases of the ovary and uterus, and infectious diseases causing early embryonic death or abortion. All of these factors result in economic losses due to reproductive failure.

Ovarian Changes During the Estrous Cycle

As described previously, the follicle in single-bearing species or several follicles that are destined to ovulate in litter-bearing species develop from a pool of primordial follicles and mature under gonadotropic stimulation to the preovulatory or Graafian stage. One to 3 days before the onset of estrus, depending on the

species, Graafian follicles directed for ovulation begin to enlarge rapidly and become turgid. The theca internal cells hypertrophy, and the oocyte, with attached *cumulus oophorus,* moves from the embedded position in the granulosa layer toward the enlarged fluid-filled antrum of the Graafian follicle (Fig. 9-14).

In most species, there is a positive correlation between anterior pituitary gonadotropin output and ovarian follicular growth and activity. Additionally, other hormones, e.g., growth hormone, and factors, e.g., insulin-like growth factor-1, are needed for follicular maturation. The follicles of most mammals enlarge very little during the luteal phase, though in several species, waves of follicular growth occur during diestrus. Follicles set to ovulate undergo a surge of growth 1 to 3 days before ovulation (Fig. 9-20).

Ovulation

There are species differences in the number of follicles that reach the preovulatory stage and in the number of days needed in each estrous cycle to reach this stage. The existence of waves of follicular growth during the estrous cycle, as opposed to the continued development of follicles, is either postulated or shown to occur for most of the domestic species. These will be discussed for each of the domestic species in the corresponding chapter on pattern of reproduction. However, as an introductory generaliza-

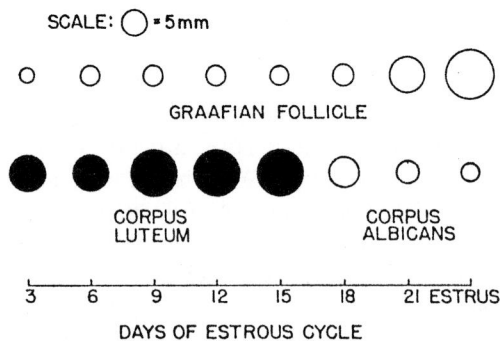

Fig. 9-20. Relative morphologic changes in the ovarian follicles during the estrous cycle of the sow. Note the rapid increase in follicular size shortly before ovulation. Also, corpora albicantia regress in size rather rapidly but are still evident at the subsequent estrus. (From: E. S. E. Hafez, *In:* Reproduction in Farm Animals, 5th ed. Philadelphia, PA, Lea & Febiger, 1987).

tion, there are species such as primates and pigs in which the dominant follicles that are destined or directed to ovulate develop only in the follicular phase of the cycle. In the cow, sheep, and mare, follicles grow in waves during the estrous cycle, but only those follicles that become dominant during the follicular phase of the cycle progress toward ovulation.

Ovulation involves the breakdown of the wall of the ovarian follicle and the release of its contents, including the maturing oocyte. A transparent area appears in the follicular wall near the apex when ovulation is impending. The point of ovulation can be seen in the resulting corpora lutea for days after ovulation in most of the species. Hemorrhagic areas develop in the vascular network of the follicular membrane, and there is extravasation of blood into the *liquor folliculi* near the time of ovulation. The granulosa cells lose cell-to-cell contact as the follicle approaches ovulation, probably by dissociation of the intercellular gap junctions. The oocyte and the cells of the *cumulus,* which at this time are projected into the follicular *antrum,* separate from the pedicle of the *cumulus* and become freed into the follicular fluid of the *antrum.* Cells from the granulosa layer reveal signs of luteinization due to gonadotropic, mainly LH stimulation. Follicular secretion of preovulatory progesterone occurs in a number of species, and in addition to the stimulation provided to the follicular cells by the ovulatory surge of LH, interleukin-1α may be involved in the process of preovulatory synthesis of progesterone. The connective tissue of the thecal layers dissociates during the preovulatory period, and the outer, thecal layers separate during the final preovulatory changes. An avascular stigma or papilla is macroscopically recognizable on the apical surface of the follicle when ovulation is imminent. As the protrusion of the papilla progresses, the layers of the follicular wall, including the adjacent superficial epithelium of the ovary, stretch and thin until the follicular wall breaks and the follicular contents are released (Fig. 9-21).

The participation of myoid cells of the follicular wall and the significance of follicular contractility in the process of ovulation remains a controversial issue. It has long been known that the mammalian ovarian tissues display contractile activity, probably under the control of autonomic nerves extending to the ovary and to the action of catecholamines, which are present in the follicular wall and fluid of some species. Several lines of evidence suggest that the contraction of myoid elements in the follicular wall may be a contributing factor to dissociate the thecal tissue at the stigma and to provide the force for the mechanical rupture of the follicular wall. The oocyte appears to passively flow out of the rupturing follicle rather than being expelled out by contraction of the follicular wall. Because ovulation is a traumatic process of rupture of tissue and subsequent hemorrhage occurs, the myoid elements may also participate in the postovulatory process of tissue repair.

In the domestic species, with the exception of the mare, ovulation occurs within 24 to 40 hours following the ovulatory surge of LH. In the mare, ovulation occurs, prior to the peak of LH, while LH levels in the blood are rising.

At the cellular level, a mature follicle possesses the appropriate hormone receptors and metabolic components needed to respond to an ovulatory surge of LH. A model[59] based on the hypothesis that the ovulatory surge of LH induces inflammatory changes in the follicular wall has been proposed. According to this model, thecal fibroblasts are in a quiescent "stationary" phase of activity before the ovulatory surge of LH. The fibroblasts secrete a procollagenase, which must be activated to collagenase to digest the extracellular collagen matrix. Gonadotropin stimulation rapidly increases the synthesis of cyclic AMP in the follicle and accelerates steroidogenic activity in the theca interna. The rising level of steroids, particularly estradiol-17β, and prostaglandins in the follicle serve to transform the fibroblasts from the stationary to the proliferative state. These proliferating fibroblasts produce collagenase, which in turn initiates collagenolysis in the follicular wall. The modified proteins that are released by this degradative process induce an acute inflammatory reaction which results in histamine release, leukocyte migration, and further release of prostaglandins. The prostaglandins then stimulate a second phase of cyclic AMP synthesis and elevate the blood flow

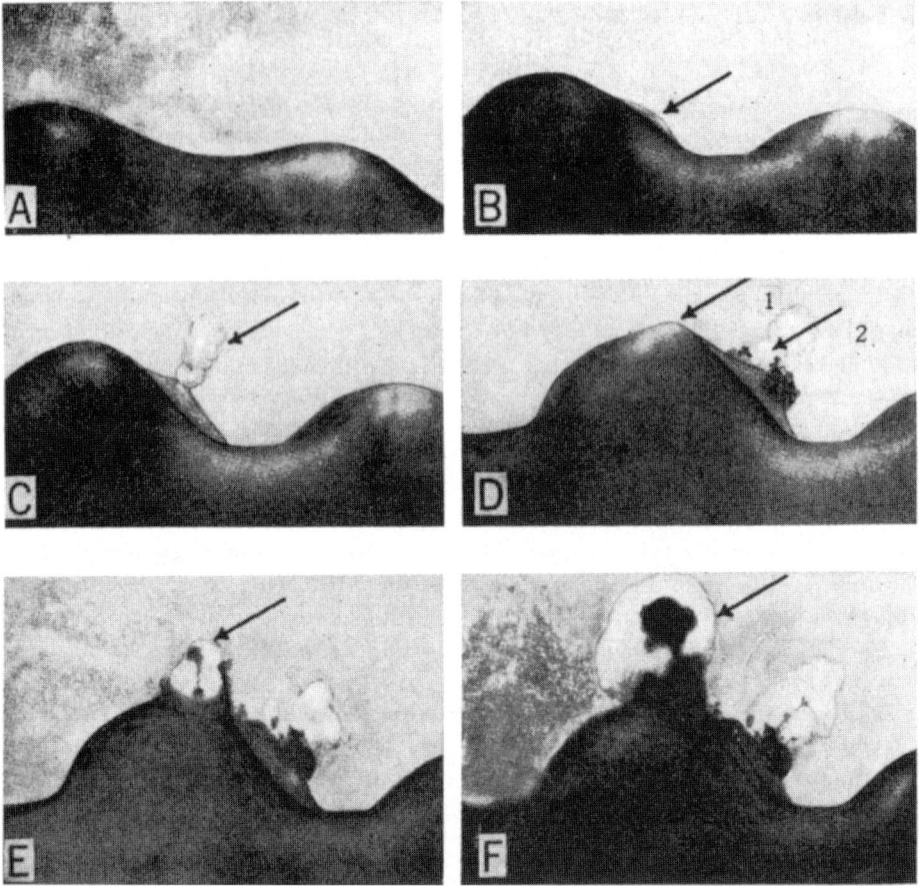

Fig. 9-21. Enlargements of single frames of a time-lapse motion picture showing ovulation in the rabbit. (From: Hill, Allen, and Kramer, Anat. Rec., 63, 1935.) **A.** Profile view of two follicles about 1½ hours before rupture. **B.** Same follicles about 1/2 hour before rupture. **C.** Exudation of clear fluid in early phases of rupture. **D.** At **arrow 1,** a new follicle becomes conical as the time of its rupture approaches. At **arrow 2,** the exudate from the follicle shown starting to rupture in **C** has become more abundant and contains some blood (dark). **E.** The follicle indicated by **arrow 1** in **D** is now beginning to rupture. The blood-tinged exudate from the follicle, which started to rupture in **C** and showed more vigorous exudation in **D** (**arrow 2**), can be seen partly behind the more recently rupturing follicle. **F.** The rupture of the follicle, which is indicated by the arrow in **E.** Time elapsed between the photographs shown in **E** and **F** is 8 seconds. The oocyte is carried out with this final gush of fluid from the ruptured follicle. (B. M. Patten, *In:* Foundations of Embryology. New York, NY, McGraw-Hill Book Co., 1958).

through the inflamed region. Not all mature ovarian follicles are destined to ovulate. In several species, but particularly in the cow, follicles often become luteinized without ovulation. This condition, clinically termed **cystic corpora lutea,** can be experimentally induced in ewes by treatment with indomethacin, which is an inhibitor of prostaglandin synthesis. This response emphasizes the role of prostaglandins in ovulation.

As ovulation approaches, there is a gross reduction in the tensile strength of the collagenous layers which encapsulate the follicle. The thin region at the apex of the follicle is the area most susceptible to distention under the stress of even a small intrafollicular pressure. Rupture is imminent as the degraded follicle wall begins to dissociate under this stress. By the time of rupture, the enzymatic activity has depolymerized the ground substance in the *cumulus oophorus* to the extent that the *corona radiata* is dislodged from the *cumulus* so that the oocyte can be expelled from the follicle.

Corpus Luteum (CL) Development

The **corpus luteum** (plural, **corpora lutea**) is a temporary endocrine organ which, for most of the domestic species, functions for only a few days during diestrus in the cycling, nonpregnant animal. During the diestrual phase of the cycle, the corpus luteum produces maximal amounts of progesterone. If a viable embryo(s) is (are) not present in the uterus by diestrus day 11 or 12 in the sow, day 13 in the ewe, day 14 in the mare, day 16 or 17 in the goat, and day 16 in the cow, the corpus luteum undergoes luteolysis and regresses as reflected by a pronounced decrease in the blood levels of progesterone. As examples, see Figure 9-22 for the sow and Figure 9-23 for the cow. Luteal regression is prevented by pregnancy in seasonally or continuous polyestrus species such as ewes, cows, goats, mares, and sows. However, for these species the corpus luteum is maintained in the animal that becomes pregnant (see Fig. 9-22 for

the sow). Among the domestic species, the bitch and pseudopregnant queen are exceptional in that the presence of a viable embryo is not necessary for diestrual luteal maintenance (see Chapters 16 and 17).

Following ovulation there is enough hemorrhage into the follicular cavity, especially in the mare and cow, for a blood clot to develop. The blood-filled follicle now devoid of the oocyte is commonly referred to as a **corpus hemorrhagicum.** This clot of blood serves as a physical framework and a nutrient medium for the rapid proliferation of the granulosa and thecal cells, which by differentiating into luteal cells, are mainly responsible for the secretion of progesterone and rapid development of the corpus luteum.

The growth of the luteal cells is one of the fastest events known in biology. Within 3 to 4 days, the blood clot is invaded by the new luteal cells so that the blood-filled cavity loses its dark

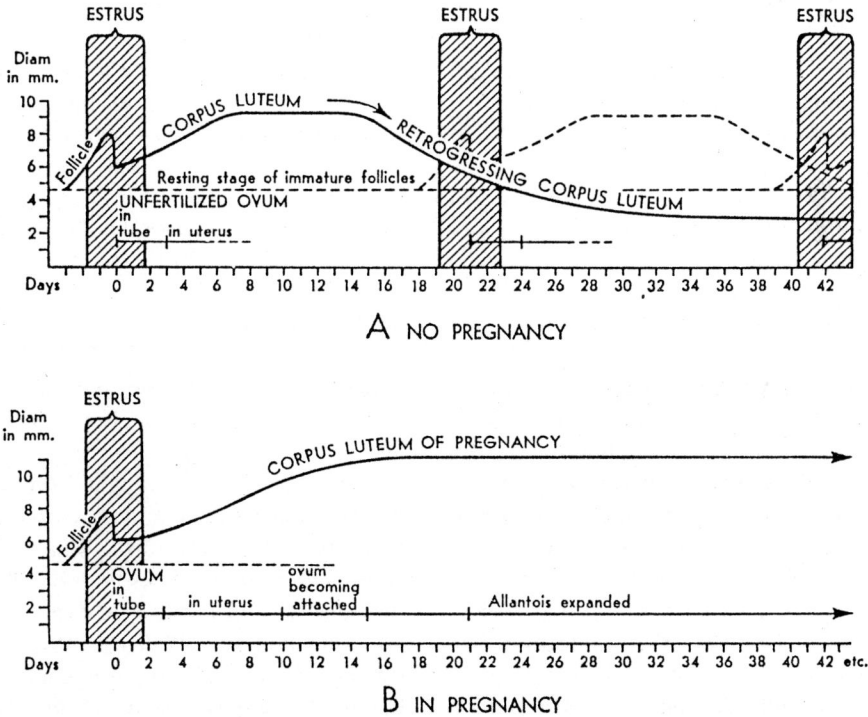

Fig. 9-22. Graphs showing the difference in history of the corpus luteum of ovulation and the corpus luteum of pregnancy in the sow. (From: B. M. Patten, *In:* Foundations of Embryology, 1st ed. New York, NY, McGraw-Hill Book Co., 1958).

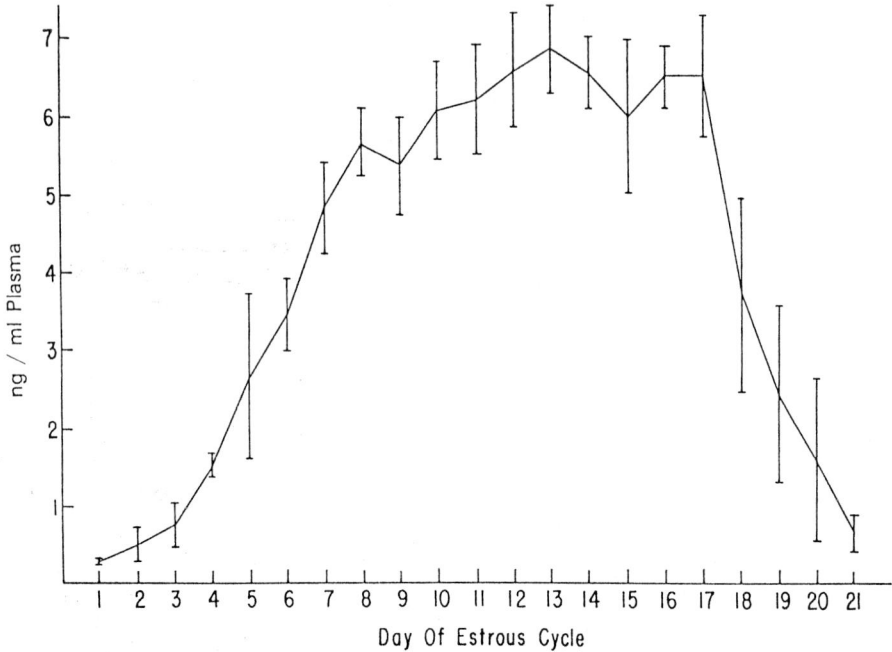

Fig. 9-23. Progesterone concentration in jugular venous plasma from four cows with 21-day estrous cycles. Vertical bars represent the standard error of the mean. (From: G. H. Stabenfeldt, L. L. Ewing, and L. E. McDonald, J. Reprod. Fertil. *19*:433, 1969).

coloration. Following ovulation, the granulosa cells remaining in the collapsed follicle and thecal cells carried from the theca interna by invading capillaries begin to hypertrophy, uptake lipid material, and become the lutein or luteal cells of the mature corpora lutea.

The corpus luteum is one of the most vascularized organs of the body. Columns of luteal cells are separated by vessels which must nourish this newly formed organ during its metabolic activity and steroid synthesis. This newly formed endocrine organ is termed a **corpus luteum verum** if the animal becomes pregnant and the corpus continues to function. In the cycling nonpregnant animal, the newly formed organ is termed a **corpus luteum spurium** because it is destined to regress.

The corpus luteum of an infertile cycle, either because of mating with a sterile animal or simply because the lack of mating, will also undergo regression by the end of diestrus. The retrogressive luteal changes are first microscopic and then grossly visible. The lutein cells degenerate rapidly, showing cytoplasmic vacuolation

and pyknotic nuclei. Progesterone production plummets sharply, even more dramatically than the anatomic changes. Corpora lutea then decrease in size along with degeneration of capillaries. Gradually the lutein cells are replaced by fibroblasts, and the other cells become enmeshed in the forming of connective tissue. The degenerating avascular nonfunctional corpus is termed a **corpus albicans** (white). Slow physical degeneration occurs, usually taking 2 to 3 weeks. A visible connective tissue scar remains on the ovary for several additional estrous cycles.

In the sow, ovarian weight increases after day 3, and the diameter of the CL reaches a peak by day 10 of the estrous cycle (Fig. 9-22). This weight increase also occurs in the other domestic species and is attributed to luteal cell growth and production of progesterone. Similarly, the size and weight of the corpus luteum of the cycling cow increases and reaches maximal weight at the time is secreting maximal amounts of progesterone, as reflected by the levels of progesterone in the blood (Fig. 9-23). Luteal tissue gradually changes from a dark red (hemorrhagic) color to a pale purple by day 15 (Fig. 9-24). Following day 15, the corpora lutea rapidly change from pale purple to a yellowish cream color and then to a white color by day 18 in the nonpregnant sow. The change in color is due to the decrease in vascularity during this regressive phase. The size of the corpora lutea decreases rapidly after day 18, and within 3 weeks most have regressed completely (Figs. 9-22 through 9-24).

Gross and histological ovarian changes in the cow and the ewe before, during, and after ovulation are somewhat different from those in the sow due to the number and location of corpora lutea within the ovary. The corpora lutea of sheep reach maximum size by day 13 and at this time are reddish-pink. Corpora lutea become pale as diestrus progresses, and after day 14, degeneration is rapid because the estrous cycle of the ewe is shorter than that of the sow. After ovulation in the cow, the granulosa cells hypertrophy and become filled with droplets of yellow lipids as the corpus luteum forms. Maximum size of the bovine corpus luteum is attained by days 11 to 16; then it degenerates rapidly. The bovine corpus luteum changes from a light brown to gold color by day 7, then to a golden yellow by day 14. Between days 14 and 20, the corpus luteum progressively changes from yellow to orange to a brick red. The changes in color of the corpus luteum of the cow correlate well with luteal weight and levels of progesterone in the blood.[63] The brick red color remains for several cycles as the old corpus luteum gradually regresses. The color of the corpus luteum of the cow or mare is more intense than that of the other species because of lutein, a yellow pigment. The corpora lutea of the ewe and sow are devoid of this lipochromic pigment, hence the lighter color.

Corpus Luteum Function

The production of progesterone by the CL is best estimated by determining the levels of progesterone in the peripheral plasma of the animal (Fig. 9-23). This gives an indication of the level of hormone that the entire body, including the target organs of the reproductive system, is subjected to. Hormonal levels in the blood are dependent upon a variety of factors, including secretion and metabolic clearance rates, frequency of blood sampling, and assay system used. The values provided in Table 9-2 are to serve only as reference and general guidelines. Figure 9-23 represents the pattern of progesterone levels in the peripheral plasma of cows.

The circulating levels of progesterone for species other than for the cow are also given in Table 9-2. Notice the variability from polytocous species to monotocous species for the highest level of progesterone during diestrus. However, the levels of progesterone during the follicular phase of the cycle are quite similar for the species named in Table 9-2.

Should pregnancy ensue, then the progesterone level slowly continues to rise after midcycle in all species. The hormonal levels during pregnancy are discussed in Chapter 12-18.

GROSS OVARIAN CHANGES DURING THE ESTROUS CYCLE

Few organs change their gross appearance or even their physiological function from day to day like the cycling ovary. Figure 9-24 will help the reader to visualize these important changes as they occur in the sow, which is a polyestrous and polytocous (litter-bearing) animal. Ovarian changes in monotocous species like the cow or mare would be less dramatic because of the single follicle ovulating at each cycle. The interestrous interval for the sow ranges from 19 to 23 days. In this case, a typical ovary was selected at slaughter for each day of a 20-day estrous cycle. Unfortunately, each day is represented by a different ovary, hence the lack of ovarian uniformity.

Day 1, photograph 1 represents the first day of estrus, and several large fluid-filled (mature, Graafian) follicles can be seen in the lower left corner. Notice how these protrude from the surface. Fusion of follicles appears to have occurred, but the *antra* or cavities remain distinct. The centermost follicle shows some blood discoloration. The right side of the ovary shown contains several blanched corpora albicans from the previous cycle. The corpora albicans are similar to the follicles in size. There are no recent ovulation sites on this ovary.

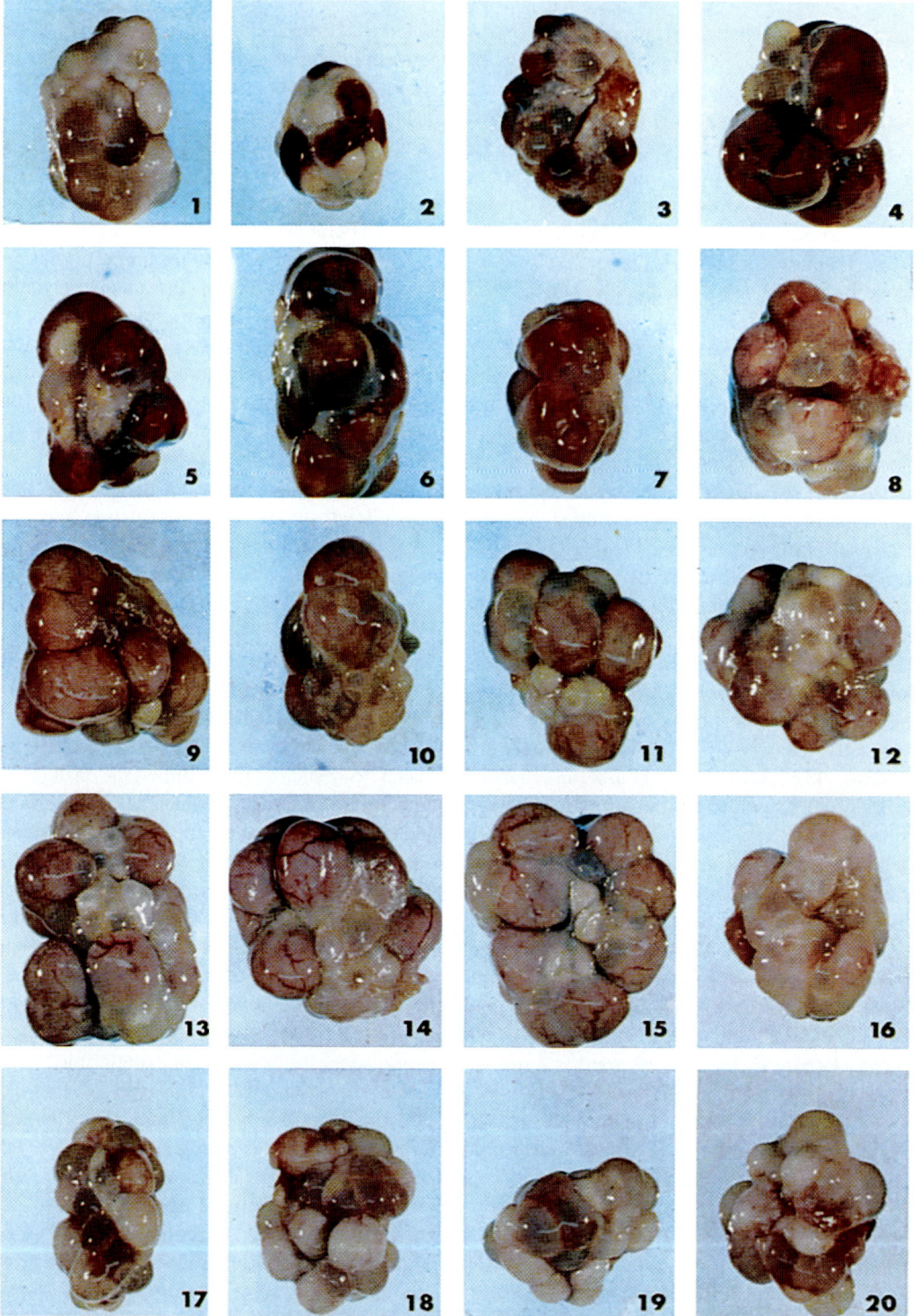

Fig. 9-24. Photograph depicting the cyclic changes in the sow ovary during a 20-day estrous cycle. Photograph **1** is the first day of estrus or day 0 of the cycle. Photographs **1** and **2** are ovaries obtained during estrus. Photographs **3** and **4** (days 3 and 4) obtained during metestrus. Photographs **5** to **16** obtained during diestrus. Photographs **17** to **20** are during proestrus. See text of this chapter for more complete discussion. (From: E. L. Akins and M. C. Morrissette, Am. J. Vet. Res. *29*:1953, 1968).

Day 2, photograph 2 shows two corpora hemorrhagica (top and left). These are the site of the first ovulations. These blood-filled and ruptured follicles are somewhat collapsed. Luteal cell growth has begun, but the new corpora lutea will not be well developed for another 2 days. Several blood-tinged follicles fill the center, and these appear ready to ovulate. The old corpora albicantia appear a bit more regressed. This is the last day of estrus.

Day 3, photograph 3 shows more ovulation sites. A few follicles have not ovulated. Ovulation sites are developing into more organized luteal masses (period of metestrus). Corpora albicantia from the previous cycle are less noticeable, very soft, and degenerate.

By **day 4**, photograph 4, the blood-clot-filled follicles have been reorganized into functional luteal tissue interspersed by a rapidly developing blood supply. The large corpora are liverlike in consistency and color. Progesterone production is rising at this time, and the period of diestrus is in full progress. A few small follicles are present which may persist until the next estrus or degenerate.

By **days 5 and 6**, photographs 5 and 6, the corpora are more distinct and have a lighter color because the blood clots have been resorbed. The corpora are still growing, and progesterone output continues to increase.

Days 7 and 8 witness corpora lutea that are more "meaty" and lighter in color. Diestrus is well underway, and the corpora lutea are fully functional.

Days 9, 10, 11, and 12 reveal a similar picture whereby the corpora lutea are fully formed, functional, distinct, encapsulated, and endowed with a good supply of blood. Most of the blood from the ovulation site has been resorbed. More small follicles are appearing, but their size is small. **Day 12** is critical in the life of the corpora lutea of the sow. If at least four viable embryos are present in the uterus to convey the signal of pregnancy, then these corpora lutea will be maintained and function normally. If there are less than four viable embryos present, these corpora lutea will initiate irreversible regression, which will then be expressed macroscopically later in the cycle.

Days 13 and 14 are similar to the previous 4 days. Macroscopic evidence of luteolysis becomes apparent by **days 15 and 16**, and some blanching of the corpora luteal vessels may be seen on day 15. Progesterone production has fallen dramatically by day 15. By day 16, the corpora lutea have lost most of their vascularity, shrinkage in size has begun, and the ovary is smaller.

By **day 17**, there is marked follicular enlargement and hyperemia. The phase of proestrus for the next estrous cycle has begun, and the follicular or estrogenic phase of the cycle will last for the next 2 to 5 days. The waning corpora are evident, and their white color and soft texture signal the end of their function. Although complete regression of these corpora albicantia will take another 15 to 20 days, they are at this time functionless.

Days 19 to 20, fluid continues to accumulate within the growing follicles. Secretions from these growing follicles increase estrogen levels in the blood.

One should recall that other cyclic changes are occurring in the genital tract concomitant with these dramatic ovarian changes. The most marked changes occur in the uterus, but epithelial and glandular changes also occur throughout the reproductive tract.

The ovaries of other litter-bearing animals, such as the bitch, resemble to some degree the grape-cluster appearance of the ovaries of the sow, but those of the bitch usually have fewer ovulation sites. The monotocous animals like the cow, ewe, and mare would usually have only one ovary involved in each cycle, but the individual growth and regression of the follicle and corpus luteum resembles that of a single follicle in the sow.

Uterine Changes During the Estrous Cycle

The steroid hormone-dependent organs of the female reproductive system undergo profound changes in growth and differentiation as puberty approaches. Once puberty is reached and estrous cycles occur, the tubular genital tract is sequentially exposed during each cycle to estrogens in general and to estradiol-17β, the dominant hormone during the follicular phase of the cycle, and

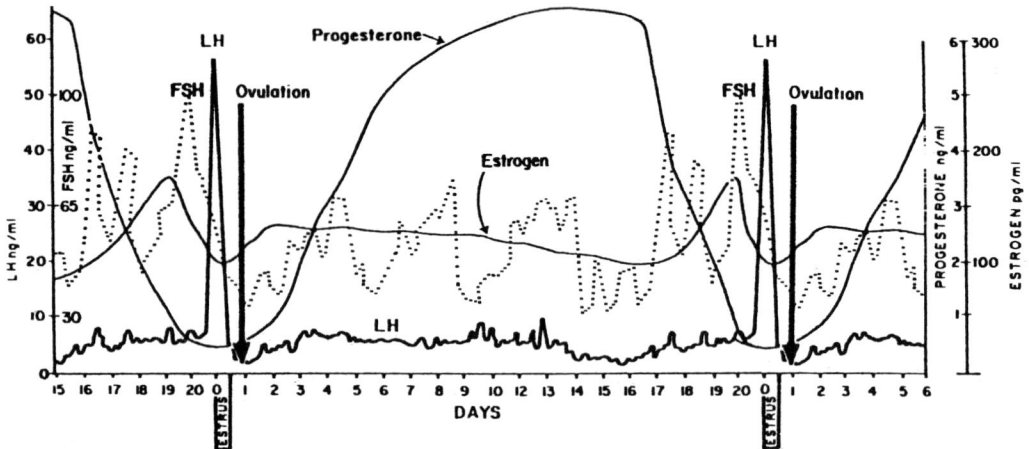

Fig. 9-25. Cyclic hormonal changes in the cow.

then to progesterone, the dominant hormone during the luteal phase of the cycle, or to both hormones, acting in synergy, during the overlapping parts of the follicular with the luteal phases of the cycle. The reproductive organs of the female undergo macro- and microscopic changes, which are induced by either estrogens or progesterone. At the end of the follicular phase and the beginning of the luteal phase of the cycle, as well as at the end of the luteal phase and beginning of the subsequent follicular phase, the reproductive organs respond to the transitional dominance from estrogens to progesterone and back to estrogens with changes that reflect the combined effects of both hormones.

Estrogen Influence

Estrogens favor retention of water and electrolytes throughout the genital tract (Table 9-4). The most prominent morphological changes noted in the uterus during the estrous cycle are in the endometrium and its associated glands. During estrus, increased estrogenic secretion (Fig. 9-25) stimulates the endometrial cells to increase in height and show intense mitotic activity, and the glandular elements of the endometrium secrete a fluid mucus which flushes the tract. Under estrogenic influence, the capillary bed in the endometrium and the general vasculature of the uterus grows, increasing the blood supply to the uterus. The increase in blood supply results in further growth and thick-

ening of the endometrium due to cell proliferation and edema. Similar changes occur in the oviductal mucosa and musculature.

Progesterone Influence

As the corpus luteum develops after ovulation and begins to secrete progesterone (Fig. 9-25), the superficial endometrial cells further increase in size and the glandular elements of the endometrium multiply and secrete. This period is sometimes called the "secretory phase" because the uterine glands respond to progesterone by glandular development and secretion of a thick material, "uterine milk", into the uterine lumen to nourish the preimplantation embryo. The subepithelial layer becomes infiltrated with neutrophils and eosinophils as the cycle progresses, and the edema lessens. By midcycle, high columnar cells predominate in the surface epithelium, and invasion of the superficial stroma with eosinophilic leukocytes becomes maximal.

Falling Progesterone and Rising Estrogen Influence

If a viable embryo (or embryos for some species) is (are) not present by the end of diestrus, the corpus luteum initiates retrogressive changes, and the synthesis of progesterone is severely impaired. Concurrently, the progesterone-receptors are down-regulated in favor of prevalence for estrogen-receptors. The increasing estrogenic influence is reflected in the tubular genitalia by changes in the surface epithelium, which becomes low and cuboidal. Marked vacuolar degeneration of the epithelial cells is a characteristic effect of the declining progesterone at this stage of the cycle. Thus, the major changes noted during the estrous cycle appear to be the cyclic manifestations of stromal edema, neutrophilic and eosinophilic infiltrations of the subepithelial areas, and changes in the growth of surface and glandular epithelia.

THE ANTERIOR PITUITARY AND THE OVARY

Two separate gonadotropins that specifically stimulate the ovary are present in the anterior pituitary. One, called follicle-stimulating hormone (FSH), promotes follicular growth in the ovary, whereas the second gonadotropin, called luteinizing hormone (LH), acts on an ovary previously stimulated by FSH (see Chapter 2).

The ovarian follicles in mammals are dependent upon FSH and LH for follicular growth and maturation. Both FSH and LH are essential for the synthesis of estrogen. Rising blood levels of estrogen suppress the pituitary release of FSH and facilitate release of LH. Purified LH in itself has no conspicuous effects on the initial growth of growing ovarian follicle. Thus, it is now well established that FSH promotes ovarian growth, but FSH in synergy with LH is needed to promote follicular maturation. LH is essential for synthesis of estrogen, ovulation, and for the initial development of the corpus luteum in most species. Prolactin, considered a third pituitary gonadotropin, stimulates the corpora lutea of the rat and possibly of other species to produce progesterone.

Estrogens in pharmacological doses inhibit FSH secretion. Large quantities of estrogen completely inhibit the secretion of gonadotropic hormones. Low physiological levels of estrogen cause in some species a positive feedback on gonadotropin output. Injection of low doses of certain estrogenic substances can facilitate ovulation in cattle, sheep, rabbits, and rats. It also has been reported that progesterone, in a low dosage, can stimulate the release of LH. Thus, it seems that both steroids may be essential to the ovulatory process in mammals.

Apparently FSH and LH are synthesized continuously and stored in the pituitary gland from where they are released throughout the estrous cycle. The proportions and levels of each of these gonadotropins change during the different stages of the cycle (Fig. 9-25). In relation to the amount of hormone released, the levels reached in the peripheral circulation, and the periodicity of the release of these hormones, one can distinguish at least three major forms: Basal levels, pulses, and surges. **Basal levels** refer to a low and relatively constant level of the hormone in the blood. **Pulses** refer to a sharp and increased concentration of the hormone in the blood above the preceding plasma concentration, lasting for short periods, usually less than 1 hour. A **surge** is defined as a large, statistically significant increase in the concentration of a hormone in the blood above the basal level, lasting for more than 1 hour. A brief recapitulation of the hormonal changes during the cycle is in order. Figure 9-25 shows hormonal levels during a typical cycle in the cow. On day 16, a luteolysin (likely prostaglandin $F_{2\alpha}$) from the nonpregnant endometrium reaches the ovary by a local route and induces luteolysis. Progesterone levels plummet, thereby allowing an outpouring of FSH, since the progesterone block on the pituitary is released. The FSH levels are pulsatile, but the clearest and most peaks are on days 17 and 18. FSH, in synergy with LH, facilitates follicular growth and estrogen production. The declining levels of progesterone and rapidly rising levels of estrogen induce behavioral estrus in most of the domestic species. Rising estrogen triggers the release of the "ovulatory surge" of LH on the day of estrus. Estrogen levels then decline, but the new CL starts progesterone production, which rises during the next few days and holds gonadotropin release at low levels. If embryonic luteotropic signals are not given at the appropriate time, the CL irreversibly regresses and a new cycle will follow.

PROSTAGLANDINS

Swedish Nobel Laureate von Euler coined in 1934 the name **prostaglandin** (PG) for a substance found in human semen. Since 1960, considerable interest has been shown in this group

Fig. 9-26. $PGF_{2\alpha}$ has an hydroxyl at carbon 9, whereas PGE has a ketone. Both arise (steps not shown) from the essential dietary linoleic (18-carbon) and arachidonic (20-carbon) fatty acids.

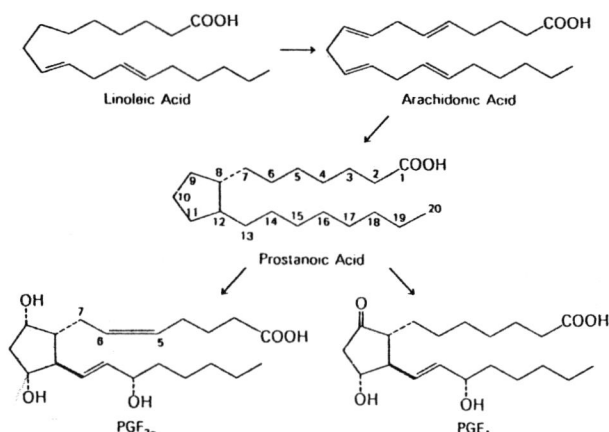

of 20-carbon unsaturated fatty acids, which have been found in many mammalian tissues. The precursors of PG are essential dietary fatty acids. The trivial names of the PGs are followed by letter and subscript number as shown in Figure 9-26. Prostaglandins have a wide variety of actions as follows: $PGF_{2\alpha}$ (induction of labor, abortion, and destruction of the corpus luteum or luteolysis); PGA_1 (inhibition of gastric secretion); PGE_1 and PGE_2 (bronchial dilation); PGA_1 (vasodilation and diuresis); and PGE_1 (inhibition of platelet aggregation). PGF and PGE differ only in a ketone or hydroxyl group at C-9 and a double bond between C-5 and C-6. Consideration will be given primarily to the role of $PGF_{2\alpha}$ in animal reproduction. PGF was assigned the letter F because it was found to be soluble in phosphate (spelled *fosfat* in Swedish), whereas PGE was found to be soluble in ether.

Prostaglandins in general and $PGF_{2\alpha}$ in particular are rapidly metabolized in the body, namely in the lungs. However, there are species differences in the degree and rate of metabolism of exogenous prostaglandins. For instance, in the ewe, regardless of the stage of the cycle, 99% of the $PGF_{2\alpha}$ that was injected in the pulmonary artery was metabolized during a single passage through the lungs, whereas in the sow, only about 18% of exogenous prostaglandin was metabolized during a single passage through the lungs.[41] Interestingly, as will be discussed later in this chapter,

the luteolytic activity of uterine $PGF_{2\alpha}$ is exerted through local utero-ovarian pathways in the sheep, a species in which most of the $PGF_{2\alpha}$ is metabolized during a single passage through the lungs, while the luteolytic activity of uterine $PGF_{2\alpha}$ is mainly systemic in the sow. It is tempting to speculate that in the mare, little if any of the $PGF_{2\alpha}$ is metabolized during a single passage through the lungs, because $PGF_{2\alpha}$ is a very effective luteolysin even when given in small doses, and the pathway of uterine luteolytic control is systemic in mares.

Prostaglandins in Luteolysis

It is now accepted that $PGF_{2\alpha}$ is the natural **luteolysin** for the majority of the domestic species. Indomethacin, a potent inhibitor of prostaglandin synthesis, extends the functional lifespan of the corpus luteum in several species if given at that time of diestrus when prostaglandins are secreted by the uterus. Oxytocin may also be involved in the release of $PGF_{2\alpha}$ by the uterus. Exogenous oxytocin given to heifers early in diestrus induces luteal regression and shortens the length of the estrus cycle, whereas the administration of antibodies to oxytocin delays luteolysis. Figure 9-27 displays a postulated mechanism by which estradiol-17β induces the formation of oxytocin receptors in the endometrial cells. Oxytocin would then activate

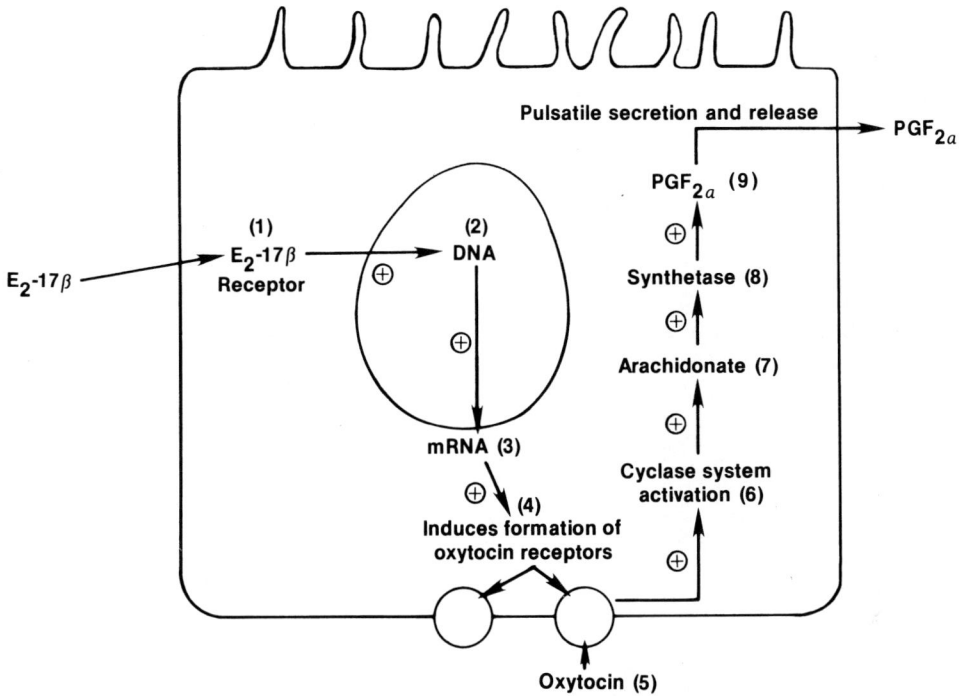

Fig. 9-27. Receptor regulation of pulsatile secretion and release of **PGF$_{2\alpha}$** from the uterus at the end of the luteal phase of the cycle in (Drawn and adapted from: J. A. McCracken, Res. Reprod. *16*:1, 1984).

these receptors, resulting in the synthesis, secretion, and pulsatile release of PGF$_{2\alpha}$.

Several mechanisms have been proposed to explain the luteolytic activity of PGF$_{2\alpha}$. Among these are:

1. prostaglandin-induced constriction of the utero-ovarian vessels causing ischemia and starvation of the luteal cells;
2. interference with progesterone synthesis;
3. competition with LH for the receptor site; or
4. destruction of LH receptor sites.

For all the species so far studied, including the domestic species, the ovarian artery is coiled and follows a tortuous course along the major (ewe and cow) or minor (mare, sow, bitch, queen) branches of the utero-ovarian vein draining the uterus. The ovarian artery is intertwined and in close apposition with a complex vascular network of venules from the utero-ovarian vein (Fig. 9-28). This vascular arrangement favors the passage of substances from the venous blood draining the uterus to the arteries supplying the ovary. In fact, luteolytic substances from the uterus, likely PGF$_{2\alpha}$, are now generally believed to reach the ovary in species such as the ewe and cow by transfer, diffusion, or some other means, from the venous efferent to the arterial afferent circulation. For these two species, the uterine horn controls the corpus luteum on the ipsilateral ovary through a local luteolytic pathway in the nonpregnant animal and through a local luteotropic pathway when a viable embryo is present in the ipsilateral horn of the gestating animal (Fig. 9-29). The local utero-ovarian pathway demonstrated for the cow and ewe (Fig. 9-28) has not been established for the goat. Furthermore, intrauterine devices, which induce luteolysis through a local pathway in cows and ewes, appear to act by a systemic route in goats.

The reader is encouraged to review the vascular anatomy of the uterus and ovaries for the

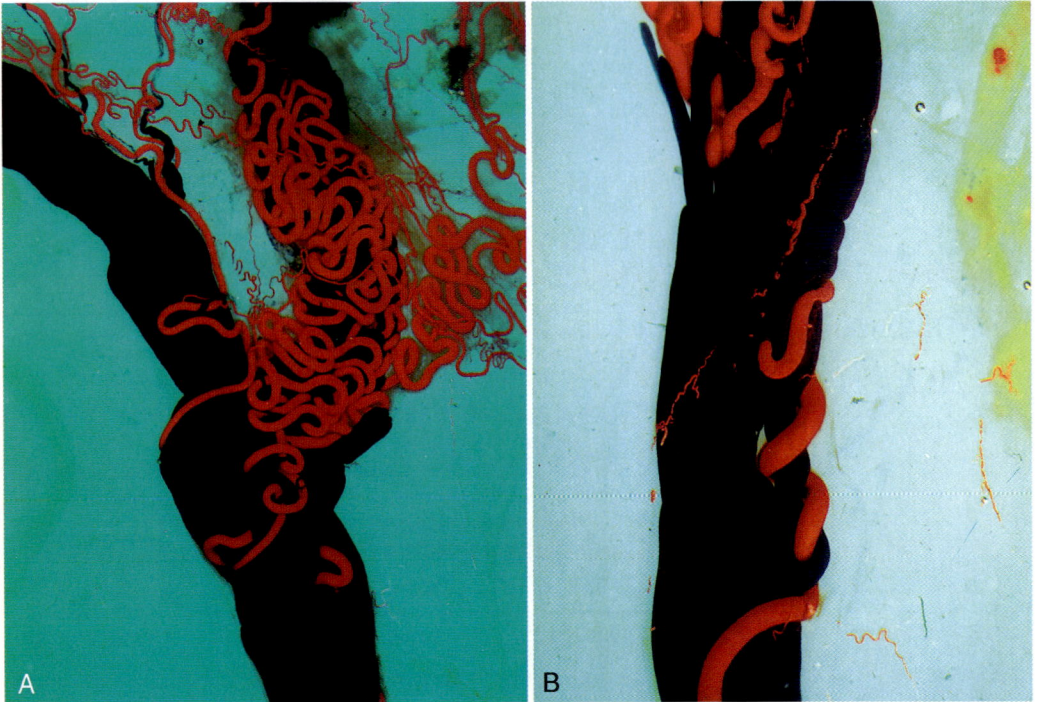

Fig. 9-28. Angioarchitecture of the uterus and ovaries at the ovarian pedicle in the ewe. **A.** Notice the rich network of veins and venules (**blue**) draining the uterus and their apposition to highly coiled arteries (**red**) carrying blood to the ovary. **B.** The ovarian artery is not only coiled on the surface and around the uterine and ovarian veins but is also intensively intertwined and penetrates through "handle-like" formation of the vein. This type of association and apposition favors the transfer of luteolysins from the uterine vein draining the uterus to the arteries carrying blood to the ovary. (Courtesy of Dr. C. H. Del Campo,[42-46] Laboratorio de Reproducción Animal, Universidad Austral de Chile, Valdivia, Chile).

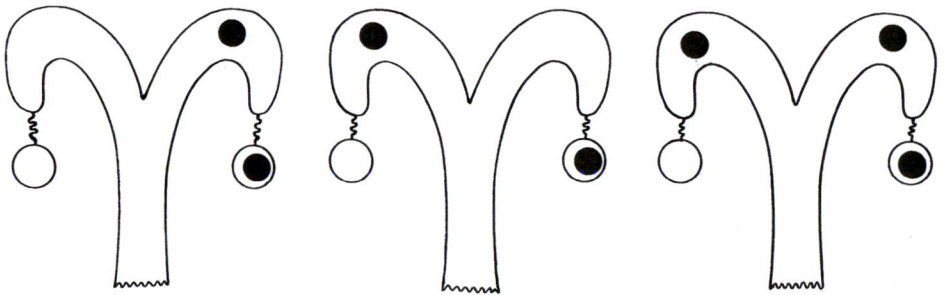

PERCENTAGE OF EMBRYO SURVIVAL

Day of pregnancy	Ipsilateral	Contralateral	Bilateral
< 30	73	33	67
110	67	13	27

Fig. 9-29. Embryo survival in heifers when a single embryo (**black dot in the horn**) is transferred to the horn ipsilateral or contralateral to the ovary carrying the corpus luteum (**black dot in the ovary**), or when a single embryo is transferred to each horn. (Adapted from: M. R. Del Campo et al., Reprod. Nutr. Develop. *23*:303, 1983).

domestic species published in Veterinary Scope[73] or in the pertinent articles listed in the Reference section of this chapter.

PGF$_{2\alpha}$ induces abortion when given during early pregnancy and will induce labor when given during late pregnancy in most species. Abortion during the early periods of pregnancy is probably due to luteolysis since progesterone production Falls sharply. Induction of labor during late pregnancy may depend on the action of PGs on the myometrium in addition to possible effects on the corpus luteum.

The ability of PGF$_{2\alpha}$ to induce luteolysis in cattle, sheep, mares, and other species has stimulated study of its use and the development of synthetic prostaglandins to control and synchronize estrus and general reproductive management in livestock species.

MAINTENANCE OR REGRESSION OF THE CORPUS LUTEUM

In polyestrous domestic animals, corpora lutea develop after ovulation and function depending on the species for only 13 to 16 days unless pregnancy occurs to signal the corpora lutea to continue functioning. The question then raised is **how does the corpus luteum 'know' that a 2-week-old, often unattached or unimplanted blastocyst is in the uterus?**

There appear to be marked species differences in the control of luteal function. Much of the early work was done on the rat, which now appears to be an atypical species. For purposes of simplicity this discussion will be confined to the sow, mare, goat, ewe, and cow. The bitch and queen are also atypical species. Corpora lutea of nonpregnant bitches continue to function for approximately the same length of time as for the pregnant bitch, a condition termed **pseudopregnancy.** In the bitch, PGF$_{2\alpha}$ does not induce complete regression of the corpus luteum when given in single doses, even when given at doses which are toxic or lethal to the bitch. The corpora lutea of the queen are also resistant to PGF$_{2\alpha}$. This phenomenon is discussed in Reproductive Patterns of Dogs (Chapter 16) and Cats (Chapter 17).

The study of the factors that control the formation, functional life, secretory activity, and regression of the corpus luteum in the cycling animal must include both the **luteotropic** and **luteolytic** influences or signals and also the temporal, sequential interplay of these influences. Luteotropic influences to the corpus luteum are provided by pituitary gonadotropins, mainly luteinzing hormone and after a fertile mating has occurred, by the embryo in most species.

Pituitary Effect

The pituitary in most species produces luteotropin at ovulation to form the corpus luteum. Luteinizing hormone is considered the luteotropic hormone for most domestic animals, although the mere act of ovulation induced by the ovulatory surge of LH favors luteal development in most species. For species in which hypophysectomy has been successfully performed, the corpus luteum does not form when hypophysectomy is done before the ovulatory surge of LH. If hypophysectomy is performed after the ovulatory surge of LH, the corpus luteum forms and, depending upon the species, either remains functional for a few days to regress early in diestrus (ewe, heifer) or remains functional for the length of the diestrus to regress at the expected time (sow). Administration of LH or LH-like hormones, such as hCG, at appropriate times during diestrus to ewes, heifers, goats, mares, and sows prolongs the functional lifespan of the corpus luteum of the cycle. On the other hand, the administration during mid-diestrus of antiserum containing high titers of biologically active antibodies to LH shortens the lifespan of the corpus luteum, and luteal regression is induced in ewes, goats, heifers, and mares, but not in the sow. The corpora lutea of the cycle in the sow are somehow independent of further pituitary LH luteotropic control once the initial luteotropic stimulus is given by the ovulatory surge of LH. However, antibodies to LH when given in early pregnancy can induce luteal regression in the sow. Antiserum to LH also interferes with luteal function in the bitch, and drugs that block the release of prolactin from the pituitary also suppress corpus luteum activity in this species, suggesting that the corpora lutea of the bitch are under the control of both pituitary hormones. There is no information available for the queen regarding pituitary control of CL function, though one can anticipate that LH is also luteotropic for the queen.

Uterus Effect

Loeb demonstrated in 1923 that the uterus exerted some form of control on ovarian function by studying the effects of hysterectomy on corpus luteum maintenance in the rabbit. A wealth of experimental evidences have accumulated since 1923 that point to the uterus as the center that controls the lifespan of the corpora lutea during the estrous cycle. Studies in several domestic species indicate that the nonpregnant uterus produces a substance, likely $PGF_{2\alpha}$, which has a "lytic" influence on the corpus luteum. With the exception of the bitch, which is a special case to be discussed in Chapter 16, and the queen, for which no information was available at the time of the writing of this chapter, the complete removal of the uterus during mid-diestrus in the cycling cow, ewe, goat, mare, and sow prolongs the lifespan of the corpus luteum of that cycle for a length of time approaching that of pregnancy for the species. Another interesting aspect of the utero-ovarian relationship in relation to the mechanisms of uterine control of corpus luteum function in the domestic species is the local pathway of uterine control for some of the species versus the systemic pathway of control for the others. In mares, total but not partial removal of the uterus prolongs the lifespan of the corpus luteum of the cycle. This is attributable to the vascular anatomy of the uterus and ovaries for this species, which favors the systemic distribution of the uterine luteolytic factors to the ovary carrying the corpus luteum. The uterus as a whole contributes the amount of uterine luteolysin necessary to cause regression of the corpus luteum. In the cow and ewe there is a local relationship and effect of the uterus on the corpus luteum and unilateral hysterectomy, implying the removal of only one of the uterine horns during mid-diestrus will or will not prolong the lifespan of the CL, depending on which of the uterine horns is removed with respect to

the location of the ovary carrying the corpus luteum. If the horn removed was adjacent or **ipsilateral** to the ovary carrying the corpus luteum, the corpus luteum will be maintained functional, as it would after total removal of the uterus. If the horn removed is on the side **contralateral** to the ovary carrying the corpus luteum, the corpus luteum regresses at the expected time in the cycle, as it would in the nonhysterectomized, intact animal. This differential response to the total or to the partial hysterectomy is also attributable to the vascular anatomy of the uterus and ovaries, which in these two species favors the local transfer of uterine luteolysin to the ipsilateral ovary via a local, venous-arterial pathway (Fig. 9-28).

In sows, both the systemic (as in mares) and the local (as in ewes and cows) pathways of uterine control participate in the regression of the corpora lutea. Experimental evidence indicates that a minimal amount of uterine tissue is needed in both horns for bilateral luteal regression. If as little as one-fourth of the ovarian end of each horn is left intact and *in situ* and the vascular connections have not been impaired, the corpora lutea of both ovaries will regress, even though three-fourths of each horn was removed and therefore, contributed no luteolysin. On the other hand, if unilateral, partial hysterectomy is performed and a complete horn is extirpated or less than one-fourth of that uterine horn is left *in situ,* while the horn in the other side is left intact, the corpora lutea in the **ipsilateral** ovary will initially be maintained; whereas the corpora lutea in the other ovary, **ipsilateral** to the intact horn, will regress. Due to the systemic distribution component of uterine luteolysis in the sow, the CLs present in both ovaries will regress in time.

In the control of the estrous cycle, the mechanism that "turns off" the corpus luteum appears to be of much greater practical significance than the pituitary mechanism(s) that "turns on" ovulation as well as initiates growth and function of the corpus luteum.

It may be concluded, therefore, that luteolysin(s), likely $PGF_{2\alpha}$ from the nonpregnant uterus, induces the apoptotic regression of the corpus luteum at the end of the cycle. Luteal degeneration can be shown through morphological studies of luteal cell degeneration as well as through analysis of their progesterone content and by the declining levels of progesterone in the blood. The uterus manifests its maximal "luteolytic" influence on the corpus luteum when it is under maximal influence of progesterone from the corpus luteum.

Exogenous $PGF_{2\alpha}$ effectively induces luteal regression and shortens the length of the estrous cycle only when the corpus luteum is fully formed and secreting progesterone. Exogenous $PGF_{2\alpha}$ does not induce luteal regression when given during the first 4 to 5 days of diestrus in cows, ewes, goats, and mares. The sow is a particular case in that $PGF_{2\alpha}$ induces luteal regression only on days 11 and 12 of diestrus, at a time when the corpora lutea of the sow are to begin retrogressive changes if viable embryos are not present in the uterus by this time. On this basis, the use of $PGF_{2\alpha}$ has no practical application in the cycling sow because the sow will come to estrus at the expected time 8 to 10 days later, regardless whether $PGF_{2\alpha}$ was administered or not. However, repeated treatment with $PGF_{2\alpha}$ may induce luteolysis in the sow (See Chapter 15).

Corpora lutea can be made to regress not only by the abrupt effect of $PGF_{2\alpha}$, but also by a lack of pituitary-tropic effect on the corpus luteum, as previously discussed. Regression of luteal tissue in the latter case is gradual.

There also appears to be a third way in which corpora lutea may regress. In hysterectomized ewes, retained corpora lutea diminish in progesterone concentration by 150 days, which is the length of gestation in the intact ewe. If hysterectomized ewes are made to ovulate and new corpora lutea form, then these will also persist but will diminish in progesterone content in another 120 days. This effect suggests that "aging" may be a factor in corpora luteal regression. The corpora lutea of the bitch appear to be independent of uterine control insofar as their regression is concerned. Bilateral hysterectomy in diestrual bitches does not prolong the lifespan of the corpora lutea, and the corpora lutea of pregnant, nonpregnant, mated, or nonmated bitches regress at about the same time, suggesting again that aging or the lack of extrauterine luteotropic stimuli may be contributing factors to their demise by the end of pregnancy or pseudopregnancy.

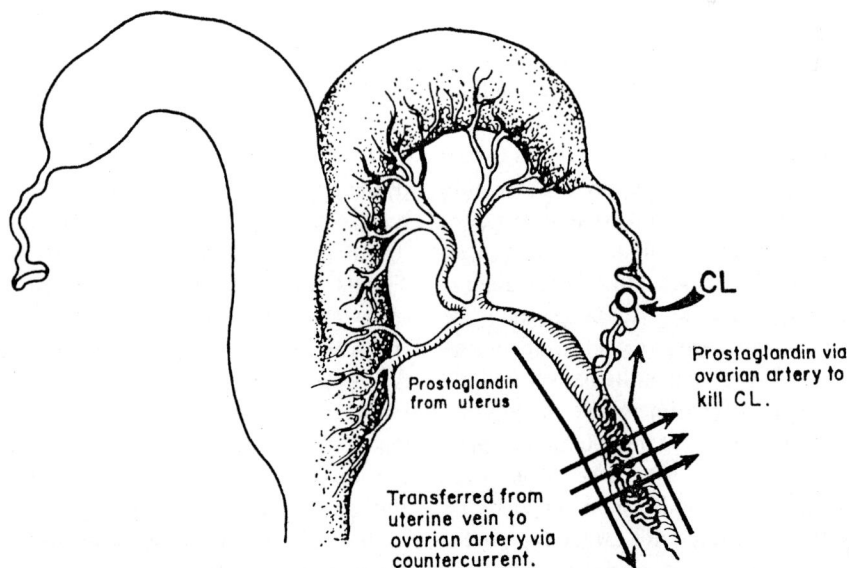

Fig. 9-30. Prostaglandins transfer from the uterus to the uterine vein, then by countercurrent transfer to the ovarian artery, and thence to the corpus luteum in the ewe and possibly other species.

Local Uterus-Corpus Luteum Relationships

Progesterone production in the ewe plummets on day 15 much like the decrease on day 17 in the cow. This decrease is attributed to the release of $PGF_{2\alpha}$ from the nonpregnant progesterone-dominated endometrium. By local circulation, the $PGF_{2\alpha}$ is transferred from the uterine vein to the ovarian artery by the countercurrent pathway shown in Figure 9-30. Figure 9-31 shows the effects of unilateral and bilateral hysterectomy in the ewe. Similar responses also occur in the cow. In subfigure *a,* the normal corpus luteum of a nonpregnant cycle lasts until day 15 with an intact uterus. In subfigure *b,* total hysterectomy prolongs the function of the corpus luteum for approximately 5 months because the source of $PGF_{2\alpha}$ has been removed. Subfigure *c* shows that transplantation of the ovaries to the neck prolongs the life of the corpus luteum for many weeks because the $PGF_{2\alpha}$ countercurrent system has been interrupted. In subfigure *d,* the same principle is shown; because removal of the uterine horn adjacent to the ovary carrying the CL causes the corpus luteum to live for at least the length of one cycle because the local transfer of $PGF_{2\alpha}$ is interrupted and a less efficient systemic route must be utilized. Finally in subfigure *e,* removal of the uterine horn contralateral to the ovary carrying the CL does not affect corpus luteal life because the uterine horn ipsilateral to the ovary carrying the CL produces $PGF_{2\alpha}$, which reaches the corpus luteum by the local route as shown in subfigure *a.* Available evidence lends support to this route in the ewe, sow, and cow. The pattern of utero-ovarian, vascular relationships in South American camelids (see Fig. 18-4) may help to understand the prevalence of pregnancies in one of the uterine horns. Most of pregnancies in llamas and alpacas occur in the left uterine horn, which is distinctly larger than the right uterine horn even in fetal and newborn animals (see Fig. 18-5). It appears that the side of ovulation, whether in the right or left ovary, does not affect the prevalence of pregnancies in the left uterine horn.

A recent report[46] indicates that there is a crossing-over of arteries from the right horn to supply blood and possibly larger amounts of nutrients to the left uterine horn. The venous drainage from the right uterine horn is closely intertwined with ovarian arteries supplying blood to the right ovary such that luteolysins produced by the endometrium of the right horn may cause luteolysis of corpora lutea in the right ovary, in a local type of pathway similar to that described for ewes and cows. What is most perplexing is that there is also a crossing-over of large veins from the left uterine horn to the right horn in an angioarchitectural arrangement that favors the local passage of luteolysins from the left horn to the right ovary, such that the left uterine horn may influence luteolysis in both ovaries.

Understanding of both the local and systemic pathways of uterine control of luteal function has physiologic and pharmacologic implications for the veterinary clinician. For instance, the mare, which has a systemic pathway of uterine control of luteal function, requires much smaller doses of $PGF_{2\alpha}$, regardless of the route of administration, to effectively induce luteolysis than does the cow. However, if $PGF_{2\alpha}$ is infused into the uterus of the cow, which has a local pathway of uterine control, the required dose of $PGF_{2\alpha}$ is about 10 times lower than that needed when the parenteral route is used. In this case, the effective dose of $PGF_{2\alpha}$ for the cow is about the same as that needed for the mare.

It is not clear whether the interaction of the embryo with the endometrium prevents the secretion and/or release of the uterine luteolysin or the embryo produces a luteotropin that counteracts, at the ovarian level, the luteolytic activity of uterine factors. In sheep, luteotropic signals from the embryo reach the ipsilateral ovary through a local venous-arterial pathway (Figs. 9-28 and 9-30) similar to that described for the luteolytic activity of $PGF_{2\alpha}$. Furthermore, the experimental transfer of embryos to the uterine horn ipsilateral to the ovary carrying the corpus luteum results in luteal maintenance and pregnancy in sheep and heifers, whereas the transfer of embryos to the horn contralateral to the ovary with the corpus luteum often results in embryonic mortality (Fig. 9-29). Embryos from some species at certain stages of embryonic de-

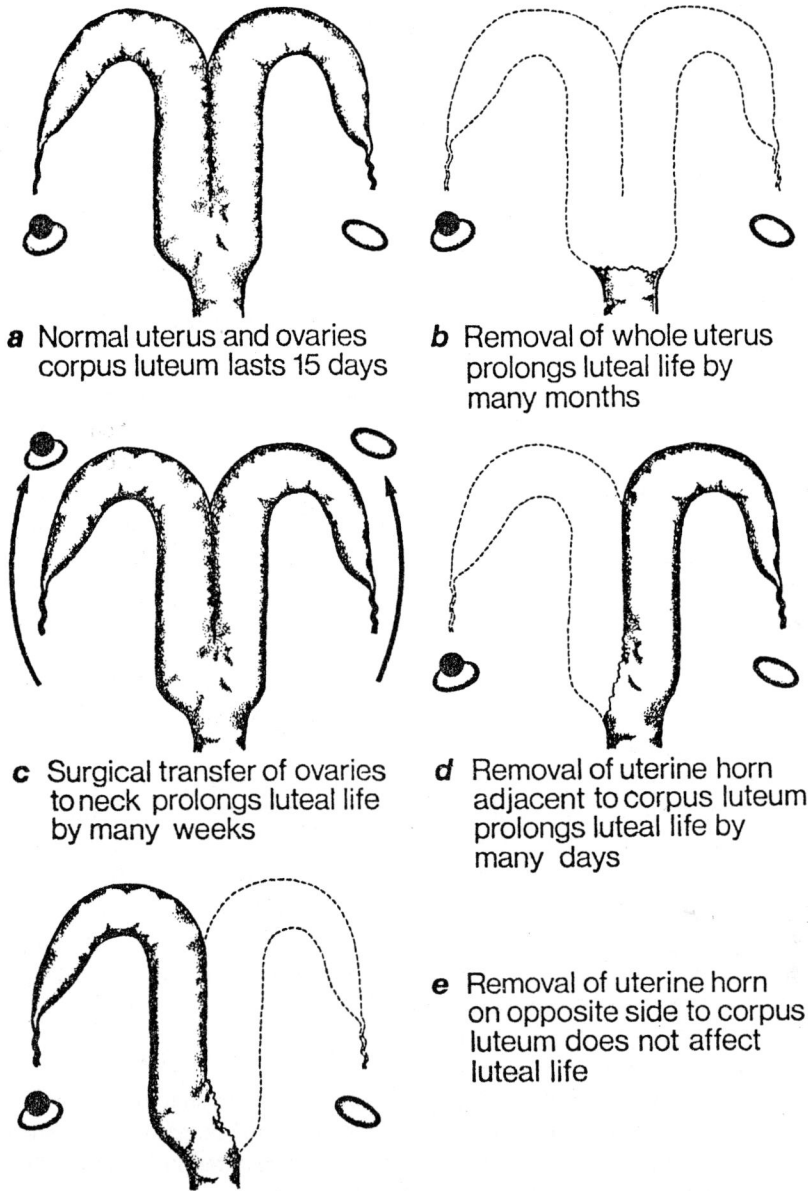

Fig. 9-31. The local lytic effect of the uterus on the corpus luteum in sheep. For the sake of simplicity, the corpus luteum is always shown in the left ovary. (From: C. R. Austin and R. V. Short, eds. *In:* Reproduction in Mammals. Cambridge, England, Cambridge University Press, 1972).

velopment are known to produce LH-like factors, while embryos from other species are known to secrete estrogens, which are needed for implantation. These may form part of the embryonic luteotropic signal that counteracts the uterine luteolysin or prevents its activity. Furthermore, intrauterine infusion of embryonic extracts prolongs luteal maintenance in some species. Also, there is evidence to suggest that the embryo may suppress the pulsatile release of ovarian oxytocin and as a consequence interferes with and prevents the release of $PGF_{2\alpha}$ from the uterus (see Fig. 9-27).

As discussed previously in this chapter, the presence of a viable embryo in the uterus is needed in single-bearing species at a critical time, before the end of diestrus, to prevent luteal regression. In mares, the embryo at the preimplantation stage of development promotes increased uterine tone and contractility, facilating the preimplantation intrauterine displacement of the embryo, which is characteristic for this species. In the sow, and probably in other litter-bearing species, more than four embryos are required to establish and maintain pregnancy. Apparently, four embryos or less are unable to overcome completely the luteolytic effect normally exerted by a nongravid porcine uterus. It is possible that when fewer than four embryos are present during the second to third weeks of pregnancy, more than one-fourth of the internal uterine surface is not occupied by the trophoblasts; and thus, the ensuing production of $PGF_{2\alpha}$ causes luteolysis. It has also been shown experimentally in swine that if embryos are confined to one uterine horn, the unilateral pregnancy so established is not maintained unless the nonpregnant horn is removed before the fourteenth day of pregnancy.

Other Uterine Effects

Chronic uterine infections prevent luteal regression in the ewe and cow. Perhaps uterine infections mimic pregnancy and cause persistent corpora lutea by preventing secretion of $PGF_{2\alpha}$ from the endometrium. In the mare, chronic uterine infections cause prolonged luteal function, but acute uterine infections trigger corpus luteum degeneration and cycle shortening.

Other lines of evidence for uterine involvement in luteal life have been shown by studies with intrauterine devices (IUD) in sheep, goats, cattle, and swine and the effects of intrauterine infusion of saline in mares. The IUDs were similar to the contraceptive devices used in the human female. Estrous cycles were shortened by IUDs in cattle and sheep but were not affected in goats and swine. It has been shown that these devices cause luteal degeneration

through local mechanisms operating directly between the uterine horn and the adjacent ovary. For years, equine practitioners have used intrauterine infusion of 500 to 1,000 ml of sterile, physiological saline solution to initiate estrus in anestrous mares. Estrus usually follows in 2 to 4 days after the infusion of saline. The mechanism is not known but may be similar to that postulated for the effects of an IUD.

OVARIAN HORMONES

The ovary produces two main steroid hormones (Table 9-3), estradiol-17β and progesterone, which bring about changes in the genital tract and some other parts of the body. There are several pathways, precursors, and metabolites in the process of steroid biosynthesis (Fig. 9-32). In this chapter, the discussion will be restricted to the major end-products of ovarian steroid biosynthesis: Estradiol-17β, the natural estrogenic hormone, and progesterone, which is the hormone secreted by the corpus luteum. Two physiologically important circulating metabolites of estradiol-17β, estriol and estrone, will be also discussed. These steroids are generically classified as estrogens. Figure 9-33 shows the structure of several natural steroids and of a synthetic steroid, diethylstilbestrol (DES). Notice that estrogens have 18 carbons (C18); androgens (testosterone) are C19; progesterone is C21; and DES, a synthetic estrogen, is also a C18 compound.

Peptide Factors Produced by the Ovary

In addition to steroid hormones, the ovary is involved in the secretion of peptide factors such as oocyte maturation inhibitor (OMI), inhibin, gonadocrinin, relaxin, and possibly MIH (Table 9-3). Oocyte maturation inhibitor is secreted by the granulosa cells of primordial and developing follicles and is responsible for maintenance of the oocyte at the arrested, dictyate stage of meiosis. It is not yet clear whether the ovulatory surge of LH inhibits the production of OMI or blocks its transfer from the cells of the *cumulus* to the oocyte (see Fig. 7-10 in Chapter 7). Inhibin is a dimeric polypeptide factor produced by the granulosa cells which selectively controls and inhibits the secretion and release of

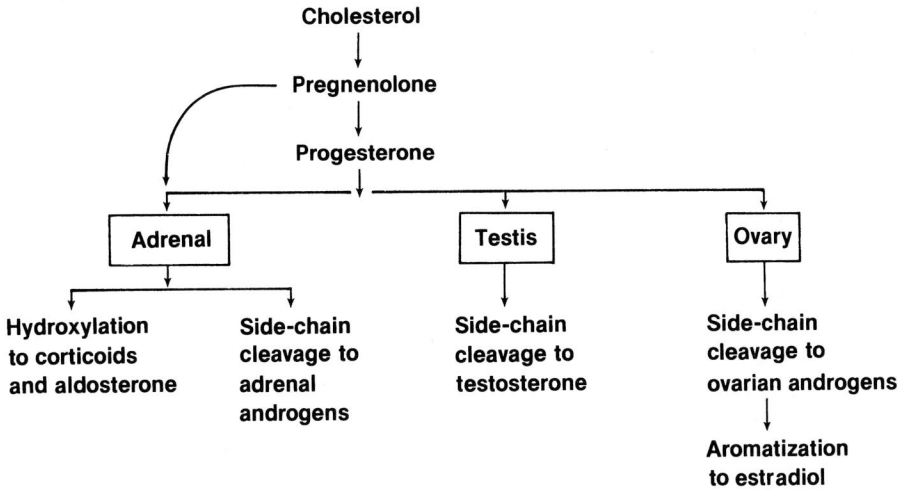

Fig. 9-32. Unified concept of steroid formation. Notice the common precursors and side-chain cleavages to originate end-products. (Adapted from: K. J. Ryan, Steroid hormones and Prostaglandins. *In:* Principles and Management of Human Reproduction, D. E. Reid et al., eds. Philadelphia, PA, W. B. Saunders Co., pp. 4–27, 1972).

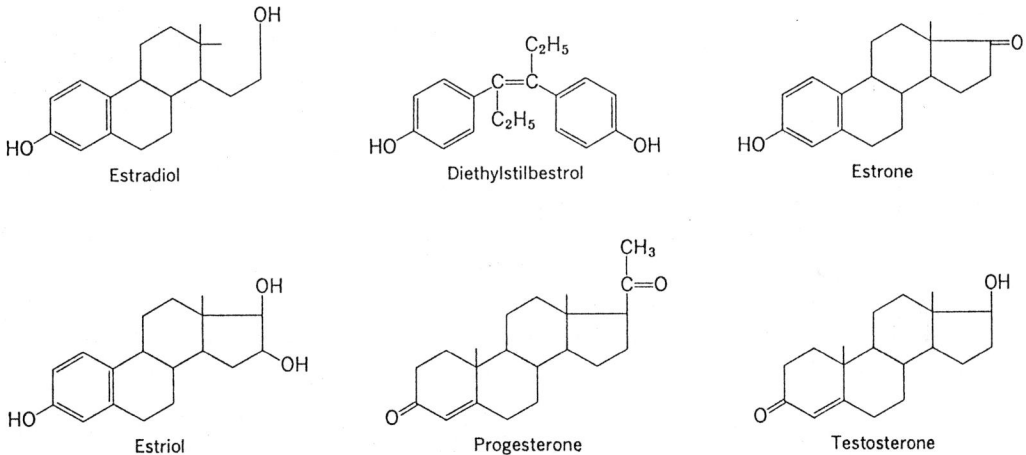

Fig. 9-33. The structure of some steroid hormones.

FSH by the adenohypophysial cells. Thus, inhibin is indirectly involved in the regulation of the growth of ovarian follicles. Gonadocrinin is a small peptide, similar to GnRH in activity but produced locally in the ovarian follicle by the granulosa cells (see Chapter 8, Fig. 8-4). The physiologic role of gonadocrinin has not been clearly determined, and specific receptors for GnRH have not been found in the follicles of cows, ewes, and sows. However, experimental evidences in other species suggest that gonadocrinin would, in a paracrine fashion, play an antigonadotropic role and locally control steroidogenesis by the thecal cells (see Fig. 8-4) by decreasing LH receptors and by interfering with the cAMP system of the follicular cells.

The insulin-like growth factor 1 (IGF-1), apparently also produced by the granulosa cells, has been recently implicated in the rat as an internal paracrine controller of steroidogenesis by amplifying the binding of gonadotropins on granulosa and thecal cells. The site for gene expression for IGF-1 in rats appears to be located only on granulosa cells. However, receptors for

Table 9-5   Estrogens Found in Endocrine Organs of Female Mammals

Species	Organ	Estrone	Estradiol-17β	Estradiol-17α	Estriol	Estradiol-17β 6-α-OH
Sow	Ovary	+	+	––	––	––
Cow	Ovary, follicular fluid	7.3	68.5	––	––	––
Mare in estrus	Ovary, follicular fluid	16.9	252	––	––	––
	Ovary	+	+	––	––	+
Woman	Ovary, luteal tissue of pregnancy	24–89	7–64	––	24	––
Sow	Placenta	+	––	––	––	––
Cow	Placenta	+	+	+	––	––
Ewe	Placenta	––	––	+	––	––
Goat	Placenta	––	––	+	––	––
Woman	Placenta	+	+	––	+	––
Cow	Adrenal glands	+	––	––	––	––

Values shown are micrograms (μg) per 100 ml.
Reprinted with permission from: A. Van Tielnhoven, Reproductive Physiology of Vertebrates, Philadelphia, PA, W. B. Saunders Co., 1968.

IGF-1 are present in both the granulosa and thecal cells in the rat and mainly in the theca externa of sheep. Insulin-like growth factor-2 (IGF-2) has not been identified as a product of secretion of follicular cells in domestic animals.

Activin, a homodimer of inhibin and follistatin, a family of proteins derived by differential splicing and proteolysis of follicular fluid proteins, are also peptide factors produced by follicular cells which on the basis of *in vitro* studies are postulated to have a role in the local regulation of ovarian function. The specific roles of activin and follistatin on the *in vivo* functional control of the ovary awaits confirmation.

Opioid peptides, such as β-endorphin produced locally by follicular cells, may, in a paracrine or endocrine fashion, influence ovarian steroid hormone production by modulation of the hypothalamic-pituitary-gonadal axis. Oxytocin has also been detected in the corpus luteum and ovarian follicles of several domestic species, including the cow, goat, ewe, and sow. However, the granulosa cells of the preovulatory follicle in mares do not produce oxytocin; neither appears to participate in steroidogenesis by the follicular cells. Oxytocin is apparently secreted by the luteal and granulosa cells. The physiological role of oxytocin produced by the ovary has not been established, but it may exert a local, paracrine control of estrogen and progesterone secretion.

Relaxin is a polypeptide factor considered to be a hormone of pregnancy, responsible for relaxation of the pelvic structures and cervix needed for normal parturition. Relaxin is also present in significant amounts in the blood of nonpregnant gilts and sows. Granulosa cells of the ovarian follicle appear to be the source of relaxin in the nonpregnant animal. The role of relaxin in the nonpregnant animal remains unclear.

Müllerian-inhibiting hormone (MIH), the hormone produced by the fetal Sertoli cells that inhibits the development of Müllerian structures in male feti, has been immunocytochemically detected in the ovaries of fetal, prenatal, and postnatal sheep and in the adult bovine ovary. Apparently, it is produced by the granulosa cells of growing follicles; its physiological role remains to be determined.

Estrogens

Estrogens have been isolated from the ovaries, adrenals, placenta, and even the testes of the male, especially the stallion. Table 9-5 lists several forms and the concentration of estrogens in different organs of female mammals.

Estradiol-17β is the female hormone and forms part of a group of steroid hormones

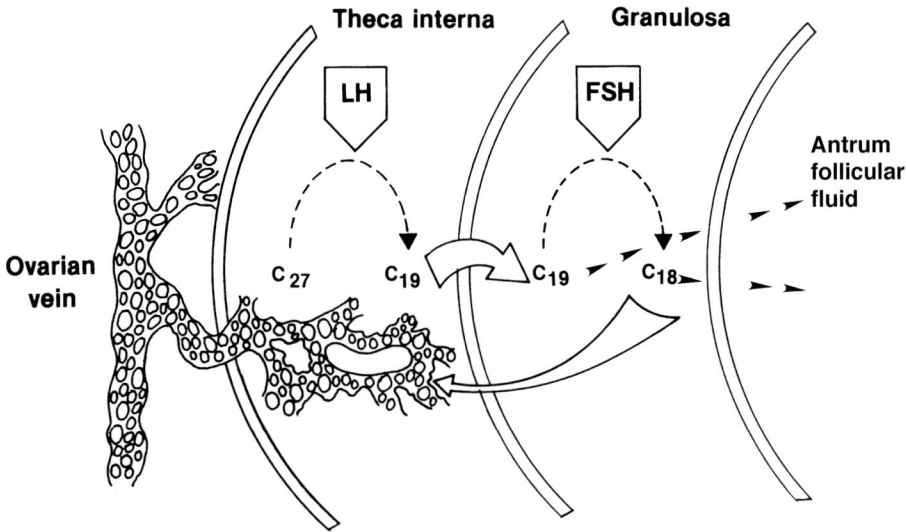

Theca interna   **Granulosa**

C_{27}=Cholesterol; C_{19}=Androgen; C_{18}=Estrogen

Fig. 9-34. Biosynthesis of estrogen in the preovulatory follicle. (Adapted from: S. G. Hillier, J. Endocrinol. *89*:3P, 1981).

named estrogens. Estrogens are produced by the theca interna and granulosa cells of the ovarian follicle under the synergistic, positive control of FSH and LH and under the negative influence of inhibin. Possibly, other intrafollicular factors such as IGF-1 and gonadocrinin participate in the secretion of estrogens. Luteinizing hormone receptors are present on the thecal and interstitial cells of the ovary, but the granulosa cells of the developing follicles appear to be the only follicular cells to have measurable receptors for FSH. As the follicle matures, LH receptors begin to develop in the granulosa cells reaching their highest concentration in the mature follicle, prior to ovulation. Thus, the appearance of receptors to LH in both thecal and granulosa cells marks a major event enabling the follicle to respond to the rising levels of LH during the preovulatory surge. The interaction between the thecal and granulosa cells is required for follicular steroidogenesis. Figure 9-34 shows an operational model for interaction between thecal and granulosa cells during steroidogenesis in the domestic species, with the possible exception of

the mare. In this model, LH stimulates the biosynthesis of androgens from cholesterol by the thecal cells. The androgens then diffuse across the basement membrane of the follicular wall, and a portion of these androgens reach the antrum. The granulosa cells uptake the androgens diffusing across the basement membrane and aromatize them to estrogens under the influence of FSH. A portion of these estrogens accumulate in the follicular fluid filling the antrum, but the majority diffuse into the rich capillary bed of the thecal layer, to be distributed into the systemic circulation. In the mare, the granulosa cells are thought to be initially the major source of preovulatory and postovulatory progesterone production, though the thecal cells may later become the major site of estrogenic biosynthesis by the follicle. Thus, the model represented by Figure 9-34 may not be applicable to the mare. Ovarian androgens, which diffuse into the capillary bed of the follicle, can be detected in the systemic circulation. Countercurrent transfer of androgens and other steroids from the venous to the arterial blood occurs at the ovarian pedicle in some species, providing additional androgenic substrate for follicular steroidogenesis and estrogen biosynthesis.

The main physiologic roles of estradiol-17β and estrogens in general are the development and maintenance of the functional structure of the female sex organs by stimulating protein synthesis and mitosis of estrogen-dependent organs. The secondary sex characteristics of the female, including changes in body conformation and growth, hair or plumage distribution, and mammary gland development are under estrogenic control. Estrogens are responsible for the induction of sexual receptivity to mating of the female. In most of the domestic species, estrogens alone or increasing blood levels of estrogen in association with declining levels of progesterone induce behavioral estrus. In the queen, the estrogenic hormone alone appears to be sufficient to induce sexual receptivity, whereas the bitch requires declining plasma levels of estrogens and increasing levels of progesterone for the full expression of behavioral standing estrus.

Perhaps the most dramatic organic changes induced by estrogens are those of the uterus, vagina, and vulva. The estrogens secreted during the cycle by the developing follicles, or the exogenous administration of pharmacological doses of estrogens, induce pronounced vascularization, increased blood flow and hyperemia, water and salt retention, and edema of the uterus, vagina, and vulva. Swelling of the vulva is an external sign of the edema of the tract associated with estrus. Estrogens also cause an increased uterine tone, which can be ascertained during the follicular phase of the cycle through rectal palpation of the uterus in large animal species. The myotropic effect of estrogens is expressed by increased myometrial contractions during proestrus and estrus. At this time, the myometrium is sensitized by estrogens to respond to oxytocin and prostaglandins. Prolonged exposure to pharmacologic doses of estrogens may cause uterine disturbances, including hyperplasia of the glandular epithelium of the uterus and excessive mucus secretion. Ewes grazed on subterranean clover in Australia develop infertility due to the high and prolonged intake of ginestein, a plant proestrogen which is converted to estrogens during ruminal digestion. Estrogens increase antibody levels in the uterus, enhance local protection against infection, and are responsible for the marked cornification of the vaginal epithelium in some the species, such as humans, rats, and bitches. Estrogens induce ductal development of the mammary glands in all of the domestic species and also induce mammary alveolar development in the heifer. Estrogens inhibit the growth of bones and favor ossification of the epiphyses, interrupting the postpubertal growth of the female.

While progesterone dominance is necessary for the maintenance of pregnancy, localized estrogenic action is necessary in some species for embryonic attachment or implantation. Blastocysts from several species, including the sheep, cow, and pig, produce estrogens. These estrogens act locally to counteract the antiinflammatory activity of progesterone at the site of implantation and create a localized hyperemic area where embryo-uterine attachment can occur.

Administration of natural or synthetic estrogens to animals is a common clinical practice for the control and treatment of a variety of conditions affecting the reproductive system. However, estrogens, like any other hormonal factor, must be used with caution, and the understanding of their actions and associated undesirable side effects is essential. Estrogens are routinely used in veterinary clinical practice for the control of mismating in bitches to prevent conception by disrupting embryo displacement toward the uterus when given before day 10 of diestrus or to induce early abortion when given after day 10 of diestrus. Implantation in bitches begins at about day 10 of diestrus and continues until day 22 of diestrus. The effectiveness of estrogens to induce early abortion in bitches declines rapidly between days 10 through 22 of diestrus (see Chapter 16). Estrogens are also used for the treatment of urinary incontinency of spayed bitches or for the treatment of hypertrophy of the prostate in dogs. However, doses given are often unnecessarily large and the treatment excessively prolonged. As a consequence, a fatal condition may develop because estrogens are myelotoxic for dogs. Dogs and particularly bitches over 5 years old are prone to react with bone marrow depression, impaired erythropoiesis conducive to aplastic anemia, thrombocytopenia, and leukopenia, conditions which are for most cases irrecoverable. To decrease the potential development of bone marrow toxicity if estrogens are to be used to control mismatings, the use of low-level estrogenic drugs such as mestranol (2-methyl, 17α-ethynyl-estradiol) is recommended. Species differences must also be considered when prescribing treatment with estrogens. For instance, estrogens are luteolytic when given in pharmacological doses during middiestrus to cows and ewes. Luteal regression occurs, and the animal returns to estrus within 3 to 7 days after estrogen treatment. In the sow, however, exogenous estrogens are luteotropic and extend the lifespan of the corpora lutea, resulting in prolonged interestrous intervals. In mares, exogenous estrogens do not affect the lifespan of the corpus luteum, but they prolong the interestrous interval by interfering with follicular development and ovulation.

The role of estrogens is especially important in ruminants because of the protein anabolic effect as seen when a small amount of a synthetic estrogen, diethylstilbestrol (DES), is fed to fattening beef cattle. The United States Food and Drug Administration banned the use of estrogenic growth promoters because of public health implications. Research is continuing in the search for other nonestrogenic anabolic substances.

Ingestion by ruminants and other herbivores of nonsteroidal dietary substances with estrogenic activity called phytoestrogens is associated with disruption of the estrous cycle and infertility. Chronic ingestion of phytoestrogens is conducive to cell differentiation resembling a pubertal pattern in the cervix, increased uterine weight, altered protein synthesis by endometrial cells, and changes in enzyme activity.

Extraovarian Sources of Estrogens

The normal adrenal glands produce estrogens in quantities that are insufficient *per se* to replace the normal ovarian production of estrogens. Thus, atrophy of the female estrogen-dependent organs invariably follows ovariectomy.

In the pregnant animal, the placenta is an important physiologic source of estrogens, as well as of other endocrine factors, including progesterone, gonadotropins, and GnRH-like factors. In the pregnant mare, estrone appears to be a major contribution from the developing fetus and placenta during early pregnancy.

Progesterone

Progesterone is the primary progestational hormone produced by the corpus luteum of the nonpregnant, cycling animal and by the corpus luteum and placenta of some species during pregnancy. Progesterone is needed for the maintenance of pregnancy in all species, whether supplied by the corpus luteum, by the placenta, or both. Abortion will ensue if progesterone is lacking or secreted in insufficient amounts to maintain pregnancy. In fact, pregnancy can be maintained in bilaterally ovariectomized animals of those species whose placenta does not produce progesterone by exogenous treatment with progesterone or synthetic progestagens.

Although progesterone has been isolated from the adrenal cortices of several species, the main source of progesterone in the cycling animal are the luteal cells of the corpus luteum.

The corpus luteum of domestic species is formed by cells with distinct morphologic characteristics. The corpus luteum of the cow, ewe, and sow contains two major cell types, large and small lutein cells, which differ in their steroidogenic capabilities, even though both types contain the same enzymatic machinery (3β-hydroxysteroid dehydrogenase) and capacity to synthetize and secrete progesterone. An emerging model (Fig. 9-35) suggests that under the influence of LH, the small lutein cells, which probably originate from the thecal cells, have the capability to uptake and store cholesterol. Upon further stimulation by LH, the small lutein cells respond by secreting progesterone in short pulses. The large lutein cells probably originate from the granulosa cells and are more attenuated than the small lutein cells in their response to LH stimulation and in the uptake cholesterol from the small lutein cells (Fig. 9-35). Thus, these cells would be able to secrete more progesterone for prolonged periods. In ewes, cytoplasmic release of progesterone from large lutein cells increases and parallels the development of the corpus luteum. Furthermore, the

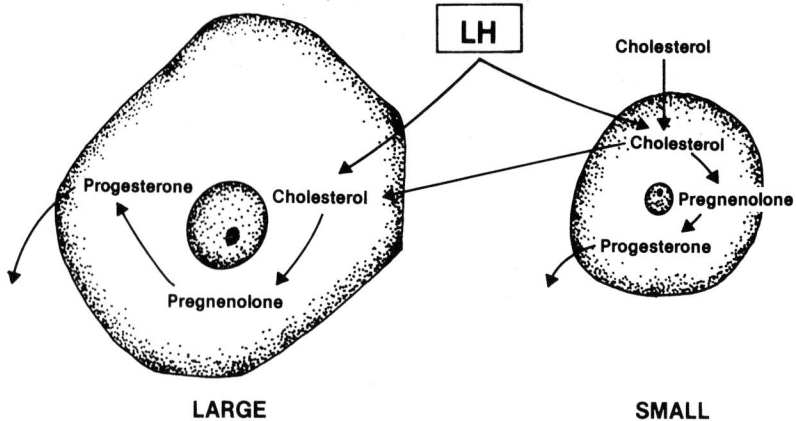

Fig. 9-35. Interaction between **LH** and **small** and **large** luteal cells in the synthesis of progesterone. (Adapted from different sources).

large lutein cells have more mitochondria than the small lutein cells. The small lutein cells are often interposed between the large lutein cells and blood capillaries. Cell-to-cell relationships, including gap junctions, may facilitate the diffusion of cholesterol and other precursors from one cell type to the other. Thus, the role of LH, at this level, would be to mobilize cholesterol stored in the small to the large lutein cells. In addition, it has been postulated that the small luteal cells would eventually become large luteal cells as the corpus luteum develops and ages. However, this view may no longer be tenable because recent evidence[218] for the ewe and cow indicates that the number of small luteal cells increases with little change in cellular volume, whereas the large luteal cells increase in size remaining relatively constant in number of cells.

The effects of progesterone are usually seen only after the target tissue has been subjected to a period of estrogen stimulation. This **priming by estrogen** leads to a synergistic response. Progesterone acts on the uterus to cause quietening of the myometrium and induces secretion of uterine milk by the endometrial glands. The uterine glands increase not only in depth but especially in branching and tortuosity.

Large doses of progesterone inhibit gonadotropin output of the pituitary gland. In some cycling animals (cow, ewe, mare, sow)

this may regulate the length of diestrus because as soon as the corpus luteum regresses and fails to secrete progesterone, a burst of FSH follows, which in synergy with LH causes the development and maturation of the ovarian follicles.

Declining blood levels of progesterone to less than 1.0 ng/ml, in synergistic action with rising levels of estrogens, brings about behavioral estrus in most of domestic species. In the prepubertal ewe and heifer, the progesterone secreted from a short-lived corpus luteum is needed to establish the postpubertal cyclic pattern of gonadotropin release. In seasonal breeders, such as the goat and ewe, progesterone is required at the beginning of the season before a full response to estrogen can be seen. This requirement may explain the silent heat in the ewe during the first estrous cycle of each breeding season. The first surge of estrogen is unable after a prolonged period of seasonal anestrus to elicit heat in the absence of exposure to progesterone from a previous corpus luteum. Progesterone also appears to facilitate the estrogen-induced behavioral receptivity in the female. The influence of progesterone on lactation is important—it acts on the mammary glandular tissue much as it acts on the uterine glands.

The most dramatic role of progesterone probably occurs during pregnancy. As the name of the steroid implies, progesterone **favors gestation** in all species. The early rise in progesterone

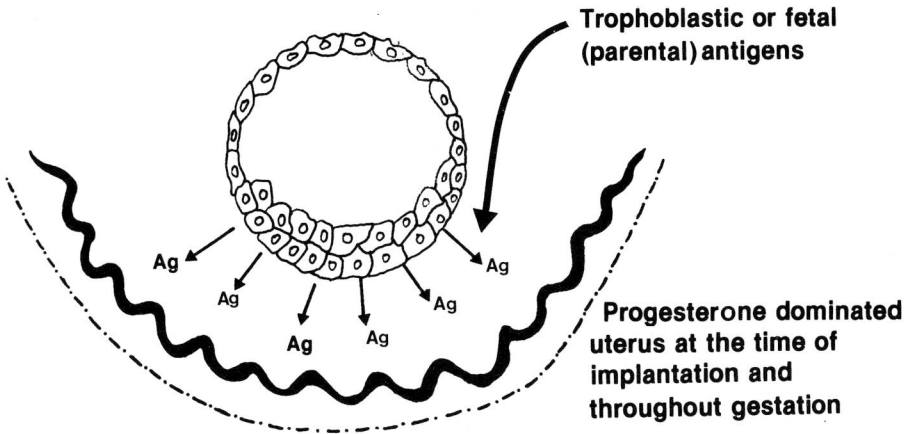

Trophoblastic or fetal (parental) antigens

Ag Ag Ag Ag Ag Ag

Progesterone dominated uterus at the time of implantation and throughout gestation

Fig. 9-36. Progesterone and probably other steroid hormones in high local concentrations exert local immunosuppressive activities in the uterus. These activities include: Anti-inflammatory reaction, inhibition of lymphocytes, and macrophage activation.

following the development of the corpus luteum prepares the uterus for pregnancy. Progesterone acts on the endometrium to inhibit myometrial activity and cause preparation for nidation regardless of whether an embryo is present.

The essentiality of progesterone production by the corpus luteum and/or placenta for pregnancy maintenance may be due to its ability to inhibit cell-mediated responses involved in tissue rejection. Progesterone may be nature's immunosuppressant of the mother's rejection mechanism of the fetus, because the fetus contains paternal antigens that would be incompatible with those of the mother (Fig. 9-36). Immunosuppression by progesterone may be likened to the immunosuppressant activity of glucocorticoids.

Progesterone favors an economy of body metabolism, and during pregnancy the female uses nutrients more efficiently. Appetite is stimulated during pregnancy, presumably due to the influence of progesterone, but there is also a tendency toward less physical activity. The combination of these effects favors weight gain in the pregnant animal. Psychic effects of progesterone favor maternal behavior in the female such as nest building. The biological half-life of progesterone is only 22 to 36 minutes in the cow. Thus, a constant secretion of progesterone

is essential to maintain circulating levels commensurate with the biological needs for maintenance of pregnancy.

Progesterone analogs that bind competitively with progesterone receptors are used as contraceptives and as abortifaciens or contragestives in humans and are proposed as contraceptives to control mismating in bitches. RU486 is a progesterone analog which quite effectively induces early or late abortion in bitches.[162] A recent study[21] on the amino acid sequencing of the progesterone receptor identified a critical amino acid, glycine, in position 527 of the binding domain of the progesterone receptor. Substitution of glycine by another amino acid blocks the receptor binding of RU486. Differences in amino acid composition and sequencing in the hormone-binding domain of the progesterone receptor may help to explain differential responses among species to treatment with progesterone analogs such as RU486. Hamsters and chickens have cysteine in the hormone-binding domain of the progesterone receptor, and they are unresponsive to RU486. The pregnant queen seems refractory to the contraceptive or abortifacient activity of RU486. Hence, it is possible that the hormone-binding domain of the progesterone receptor for the queen is lacking glycine.

Gonadal Steroid Transport and Mechanism of Action

Transport of estrogens (estradiol-17β, in particular) and progestagens (progesterone in particular) in the serum is similar. Both are weakly yet extensively bound to albumin. This accounts for most of the circulating sex steroids. Of the remainder, progesterone is strongly bound to transcortin, whereas estrogen is weakly bound to the sex steroid-binding globulin (SSBG).

Most of the steroid (90 to 95% of the estrogens) is transported in a bound form which is a protection from liver and kidney metabolism. A small amount circulates in the free form, which enters the target cell (Fig. 9-37). Actually, the free steroid enters all cells but is retained only in those which have the appropriate receptors (target cells). As the blood level of free steroid falls, bound steroid is released to maintain the free steroid level.

Once a sex steroid enters the target cell, it performs its function as depicted in Figures 9-37 and 9-38. In this model, the steroid hormone interacts with cytoplasmic receptors and then is translocated to the nucleus to stimulate or repress transcription of genes, finally leading to the specific biological effect of the hormone. This concept is now being challenged on the basis of new evidence that suggests that estradiol, progesterone, and glucocorticoid receptors are located within the nucleus and are associated with condensed chromatin. The steroid receptor diffuses into the cytoplasm and is constantly translocated between the nucleus and the cytoplasm. Once protein synthesis is induced, then the target cell will function accordingly. For example, a glandular cell could increase rate of secretion, mitosis could be stimulated in an epithelial cell, psychic estrus could be induced if the target cell was a neuron, or hypertrophy could be induced in a myometrial cell.

Gonadal Hormones During Senility

Few domestic animals except pet animals are retained until old age. Gonadal hormone production usually declines as the animal ages, and the protein anabolic effect is lost. Consequently, the addition of androgen or estrogen to "geriatric pills" may be indicated to counteract the

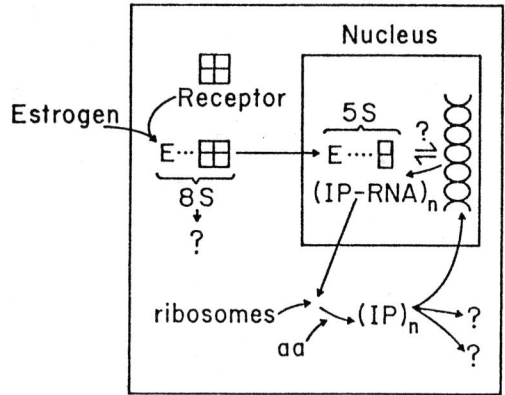

Fig. 9-37. Hypothetical model for estrogen interaction with uterine cells. **E,** estrogen; ⊞ cytoplasmic receptor; ⊟ nuclear receptor; ⋈ genetic apparatus; **IP,** induced protein; **aa,** amino acids. (Reproduced from: Handbook of Physiology, Section 7, Endocrinology. American Physiological Society, Baltimore, MD, Williams & Wilkins, 1973).

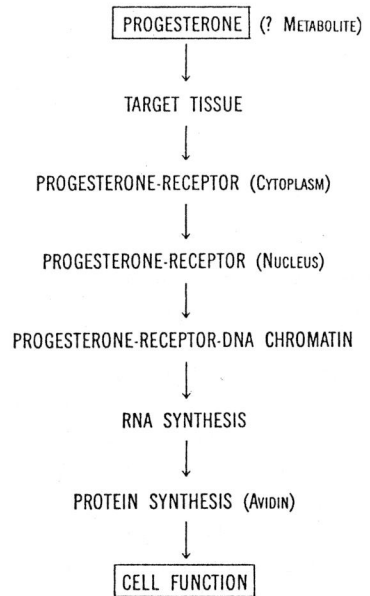

Fig. 9-38. Summary of the biochemical sequence of events occurring during progesterone action in the cells of target tissues. (Reproduced from: Handbook of Physiology, Section 7, Endocrinology. American Physiological Society, Baltimore, MD, Williams & Wilkins, 1973).

"wasting disease" of old age. Commercial efforts to synthesize androgens or estrogens possessing mainly the anabolic effects with minimal androgenic or estrogenic effects so far have been moderately successful.

ESTRUS DURING PREGNANCY

Folliculogenesis is depressed during pregnancy because of the accompanying high levels of progesterone. This is true for all domestic animals except the mare, where an unusual situation prevails, leading to follicular growth, ovulation, and formation of accessory or secondary corpora lutea while the mare is in early pregnancy. This will be described in detail in Chapter 13, Reproductive Patterns of Horses.

The placenta produces estrogen, which might account for the occurrence of sexual receptivity during pregnancy. Occurrence of estrus during pregnancy has been observed in all species but has been most studied in the cow. Natural insemination through copulation is not apt to have an adverse effect on the pregnancy, but the artificial insemination of the pregnant cow using rigid pipets should be avoided.

Estrus in the pregnant ewe is associated with follicular growth, but ovulation usually does not occur. Estrus has been reported during pregnancy in other species, but ovulation usually does not occur.

POSTPARTUM ESTRUS

Occurrence of estrus after parturition and the endocrinology controlling this event are quite different among the domestic species. Perhaps the situation in the human should be mentioned since this demonstrates an evolutionary trait which is protective of the maternal organism. The corpus luteum is maintained in postpartum women by the stimulus of lactation. The ovary usually does not grow follicles or ovulate as long as the young are suckling. The human female, in many countries but especially in primitive societies and underdeveloped areas of the world, has long and effectively utilized this approach for control of conception. The young are sometimes nursed for 4 or 5 years for this reason.

In domestic animals, the other extreme is the sow, which, for reasons not fully understood, experiences estrus within 3 to 6 days after parturition even though nursing a litter. Subsequently, follicles do not grow, ovulation does not occur, and pregnancy does not follow. Thereafter, as long as the sow nurses the piglets, the ovaries will remain inactive, and estrus does not occur until after the pigs are weaned. After weaning, the suppressive effect of lactation is removed and **estrus with ovulation** occurs within a week. This is a favorable time to breed the sow. Early weaning or loss of the litter soon after delivery is also followed by estrus and ovulation.

Most ewes are seasonal breeders; consequently, during the nonbreeding period the ovaries apparently remain inactive until the next breeding season. In the breeds which have been selected to produce two crops of lambs each year, there is need for breeding soon after lactation ceases. As soon as weaning occurs, these breeds usually show a cyclic activity in the ovaries accompanied by estrus and ovulation.

The mare ordinarily shows estrus 6 to 12 days after parturition, which is termed the "foal heat". Follicles grow, ovulation occurs, and it is possible for the mare to become pregnant if she is bred. However, the conception rate is usually poor,[132] less than 32%, because complete uterine involution does not occur for approximately 30 days, and breeding during the "foal heat" is not wise management. Breeding of mares on the second postpartum estrus usually produces satisfactory percentages (63%) of pregnancy.

The first standing estrus in the cow usually occurs 40 to 50 days after parturition, but examination of the ovaries reveals that the first ovulation usually occurs 25 to 30 days postpartum. This means that the first follicular growth and ovulation are accompanied by silent estrus. Although the cow is a nonseasonal breeding animal, there is some effect of season on the postpartum estrous interval since the Winter months lengthen and the Summer months shorten the interval.

The bitch and the cat are seasonal breeders; consequently, there is no tendency toward an early postpartum heat even after weaning. The uterus of the bitch involutes slowly, taking up to 4 months to return to the prepregnancy state.

PSEUDOMENSTRUATION

Several domestic animals shed blood from the uterus at certain phases of the estrous cycle which eventually is discharged in the vaginal secretions. It is important not to confuse this shedding of blood in animals such as in primates which undergo menstruation. For example, heifers and some cows discharge blood from the uterus after ovulation during the first day of postestrus. This is due to intensive endometrial stimulation by estrogen during proestrus and estrus, leading to fragility of the vascular system and diapedesis. A similar condition occurs in the bitch, but the blood is shed earlier, during proestrus. Again the cause is thought to be due to overstimulation of the endometrium by estrogens from the growing follicles.

FERTILITY—INFERTILITY—STERILITY—FECUNDITY—PROLIFICACY

There is considerable misuse of these terms, but the following definitions were agreed upon by a committee concerned with nomenclature of reproductive diseases.[93]

Fertility is a successful reproduction. **Infertility** is temporary loss of fertility. **Sterility** is permanent loss of fertility. **Fecundity** or **prolificacy** (usually considered to be synonymous) is the degree of reproduction appropriate for the species and is usually used in polytocous species to indicate relative litter size. Fertility, infertility, and sterility are applied to both sexes, but fecundity and prolificacy are reserved for the female of the species.

REFERENCES

1. Abe, H., Sendai, Y., Satoh, T., et al. (1995): Bovine oviduct-specific glycoprotein: A potent factor for maintenance of viability and motility of bovine spermatozoa *in vitro*. Mol. Reprod. Develop. *42*:226.
2. Abel, J. H., Jr., Verhage, H. G., McClellan, M. C., et al. (1975): Ultrastructural analysis of the granulosa-luteal cell transition in the ovary of the dog. Cell Tissue Res. *160*:155.
3. Adams, G. P., Sumar, J., and Ginther, O. J. (1991): Hemorrhagic ovarian follicles in llamas. Theriogenology *35*:557.
4. Adams, N. R. (1990): Permanent infertility in ewes exposed to plant oestrogens. Aust. Vet. J. *67*:197.
5. Adams, N. R. and Martin, G. B. (1983): Effects of oestradiol on plasma concentrations of luteinizing hormone in ovariectomized ewes with clover disease. Aust. J. Biol. Sci. *36*:295.
6. Adashi, E. Y. and Rohan, R. M. (1992): Intraovarian regulation. Peptidergic signaling systems. Trends Endocrinol. Metab. *3*:243.
7. Akbar, A. M., Reichert, L. E., Jr., and Dunn, T. G. (1974): Serum levels of follicle-stimulating hormone during the bovine estrous cycle. J. Anim. Sci. *39*:360.
8. Alila, H. W., Dowd, J. P., Corradino, R. A., et al. (1988): Control of progesterone production in small and large bovine luteal cells separated by flow cytometry. J. Reprod. Fertil. *82*:645.
9. Alila, H. W. and Hansel, W. (1984): Origin of different cell types in the bovine corpus luteum as characterized by specific monoclonal antibodies. Biol. Reprod. *31*:1015.
10. Anderson, L. L., Rathmacher, R. P., and Melampy, R. M. (1966): The uterus and unilateral regression of corpora lutea in the pig. Am. J. Physiol. *210*:611.
11. Armstrong, S. M. (1989): Melatonin and circadian control in mammals. Experientia *45*:932.
12. Aten, R. F., Ireland, J. J., Weems, C. W., et al. (1987): Presence of gonadotropin-releasing hormone-like proteins in bovine and ovine ovaries. Endocrinology *120*:1727.
13. Aten, R. F., Williams, A. T., Behrman, H. R., et al. (1986): Ovarian gonadotropin-releasing hormone-like protein(s): Demonstration and characterization. Endocrinology *118*:961.
14. Bagnell, C. A., Ayau, E., Downey, B. R., et al. (1989): Localization of relaxin during formation of the porcine corpus luteum. Biol. Reprod. *40*:835.
15. Baker, M. E. (1995): Endocrine activity of plant-derived compounds: An evolutionary perspective. Proc. Soc. Exp. Biol. Med. *208*:131.
16. Ball, G. D. and Day, B. N. (1982): Bilateral luteal maintenance in unilaterally pregnant pigs with infusions of embryonic extracts. J. Anim. Sci. *54*:142.
17. Basu, S. and Kindahl, H. (1987): Prostaglandin biosynthesis and its regulation in the bovine endometrium: A comparison between nonpregnant and pregnant status. Theriogenology *28*:175.
18. Bazer, F. W. (1992): Mediators of maternal recognition of pregnancy in mammals. Proc. Soc. Exp. Biol. Med. *199*:373.
19. Bazer, F. W., Roberts, R. M., and Thatcher, W. W. (1979): Actions of hormones on the uterus and effect on conceptus development. J. Anim. Sci. *49* (Suppl. 2):35.
20. Bellve, A. R. and McDonald, M. F. (1968): Directional flow of fallopian tube secretion in the Romney ewe. J. Reprod. Fertil. *15*:357.
21. Benhamou, B., Garcia, T., Lerouge, T., et al. (1992): A single amino acid that determines the sensitivity of progesterone receptors to RU486. Science *255*:206.
22. Botwood, N., Hamilton Fairley, D., Kiddy, D., et al. (1995): Sex hormone-binding globulin and female reproductive function. J. Steroid Biochem. Mol. Biol. *53*:529.
23. Bézard, J., Vigier, B., Tran, D., et al. (1987): Immunocytochemical study of anti-Müllerian hormone in sheep ovarian follicles during fetal and post-natal development. J. Reprod. Fertil. *80*:509.
24. Bézard, J., Vigier, B., Tran, D., et al. (1988): Anti-Müllerian hormone in sheep follicles. Reprod. Nutr. Develop. *28*:1105.
25. Blondin, P., Dufour, M., and Sirard M.-A. (1996): Analysis of atresia in bovine follicles using different methods: Flow cytometry, enzyme-linked immunosorbent assay, and classic histology. Biol. Reprod. *54*:631.

26. Bravo, P. W. (1994): Reproductive endocrinology of llamas and alpacas. Vet. Clin. North Am. *10*:265.

27. Bravo, P. W., Stabenfeldt, G. H., Lasley, B. L., et al. (1991): The effect of ovarian follicle size on pituitary and ovarian responses to copulation in domesticated South American camelids. Biol. Reprod. *45*:553.

28. Brinkley, H. J. (1981): Endocrine signaling and female reproduction. Biol. Reprod. *24*:22.

29. Brown, J. L. and Reeves, J. J. (1983): Absence of specific luteinizing hormone-releasing hormone receptors in ovine, bovine and porcine ovaries. Biol. Reprod. *29*:1179.

30. Buccione, R., Schroeder, C., and Eppig, J. J. (1990): Interactions between somatic cells and germ cells throughout mammalian oogenesis. Biol. Reprod. *43*:543.

31. Buhr, M. M., McKay, R. M., and Grinwich, D. L. (1986): Luteolytic action of prostaglandins in swine and effects of cloprostenol on luteinizing hormone receptors and membrane structure on porcine corpora lutea. Can. J. Anim. Sci. *66*:415.

32. Casida, L. E., Woody, C. O., and Pope, A. L. (1966): Inequality in function of the right and left ovaries and uterine horns of the ewe. J. Anim. Sci. *25*:1169.

33. Cavender, J. L. and Murdoch, W. J. (1988): Morphological studies on the microcirculatory system of periovulatory ovine follicles. Biol. Reprod. *39*:989.

34. Chemineau, P. (1986): Sexual behavior and gonadal activity during the year in the tropical Creole meat goat. I. Female oestrous behaviour and ovarian activity. Reprod. Nutr. Develop. *26*:441.

35. Clarke, P. G. H. and Clarke, S. (1996): Nineteenth century research on naturally occurring cell death and related phenomena. Anat. Embryol. *193*:81.

36. Claus, R., Over, R., and Dehnhard, M. (1990): Effect of male odour on LH secretion and the induction of ovulation in seasonally anoestrous goats. Anim. Reprod. Sci. *22*:27.

37. Conaway, C. H. (1971): Ecological adaptation and mammalian reproduction. Biol. Reprod. *4*:239.

38. Cooke, R. G. and Homeida, A. M. (1985): Suppression of prostaglandin F-2α releases and delay of luteolysis after active immunization against oxytocin in the goat. J. Reprod. Fertil. *75*:63.

39. Crafts, R. C. (1948): The effects of estrogens on the bone marrow of adult female dogs. Blood *3*:276.

40. Crisp, T. M. (1992): Organization of the ovarian follicle and events in its biology: Oogenesis, ovulation or atresia. Mutation Res. *296*:89.

41. Davis, A. J., Fleet, I. R., Harrison, F. A., et al. (1979): Pulmonary metabolism of prostaglandin $F_{2\alpha}$ in the conscious nonpregnant ewe and sow. J. Physiol. *301*:86P.

42. Del Campo, C. H. and Ginther, O. J. (1973): Vascular anatomy of the uterus and ovaries and the unilateral luteolytic effect of the uterus: Horses, sheep, and swine. Am. J. Vet. Res. *34*:305.

43. Del Campo, C. H. and Ginther, O. J. (1973): Vascular anatomy of the uterus and ovaries and the unilateral luteolytic effect of the uterus: Angioarchitecture in sheep. Am. J. Vet. Res. *34*:1377.

44. Del Campo, C. H. and Ginther, O. J. (1974): Vascular anatomy of the uterus and ovaries and unilateral luteolytic effect of the uterus: Histologic structure of uteroovarian vein and ovarian artery in sheep. Am. J. Vet. Res. *35*:397.

45. Del Campo, C. H. and Ginther, O. J. (1974): Arteries and veins of uterus and ovaries in dogs and cats. Am. J. Vet. Res. *35*:409.

46. Del Campo, M. R., Del Campo, C. H., and Ginther, O. J. (1996): Vascular provisions for a local uteroovarian cross-over pathway in new world camelids. Theriogenology *46*:983.

47. Del Campo, M. R., Rowe, R. F., Chaichareon, D., et al. (1983): Effect of the relative locations of embryo and corpus luteum on embryo survival in cattle. Reprod. Nutr. Develop. *23*:303.

48. Del Campo, M. R., Rowe, R. F., French, L. R., et al. (1977): Unilateral relationship of embryos and the corpus luteum in cattle. Biol. Reprod. *16*:580.

49. Douglas, R. H. and Ginther, O. J. (1973): Luteolysis following a single injection of prostaglandin $F_{2\alpha}$ in sheep. J. Anim. Sci. *37*:990.

50. Downing, S. J. and Hollingsworth, M. (1993): Action of relaxin on uterine contractions–A review. J. Reprod. Fertil. *99*:275.

51. Driancourt, M. A. (1991): Follicular dynamics in sheep and cattle. Theriogenology *35*:55.

52. Dukelow, W. R. (1978): Laparoscopic research techniques in mammalian embryology. *In:* Methods in Mammalian Reproduction, edited by J. C. Daniel. New York, NY, Academic Press, Inc., pp. 437.

53. Dyrmundsson, O. R. (1973): Puberty and early reproductive performance in sheep. I. Ewe lambs. Anim. Breed. Abst. *41*:273.

54. Eldridge-White, R., Easter, R. A., Heaton, D. M., et al. (1989): Hormonal control of the cervix in pregnant gilts. I. Changes in the physical properties of the cervix correlate temporarily with elevated serum levels of estrogen and relaxin. Endocrinology *125*:2996.

55. Ellinwood, W. E., Nett, T. M., and Niswender, G. D. (1979): Maintenance of the corpus luteum of early pregnancy in the ewe. 1. Luteotropic properties of embryonic homogenates. Biol. Reprod. *21*:281.

56. Eppig, J. J. and Downs, S. M. (1984): Chemical signals that regulate mammalian oocyte maturation. Biol. Reprod. *30*:1.

57. Erickson, B. H., Reynolds, R. A., and Murphree, R. L. (1976): Ovarian characteristics and reproductive performance of the aged cow. Biol. Reprod. *15*:555.

58. Erickson, G. F., Magoffin, D. A., Dyer, C. A., et al. (1985): The ovarian androgen-producing cells: A review of structure/function relationships. Endocrine Rev. *6*:371.

59. Espey, L. L. (1978): Ovarian contractility and its relationship to ovulation: A review. Biol. Reprod. *19*:540.

60. Faillace, L. S. and Hunter, M. G. (1994): Follicle development and oocyte maturation during the immediate preovulatory period in Meishan and white hybrid gilts. J. Reprod. Fertil. *101*:571.

61. Farin, C. E., Moeller, C. L., Sawyer, H. R., et al. (1986): Morphometric analysis of cell types in the ovine corpus luteum throughout the estrous cycle. Biol. Reprod. *35*:1299.

62. Fernandez-Pardal, J., Gimeno, M. F., and Gimeno, A. L. (1986): Catecholamines in sow Graafian follicles at proestrus and at diestrus. Biol. Reprod. *34*:439.

63. Fields, M. J. and Fields, P. A. (1996): Morphological characteristics of the bovine corpus luteum during the

estrous cycle and pregnancy. Theriogenology *45*:1295.

64. Findlay, J. K., Robertson, D. M., Clarke, I. J., et al. (1992): Hormonal regulation of reproduction–General concepts. Anim. Reprod. Sci. *28*:319.

65. Fish, B., Goldberg, I., Ovadia, J., et al. (1990): Physicochemical properties of follicular fluid and their relation to *in vitro* fertilization (IVF) outcome. J. In Vitro Fertil. Embryo Transf. *7*:67.

66. Fitz, T. A., Mayan, M. H., Sawyer, H. R., et al. (1982): Characterization of two steroidogenic cell types in the ovine corpus luteum. Biol. Reprod. *27*:703.

67. Fléchon, J. E., Pavlok, A., and Kopecny, V. (1984): Dynamics of zona pellucida formation by the mouse oocyte. An autoradiographic study. Biol. Cell *51*:403.

68. Fortune, J. E. (1994): Ovarian follicular growth and development in mammals. Biol. Reprod. *50*:225.

69. Foster, D. and Ryan, K. (1979): Mechanism governing onset of ovarian cyclicity at puberty in the lamb. Ann. Biol. Anim. Biochim. Biophys. *19*:1369.

70. Garcia-Villar, R., Toutain, P. L., Schams, D., et al. (1983): Are regular activity episodes of the genital tract controlled by pulsatile releases of oxytocin? Biol. Reprod. *29*:1183.

71. Geisert, R. D., Renegar, R. H., Thatcher, W. W., et al. (1982): Establishment of pregnancy in the pig: I. Interrelationships between preimplantation development of the pig blastocysts and uterine endometrial secretions. Biol. Reprod. *27*:925.

72. Gerena, R. L. and Killian, G. J. (1990): Electrophoretic characterization of proteins in oviduct fluid of cows during the estrous cycle. J. Exp. Zool. *256*:113.

73. Ginther, O. J. (1976): Comparative anatomy of utero-ovarian vasculature. Vet. Scope *20*:2.

74. Ginther, O. J. and Del Campo, C. H. (1974): Vascular anatomy of the uterus and ovaries and the unilateral luteolytic effect of the uterus: Cattle. Am. J. Vet. Res. *35*:193.

75. Ginther, O. J., Wiltbank, M. C., Fircke, P. M., et al. (1996): Selection of the dominant follicle in cattle. Biol. Reprod. *55*:1187.

76. Gittleman, J. L. and Thompson, S. D. (1988): Energy allocation in mammalian reproduction. Am. Zool. *28*:863.

77. Gnatec, G. G., Smith, L. D., Duby, R. T., et al. (1989): Maternal recognition of pregnancy in the goat: Effects of conceptus removal on interestrus intervals and characterization of conceptus protein production during early pregnancy. Biol. Reprod. *41*:655.

78. Gosden, R. G., Sadler, I. H., Reed, D., et al. (1990): Characterization of ovarian follicular fluids of sheep, pigs and cows using proton nuclear magnetic resonance spectroscopy. Experientia *46*:1012.

79. Griffin, P. G. and Ginther, O. J. (1992): Research applications of ultrasonic imaging in reproductive biology. J. Anim. Sci. *70*:953.

80. Griffing, P. G., Carnevale, E. M., and Ginther, O. J. (1993): Effects of the embryo on uterine morphology and function in mares. Anim. Reprod. Sci. *31*:311.

81. Guillemot, M. and Guay, P. (1982): Ultrastructural features of the cell surfaces of uterine and trophoblas-tic epithelia during embryo attachment in the cow. Anat. Rec. *204*:315.

82. Guiochon-Mantel, A., Delabre, K., Lescop, P., et al. (1996): Intracellular traffic of steroid hormone receptors. J. Steroid Biochem. Mol. Biol. *56:3*.

83. Gwynne, J. T. and Strauss III, J. F. (1982): The role of lipoproteins in steroidogenesis and cholesterol metabolism in steroidogenic glands. Endocrine Rev. *3*:299.

84. Hafez, E. S. E. (1993): Reproduction in Farm Animals, 6th ed. Media, PA, Lea & Febiger.

85. Hallford, D. M., Wettemann, R. P., and Thurman, E. J. (1975): Luteal function in gilts after prostaglandin $F_{2\alpha}$. J. Anim. Sci. *41*:1706.

86. Hansel, W., Alila, H. W., Dowd, J. P., et al. (1987): Control of steroidogenesis in small and large bovine luteal cells. Aust. J. Biol. Sci. *40*:331.

87. Haresign, W., Foxcroft, G. R., and Lamming G. E. (1983): Control of ovulation in farm animals. J. Reprod. Fertil. *69*:383.

88. Head, J. R. and Billingham, R. E. (1986): Concerning the immunology of the uterus. Am. J. Reprod. Immunol. Microbiol. *10*:76.

89. Heap, R. B., Hamon, M. H., and Allen, W. R. (1991): Oestrogen production by the preimplantation donkey conceptus compared with that of the horse and the effect of between-species embryo transfer. J. Reprod. Fertil. *93*:141.

90. Heap, R. B., Perry, J. S., Gadsby, J. E., et al. (1975): Endocrine activities of the blastocyst and early embryonic tissue in the pig. Biochem. Soc. Trans. *3*:1183.

91. Hillier, S. G. (1981): Regulation of follicular oestrogen biosynthesis: A survey of current concepts. J. Endocrinol. *89*:3P.

92. Hsue, A. J. W. and Schaeffer, J. M. (1985): Gonadotropin-releasing hormone as a paracrine hormone and neurotransmitter in extra-pituitary sites. J. Steroid Biochem. *23*:757.

93. Hubbert, W. T., Dennis, S. M., Adams, W. M., et al. (1972): Recommendations for standardizing bovine reproduction terms. Cornell Vet. *62*:216.

94. Huhtaniemi, I. T. and Warren, D. W. (1990): Ontogeny of pituitary-gonadal interactions. Current advances and controversies. Trends Endocrinol. Metab. *1*:356.

95. Hunter, R. H. F. (1980): Differentiation, puberty, and the oestrous cycle. *In:* Physiology and Technology of Reproduction in Female Domestic Animals. New York, NY, Academic Press, Inc., p. 1.

96. Hunter, R. H. F. and Wilmut, I. (1984): Sperm transport in the cow: Peri-ovulatory redistribution of viable cells within the oviduct. Reprod. Nutr. Develop. *24*:597.

97. Hunter, R. H. F. and Nichol, R. (1986): A preovulatory temperature gradient between the isthmus and ampulla of pig oviduct during the phase of sperm storage. J. Reprod. Fertil. *77*:599.

98. Hunter, R. H. F. and Nichol, R. (1988): Capacitation potential of the Fallopian tube: A study involving surgical insemination and the subsequent incidence of polyspermy. Gamete Res. *21*:255.

99. Imakawa, K., Day, M. L., Zalesky, D. D., et al. (1986): Regulation of pulsatile LH secretion by ovarian steroids in the heifer. J. Anim. Sci. *63*:162.

100. Ireland, J. J., Aten, R. F., and Behrman, H. R. (1988): GnRH-like proteins in cows: Concentrations during corpora lutea development and selective localization in granulosal cells. Biol. Reprod. *38*:544.

101. Jenner, L. J., Parkinson, T. J., and Lamming, G. E. (1991): Uterine oxytocin receptors in cyclic and pregnant cows. J. Reprod. Fertil. *91*:49.

102. Jewgenow, K. and Göritz, F. (1993): The recovery of preantral follicles from ovaries of domestic cats and their characterization before and after culture. Anim. Reprod. Sci. *39*:285.

103. Kasman, L. H., Hughes, J. P., Stabenfeldt, G. H., et al. (1988): Estrone sulfate concentrations as an indicator of fetal demise in horses. Am. J. Vet. Res. *49*:184.

104. Katzenellenbogen, B. S. (1996): Estrogen receptors: Bioactivities and interactions with cell signaling pathways. Biol. Reprod. *54*:287.

105. Kenny N., Farin, C. E., and Niswender, G. D. (1989): Morphometric quantification of mitochondria in the two steroidogenic ovine luteal cell types. Biol. Reprod. *40*:191.

106. Knickerbocker, J. J., Thatcher, W. W., Bazer, F. W., et al. (1986): Proteins secreted by day-16 to -18 bovine conceptuses extend corpus luteum function in cows. J. Reprod. Fertil. *77*:381.

107. Kotwica, J., Williams, G.L., and Marchello, M.J. (1982): Countercurrent transfer of testosterone by the ovarian vascular pedicle of the cow: Evidence for a relationship to follicular steroidogenesis. Biol. Reprod. *27*:778.

108. Lacker, H. M., Beers, W. H., Meuli, L. E., et al. (1987): A theory of follicle selection. I. Hypothesis and examples. Biol. Reprod. *37*:570.

109. Lacker, H. M., Beers, W. H., Meuli, L. E., et al. (1987): A theory of follicle selection. II. Computer simulation of estradiol administration in the primate. Biol. Reprod. *37*:581.

110. Leese, H. J. (1988): The formation and function of oviduct fluid. J. Reprod. Fertil. *82*:843.

111. Lemon, M. and Mauléon, P. (1982): Interaction between two luteal cell types from the corpus luteum of the sow in progesterone synthesis *in vitro*. J. Reprod. Fertil. *64*:315.

112. Leung, P. C. K. and Steele, G. L. (1992): Intracellular signaling in the gonads. Endocrine Rev. *13*:476.

113. Levasseur, M.-C. (1983): Utero-ovarian relationships in placental mammals: Role of uterus and embryo in the regulation of progesterone secretion by the corpus luteum: A review. Reprod. Nutr. Develop. *23*:793.

114. Linford, R. L., McCue, P. M., Montavon, S., et al. (1992): Long-term cannulation of the ovarian vein in mares. Am. J. Vet. Res. *53*:1589.

115. Lipner, H. and Cross, N. L. (1968): Morphology of the membrana granulosa of the ovarian follicle. Endocrinology *82*:638.

116. Lipschütz, A. (1928): New developments in ovarian dynamics and the Law of Follicular Constancy. Br. J. Exp. Biol. *5*:283.

117. Luey, M. C., Savio, J. D., Badinga, R., et al. (1992): Factors that affect ovarian follicular dynamics in cattle. J. Anim. Sci. *70*:3615.

118. Manabe, N., Imai, Y., Ohno, H., et al. (1996): Apoptosis occurs in granulosa cells but not cumulus cells in the atretic antral follicles in pig ovaries. Experientia *52*:647.

119. MacLusky, N. J. and Naftolin, F. (1981): Sexual differentiation of the central nervous system. Science *211*:1294.

120. Martin, G. B., Thomas, G. B., Terqui, M., et al. (1987): Pulsatile LH secretion during the preovulatory surge in the ewe: Experimental observations and theoretical considerations. Reprod. Nutr. Develop. *27*:1023.

121. McCracken, J. A. (1984): Update on luteolysis-receptor regulation of pulsatile secretion of prostaglandin $F_{2\alpha}$ from the uterus. Res. Reprod. *16*:1.

122. McDonald, L. E., McNutt, S. H., and Nichols, R. E. (1953): On the essentiality of the bovine corpus luteum of pregnancy. Am. J. Vet. Res. *14*:539.

123. McNatty, K. P., Gibb, M., Dobson, C., et al. (1981): Changes in the concentration of gonadotrophic and steroidal hormones in the antral fluid of ovarian follicles throughout the oestrous cycle of the sheep. Aust. J. Biol. Sci. *34*:80.

124. McNatty, K. P., Heath, D. A., Henderson, K. M., et al. (1984): Some aspects of thecal and granulosa cell function during follicular development in the bovine ovary. J. Reprod. Fertil. *72*:39.

125. McRae, A. C. (1988): The blood-uterine lumen barrier and exchange between extracellular fluids. J. Reprod. Fertil. *82*:857.

126. Moor, R. M. and Rowson, L. E. A. (1966): Local maintenance of the corpus luteum in sheep with embryos transferred to various isolated portions of the uterus. J. Reprod. Fertil. *12*:539.

127. Moor, R. M. and Seamark, R. F. (1986): Cell signaling, permeability, and microvasculatory changes during antral follicle development in mammals. J. Dairy Sci. *69*:927.

128. Moore, L. G. and Watkins, W. B. (1982): Embryonic suppression of oxytocin-associated neurophysin release in early pregnant sheep. Prostaglandins *24*:79.

129. Moran, C., Quircke, J. F., and Roche, J. F. (1989): Puberty in heifers: A review. Anim. Reprod. Sci. *18*:167.

130. Morbeck, D. E., Esbenshade, K. L., Flowers, W. L., et al. (1992): Kinetics of follicle growth in the prepubertal gilt. Biol. Reprod. *47*:485.

131. Mori, Y. and Kano, Y. (1984): Changes in plasma concentrations of LH, progesterone and oestradiol in relation to the occurrence of luteolysis, oestrus and time of ovulation in the Shiba goat. J. Reprod. Fertil. *72*:223.

132. Muñoz, B. and Carrillo, R. (1980): Analysis crítico de la utilización del celo del potro en la yegua F.S. de carrera. Haras y Pistas, Santiago, Chile *15*:58.

133. Murakami, T., Ikebuchi, Y., Ohtsuka, A., et al. (1988): The blood vascular wreath of rat ovarian follicle, with special reference to its changes in ovulation and luteinization: A scanning electron microscopic study of corrosion casts. Arch. Histol. Cytol. *51*:299.

134. Murdoch, W. J. (1985): Follicular determinants of ovulation in the ewe. Domestic Anim. Endocrinol. *2*:105.

135. Murdoch, W. J. (1989): Effect of indomethacin on the vascular architecture of preovulatory ovine follicles: Possible implication in the luteinized unruptured follicle syndrome. Fertil. Steril. *51*:153.

136. Murdoch, W. J. (1995): Endothelial cell death in preovulatory ovine follicles: Possible implication in the biomechanics of rupture. J. Reprod. Fertil. *105*:161.

137. Nakamura, H., Kato, H., and Terranova, P. F. (1990): Interleukin-1α increases thecal progesterone production of preovulatory follicles in cyclic hamsters. Biol. Reprod. *43*:169.

138. Niswender, G. D., Sawyer, H. R., Chen, T. T., et al. (1980): Action of luteinizing hormone at the luteal cell level. Adv. Hormone Res. *4*:153.

139. Niswender, G. D., Schwall, R. H., Fitz, T. A., et al. (1985): Regulation of luteal function in domestic ruminants–New concepts. Recent Prog. Hormone Res. *41*:101.

140. Niswender, G. D., Juengel, J. L., McGuire, W. J., et al. (1994): Luteal function: The estrous cycle and early pregnancy. Biol. Reprod. *50*:239.

141. Northey, D. L. and French, L. R. (1980): Effect of embryo removal and intrauterine infusion of embryonic homogenates on the lifespan of the bovine corpus luteum. J. Anim. Sci. *50*:298.

142. Odend'hal, S., Wenzel, J. G. W., and Player, E. C. (1986): The *rete ovarii* of cattle and deer communicates with the uterine tube. Anat. Rec. *216*:40.

143. Okkens, A. C., Dieleman, S. J., Bevers, M. M., et al. (1986): Influence of hypophysectomy on the lifespan of the corpus luteum in the cyclic dog. J. Reprod. Fertil. *77*:187.

144. Okuda, K., Miyamoto, A., Sauerwein, H., et al. (1992): Evidence for oxytocin receptors in cultured bovine luteal cells. Biol. Reprod. *46*:1001.

145. Olson, P. N., Bowen, R. A., Behrendt, M. D., et al. (1984): Concentrations of testosterone in canine serum during late anestrus, proestrus, estrus, and early diestrus. Am. J. Vet. Res. *45*:145.

146. Olson, P. N., Bowen, R. A., Behrendt, M. D., et al. (1984): Concentrations of progesterone and luteinizing hormone in the serum of diestrous bitches before and after hysterectomy. Am. J. Vet. Res. *45*:149.

147. O'Shea, J. D. (1981): Structure-function relationships in the wall of the ovarian follicle. Aust. J. Biol. Sci. *34*:379.

148. Pant, H. C., Hopkinson, C. R. N., and Fitzpatrick, R. J. (1977): Concentration of oestradiol, progesterone, luteinizing hormone and follicle-stimulating hormone in the jugular venous plasma of ewes during the oestrous cycle. J. Endocrinol. *73*:247.

149. Perkins, S. N., Cronin, M. J., and Veldhuis, J. D. (1986): Properties of β-adrenergic receptors on porcine corpora lutea and granulosa cells. Endocrinology *118*:998.

150. Pierson, R. A. and Ginther, O. J. (1988): Ultrasonic imaging of the ovaries and uterus in cattle. Theriogenology *29*:21.

151. Pope, W. F. (1988): Uterine asynchrony: A cause of embryonic loss. Biol. Reprod. *39*:999.

152. Price, C. A. (1991): The control of FSH secretion in the larger domestic species. J. Endocrinol. *131*:177.

153. Rajakoski, E. (1960): The ovarian follicular system in sexually mature heifers. Acta Endocrinol. *34* (Suppl. 52):1.

154. Re, G., Badino, P., and Novelli, A. (1995): Distribution of cytosolic oestrogen and progesterone receptors in the genital tract of the mare. Res. Vet. Sci. *59*:214.

155. Reimers, T. J., Smith, R. D., and Newman, S. K. (1985): Management factors affecting reproductive performance of dairy cows in the Northeastern United States. J. Dairy Sci. *68*:963.

156. Ricketts, A. P. and Flint, A. P. F. (1980): Onset of synthesis of progesterone by ovine placenta. J. Endocrinol. *86*:337.

157. Rodgers, R. J., O'Shea, J. D., and Findlay, J. K. (1985): Do small and large luteal cells of the sheep interact in the production of progesterone? J. Reprod. Fertil. *75*:85.

158. Romagnoli, S. E., Camillo, F., Novellini, S., et al. (1996): Luteolytic effects of prostaglandin $F_{2\alpha}$ on day 8 to 19 corpora lutea in the bitch. Theriogenology *45*:397.

159. Roser, J. F., McCue, P. M., and Hoye, E. (1994): Inhibin activity in the mare and stallion. Domestic Anim. Endocrinol. *11*:87.

160. Ross, G. T. and Lipsett, M. B. (1978): Homologies of structure and function in mammalian testes and ovaries. Int. J. Androl. (Suppl. 2):39.

161. Rothchild, I. (1981): The regulation of the mammalian corpus luteum. Recent Prog. Hormone Res. *37*:183.

162. Sankai, T., Endo, T., Kanayawa, K., et al. (1991): Antiprogesterone compound, RU486 administration to terminate pregnancy in dogs and cats. Jpn. J. Med. Sci. *53*:1069.

163. Savouret, J. F., Chauchereau, A., Misrahi, M., et al. (1994). The progesterone receptor. Biological effects of progestins and antiprogestins. Human Reprod. *9*:7.

164. Sawyer, H. R., Moeller, C. L., and Kozlowski, G. P. (1986): Immunocytochemical localization of neurophysin and oxytocin in ovine corpora lutea. Biol. Reprod. *34*:543.

165. Schams, D. and Prokopp, S. (1979): Oxytocin determination by RIA in cows around parturition. Anim. Reprod. Sci. *2*:267.

166. Schams, D., Schallenberger, E., Gombe, S., et al. (1981): Endocrine patterns associated with puberty in male and female cattle. J. Reprod. Fertil. (Suppl. 30):103.

167. Schams, D., Schallenberger, E., Menzer, C., et al. (1978): Profiles of LH, FSH and progesterone in postpartum dairy cows and their relationship to the commencement of cyclic functions. Theriogenology *10*:453.

168. Schramm, W., Einer-Jensen, N., and Schramm, G. (1986): Direct venous-arterial transfer of ^{125}I-radiolabelled relaxin and tyrosine in the ovarian pedicle in sheep. J. Reprod. Fertil. *77*:513.

169. Schramm, W., Einer-Jensen, N., Schramm, G., et al. (1986): Local exchange of oxytocin from the ovarian vein to ovarian arteries in sheep. Biol. Reprod. *34*:671.

170. Schultz, R. M. (1985): Roles of cell-to-cell communication in development. Biol. Reprod. *32*:27.

171. Schumacher M., Coirini, H., Pfaff, D. W., et al. (1990): Behavioral effects of progesterone associated with rapid modulation of oxytocin receptors. Science *250*:691.

172. Schwall, R. H., Gamboni, F., Mayan, M. H., et al. (1986): Changes in the distribution of sizes of ovine luteal cells during the estrous cycle. Biol. Reprod. *34*:911.

173. Schwall, R. H., Sawyer, H. R., and Niswender, G. D. (1986): Differential regulation by LH and prostaglan-

dins of steroidogenesis in small and large luteal cells of the ewe. J. Reprod. Fertil. *76*:821.

174. Sharpe, R. M. (1982): Cellular aspects of the inhibitory actions of LH-RH on the ovary and testis. J. Reprod. Fertil. *64*:517.

175. Sheldrick, E. L., Mitchell, M. D., and Flint, A. P. F. (1980): Delayed luteal regression in ewes immunized against oxytocin. J. Reprod. Fertil. *59*:37.

176. Siiteri, P. K., Febres, F., Clemens, L. E., et al. (1977): Progesterone and maintenance of pregnancy: Is progesterone nature's immunosuppressant? Ann. N. Y. Acad. Sci. *286*:384.

177. Siiteri, R. K. and Stites, D. P. (1982): Immunologic and endocrine interrelationships in pregnancy. Biol. Reprod. *26*:1.

178. Sirois, J., Kimmich, T. L., and Fortune, J. E. (1990): Developmental changes in steroidogenesis by equine preovulatory follicles: Effects of equine LH, FSH, and CG. Endocrinology *127*:2423.

179. Smith, J. F. (1988): Influence of nutrition on ovulation rate in the ewe. Aust. J. Biol. Sci. *41*:27.

180. Smith, M. S. and McDonald, L. E. (1974): Serum levels of LH and progesterone during the estrous cycle, pseudopregnancy and pregnancy in the dog. Endocrinology *94*:404.

181. Sokolowski, J. H., Zimbelman, R. G., and Goyings, L. S. (1973): Canine reproduction: Reproductive organs and related structures of the nonparous, parous, and postpartum bitch. Am. J. Vet. Res. *34*:1001.

182. Spicer, L. J. and Echternkamp, S. E. (1986): Ovarian follicular growth, function and turnover in cattle: A review. J. Anim. Sci. *62*:428.

183. Squires, E. L., Hillman, R. B., Pickett, B. W., et al. (1980): Induction of abortion in mares with Equimate: Effect on secretion of progesterone, PMSG and reproductive performance. J. Anim. Sci. *50*:490.

184. Stabenfeldt, G. H. (1974): Physiologic, pathologic and therapeutic roles of progestins in domestic animals. J. Am. Vet. Med. Assoc. *164*:311.

185. Stabenfeldt, G. H., Hughes, J. P., and Evans, J. W. (1972): Ovarian activity during the estrous cycle of the mare. Endocrinology *90*:1379.

186. Stock, A. E., Emeny, R. T., Sirois, J., et al. (1995): Oxytocin in mares: Lack of evidence for oxytocin production by or action on preovulatory follicles. Domestic Anim. Endocrinol. *12*:133.

187. Stormshak, F., Kelley, H. E., and Hawk, H. W. (1969): Suppression of ovine luteal function by 17β-estradiol. J. Anim. Sci. *29*:476.

188. Sumar, J. and Bravo, P. W. (1991): *In situ* observation of the ovaries of llamas and alpacas by use of a laparoscopic technique. J. Am. Vet. Med. Assoc. *199*:1159.

189. Szego, C. M. (1984): Mechanisms of hormone action: Parallels in receptor-mediated signal propagation for steroid and peptide effectors. Life Sci. *35*:2383.

190. Takahashi, S., Hayashi, M., Manganaro, T. F., et al. (1986): The ontogeny of Müllerian-inhibiting substance in granulosa cells of the bovine ovarian follicle. Biol. Reprod. *35*:447.

191. Taymor, M. L. (1996): The regulation of follicle growth: Some clinical implications in reproductive endocrinology. Fertil. Steril. *65*:235.

192. Telfer, E. and Gosden, R. G. (1987): A quantitative cytological study of polyovular follicles in mam-

malian ovaries with particular reference to the domestic bitch (*Canis familiaris*). J. Reprod. Fertil. *81*:137.

193. Tesoriero, J. V. (1984): Comparative cytochemistry of the developing ovarian follicles of the dog, rabbit, and mouse: Origin of the zona pellucida. Gamete Res. *10*:301.

194. Thatcher, W. W., Bartol, F. F., Knickerbocker, J. J., et al. (1984): Maternal recognition of pregnancy in cattle. J. Dairy Sci. *67*:2797.

195. Thibault, C., Courot, M., Martinet, L., et al. (1966): Regulation of breeding season and estrous cycles by light and external stimuli in some mammals. J. Anim. Sci. *25*:119.

196. Tilly, J. L. (1996): Apoptosis and ovarian function. Rev. Reprod. *1*:162.

197. Twagiramungu, H., Guilbault, L. A., and Dufour, J. J. (1995): Synchronization of ovarian follicular waves with a gonadotropin-releasing hormone agonist to increase the precision of estrus in cattle: A review. J. Anim. Sci. *73*:3141.

198. Tyslowitz, R. and Dingemanse, E. (1941): Effect of large doses of estrogen on blood picture of dogs. Endocrinology *29*:817.

199. Ueno, S., Kuroda, T., MacLaughlin, D. T., et al. (1989): Müllerian-inhibiting substance in the adult rat ovary during various stages of the estrous cycle. Endocrinology *111*:1562.

200. Umansky, S. R. (1996): Apoptosis: Molecular and cellular mechanisms (a review). Mol. Biol. *30*:285.

201. Van de Wiel, D. F. M., Bar-Ami, S., Tsafriri, A., et al. (1983): Oocyte maturation inhibitor, inhibin and steroid concentrations in porcine follicular fluid at various stages of the estrous cycle. J. Reprod. Fertil. *68*:247.

202. Van den Hurk, R., Bevers, M. M., and Beckers, J. F. (1997): *In-vivo* and *in-vitro* development of preantral follicles. Theriogenology *47*:73.

203. Varsano, J. S., Izhar, M., Perk, K., et al. (1990): Effect of β-endorphin on steroidogenesis by bovine luteal cells. Reprod. Fertil. Develop. *2*:237.

204. Vaux, D. L. and Strasser, A. (1996): The molecular biology of apoptosis. Proc. Nat. Acad. Sci., USA *93*:2239.

205. Voss, A. K. and Fortune, J. E. (1992): Oxytocin/-Neurophysin-I messenger ribonucleic acid in bovine granulosa cells increases after the luteinizing hormone (LH) surge and is stimulated by LH *in vitro*. Endocrinology *131*:2755.

206. Walles, B., Edvinsson, L., Owman, C., et al. (1976): Cholinergic nerves and receptors mediating contraction of the Graafian follicle. Biol. Reprod. *15*:565.

207. Wathes, D. C. (1984): Possible actions of gonadal oxytocin and vasopression. J. Reprod. Fertil. *71*:315.

208. Wathes, D. C. and Hamon, M. (1993): Localization of oestradiol, progesterone and oxytocin receptors in the uterus during the oestrous cycle and early pregnancy of the ewe. J. Endocrinol. *138*:479.

209. Wathes, D. C., Kendall, P. A. D., Perks, C., et al. (1992): Effects of stage of the cycle and estradiol-17β on oxytocin synthesis by ovine granulosa and luteal cells. Endocrinology *130*:1009.

210. Wathes, D. C., Smith, H. F., Leung, S. T., et al. (1996): Oxytocin receptor development in ovine uterus and cervix throughout pregnancy and parturition as determined by *in situ* hybridization analysis. J. Reprod. Fertil. *106*:23.

211. Wathes, D. C., Swan, R. W., and Pickering, B. T. (1984): Variations in oxytocin, vasopressin and neurophysin concentrations in the bovine ovary during the oestrous cycle and pregnancy. J. Reprod. Fertil. *71*:551.

212. Weems, C. W., Weems, Y. S., Lee, C. N., et al. (1989): Progesterone in uterine and arterial tissue and in jugular and uterine venous plasma of sheep. Biol. Reprod. *41*:1.

213. Wei, L. L. and Horwitz, K. B. (1985): The structure of progesterone receptors. Steroids *46*:677.

214. Wenzel, J. G. W. and Odend'hal, S. (1985): The mammalian *rete ovarii:* A literature review. Cornell Vet. *75*:411.

215. Wenzel, J. G. W., Odend'hal, S., and Player, E. C. (1987): Histological and histochemical characterization of the bovine *rete ovarii* through the estrous cycle and gestation. Anat. Histol. Embryol. *16*:124.

216. Wheeler, A. G., Walker, M., and Lean, J. (1987): Influence of adrenergic receptors on ovarian progesterone secretion in the pseudopregnant cat and oestradiol secretion in the oestrus cat. J. Reprod. Fertil. *79*:195.

217. Wiltbank, J. N., Kasson, C. W., and Ingalls, J. E., (1969): Puberty in crossbred and straightbred beef heifers on two levels of feed. J. Anim. Sci. *29*:602.

218. Wiltbank, M. C. and Niswender, G. D. (1992): Functional aspects of differentiation and degeneration of the steroidogenic cells of the corpus luteum in domestic ruminants. Anim. Reprod. Sci. *28*:103.

219. Wolfenson, D., Thatcher, W. W., Drost, M., et al. (1985): Characteristics of prostaglandin F measurements in the ovarian circulation during the oestrous cycle and early pregnancy in the cow. J. Reprod. Fertil. *75*:491.

220. Wolff, L. K. and DeMonty, D. E., Jr. (1974): Physiologic response to intense Summer heat and its effect on the estrous cycle of nonlactating and lactating Holstein-Friesian cows in Arizona. Am. J. Vet. Res. *35*:187.

221. Wolgemuth, D. J., Celenza, J., Bundman, D. S., et al. (1984): Formation of the rabbit zona pellucida and its relationship to ovarian follicular development. Develop. Biol. *106*:1.

222. Woods, G. L. and Ginther, O. J. (1983): Intrauterine embryo reduction in the mare. Theriogenology *20*:699.

References Added in Proof

223. Adams, G. P. (1999): Comparative patterns of follicle development and selection in ruminants. J. Reprod. Fertil. (Suppl. 54):17.

224. Almeida, F., R., C., L., Novak, S. and Foxcroft, G. R. (2000): The time of ovulation in relation to estrus duration in gilts. Theriogenology *53*:1389.

225. Asselin, E., Xiao, C. W., Wang, Y. F., et al. (2000): Mammalian follicular development and atresia: Role of apoptosis. Biol. Signals Receptors *9*:87.

226. Cunningham, M. J., Clifton, D. K., and Steiner, R. A. (1999): Leptin's actions on the reproductive axis: Perspectives and mechanisms. Biol. Reprod. *60*:216.

227. D'Occhio, M. J., Fordyce, G., Whyte, T. R., et al. (2000): Reproductive responses of cattle to GnRH agonists. Anim. Reprod. Sci. *2*:433.

228. Ireland, J. J., Mihm, M., Austin, E. et al. (2000): Historical perspective of turnover of dominant follicles during the bovine estrous cycle: Key concepts, studies, advancements, and terms. J. Dairy Sci. *83*:1648.

229. Keisler, D. H., Daniel, J. A., and Morrison, C. D. (1999): The role of leptin in nutritional status and reproductive function. J. Reprod. Fertil. (Suppl. 54):425.

230. Lackey, B. R., Gray, S. L., and Henricks, D. M. (1999): The insulin-like growth factor (IGF) system and gonadotropin regulation: Actions and interactions. Cytokine Growth Factor Rev. *10*:201.

231. Lucy, M. C. (2000): Regulation of ovarian follicular growth by somatotropin and insulin-like growth factors in cattle. J. Dairy Sci. *83*:1635.

232. Mather, J. P., Moore, A., and Li, R-H. (1997): Activins, inhibins, and follistatins: Further thoughts on a growing family of regulators. Proc. Soc. Exp. Biol. Med. *215*:209.

233. Peng, C. and Mukai, S. T. (2000): Activins and their receptors in female reproduction. Biochem. Cell Biol. *78*:261.

234. Sutovsky, P., Moreno, R. D., Ramalho-Santos, J. et al. (2000): Ubiquitinated sperm mitochondria, selective proteolysis, and the regulation of mitochondrial inheritance in mammalian embryos. Biol. Reprod. *63*:582.

235. Wood, R. I. and Foster, D. L. (1998): Sexual differentiation of reproductive neuroendocrine function in sheep. Rev. Reprod. *3*:130.

Artificial Insemination

S. M. Hopkins and L. E. Evans

10

INTRODUCTION

Artificial insemination (AI) in the broadest sense is the use of a technological process involving semen collection for the obtainment, pro- cessing, and deposition of male gametes in the female genitals to fertilize the oocyte(s), thereby bypassing semen deposition by natural mating. Typically, one component of the process involves the insemination of the female, or cultured oocyte(s) with freshly ejaculated, extended or frozen-thawed semen. The other element of AI programs encompasses the examination of the male for normal structural development, ejaculation capability, and analysis of seminal samples for quality and as well as for processing the ejaculate for short or long term storage. Together the two components can provide for the collection and transfer of acceptable numbers of normal spermatozoa to ensure fertilization of the oocyte.

In vitro fertilization and insertion of spermatozoa into the oocyte remain in the developmental/ research stage and have only limited domestic animal application. Due to the highly specialized nature of the processes, this type of assisted reproductive technology is beyond the scope of this chapter.

The driving force behind commercial AI is to disseminate superior genes with genetic merit into the population at an affordable cost. The important genetic traits, depending on the species, include the rate of muscle production, milking gains, athletic performance, and correct conformation.

The cattle industry relies extensively on the use of frozen semen, whereas the other domestic species are more commonly inseminated with fresh or cooled, extended semen. This is due to economic and technical constraints to the widespread use of cryopreserved semen. First, the use of frozen semen significantly decreases fertilization rates and/or is difficult to perform when compared to the results of AI with non-frozen semen. Secondly, the resultant offspring may not command a price which makes research for the improvement of the technology economically important to the industry. An example would be the canine breeds which can be inseminated with either nonfrozen or frozen semen. The economic return to those involved with collection, processing, and distribution of the frozen canine semen generally has been insufficient to support significant research and protocol development to increase pregnancy rates. Additionally, the conception rates with the available technology are erratic, further limiting economic return.

One of the potential limitations for AI in any species involves the identification of genetic merit. The dairy and swine industries collect data on progeny production which is used to predict genetic potential. Since these indices are based on large numbers of production records rather than pedigree or body type, they can identify true genetic merit. Unless the industries dealing with the other species develop comparable means of identifying individuals of superior genetics, there is no reasonable assurance that their offspring will perform above average. This also includes identifying potentially lethal or defective genes before they are seeded into the population.

There is the potential for advancement to be made within the AI industries in all species. There must, however, be sufficient funding, guidelines, and controls to make the venture economically feasible and genetically sound.

DISEASE CONTROL THROUGH ARTIFICIAL INSEMINATION (AI)

Artificial insemination when done properly, reduces or eliminates the spread of diseases between breeding animals. This protection encompasses not only the venereal and reproductive diseases which are transmittable through mating, but other pathogens spread via contact. These include a wide variety of protozoal, viral, and bacterial organisms, which could be parasitic and pathogenic.

The cattle industry had established guidelines to minimize the transfer of significant pathogens through AI. These guidelines take three approaches:

1. identification of specific pathogen-free males,
2. sanitary collection procedures, and
3. the treatment of semen with antibiotics.

The National Association of Animal Breeders (NAAB) established governing rules for member organizations for the isolation and testing of bulls in order to provide assurance that the semen is free from specific viral, bacterial, and protozoal organisms. The tests currently performed are brucellosis, campylobacteriosis, leptospirosis, trichomoniasis, tuberculosis, and for the detection of bovine virus diarrhea. Preparing semen for export, however, frequently requires that the bull undergoes additional tests which have been established by the regulatory agencies of the particular country. Unfortunately, there is not a standard series of tests applicable to all countries.

Antibiotics are added first to the freshly collected ejaculates as a safeguard against some diseases borne by bull semen. The combination of antibiotics such as gentamicin, tylosin, lincomycin, and spectinomycin have been tested for efficacy against campylobacteriosis, ureaplasmosis, *Hemophilus somnus,* and mycoplasmosis. Dilution of the semen during the process of extension provides additional nonspecific protection against disease transmission. Dilution may lower the number of pathogenic organisms to a level below that required for host infection.

In the cattle industry, the use of disease testing, addition of antibiotics, and proper hygiene during collection and processing of the semen have made the likelihood of pathogen transmission from semen extremely remote.

There are no definite testing requirements established for AI in the other domestic species, although many organizations routinely add antibiotics to the semen in a similar fashion as done for the cattle industry. There has been a lack of adequate information in these species regarding the efficacy of adding antibiotics to semen to prevent the spread of disease. Also, the direct effect of the antibiotics on spermatozoal viability have largely been empirical.

SEMEN COLLECTION

The collection of semen from domestic animals typically employs the use of an **artificial vagina** (AV), **electroejaculation** (EE), or **digital manipulation** (DM).

Artificial Vagina

Each species requires its own type of AV; however, the basic construction, preparation, and usage have many common traits (Figs. 10-1, 10-2, and 10-3). The temperature of the interior of the AV is maintained by placing warm water between an interior liner and outer casing. The inner liners are generally made of latex and have a smooth to coarse texture depending on the species from which the semen is to be collected and the individual male's preference. The outer casing can be either rigid or soft. Water at the appropriate temperature is placed into the AV through a valve, then air is added to create the proper level of pressure.

The AV is lubricated with sterile jelly to permit atraumatic intromission of the penis into the AV. The collection end of the AV has a director cone to which the semen collection vial is attached. Depending on ambient conditions, the collection vial is frequently protected with a water jacket and/or insulating cover to prevent temperature shock to the spermatozoa.

Electroejaculation

There are different types of commercially available electroejaculators with automatic and/or manual electrical controls and rectal probes designed for the individual species (Figs. 10-4 and 10-5). The power supply to the control units may be generated by either alternating (AC) or direct (DC) current sources.

Digital Manipulation (DM)

Digital manipulation is the procedure of choice for collection of semen from the boar or dog and in general, involves imitation of the pressure exerted by the female cervical or vaginal components on the penis. Erection and extension of the penis of the boar is typically obtained by teasing the male with an estrous, or with a nonestrous, but restrained female. Frequently boars can be trained to mount and ejaculate on a padded "dummy" sow. Dogs may need teasing bitches but some dogs will ejaculate without the presence of a female.

If performed properly, the typical ejaculatory pattern that would occur during natural mating will also take place under digital manipulation.

COLLECTION TECHNIQUES

Bovine

From a practical standpoint and based on predictability of response, collection of semen from bulls is performed by EE or the use of an AV. Digital massage of the accessory glands through the rectum produces erratic responses, semen of variable quality, and is infrequently employed.

Electroejaculation is widely used for performing breeding soundness examinations and evaluation of breeding health under field conditions. An AV, however, is preferred for semen collection where the ejaculate is to be processed and frozen for use in AI.

The characteristics of bull semen collected by EE differ from those of semen collected with the AV. EE usually produces samples of greater volume, higher pH, and lower concentrations of spermatozoa and fructose per ml of semen. The characteristics of the three fractions of bull semen collected by EE or AV are shown in Table 10-1. Electroejaculation stimulates the release of additional accessory gland fluids along with the sperm-rich fraction, while semen collected with a standard AV protocol is more concentrated. Occasionally, semen for AI with frozen semen is collected by EE from superior bulls which are physically unable to mount and ejaculate in the AV.

Collection of semen by electroejaculation requires a minimum of practice and is simple to perform. Most commercially available ejaculators are suitable for EE of bulls (Fig. 10-4). Newer electroejaculation units are computer controlled and can be programmed to regulate the rate of stimulus application, 'steps' of increasing voltage, and number of stimuli applied. There are differences in the size of rectal probes, number of electrodes, and electrode orientation. A probe with three ventrally located

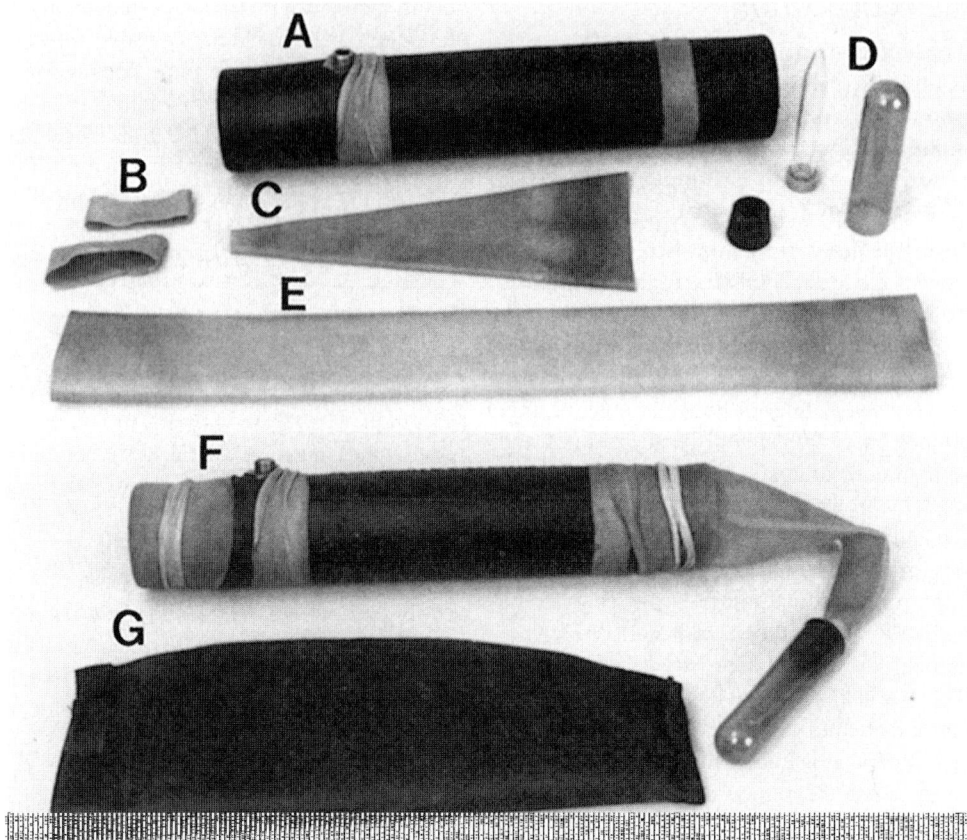

Fig. 10-1. Unassembled and assembled bovine artificial vagina (AV) and insulating cover. **A.** Molded, rubber casing. **B.** Rubber bands used to attach coarse liner (**E**) and directing cone (**C**) to the casing. **D.** Sterile test tube and insulating water jacket. **F.** Assembled AV. **G.** Insulating cover.

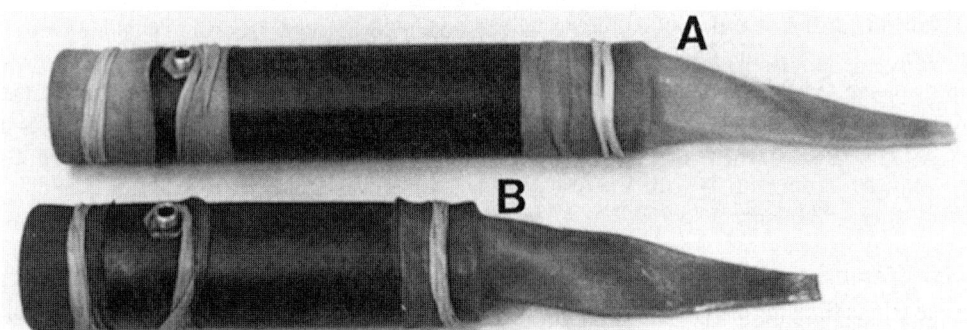

Fig. 10-2. Assembled: **A,** standard-length bovine AV and **B,** shortened AV.

electrodes, is considered superior to a four electrode model (Fig. 10-5) because of the focused stimulation of the reproductive tract, less muscular rigidity, and a firmer foot placement.

Procedures for the collection of semen by electroejaculation may vary somewhat between bulls due to their temperament and physical condition. Usually the bull is restrained in a chute

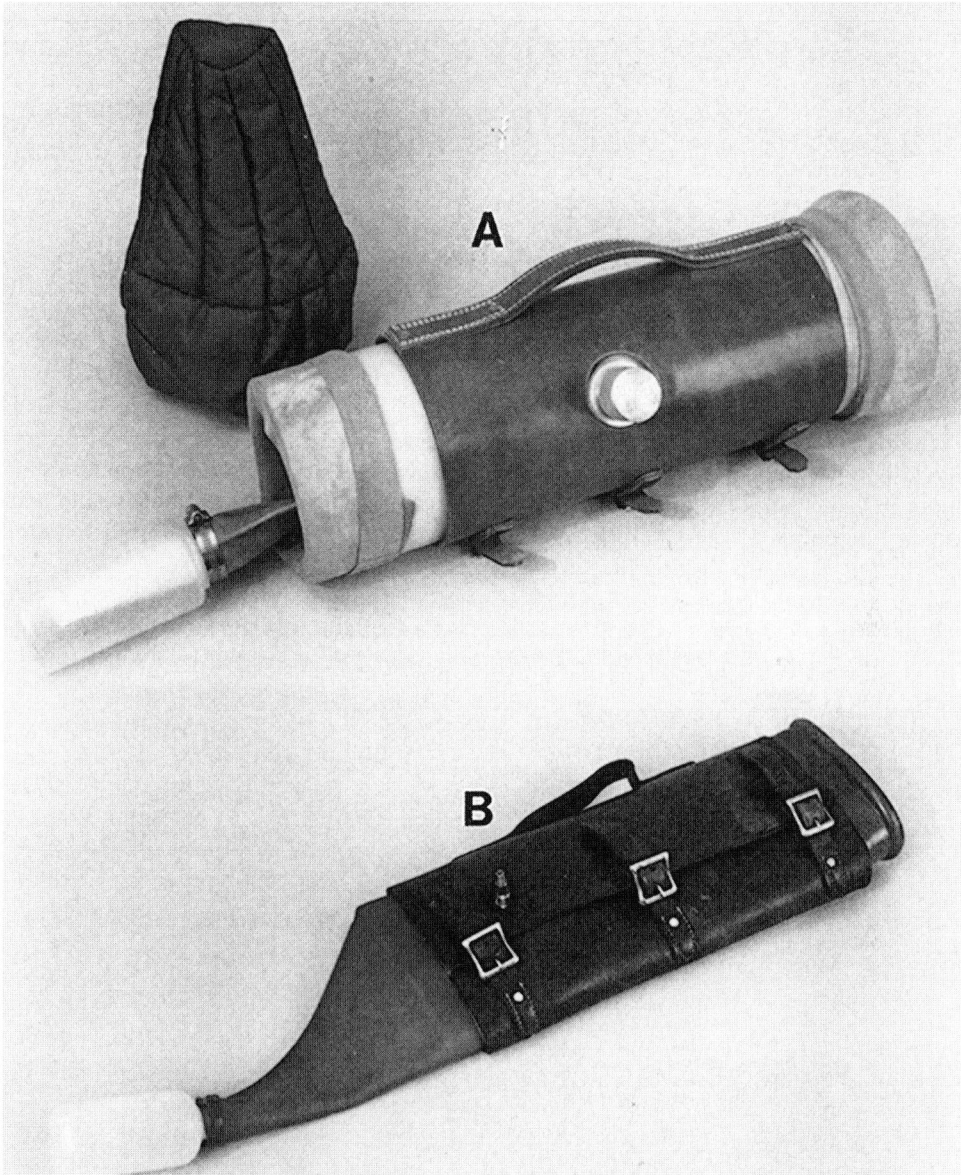

Fig. 10-3. Assembled: **A,** rigid equine AV and **B,** molded rubber equine AV.

capable of handling these powerful animals. The animal should then be identified by tattoo, metal ear tag, or brand if possible. The probe is then lubricated, inserted into the evacuated rectum and an assistant holds the yoke to prevent the bull from expelling the probe.

The person who gives the electrical stimulation to the bull may also collect the ejaculate in a sterile container that maintains the semen at 30 to 35°C.

A regimen of stimulation[39] used to collect semen from bulls with an electroejaculation unit that incorporates a power control knob with "fixed" voltage steps and a rheostat to provide variable voltages from 0 to the maximum of each step is as follows:

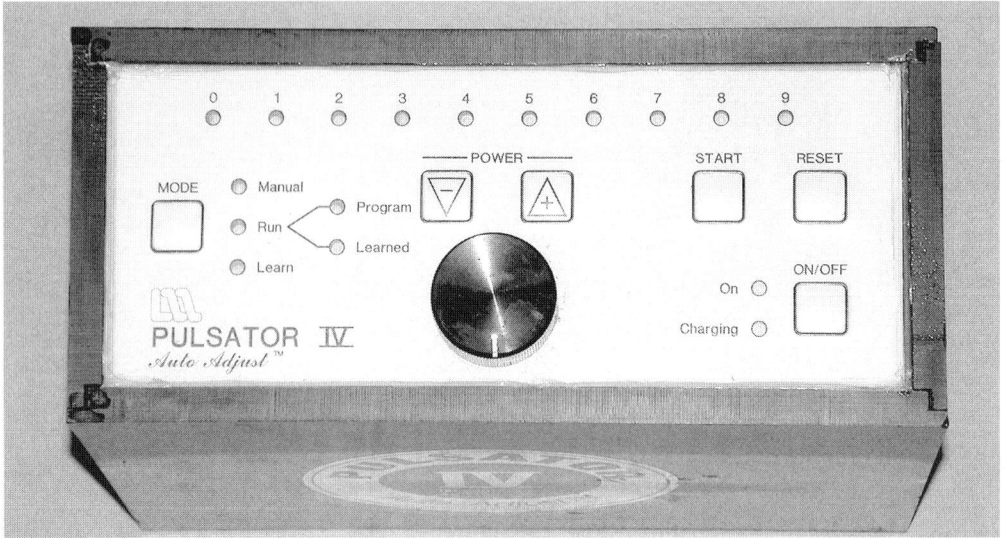

Fig 10-4. Commercial electroejaculator for use in farm animals (Pulsator IV, Lane Manufacturing Inc., Denver, CO). The electroejaculation unit can be operated with alternating (AC) or direct (DC) current sources. To collected semen, the operator selects to manually control the application of electrical stimuli via the large circular knob on the front of the unit or using the automatic (programmable) mode of operation.

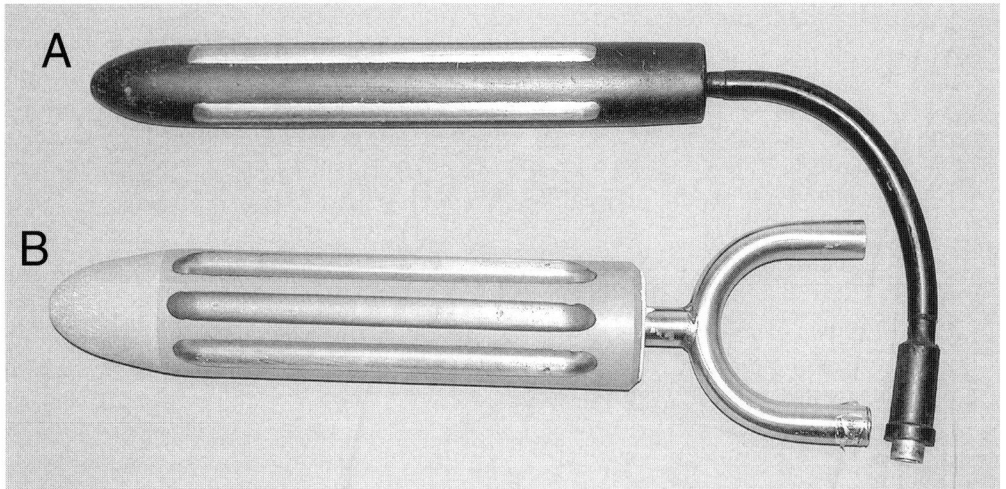

Fig. 10-5. Bovine rectal probes. **A.** Four-electrode model, only two electrodes are depicted. **B.** Three-electrode model.

1. Set the fixed voltage knob on the electroejaculation unit to 10 volts.

2. Initiate electrical stimulation using the rheostat to smoothly apply a 1 to 2 volt electrical stimulus (approximately 20% of the power range) for 2 to 3 seconds,

3. return the rheostat smoothly back to 0 volts for a rest interval of 1 to 2 seconds,

4. repeat this process at 2 volt-increments (40, 60, and 80% of the 10 volt setting) until the maximum of 10 volts (100%) is reached.

5. Then, quickly switch the fixed voltage knob to 15 volts and

6. continue to apply electrical stimulation by providing a 0 to 3 volt (20%) stimulation, followed by another rest interval of 1 to 2 seconds.

Table 10-1   Characteristics of Three Fractions of Bull Semen Collected with an Artificial Vagina (AV) or by Electroejaculation (EE)

Parameter	Presperm		Sperm-rich		Postsperm	
	AV	EE	AV	EE	AV	EE
Sperm count (millions/ml)	4 ± 2	8 ± 4	$1{,}062 \pm 124$	572 ± 80	19 ± 8	132 ± 85
No. samples	18	9	16	9	5	9
Fructose (mg/dl)	3 ± 2	76 ± 38	602 ± 50	444 ± 77	139 ± 64	503 ± 85
No. samples	18	9	16	9	5	9
Nitrogen (μg/ml)	11 ± 3	27 ± 6	59 ± 13	48 ± 10	38 ± 13	49 ± 11
No. samples	18	9	15	9	4	9
Free amino acids (mg/dl)	17.4 ± 6.9	27.2 ± 8.5	86.0 ± 11.1	67.6 ± 13.3	47.6 ± 7.0	50.4 ± 13.1
No. samples	14	9	12	9	4	9
pH	7.45 ± 0.1	7.97 ± 0.5	6.73 ± 0.09	7.30 ± 0.11	7.80 ± 0.05	7.63 ± 0.16
No. of samples	18	9	16	9	5	9

Data are presented as mean $\pm$ SD.
Adapted from: L. C. Faulkner, et al., J. Dairy Sci. *47*:824, 1964.

7. The pattern of stimulation continues at 3 volt increments (6V, 9V, and 12V) to finally reach the maximum setting of 15 volts. The process of dividing each fixed voltage setting into 20% 'substeps' of the maximal voltage continues until ejaculation occurs or the maximal voltage is reached. If ejaculation does not occur by the time the maximal voltage is given, the bull may not be suitable for collection of semen by EE. In some cases, for bulls producing oligo- or azoospermic electroejaculates, the procedure is repeated after a 10 to 15 minute period of rest.

The penis of the normal bull erects and extends past the preputial orifice during the initial (lower voltage) electrical stimulations. This allows the collection of an ejaculate with minimal contamination. If the bull fails to protrude his penis, extension may be assisted by pushing and straightening the distal sigmoid flexure. There are organic diseases, however, such as traumatic adhesions, corpus cavernosus shunts, and other anatomic defects which may prevent extension of the penis.

To prevent cold shock, the ejaculate should be maintained at 30 to 35°C in an isothermal, insulated container during the seminal collection and evaluation process. Specific criteria for semen analysis will be discussed later in this chapter.

Collection of semen by an AV requires a tractable animal and more extensive facilities for handling both the bull and mount steer.

The AV should be selected for proper length. It is necessary for the bull to ejaculate while the tip of the penis is within the directing cone rather than on the liner. The higher temperature of the liner can be lethal to spermatozoa. Conversely, if the casing is too short, the bull's penis may dislodge the collection vial resulting in loss of the ejaculate. A standard bovine casing suitable for mature animals is 41 cm $\times$ 7.5 cm in length and width, respectively (Fig. 10-1). The collection of semen with an AV from younger bulls should be done with an AV made from a casing and liners which have been shortened ($^1/_2$ to $^2/_3$ of the length for mature bulls as shown in Fig. 10-2). To prepare the AV, the space between the liner (see Fig. 10-1E) and the rigid rubber casing (see Fig. 10-1A) is partially filled with warm water to ensure a temperature of 42 to 46°C at the time of semen collection. Time elapsed from filling the AV to semen collection and the ambient temperature conditions determine the temperature of the water used to fill the AV. The first 10 to 15 cm of the AV is lubricated with a nonspermicidal lubricant and the fluid reservoir between the outer casing and the liner is pressurized with air introduced through a valve in the outer casing. Air is used to establish the correct amount of pressure on the bull's penis during "intromission" with the AV. An insulated cover (see Fig. 10-1G) is commonly placed over the directing cone, sterile test tube, and water jacket in order to prevent sudden changes in temperature (thermal shock) of semen following collection. Thermal shock irreparably damages or kills the spermatozoa.

The bull must be prepared by "teasing" before the actual collection takes place in order to maximize ejaculate output (volume and concentration of the sperm-rich fraction). This includes psychic stimulation by walking the bull to be collected past other bulls or restraining the male in close proximity to another bull. In addition, the bull is allowed to mount 1 to 3 times before the semen is collected. When the bull is firmly on the mount steer, the penis is deviated as the bull thrusts. During these initial thrusts made by the bull, no attempt is made to collect the seminal fluid that is ejected. This procedure increases the spermatozoal concentration in the ejaculate collected within the AV, and is used because oligospermic ejaculates produce too few units of processed semen to warrant their use for commercial production.

Once the bull has eliminated seminal fluid during these false mounts, the bull is then allowed to mount the steer, the penis is again deviated and directed into the AV. If the pressure, temperature, and consistency of the liner are correct, the bull will lunge, complete intromisssion, and ejaculate within a few seconds.

If additional ejaculates are desired, the bull should be rested for a minimum of 10 to 15 minutes and the process repeated with a new AV. The AV is changed at each collection to prevent contamination of the ejaculate by bacteria, debris, and dead cells.

Equine

Semen is routinely obtained from the stallion with an AV for semen evaluation, for breeding soundness examination, and for AI with fresh-extended, chilled or frozen semen. Stallions do not tolerate electroejaculation and condoms have been used in the past and are still available, but are rarely used in clinical situations.

There are two styles of equine AVs available but the collection responses are similar so the model to be used is based on the collector's personal preference.

One type of AV consists of a rigid outer casing while the other type has two layers of soft rubber with a small leather harness for carrying support (Fig. 10-3). The rigid AV use rubber or disposable liners and collecting cones, whereas the cone is an integral component of the soft AV. The rigid models are assembled as for the bovine AV in that the rubber liner and cones are secured to the exterior casing, then the AV is filled with water, lubricated, and air is added to achieve the proper pressure. The recommended water temperature at the time of collection of semen for the 2 models is between 45° to 50°C. Water and lubricant are placed in the soft AV. Then, the leather carrying harness is attached and air is added to achieve the proper pressure.

Sterile plastic bottles can be used to collect the ejaculate with or without an integral filter which removes the gel fraction of the ejaculate. An insulating cover is placed over the cone and bottle to control thermal changes in the ejaculate.

A mount mare, or a mounting phantom to which the stallion is conditioned to mount, is generally needed for the collection of semen with AV. The phantom is a padded horizontal tube on which the stallion is trained. The training process requires variable periods of training and can be a time-consuming effort, but is useful when frequent collections of stallion semen are anticipated or required. The mount mare should be very passive or in estrus in order to provide a controllable animal, willing to stand to be mounted by the stallion. The mare is prepared by clipping or wrapping the tail for sanitation and to prevent penile abrasions during seminal collection. This is followed by thoroughly washing, rinsing, and drying of the perineal area. After preparation, the mare is restrained while the stallion is allowed to "tease" her. Teasing allows additional evaluation of the mount mare's response to a particular stallion and generally produces a favorable response in the male resulting in a greater volume of ejaculate and increased sperm output. During teasing, most stallions undergo erection and extension of the penis. After the stallion has been stimulated, he may be backed away from the mare and the erect penis washed. Washing involves grasping the penis behind the glans and gently cleaning the distal half of the penis with wet cotton pledgets. The smegma from the preputial diverticulum is also removed and the penis rinsed liberally with clean water. Washing the penis of the stallion requires a period of training and should always be approached cautiously.

The actual seminal collection involves moving the mare to an open area and restraining her. In addition, a foreleg may be held up to hinder kicking. After the stallion mounts, the foreleg is dropped so that the mare can support herself and the male.

Once the mare is appropriately restrained, the stallion is allowed to approach the mare from the rear and slightly toward her left side. The semen collector follows the stallion handler as the stallion approaches the mare. After the stallion mounts, the collector deviates the penis towards the AV by grasping the shaft of the penis rather than the sensitive glans.

As the stallion moves further onto the mare, the penis is guided into the AV and the stallion will begin thrusting motions in order to complete intromission. At ejaculation, "flagging," an up and down motion of the stallion's tail generally occurs. This motion ceases after ejaculation and the stallion begins to dismount. The head of the mare is turned partially toward the stallion as he dismounts, so that the mare's hindquarters are turned away from the stallion in order to prevent injury if the mare should kick.

Ovine

Semen is collected from rams by EE or with an AV, depending on their previous training. Rams can readily be taught to service an AV while mounting a ewe. Electrojaculation is more commonly employed in clinical practice because it is easier to obtain semen by EE from rams untrained to ejaculate in an AV. To collect semen by EE, a three-electrode rectal probe is inserted into the rectum of the ram and semen is collected as in the bull.

To electroejaculate a ram, two different approaches may be considered. One approach allows the ram to remain standing within a crate with removable boards designed to limit forward, backward, and lateral movements of the ram. A variation of this approach is to have the ram standing behind a gate, restrained by an assistant. Should the ram fail to expose or extend the penis, ejaculation within the preputial sheath may result. Extension failure with ejaculation produces a sample of low volume which is heavily contaminated with bacteria, preputial epithelial cells, and debris.

A second method is the lateral recumbency approach. This allows easy exteriorization of the penis but requires more physical restraint by assistants. Basically, the ram is cast so that he is sitting on his haunches with his shoulders held between the standing holder's knees. The increased abdominal pressure helps the operator to gently exteriorize the penis by retracting the prepuce. Once the tip of the penis is exposed, it is grasped with a piece of gauze and the ram is then moved to lateral recumbency. Next, the probe is inserted into the rectum and stimulation applied. The operator holding the penis collects the semen into a suitable warm sterile container. Rams generally electroejaculate using stimuli ranging from 0V to a maximum of 6V. These voltages are lower than those needed to collect semen from a bull. For additional details on the methodology and EE protocol for the collection of semen from rams see references 39, 59, and 68 at the end of this Chapter.

To collect semen with an AV, the ewe is placed in a stanchion, which consists of a head catch and side restraining bars. The mount ewe need not be in estrus for collection of semen from a trained ram. The ram will respond to an immobile ewe, whether due to restraint or standing estrus. The ram is allowed to approach from the rear with minimal handling and mount the female. The AV is similar in design to that used on bulls except that it is of smaller diameter (5.5 cm) and shorter (20 cm). Some models have an attachment for a rubber bulb for the addition of air in order to obtain the correct pressure. Generally, the temperature of the AV liner should be between 40° and 45°C. The collection procedure used in the ram is similar to that described for the bull.

Caprine

Collection of semen from a buck by EE is primarily used for semen evaluation, whereas semen for AI is generally obtained with an AV.

Electroejaculation requires that the buck be restrained and the rectum emptied of contents by gentle lavage using warm water. The procedure may be performed standing or in lateral recumbency; however, both techniques require adequate restraint due to movement and extreme vocalization.

The electroejaculation method used for bucks is comparable to procedures used for rams. To collect semen, the probe is placed into the rectum with the three electrodes directed ventrally and the buck is stimulated for 2 to 4 seconds, followed by a rest phase of 2 to 3 seconds. Increasing levels of voltages, from 0V to 6V are administered; with successive stimuli, the penis is extended and ejaculation takes place.

The AV used for bucks is similar to those for the ovine species. The construction includes the molded rubber housing with an inner liner, director cone, collection tube, insulating water jacket, and outer covering. The unit is filled so that the internal temperature of the AV is between 40° and 45°C at the time of collection. Air is used to provide the proper pressure.

In most cases, an untrained buck requires the use of a doe in estrus. Trained bucks, however, will readily mount a restrained, nonestrual doe. The collector stands to one side as the buck is led up to the doe. After sniffing and testing the female, the buck mounts and extends the penis. At this time, the collector grasps the prepuce and deviates the penis laterally into the AV. At the time of ejaculation, the buck produces a pronounced pelvic thrust followed by dismount. The AV should be maintained on the penis during the dismount due to the continued expulsion of the sperm rich fraction.

Porcine

Swine semen may be collected for evaluation, insemination, or freezing by either EE, DM with the fingers of a gloved hand, or with an AV. Generally DM is the preferred technique and the collection of semen with an AV is not commonly done in swine. DM gives equivalent results, when compared to the AV, and is also easier to perform.

The DM or gloved-hand technique involves collection of boars on a mount sow or a phantom (Fig. 10-6). Training the boar for seminal collection using a phantom requires replacement of the teaser, estrous sow or gilt, with the phantom, usually after several successful collections, or to allow the boar to observe another boar mounting the phantom. Frequently, the presence of another boar's scent (pheromones) will help untrained boars to mount the phantom.

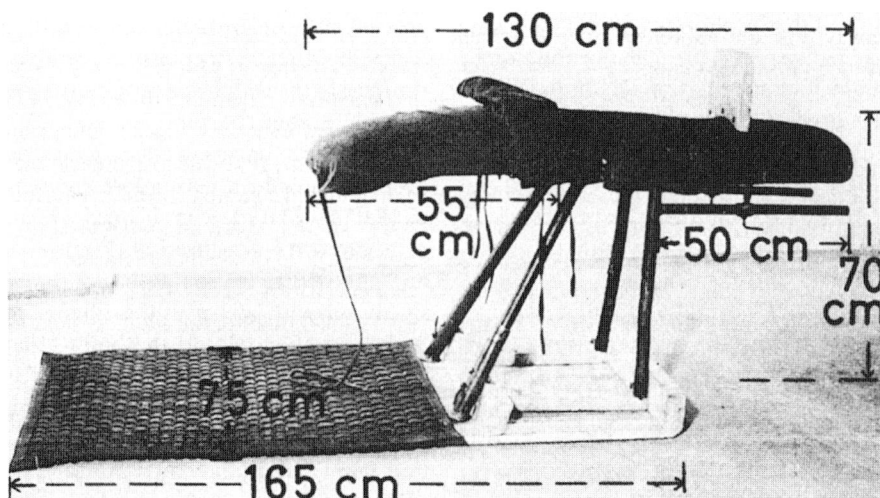

Fig. 10-6. Dummy sow, made of galvanized iron, has a changeable cover. The adjustable wooden block, **top right,** prevents the boar from getting too far forward during collection of semen. (From: J. Aamdal, Swine. *In:* The Artificial Insemination of Farm Animals, 3rd ed., edited by E. J. Perry. New Brunswick, NJ, Rutgers University Press, 1960, p. 261).

After the boar mounts, the spiral portion of the glans penis is firmly grasped using a vinyl glove. Latex gloves are not recommended because latex is spermicidal. The gloved hand of the collector mimics the pressure and stimulation of the sow's cervix on the glans penis. The semen is directed into an insulated container once ejaculation of the sperm-rich fraction begins.

The AV for collection of semen from boars is similar to those used with other species. The casing is 22.5 cm × 3.75 cm in length and width and commonly uses a latex rubber liner. The casing is filled with water and air so at the time of collection, the interior of the AV is between 45° to 50°C. The boar is "locked" into the AV by grasping the spiral tip through the long rubber collection cone. Ejaculation may last up to 15 minutes. Boars ejaculate large volumes, so the collection bottle should be large enough to hold 450 to 500 ml of semen. After ejaculation is complete, the hand pressure applied to the glans is released and the boar will dismount.

The collection of boar semen by EE requires the use of general anesthesia, since physical restraint would be inadequate to control the boar and to exteriorize the penis. The most frequently used anesthetic is thiopental (Pentothal®), an ultra-short acting barbiturate. Thiopental is safe when administered in the proper dose (7.4 mg per kg, IV) to a normal animal. Deaths, however, have been reported in boars with lung damage due to chronic respiratory disease or in genetic carriers of porcine stress syndrome.

To administer the anesthetic, the animal is restrained with a nose rope or snare and thiopental is administered into an ear vein or the anterior vena cava. The anesthetic is given as a bolus and the animal becomes recumbent within seconds.

Fecal material is removed from the rectum with the fingers of a gloved hand prior to probe insertion. The boar probe depicted in Figure 10-7 has circular rather than longitudinal electrodes. Newer rectal probes, similar to those used in rams, have linear electrodes, except that they are larger in diameter and have a longer handle. After placement of the probe within the rectum, the operator applies a light level of stimulation. This provides some penile erection and facilitates exteriorization. To complete exteriorization, a long atraumatic forceps is inserted into the prepuce, the glans penis is engaged and gently exteriorized. Immediately after the penis has been extended, it is grasped with a hand-held gauze and the tip is directed into a collection container. The container is usually a warm thermos containing a sterilized plastic bag to hold the ejaculate and the mouth of the thermos is covered by gauze in order to filter out the gel portion of the boar ejaculate. The duration and number of electrical stimulations to ejaculate a boar differ from that used in other species in that power is administered for 5 to 7 seconds followed by a rest phase of 5 to 10 seconds. The

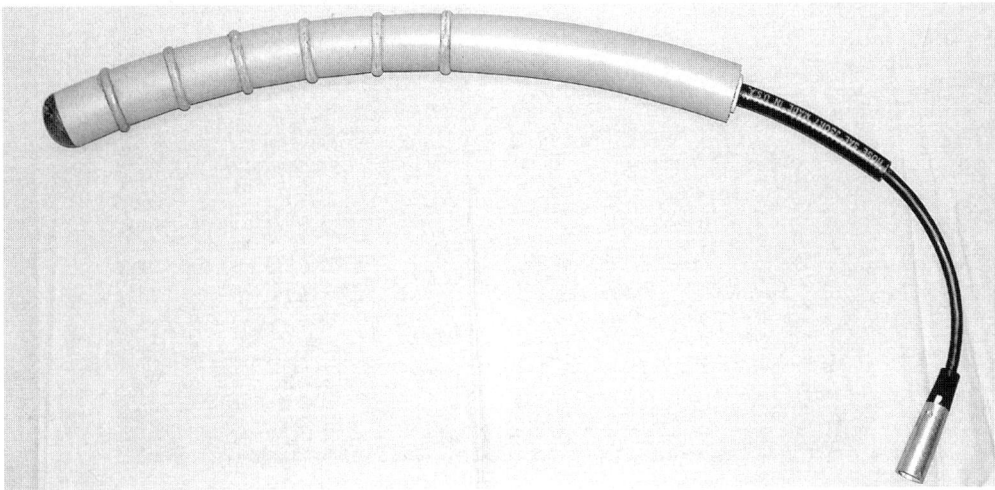

Fig. 10-7. Boar rectal probe with circular electrodes for electroejaculation.

long rest period becomes necessary because the progressively higher stimulations interfere with the intercostal muscles and respiration.

The boar will normally ejaculate sperm-poor fluids during the initial stimulations which is discarded. The sperm-rich fraction intermixed with gel follows next and the total volume to be collected will depend on whether the sample is for analysis, insemination, or freezing.

Canine

Semen collection for the canine species most commonly involves DM of the penis and less frequently the use of an AV. With either technique, collection of semen is often facilitated by the presence of an estrous bitch. The female is restrained to prevent movement in an area which provides secure footing. The male is brought up to the female on a short leash and allowed nasal-genital contact.

Initially, the penis may be massaged through the prepuce in order to stimulate erection. After partial erection has commenced, the sheath is gently retracted behind the bulbus glandis and the penis cleaned with a cotton pledget saturated with warm water. Digital pressure is then applied behind the bulbus glandis to complete erection. The male frequently begins to ejaculate while the penis is being handled, however, some dogs may require additional stimulation for ejaculation. Gentle massage of the tip of the glans penis may elicit further erection leading to ejaculation.

There are three fractions to the ejaculate (Fig. 10-8). The first fraction is clear and nearly sperm-free, the second fraction is sperm-rich and the final portion is watery and sperm-poor. The sperm-rich fraction can be collected in a warm funnel attached to a sterile test tube. A new Styrofoam cup makes a useful insulated collection receptacle. The ejaculate should not be cold-shocked during collection or evaluation.

Following ejaculation, the male should be checked periodically to be sure that detumescence and retraction of the penis has taken place.

A procedure[57] to collect semen from dogs that has gained considerable acceptance is to use a latex directing cone attached to a plastic tube to collect the ejaculate (Fig. 10-9). The directing

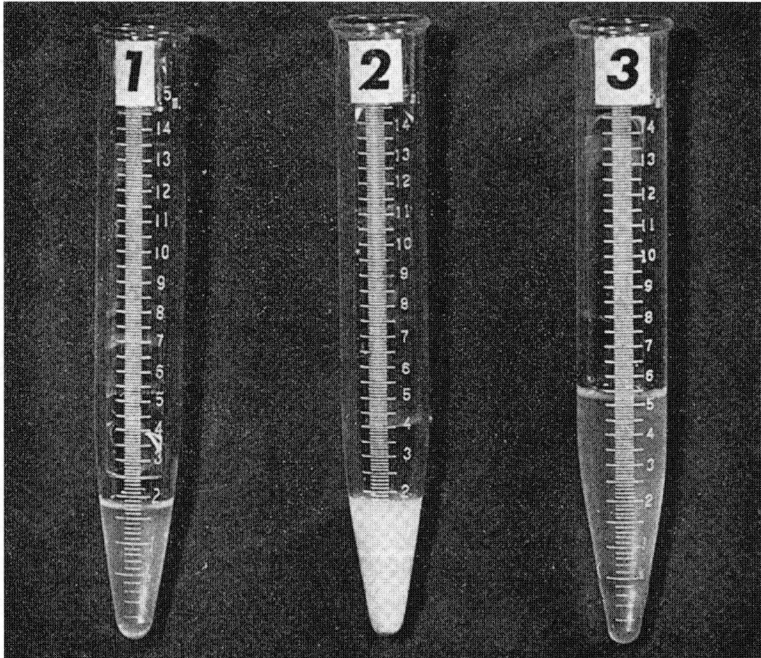

Fig. 10-8. The three fractions of the dog's ejaculate shown are from left to right: **1**, first, presperm fraction, **2**, second, sperm-rich fraction, **3**, third, postsperm fraction. (From: J. H. Boucher, et al., Cornell Vet. *48*:73, 1958).

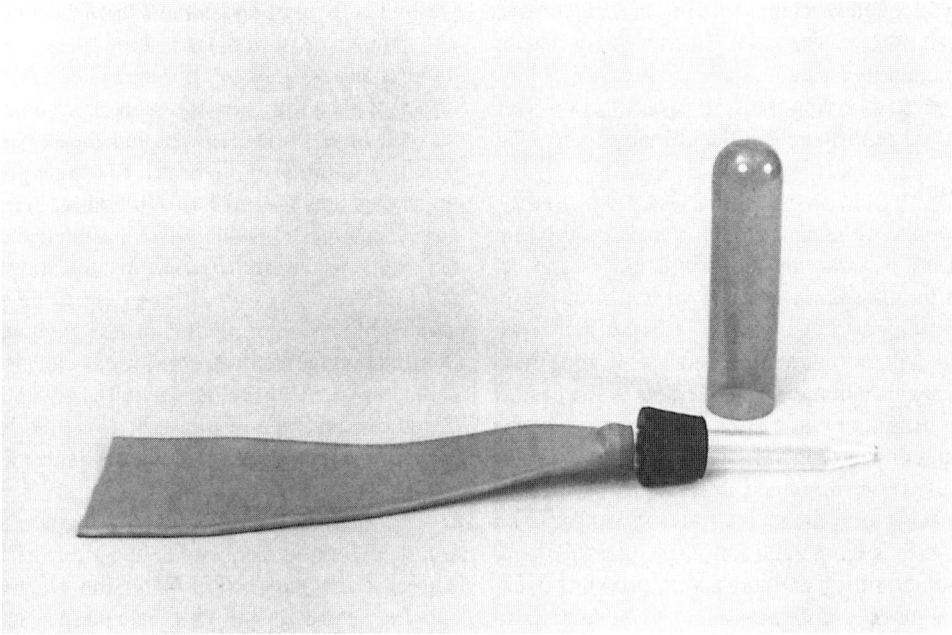

Fig. 10-9. Directing cone and collection tube including protective waterjacket for semen collection by digital manipulation (DM) from dogs.

cone is placed over the exposed tip of the penis and is used to push the prepuce behind the bulbus glandis. The collection of semen then continues as described for seminal collecting by DM, except that, in this case, the collector's hand applies pressure over the latex cone behind the bulbus glandis. The ejaculation pattern is identical as described for the collection of semen by DM, and frequently the first and the second (sperm-rich) fractions are collected together.

Semen is seldom collected from dogs with an AV. Dogs need to be trained to ejaculate in the AV and in addition, artificial vaginas for dogs are not commercially available. Furthermore, several artificial vaginas of different sizes would have to be available to accommodate the variation in the size of the penis of dogs of different breeds and ages. The cleaning, sterilizing and assembling of the AV is time consuming and adds to the costs associated with the collection of dog semen with an AV.

Feline

Semen can be collected from felines by EE or with an AV. There has not been a great de-

mand for the collection of feline semen from domestic toms so the techniques, although adequate, are not routinely employed in the clinical practice. However, collection of semen by EE from wild felids is routinely practiced in zoological gardens engaged in programs to increase the population of endangered wild cat species. Some of these species are on the verge of extinction. Also, some zoos have programs to artificially inseminate wild cats, raise the young in captivity and then use these animals to repopulate areas in the world from where these animals became extinct.

To collect semen by EE, the tom is anesthetized, then placed in lateral recumbency. The electronic control unit and probes are usually custom made because there is not a commercial source of this equipment. After insertion of the probe, the collection tube is placed on the exposed penis and electrical stimulation is applied in a series of stimuli. A rest phase is permitted between the pulse series, then stimulation is reapplied at a higher power setting. The specifics for EE in the tom are now established (see Chapter 17).

Collection with an AV requires a trained tom and an estrous queen. See Chapter 17 for details. The feline AV can be made from a rubber bulb and glass tube (Fig. 10-10). The AV is directed over the penis to collect the ejaculate.

Avian

Digital massage is the preferred method for collecting semen from poultry. Collection begins by massaging the back of the bird, beginning behind the wings and stroking gently toward the tail with the thumb and forefinger making a slight upward movement at the base of the tail. This motion stimulates erection of the copulatory organ. Repetitive stroking may be required on untrained birds. An alternative method is to massage the bird's abdomen. In either case, a thumb and forefinger part the feathers around the vent and gentle pressure is exerted on the ejaculatory ducts. Collection of semen from the turkey is essentially the same as for the rooster.

MAINTENANCE OF THE COLLECTION EQUIPMENT

Depending on the species there may be many disposable products used with AV collections, eliminating the need for post-use cleaning. These include plastic test tubes, directing cones, and inner liners. Latex items must be cleaned and sanitized after each use. First the liner is rinsed and scrubbed to remove gross contamination, then washed with a mild detergent. After

washing, the liners and cones are rinsed with tap and then with distilled water. Finally, the equipment is rinsed with alcohol and allowed to air dry in a dust-free environment. Glassware is washed in a similar fashion and then dry-heat sterilized (160°C for 2 hours). Reusable plastic items which withstand exposure to high temperatures are cleaned and sterilized with alcohol or dry-heat. Steam sterilization is not routinely used due to the possibility of depositing salts which may be spermicidal on the containers. Sterilization with ethylene oxide gas can also be used, but is expensive, and requires airing time to remove all trace of this very toxic oxide. In addition, availability of ethylene oxide gas is not assured.

The rectal probes used in electroejaculation and the EE equipment is cleaned after the final collection. Mucus build-up on the electrodes can be removed by lightly cleaning with an abrasive cleanser or better, by polishing with fine steel wool.

ANALYSIS OF SEMEN

The semen is brought to the laboratory and the collection container is placed in a waterbath, incubator, or dri-block heater at 35° to 37°C for temperature stability. In general, the ejaculate will be first examined for motility and normal morphology. Semen should be stored and handled in an isothermal environment until analysis is completed and processing begins. Some species release semen that tolerate cooling bet-

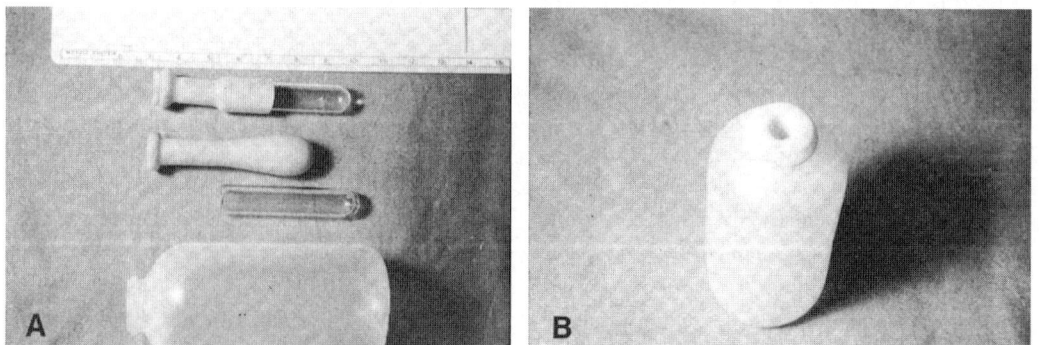

Fig. 10-10. Equipment for semen collection with an artificial vagina (AV) from the cat. **A.** Components of the AV. **B.** Assembled AV. (From: N. J. Sojka, et al., Lab. Anim. Care *20*:199, 1970).

ter than others; for example, semen from the dog and pig, if allowed to cool slowly, can be held at room temperature for several hours without addition of extenders. Sensitivity of spermatozoa to temperature change is governed by the protective action of the components of the seminal plasma and by the integrity of the spermatozoal cell membrane. Integrity of the membrane at different temperatures is strongly influenced by its basic lipid-protein composition and the ratio of cholesterol to phospholipids forming the membrane bi-layer.

To date, the most comprehensive protocols and standards have been developed for the analysis of bovine semen. The analysis of semen from other species is similar to that used for bovine; however, the parameters have not been as critically assessed. Semen evaluations *per se* cannot guarantee fertility or rank individuals.

Rather, evaluation procedures are used to identify ejaculates that have a high probability of being substandard.

The motility of the spermatozoa is estimated by microscopic examination at 40 to 100X. Normally, concentrated bovine semen samples will display rapidly swirling patterns with 75% or more of the cells in vigorous forward motion. The subjective estimation of the gross microscopic pattern of motility (swirls) within an ejaculate is dependent on spermatozoal activity (motility) and concentration. If large amounts of accessory gland secretions are released by a bull and discarded prior to collection of semen with an AV or by EE, then the spermatozoal concentration of the sample will be greatly increased. On the other hand, if large volumes of seminal fluid are collected along with the sperm-rich fraction, the sample will be diluted and may not display strong wave patterns. To help overcome the influence of marked variations in spermatozoal concentration on subjective estimates of motility, a 5 μl drop of the sample can be placed on the slide, cover-slipped and evaluated for the percentage of progressively motile cells. Highly concentrated samples can be diluted with buffered saline before examination.

Some breed organizations have advocated minimally acceptable spermatozoal motility lev-

els for fresh ejaculates, though these can be as low as 30%. Samples that fall below the suggested standards for use in AI are discarded.

Spermatozoal morphology is commonly assessed by microscopic examination of a small drop of semen which has been mixed with a drop of stain, smeared on a slide, and air dried. Eosin-nigrosin is the most common stain used for spermatozoal examination; however, other simple, acceptable stains include India ink or Wright's.

Historically, spermatozoal abnormalities from bulls were classified as primary (major abnormalities such as head shapes) or secondary (minor abnormalities such as bent tails) according to their perceived importance relative to fertility. Depending on the total number of primary and secondary abnormalities, the morphology score was calculated and the ejaculate was rated as satisfactory or unsatisfactory. Current recommendations for bulls suggest that a minimum normal morphology score of 70%, without distinguishing between types of abnormalities, constitutes a satisfactory score.

Photomicroscopy, videomicroscopy, and automated spermatozoal analyzers may be used to further assess spermatozoal morphology and the quantitative and qualitative levels of motility for individual cells.

Although not routinely performed as part of a breeding soundness examination, AI centers may evaluate the acrosomal integrity of spermatozoa in samples of frozen-thawed semen before the semen is released for commercial application. Excessive premature acrosomal activation or damage have been associated with substandard conception rates. Hence, evaluation of spermatozoa with a phase-contrast or differential interference contrast microscope can be performed to detect these morphologic abnormalities. For some species, spermatozoa are incubated with fluorescent dyes and acrosomal integrity is assessed using a fluorescent microscope.

Scrotal circumference is assessed in the bull as part of the breeding soundness evaluation. The scrotal circumference provides an estimate of the bull's capacity to produce spermatozoa, because spermatozoal production per gram of testes is fairly constant and correlates well with spermatozoal output. Bulls with extremely small testes produce few normal spermatozoa and they are considered subfertile or sterile. Also, a bull with small testes as a yearling will increase the scrotal circumference as he grows, but will continue to produce fewer spermatozoa. If an animal does not have a minimum satisfactory scrotal circumference by 16 to 18 months of age, he should not be used for breeding. Bulls with a large scrotal circumference undergo puberty earlier and develop a greater capacity to service more cows. These are desirable heritable characteristics, and things being equal, should be preferentially selected over bulls with a smaller scrotal circumference (Table 10-2)

Breeding soundness examination of boars, including seminal analysis is similar to the analysis applied to the evaluation of semen from bulls. The principal difference is that the scrotal size is determined by measuring the length and width of individual testes. A yearling boar should have a testicular size of at least 11 cm in length by 7 cm in width for each testis. A spermatozoal motility estimate of 75% or greater is considered satisfactory. A total of 20% or more of 'primary' abnormalities or greater than 40% 'secondary' abnormalities would render the boar as suspect and potentially of reduced fertility.

Semen analysis in the stallion is based on spermatozoal motility, morphology, and concentration. Measurement of testicular size is not routinely done because untrained stallions may react violently to scrotal palpation. In addition, scrotal size does not correlate well with the quality of semen and fertility of the equine ejaculate.

Unless the stallion semen was collected into an AV with a filter, the gel fraction should be removed from the ejaculate by syringe aspiration or filtration. This is necessary to prevent trapping of the spermatozoa in the gel and hindering the estimation of motility.

Spermatozoal concentration can be determined by employing a hemocytometer to count cells/unit area of diluted semen and then with appropriate formulas determine concentration of spermatozoal/ml of the ejaculate. Alternately, a densitometer can be used to estimate the concentration of a sample in field conditions.

Generally, stallion ejaculates are not as dense as bovine samples, so motility estimates can be performed with undiluted samples of semen on a warm slide with a coverslip placed over the sample. The percentage of motile sperm are then estimated, with greater than 75% motile considered desirable. The ejaculate should also have at least 70% morphologically normal cells.

Analysis of the ram ejaculate is based on motility and morphology, in addition to satisfactory scrotal circumferences. General guidelines require that a ram evaluated during the breeding season have greater than 75% motility and less than 25% major morphologic abnormalities. Evaluations performed out of the breeding season will generally show an increase in abnormal cells, and decreases in spermatozoal motility and scrotal circumference.

Seminal parameters in the buck are similar to that of the ram. A satisfactory ejaculate has a motility estimate of at least 75% with less than 25% major morphological defects.

Analysis of semen for breeding soundness examination of dogs are based on spermatozoa motility with at least 75% of the spermatozoa displaying a rapid forward motion and a morphologic estimate of not more that 25% major abnormalities.

There are no specific recommendations for semen analysis to estimate breeding soundness of the feline species other than to estimate the percentage of progressively motile spermatozoa.

SEMEN EXTENSION AND CRYOPRESERVATION

Diluting semen in a buffered extender helps to maintain sperm viability for short-term storage which may vary, according to the species,

Table 10-2   Minimally Acceptable Scrotal Size by Age for Bulls of Common Breeds

Age (months)	Scrotal Size (cm)
12 to 15	30
16 to 18	31
19 to 21	21
22 to 24	33
over 24	34

from hours to days before insemination or for long-term storage and freezing. Bitches are routinely inseminated with fresh, non-extended semen, though the use of AI with frozen extended semen is increasing.

Extenders differ in composition depending upon the species, intended use, storage temperature, and the desired duration of storage. All extenders are based on a particular buffer. Buffers modulate the change in extender pH due to the metabolic products of the stored spermatozoa. In addition, carbohydrates are added to provide an energy source for sperm glycolysis. Egg yolk or milk-based fractions are added to promote membrane stabilization at cooler temperatures and limit premature acrosomal membrane activation.

Some extenders will maintain spermatozoal viability at 20°C while others are effective at 4° to 5°C, temperatures at which the metabolic rate of the spermatozoa is lower. In addition these temperatures control bacterial growth. Extenders to be used in the cryopreservation of semen contain freezing point depressing compounds, which inhibit ice formation, dehydrate the cells, and protect cellular structures. Although the basic freezing principles are applicable across the species, each group may have several acceptable protocols. Specific procedures have been published and should be consulted for detailed descriptions of freezing techniques.

Bovine

Freezing of semen has been used for AI in the bovine species for decades and has served as a basic model for processing semen of other species. There are, however, acceptable variations in bovine extenders an freezing rates. The information concerning the optimum parameters for semen cryopreservation are not standardized and different sources conflict over the best techniques. The procedure described herein is employed on a commercial basis in our laboratory at Iowa State University.

First the fresh bovine ejaculate is evaluated for volume, motility, and morphology. To be satisfactory for further processing, the sample must have an initial minimum of 75% progressive motility and 70% or grater of normal morphology. Samples of lower quality are discarded.

An aliquot of semen is diluted 100-fold with normal saline solution and the concentration of cells/ml is determined by optical density with a calibrated spectrophotometer. Alternately, automated densitometers can be used to measure the concentration of a sample. Antibiotics are added to seminal samples of acceptable quality for pathogen control. The antibiotic-semen mixture is then incubated prior to extension. This approach is used because the antimicrobial activity of antibiotics is hindered by the presence of milk or egg-yolk phospholipids commonly used in semen extenders.

After equilibration with the antibiotics, the semen is added to isothermal extender. The initial extension is only half the final desired dilution. The extended semen is then placed in an isothermal water jacket, which is in turn placed into a 5°C cold cabinet and allowed to cool over a period of several hours. At the end of the cooling phase, the samples are removed from the water jackets and maintained at 5°C.

After the semen has been held at 5°C, it is then diluted to the final desired concentration with a glycerolated extender. The semen is then packaged into 0.5-ml plastic french straws, sealed, and frozen for 10 minutes in static nitrogen vapor at a starting temperature of –160°C.

After freezing, the straws are immersed into liquid nitrogen until the time of thawing. Thawing is achieved by placing the straw into a 35°C waterbath for 30 to 60 seconds. All post-thaw evaluations are performed at 35°C. Semen samples are classified as acceptable for commercial distribution if they meet or exceed the criteria listed in Table 10-3.

Table 10-3 Post-Thaw Analysis: Minimum Standards

	Time of Assay	
Spermatozoal End Point	**0 hr.**	**2 hr.**
Motility (%)	25	15
Spermatozoal Progressive Linear Motility (PLM)	3	2
Intact Acrosomes (%)	60	40

PLM is a subjective estimate of the rate of forward motion. The range is from 0 to 5 with 0 assigned to no motion and 5 indicating extremely rapid progressive linear movement.

Equine

Stallion semen may be diluted with egg-yolk buffer or milk solids-glucose extenders, then either used immediately or slowly cooled to 5°C and stored at that temperature for AI of mares which are within 24 to 48 hours of ovulation. Special containers such as Equitainer® have been developed for shipping chilled semen overnight.

Frozen stallion semen is used commercially only on a limited basis. Freezing uniformity, packaging systems, and conception rates are variable. Particularly the conception rates are erratic.

In one freezing method, the semen is centrifuged to remove the seminal plasma and concentrate the sample. The soft pellet is then extended at 20°C in a sodium-citrate-ethylene diamine tetraacetic acid (EDTA) lactose-egg yolk medium containing the cryoprotectant, glycerol. The final extended semen should have a concentration sufficient to provide at least 200 $\times$ 10^6 motile, normal cells after thawing. The semen is packaged into plastic straws ranging in volume from 0.5 ml to 5.0 ml.

Freezing is accomplished in a passive or mechanically forced nitrogen vapor unit. The frozen straws are then immediately immersed in liquid nitrogen for storage at −196°C.

Thawing techniques depend on the type of straw used and specific recommendations are provided by the organization that processes the semen. Currently, thawing protocols for AI with frozen equine semen are not standardized.

Ovine

As in the equine species, ram semen can be extended for fresh insemination, cooled for short term storage (24–48 hours) or stored frozen for long-term preservation. There are several variations in the protocol for freezing ram semen, including spermatozoal concentration, percentage of glycerol, equilibration times, and rate of freezing.

One technique involves the use of tris-glucose extender at a dilution rate of 1 part semen to 2 parts extender. The extended semen is then cooled slowly to 5°C over 2 hours before placing into 0.5 ml french straws and freezing in liquid nitrogen vapor at a starting temperature of −120°C. After freezing, straws are stored in liquid nitrogen at −196°C. Thawing is done by placing the straws in 35°C water for at least 30 seconds.

Caprine

Goats are inseminated with fresh extended, cooled, or with frozen semen.

Cryopreservation of buck semen employs milk or tris-citrate-egg yolk extenders, glycerol, and packaging in 0.5-ml french straws. A low level of egg yolk (4–5%) is used due to the detrimental effects of higher levels on viability. Initial cooling is to 5°C in non-glycerolated extender. The glycerolated portion is then added slowly and the mixture is allowed to equilibrate over 2 hours before freezing in nitrogen vapor and storage at −196°. Thawing is accomplished by placing the straw in a 35°C waterbath for 30 seconds prior to insemination.

Porcine

Increasingly larger numbers of swine in the United States are now bred by AI. In 1996 approximately 15% of the females were bred by artificial means, and this number is expected to rise sharply in the next decade. The vast majority of these breedings were done using fresh-extended or chilled-extended semen rather than with frozen-thawed semen. The typical chilled extender is designed to maintain adequate fertility at 17° to 19°C for 3 to 7 days, depending on the initial quality of the ejaculate and spermatozoal viability. Best results, however, are obtained when stored semen is utilized within 72 hours of collection. Specific advantages of AI in sows include reduced labor and lower boar-to-sow ratios.

Freezing of swine semen is a multistep process due to the sensitivity of the spermatozoal membranes to temperature fluctuations and the depressing effect of glycerol on fertility. Specifics are beyond the scope of this chapter; however, highlights of one commercial method will be described.

The collected ejaculate is added to a predilution extender and cooled to 18°C over 4 hours. The semen is then centrifuged for 10 minutes at 18°C and the pellet resuspended in a cooling diluter containing egg yolk. The semen is then cooled from 18° to 5°C. Prior to freezing, the semen is diluted to a final concentration of 1.2 × 10⁹ spermatozoa/ml in a deep-freeze diluter at 4% glycerol. The semen is then frozen in 5-ml plastic tubes.

The freezing program involves four different cooling rates to –100°C followed by immersion into liquid nitrogen (–196°C). Thawing recommendations are to use water at 52°C for 50 seconds.

As a rule, frozen boar semen results in lower pregnancy rates and litter sizes compared to breeding with chilled extended semen.

Canine

Canine ejaculates can be extended, chilled to 5°C, and stored or shipped to breeders for use within 24 to 48 hours of collection. Commercial extenders have been developed for this type usage. The primary advantage of AI in dogs is that an estrous bitch does not have to be shipped somewhere for breeding.

Canine semen can also be frozen and its use is recognized by the American Kennel Club. The highest and most consistent pregnancy rates obtained with canine frozen-thawed semen are those obtained with transcervical or surgical intrauterine insemination.

In our laboratory, the ejaculate is equilibrated and diluted with pipes-citrate-egg yolk extender to a concentration of 225 × 10⁶ spermatozoa/ml then cooled to 5°C over 60 minutes. Additional isothermal extender containing 9% glycerol, is added, one part to two parts of equilibrated

semen, and held for an additional 30 minutes. The semen is loaded into 0.5 ml french straws and frozen in nitrogen vapor at –120°C.

To thaw, the straws are placed in 35°C water for 30 to 60 seconds. Insemination should be performed within 10 minutes of thawing.

Feline

The use of frozen feline semen for the artificial insemination of domestic queens has not been adequately documented. However, many zoological gardens in the United States and other countries have established successful, interzoo-collaborative programs for artificial insemination with frozen semen of wild cats, as a way to increase the population of endangered species or to replenish those that have become extinct in their natural habitat.

INSEMINATION PROCEDURES

The objective of artificial insemination is to deposit an adequate number of normal, motile spermatozoa in the female tract so they reach the oocyte at the most favorable time to ensure spermatozoal capacitation and fertilization (Table 10-4).

Most domestic species, except the queen, are transcervically inseminated into the uterus with fresh-cooled or with frozen-thawed semen. Bitches were frequently inseminated in the anterior vagina because of the presence of a pseudocervix (see Chapter 16). However, fiberoptic techniques are now available to allow visualization of the external os of the cervix of the bitch,

---

Table 10-4   Some Seminal Parameters and Time of Insemination for Domestic Mammals

Parameters	Bovine	Equine	Ovine	Caprine	Porcine	Canine	Feline
Volume (ml)	5	60	1	0.8	225	10	0.06
Spermatozoal concentration (10⁹/ml)	1.2	0.15	3.0	2.4	0.20	0.3	1.7
Total number of spermatozoa per ejaculate (10⁹)	6.0	9.0	3.0	1.9	45	3.0	0.1
Time of insemination, relative to day of estrus	Middle to end	Third day	Toward end	Toward end	First or second day	Second and fourth day	During estrus

In the mare, insemination is repeated at 48-hour intervals until ovulation.

Gilts are to be inseminated on the first day, sows on the second day. Repeat inseminaiton if gilts and sows are still standing to be mounted within 12 hours after the last insemination.

For the cat, ovulation is induced with gonadotropins after insemination.

facilitating the transcervical passage of the insemination catheter. Artificial insemination with frozen-thawed canine semen requires either transcervical or surgical intrauterine insemination for successful pregnancies.

Bovine

Semen for the AI of cattle is generally packaged into 0.25 or 0.5 ml plastic french straws (Fig. 10-11). The bovine AI industry has primarily phased out the use of ampules and replaced them with plastic straws due to more efficient storage capabilities and improved insemination instruments.

Regardless of the packaging, the semen can be stored on the farm in small liquid nitrogen tanks (Fig. 10-12). These tanks have a static loss (low level of evaporation) of nitrogen and must be periodically refilled to maintain proper cryogenic temperatures. The maximal length of time spermatozoa can remain viable, if properly stored, is unknown, but AI with bovine semen collected over 40 years ago still provides ac-

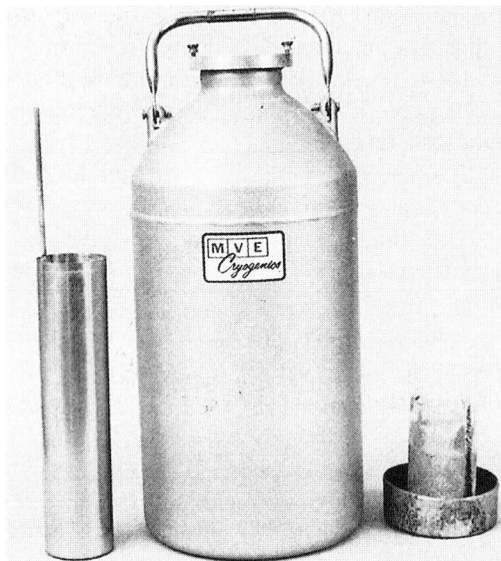

Fig. 10-12. Liquid nitrogen tank for shipping or for temporary storage of semen.

ceptable fertility. There is, however, a gradual decrease in viability for spermatozoa stored even at this low temperature.

When handling stored semen, whether for the transferring of straws from tank to tank or for removing a unit from a goblet, the exposure time to the elevated room temperature must be limited to seconds. If the semen is allowed to warm to above –80°C, recrystallization, which damages the spermatozoa, can occur.

Straws are generally thawed out rapidly in a 35°C waterbath for 30 to 60 seconds. The physical chemistry involved in freezing and thawing of semen is outside the scope of this chapter, but involves rate of freezing, size of intracellular ice crystals, changes in intracellular osmolarity during freezing and thawing, and the degree of dehydration of the cell. Generally, if freezing is fast, then thawing must be fast.

Once a straw is thawed, it is removed from the warm water and dried. The straw was identified prior to freezing and remains marked while still in the liquid nitrogen tank and is now double-checked to ensure insemination with the right bull's semen.

Straws are loaded into an insemination gun after the sealed tip has been removed (Fig. 10-13). A rigid plastic sheath is placed over the gun, followed by a sanitary sheath. While load-

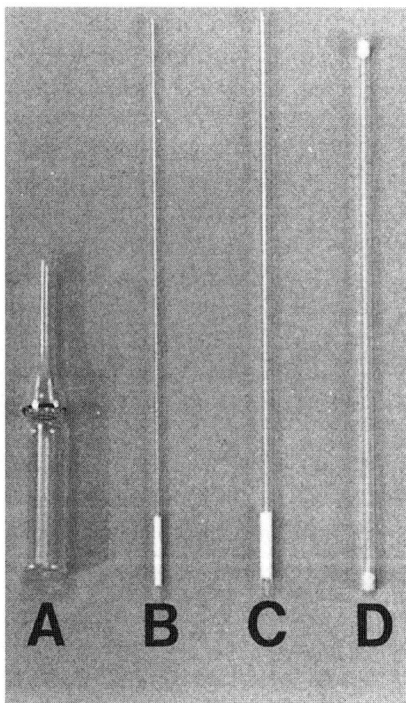

Fig. 10-11. A. 1.0 ml glass ampule. **B.** 0.25 ml french straw **C.** 0.5 ml french straw **D.** Continental straw.

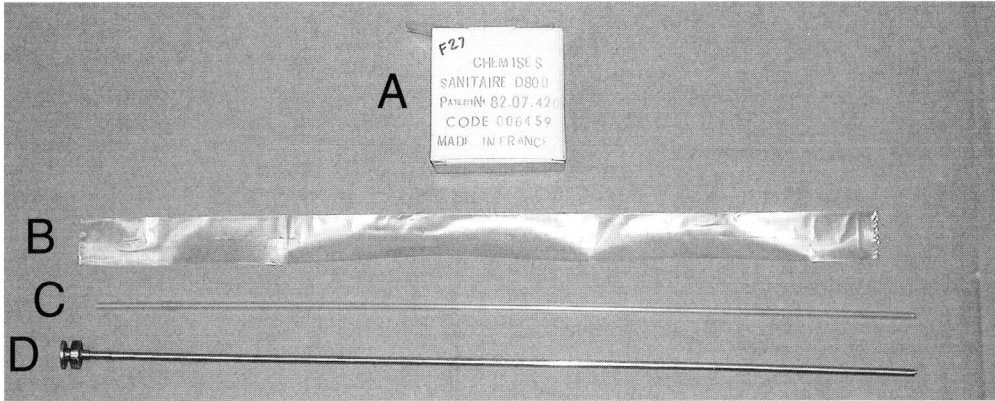

Fig. 10-13. Insemination gun for french straws containing frozen semen. After thawing, the straw (not shown in figure) is inserted into the stainless steel gun (**A**) and a rigid plastic tube (**B**) is placed over the gun to hold the straw in place. A thin plastic protective sheath or Chemise® (**C**) is then placed over the assembled unit to prevent vaginal contamination of the plastic tube and french straw. (**D**) Box containing additional protective sheaths.

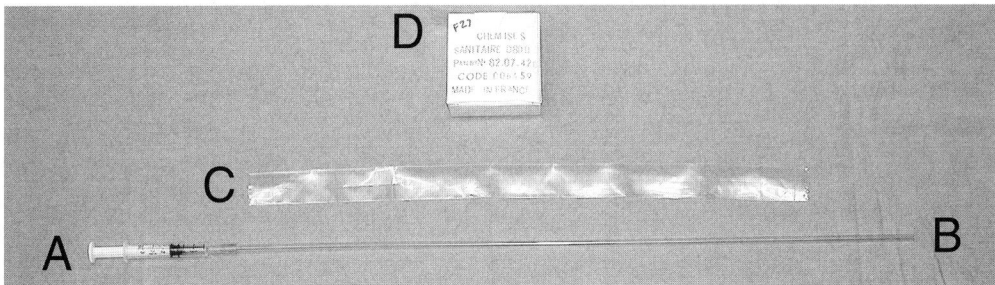

Fig. 10-14. A 3 ml plastic syringe (**A**) is connected to a disposable insemination pipette (**B**, Infuzee®) for AI of semen stored in glass ampules (ampule is not shown). After the thawed semen has been aspirated into the pipette, a sanitary sheath (**C**, Chemise®) is placed over the insemination pipette to prevent contamination. Box containing additional plastic sheaths is also shown (**D**).

ing the gun, transporting it to the breeding site, and manipulating the gun into the vagina, the semen should not be exposed to severe temperature changes or to rapid temperature fluctuations. A temperature range of 15°C to 37°C for post-thaw semen is compatible with satisfactory pregnancy rates. A rigid pipette attached to a small syringe is used for AI of semen contained in ampules. The minimum number of spermatozoa per insemination dose of freshly collected, extended semen for AI of heifers and cows is 5×10^6 of normal and progressively motile spermatozoal. The minimal recommended dose for frozen semen is 10×10^6 spermatozoa.

The insemination procedure involves passing the AI gun through the cow's vagina, while manipulating the cervix through rectal palpation with one hand (Fig. 10-15). Once the pipette reaches the external cervical os, the AI gun is

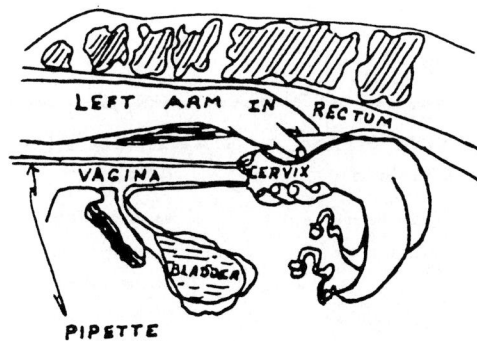

Fig. 10-15. The rectovaginal approach for cervical insemination of the cow.

pushed through the sanitary sheath and guided past the 3 to 5 cervical rings. The site of deposition is at the level of the internal cervical os. Depositing the semen only part way through the cervix significantly decreases conception rates.

The success of AI within any breeding program depends upon several factors including the accuracy of estrus detection, semen quality, individual fertility of sires and dams, and the expertise of the AI technician.

Estrus detection is one of the major factors controlling conception rates with AI. For example, if 95% of the animals are accurately detected in heat and bred at the appropriate time and the fertility level of the herd is 70% (first service conception rate), then 67 of 100 heifers will become pregnant. If, however, only 50% of the animals are properly detected as in estrus only 35 of the 100 heifers will become pregnant.

For dairy cattle, the goals are to achieve an estrus detection rate of 85% for cows and 95% for heifers within a 24-day period of observation.

A cow in estrus will stand to be mounted by other cows, prepared teasers, or a bull. Accompanying the standing to be mounted behavior are variable degrees of restlessness, vocalization, mucus discharge, and edema of the vulva. These ancillary signs develop as the animal approaches estrus, become more frequent and intense during estrus, and then decline after estrus. The only accurate way to assess estrus is to note when the cow stands to be mounted. Generally, the acceptable breeding period ranges from 10 to 24 hours after the cow begins to stand (Fig. 10-16). Aids in estrus detection include observation of nonstanchioned cows 2 to 3 times daily, the use of pressure sensitive devices, and estrus detecting animals such as teaser bulls or androgenized cows. Milk or serum progesterone assays and electronic devices that measure the conducting potential of the vaginal mucus have been used, with poor to erratic results.

Estrus synchronization procedures that shorten the interval that females must be observed for estrus, or that allow for timed matings, have also been successfully used with AI of cattle.

Heifers are generally bred at an approximate body weight and age that is particular for the breed. Postpartum dairy cows are usually rebred the first time between 45 and 60 days after calving and beef cows at 50 to 80 days after calving.

WHEN TO BREED — *"Timing Guide" for the average cow*

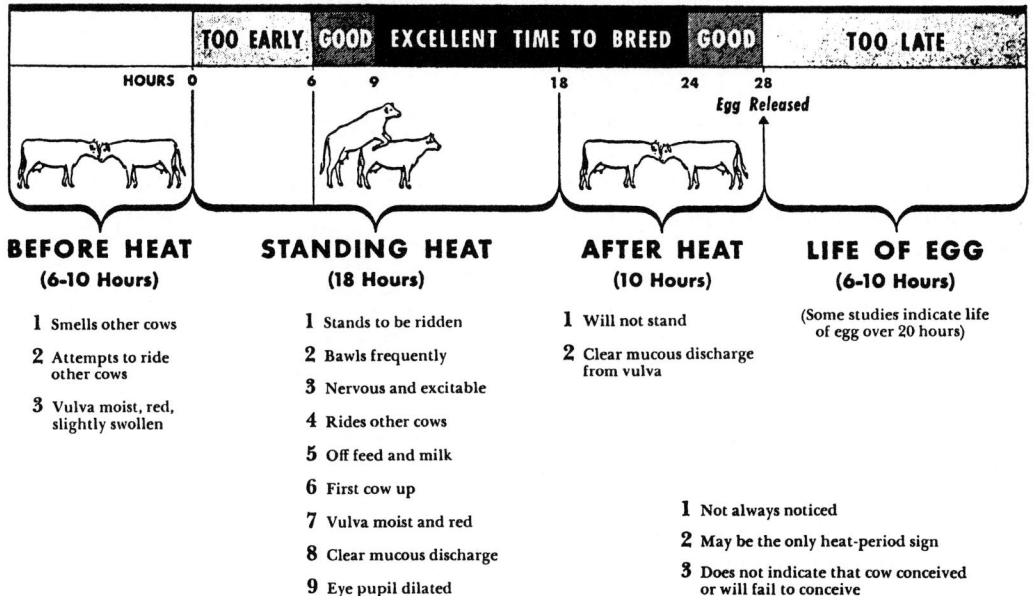

| TOO EARLY | GOOD | EXCELLENT TIME TO BREED | GOOD | TOO LATE |

HOURS   0   6   9   18   24   28
                                                 Egg Released

BEFORE HEAT (6-10 Hours)

1 Smells other cows

2 Attempts to ride other cows

3 Vulva moist, red, slightly swollen

STANDING HEAT (18 Hours)

1 Stands to be ridden

2 Bawls frequently

3 Nervous and excitable

4 Rides other cows

5 Off feed and milk

6 First cow up

7 Vulva moist and red

8 Clear mucous discharge

9 Eye pupil dilated

AFTER HEAT (10 Hours)

1 Will not stand

2 Clear mucous discharge from vulva

LIFE OF EGG (6-10 Hours)

(Some studies indicate life of egg over 20 hours)

1 Not always noticed

2 May be the only heat-period sign

3 Does not indicate that cow conceived or will fail to conceive

Fig. 10-16. Example of a "timing guide" to assist cattle breeders. (From: E. J. Perry, Cattle. *In*: The Artificial Insemination of Farm Animals, 3rd ed. New Brunswick, NJ, Rutgers University Press, 1960, p. 140).

Equine

The minimum number of spermatozoa per insemination dose of freshly collected semen for AI of mares is 500×10^6 progressively motile, normal spermatozoa. The recommended dose for chilled semen is 1 billion motile sperm per insemination dose while frozen-thawed insemination doses are at least 200×10^6 motile spermatozoa.

Estrus detection in mares requires the use of a teaser stallion in order to elicit the standing estrual response. The average estrous cycle is about 20 to 21 days long during the breeding season. The luteal phase (progesterone dominance) lasts about 15 days and the follicular phase (estrogen dominance) has an average duration of 5.5 days. As the mare approaches late diestrus—early estrus, her reaction to the stallion progressively changes from rejection to acceptance. Estrual signs include raising of her tail, squatting, urinating, and vulvar "winking" when being teased by the stallion. Additionally, rectal palpation of the ovaries will reveal follicular growth with a soft follicle(s), >35 mm in diameter, an edematous uterus, and a relaxed cervix. Ultrasound examination usually shows a characteristic echogenicity pattern and an irregularly shaped follicle(s). The mare ovulates 24 to 48 hours before the end of estrus. Consequently, most management systems begin breeding on the 2nd or 3rd day of estrus. The minimal expected lifespan of normal stallion spermatozoa in the oviduct is estimated to be 48 hours, so mares are inseminated with fresh semen every 2 days until estrus ceases or ovulation is detected by rectal palpation or ultrasonography. Insemination with chilled semen should take place within 24 hours of ovulation while breeding with frozen-thawed semen should take place within 12 hours before to 6 hours after ovulation.

The mare is prepared for insemination by securing her in a set of stocks. The tail is wrapped and tied out of the way or held by an assistant. Wrapping helps prevent tail hairs from being pulled into the vagina during insemination. Next the perineal area is washed and rinsed with water. Generally a minimum of 3 to 5 wash-rinse cycles are necessary for proper hygiene.

While the mare is being cleaned, an assistant aspirates semen into a non-spermicidal syringe. The inseminator puts on a sterile plastic shoulder-length glove, applies sterile lubricant to the glove, and passes the insemination pipette (Fig. 10-17) through the vagina and guides the tip of the pipette through the cervix. The semen is then gently expelled into the uterus over a period of 15 to 30 seconds. In special circumstances, the AI of mares with surgically corrected anatomical defects are typically inseminated by manipulating the pipette to and through the cervix using a vaginal speculum.

Ovine

Most ewes are bred by natural service with the ewes kept in pastures, or in semi-confinement, together with rams. However, there are sheep producers that AI their ewes using fresh extended or, less frequently, frozen ram semen. The semen which is frozen in straws or pellets is usually processed on a "custom" basis where the ram is brought to an AI center for seminal collection and returned after the requested number of units are produced and cryopreserved.

A major limitation to successful AI in sheep is the difficulty of traversing or bypassing the cervix with inseminating instruments. Vaginal or shallow cervical deposition results in low pregnancy rates, whereas intrauterine deposition through he cervix of fresh semen or laparoscopic intrauterine insemination can reach levels similar to natural breeding.

The nonsurgical insemination process requires a vaginal speculum and a light source for cervical visualization. The insemination is performed on a restrained standing ewe or one placed on a tilt table which elevates the hindquarters. The AI gun is specifically designed for use in sheep and consists of a stainless steel tube with plunger. The unit of semen is placed in the stainless steel tube over which a plastic sheath with a bendable tip is added. The tip is slightly bent for use in virgin ewe lambs and more severely bent in older animals. The bent tip helps in threading of the cervix in a higher proportion of the females.

Estrus detection is critical in a sheep AI program. A vasectomized teaser male is commonly used to identify the standing estrous females. The teaser has a marking harness (Fig. 10-18) or grease paint on the chest, which leaves a colored dye on the ewe's wool. Insemination should be done 12 to 24 hours after the onset of estrus.

In large herds, ewes are synchronized so that the majority are in estrus within a specified interval and then, AI can be performed at a preset time.

Caprine

Goats can be successfully inseminated with fresh, extended or with frozen semen. However, AI is not widely used in goats. Restraint is necessary, the degree of which depends on the animal's temperament. This will vary from the use of a collar to a tilt table. On special occasions, some goats will need to be tranquilized.

The perineal area is cleaned with water and a lubricated speculum is passed into the vagina.

Mucus that is cloudy or turbid indicates the doe is in late estrus, which is the optimum time for insemination.

The type of instrument used for insemination depends on the packaging of the semen. A shortened plastic pipette is used for ampules, or pellets while the sheep AI gun is suitable for straws.

The cervical os is located with the aid of a light and the tip of the AI gun is entered into the os. Gentle pressure is used to pass the gun past the cervical rings. Frequently, penetration of the cervix is not possible, so the semen is then deposited intracervically.

Conception rates are generally lower than those obtained with natural service, but a 60% conception rate is possible when AI is done under optimal conditions. As with sheep, laparoscopic intrauterine insemination is used in special cases, resulting in satisfactory pregnancy rates.

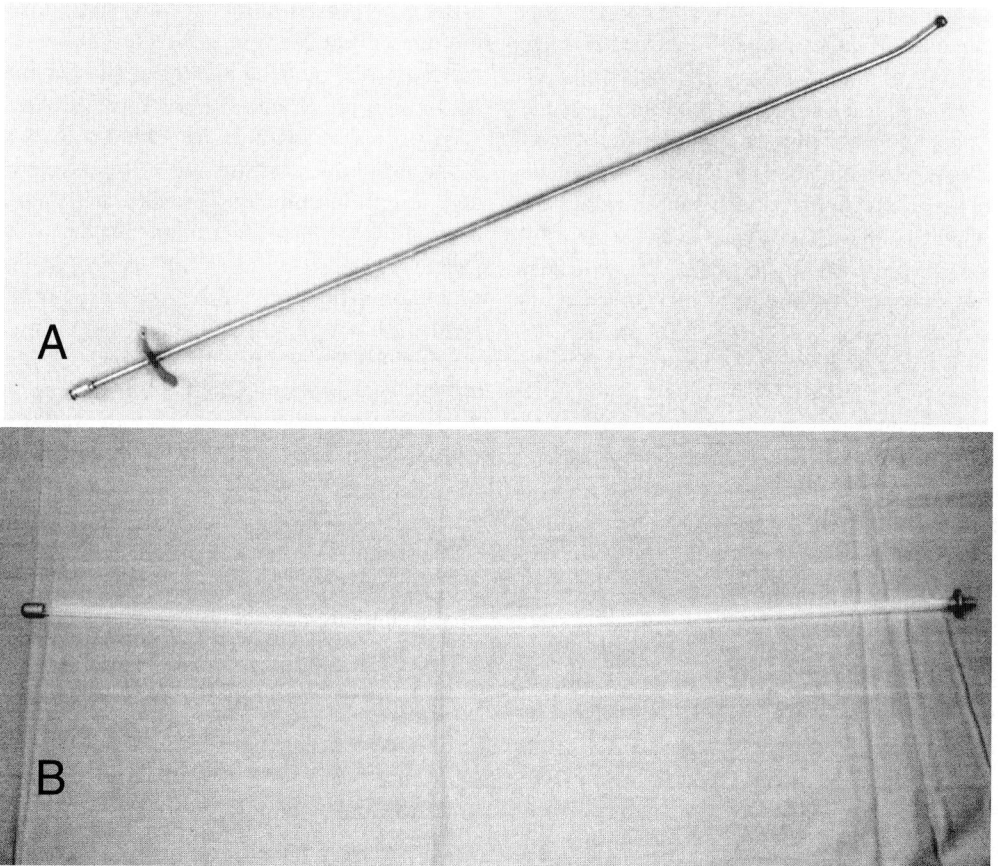

Fig. 10-17. A. Reusable Chambers' catheter used for artificial insemination (AI) of mares. **B**. Disposable plastic catheter (Minitüb®, Minitube of America, Verona, WI) commonly used for equine AI in the United States.

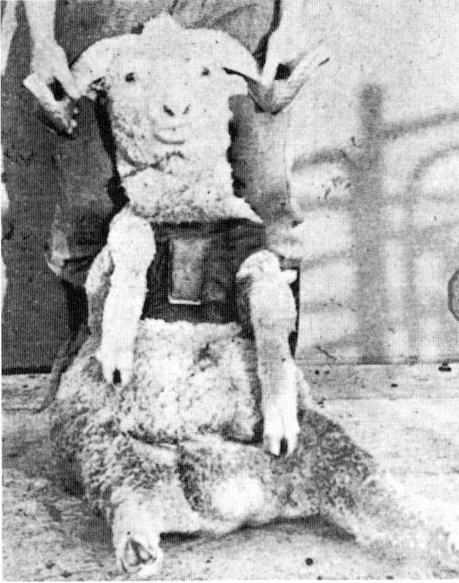

Fig. 10-18. Ram with a removable ewe-marking crayon (From: R. H. Watson and H. M. Radford, Aust. Vet. J. *11*:65, 1960).

Porcine

Sows and gilts are inseminated with either fresh extended, cooled, or frozen semen. With an accurate program of estrus detection and selection of optimal breeding time, the conception rate of AI with fresh extended semen equals that obtained with natural breeding. AI with frozen semen usually results in a lower conception rate and litter size.

Normally the sow or gilt is inseminated with 2 to 4 $\times$ 10^9 motile spermatozoa using fresh semen extended to a volume of 80 to 100 ml. If frozen-thawed semen is used, the number of spermatozoa inseminated is increased to 6 to 12 $\times$ 10^9 motile spermatozoa.

The proestrous female displays increased sexual activity and will stand for mounting at the onset of estrus. Standing estrus lasts 24 to 36 hours with gilts and 30 to 60 hours with sows. Gilts should be mated 12 to 18 hours after the onset of estrus and again 12 hours later, if still standing to be mounted. Sows are bred 24 hours from the onset of estrus and again 12 to 18 hours later. To facilitate estrus detection, a boar is walked by or allowed into the pen with the females to identify those which will stand to be mounted or stand to back pressure applied by the handler.

Insemination involves the use of a spirette, or a disposable pipette with a small form rubber tip (Fig. 10-19). The vulva is cleaned with a paper towel and the lubricated spirette is inserted along the dorsal vaginal wall to the external cervical os. When resistance is detected with the spirette, it is gently rotated counter clockwise so that the spiral end advances and locks into the cervix (Fig. 10-20). A pipette will advance past one or two cervical rings with manipulation and will lock into the cervix. The semen is injected slowly into the uterus with a collapsible plastic bottle or bag. The expulsion of the semen should take place over a period of at least 3 minutes.

Canine

Artificial insemination in the canine is mostly based on the use of unextended fresh, or chilled extended semen. In this case, the entire

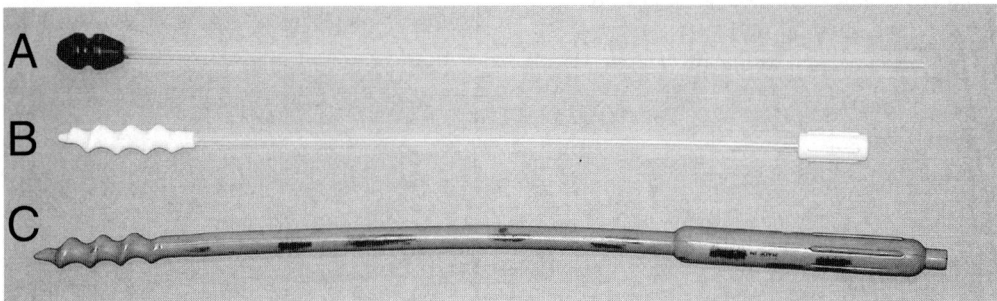

Fig. 10-19. Disposable (**A,B**) and reusable (**C**) pipettes for porcine artificial insemination (AI). **A.** Disposable sponge-tipped insemination pipette. The spiral tips on the disposable (**B**) and reusable (**C**) pipettes are designed 'fix' or 'lock' the insemination pipette within the cervix of the gilt or sow during the introduction of freshly collected or extended semen.

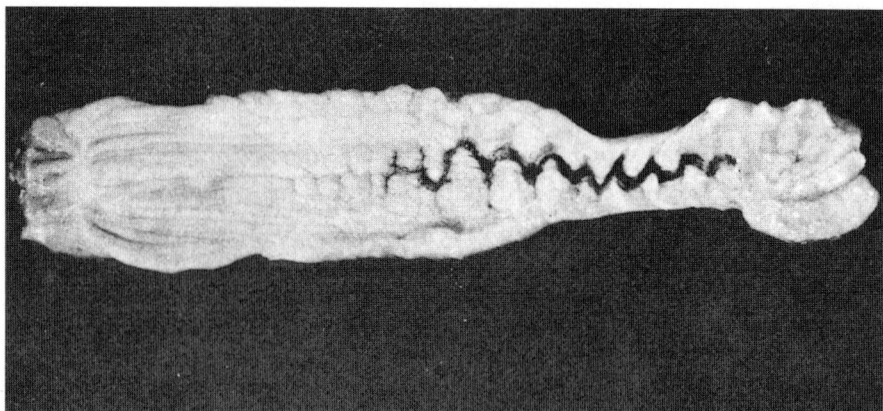

Fig. 10-20. Longitudinal section through the vagina (**left**) and cervix of a sow. The curved course of the cervical canal is stained. (From: J. Aamdal, Swine. *In*: The Artificial Insemination of Farm Animals, 3rd ed., edited by E. J. Perry. New Brunswick, N.J, Rutgers University Press, 1960, p. 265).

sperm rich fraction is deposited, using a plastic pipette, into the anterior vagina of the estrous bitch. The pipette is directed to pass the pseudo-cervix to deposit the semen in the anterior fornix of the vagina. Intracervical or intrauterine insemination via the vagina without the aid of fiberoptic equipment is nearly impossible (see Chapter 16). The semen is slowly injected, followed by elevation of the bitch's hindquarters for 5 minutes. Elevation helps prevent the premature loss of semen from the vaginal tract. Vaginal stimulation with a gloved finger may aid in the transport of semen into the uterus via genital contractions and altering vaginal pressures. Artificial insemination with chilled semen follows the same process and the inseminating dose is 400 to 600 × 10⁶ spermatozoa/ml.

The use of transvaginal insemination with frozen semen has produced extremely erratic results in conception rate and litter size. Transcervical or intrauterine insemination via the vagina is now possible with the aid of a rigid laparoscope. The most consistent results are obtained by the intrauterine insemination of frozen-thawed semen containing at least 100×10^6 motile spermatozoa per inseminating dose.

The timing of insemination is extremely important with the use of chilled or frozen semen. Timing can be facilitated with vaginal cytology, however, due to the prolonged duration of estrus in the bitch the operator cannot anticipate the time of ovulation through the examination of vaginal smears. The optimal fertility period is best predicted by detecting the ovulatory surge of luteinizing hormone or by determining blood levels of progesterone as a sign that the bitch has ovulated.

Feline

The queen is inseminated in the anterior vagina with a minimum of 5×10^6 spermatozoa. The insemination pipette is passed through the vagina to the anterior fornix, and the insemination dose is expelled. The time of breeding coincides with the maximum hypertrophy of the vaginal epithelial cells. Consequently, a vaginal wash is performed to check that the queen is in estrus prior to insemination.

After insemination, the queen must be given LH or hCG to induce ovulation.

Avian

The recommended insemination dose of neat semen is 0.1 ml for chickens and 0.025 ml for turkeys with a minimum total number of 300×10^6 spermatozoa. For AI, the vagina of the hen is everted, the inseminating syringe is inserted to a depth of about 3 cm and the semen is deposited (Fig. 10-21). Pressure on the abdomen is released and the vagina is allowed to retract. The inseminator gently blows on the vent to induce rhythmic contractions of the vaginal wall. The recommended time for insemination is late

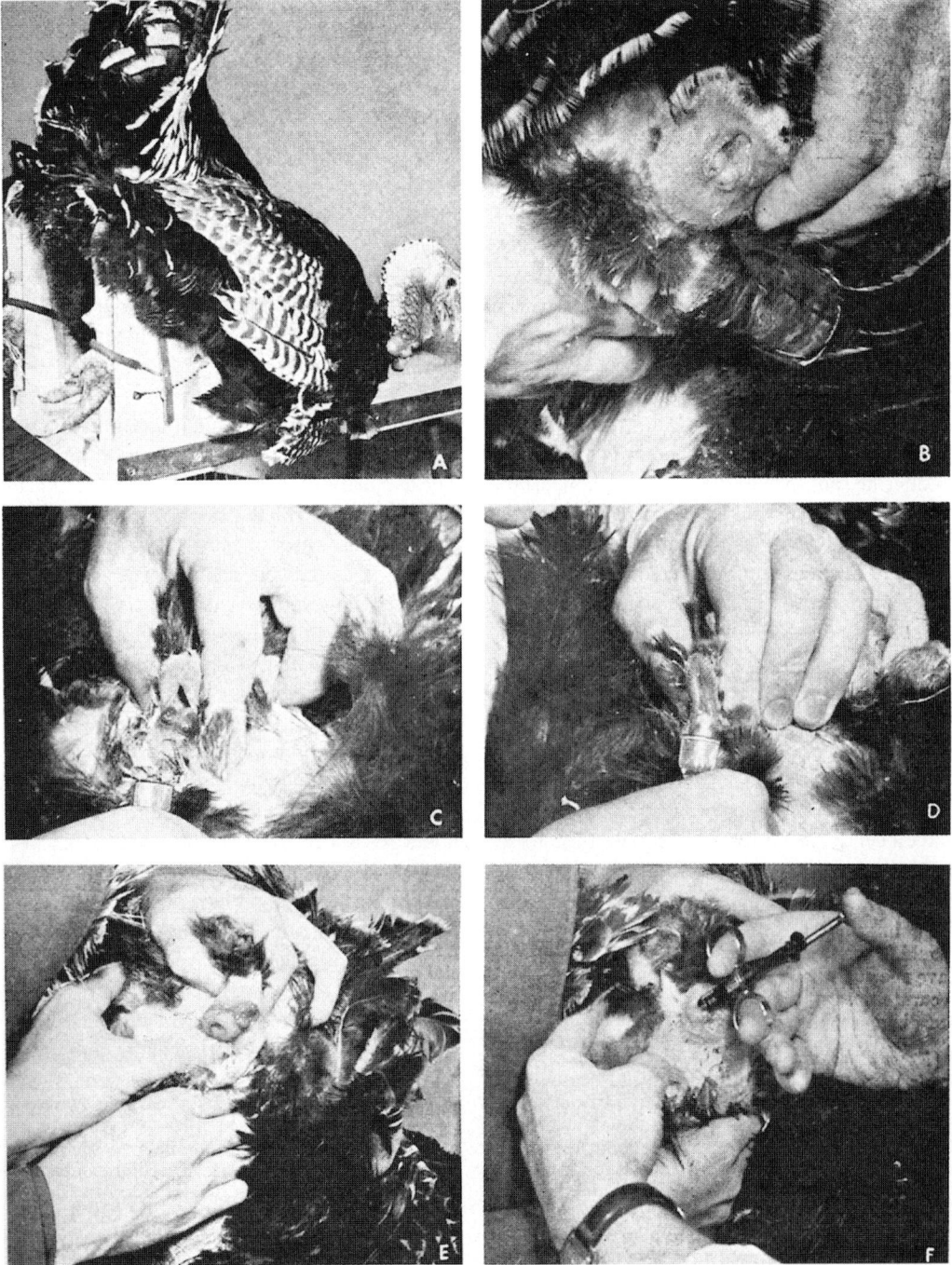

Fig. 10-21. Steps in the collection of semen and artificial insemination of turkeys. **A.** The male (tom) is secured on a special stand. As an alternative the tom may be held on a table or suitable support. **B.** Position of hands for stimulating the ejaculatory reflex in toms. **C.** The tom is ready to ejaculate: The vent becomes partly everted, revealing the turgid phallic and lymph folds. Massaging should now stop. **D.** The semen is being collected into a vial. **E.** Left oviduct of a laying hen is everted with moderate pressure from below the cloacal region. **F.** After the syringe is inserted into the oviduct, the vagina and the cloaca should be allowed to become withdrawn to their normal position. (Canadian Department of Agriculture: Artificial Insemination of Turkeys. Publ. No. 897, 1953).

in the afternoon in order to avoid the presence of a hard-shelled egg in the oviducts.

Insemination is repeated at weekly intervals in chickens and every 2 to 3 weeks in turkeys. The inseminated spermatozoa enter the utero-vaginal host gland where they are stored and released over time, providing the capability for 1 to 3 weeks of normal fertilization. Though spermatozoa may remain viable longer than the period recommended between breedings, the fertility level begins to decline when the interval between inseminations is extended. Inseminating equipment for avian species is depicted in Figure 10-22.

AGING OF GAMETES

The physiological basis pertaining to neural, endocrine, and behavioral patterns concerning the release of male and female gametes has been presented in Chapters 7–9 and in each of the chapters dealing with Patterns of Reproduction for a particular species. The male and female gametes tend to be released in a synchronized manner to ensure the successful encounter and gametic interaction. The female must be in the proper stage of her estrous cycle and a sufficient number of spermatozoa must be deposited into the female tract at the appropriate time.

The spermatozoa of domestic species must have been exposed for an adequate time to secretions from the female tract to undergo capacitation (see Chapter 7, Table 7-5). In addition the oocyte has only a limited lifespan within the oviduct, during which it can be fertilized (Table 10-5).

Any influence which disrupts normal reproductive patterns can prevent conception. This is a factor of importance when using AI because the female may be inseminated at a suboptimal time and with a number of spermatozoa in the inseminating dose lower than in the semen released during a natural mating. Most commonly, the effects of suboptimal timing are expressed in failure of conception. The female undergoes an infertile cycle and the return to estrus if a polyestrous species. In some cases, though fertilization may occur, the resulting embryo does not develop to term due to aging (Table 10-6).

Correct timing of insemination depends on accurate estrous detection or repetitive insemi-

nations until ovulation takes place. The major disadvantages of the routine use of repetitive inseminations lies in the increased costs of semen, labor, and the repeated challenges to the uterine defense mechanisms. However, animals given superovulatory treatments may need to be inseminated multiple times during estrus to ensure that all of the oocytes released are fertilized (see Chapter 19). The use of estrous synchronization programs to time inseminations invariably result in lower conception rates, when compared to natural breeding, or insemination after the detection of estrus.

In cattle, the "ideal" animal is in estrus for 12 to 18 hours with the optimum insemination time being 10 to 24 hours after the onset of estrus. The majority of cows begin estrus during the evening hours, which makes it difficult to ascertain the exact onset of estrus. Frozen bull semen that has been thawed, has a shorter lifespan for fertility. Consequently, one bull's semen may work successfully if used 10 hours after the onset of heat, whereas another bull's spermatozoa may fertilize the oocyte only when used 20 to 24 hours after the beginning of estrus.

Stallion spermatozoa do not withstand extension, and particularly, storage. As a result, AI with chilled semen stored for more than 24 to 36 hours results in lower conception rates. Also, mares inseminated with viable semen more than 6 hours post-ovulation have a very high rate of early embryonic death. In these cases, the mare may produce a detectable pregnancy, only to lose it in the first or second month of gestation.

Due to the impossibility to accurately predict the time of ovulation in the mare, multiple inseminations with fresh-extended semen were the rule. However, excessive breeding can be detrimental, due to the repetitive challenges to the mare's uterine defense mechanisms by contaminants in stallion semen. Currently, multiple palpations and ultrasound scans to predict the time of ovulation are being used in conjunction with the AI of mares. This approach reduces the number of inseminations to achieve pregnancy and maximizes the likelihood that the pregnancy will be maintained to term.

Similar situations affecting gamete aging and survival exist in the other domestic species.

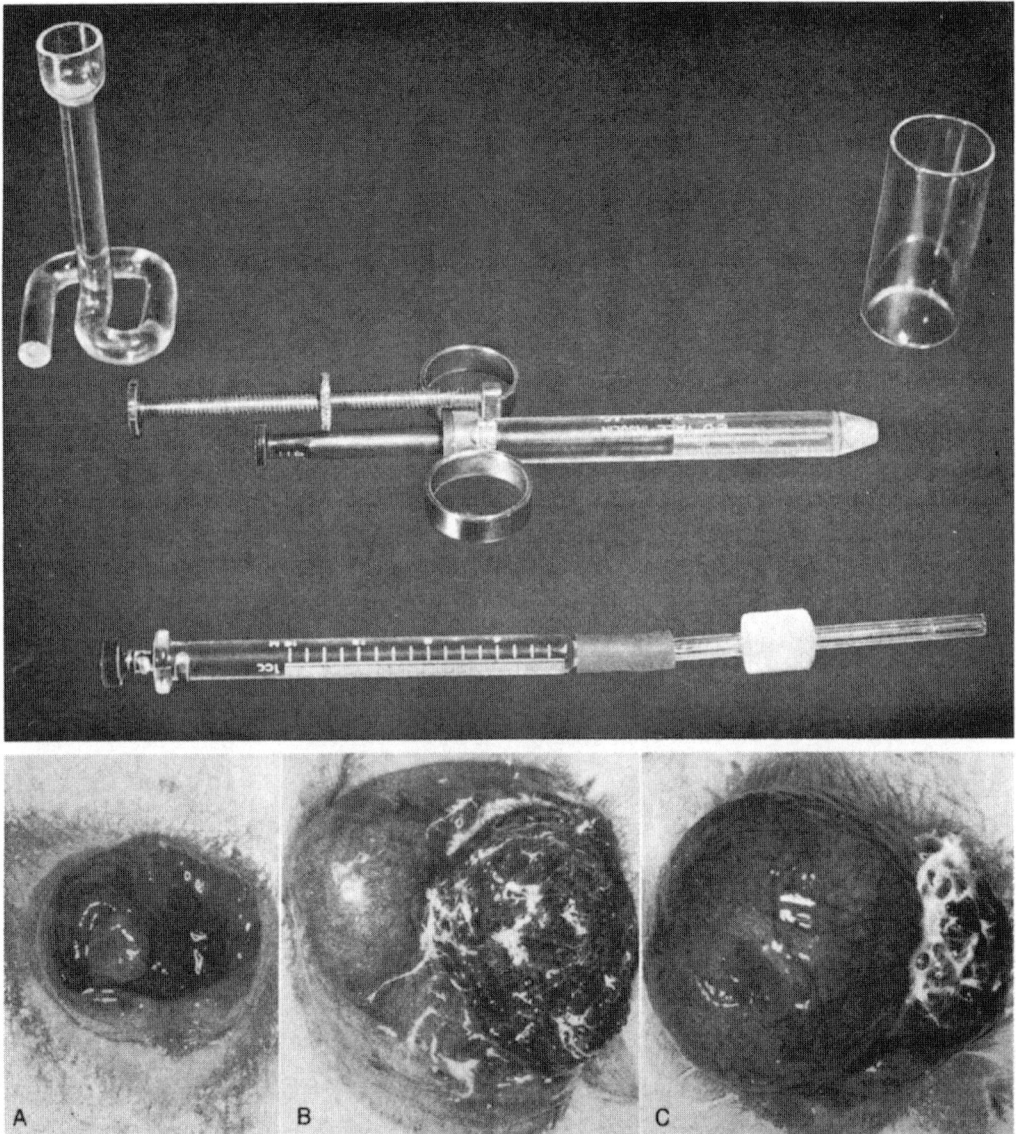

Fig. 10-22. Top picture, equipment used in artificial insemination of chickens and turkeys. Either of the two types of beakers shown should prove to be satisfactory for relatively small flocks. The two types of syringes have specific uses. The nut on the threaded rod and metal grips of upper syringe facilitate delivery of accurate dosage in mass-inseminated flocks. The detached glass tube on the lower syringe is useful in pedigree breeding such that each tube contains semen from an individual male. (Canadian Department of Agriculture: Artificial Insemination of Turkeys. Publ. No. 897, 1953). **Bottom pictures,** oviductal occluding plate in female turkeys. The establishment of a satisfactory level of fertility in the turkey breeding flock may be impaired or even prevented by the oviductal occluding plate. This plate is present in a high proportion of females at the time of the initial mating or AI. The oviductal occluding plate is a membranous tissue, located between the vaginal and the shell-gland portions of the oviduct and forms a physical barrier to the spermatozoa. In the female turkey nearing sexual maturity, the plate is at first small and inconspicuous (**A**), then light-colored tissue on the left, balloons (**B**), and finally becomes perforated (**C**) just before the laying of the first egg. (From: J. A. Harper, Poultry Sci. *42*:482, 1963).

Table 10-5　Effects of Aging on the Fertility of Bovine Oocytes

Hours from Ovulation to Insemination	Percentage of Cows with Fertilized Oocytes on Days 2–4 Post-insemination	Percentage of Cows with Normal Embryos or Feti; Days 21–290 of Gestation
2–4	75	75
6–8	75	30
9–12	60	31
14–16	25	0
18–20	40	17
22–28	0	0

Adapted from: G. R. Barrett, Time of Insemination and Conception Rates in Dairy Cows, PhD Thesis, Univ. of Wisconsin, Madison, WI, 1948.

Table 10-6　Postovulatory Aging of Porcine Oocytes in the Oviduct and Effects on Fertilization and Embryonic Survival at Day 25 Post-insemination

Estimated Age (Hours) of Oocyte at Fertilization	Percentage of Fertilized Oocytes	Percentage of Viable Embryos
0	90.8 ± 4.5	87.9 ± 2.9
4	92.1 ± 2.7	72.9 ± 14.9
8	94.6 ± 2.3	60.5 ± 13.2
12	70.3 ± 7.8	53.3 ± 15.7
16	48.3 ± 8.4	27.9 ± 14.5
20	50.9 ± 7.5	32.3 ± 15.2

Data are presented as mean ± SEM.
Adapted from: R. H. Hunter, Br. Vet. J. *133*:461, 1977.

The improvement of techniques for estrous detection and prediction of ovulation time would enhance the use of AI in all the domestic species. Improved procedures for semen cryopreservation and insemination are necessary for breeders of the other species to achieve results comparable to those routinely obtained by the AI of cattle.

REFERENCES

Disease Control

1. Anderson, J. B. and Warming, M. (1980): Danish legislative measures for the prevention and control of disease transmission through A.I. in cattle. Proc. 9th Int. Congr. Anim. Reprod. A.I., Madrid, Spain, June 16–20, 1980 Vol. III, p. 228.
2. Back, D. G., 1980, Pickett, B. W., Voss, J. L., et al. (1975); Effect of antibacterial agent on the motility of stallion spermatozoa at various storage times, temperatures and dilution ratios. J. Anim. Sci. *41*:137.
3. Bowne, J. M. (1986): Venereal diseases of stallions. *In*: Current Therapy in Equine Medicine, 2nd ed., edited by N. E. Robinson. Philadelphia, PA, W. B. Saunders, p. 508.
4. Bowen, R. A., Howard, T. H., Entwistle, K. W. et al. (1983): Seminal shedding of Bluetongue virus in experimentally infected mature bulls. Am. J. Vet. Res. *44*: 2268.
5. Brickon, R. D., Luedke, A. J., and Walton, T. E. (1980): Bluetongue virus in bovine semen: Viral isolation. Am. J. Vet. Res. *41*:439.
6. Cameron, R. D. A. (1976): Characteristics of semen changes during *Brucella ovis* infection in rams. Vet. Rec. *99*:231.
7. Carmichael, L. E. (1976): Canine brucellosis. An annotated review with selected cautionary comments. Theriogenology 6:105
8. Dubey, J. P. and Sharma, S. P. (1980): Prolonged excretion of *Toxoplasma gondii* in semen of goats. Am. J. Vet. Res. *41*:794.
9. Hall, C. E. and McEntee, K. (1981): Reduced post-thawing survival of sperm in bulls with mycoplasmal vesiculitis (*Mycoplasma bovigenitalium*). Cornell Vet. *71*:111.
10. Harbi, M. S. A. A., Elhassan, S. M., and Ahmed, M. A. (1983): Isolation and identification of *Mycoplasma bovigenitaluim* from imported semen of bulls. Vet. Rec. *113*:114.
11. Hashimoto, K., Kishma, M., Nakano, Y., et al. (1981): Isolation of Ureaplasmas sp. from bovine frozen semen, preputial washings and cervicovaginal mucus. Nat. Inst. Anim. Health Quart., Japan *21*:189.

12. Herman, H. A., Mitchell, J. R., and Doak, G. A. (1994): Extenders and extension of semen. *In*: Artificial Insemination and Embryo Transfer of Dairy and Beef Cattle, 8th ed. Interstate Publishers, Inc., Danville, IL, p. 101.

13. Humphrey, J. D., Little, P. B. Barnum, D. A., et al. (1982): Occurrence of *Haemophilus somnus* in bovine semen and in the prepuce of bulls and steers. Can. J. Comp. Med. *46*:215.

14. Kahrs, R. F., Gibbs, E. P. J., and Larsen, R. E. (1980): Diagnostic techniques for identifying viruses in bovine semen. Proc. 2nd Int. Symp. Vet. Lab. Diagnosticians, Lucerne, Switzerland, June 24–26, 1980, Vol. II, p. 274.

15. Kaja, R. W. and Olson, C. (1982): Non-infectivity of semen from bulls infected with bovine leukosis virus. Theriogenology *18*:107.

16. Kirkland, P. D., Mackintosh, S. G., and Moyle, A. (1984): The outcome of widespread use of semen from a bull persistently infected with pestivirus. Vet. Rec. *135*:527.

17. Kobisch, M. and Goffaux, M. (1980): Isolation of mycoplasma from boar semen. Proc. Int. Congr. Pig Vet. Soc., Copenhagen, Denmark, p. 217.

18. Krogh, H. V., Pedersen, K. B., and Blom, E. (1983): *Haemophilus somnus* in semen from Danish bulls. Vet. Rec. *112*:460.

19. LaFaunce, R. E. and McEntee, K. (1982): Experimental *Mycoplasma bovis* seminal vesiculitis in the bull. Cornell Vet. *72*:150.

20. Larsen, R. E. and Leman, A. D. (1980): Effect of pseudorabies on semen quality in the boar. Proc. 9th Int. Congr. Anim. Reprod. A. I., Madrid, Spain, June 16–20, 1980, Vol. III, p. 224.

21. Larsen, R. E., Shope, R. E. Jr., Leman, A. D., et al. (1980): Semen changes in boars after experimental infection with pseudorabies virus. Am. J. Vet. Res. *41*:733.

22. Larsen, A. B., Stalheim, O. H. V., Hughes, D. E., et al. (1981): *Mycobacterium paratuberculosis* in the semen and genital organs of a semen-donor bull. J. Am. Med. Assoc. *179*:169.

23. Nash, J. W. and Hanson, L. A. (1995): Bovine immunodeficiency virus in stud bull semen. Am. J. Vet. Res. *56*:760.

24. Rae, A. G. (1982): Isolation of mycoplasma from bovine semen. Vet. Rec. *111*:462.

25. Rideout, M. I., Burns, S. J., and Simpson, R. B. (1982): Influence of bacterial products on the motility of stallion spermatozoa. J. Reprod. Fertil., (Suppl. 32):35.

26. Romanowski, W., Marre, H., and Pfeilsticker, J. (1980): Hygiene at A. I. centers in special consideration of leucosis (sic). Proc. 9th Int. Congr. Anim. Reprod. A. I., Madrid, Spain, June 16–20, 1980, Vol. III, p. 258.

27. Rutherford, R. N. and Curnock, R. M. (1984): The use of sheep artificial insemination as an aid to the control of scrapie. Animal Production *38*:547, Abstract.

28. Scott, P. R. (1994): Control of venereal campylobacteriosis in a beef herd. Vet. Rec. *135*:162.

29. Sellers, R. F. (1983): Transmission of viruses by artificial breeding techniques: A review. J. Royal Soc. Med. *76*:772.

30. Sone, M., Ohmura, K., and Bamba, K. (1982): Effects of various antibiotics on the control of bacteria in boar semen. Vet. Rec. *111*:11.

31. Spire, M. F. (1995): Health management of beef bulls. Vet. Med. *90*:777.

32. Storz, J., Carroll, E. J., Stephenson, E. H., et al. (1976): Urogenital infection and seminal excretion after inoculation of bulls and rams with chlamydiae. Am. J. Vet. Res. *37*:517.

33. Thibier, M. and Nibart, N. (1987): Disease control and embryo importations. Theriogenology *27*:37.

34. Truscott, R. B. (1983): Factors associated with the determination of antibiotic activity in bovine semen. Can. J. Comp. Med. *47*:480.

35. Van der Schalie, J. and Evermann, J. (1989): Equine viral arteritis alert—Status in the Northwest. Equine Vet. Sci. *10*:14.

36. Van Oirschot, J. T. (1995): Bovine herpesvirus I in semen of bulls and the risk of transmission: A brief review. Vet. Quart. *17*:29.

Collection of Semen

37. Aamdal, J. (1960): Cattle. *In*: The Artificial Insemination of Farm Animals, 3rd., edited by E. J. Perry. New Brunswick, NJ, Rutgers University Press, p. 258.

38. Almquist, J. D., Branas, R. J., and Barber, K. A. (1976): Post-puberal changes in semen production of Charolais bulls ejaculated at high frequency and the relation between testicular measurements and sperm output. J. Anim. Sci. *42*:670.

39. Ball, L. (1976): Electroejaculation. *In*: Applied Electronics for Veterinary Medicine and Animal Physiology, edited by W. R. Klemm. Springfield, IL, Charles C. Thomas, p. 394.

40. Bongso, T. A., Jainudeen, M. R., and Zahrah, S. (1982): Relationship of scrotal circumference to age, body weight and spermatogenesis in goats. Theriogenology *18*:513.

41. Boucher, J. H., Foote, R. H., and Kirk, R. W. (1958): The evaluation of semen quality in the dog and the effects of frequency of ejaculation upon semen quality, libido, and depletion of sperm reserves. Cornell Vet. *48*:67.

42. Braun, W. F., Thompson, J. M., and Ross, C. V. (1980): Ram scrotal circumference measurements. Theriogenology *13*:221.

43. Chenoweth, P. J. (1989): Update on the breeding soundness examination of bulls. Beef Science Cattle Handbook. Lang Printing, Inc., Bryan, TX, *23*:125.

44. Crump, J., Jr. and Crump, J. (1989): Stallion ejaculation induced by manual stimulation of the penis. Theriogenology *31*:341.

45. Dowsett, K. F. and Pattie, W. A. (1980): Collection of semen from stallions at stud. Aust. Vet. J. *56*:373.

46. Elmore, R. G., Bierschwal, C. J., and Youngquist, R. S. (1976): Scrotal circumference measurements in 764 beef bulls. Theriogenology *6*:485.

47 Faulkner, L. C., Masken, J. F., and Hopwood, M. L. (1964): Fractionation of the bovine ejaculate. J. Dairy Sci. *47*:823.

48. Hafez, E. S. E. (1993): Artificial insemination. *In*: Reproduction in Farm Animals, 6th ed. Philadelphia, PA, Lea & Febiger, p. 424.

49. Hillman, R. B., Olar, T. T., Squires, R. L., et al. (1980): Temperature of the artificial vagina and its effect on seminal quality and behavioral characteristics of stallions. J. Am. Vet. Med. Assoc. *177*:720.

50. Kumi-Diaka, J., Nagaratnam, V., and Rwuaan, J. S. (1980): Seasonal and age-related changes in semen quality and testicular morphology of bulls in a tropical environment. Vet. Rec. *198*:13.

51. Morrow, D. (1980): Breeding soundness evaluation in bulls. *In*: Current Therapy in Theriogenology, 2nd ed., edited by D. A. Morrow. Philadelphia, PA, W. B. Saunders Co., p. 330.

52. Morton, D. B. and Bruce, S. G. (1989): Semen evaluation cryopreservation, and factors relevant to the use of frozen semen in dogs. J. Reprod. Fertil. (Suppl. 39):311.

53. Ott, R. S. (1986): Breeding soundness examination of bulls. *In*: Current Therapy in Theriogenology, Vol. 2, edited by D. A. Morrow. Philadelphia, PA, W. B. Saunders Co., p. 125.

54. Ott, R. S. and Memon, M. A. (1980): Breeding soundness examination of rams and bucks. A review. Theriogenology *13*:155.

55. Pickett, B. W. and Back, D. G. (1982): Procedures for preparation, collection, evaluation and insemination of stallion semen. Colorado State Univ. Exp. Sta. Anim. Reprod. Lab., Gen. Series Bulletin No. 935.

56. Pickett, B. W., Gebauer, M. R., Seidel, G. E., Jr., et al. (1974): Reproductive physiology of the stallion: Spermatozoal losses in the collection equipment and gel. J. Am. Vet. Med. Assoc. *165*:708.

57. Pineda, M. H. (1977): A simple method for collection of semen from dogs. Canine Pract. *4*:14.

58. Pineda, M. H., Dooley, M. P., Hembrough, F. B., et al. (1987): Retrograde flow of spermatozoa into the urinary bladder of rams. Am. J. Vet. Res. *48*:562.

59. Pineda, M. H. and Dooley, M. P. (1991): Effect of method of seminal collection on the retrograde flow of spermatozoa into the urinary bladder of rams. Am. J. Vet. Res. *52*:307.

60. Platz, C. C., Wildt, D. E., and Seager, S. W. J. (1978): Pregnancy in the domestic cat after artificial insemination with previously frozen spermatozoa. J. Reprod. Fertil. *52*:279.

61. Society for Theriogenology (1976): A Compilation of Current Information on Breeding Soundness Evaluation, and Related Subjects. Vol. VII, 2nd Edition, September, 1976.

62. Sojka, N. J., Jennings, L. L., and Hamner, C. E. (1970). Artificial Insemination of the Cat (*Felis catus* L.) Lab. Anim. Care *20*:199.

63. Tischner, M., Kosiniak, K., and Bielanski, W. (1974): Analysis of the pattern of ejaculation in stallions. J. Reprod. Fertil. *41*:329.

Analysis of Semen

64. Berger, T., Drobnis, E. Z., Foley, L., et al. (1994): Evaluation of relative fertility of cryopreserved goat semen. Theriogenology 41:711.

65. Bielanski, W. (1975): The evaluation of stallion semen in aspects of fertility control and its use for artificial insemination. J. Reprod. Fertil. (Suppl. 23):19.

66. Brown, K. I. and Graham, E. F. (1971): Effect of semen quality on fertility in turkeys. Poultry Sci. *50*:295.

67. Buckland, R B. (1971): Comparison of chicken semen diluents and evaluation of various methods of estimating fertility. Can. J. Anim. Sci. *51*:252.

68. Cochran, R. C., Judy, J. K., Parker, C. F., et al. (1985): Prefreezing and post thaw semen characteristics of five ram breeds collected by electro-ejaculation. Theriogenology *23*:431.

69. Dott, H. M. (1975): Morphology of stallion spermatozoa. J. Reprod. Fertil. (Suppl. 23):41.

70. Dowsett, K. F., Osborne, H. G., and Pattie, W. A. (1984): Morphological characteristics of stallion spermatozoa. Theriogenology *22*:463.

71. Dowsett, K. F. and Pattie, W. A. (1982): Stallion semen characteristics and fertility. J. Reprod. Fertil. (Suppl. 32):1.

72. Gibson, C. D. (1983): Clinical evaluation of the boar for breeding soundness: Physical examination and semen morphology. Compend. Cont. Educ. Pract. Vet. *5*:S244.

73. Hammitt, D. (1985): The relationship between heterospermic fertility *in vivo* and *in vitro* tests of spermatozoan quality and function. Ph.D. Thesis, Iowa State University, Ames, IA.

74. Harasymowycz, J., Ball, L., and Seidel, G. E., Jr. (1976): Evaluation of bovine spermatozoal morphologic features after staining or fixation. Am. J. Vet. Res. *37*:1053.

75. Hulet, C. V. (1977): Prediction of fertility in rams: Factors affecting fertility, and collection, testing and evaluation of semen. Vet. Med./Small Anim. Clin. *72*:1363.

76. Johnson, L., Berndtson, W. E., and Pickett, B. W. (1976): An improved method for evaluating acrosomes of bovine spermatozoa. J. Anim. Sci. *42*:951.

77. Linford, E., Glover, F. A., Bishop, C., et al. (1976): The relationship between semen evaluation methods and fertility in the bull. J. Reprod. Fertil. *47*:283.

78. Pickett, B. W., Sullivan, J. J., and Seidel, G. E., Jr. (1975): Reproductive physiology of the stallion. V. Effect of frequency of ejaculation on seminal characteristics and spermatozoal output. J. Anim. Sci. *40*:917.

79. Pickett, B. W., Voss, J. L., and Squires, E. L. (1983): Factors affecting quality and quantity of stallion spermatozoa. Compend. Cont. Educ. Pract. Vet. *5*:S259.

80. Swierstra, E. E. (1973): Influence of breed, age, and ejaculation frequency on boar semen composition. Can J. Anim. Sci. *53*:43.

81. Taha, M. B., Noakes, D. E., and Allen, W. E. (1981): The effect of season of the year on the characteristics and composition of dog semen. J. Small Anim. Pract. *22*:177.

82. Taha, M. B., Noakes, D. E., and Allen, W. E. (1983): The effect of the frequency of ejaculation on seminal characteristics and libido in the Beagle dog. J. Small Anim. Pract. *24*:309.

83. Voss, J. L., Pickett, B. W., and Squires, E. L. (1981): Stallion spermatozoal morphology and motility and their relationship to fertility. J. Am. Vet. Med. Assoc. *178*:287.

Semen Extension and Cryopreservation

84. Almquist, J. O. and Rosenberger, J. L. (1979): Effect of thawing time in warm water on fertility of bovine spermatozoa in plastic straws. J. Dairy Sci. *62*:772.

85. Berndtson, W. E. and Pickett, B. W. (1980): Evaluation of frozen semen. *In*: Current Therapy in Theriogenology, 2nd ed., edited by D. A. Morrow. Philadelphia, PA. W. B. Saunders Co., p. 347.

86. Brown, J. L., Senger, P. L., and Hillers, J. K. (1982): Influence of thawing time and post-thaw temperature on acrosomal maintenance and motility of bovine spermatozoa frozen in .5-ml french straws. J. Anim. Sci. *54*:938.

87. Cochran, J. D., Amann, R. P., Fromon, D. P., et al. (1984): Effects of centrifugation, glycerol level, cooling to 5°C freezing rate and thawing rate on the post-thaw motility of equine sperm. Theriogenology *22*:25.

88. Colas, G. (1975): Effect of initial freezing temperature, addition of glycerol and dilution on the survival and fertilizing ability of deep frozen ram semen. J. Reprod. Fertil. *42*:277.

89. Cristanelli, M. J., Squires, E. L., Amann, R. P. et al. (1984): Fertility of stallion semen processed, frozen and thawed by a new procedure. Theriogenology *22*:39.

90. Critser, J. K. (1999): Semen Cryopreservation and Artificial Insemination. Proc. Soc. Theriogenology Annu. Meeting, September 22–24, 1999, Nashville, Tennessee, p. 241.

91. Darin-Bannett, A. and White, I. G. (1977): Influence of cholesterol content or mammalian spermatozoa on susceptibility to cold shock. Cryobiology *14*:466.

92. DeAbreu, R. M., Berndtson, W. E., Smith, R. L., et al. (1979): Effect of post-thaw warming on viability of bovine spermatozoa thawed at different rates in french straws. J. Dairy Sci. *62*:1449.

93. Entwistle, K. W. and Martin, I. C. A. (1972): Effects of the number of spermatozoa and of volume of diluted semen on fertility in the ewe. Aust. J. Agric. Res. *23*:467.

94. Hammerstedt, R. H., Graham, J. K., and Nolan, J. P. (1990): Cryopreservation of mammalian sperm: What we ask them to survive. J. Androl. *11*:73.

95. Holt, W. V. and North, R. D. (1985): Determination of lipid composition and thermal phase transition temperature in an enriched plasma membrane fraction from ram spermatozoa. J. Reprod. Fertil. *73*:285.

96. Larsson, K. (1978): Deep-freezing of boar semen. Cryobiology *15*:352.

97. Lee, A. G. (1977): Lipid phase transitions. Biochem. Biophys. Acta *472*:237.

98. Loomis, P. R., Amann, R. P., Squires, E. L., et al. (1983): Fertility of stallion spermatozoa frozen in EDTA-lactose egg yolk extender and packaged in 0.5 ml straws. J. Anim. Sci. *56*:687.

99. Lundgren, B. (1980): Influence of long-term storage on fertility of deep frozen bull semen. Nordisk Vet. *32*:427.

100. Moore, H. D. M. and Hibbitt, K. G. (1977): Fertility of boar spermatozoa after freezing in the absence of seminal vesicular proteins. J. Reprod. Fertil. *50*:349.

101. Morris, G. R., Burtan, L. J., and Pitt, C. J. (1984): Sperm losses during deep-freeze processing of bull semen. Theriogenology *21*:1001.

102. Pickett, B. W. and Voss, J. L. (1975): The effect of semen extenders and sperm number on mare fertility. J. Reprod. Fertil. (Suppl. 23):95.

103. Pistenma, D. A., Snapir, N., and Mel, H. C. (1971): Biophysical characterization of fowl spermatozoa. I. Preservation of motility and fertilizing capacity under conditions of low temperature and low sperm concentrations. J. Reprod. Fertil. *24*:153.

104. Pope, C. E., Turner, J. L., Quatman, S. P., et al. (1991): Semen storage in the domestic felid. A comparison of cryopreservation methods and storage temperatures. Biol. Reprod. *44* (Suppl. 1):117.

105. Province, C. A., Amann. R. P., Pickett, B. W., et al. (1984): Extenders for the preservation of canine and equine spermatozoa at 5°C. Theriogenology *22*:409.

106. Quinn, P. J. (1989): Principles of membrane stability and phase behavior under extreme conditions. J. Bioenerg. Biomembr. *21*:3.

107. Robbins, R. K., Saacke, R. G., and Chandler, P. T. (1976): Influence of freeze rate, thaw rate and glycerol level on acrosomal retention and survival of bovine spermatozoa in straws. J. Anim. Sci. *42*:145.

108. Rodriguez, O. L., Berndtson, W. E. Ennen, B. D., et al. (1975): Effects of the rates of freezing, thawing and level of glycerol on the survival of bovine spermatozoa in straws. J. Anim. Sci. *41*:129.

109. Salamon, S. and Visser, D. (1974): Fertility of ram spermatozoa frozen-stored for 5 years. J. Reprod. Fertil. *37*:433.

110. Senger, P. L., Becker, W. C., and Hillers, J. K. (1976): Effect of thawing rate and post-thaw temperature on motility and acrosomal maintenance in bovine semen frozen in plastic straws. J. Anim. Sci. *42*:932.

111. Senger, P. L., Mitchell, J. R., and Almquist, J. O. (1983): Influence of cooling rates and extenders upon post-thaw viability of bovine spermatozoa packaged in .25 and .5 ml french straws. J. Anim. Sci. *56*:1261.

112. Smith, F. (1984): Update in freezing canine semen. Proc. Soc. Theriogenology Annu. Meeting, Sept. 26–28, 1983, Denver, CO., p. 61.

113. Sullivan, J. J. (1978): Characteristics and cryopreservation of stallion spermatozoa. Cryobiology *15*:355.

114. White, I. G. and Darin-Bennett, A. (1976): The lipids of sperm in relation to cold shock. Proc. 8th Int. Congr. Anim. Reprod. A.I., Cracow, Poland, July 12–16, 1976, Vol. 4, p. 951.

115. Wilmut, I. and Polge, C. (1977): The low temperature preservation of boar spermatozoa. 1. The motility and morphology of boar spermatozoa frozen and thawed in the presence of permeating protective agents. Cryobiology *14*:471.

116. Wilmut, I. and Polge, C. (1977): The low temperature preservation of boar spermatozoa. 2. The motility and morphology of boar spermatozoa frozen and thawed in diluent which contained only sugar and egg yolk. Cryobiology *14*:479.

117. Wilmut, I. and Polge, C. (1977): The low temperature preservation of boar spermatozoa. 3. The fertilizing capacity of frozen and thawed boar semen. Cryobiology *14*:483.

Insemination Procedures

118. Aamdal, J. (1960): Cattle. *In*: The Artificial Insemination of Farm Animals, 3rd ed., edited by E. J. Perry. New Brunswick, NJ, Rutgers University Press, p. 264.

119. American Breeders Service (1986): Straw insemination procedure. *In:* A. I. Management Manual, 2nd ed., edited by W. R. Grace Co., DeForest, WI, p. 48.

120. Asbury, A. C. (1984): Uterine defense mechanisms in the mare: The use of intrauterine plasma in the management of endometritis. Theriogenology *21*:387.

121. Bailey, M. T., Bott, R. M., and Gimenez, T. (1995): Breed registries' regulations on artificial insemination an embryo transfer. J. Equine. Vet. Sci. *15*:60.

122. Ball, G. D., Leinfried, M. L., Lenz, R. W., et al. (1983): Factors affecting successful *in vitro* fertilization of bovine follicular oocytes. Biol. Reprod. *28*:717.

123. affecting fertility: Artificial insemination program for beef cattle. Bov. Pract. *1*:35.

124. Chenoweth, P. J., Spitzer, J. C., and Ramge, J. C. (1980): Beef cattle breeding programs employing synchronization of estrus and artificial insemination. Southwestern Vet. *33*:31.

125. Christenson, R. K. (1989): Breeding management of swine. In: Sow Manual, Society for Theriogenology, Vol. 17, p. 17.

126. Cooper, W. L. (1980): Artificial breeding of horses. Vet. Clin. North Am., Large Anim. Pract. *2*:267.

127. Douglas-Hamilton, D. H., Osol, G., et al. (1984):A field study of the fertility of transported equine semen. Theriogenology *22*:291.

128. Edwards, D. F. and Aizinbud, E. (1980): Bibliography on the timing of artificial insemination in cattle, sheep and pigs by measurement of vaginal conductivity. Bibliography Reprod. *36*:425 and 549.

129. Foote, R. H. (1996): Review: Dairy cattle reproductive physiology research and management—past progress and future prospects. J. Dairy Sci. *79*:980.

130. Gomez, W. R. (1977): Artificial insemination. In: Reproduction in Domestic Animals, 3rd ed., edited by H. H. Cole and P. T. Cupps. New York, NY, Academic Press, Inc. p. 257.

131. Goodrowe, K. L. (1992): Feline reproduction and artificial breeding technologies. Proc. 12th Int. Congr. Anim. Reprod. A.I., The Hague, Netherlands, August 23–27, 1992. Reprinted from: Anim. Reprod. Sci. *28*:389, 1992.

132. Huhtinen, M., Koskines, E., Skidmore, J. A., et al. (1996): Recovery rate and quality of embryos from mares inseminated after ovulation. Theriogenology *45*:719.

133. Hunter, R. H. F. (1977): Physiological factors influencing ovulation, fertilization, early embryonic development and establishment of pregnancy in pigs. Br. Vet. J. *133*:461.

134. Husein, M. Q., Ababneh, M. M., Crabo, B. G., et al. (1996): Out-of-season breeding of ewes using transcervical artificial insemination. Sheep Goat Res. J. *12*:39.

135. Kenney, R. M., Bergman, R. V., Cooper, W. L., et al. (1975): Minimal contamination techniques for breeding mares: Technique and preliminary findings. Proc. Am. Assoc. Equine Pract., Boston, MA, Dec. 1–3, 1975, p. 327.

136. Manothaiudom, K., Johnston, S. D., Hegstad, R. L., et al. (1995): Evaluation of the ICAGEN-target canine ovulation timing diagnostic test in detecting canine plasma progesterone concentrations. J. Am. Anim. Hosp. Assoc. *31*:57.

137. Nicholas, F. W. (1996): Genetic improvement through reproductive technology. Anim. Reprod. Sci. *42*:205.

138. Ott, R. S. (1981): Use of a teaser bull in a beef cattle artificial insemination program. J. Am. Vet. Med. Assoc. *179*:694.

139. Park, Y. W. and Hunter, A. G. (1977): Effect of repeated inseminations with egg yolk semen extender on fertility in cattle. J. Dairy Sci. *60*:1645.

140. Perry, E. J. (1960): Cattle. In: The Artificial Insemination of Farm Animals, 3rd ed., edited by E. J. Perry. New Brunswick, NJ, Rutgers University Press, p. 113.

141. Pickett, B. W. and Back, D. G. (1973): Procedures for Preparation, Collection, Evaluation, and Insemination of Stallion Semen. Information Series No. 2-1, Anim. Reprod. Lab., Colorado State University, Fort Collins, CO, p. 19.

142. Rossdale, P. D. and Ricketts, S. W. (1980): The stallion. In: Equine Stud Farm Medicine, 2nd ed. London, England, Bailliere Tindall, p. 158.

143. Schams, D., Schallenberger, E., Hoffman, B., et al. (1977): The oestrous cycle of the cow: Hormonal parameters and time relationships concerning oestrus, ovulation and electrical resistance of the vaginal mucus. Acta Endocrinol. *86*:180.

144. Schindler, H. and Amir, D. (1973): The conception rate of ewes in relation to sperm dose and times of insemination. J. Reprod. Fertil. *34*:191.

145. Seager, S. W. J. and Platz, C. C. (1977): Artificial insemination and frozen semen in the dog. Vet. Clin. North Am. *7*:757.

146. Seager, S. W. J., Platz, C. C., and Fletcher, W. S. (1975): Conception rates and related data using frozen dog semen. J. Reprod. Fertil. *45*:18.

147. Smith, R. D. (1986): Estrous detection. In: Current Therapy in Theriogenology, 2nd ed., edited by D. A. Morrow. Philadelphia, PA, W. B. Saunders Co., p. 153.

148. Stover, D. G. and Sokolowski, J. H. (1978): Estrous behavior of the domestic cat. Feline Pract. *8*:54.

149. Sturman, H., Bakhar, A., and Ben-Smuel, Z. (1980): The rate of incidence and damage caused by insemination of cows not in estrus in large dairy herds in Israel. Proc. 9th Int. Congr. Anim. Reprod. A. I., Madrid, Spain, June 16–20, 1980, Vol. III, p. 236.

150. Watson, E. D. and MacDonald, B. J. (1984): Failure of conception in dairy cattle: Progesterone and oestrdiol-17B concentration and the presence of ovarian follicles in relation to the timing of artificial insemination. Br. Vet. J. *149*:398.

151. Watson, R. H. and Radford, H. M. (1960): The influence of rams on onset of oestrus in Merino ewes in the spring. Aust. J. Agric. Res. *11*:65.

152. Wenkoff, M. (1986): Estrous synchronization in cattle. In: Current Therapy in Theriogenology, 2nd ed., edited by D. A. Morrow. Philadelphia, PA, W. B. Saunders Co, p. 158.

153. Woodard, A. E. and Abplanalp, H. (1975): The effects of three systems of housing turkey breeder males on semen quality and quantity. Poultry Sci. *54*:872.

Aging of Gametes

154. Barrett, G. R. (1948): Time of insemination and conception rates in dairy cows. Ph.D. Thesis, University of Wisconsin, Madison, WI.

155. Eppig, J. J. and O'Brien, M. (1995): *In vitro* maturation and fertilization of oocytes isolated from aged mice. A strategy to rescue valuable genetic resources. J. Assist. Reprod. Genet. *12*:269.

156. Hunter, R. H. F. (1991): Oviduct function in pigs with particular reference to the pathological condition of polyspermy. Mol. Reprod. Develop. *29*:385.

157. Hunter, R. H. (1977): Physiological factors influencing ovulation, fertilization, early embryonic development and establishment of pregnancy in pigs. Br. Vet. J. *133*:461.

158. Kim, N. H., Moon, S. J., Prather, R. S., et al. (1996): Cytoskeletal alterations in aged porcine oocytes and parthenogenesis. Mol. Reprod. Develop. *43*:513.

159. Longo, F. J. and So. F. (1982): Transformations of sperm nuclei incorporated into aged and unaged hamster eggs. J. Androl. 3:420.

160. Vander Vliet, W. L. and Hafez, E. S. E. (1974): Survival and aging of spermatozoa: A review. Am. J. Obstet. Gynecol. 118:1006.

References Added in Proof

161. Hohenboken, W. D. (1999): Applications of sexed semen in cattle production. Theriogenology *52*:1421.

162. Lopez-Gatius, F. (2000): Site of semen deposition in cattle: A review. Theriogenology *53*:1407.

Patterns of Reproduction

M. P. DOOLEY AND M. H. PINEDA

11

INTRODUCTION

The patterns of reproduction of animals vary between and within species, particularly in relation to breeds and nutritional status. This chapter presents summarized interspecies information, identifies environmental factors that affect reproduction, and introduces the reader to the chapters that describe the reproductive patterns of domestic animals. Table 11–1 summarizes some pertinent facts concerning the female reproductive patterns of wild mammals, including exotic and marsupial species and Table 11–2 contains data for laboratory animal species. A detailed description of the reproductive patterns of wild mammals and laboratory animal species is beyond the scope of this textbook. Regarding domesticated species, the onset of reproductive activity, patterns of estrous cyclicity, and ovulatory responses of cattle, horses, sheep, goats, swine, dogs, cats, alpacas, and llamas are summarized in Table 11–3. The reproductive patterns and physiology of these species are described in greater detail in Chapters 12 through 18.

The reproductive patterns of animals in their natural environments differ greatly from those of domesticated animals which have become adapted to a protected environment. However, the reproductive activities of animals in their natural habitat and given time, those of domestic animals that are removed from a protected environment, always tend toward a pattern which will result in the birth of the young during the period of the year when temperature and feed are optimal and chances of survival, greater.

Man's Dependency on Animal Products

Man's dependency on animal products has created a continuous demand for the selection of animals to ensure an available supply of milk, meat, eggs, and fiber to meet the needs of an ever-increasing human population.

The selection for productivity through animal breeding is slowed because of the length of the gestation period, the time required for animals to reach puberty, and the need to test for desirable traits in the offspring. Furthermore, in biparental sexual reproduction, the expression of the genotype transmitted to the offspring by the dam and sire is not totally predictable. Each offspring receives only half of the somatic chro-

Table 11-1 Summary of Reproductive Patterns of Selected Non-domesticated Species

Species	Puberty (months)	Inter-estrous Interval (days)	Estrus Duration (days)	Ovulation Time Relative to Estrus	Gestation Length (days)	Litter Size	Breeding Season[a]
Antelope, roan	—	—	—	—	300	1	non-seasonal
Ass, donkey	12	21–28	2–7	—	365	1	Mar.–Aug. (N)
Bear, N. Am., black	36	—	1–3	last 1/3	~210	1–4	May–June (N)
Beaver, Am.	24	—	—	postcoitus	~90	1–6	Jan.–Feb. (N)
Bison, Am. buffalo	24	21	2	—	270	1	July–Sept. (N)
Bobcat	12–24	44	—	—	~55	1–6	Feb.–Apr. (N)
Camel, two-humped	36	10–20	1–7	32–40 h (M)	402	1	Dec.–April (N)
Cheetah	24	27	—	—	90–95	1–4	non-seasonal
Chimpanzee	8–11	27	—	—	227	1	non-seasonal
Chinchilla	6–8	38	2–3	—	111	1–3	Dec.–May (N)
Chipmunk, western	< 12	—	—	—	28–30	5	April (N)
Coyote, northern	9–10	—	10	—	60–63	5–7	Jan.–Mar. (N)
Deer, mule	12–24	~28	—	—	204	1–2	Oct.–Nov. (N)
Elephant, African	96–144	42	3–4	—	660	1	non-seasonal
Elk, moose	16–24	30	—	—	245	1–2	Sept.–Oct. (N)
Fox, red or silver	12–14	—	2–4	first 1/2	52	4–5	Dec.–Mar. (N)
Giraffe	36–48	14	1	—	435	1	non-seasonal
Gorilla	60–84	32	1	—	258	1	non-seasonal
Ground hog, woodchuck	24	—	—	—	32	4	Feb.–Mar. (N)
Guanaco	12–24	—	—	—	350	1	Nov.–Jan. / July–Aug. (S)
Hippopotamus	48	30	4–7	—	237	1–2	non-seasonal
Hyena	18–24	40–50	1–4	—	90–95	2–4	non-seasonal
Jaguar	—	44	11	—	109	1–4	Jan.–Mar. (S)
Kangaroo, gray	20–22	35	6	—	31	1	Oct.–Mar. (S)
Leopard	28–32	43	7	—	90–100	2–4	non-seasonal
Lion	40	51	7	—	108	2–4	non-seasonal
Marmot	—	—	0.5	—	33	7	Apr. (N)
Mink	10	2	—	40–48 h (M)	46–70 (D)	4–5	Feb.–Apr. (N)
Mole, Am.	—	12	—	postcoitus	28	4	Feb.–Mar. (N)
Monkey, S. Am. spider	—	—	—	—	139	1–2	non-seasonal

Muskrat	5–12	28	3–5	—	28	6–7	Apr.–July (N)
Opossum, common Va.	6	28	1–2	first ¹/₂	12	5–13	Jan.–Nov. (N)
Panda	72–90	—	4–14	—	140	1–2	Mar.–May (N)
Porcupine, N. Am.	15	29	0.5	—	210	1	Sept.–Nov. (N)
Porpoise	14	—	—	—	300–330	1	July–Aug. (N)
Prairie dog	12	—	—	1	30	3–5	Feb.–Mar. (N)
Rabbit, cottontail	5–7	—	—	—	25–30	2–7	Jan.–June (N)
Raccoon	10	3	—	postcoitus	63	3–4	Jan.–Mar. (N)Reindeer,
caribou	18	—	—	—	225	1	Sept.–Oct. (N)
Rhinoceros, black	48–72	28–35	2–3	—	460	1	non-seasonal
Sheep, bighorn	18–24	—	—	—	180	1	July–Dec. (N)
Skunk	10	—	—	—	62	4–6	Apr. (N)
Squirrel, Am. red	10–12	—	—	—	33–38	3–5	Feb.–July (N)
Tiger	36–48	51	7	—	105–110	2–5	Mar.–Apr. (N)
Vicuña	24	9–10	—	—	340	1	Nov.–Jan. (S)
Walrus	60–72	—	—	—	330	1	Jan.–Apr. (N)
Whale, sperm	8–15	—	—	—	445–500	1	Mar.–May (N)
Wildebeest (Gnu)	16–18	—	—	—	240	1	Jan.–May (N)
Wolf	24	—	—	—	61	2–7	Jan.–Mar. (N)
Wolverine	12–24	—	—	—	—	2–4	Apr.–Oct. (N)
Zebra	12–13	21	3–6	—	362	1	Nov.–Feb. (S)

— = Not applicable or data not available.

[a]Breeding season for animals in their natural habitat; where indicated, data is for animals in northern (N) or southern (S) hemisphere.

(D = Delayed implantation / embryonic diapause; h = hour; M = Ovulation time in relation to time of mating = hours postcoitus).

Adapted mainly from: V. Hayssen, A. van Tienhoven, and A. van Tienhoven, Asdell's Patterns of Mammalian Reproduction: A Compendium of Species-Specific Data, Ithaca, N.Y., Cornell University Press, 1993; and from other sources including; S. A. Asdell, Patterns of Mammalian Reproduction, 2nd. ed. Ithaca, N. Y., Comstock-Cornell Press, 1964; G. E. Lamming, Marshall's Physiology of Reproduction, Vol. 1, Reproductive Cycles of Vertebrates, 4th ed. New York, N.Y., Churchill Livingstone, 1984.

Table 11-2   Summary of Reproductive Patterns of Selected Laboratory Animal Species

Species	Puberty (months)	Inter-estrous Interval (days)	Estrus Duration (days)	Ovulation Time Relative to Estrus	Gestation Length (days)	Litter Size
Ferret	7–12	—	3–5	30 h (M)	42	6–10
Gerbil, Mongolian	1–2	4–6	0.5	—	24–26	4–5
Guinea pig	3	16.5	0.5	last $^1/_4$	68	4
Hamster, Golden	1–2	4	1	last $^1/_2$	16	6–7
Mouse, albino	2	4–5	0.5	first $^1/_3$	21	12
Rabbit, albino	6–9	—	—	11–12 h (M)	31	4–7
Rat, albino	2–3	4–5	0.5	last $^1/_3$	22	10

— = Not applicable or data not available.
(h = hour; M = Ovulation time in relation to time of mating = hours postcoitus).
Adapted mainly from: V. Hayssen, A. van Tienhoven, and A. van Tienhoven, Asdell's Patterns of Mammalian Reproduction: A Compendium of Species-Specific Data, Ithaca, N.Y., Cornell University Press, 1993; and G. E. Lamming, Marshall's Physiology of Reproduction, Vol. 1, Reproductive Cycles of Vertebrates, 4th ed. New York, N.Y., Churchill Livingstone, 1984.

Table 11-3   Characteristics of the Estrous Cycle in Domestic and Domesticated Species

Species	Puberty (months)	Interestrous Interval	Breeding Season[a]	Estrus (days)	Type of Ovulation	Time of Ovulation
Alpaca	6–12	Recurring waves of follicular growth every 8 to 12 days, if not mated	Nov.–Mar.	Continuous	Induced by coitus	24 to 48 hours after mating
Bitch	9–16	Bitches are monoestric; with an interestrous interval of 7.4 months	NS	9 to 12	Spontaneous	During the first 3 days of standing estrus
Cat	8–13	Nonmated queens display a series of nonovulatory estruses	Jan.–Mar./ Aug.–Sept	7 to 10	Induced by coitus	24 to 48 hours after mating
Cow	9–11	20 to 22 days	NS	0.6 to 0.8	Spontaneous	12 to 18 hours after the end of estrus
Ewe	6–7	16 to 17 days	Sept.–Jan.	1 to 2	Spontaneous	By the end of the 2nd day of estrus
Goat	4–8	21 days; shorter cycles may occur at beginning and end of breeding season	Aug.–Dec.	1 to 3	Spontaneous	30 to 36 hours after the onset of estrus
Llama	6–12	Recurring waves of follicular growth every 11 to 18 days, if not mated	Nov.–Mar.	Continuous	Induced by coitus	26 to 48 hours after mating
Mare	12–24	20 to 23 days	Mar.–Aug.	4 to 8	Spontaneous	24 to 48 hours before end of standing estrus
Sow	6–7	21 days	NS	2 to 3	Spontaneous	By the end of 2nd or 3rd day of estrus

NS = Nonseasonal.
[a]Months shown for breeding season are for animals in the northern hemisphere.
Summary of information provided in Chapters 12 through 18 of this textbook.

mosomes and one sex chromosome from each parent. In addition, the heritability of productivity traits for milk, meat, and fiber is low and oftentimes, sexual reproduction becomes economically inefficient, particularly when these productive traits are associated with undesirable characteristics, such as low survival rate, decreased resistance to disease, and infertility due to the inbreeding associated with the selection for desirable traits.

Many approaches and techniques for enhancing the reproductive capacity and number of offspring sired by individual animals have been developed in the last 40 years. These include artificial insemination, estrous synchronization and superovulatory treatments, embryo recovery and manipulation, including *in vitro* or *in vivo* culture, *in vitro* fertilization, embryo splicing, gene-insertion, cryopreservation, embryo transfer, twinning, and cloning. Without a doubt, the application of these technologies have and will continue to enhance the production of fiber and animal proteins used for human consumption.

BREEDING AND PATTERNS OF REPRODUCTION

As discussed in Chapter 7, sexual reproduction and internal fertilization requires that the mating partners receive internal and external cues to elicit behavioral responses and stimuli which synchronize the release of spermatozoa and oocytes. For most species, the courtship activities which lead to ejaculation and the release of spermatozoa and ovulation of oocytes must occur within a matter of hours of each other to ensure a successful fertilization and pregnancy.

Frequently, males have to overcome a number of obstacles, including fighting with other males to find and successfully inseminate females in standing estrus. The typical male attempts to copulate and mate with as many females as available. Many times, males will attempt to copulate with females that have already been mated and therefore, received all of the spermatozoa that are needed to ensure fertilization of the oocytes. Females, on the other hand, act more selectively in accepting several matings with a given male, while refusing to

stand to copulate with other males. These traits are still present in domesticated animals, though they are more pronounced in wild or semi-wild species, in which the reproductive activities are restricted to a particular month or months of the year.

Years of exposure to controlled environmental conditions, including feeding of balanced diets, and the selection for specific production traits, such as milk, meat, and wool have imposed further burden on the females of domesticated species. As a consequence of these selective pressures, the nonpregnant cycle, which is an oddity in wild species, becomes the norm in species selected for high productivity (Table 11–3). For example, high milk-producing cows are difficult to settle and require several natural or artificial inseminations to become pregnant and, in addition, have a prolonged, infertile postpartum period. Wild Bovidae are essentially monoestric, become pregnant as a result of mating in a single estrus, and produce just enough milk to feed the calf, whereas, a high milk-producing cow can produce thousands of pounds of milk during a single lactation period. Thus, these cows could feed many calves everyday, even though they normally give birth to a single calf. The selection pressure and demands for high productivity in farm animal species requires provision of all needed nutrients at levels that become costly, in addition to the costs associated with the protection of animals from harsh environmental conditions.

Motivational Force for Mating

To postulate that animals, from insects to mammals, mate to perpetuate the species seems at odds and actually, very unlikely. Nevertheless, the urge to copulate—as the driving force—and its derived consequence, to reproduce, is very strong among all animal phyla. Males from many species, particularly those from wild species, go to extreme efforts of endurance and travel large distances in search of a receptive female. In the process they may fight with other males to protect their territory and keep other potential suitors at bay. On occasion, one or more of the combatants is mortally wounded and perishes. The male praying mantis 'loses' his head during mating because the female mantis bites the head off. This is not a deterrent, because the decapitated male continues to ejaculate and when copulation is completed, the female praying mantis eats the body of the male.

Females in season, from insects to mammals, use behavioral stances and release pheromones to announce to potential suitors that they are receptive and willing to accept the amorous advances of the male for mating. All of these activities, particularly for wild mammals, are highly demanding in energy and exhaustive of the stored energy needed to survive in lean times, such as during Winter or during extended periods of drought.

Whatever generates the strong urge to mate and engage in sexual reproduction between partners is controlled by internal and external signals, including endocrine and certain exocrine secretions, such as pheromones. These result in behavioral cues, all exquisitely coordinated by the mammalian nervous system. Many of these factors have been discussed in Chapters 7, 8, and 9. However, a puzzling question still remains unanswered: Why do animals, from invertebrates to mammals, spend so much time, energy, and effort to mate and, as a derived consequence, to reproduce? To suggest that males have the instinctive desire to spread their genes, and that they are willing to succumb in the process, for the good of the species, is difficult to accept as the motivational force for the behavior of the individual. Let us return to the praying mantis and assume the male mantis did not know what was coming to him. Obviously, the motivating force for the male was not to sacrifice his own body. It is even more difficult to accept that the male had the altruistic purpose of self-sacrifice by offering the female his own body proteins and other nutrients, as a postcoital and posthumous banquet for the good of the population of mantises. Further, some male spiders, somehow know or anticipate they are at risk of being killed, and perhaps eaten, while attempting to mate with the female spider. Hence, during evolution, males of certain spider species must have 'learned' something, because they go to extremes of caution and use a variety of approaches to ensure the female is really receptive and that she will not kill and eat them, during or after copulation. The male mantis may have not had the opportunity to 'learn' anything because the female mantis removes the male's head early in the process of copulation.

What is the motivational force, the urge for mating that drives males of all species from insects to mammals to seek, fight for, and even die for the opportunity to copulate with a receptive female? Some male birds go to extremes of beautiful displays of color and sound to entice the female to accept them as a partner. Could it be that copulation and associated sexual activities are highly pleasurable for the copulating partners of all species? Perhaps, the urge to copulate, though internally controlled by hormones and externally by pheromones, is a learned process. If this is true, then males of all species eventually succumb to the instinctive desire to seek the enjoyment to copulate, regardless of the risks involved in the process, as appears to be the case.

Control of Mating Behavior

For several species, a primary period of estrogen exposure followed by exposure to progesterone or progestagens is needed to induce behavioral receptivity and postural adjustment for mating in intact or ovariectomized females. Similar sequences of exposure to estrogens first, followed by ovulation and secretion of progesterone is the norm in most of the domestic species.

The domestic cat and South American camelids, as induced-ovulators, seem to be the exception in that the queen and female camelids develop receptive behavior and mating stance in response to priming by estrogens alone, without the need for a subsequent exposure to progesterone. In fact, significant levels of progesterone in the blood of queens and South American camelids are detected only after ovulation and the associated luteinization of follicular cells induced by mating(s) which is conducive to the formation of the corpus luteum.

In all species, levels of progesterone or progestagens above the basal level are associated with anestrus, particularly during pregnancy.

GEOPHYSICAL AND BIOLOGICAL CYCLES

Domestic animals have evolved in constant interaction with cues from the physical environment and from their association and dependence on plant and other animal species including man. Those animals that survived major geologic changes have developed mechanisms to sense, undergo physiological adaptation, and respond to environmental patterns of light and dark, and to seasonal changes affecting the habitat and availability of nutritional resources. Hence, it should not be surprising that biological organisms also display various elements of periodicity in physiologic processes as they pro-

ceed through the cycle of life and reproduction (Fig. 11–1).

Across species, the acquisition of reproductive capability is eventually followed by a decline in reproductive capacity or reproductive senescence, and death (Fig. 11–1). Domestic animals which are used for food and fiber, seldom reach an age of senescence, as can be seen in pet animals. These animals are culled when their productivity declines to noneconomical levels; oftentimes long before the onset of reproductive senescence.

Despite the marked variations in size, form, and utilization of nutritional resources, animals of all species, and plants for that matter, gener-

The Cycle of Life in Domestic Animals

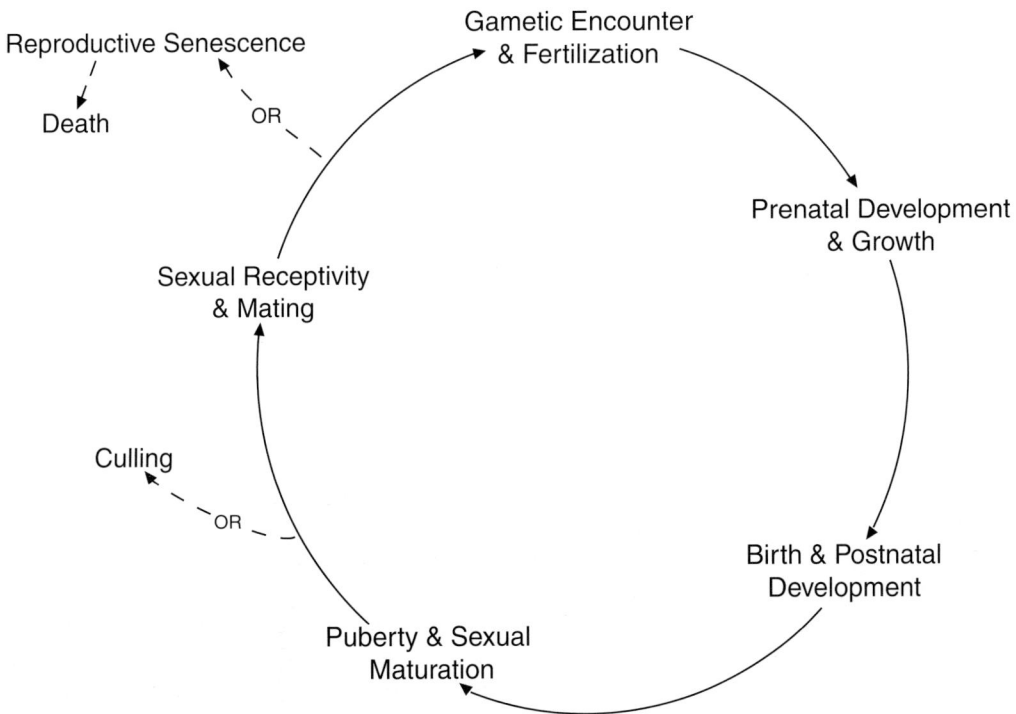

Fig. 11–1. The genetic make-up of an individual is established at fertilization and the germinal cells of the individual are established during the period of prenatal development. Animals acquire the capability of producing and releasing the gametes which give rise to the next generation after an extended period of postnatal growth and development, puberty, and sexual maturation. Hence, the repetition and fidelity of this cyclical pattern of gametic encounter and fertilization, development, growth, and sexual maturation of the organism is essential for the generation of new individuals and the survival of the species. The timing and periodicity of events, particularly the onset of puberty and the intermittent periods of sexual receptivity of females, are influenced by nutritional resources, social interactions, and environmental cues.

ate new individuals through events which can be related to the mitotic regulation of cell growth and division, cellular interactions, and the differentiation of cells, tissues, and organs. Processes that are the result of biologic mutation and evolutionary pressures. Through various mechanisms, animals have developed the ability to communicate and sense events within their natural environment. Thus, in response to environmental stresses or seasonal changes, animals undergo physiologic adaptations that maximize the likelihood of survival and ensure the successful reproduction of new individuals.

Among mammalian species, these adaptations include the development of sexual, internal reproduction and the partitioning of reproductive processes among male and female animals. Developmental differences among males and females, the lengthy interval from birth to the attainment of adult size and form and the assumption of reproductive capability, social interactions of individuals within and between sexes, and the distribution of responsibilities for nurturing offspring among parents or within males and females of a social group, are direct consequences of heterogamy and the sexual differentiation of individuals (see Chapter 7).

Geophysical Cycles

The nature of environmental variations to which animals are exposed has varied over geologic time. Existing species undoubtedly have developed evolutionary strategies and adaptive schemes for survival. The earth's environment varies day to day, month to month, and year to year, with respect to the earth's coordinates, including the distance from the equator. Animals and species that have survived to this point in time are the winners of the intra- and interspecific competition for resources and habitat. Due to those events that can be related to the rotation of the earth about its axis, the orbit of the earth around the sun, and the orbit of the moon around the earth and its relationship to the sun, various elements of geophysical periodicity have been identified (Table 11–4). For the sake of discussion, sidereal events are defined as temporal elements that can be related to the relative position of the stars and constellations and can be broadly

subdivided into: Ultradian, Circadian, and Infradian rhythms (Table 11–4). **Ultradian** rhythms are repeated at intervals that are less than the sidereal day of 23 hours, 56 minutes, and 4.09 seconds. **Circadian** rhythms are repeated at intervals which approximate the sidereal day, i.e., the time for the earth to complete a single rotation about its axis. **Infradian** rhythms are repeated at intervals which exceed the sidereal day, and include periods which may last for only a few days, to several months, or to a full year, the time required for the earth to complete a single rotation of its orbit around the sun.

The earth's axis is tilted with respect to the sun, hence, as the earth completes a single rotation about the sun, most areas of the earth's surface (including much of the northern and southern hemispheres) are sequentially exposed to periods of light and darkness which are repeated at approximately 24-hour intervals. As a consequence of this tilt of the earth's axis with respect to the sun, regions of the earth's surface experience considerable variation in the duration of illumination, the intensity of solar energy, and ambient temperatures. These variations in the duration and intensity of solar illumination over time result in the seasons of the year in temperate zones and account for the annual variations with respect to the length of periods of light and dark at a given latitude in the hemisphere. Near the poles, conditions are so extreme that there are prolonged periods of continuous daylight and darkness, each lasting for several months and again, conditions alternate over time for a given region within the respective hemispheres. Midway between these polar extremes are the equator and equatorial regions of the earth which are subjected to relatively constant levels of solar illumination as the earth orbits around the sun. Thus, day length and temperature fluctuations are minimal near the equator and result in moderate fluctuations in temperature and related climatic conditions over time. In these areas, referred to as the tropical and subtropical regions of the earth's surface, the associated growing seasons and rainfall produce a relatively constant environment and species that are seasonal breeders tend to become continuous breeders and reproduce the year-round.

Table 11-4   Elements of Geophysical Periodicity and Biological Cycles in Mammals

Source	Ultradian (< 1 day)	Circadian (~ 1 day)	Infradian (> 1 day)
Geophysical	Tidal cycles (12.4 h) (semi-diurnal tides)	Day / night (24 h)	Circannual (~ 365 d)
		Tidal cycle (24.8 h) (diurnal tide)	Lunar cycle (29.5 d)
			Season (90 d)
			Semi-lunar cycle (14.7 d)
Biological	Brain waves (< 1 s)	Hormone Levels: Glucocorticoid Mineralocorticoid	Annual breeding season (365 d)
	Cardiac cycle (~ 1 s)	Melatonin	Cell cycle of the oocyte (60 d - >20 yr)
	Cell cycle (min - h) (lymphocytes)	Sleep / wake	Estrous cycle (4 - 180 d) (depending on species)
	Respiratory (5 s)	Body temperature	Generation cycle (60 d - 15 yr)
		Urine excretion	Cycle of the seminiferous epithelium (~ 4 d)
		Cell cycle (testis)	Spermatogenic cycle (40 - 60 d) (for most species)

h = Hour; d = Day; s = Second; min = Minute; yr = Year.

Compiled from different sources, including: J. W. Hastings, B. Rusak, and Z. Boulos, *In*: Neural and Integrative Animal Physiology. Comparative Animal Physiology, Fourth Edition, edited by, C. L. Prosser. New York, NY, John Wiley & Sons, Inc., p. 435, 1991; D. S. Saunders, An Introduction to Biological Rhythms. New York, NY, John Wiley and Sons, 1977.

Biological Cycles

Biological processes evidence cyclical patterns and many of these can be related directly to the intervals of geophysical periodicity affecting environmental conditions. Environmental cycles which influence biological rhythms in animals and plants include: Circadial, circatidal, circalunar, and circannual events.

Not surprisingly, both, simple organisms that reproduce through recurring cell cycles to generate new individuals, and complex organisms composed of groups of differentiated cells and tissues, function with elements of periodicity, either in response to environmental stresses or to cues and conditions suited to meet the metabolic demands of the organism and species. In mammals, cells and tissues function within cycle intervals, which range (Table 11–4) from ultradian periods as short as a second or less, to circadian periods of approximately 24 hours, or infradian periods of up to a year. Circadian

events include the diurnal variations in the secretion of hormones, metabolic activities, and their relationship to the sleep/wake and activity cycles of animals. Examples of infradian cycles include the interval between successive estrous periods in the female (see Chapter 9) or the recurring spermatogenic cycles of male mammals (see Chapter 8).

Patterns of sexual receptivity vary among species (Table 11–5) and within a species among those female mammals that have reached adulthood. For many of the domesticated species, females display a monophasic pattern of recurring periods of sexual receptivity repeated at regular intervals (Table 11–3; see also Chapter 9), unless interrupted by mating and/or the establishment of pregnancy. Among domesticated and laboratory animal species, the interestrous intervals may range from a few days (e.g., rats; mice), to periods of several weeks (e.g., cattle; pigs), or

Table 11-5   Female Reproductive Characteristics and Patterns of Receptivity of Selected Species

---

I. SPONTANEOUS OVULATION

Seasonal Breeders
  Polyestrous—several estrous cycles during each breeding season
    Horse; Donkey (Long-day breeders) — Mare is receptive in Spring through early Fall
    Sheep; Goat (Short-day breeders)   — Ewe and doe are receptive in late Summer to early Winter

  Monoestrous—one estrous cycle per breeding season
    Dog (bitches may display 2 breeding seasons per year)

Nonseasonal Breeders
  Polyestrous —cycle year-round at regular intervals
    Cattle (cow; heifer); Pig (sow; gilt)

II. INDUCED (REFLEX) OVULATION

Seasonal Breeders—recurring periods of receptivity during each breeding season
  Cat (feral)   — Display 2 clear breeding seasons per year; early Spring and early Fall
  Cat (colony)— Maintained in controlled light and temperature cycle year-round; tend to display
          nonbreeding season or decreased receptivity from October through December.

Seasonal Breeders—continuously receptive during breeding season until mated
  Alpaca; Llama

---

even several months in length such that for the female dog. Sexual cyclicity and receptivity occur as a biannual event for most female dogs, or as an annual event for a few breeds of domestic dogs and for most wild Canidae. Furthermore, species such as the equine and ovine display a diphasic pattern in their periodic onset and cessation of cycles of sexual receptivity. In these species, the breeding season occurs at a similar time of the year within a hemisphere, and during the breeding season, each female displays recurring periods of sexual receptivity (estrus), which continue until the female is bred and becomes pregnant. In the absence of mating and pregnancy, these periods of sexual receptivity cease to occur at the end of the breeding season. Animals that have several cycles during specific times of the year are termed seasonally polyestrous (Table 11–5; see also Chapters 9, 13, and 14). Spermatogenesis continues throughout the year in males of these species, although they also undergo seasonal changes in the quality of semen and libido.

Circadian Rhythms

Circadian rhythms or 'clocks' are prominent and pervasive elements of plant and animal physiology.[27] The circadian 'clock' refers to the endogenous oscillator(s) of plants and animals which regulate biological processes with a periodicity that approximates the rotation of the earth about its axis. Endogenous circadian oscillators are self-sustaining. Among both animal and plant species, the endogenous oscillator (also called free-running period or **Zeitgeber**) regulating a physiological event can be synchronized by external influences such as light, temperature, and tidal cycles common to the external environment.[27] It appears that most complex organisms have a specific photoreceptor which regulates the circadian clock and a photic input that influences the response of animals to patterns of light and darkness has been identified in mammals. The elements which influence this circadian clock include retinal photoreceptors, the neural connections and fibers of the retinohypothalamic tract, the suprachiasmatic nucleus of the hypothalamus, neural pathways involving the hindbrain, spinal cord, and superior cervical ganglion, and the pineal gland (Fig. 11–2).

Circannual Rhythms

Circannual patterns of periodicity are evident in physiological processes of many domesti-

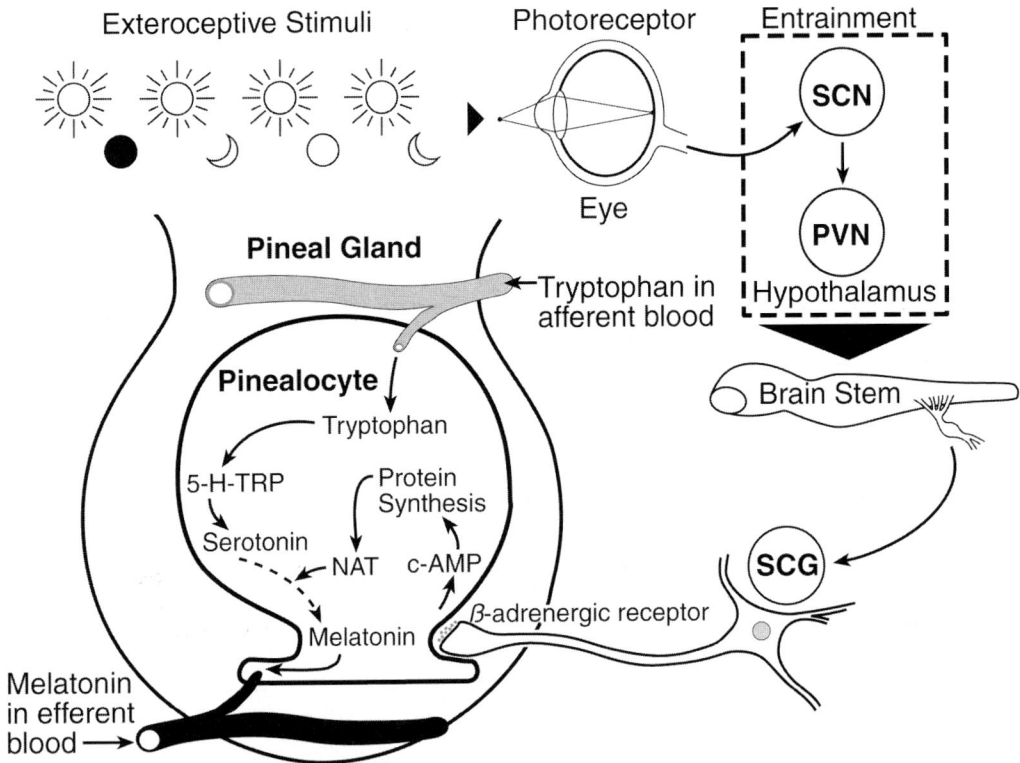

Fig. 11–2. Exteroceptive signals influence neural centers involved with circadian rhythms to influence the neuroendocrine regulation of reproductive processes. In adult mammals, seasonal reproductive activities are synchronized by the patterns of secretion of melatonin from pinealocytes. The mammalian **pinealocyte** acts as neuroendocrine transducer of environmental changes in day length through the activity of N-acetyltransferase (**NAT**) which converts serotonin to N-acetylserotonin and is the key regulatory enzyme for melatonin secretion. Melatonin synthesis is stimulated by the release of norepinephrine (NE) from sympathetic nerve fibers extending from the superior cervical ganglion (**SCG**). Norepinephrine binds to β-adrenergic receptors on pinealocytes and induces the formation of cyclic adenosine monophosphate (**c-AMP**) which promotes protein synthesis and the formation of NAT. The conversion of serotonin to N-acetylserotonin and the release of melatonin into the circulation increase markedly during the hours of darkness (**PVN** = paraventricular nucleus; **SCN** = suprachiasmatic nucleus; **5-H-TRP** = 5-hydroxy-tryptophan). (Adapted from: J. Arendt, Rev. Reprod. *3*:13, 1998 and R. J. Reiter, Psychoneuroendocrinology *8*:31, 1983).

cated and non-domesticated species. Although the biologic timing mechanisms that govern circannual patterns of rhythmicity have not been determined, an 'annual clock' is evident, even for animals that are isolated from synchronizing environmental influences. This 'clock' typically runs faster than when environmental cues are provided. Examples of infradian periodicity in animals maintained under conditions of controlled light and temperature include changes in body weight, estrous behavior, and hibernation in some species, molting in birds, udder development and milk production, changes in testicu-

lar size, prolactin levels, and breeding activity.[24] Typically the periodicity of successive events ranges from 8 to 13 months, depending on the species, the individual animal, and the physiological process that is measured. There is considerable similarity between the regulatory events associated with these annual cycles and the clock-like patterns associated with circadial rhythms.

The evolution of an endogenous timing mechanism in animals, such as hibernation, provides a selective advantage for animals to cope with the temporal variations which are related to the orbit of the earth about the sun. When animals are isolated from the synchronizing cues of the natural environment, changes in photoperiod and temperature affect the timing of events.

THE TIMING OF BIOLOGICAL CYCLES

Circadian rhythms and seasonal variations in the length of daylight are fundamental coordinating components of the reproductive activities of both, males and females of many animal species, including domesticated species. Animals of all phyla have developed a definite response to circadian rhythms and to seasonal variations in the daily changes in the length of day-light and night-darkness hours. These circadian and circannual rhythms, either by evolutionary or genetic selection pressures, regulate the activities of the male and the reproductive cyclicity of the female to coordinate receptivity and mating and ensure that ovulation and fertilization occur at the most appropriate time for normal embryonic development, gestation, and delivery of young during the season of the year which is most propitious for the offspring to survive environmental stresses and predatory animals.

Obviously, at one time or another, there was an evolutionary selective pressure for the survival of those wild animals that had keyed-in biological, well-tuned, circadian and circannual rhythms. So fine-tuned are the circadian and circannual clocks that it does not take long for animals translocated from the northern to the southern hemisphere, where the seasons are reversed, to adapt and respond to these new environmental conditions. Seasonal breeders initiate estrous cycles at the appropriate time, warranting the survival of the offspring.

Primitive, human societies in Europe, Asia, Africa, and the North, Central, and South American continents were quite advanced and capable of using and extending, even in those early, primeval times, the circadian clock to time the circannual cycle and to exploit seasonal variations in the length of the photoperiod for all kinds of human activities: Agricultural, societal, and reproductive.

As previously discussed, the orbiting of a tilted earth around the sun causes 'circadian' changes in the length of daylight or photoperiod at the different seasons of the year. These seasonal changes in the photoperiod are more pronounced at the North and South polar regions than in the equatorial region, where photoperiodic variations between seasons are hardly noticeable. Mares, for instance, are 'long-day' breeders' because they initiate estrous cycles during the Spring, when the photoperiod increases steadily in length, and, if not mated or mated with infertile stallions, continue to cycle during the Summer and early Fall, precisely during the period of long daylight. Mares will have a more restricted and a definitely shorter breeding season as the distance from the equator increases, North or South. On the other hand, mares in the subequatorial and equatorial regions tend to have prolonged breeding seasons, approaching that of continuously polyestrous species, which do not have a definite breeding season and cycle regularly during the year (Table 11–5). Some other species are 'short-day' breeders and respond to a decrease in the intensity and length of the photoperiod with the onset of sexual receptivity and mating. Sheep and goats begin to cycle in late Summer and their estrous cycling activity may extend to early Winter if a fertile mating has not occurred. If pregnancy ensues from matings during the periods of decreasing photoperiod, offspring are born in the following Spring when forage is readily available for the young. Rams and billy goats, though capable of producing and ejaculating fertile spermatozoa year-round, also experience variations in the quality of their semen. As could be expected, the quality of semen for rams and billy goats is highest during the months of decreasing or short photoperiod, corresponding with the months in which female sheep and goats are sexually receptive.

Continuously polyestrous species, like the cow, cycle year-round with no pronounced or definite seasonal variations. It is suspected but not really known, that domestication, selection for high production traits, and possibly for regularity in estrous cyclicity may have freed heifers and cows from the timed-biological clocks of circadian or circannual rhythms. In fact, non-domesticated, wild Bovidae have very definite breeding seasons. Due to the length of gestation, wild Bovidae have also adapted matings to occur at times of the year such that parturition would occur during late Spring, Summer, and early Fall. However, domesticated cows cycle, gestate, and undergo parturition year-round. In this case, some argue that these animals do not need to time their reproductive activity to ensure the birth of their young during the most appropriate months of Spring and Summer because they are well-managed and provided with an adequate quantity and quality of nutritional components in their diets. In a way this may be plausible, because in regions too far North or South from the equator, where the climatic and environmental conditions are harsh, these non-seasonal breeders tend to cycle, mate, and deliver young when the climatic conditions are favorable. Others argue that many wild and domesticated Bovidae originated ancestrally from equatorial areas, therefore, they have the genetic machinery for a nonseasonal mode of breeding.

Changes in the length of the photoperiod are associated with fluctuations in environmental temperature, climatic variation, and the availability and quality of feed. These factors act as bioregulators of reproduction and fertility among animals of all species.

Humans and large apes, in general, somehow have become independent of circadian and circannual rhythms affecting reproduction, and hence, photoperiod does not appear to restrict reproductive activities and matings to a definite season. The use of the term reproductive activities, however, must be used cautiously when applied to humans because it requires one to recognize that in humans, sexual activities or sexual behavior are not necessarily related or contributing solely to reproduction. Though there are no clearly discernible effects of photoperiod in humans and apes, there are nevertheless circadian rhythms in the pattern of secretion and release of hypothalamic releasing hormones and adenohypophyseal hormones, namely gonadotropins. However, it seems that the major biological regulator of reproduction in humans and apes is the lactationally-induced amenorrhea. Members of primitive societies have known for centuries that women who breast

feed their young do not undergo menstrual cycles while lactating. This lactationally-induced amenorrhea may last for up to 4 years and during this period, gonadotropic secretion is reduced or absent and follicular development in the ovaries is arrested.

Circannual changes in photoperiod affect spermatogenesis and libido in domesticated and non-domesticated species and it is well-known and established that the quality of ejaculated semen is best when the females of the species are also undergoing seasonal, estrous cyclicity. In general, males of the seasonal-breeding species do not arrest their reproductive activity including spermatogenesis and libido, as for the female of the species. However, the daily sperm output and production, as well as the quality of the ejaculate, is considerably reduced during the non-breeding months for males of seasonal-breeding species, such as the goat, sheep, and horse.

Neural Control

It is now established that the central nervous system, the hypothalamus, the adenohypophysis, and the pineal gland are major elements coordinating for each animal the circadian and the circannual rhythms, insofar as related to seasonal breeding. The role of the pineal gland in the timing of the circadian and circannual rhythms is a controversial subject that has been debated for years. However, evidence gathered in the last 25 years has clearly established that the pineal gland acts as a functional neuroendocrine transducer, translating the environmental seasonal changes of the photoperiod into neural impulses that coordinate the responses of the endocrine system in males and females, particularly those related to hypothalamic releasing- factors and gonadotropins. The major product of the pineal gland is melatonin. Melatonin released from pinealocytes passes into the capillaries and peripheral circulation in mammalian species (Fig. 11–2). Melatonin synthesis and secretion is highest during the hours of darkness. Cows display a typical pattern of melatonin release, melatonin levels begin to rise near dusk and the highest amplitude pulses of melatonin occur during scotophase or the hours of darkness. Furthermore, for many species the nocturnal release of melatonin is independent in its effects, whether the species is diurnal or nocturnal in its behavioral activity.

The peripheral concentrations of melatonin also fluctuate in a pattern that mimics the seasonal variations in the photoperiod and these changes in melatonin secretion are known to affect reproductive activities, particularly in species that are seasonal breeders. It seems that melatonin and possibly other non-identified but suspected factors from the pineal gland inhibit the pulsatile release of the gonadotropin-releasing hormone of males and females. However, as mentioned earlier, the response of the male is less pronounced than that of the female of the species.[67] The mechanisms participating in the inhibitory activity of melatonin from the pineal gland are not yet fully determined. However, it is believed that environmental stimuli, mainly intensity and duration of light (photoperiod) alter the secretion of melatonin by pinealocytes. Hence, it is the pattern and duration of secretion of melatonin by the mammalian pineal gland that regulates circannual rhythms in reproductive processes. Melatonin reaching the suprachiasmatic nucleus in the hypothalamus and the adenohypophysis would inhibit the frequency and magnitude of the pulsatile discharge of the hypothalamic, gonadotropic releasing-hormones which regulate the release of pituitary gonadotropins (see Chapter 2). This pattern of neuroendocrine modulation influenced by external light and via the pineal gland through the secretion of melatonin appears to be responsible for the initiation of reproductive activities in animals such as the goat and sheep that are short-day, seasonal breeders, precisely at the time of the year when days are becoming shorter and the photoperiod decreases during late Summer to late Fall.

The pineal gland also seems to exert an inhibitory influence on the pulsatile release of hypothalamic hormones and gonadotropins in animals that are classified as long-day breeders, such as mares, stallions, and the other equids that mate during the months of Spring and Summer. However, in these long-day breeder species, the major inhibitory effects of the pineal gland occur during the short days of late Fall and Winter, such that these animals enter and remain in a seasonal anestrus. As the length of the photoperiod increases, the pineal becomes less active and the secretion of melatonin is considerably reduced. Increased photoperiod results in a decrease and eventually a release from the hypothalamic inhibition caused by the synthesis and release of melatonin by the pineal gland of mares and stallions. This reduction in melatonin levels liberate the hypothalamus to release gonadotropin-releasing hormones which stimulate the pituitary gland to secrete and release gonadotropins. The result of these interactions between exteroceptive stimuli and regulatory factors affecting the pineal gland, hypothalamus, and the pituitary gland is the initiation of seasonal cycling (estrous) and ovulation in mares and the production of ejaculates of high fertility by stallions.

Interestingly, it seems that the initiation of reproductive activities, mainly in female sheep and goats, but also to a lesser degree in rams and billy goats cannot be stimulated simply by exposure to a short-day photoperiod. Nor can mares be induced to cycle and ovulate simply by exposure to a long-day photoperiod. In fact, prolonged exposure to light makes these animals refractory to cycle. It appears that animals that are short-day breeders need a prior exposure to the photoperiod associated with long-days and animals that are long-day breeders must be initially exposed to a short-day photoperiod. These considerations have relevance to schemes designed for the control of reproduction by application of artificial light to males and females of species that belong to the category of seasonal breeders (Table 11–5).

Control of reproductive cycles by introducing changes in photoperiod to expand the breeding season of seasonal-breeding species is becoming economically important for sheep and horse breeders at large and for the breeders of nonseasonal breeding species, as well. The presence of melatonin-binding receptors in the hypothalamus and pituitary gland of the horse and donkey should not be surprising because these two species are seasonal breeders, but it is puzzling that binding sites for melatonin are also found in the hypothalamus and pituitary gland of the bovine, a species that is not a seasonal breeder. Also, the domestic dog, usually a biestric species, has melatonin receptors in the brain and expresses rhythms in melatonin levels in the peripheral blood. The pinealocytes of the sow, which is not seasonal, but like the bovine, is a continuous polyestrous species, display cytological changes indicative of increased or decreased secretory activity. The causes and implications for a potential role of the pineal gland and melatonin in nonseasonal breeders remains to be determined.

Photoreceptors

It is now well-established that the mammalian eye contains photoactive molecules called photopigments that are responsible for vision and that these or other retinal factors are involved with the photoresponsiveness of the animal. In mammals and lower animals, photoreceptors in the eye appear to perform a dual role: Visual responses essential for imaging of objects and circadian and circannual responses including essential elements for reproduction.

Circadian and circannual responses appear to depend on the photoactivation of vitamin B_2-based pigments associated with blue-light, retinal receptors. The retinal receptors found in mice and humans appear to be homologous to the cryptochrome pigments of plants and lower animal forms. In mice, cryptochromes identified as CRY1 and CRY2 are expressed in ganglion cells and in the inner layers of the mouse retina and the levels of expression of the CRY1 gene in cells of the suprachiasmatic nucleus of the hypothalamus oscillate in a circadian manner.[39] The timing of physiological processes in man and animals, including reproductive activities, may rely on the neural input resulting from the activation of these retinal photopigments.

Although speculative at this time, it would be understandable that those animals and plants that have co-evolved within the earth's biosphere, could have a high degree of conservation of light-sensitive pigments, such as cryptochromes, which these species then use to monitor circadian and circannual patterns of illumination. Organisms may use day-length or the intensity of illumination at distinct periods of the day to interface biological events with the corresponding geophysical elements of the environment. The capability to coordinate physiological processes with geological variables which are dependent on the periodic oscillations caused by the rotation of the earth and the orbital displacement of the earth and moon within the solar system would confer a survival advantage to the organism.

RECAPITULATION

Considering the magnitude of the expenditures of bodily energy and resources by the female of the species in the fulfilment of reproductive activities, it should not be surprising that the success or failure to cycle regularly, be inseminated, become pregnant, carry the embryo and fetus to term, and produce a viable offspring is closely related to and ultimately depends on favorable environmental conditions. Natural selection has resulted in well-defined seasons for certain species to breed. Depending on the length of gestation, some females breed during the 'short-days' of late Summer and Fall so that their offspring are born in the next Spring (sheep, goat). Others, breed during the 'long-days' of late Spring, Summer, and early Fall, so that their offspring are also born in the Spring (horse, jack ass).

Males of these seasonal-breeding species produce and release spermatozoa in their ejaculates, display libido, mount, and copulate with females that are artificially induced to cycle during the non-breeding season. However, the fertility and overall quality of ejaculates are considerably reduced and, characteristically, the male jack ass, goat, sheep, and horse produce their poorest-quality ejaculates while the females are gestating or going through the months of the nonbreeding season.

REFERENCES

1. Arendt, J. (1995): Melatonin and the Mammalian Pineal Gland. New York, NY, Chapman & Hall, p. 110.
2. Arendt, J. (1998): Melatonin and the pineal gland: Influence on mammalian seasonal and circadian physiology. Rev. Reprod. *3:*13.

3. Arendt, J., Symons, A. M., English, J., et al. (1988): How does melatonin control seasonal reproductive cycles? Reprod. Nutr. Develop. *28:*387.

4. Argo, C. M., Cox, J. E., and Gray, J. L. (1991): Effect of oral melatonin treatment on the seasonal physiology of pony stallions. J. Reprod. Fertil. (Suppl. 44):115.

5. Armstrong, S. M. (1989): Melatonin and circadian control in mammals. Experientia *45:*932.

6. Asdell, S. A. (1964): Patterns of Mammalian Reproduction, 2nd, edition. Ithaca, NY, Comstock-Cornell Press.

7. Bartle, S. J., Males, J. R., and Preston, R. L. (1984): Effect of energy intake on the postpartum interval in beef cows and the adequacy of the cow's milk production for calf growth. J. Anim. Sci. *58:*1086.

8. Berthelot, X., Laurentie, M., Revault, J. P., et al. (1990): Circadian profile and production rate of melatonin in the cow. Domestic Anim. Endocrinol. *7:*315.

9. Bruce, H. M. (1966): Smell as an exteroceptive factor. Environmental influences on reproductive processes. J. Anim. Sci. *25* (Suppl):83.

10. Chemineau, P., Malpaux, B., Delgadillo, J. A. et al. (1992): Control of sheep and goat reproduction: Use of light and melatonin. Anim. Reprod. Sci. *30:*157.

11. Christenson, R. K. (1980): Environmental influences on the postpartum animal. J. Anim. Sci. *51* (Suppl. 2):53.

12. Clay, C. M. and Squires, E. L. (1987): Influences of season and artificial photoperiod on stallions: Testicular size, seminal characteristics and sexual behavior. J. Anim. Sci. *64:*517.

13. Conaway, C. H. (1971): Ecological adaptation and mammalian reproduction. Biol. Reprod. *4:* 239.

14. Cozzi, B., Morel, G., Ravault, J. P., et al. (1991): Circadian and seasonal rhythms of melatonin production in mules (*Equus asinus* x *Equus caballus*). J. Pineal Res. *10:*130.

15. D'Occhio, M. J. and Suttie, J. M. (1992): The role of the pineal gland and melatonin in reproduction in male domestic ruminants. Anim. Reprod. Sci. *30:*135.

16. Dunn, T. G. and Kaltenbach, C. C. (1980): Nutrition and the postpartum interval of the ewe, sow and cow. J. Anim. Sci. *52* (Suppl. 2):29.

17. Dutt, R. H. (1960): Temperature and light as factors in reproduction among farm animals. J. Dairy Sci. *43* (Suppl.):123.

18. Edmunds, L. N., Jr. (1984): Cell Cycle Clocks. New York, NY, Marcel Dekker, Inc.

19. Edmunds, L. N., Jr. (1988): Cellular and Molecular Bases of Biological Clocks. New York, NY, Springer-Verlag.

20. England, B. G., Foote, W. C., Matthews, D. H., et al. (1969): Ovulation and corpus luteum function in the llama (*Lama glama*). J. Endocrinol. *45:*505.

21. Evered, D. and Clark, S. (1985): Photoperiodism, Melatonin, and the Pineal. London, England, Pitman Publishing Ltd.

22. Fernandez-Baca, S., Madden, D. H. L., and Novoa, C. (1970): Effect of different mating stimuli on induction of ovulation in the alpaca. J. Reprod. Fertil. *22:*261.

23. Griffin, E. A., Jr., Staknis, D., and Weitz, C. J. (1999): Light-independent role of CRY1 and CRY2 in the mammalian circadian clock. Science *286:*768.

24. Gwinner, E. (1986): Circannual Rhythms. New York, NY, Springer-Verlag

25. Hale, E. B. (1966): Visual stimuli and reproductive behavior in bulls. J. Anim. Sci. *25* (Suppl.):36.

26. Hall, J. C. (1995): Tripping along the trail to the molecular mechanisms of biological clocks. Trends Neurosci. *18:*230.

27. Hastings, J. W., Rusak, B., and Boulos, Z. (1991): Circadian rhythms: The physiology of biological timing. *In:* Neural and Integrative Animal Physiology. Comparative Animal Physiology, Fourth Edition, edited by, C. L. Prosser. New York, NY, John Wiley & Sons, Inc., p. 435.

28. Hayssen, V., van Tienhoven, A., and van Tienhoven, A. (1993): Asdell's Patterns of Mammalian Reproduction: A Compendium of Species-Specific Data. Ithaca, N.Y., Cornell University Press.

29. Illius, A. W., Haynes, N. B., and Lamming, G. E. (1976): Effects of ewe proximity on peripheral plasma testosterone levels and behavior in the ram. J. Reprod. Fertil. *48:*25.

30. Karasek, M. (1983): Ultrastructure of the mammalian pineal gland: Its comparative and functional aspects. *In:* Pineal Research Review, edited by R. J. Reiter. New York, NY, Alan R. Liss, p. 1.

31. Karasek, M. (1985): Ultrastructural study of the pineal-hypothalamo-hypophysial-gonadal axis in mammals. *In:* The Pineal Gland, edited by B. Mess, C. Ruzsas, L. Tima, and P. Pevet. Budapest, Hungary, Akademiai Kiado, p. 35.

32. Kiddy, C. A., Mitchell, D. S., Bolt D. J., et al. (1978): Detection of estrus-related odors in cows by trained dogs. Biol. Reprod. *19:*389.

33. Korf, H. W. (1994): The pineal organ as a component of the biological clock. Phylogenetic and ontogenetic considerations. Ann. N. Y. Acad. Sci. *719:*13.

34. Lamming, G. E. (1984): Marshall's Physiology of Reproduction, Vol. 1, Reproductive Cycles of Vertebrates, 4th ed. New York, NY, Churchill Livingstone.

35. Lincoln, G. A. and Peet, M. J. (1977): Photoperiodic control of gonadotropin secretion in the ram: A detailed study of the temporal changes in plasma levels of follicle-stimulating hormone, luteinizing hormone and testosterone following and abrupt switch from long to short days. J. Endocrinol. *74:*355.

36. Lincoln, G. A. and Short, R. V. (1980): Seasonal breeding: Nature's contraceptive. Recent Prog. Hormone Res. *36:*1.

37. Love, R. J., Evans, G., and Klupiec, C. (1993): Seasonal effects on fertility in gilts and sows. J. Reprod. Fertil. Suppl. *48:*191.

38. Marshall, F. H. A. (1937): On the change over in the oestrous cycle in animals after transference across the equator, with further observations on the incidence of the breeding seasons and the factors controlling sexual periodicity. Proc. Royal Soc., [B], London, England *122:*413.

39. Miyamoto Y. and Sancar, A. (1998): Vitamin B2-based blue-light photoreceptors in the retinohypothalamic tract as the photoactive pigments for setting the circadian clock in mammals. Proc. Nat. Acad. Sci., USA *95:*6097.

40. Nonno, R., Capsoni, S., Lucini, V., et al. (1995): Distribution and characterization of the melatonin recep-

tors in the hypothalamus and pituitary gland of three domestic ungulates. J. Pineal Res. *18:*207.

41. O'Callaghan, D., Karsch, F. J., Boland, M. P. et al. (1992): Variation in the timing of the reproductive season among breeds of sheep in relation to differences in photoperiodic synchronization of an endogenous rhythm. J. Reprod. Fertil. *96:*443.

42. Pepelko, W. E. and Clegg, M. T. (1965): Influence of season of the year upon patterns of sexual behavior in male sheep. J. Anim. Sci. *24:*633.

43. Przybylska, B., Wyrzykowski, Z., Wyrzykowska, K., et al. (1990): Ultrastructure of pig pinealocytes in various stages of the sexual cycle: A quantitative study. Cytobios *64:*7.

44. Ritar, A. J. (1991): Seasonal changes in LH, androgens and testes in the male angora goat. Theriogenology *36:*959.

45. Reiter, R. J. (1974): Circannual reproductive rhythms in mammals related to photoperiod and pineal function: A review. Chronobiologia *1:*365.

46. Reiter, R. J. (1983): The pineal gland: An intermediary between the environment and the endocrine system. Psychoneuroendocrinology *8:*31.

47. Reiter, R. J. (1987): The melatonin message: Duration versus coincidence hypotheses. Life Sci. *40:*2119.

48. Reiter, R. J. (1991): Pineal melatonin: Cell biology of its synthesis and of its physiological interactions. Endocrine Rev. *12:*151.

49. Reiter, R. J. and Fraschiny, F. (1969): Endocrine aspects of the mammalian pineal gland: A review. Neuroendocrinology *5:*219.

50. Reiter, R. J. and Sorrentino, S. Jr. (1970): Reproductive effects of mammalian pineal. Am. Zool. *10:*247.

51. Sancar, A. (2000): Cryptochrome: the second photoactive pigment in the eye and its role in circadian photoreception. Annu. Rev. Biochem. *69:*31.

52. Saunders, D. S., (1977): An Introduction to Biological Rhythms. New York, NY, John Wiley and Sons, p. 9.

53. Schanbacher, B. D. and Ford, J. J. (1979): Photoperiodic regulation of ovine spermatogenesis: Relationship to serum hormones. Biol. Reprod. *20:*719.

54. Seidel, G. E., Jr. and Brackett, B. G. (1981): Perspectives on animal breeding. *In:* New Technologies in Animal Breeding, edited by B. G. Brackett, G. E. Seidel, Jr., and S. M. Seidel. San Diego-San Francisco, CA, Academic Press, Inc., p. 3.

55. Sharp, D. C., Davis, S. D., and Cleaver, B. D. (1993): Photoperiod. *In:* Equine Reproduction, edited by J. L. Voss and A. O. McKinnon. Philadelphia, PA, Lea and Febiger, Inc., p. 179.

56. Shearman, L. P., Sriram, S., Weaver, D. R., et al. (2000) : Interacting molecular loops in the mammalian circadian clock. Science 288:1013.

57. Short, R. V. (1981): Reproductive regulation. *In:* Bioregulators of Reproduction, 1st edition, edited by G. Jagiello and J. J. Vogel. New York, NY, Academic Press, Inc., p. 1.

58. Shorey, H. H. (1976): Animal Communication by Pheromones. New York, NY, Academic Press, Inc.

59. Spicer, L. J. and Echternkamp, S. E. (1986): Ovarian follicular growth, function and turnover in cattle: A review. J. Anim. Sci. *62:*428.

60. Stankov, B., Cozzi, B., Lucini, V., et al. (1991): Characterization and mapping of melatonin receptors in the brain of three mammalian species: Rabbit, horse and sheep. A comparative *in vitro* binding study. Neuroendocrinology *53:*214.

61. Stankov, B., Moller, M., Lucini, V., et al. (1994): A carnivore species (*canis familiaris*) expresses circadian melatonin rhythm in the peripheral blood and melatonin receptors in the brain. Europ. J. Endocrinol. *131:*191.

62. Sweeney, T., Donovan, A., Karsch, F. J., et al. (1997): Influence of previous photoperiodic exposure on the reproductive response to a specific photoperiod signal in ewes. Biol. Reprod. *56:*916.

63. Taymor, M. L. (1996): The regulation of follicle growth: Some clinical implications in reproductive endocrinology. Fertil. Steril. *65:*235.

64. Thibault, C., Courot, M., Martinet, L. et al. (1966): Regulation of breeding season and estrous cycles by light and external stimuli in some mammals. J. Anim. Sci. 25 (Suppl):119.

65. Thrun, L. A., Moenter, S. M., O'Callaghan, D. et al. (1995): Circannual alterations in the circadian rhythm of melatonin secretion. J. Biol. Rhythms *10:*42.

66. Williamson, G. and Payne, W. J. A. (1978): The effect of climate, Chapter 1. *In:* Animal Husbandry in the Tropics, Third Edition. New York, NY, Longman, Inc., p.2.

67. Wood, R. I., Ebling, F. J. P., I'Anson, et al. (1991): The timing of neuroendocrine sexual maturity in the male lamb by photoperiod. Biol. Reprod. *45:*82.

68. Woodfill, C. J., Robinson, J. E., Malpaux, B., et al. (1991): Synchronization of the circannual reproductive rhythm of the ewe by discrete photoperiodic signals. Biol. Reprod. *45:*110.

Reproductive Patterns of Cattle*

S. M. HOPKINS

12

INTRODUCTION

The postpubertal, domestic bovine (Bos taurus) female is a nonseasonally polyestrous animal. Estrus normally occurs at approximately 21-day intervals for cows and 20 days for heifers (modal range 17 to 25 days, Fig. 12-1).

Based on the endocrine profile and presence of ovarian cyclic structures such as follicles and

*Much information concerned with reproduction in cattle has been presented in Chapter 2 (The Pituitary Gland), Chapter 7 (The Biology of Sex), Chapter 8 (Male Reproductive System), Chapter 9 (Female Reproductive System), Chapter 10 (Artificial Insemination), and Chapter 11 (Patterns of Reproduction). The reader is encouraged to refer to these chapters in order to permit conciseness.

corpora lutea, uterine and vaginal changes, and overt behavioral responses, the estrous cycle of heifers and cows is conventionally divided into four phases: Estrus (Day = 0), metestrus (Day = 1 to 4), diestrus (Day = 5 to 18), and proestrus (Day = 19 to onset of estrus).

During estrus, also termed heat, the female displays behavioral manifestations indicating sexual receptivity. The ovaries contain one and occasionally two Graafian follicles which have matured to preovulatory size. The **corpus luteum** (CL) of the preceding cycle has become a **corpus albicans** (CA), which is nonsecretory. During estrus, the uterus shows a marked turgidity and is edematous. Concurrently, the vaginal mucosa is congested and the mucosal cells of the vagina and cervix have high levels of secretory activity.

Ovulation occurs during metestrus, when the behavioral manifestations of estrus have abated and the animal no longer stands for mating (Fig. 12-2).

In addition to the recently ovulated follicle, there may also be anovulatory follicles which were functionally immature and failed to ovulate during the preceding cycle. The walls of the ovulated follicle collapse, forming an ovulatory depression which can be detected through rectal palpation of the ovaries. The theca and granulosa cells proliferate, undergo hypertrophy, and initially form a **corpus hemorrhagicum** (CH), which matures into an actively secreting CL.

During diestrus the CL continues to increase in mass and reaches a mature size by day 7. Follicular development and regression occur in distinct waves throughout the phase of diestrus,

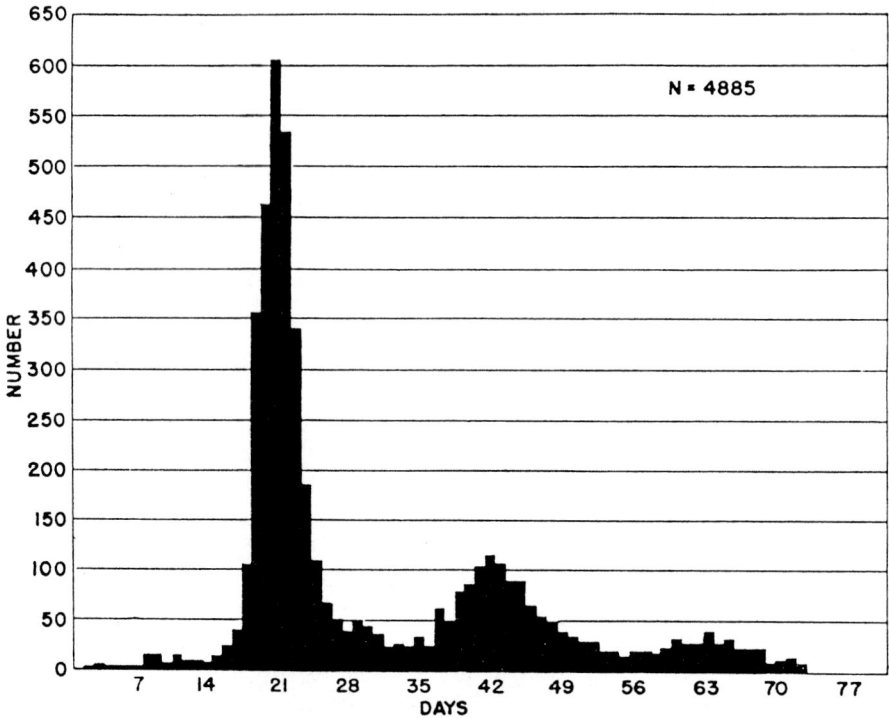

Fig. 12-1. Histogram of the length of the estrous cycle in cows, as determined by the interval between services in artificial insemination. (Reprinted with permission from: K. Moeller and N. L. VanDemark, J. Anim. Sci. *10:*987, 1951).

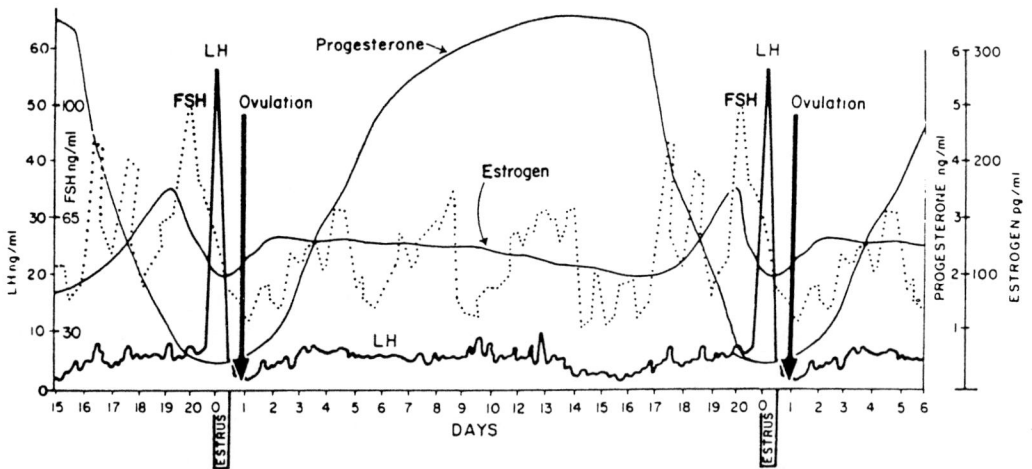

Fig. 12-2. Hormonal levels during the estrous cycle of the cow. (FSH values from: D. Schams et al., Acta Endocrinol. *86:* 180, 1977, Theriogenology *10:* 453, 1978).

which can be detected through ultrasonic evaluation. It is only after the CL of the cycle regresses during proestrus that the follicle destined to ovulate following the next estrus begins its final maturation.

In relationship to their spermatogenic activity, bulls are noncyclic. Depending on the geographic area, however, there may be periods of decreased spermatozoal motility and abnormal spermatozoal morphology and concentration accompanied by changes in the biochemical characteristics of the ejaculate. These changes are often related to heat stress and observed during periods of high temperature and humidity. The degree of spermatogenic depression varies among individuals and breeds, and with the level and duration of the stress.

PUBERTY AND SEXUAL MATURITY

Puberty in the female is defined as the age at which the heifer initiates reproductive cyclicity; in the male, it is defined as the age at which bull calves first have spermatozoa in their ejaculates. Puberty is also defined for dairy bulls to be used in centers of artificial insemination as the age at which a bull produces ejaculates containing 50 million or more spermatozoa/ml, of which at least 10% display progressive motility. Puberty is the consequence of somatic growth and a series of cumulative hormonal events in both males and females (see Chapters 8 and 9). In the bovine species, the onset of puberty is more closely correlated to body weight rather than to age. Both bull and heifer calves reach their breed average weight (about 50% of their adult weight) before puberty ensues. Males undergo pubertal changes earlier than heifers of the same breed.

Female

The ovaries of prepubertal heifers are steroidogenically active and contain growing follicles before the heifer displays overt estrual activity. These follicles usually regress and become atretic. Waves of follicular development and regression continue until puberty. Prior to puberty, the resultant follicular estrogens are unable to stimulate the release of hypothalamic gonadotropin-releasing hormones due to the high threshold for estrogens in the hypothalamus of the immature heifer. As the heifer ages, however, the hypothalamic threshold for estrogenic stimulation of secretion of releasing hormones decreases and, as a consequence, LH is released from the pituitary in a pulsatile pattern (see Chapter 9).

The onset of puberty is regulated by the maturity of the hypothalamic-adenohypophyseal axis rather than by the ability of the pituitary to produce gonadotropins or as a result of ovarian insensitivity to their effects (see Chapter 9). As puberty approaches, the frequency of LH peaks increases, followed by a transient rise in progesterone levels. After this brief progesterone priming, the pubertal preovulatory surge of LH occurs and is associated with behavioral estrus.

The initiation of puberty is strongly influenced by the nutritional level received during the prepubertal period after weaning. At low energy levels, the onset of puberty is significantly delayed. The onset of puberty may range from 5 to 20 months, with an average range of 9 to 11 months. Holstein heifers maintained at a high level of energy intake had their first estrus at 7 to 10 months of age, 6 to 9 months earlier than for heifers of the same breed that were provided a low nutritional intake (Table 12-1). Poorly fed animals have delayed puberty and do not display estrus until they reach a body weight similar to the body weight at first estrus observed in well-fed animals of that breed (Table 12-1).

THE ESTROUS CYCLE

The four phases of the bovine estrous cycle– **proestrus**, **estrus**, **metestrus**, and **diestrus**

Table 12-1   Age and Weight at First Estrus in Holstein Heifers Fed at Three Energy Levels

	Age in Weeks and Months at First Estrus				Weight in Pounds at First Estrus[a]	
TDN Intake	Range	Avg.	Range	Avg.	Range	Avg.
Low (60%)	59–80	72	13.6–18.5	16.6	430–575	540
Normal (100%)	37–55	49	8.5–12.7	11.3	440–650	580
High (140%)	29–43	37	6.7–9.9	8.5	460–640	580

[a] Estimated from growth curves.
TDN = Total digestible nutrient
Adapted from: A. M. Sorensen, et al., Cornell Univ. Agric. Exp. Sta. Bull. No. 936, 1959.

reflect parallel cyclic changes in the endocrine profile of the animal.

Endocrine Profile

The cycle is controlled by the interactions of the hypothalamic-pituitary axis in concert with the cyclic ovarian structures and uterus. A functional CL from a postpubertal animal produces progesterone and the peptide hormone oxytocin. Thus, a CL can participate in controlling the expression of estrus and subsequent ovulation. The absence of a viable embryo and the maternal recognition of pregnancy after day 14 of the cycle results in the pulsatile release of prostaglandin $F_{2\alpha}$ from the uterus. The prostaglandin enters the utero-ovarian vein and passes into the ovarian artery and subsequently to the CL. Prostaglandin $F_{2\alpha}$ then stimulates the release of luteal oxytocin, which impacts the uterus, resulting in a reciprocal release of another $PGF_{2\alpha}$ pulse (See Chapter 9, Fig. 9-27). This $PGF_{2\alpha}$-oxytocin release pattern continues until the depletion of the luteal oxytocin. Concurrently, the corpus luteum regresses and ceases to produce progesterone.

Follicular growth and regression continues in distinct waves throughout the estrous cycle in response to FSH secretion. Each wave consists of a cohort of follicles, of which one becomes dominant and the others remains subordinate. Cattle typically have two or three follicular waves per estrous cycle. In the presence of high progesterone levels, the dominant follicle of the cohort increases in size, plateaus, which is then followed by a size decrease, reflecting atresia. The remaining cohort of follicles do not have a significant growth phase and undergo atresia. These follices produce estradiol, which synergizes with the high progesterone levels to suppress the gonadotropin-releasing hormone-induced release of LH. A follicular wave associated with a natural or induced regression of the CL, produces a dominant follicle destined to complete follicular maturation and ovulation. Concurrent with the development of this preovulatory follicle and a decline in progesterone levels is a rise in the basal LH levels. Hypothalamic gonadotropin-releasing hormones induce the release of LH in a pulsatile fashion. The pulse frequency increases from approximately one pulse per 4 hours to one or more pulses per hour. The increasing LH levels promote a continual increase in estradiol secretion from the theca and granulosa cells of the dominant follicle, beginning about 4 days prior to estrus. Once the estradiol levels reach a threshold level, a preovulatory surge of LH and FSH is triggered. This gonadotropin surge causes the maturation of the Graafian follicle and ovulation 27 to 30 hours later. The onset of behavioral estrus also begins near the time of the gonadotropin surge. Immediately following ovulation, the theca and granulosa cells proliferate and differentiate into small (less than 23 μm) and large (greater than 23 μm) luteal cells, respectively. Both types of luteal cells secrete progesterone; however, they differ in their LH and prostaglandin receptor content. Small luteal cells contain most of the LH receptors and are more sensitive to LH stimulation, leading to increased progesterone production. Large luteal cells overall, secrete the majority of the progesterone, have few of the LH receptor sites, and most of the prostaglandin receptors. Large luteal cells also produce and store oxytocin. Even though the prostaglandin receptor levels remain relatively constant, the CL is refractory to endogenously or exogenously prostaglandin-induced regression until about the fifth day of the cycle.

This dynamic pattern of follicular and luteal development and regression continues in subsequent cycles until the maternal recognition of pregnancy occurs and gestation ensues.

Following conception, the progesterone levels increase initially as in an unbred cycle. If the developing embryo is viable past day 14 to 15, then the leutolytic cascade is blocked. The embryo can produce prostaglandins, steroid hormones, and bovine trophoblastic protein-1 (bTP-1), which may play a role in preventing luteal demise. The cow requires a functional CL for the first 200 to 220 days of gestation. Many cows ovariectomized after day 200 maintain the pregnancy to term due to progesterone secretion by the adrenal glands. However, there is an increase in retained placentas and losses of calves, suggesting that bilateral ovariectomy during late gestation is not compatible with normal parturition.

After parturition, FSH levels begin to increase, and significant follicular activity has been demonstrated as early as day 10 to 14 postpartum. Levels of LH begins also a gradual increase, and the pulse frequency eventually becomes about one per hour. The frequent LH release associated with significant follicular growth leads to estrogen production and ovulation. The first postpartum ovulation, termed "silent heat," is not associated with an overt estrus. Typically, this early luteal phase is shorter, less than 10 to 12 days, and the CL is subfunctional compared to that of subsequent cycles.

Factors which inhibit the postpartum return to estrous cyclicity are numerous and primarily relate to the energy demands of lactation. As a result, management goals are directed towards the provisions of balanced diets in energy and proteins.

Sexual Behavior

The behavioral changes in the nonstressed estrous cow are short in duration–12 to 22 hours (range 2 to 50 hours)–but high in intensity. The heifer is in heat fewer hours than the mature cow. During the period of estrus, the female bellows and, though attempts to mount other cows or bulls, will stand to be mounted by bulls or cows. The latter is the usual criterion (gold standard) to consider a cow or heifer to be in estrus.

Appetite declines in estrous cows, and milk production may drop. This period of frenzied activity varies among cows and usually is more dramatic and intense in the bovine than in other farm species.

The bull detects the estrous cow by pheromones released from the vaginal secretions, by auditory communication from the bellowing cow, or by visual communication when he observes increased activity of the estrous cow, including the mounting of other cows. Upon approaching the estrous cow, the experienced bull nuzzles the external genitalia and rear quarters for several minutes and then reacts by standing rigidly with the head extended and the upper lip raised, displaying the "Flehmen reaction." Often the bull will approach the cow at a right angle and rest his head over the middle of the cow's back, whereupon the estrous cow re-

acts by standing quietly. After several minutes of such activity, the bull approaches the rear quarters of the cow, mounts, presses his forelimbs into her flanks, presses the chin firmly on the cow's back, and makes a single pelvic and ejaculatory thrust during intromission. The cow usually arches her back and elevates the tail to facilitate weight bearing and intromission. The bull dismounts shortly after ejaculation and often leaves the cow at this point. The actual act of copulation lasts only a few seconds, during which the bull's rear feet may have momentarily left the ground during the pelvic thrust. Depending on the bull, a refractory period usually follows, during which the male shows little interest in the estrous cow. Some bulls have an enormous capacity for frequent copulations, particularly if there is additional stimulation from other estrous cows. A single breeding or insemination near the end of estrus is satisfactory for a good conception rate, although several breedings often occur during unrestricted natural matings.

Estrus Detection

Overt signs of estrus in the female can be classified into pre-estrual, estrual, and postestrual manifestations. These signs include mucus discharge, vulvar edema, vocalization, increased activity, decreased milk production, and the mounting of other cows. The cow in estrus will stand to be mounted by bulls, steers, or other cows or heifers. Artificial insemination based only on signs such as mucus discharge, vulvar edema, and vocalization yields significantly lower pregnancy rates as compared to timing the breeding of the cow on the basis of standing to be mounted.

For the purpose of artificial insemination, females that are open or not pregnant should be observed at least twice daily. This will potentially allow for detection of estrus in 90% of these animals. However, this percentage may vary considerably depending on the environment and on the knowledge and ability of the observer. Also, 60 to 70% of this estrual activity takes place between 6 PM and 6 AM if the cows are allowed to roam freely. Consequently, aids to detect estrual activities have been developed to supplement visual observation. These aids include pressure-sensitive devices, sexually aggressive "teaser" animals, electronic probes, pedometers, and videotapes. The pressure devices are placed on the tailhead of the female. When she stands to be mounted, the indicator smears or changes color, indicating that standing and mounting has occurred. Another pressure-sensitive device interfaces automatically with a computer through receivers positioned near the cows. Mounting activity is continuously monitored and stored, allowing for the interpretation of daily estrous activity. Similarly, teaser males or testosterone-primed females, which display libido similar to that of an intact male, can be used to seek out receptive females by their acceptance to be mounted. A chin ball marker attached to a teaser male or female will leave an ink mark upon the withers of ridden cows, indicating that standing and acceptance to mounting have occurred.

Electronic vaginal probes have been advocated for the measurement the electrical conductivity of the cervical mucus. There is a decrease in the resistance of the cervical mucus around the time of estrus when compared to the resistance during the remainder of the cycle. This technique has merit only if the normal electrical pattern of each animal is established during one or two previous cycles. There is simply too much individual variation to accurately assign a minimum level of vaginal mucus resistance for all animals relative to the optimum breeding time.

The increase in levels of activity in cows approaching estrus can be monitored with a pedometer. A diestrual animal has a typical daily pattern of eating, moving, and resting. Any increase in the amount of mobility often indicates which animals should be preferentially observed for standing behavior.

Video monitors and recorders can also be used on animals which are allowed to roam within a confined area. The videotapes can be reviewed to identify those animals which stood to be mounted within a given period. This system works effectively but is expensive and requires visible identification tags on the cows which are clearly recognizable on the video monitor.

Estrus synchronization procedures can be incorporated into management programs. The timely use of injectable prostaglandins alone or in concert with progestogens can induce estrus over a relatively narrow time period. Depending on the program, breeding can be set at a certain time or following estrus detection. A recent estrus synchronization program is based on the understanding of dominant follicles and follicular waves. Synthetic gonadotropin-releasing hormone, GnRH, is injected into cyclic animals on random days of the cycle to induce the LH surge and to ovulate mature follicles. Seven days later, a luteolytic dose of prostaglandin $PGF_{2\alpha}$(s) is given to regress the CL(s). Forty-eight hours later, GnRH is readministered to cause ovulation, followed by breeding within 24 hours.

The average cycle length is 20 to 21 days, so on any given day of the month, 1/20 or 5% of randomly cycling animals should be in estrus. The estrus detection efficiency for a herd can be calculated by dividing the number of cows found in estrus over a 24-day period by the total number of eligible cows. Estrus detection is of fundamental importance since the optimal time for breeding cattle by artificial insemination is during the last half of standing estrus.

Duration of Estrus

The length of estrus averages 17.8 hours in dairy cows and 15.3 hours in dairy heifers. Animals which first show estrus in the afternoon remain in heat for 2 to 4 hours longer than those animals that first show estrus in the morning.

Genital tract stimulation also affects the length of estrus and ovulation time. Breeding estrous heifers to a vasectomized bull shortens estrus to about 8 hours, as compared to 10 hours for nonbred heifers. Stimulation of the clitoral area during artificial insemination can have a similar effect. Copulation causes oxytocin release, and lactating cows may have a let-down of milk. Dripping of milk is particularly noticeable in the dairy cow.

Fertilization Time

The cow has such a short period of sexual receptivity that breeding or artificial insemination times are restricted relative to the time of ovula-

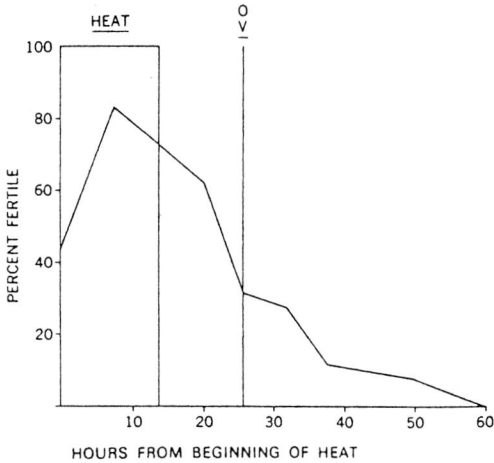

Fig. 12-3. The effect of the time of insemination upon the chance of conception in the cow. The duration of estrus (**heat**) and the time of ovulation (**OV**) are shown. (From: S. A. Asdell, Patterns of Mammalian Reproduction. Ithaca, NY, Comstock Publishing Associates, 1964, p. 587).

Table 12-2 The Effect of Inseminating Cows at Different Times on Fertility

Time of Insemination	% Fertile
Beginning of estrus	44.0
Middle of estrus	82.5
End of estrus	75.0
6 hours after end	62.5
12 hours after end	32.0
18 hours after end	28.0
24 hours after end	12.0
36 hours after end	8.0
48 hours after end	0

Data from: G. W. Trimberger and H. P. Davis, Nebraska Agric. Exp. Sta. Res. Bull. No. 129, 1943.

Table 12-3 The Effect of Ovulation Time on Fertility (Cows)

Time of Insemination	% Fertile
Over 24 hours before ovulation	53.3
19 to 24 hours before ovulation	73.3
13 to 18 hours before ovulation	85.7
7 to 12 hours before ovulation	78.5
6 hours or less before ovulation	57.1
2 hours or less after ovulation	30.0
6 hours after ovulation	40.0
12 hours after ovulation	25.0

Data from: S. A. Asdell, Patterns of Mammalian Reproduction. Ithaca, NY, Comstock Publishing Associates, 1964, p. 587.

tion (Fig. 12-3). Artificial Insemination (AI) is most successful when performed from mid-estrus up to a few hours after the end of estrus (Table 12-2). Table 12-3 shows that fertility is maximal when insemination occurs 13 to 18 hours before ovulation. Because the majority of AI programs now use frozen-thawed semen, which has a shorter viability span than for fresh semen, breeding too early can result in fewer sperm capable of fertilizing the oocyte. As ovulation approaches, artificial insemination becomes less successful due to the lack of sufficient time for capacitation of inseminated spermatozoa. The oocyte must be fertilized within 6 hours after ovulation if a high rate of fertility is to occur. Aging of spermatozoa for 15 to 20 hours is not as critical as the aging of oocytes, as evidenced by data in Table 12-3, and it profoundly decreases the fertilizability of the oocyte, resulting in lower percentages of pregnancy.

The embryo or the unfertilized oocytes enter the uterus 72 to 96 hours from the onset of estrus.

Estrous Cycle Length

The length of the estrous cycle is variable but averages 21 days in the cow with a standard de-

viation of 4 days. The length of the cycle is slightly shorter for heifers; it lasts 20 days with a standard deviation of 3 days. These data are similar for both dairy and beef cattle.

There are reports which indicate that up to 30% of all estrous cycles are less than 17 days or greater than 25 days in length. As shown in Figure 12-1 considerable variations in the length of estrous cycles should be expected.

Uterine Therapy and Cycle Length

The length of the estrous cycle can be shortened or lengthened by uterine infusions of irritating solutions or antibiotics, such as tetracycline, when given on different days of the estrous cycle. Uterine infusion given during days 3 to 9 of the cycle (estrus = day 0) may significantly shorten the time for the female to return to estrus, whereas treatment on days 14 to

17 prolongs the luteal period. Uterine irritants cause endometrial damage and probably favor prostaglandin release about 3 days after infusion. The CL is generally refractory to prostaglandin-induced lysis from the time of ovulation to day 5 of the cycle. Irritating intrauterine infusions on day 4 of the cycle result in luteolysis on day 7, whereas infusions earlier than day 3 generally fail to induce luteolysis (Fig. 12-4). Intrauterine infusion on day 15 would interfere with the normal prostaglandin release, resulting in a lengthening of the current luteal phase. These results suggest that the uterus contributed to the decline in progesterone by producing luteolytic factors. The declining progesterone levels are usually followed by the release of LH, due to the removal of the negative feedback of progesterone (Fig. 12-5).

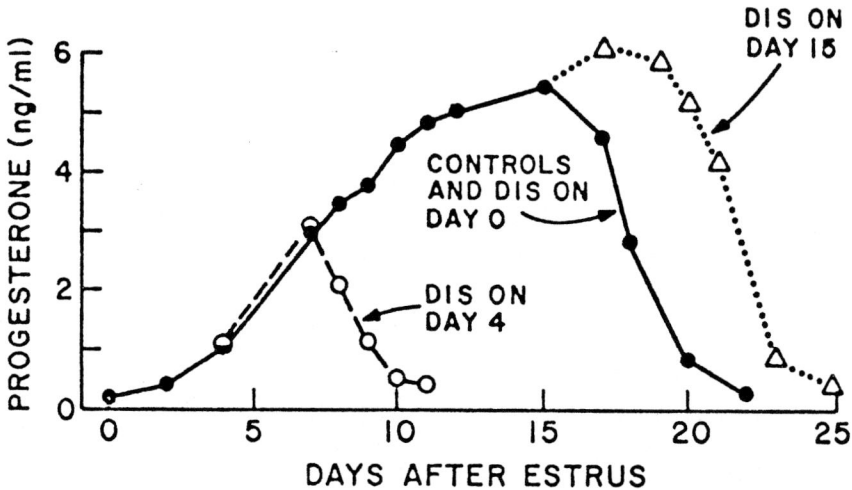

Fig. 12-4. Serum progesterone concentrations in cows given intrauterine injection of dilute iodine solution (**DIS**) on days **0**, **4**, or **15** of the estrous cycle. (From: B. E. Seguin et al., Am. J. Vet. Res. *35*:57, 1974).

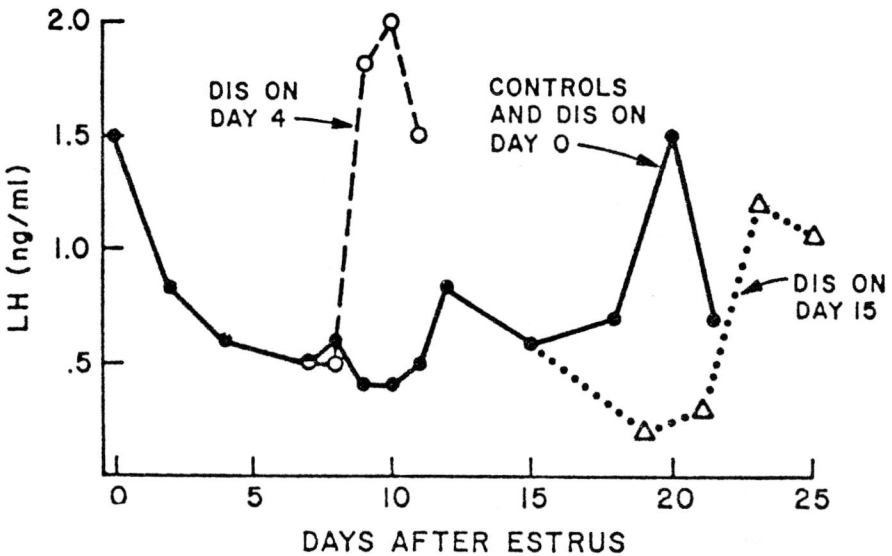

Fig. 12-5. Serum luteinizing hormone (LH) values in cows given intrauterine injection of dilute iodine solution (**DIS**) on days **0**, **4**, or **15** of the estrous cycle. (From: B. E. Seguin et al. Am. J. Vet. Res. *35*:57, 1974).

OVARY

Oogenesis with the oocyte arrested at the dictyate stage of meiosis is completed by the time of birth. The newborn heifer has approximately 75,000 oocytes within each ovary. This number declines during the prepubertal period. The mature cow may have only 60,000 oocytes in the ovaries, and an aged cow may have as few as 1,000. Most oocytes are lost during follicular atresia or degenerate during the reproductive life of the cow. Only a small number of oocytes are lost through ovulation of animals that are not bred.

Prepubertal heifers may have rather large follicles on the ovary; some follicles may be as large as 12 mm in diameter. After puberty, follicles reach diameters greater than 16 mm, and only one oocyte will normally be shed at each estrous period. Antral follicles in adult cows generally range between 5 to 20 mm in diameter.

At the time of ovulation, there is slight hemorrhage at the point of rupture, and the ruptured walls of the follicle protrude. Most of the liquor and the cumulus cells leave the follicle, but blood clots and the granulosa and thecal cells that formed part of the follicular wall remain intact within the crater.

Immediately after ovulation, the small, soft corpus hemorrhagicum (CH) begins to organize and develop. Cells from the theca interna and the granulosa layers begin rapid division and growth. Organizational changes continue during the first week of the life of the CL. A considerable amount of progesterone is produced and released from the CL beginning on day 3 or 4 of the cycle. Between day 8 to day 16, the physical changes are minimal, the CL is large and firm, and the output of progesterone by the CL is maximal. Degenerative changes begin to develop by day 17 unless the "pregnancy recognition factor" is provided by the embryo. The secretory activities cease, and the regressing CL becomes a small and hard corpus albicans (CA). The nonfunctional CA of the previous cycle sometimes is nearly as large as the newly formed CH, and often the ovary will contain CAs from previous cycles in varying stages of physical degeneration and resorption.

The mature CL is round or ovoid, solid or with a fluid-filled center, usually about 20 to 25 mm in diameter, and weighs about 5 g. As much as one-half of the luteal mass may protrude above the surface of the ovary. During pregnancy, there is little increase in weight or size of the CL over that of a nonpregnant cycle. The CL is encapsulated but highly vascularized. Manual enucleation of the CL from the ovary may result in considerable hemorrhage conducive to periovarian adhesions.

The mature CL of the cow contains a yellow lipochromic pigment which gives it a light brown to yellow appearance. Because of this coloration, the CL is frequently referred to as the 'yellow body'. As the CL ages and begins degeneration, the color darkens until it finally becomes deep orange to brown. After complete degeneration, the CA becomes white in color.

OVIDUCT

The oviduct of the cow is approximately 25 cm in length. The fimbria and funnel shape of the ovarian end enhance the ability of the oviduct to capture follicular fluid and oocytes at the time of ovulation. The secretory and muscular activities of the oviduct are influenced by the gonadal hormones. The oocyte enters the *ampulla* within 2 hours after ovulation but spends approximately 40 to 80 hours moving along the length of the oviduct. Fertilization occurs within the upper or middle regions of the *ampulla*.

Folds of mucus membranes of the oviduct tend to act as a sphincter-like constriction, termed the utero-tubal junction, at the junction of the oviduct and uterus. Gonadal hormones influence the muscular activity of the isthmus and probably control transport of the embryo to the uterus. Elevated progesterone levels due to multiple ovulations or after exogenous progesterone administration appear to hasten embryo entry into the uterus.

UTERUS

Gonadal hormones induce cyclic changes in the epithelium of the uterus. Under the influence of estrogen, there is congestion and edema of the uterine mucosa with a predominance of mucin-filled columnar epithelial cells. On the day after estrus, edema of the mucosa lessens, but a breakdown occurs in some of the congested uterine blood vessels. This allows an extravasation of blood or diapedesis of erythrocytes, which may cause a blood-tinged vaginal mucus. This postestrual hemorrhage is commonly observed in heifers but seldom in the cow. The appearance of blood-tinged mucus on the tail 1 to 3 days after estrus in the heifer is due to the postestrual hemorrhage. The postestrual hemorrhage of the bovine is not related to the menstruation of primates and should not be referred to as such. Some cattle breeders believe that the appearance of this blood-tinged mucus indicates fertilization failure. There is no scientific basis for such a belief.

Marked glandular development of the uterus is associated with estrus. Under the influence of estrogens, during proestrus and estrus there is a period of straight luminal growth of the endometrial glands, often referred to as the proliferative phase. Within 3 to 5 days after estrus, progesterone rises and stimulates the endometrial glands to grow, branch, coil, and secrete. This period is often referred to as the secretory phase. The uterus normally has 80 to 125 caruncles which are devoid of glands.

Following ovulation, progesterone produced by the CL acts on the estrogen-primed uterus to prepare it for pregnancy. The growth processes of uterine muscles, glands, vasculature, and epithelium are stimulated. This process is repeated every 3 weeks unless interrupted by pregnancy.

If pregnancy occurs, the uterine gland secretions nourish the preimplantation embryo for the first 30 days of its uterine life. At about 35 days of gestation, the chorioallantoic membranes gradually begin to establish a weak attachment to the uterus. Until attachment, the embryo survives on the uterine luminal fluids or "uterine milk." The uterine fluid contains proteins, salts, hormones, mucus from the uterine glands, desquamated epithelial cells, and some blood cells. It is a nutritious medium for the young developing embryo. Unfortunately, it is also a good medium for the growth of many microorganisms, and the uterus can serve as a perfect incubator for pathogenic organisms.

CERVIX

The cervix is the port of entrance from the vagina to the uterus. It is closed during diestrus or pregnancy but is a potential opening during estrus. Closure is only relative since it is occluded by a thick mucous secretion stimulated by progesterone. Under the influence of estrogen at estrus there is a relaxation of the cervical folds. Liquefaction of the cervical mucus during estrus permits uterine drainage, the insertion of an insemination pipet, or the displacement of spermatozoa and seminal plasma of the ejaculate after copulation. It should be remembered that the cervix establishes the transition from the frequently contaminated vagina to the semisterile environment of the uterus. In addition, the cervix serves as a barrier to abnormal spermatozoa from the ejaculate following natural breeding.

VAGINA AND VULVA

The secretory and epithelial changes of the vagina are cyclic, responding to varying levels of estrogen and progesterone in a fashion similar to that of other parts of the tract. Attempts to identify the stages of the estrous cycle in the cow by a vaginal smear or biopsy have met with little success.

The vulva responds to the varying levels of estrogen and progesterone. During proestrus and estrus, under estrogen domination, the vulva is slightly swollen and congested. This edema recedes after estrus, and the vulva becomes small during early pregnancy when progesterone is dominant. As parturition approaches, the vulva again becomes edematous and relaxed. This response is associated with rising levels of placental estrogen and relaxin from the CL.

CLINICAL OVARIAN DYSFUNCTION

It is not within the scope of this chapter to cover clinical aspects of reproduction, but at this point an understanding of the reproductive cycle may be enhanced by a brief description of some common ovarian abnormalities in the cow. Ovarian dysfunction may be classified into three general groups: Anestrus; subestrus; and pathologic ovarian changes.

Anestrus

Anestrus, or the lack of cyclicity, is normal in the prepubertal, pregnant, or early postpartum animal. Only when anestrus extends past the normal time of puberty, or exceeds the normal postpartum interval, it is considered to be abnormal. These animals are classified as anestrous because of the lack of reproductive cyclicity, which is necessary in order to breed the female. Pregnancy is the most frequent and normal cause of anestrus in the mated cow or heifer.

The two major causes of pathological anestrus in heifers are developmental abnormalities of the reproductive tracts and nutritional deficiencies. The nutritional component has been discussed previously in this chapter under puberty. The best therapy for pubertal anestrus is to provide adequate nutrition to the heifers. If, however, the heifer is near the breed-weight average for puberty, she could be induced to undergo her pubertal estrus by treatment with exogenous hormones. Progestagens, also called progestins (synthetic progesterone), are given orally or as implants in order to mimic the progesterone increase which usually occurs prior to the pubertal estrus. The progestagen is then withdrawn, resulting in a gonadotropin surge similar to that of normal pubertal heifers. If these induced-puberty heifers are bred, however, without attaining sufficient body size, dystocia can result.

The percentage of animals which have abnormal reproductive tracts is generally small. These animals are identifiable by rectal palpation of the uterus and oviducts and should be eliminated from the breeding herd.

A major cause of anestrus in cows is associated with prolonged postpartum intervals. These animals have calved and their uteri have involuted; however, they do not initiate follicular activity leading to ovulation. As a result, they are not rebred in a timely fashion and constitute a major direct economic loss to the producer.

Lactation usually exacerbates the problems caused by a poor diet and can directly influence the length of the anestrous period. Mastectomized postpartum cows will return to cyclicity within a few weeks. A lactating animal will normally have a longer anestrous period unless milking or suckling ceases. It appears that, either through machine milking or the suckling of the calf, there is a negative influence on the release of gonadotropic hormones. The negative effect appears to be associated with the amount of udder stimulation and has been shown to relate directly to a lower frequency of the pulsatile release of LH.

Another pathologic condition common in dairy cows is cystic follicular degeneration or cystic ovarian disease. Although the exact mechanism is still not well defined, the follicles which develop in a cycle fail to ovulate and continue to enlarge, sometimes reaching 5 to 6 cm in diameter. The normal preovulatory follicle is less than 2.5 cm in diameter. Cystic follicular degeneration can be successfully treated with exogenous hormones. Thin-walled or follicular cysts are treated with GnRH, LH, or LH-like hormones such as human chorionic gonadotrophin to promote luteinization. If adequate levels of luteinization occur within the cyst, it will act like a CL and regress in about a normal cycle length. Prostaglandin treatment could be incorporated after luteinization to hasten the return to estrus. Thick-walled or luteal cysts can be treated directly with prostaglandin for a more rapid return to estrus. There is, however, a heritable component to this disease, and routine treatment of the cystic follicular degeneration could contribute to increase the incidence of this disease within the herd.

Silent Estrus

Unobserved or silent estrus are terms indicating the failure to identify cows that are in estrus or cows which cycle but fail to express overt, detectable signs of estrus. The economic importance is obvious when artificial insemination is contemplated since these cows are not bred, and the number of days they remain open (time from calving to the next conception) increases. In many cases, the major cause is failure to detect estrus, mainly due to inadequate observation times. As a consequence, short estruses are missed. Observation failure is further hampered by the fact that the natural mounting behavior is brief and freely roaming cattle display most estrual activity at night.

Cows that frequently display silent estrus may have significantly shorter periods of estrus than the average cow. Some cows have an estrous period of less than 16 hours, and up to 25% of these animals may be in heat for 8 hours or less. These animals often display mounting behavior but are not detected due to the shorter estrual period.

Of special consideration is the effect of high ambient temperature and humidity on cyclicity. Thermal stress causes a pronounced decrease in the duration of estrus and in the intensity of behavioral changes. These animals cycle but are much more difficult to detect as in estrus and inseminate artificially. An additional component is that high thermal stress has a negative effect on the male and on the normal development of the embryo. During the hot summer months, thermal stress can have an extremely pronounced detrimental effect on cattle reproduction. Other factors such as undernutrition and environment (footing) may also play a role.

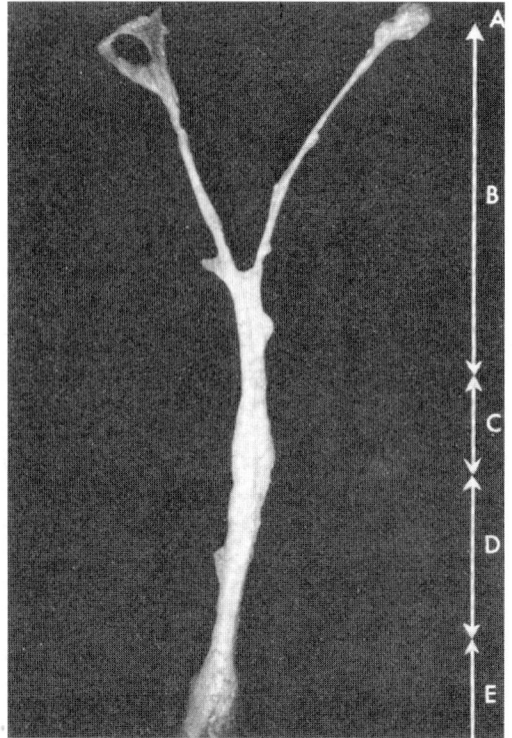

Fig. 12-6. Freemartin. **A.** Rudimentary gonad. **B.** Oviduct and horn. **C.** Body and cervix. **D.** Vagina. **E.** Anterior segment of vestibulum. (From: R. Zemjanis, *Diagnostic and Theraputic Techniques in Animal Reproduction.* Baltimore, MD, Williams & Wilkins, 1962, p. 50).

FREEMARTINISM

A **freemartin** is a sterile heifer which has been born twin to a bull calf. Sterility occurs in greater than 90% of these heifers. The male is fertile, although there is evidence of lowered fertility. The physical cause of infertility is the repressed or interrupted development of the female genital tract (Fig. 12-6). Fetal Sertoli cells from the male fetus secrete Müllerian-inhibiting hormone (MIH), also called anti-Müllerian hormone (AMH), which induces regression of the Müllerian ducts. Other factors from the male co-twin also participate and prevent or alter development of reproductive organs in the co-twin heifer (see Chapter 7). In the case of heterosexual twins, areas of placental vascular anastomosis allow the AMH to impact the female reproductive tract as early as day 40 of gestation. The anastomosis also allows the feti to become chimeras. The external genitalia may resemble those of the normal female, although the vagina is usually shorter. The gonads, when present, are more testicular than ovarian and are frequently nonfunctional; consequently, a freemartin heifer typically displays prolonged periods of anestrus. The clitoris is sometime overly developed and the mammary glands fail to develop. All freemartins have small seminal vesicles located laterally to the incompletely developed cervix. These are diagnostic aids for this condition if the animal is large enough to be palpated.

Since the majority of the heifers born twin to a bull are sterile, the possibilities of a potentially fertile heifer arising from twinning is less than 1 in 10. Freemartinism is a congenital abnormality rather than heritable. Hence, it may be important to know if a specific, genetically valuable heifer is potentially fertile. Caution must be exercised when planning to breed such females because twinning is an undesirable heritable trait in cattle.

The appearance of the external genitalia of the newborn freemartin heifer can be relatively normal, yet the internal genitalia are abnormal. A diagnosis can be made in several ways. One method is to insert a 10-ml test tube into the vagina of the newborn heifer. If the tube can be introduced only 5 to 7.5 cm into the vagina, the heifer is probably a freemartin. In a normal newborn heifer, the test tube can be inserted into the vagina for its full length. Observation should also be made of the clitoris, since it is often enlarged in the freemartin.

A definitive diagnostic test is to send blood samples from the female to a karyotyping laboratory to determine if the animal is an XX/XY chimera. If the heifer is mature enough to permit rectal examination of the genital tract, this should indicate whether the internal components of the tract are properly developed.

THE MALE

In the bull, puberty is earliest in the dairy breeds and occurs relatively later in the beef breeds. A range of 5 to 7 months would cover the onset of puberty in most well-nourished bulls. Puberty is delayed by undernutrition in the male as in the female. Underfeeding delays the onset of puberty, but it is difficult to completely prevent puberty by starvation. Bulls on a total digestible nutrient (TDN) intake of only 60 to 70% (Table 12-4) reached puberty at 14 to 15 months of age or older.

Young bulls are typically evaluated for breeding soundness at about 12 months of age. Future use is then projected based on the ejaculate quality and scrotal size. Maximal semen production and reproductive capacity are reached by 4 years of age and begin to decline after 7 years of age. Few bulls remain in the breeding herd beyond 8 to 10 years of age, although some bulls have been reported to remain fertile until 20 years of age.

Erection and copulation in the bull are associated with enormous increases in the blood pressure within the penis, as discussed in Chapter 8. The correlations between testicular size and spermatozoal production (quantity and quality) of bulls are described in Chapter 10.

Prepubertal bull calves show an increase in the amplitude of LH peaks up to about 3 months of age, when the amplitude of these LH peaks begins to decline. The frequency of LH pulses increases until 4 months of age. From 7 through 13 months of age, the plasma levels of LH increase in a linear fashion. Initially, the Leydig

Table 12-4 *Age and Physical Measurements of Holstein Bulls on Low-, Medium-, and High-Energy Intakes at the Time the First Ejaculate Contained Motile Spermatozoa*

Source	Feeding Level (% Required TDN)	No. Bulls	Age (weeks)	Weight (lb)
Cornell	60	3	56	503
	75	6	47	526
	100	12	43	578
	140	6	36	599
	160	6	39	688
Pennsylvania	70	8	61	523
	100	8	45	643
	115	6	41	675
	130	8	44	784
Illinois	60	6	52	352
	100	6	45	588

TDN = Total digestible nutrient
Adapted from: G. W. Salisbury and N. L. VanDemark, Physiology of Reproduction and Artificial Insemination of Cattle. San Francisco, CA, W. H. Freeman and Co., 1964, p. 600.

cells require a high level of LH for testosterone secretion. This threshold begins to decline at about 6 months of age. Leydig cells are steroidogenically active after about 3 months of age for androstenedione production, and by 7 months, testosterone production ensues. Apparently, there is an interaction between these testicular steroids and the hypothalamic-hypophysial axis which results in increased sensitivity to LH through maturation. The roles of follicle-stimulating hormone and prolactin relative to the onset of puberty in the male have not yet been defined.

The process of spermatogenesis in the prepubertal bull has been described to consist of four stages which occur between 2 and 11 months of age. The infantile phase from birth to 2 months of age is characterized by solid sex cords and undifferentiated supporting cells. The second or proliferation phase follows and is completed by 5 to 6 months of age. Spermatogonia appear during this time in all the tubules. The next or prepubertal phase lasts until approximately the end of the 8th month. The Sertoli cells and seminiferous tubule lumens are formed. Over this period, spermatogonia, primary and secondary spermatocytes, and spermatids develop and spermatozoa are detectable by the end of the third phase. The final period is the pubertal phase, lasting until approximately the 11th month of age, at which time puberty ensues. Following puberty, changes in spermatogenesis are primarily qualitative. After the onset of puberty, seminal evaluation reveals an increase in spermatozoal motility, concentration, and the percentage of normal spermatozoa in ejaculates obtained over time during the postpubertal period. Concurrently, there is also a decline in the number of spermatozoa with proximal cytoplasmic droplets.

Testicular development and scrotal circumference are closely associated with the onset of puberty. In bulls, puberty is associated with a scrotal circumference of 25.9 to 26.3 cm. This relationship seems to be consistent across various breeds. The normally developing testes reach 90% of their adult size by 24 months of age.

Nutrition influences the onset of puberty of the male (Table 12-4) in a similar fashion as described for the female. Balanced high-energy diets fed until puberty appear to be beneficial, resulting in bulls which can produce acceptable numbers of spermatozoa and seminal quality. However, high-energy diets given to bulls after puberty can be detrimental and cause decreases in both spermatozoal reserves and ejaculate quality.

REFERENCES

1. Abdel-Raouf, M. (1960): The postnatal development of the reproductive organs in bulls with special reference to puberty. Acta Endocrinol. (Suppl.) *49*:9.
2. Alila, H. W., Dowd, J. P., Corradino, R. A., et al. (1988): Control of progesterone production in small and large bovine luteal cells separated by flow cytometry. J. Reprod. Fertil. *82*:645.
3. Anderson, L. L. (1982): Relaxin localization in porcine and bovine ovaries by assay and morphologic techniques. Adv. Exp. Med. Biol. *143*:1.
4. Archbald, L. F., Schultz, R. H., Fahning, M. L., et al. (1973): Sequential morphologic study of the ovaries of heifers injected with exogenous gonadotropins. Am. J. Vet. Res. *34*:21.
5. Asdell, S. A. (1964): Domestic cattle. *In:* Patterns of Mammalian Reproduction, 2nd ed., edited by S. A. Asdell. Ithaca, N.Y., Comstock Publishing Associates, p. 587.
6. Batta, S. K. (1975): Effect of prostaglandin on steroid biosynthesis. Steroid Biochem. *6*:1075.
7. Beck, T. W. and Convey, E. M. (1977): Estradiol control of serum luteinizing hormone concentrations in the bovine. J. Anim. Sci. *45*:1096.
8. Beckett, S. D., Walker, D. F., Hudson, R. S., et al. (1974): Corpus cavernosum penis pressure and penile muscle activity in the bull during coitus. Am. J. Vet. Res. *35*:761.
9. Brewster, J. E. and Cole, C. L. (1941): The time of ovulation in cattle. J. Dairy Sci. *24*:111.
10. Brown, B. W. (1994): A review of nutritional influences on reproduction in boras, bulls and rams. Reprod. Nutr. Develop. *34*:89.
11. Butler, W. R. and Smith, R. D. (1989): Interrelationships between energy balance and postpartum reproductive function in dairy cattle. J. Dairy Sci. *72*:767.
12. Carruthers, T. D. and Hafs, H. D. (1980): Suckling and four-times daily milking: Influence on ovulation, estrus and serum luteinizing hormone, glucocorticoids and prolactin in post-partum Holsteins. J. Anim. Sci. *50*:919.
13. Chenault, J. R., Thatcher, W. W., Kalra, P. S., et al. (1975): Transitory changes in plasma progestin estradiol, and luteinizing hormone approaching ovulation in the bovine. J. Dairy Sci. *58*:709.
14. Committee on Bovine Reproductive Nomenclature (1972): Recommendations for standardizing bovine reproductive terms. Cornell Vet. *62*:216.
15. Convey, E. M., Beck, T. W., Neitzel, R. R., et al. (1977): Negative feedback control of bovine serum luteinizing hormone (LH) concentration from completion of the preovulatory LH surge until resumption of luteal function. J. Anim. Sci. *45*:792.

16. Convey, E. M., Kesner, J. S., Padmanabhan, V., et al. (1981): Luteinizing hormone releasing hormone-induced release of luteinizing hormone from pituitary explants of cows killed before or after oestradiol treatment. J. Endocrinol. *88*:17.

17. Dixon, S. N. and Gibbons, R. A. (1979): Proteins in the uterine secretions of the cow. J. Reprod. Fertil. *56*:119.

18. Eley, R. M., Thatcher, W. W., and Bazer, F. W. (1979): Luteolytic effect of estrone sulfate on cyclic beef heifers. J. Reprod. Fertil. *55*:191.

19. Erickson, B. H. (1966): Development and senescence of the postnatal bovine ovary. J. Anim. Sci. *25*:800.

20. Erickson, B. H., Reynolds, R. A., and Murphree, R. L. (1976): Ovarian characteristics and reproductive performance of the aged cow. Biol. Reprod. *15*:555.

21. Estergreen, V. L., Frost, O. L., Gomes, W. R., et al. (1967): Effect of ovariectomy on pregnancy maintenance and parturition in dairy cows. J. Dairy Sci. *50*:1293.

22. Farris, E. J. (1954): Activity of dairy cows during estrus. J. Am. Vet. Med. Assoc. *125*:117.

23. Fields, M. J., Fields, P. A., Castro-Hernandez, A., et al. (1980): Evidence for relaxin from corpora lutea of late pregnant cows. Endocrinology *107*:869.

24. Fields, M. J., Bannos, C. M., Watkins, W. B., et al. (1992): Characterization of large luteal cells and their secretory granules throughout the estrous cycle of the cow. Biol. Reprod. *46*:535.

25. Fields, M. J., LaRosa, D. V., Chang, S., et al. (1992): Immunolocalization of oxytocin and neurophysin in large luteal cells of the early pregnant cow. Biol. Reprod. *46*:152 (Abstract).

26. Fortune, J. E. (1991): Bovine theca and granulosa cells interact to promote androgen production. Biol. Reprod. *35*:292.

27. Fuchs, A. R., Behrens, O., Helmer, H., et al.(1990): Oxytocin and vasopressin receptors in bovine endometrium and myometrium during the estrus cycle and early pregnancy. Endocrinology *127*:629.

28. Geisert, R. D., Morgan, G. L., Short, E. C., et al. (1992): Endocrine events associated with endometrial function and conceptus development in cattle. Reprod. Fertil. Develop. *4*:301.

29. Ginther, O. J. and Meckley, P. E. (1972): Effect of intrauterine infusion on length of diestrus in cows and mares. Vet. Med. Small Anim. Clin. *67*:751.

30. Ginther, O. J., Knopf, L., and Kastelic, J. P. (1989): Temporal associations among ovarian events in cattle during oestrous cycles with two or three follicular waves. J. Reprod. Fertil. *87*:223.

31. Ginther, O. J., Wiltbank, M. C., Fricke, P. M., et al. (1996): Selection of the dominant follicle in cattle. Biol. Reprod. *55*:1187.

32. Goodsaid-Zalduondo, F., Rintoul, D. A., Carlson, J. C., et al. (1982): Luteolysis-induced changes in phase composition and fluidity of bovine luteal cell membranes. Proc. Nat. Acad. Sci., USA *79*:4322.

33. Hansel, W. and Convey, E. M. (1983): Physiology of the estrus cycle. J. Anim. Sci. *57* (Suppl. 2):404.

34. Hansel, W. and Snook, R. B. (1970): Pituitary ovarian relationship in the cow. J. Dairy Sci. *53*:945.

35. Hixon, J. E. and Hansel, W. (1979): Effects of prostaglandin $F_{2\alpha}$ estradiol and luteinizing hormone in dispersed cells preparations of bovine corpora lutea. *In:* Ovarian Follicular and Corpus Luteum Function,

edited by C. P. Channing and J. M. Marsh. New York, NY, Plenum Publishing Corp., p. 613.

36. Horton, E. W. and Poyser, N. L. (1976): Uterine luteolytic hormone: A physiological role for prostaglandin $F_{2\alpha}$. Physiol. Rev. *56*:595.

37. Jost, A. (1970): Hormonal factors in the sex differentiation of the mammalian foetus. Phil. Trans. Royal Soc. [B], London, England *259*:119.

38. Kastelic, J. P. (1994): Understanding ovarian follicular development in cattle. Vet. Med. *89*:64.

39. Kesner, J. S. and Convey, E. M., (1982): Interaction of estradiol and luteinizing hormone-releasing hormone on follicle-stimulating hormone release in cattle. J. Anim. Sci. *54*:817.

40. Kesner, J. S., Convey, E. M. and Anderson, C. R. (1981): Evidence that estradiol induces the preovulatory LH surge in cattle by increasing the pituitary sensitivity to LHRH and then increasing LHRH release. Endocrinology *108*:1386.

41. Killian, G. J. and Amann, R. P. (1972): Reproductive capacity of dairy bulls, changes in reproductive organ weights, and semen characteristics of Holstein bulls during the 1st 30 weeks after puberty. J. Dairy Sci. *55*:1631.

42. Kindahl, H., Granstrom, E., and Edqvist, L. E. (1977): Progesterone and 15-keto-13,14-dihydroprostaglandin $F_{2\alpha}$ levels in peripheral circulation after intrauterine iodine infusions in cows. Acta Vet. Scand. *18*:274.

43. Knickerbocker, J. J., Wiltbank, M. C., and Niswender, G. P. (1988): Mechanism of luteolysis in domestic livestock. Domestic Anim. Endocrinol. *5*:91.

44. Laing, J. A. (1970): Anoestrus and suboestrus in cattle. I. Functional abnormalities causing infertility in cattle. Vet. Rec. *87*:34.

45. Lamond, D. R., Dickey, J. R., Hendrick, D. M., et al. (1971): Effect of a progestin on the bovine ovary. J. Anim. Sci. *33*:77.

46. Leclerc, A., Guay, P., Malo, R., et al. (1972): Relationship between reproduction and the presence of microorganisms in the external opening of the cervix in the cow. Can. Vet. J. *13*:234.

47. Lineweaver, J. A. and Hafez, E. S. E. (1970): Ovarian responses in gonadotropin-treated calves. Am. J. Vet. Res. *31*:2157.

48. Liptrap, R. M. and McNally, P. J. (1976): Steroid concentration in cows with corticotropin-induced cystic ovarian follicles and the effect of prostaglandin $F_{2\alpha}$ and indomethacin given by intrauterine injection. Am. J. Vet. Res. *37*:369.

49. Lombard, L., Morgan, B. B., and McNutt, S. H. (1950): The morphology of the oviduct of virgin heifers in relation to the estrous cycle. J. Morphol. *86*:1.

50. McDonald, L. E., Nichols, R. E., and McNutt, S. H. (1952): Studies on corpus luteum ablation and progesterone replacement therapy during pregnancy in the cow. Am. J. Vet. Res. *13*:446.

51. McLaren, A. (1976): Mammalian Chimaeras. New York, NY, Cambridge University Press, p. 39.

52. Matton, P., Adelakoun, V., Couture, Y., et al. (1981): Growth and replacement of the bovine ovarian follicles during the estrous cycle. J. Anim. Sci. *52*:813.

53. Marion, G. B., Smith, V. R., Wiley, T. E., et al. (1950): The effect of sterile copulation on time of ovulation in dairy heifers. J. Dairy Sci. *33*:885.

54. Moeller, K. (1970): A review of uterine involution and ovarian activity during the postparturient period in the cow. N. Z. Vet. J. *18*:83.

55. Moeller, K. and VanDemark, N. L. (1951): The relationship of the interval between inseminations to bovine fertility. J. Anim. Sci. 10:987.

56. Moran, C., Quirke, J. F., and Roche, J. F. (1989): Puberty in heifers: A review. Anim. Reprod. Sci. *18*:167.

57. Morrow, D. A., Roberts, S. J., and McEntee, K. (1969): Postpartum ovarian activity and involution of the uterus and cervix in dairy cattle. I. Ovarian activity. II. Involution of uterus and cervix. III. Days nongravid and services per conception. Cornell Vet. *59*:173.

58. Morrow, D. A., Swanson, L. V., and Hafs, H. D. (1970): Estrous and ovarian activity in pubertal heifers. J. Anim. Sci. *31*:232.

59. Morrow, D. A., Swanson, L. V., and Hafs, H. D. (1976): Estrous behavior and ovarian activity in prepubertal heifers. Theriogenology 6:427.

60. Nadaraja, R. and Hansel, W. (1976): Hormonal changes associated with experimentally produced cystic ovaries in the cow. J. Reprod. Fertil. *47*:203.

61. Nakahara, T., Domeki, I., and Yamauchi, M. (1971): Synchronization of estrous cycle in cows by intrauterine injection with iodine solution. Nat. Inst. Anim. Health Quart., Japan *11*:219.

62. Nebel, R. L., Walker, W. L., McGilliard, M. L., et al. (1994): Timing of artificial insemination of dairy cows: Fixed time once daily versus morning and afternoon. J. Dairy Sci. 77:3185.

63. Northey, D. L. and French, L. R. (1980): Effect of embryo removal and intrauterine infusion of embryonic homogenates on the lifespan of the bovine corpus luteum. J. Anim. Sci. *50*:298.

64. Oxenreider, S. L. and Wagner, W. C. (1971): Effect of lactation and energy intake on postpartum ovarian activity in the cow. J. Anim. Sci. *33*:1026.

65. Padmanabhan, V., Leung, K., and Convey, E. M. (1982): Ovarian steroids modulate the self-priming effect of luteinizing hormone-releasing hormone on bovine pituitary cells *in vitro.* Endocrinology *110*:717.

66. Parsley, J. R., Mee, M. O., and Wiltbank, M. C. (1995): Synchronization of ovulation in dairy cows using PGF$_{2\alpha}$ and GnRH. Theriogenology *44*:915.

67. Patterson, D. J., Kinacofe, G. H., Stevenson, J. S., et al. (1989): Control of the bovine estrous cycle with melengestrol acetate (MGA): A review. J. Anim. Sci. 67:1895.

68. Putney, D. L., Drost, M., and Thatcher, W. W. (1988): Embryonic development in dairy cattle exposed to elevated ambient temperature between days 1 to 7 post insemination. Theriogenology 30:195.

69. Plasse, D., Warnick, A. C., and Koger, M. (1970): Reproductive behavior of *Bos indicus* females in a subtropical environment. IV. Length of oestrous cycle, duration of estrus, time of ovulation, fertilization and embryo survival in grade Brahman heifers. J. Anim. Sci. *30*:63.

70. Radford, H. M., Nancarrow, C. D., and Mattner, P. E. (1978): Ovarian function in suckling and nonsuckling beef cows post partum. J. Reprod. Fertil. *54*:49.

71. Rahe, C. H., Owens, R. E., Fleeger, J. L., et al. (1980): Pattern of plasma luteinizing hormone in the cyclic cow: dependence upon the period of the cycle. Endocrinology *107*:498.

72. Rao, A. V. and Kesava, M. A. (1971): Variation of body temperature in cows during certain stages of estrus cycles. Indian Vet. J. *48*:1237.

73. Roberts, R. M., Malathy, P. V. Hansen, J. R., et al. (1990): Bovine conceptus products involved in pregnancy recognition. J. Anim. Sci. *68* (Suppl. 2):28.

74. Roche, J. F. and Prendville, D. J. (1979): Control of estrus in dairy cows with a synthetic analogue of prostaglandin F$_2$ alpha. Theriogenology *11*:153.

75. Rosati, P. and Pelagalli, G. V. (1970): Blood supply of the ovary with reference to the developing Graafian follicle and corpus luteum research in *Bos taurus.* Acta Soc. Ital. Sci. Vet. *23*:260.

76. Saiduddin, S., Rowe, R. F., Thompson, K. W., et al. (1971): Effect of ovariectomy on pituitary gonadotrophins in the cow. J. Dairy Sci. *54*:432.

77. Salisbury, G. W. and VanDemark, N. L. (1964): Physiology of Reproduction and Artificial Insemination of Cattle. San Francisco, CA, W. H. Freeman and Co., p. 600.

78. Schams, D., Schallenberger, E., Hoffmann, B., et al. (1977): The oestrous cycle of the cow: hormonal parameters and time relationships concerning oestrous, ovulation and electrical resistance of the vaginal mucus. Acta Endocrinol. *86*:180.

79. Schams, D., Schallenberger, E., Menzer, C., et al. (1978): Profiles of LH, FSH and progesterone in postpartum dairy cows and their relationship to the commencement of cyclic functions. Theriogenology *10*:453.

80. Seguin, B. E., Morrow, D. A., and Louis, T. M. (1974): Luteolysis, luteostasis, and the effect of prostaglandin F$_{2\alpha}$ in cows after endometrial irritation. Am. J. Vet. Res. *35*:57.

81. Seguin, B. E., Morrow, D. A., and Oxender, W. D. (1974): Intrauterine therapy in the cow. J. Am. Vet. Med. Assoc. *164*:609.

82. Senger, P. L. (1994): The estrus detection problem: New concepts, technologies, and possibilities. J. Dairy Sci. 77:2745.

83. Shemesh, M. and Hansel, W. (1975): Levels of prostaglandin F (PGF) in bovine endometrium, uterine venous, ovarian arterial and jugular plasma during the estrous cycle. Proc. Soc. Exp. Biol. Med. *148*:123.

84. Shemesh, M. and Hansel, W. (1975): Arachidonic acid and bovine corpus luteum function. Proc. Soc. Exp. Biol. Med. *148*:243.

85. Short, R. E., Bellows, R. A., and Wiltbank, N. H. (1970): Unilateral ovariectomy and CL removal in the bovine. J. Anim. Sci. *31*:230.

86. Short, R. E., Bellows, R. A., Staigmiller, R. B., et al. (1990): Physiological mechanisms controlling anestrus and infertility in postpartum beef cattle. J. Anim. Sci. *68*:799.

87. Stafford, M. J. (1972): The fertility of bulls born co-twin to heifers. Vet. Rec. *63*:146.

88. Tan, G. J. S., Tweedale, R., and Biggs, J. S. G. (1982): Effects of oxytocin on the bovine corpus luteum of early pregnancy. J. Reprod. Fertil. *66*:75.

89. Trimberger, G. W. and Davis, H. P. (1943): Conception rate in dairy cattle by artificial insemination at

various stages of estrus. Nebraska Agric. Exp. Sta. Res. Bull. No. 129.

90. Trimberger, G. W. (1948): Breeding efficiency in dairy cattle from artificial insemination at various intervals before and after ovulation. Nebraska Agric. Exp. Sta. Res. Bull. No. 153.

91. Trimberger, G. W. and Fincher, M. G. (1956): Regularity of estrus, ovarian function and conception rates in dairy cattle. Cornell Univ. Agric. Exp. Sta. Bull. No. 911.

92. Vandeplassche, M. M. (1990): Fertility and infertility in the bull. Vet. Annu. *30*:37.

93. Veis, A. (1980): Cervical dilatation. A proteolytic mechanism for loosening the collagen fiber network. *In:* Dilation of the Uterine Cervix, edited by F. Naftolin and P. G. Stubblefield. New York, NY, Raven Press, p. 195.

94. Villa-Godoy, A., Ireland, J. J., Wortman, J. A., et al. (1981): Luteal function in heifers following destruction of ovarian follicles at three stages of diestrus. J. Anim. Sci. *52* (Suppl. 1):372.

95. Wagnon, K. A., Rollins, W. C., Cupps, P. T., et al. (1972): Effects of stress factors on the oestrous cycles of beef heifers. J. Anim. Sci. *34*:1003.

96. Walker, W. L., Nebel, R. L., and McGilliard, M. L. (1996): Time of ovulation relative to mounting activity in dairy cattle. J. Dairy Sci. *79*:1555.

97. Whisnat, C. S., Kiser, T. E., Thompson, F. N., et al. (1986): Opioid inhibition of luteinizing hormone secretion during the postpartum period in suckled beef cows. J. Anim. Sci. *63*:1445.

98. Whitmore, H. L., Tyler, W. J., and Casida, L. E. (1974): Incidence of cystic ovaries in Holstein-Friesian cows. J. Am. Vet. Med. Assoc. *168*:693.

99. Williamson, N. B., Morris, R. S., Blood, D. C., et al. (1972): A study of oestrus detection methods in a large commercial dairy herd. I. The relative efficiency of methods of oestrus detection. II. Oestrus signs and behavior patterns. Vet. Rec. *91*:50.

100. Wishart, D. F. and Snowball, J. B. (1973): Endoscopy in cattle: Observation of the ovary *in situ.* Vet. Rec. *92*:139.

101. Wolfenson, D., Thatcher, W. W., Badinga, L., et al. (1995): Effect of heat stress on follicular development during the estrous cycle in lactating dairy cattle. Biol. Reprod. *52*:1106.

102. Wordinger, R. J., Ramsey, J. B., Dickey, J. F., et al. (1973): On the presence of a ciliated columnar epithelial cell type within the bovine cervical mucosa. J. Anim. Sci. *36*:936.

103. Zemjanis, R. (1962): Diagnostic and Theraputic Techniques in Animal Reproduction, 2nd ed., edited by R. Zemjanis. Baltimore, MD, Williams & Wilkins, p. 50.

References Added in Proof

104. Hohenboken, W. D. (1999): Applications of sexed semen in cattle production. Theriogenology *52*:1421.

105. Lopez-Gatius, F. (2000): Site of Semen Deposition in Cattle: A Review. Theriogenology *53*:1407.

106. Royal, M., Mann, G. E., and Flint, A. P. (2000): Strategies for reversing the trend towards subfertility in dairy cattle. Vet J. *160*:53.

Reproductive Patterns of Horses*

S. M. HOPKINS AND G. C. ALTHOUSE

13

*Much information concerned with reproduction in horses has been presented in Chapter 2 (Pituitary Gland), Chapter 7 (The Biology of Sex), Chapter 8 (Male Reproductive System), Chapter 9 (Female Reproductive System), Chapter 10 (Artificial Insemination), and Chapter 11 (Patterns of Reproduction). The reader is encouraged to refer to these chapters to permit conciseness.

INTRODUCTION

Domestic mares are seasonally polyestrous breeders, with the onset and cessation of the ovulatory estrous cycles primarily influenced by the length of daylight (photoperiod). Additionally, general modifying factors include nutritional resources and climatic effects.

In the Northern Hemisphere, folliculogenesis is erratic in mares in the early Spring, during the period of Vernal transition, which may last for several weeks. During this period, multiple follicles develop and then regress without ovulation. At the end of this transitional period, during late Spring or early Summer, mares initiate their cyclic ovulatory activity until becoming anovulatory in the Fall. At this stage, which is called Fall or Autumn transition, some mares may display weak estruses but seldom ovulate. Fall transition is followed by Winter anestrus, characterized by complete reproductive quiescence. Winter anestrus continues until photostimulation increases, leading to the Vernal transition first, followed by full estrual cyclicity. The relative duration of each period is dependent on the individual mare and the latitude of her location. In areas of temperate and tropical climates, mares display long, ovulatory estrous cycles. Under these conditions, a small proportion of mares (15 to 20%) remain polyestrous throughout the year. These mares do not have a period of Fall transition leading to Winter anestrus.

Although not as evident as with the mare, stallions also undergo seasonal reproductive changes. Maximal values of volumes of ejaculate

413

and sperm-rich fractions, spermatozoal concentration in semen, libido, and gonadotropin levels occur during the longest periods of photostimulation, and they are minimal during the shortest periods of photostimulation. The stallion, however, does not undergo seasonal reproductive quiescence as do most mares.

THE FEMALE

Anatomy of the Reproductive Organs

The female reproductive tract consists of the paired ovaries and oviducts (uterine tubes), uterus including cervix, vagina, vestibule, and vulva. The tubular portion of the reproductive tract of the nonpregnant mare changes position. The magnitude of the positional change depends on the distention and movement of the abdominal viscera. The ovaries are suspended by the cranial portion of the broad ligament, or mesovarium, and the uterus is suspended by the caudal portion, or mesometrium. The somatic attachment of the broad ligament is to the dorsal sublumbar area. Currently, clinical examination and evaluation of these organs may involve rectal palpation, ultrasonography, vaginoscopy, digital examination of the cervix, uterine cytology, culture, biopsy, and hysteroscopy. Operators who will do rectal palpation in mares must be aware of the rectogenital pouch, which is a reflection of the peritoneum located between the rectum and genital tract. This peritoneal reflection extends to within approximately 15 cm of the anus. Rectal tears can occur because rectal examination generally takes place more than 25 cm cranial to the anus. These tears can penetrate through the intestinal mucosa and peritoneum into the pouch, leading to fecal-induced peritonitis and death. Consequently, the operator must be cognizant of the rectogenital pouch. Though rectal palpations are routinely performed in clinical practice for the equine species, they must be done with caution and finesse.

Ovaries

The ovaries resemble kidney beans in shape, and the mesovarium attaches to the dorsal convex surface. The concave ventral border contains the ovulation or ovulatory fossa. In the equine species, ovulations normally occur in the ovulatory fossa. During fetal development, the ovary develops into an outer connective tissue capsule and an inner parenchymatous area which reaches the ovarian surface only at the fossa. Full antral follicular growth occurs in the parenchymatous tissue with the apical wall of the Graafian follicle ultimately developing towards the fossa for ovulation. The overall size of the ovaries depends on the breed of the mare, season, and her cyclicity status. Mares in Winter anestrus lack significant follicular development, so the ovaries are small and firm compared to mares at the beginning of the breeding season.

Oviducts

The oviduct of the mare is convoluted and 20 to 30 cm in length, approximately 6 mm in external diameter at the *ampulla* and about 3 mm in diameter at the isthmus. The isthmus opens into the tip of the uterine horn through a small papilla. Fertilization, like in most females, occurs in the ampullar region of the oviduct, and the embryo takes 5 to 6 days to traverse the entire length of the oviduct to enter the uterus. Unfertilized oocytes are retained in the oviducts for several months, slowly degenerating. The mechanisms controlling the oviductal retention of unfertilized oocytes but allowing the passage through the oviduct of fertilized oocytes are unknown.

Uterus

The uterus of the mare can be divided into two major components, the body and two paired horns. The uterine body of a Quarter Horse, e.g., is about 20 cm in length, while each horn is 20 to 25 cm long. The uterine wall is formed by the following layers: Endometrium, which has an internal surface epithelium, a compact and then spongy lamina propria, and connective tissue, followed by myometrium and, finally, perimetrium. Uterine glands traverse the compact and spongy lamina propria. The endometrium and connective tissue are arranged into 12 to 15 longitudinal folds. The cavity or lumen of the uterus is not readily detectable by ultrasound unless distended with fluid during pregnancy or by inflammatory exudates or by air introduced in the uterus during breeding soundness examinations. Uterine glands can be evaluated by biopsy for the diagnosis of fibrosis. Increasing layers of periglandular fibrosis have been associated with a decrease in the ability of a mare to carry a foal to term. Additionally, inflammation or infections may be detected in the biopsy.

Cervix

The cervix of the mare changes dramatically in consistency, length, and diameter depending on the stage of the estrous cycle or pregnancy. The cervix is composed of connective tissue and smooth muscle, with the cervical canal connecting the external to the internal cervical os. The longitudinal cervical folds of the canal are continuous with the endometrial folds of the uterus. The cervix is clinically evaluated for color and consistency by visualization with a vaginal speculum and/or by digital palpation for the presence of adhesions, inflammation, or structural defects. Functionally, the cervix forms the last physical barrier to uterine infections in the nonestrous mare.

Vagina

The vagina of the mare is largely retroperitoneal except at the cranial portion, and rectovaginal tears do occur at foaling in some mares. However, these tears, although dramatic, are generally not life threatening. The vagina is demarcated by the transverse fold at the caudal juncture with the vestibule to the cranial confluence with the cervical portion of the vagina. The stratified squamous epithelium lining the vagina does not change significantly during the estrous cycle. Hence, vaginal smears as a means to diagnose the stage of the cycle are of no value. Typically, the vagina is examined though a speculum for anatomical configuration and signs of hyperemia or inflammation, suggestive of a concurrent endometritis.

Vestibule

The stratified squamous epithelium of the vagina is contiguous with that of the vestibule. The junction between the vagina and vestibule, the transverse fold, is derived from a hymenal remnant. This fold is part of the "pseudosphincter" or second physical barrier which helps to prevent pneumovagina caused by the aspiration of air into the vagina. Vaginitis could eventually lead to the development of endometritis, thus preventing the establishment of pregnancy. The external urethral orifice opens just caudal to the fold. The posterior limit of the vestibule is the labia of the vulva.

Vulva

The vulva is comprised of the paired labia, with the clitoris located ventrally in the inferior commissure of the vulva. In the normal, healthy mare, the labia are in tight apposition, forming the vulvar cleft. The labia are also part of the "pseudosphincter" system. The closure of the labia becomes an important consideration in the assessment of breeding soundness examinations in older, pluriparous or in mares with defective external genitalia. Inadequate labial conformation frequently leads to the necessity for a Caslick surgery to reestablish the closure of this portion of the anatomical "pseudosphincter."

Synopsis of Reproductive Endocrinology

The pineal gland, hypothalamus, and pituitary form the major neuroendocrine controlling axis, which is involved in puberty, reproductive cyclicity, and pregnancy.

In the postpubertal mare, the epithelial cells of the pineal secrete melatonin in amounts inversely proportional to the magnitude of white-light stimulation. Melatonin is antigonadotropic, and the effect appears to be mediated through the pituitary, which contains specific melatonin binding sites (Fig. 13-1). Long periods of light limit melatonin production and permit the release of follicle-stimulating hormone (FSH) and luteinizing hormone (LH) from the pituitary in response to stimulation by releasing hormones. The consequence is a stimulatory effect on follicular development which culminates in ovulation (Fig. 13-1).

Photoperiodic Signal ─────────┐
                                              (−)
        │   │
        ▼   ▼
Suprachiasmatic Nucleus   Pineal
              │ (+)   │
              ▼   Low Melatonin
        Hypothalamus   │
              │ GnRH   │
              ▼   │
        Pituitary ←── ──_(?)_── ── ┘
         (+) FSH - LH
Inhibin(−) FSH
        Dominant Follicle
              │
              ▼
        Estrogen ──────→ (+) Sexual Receptivity (Estrus)
                  ──────→ Uterus ┌─→ Edema
                                  └─→ Cervical Relaxation
                  ──────→ (+) Follicular LH Receptors

        Graafian Follicle ←──────
              │
              ▼
        ── Ovulation
              │
              ▼
Oocyte   Luteal Tissue (CL)
  │   │
  ▼   ▼
Fertilization
(if bred) Progesterone ───→ (−) Sexual Receptivity (Diestrus)
  │   │
  ▼   │
Uterus ←───────┘

        ├─→ Tone, cervical organization

        ├─→ (+) Pregnancy Recognition ⇢ CL Maintained

        └─→ (−) Pregnancy Recognition ⇢ CL Regressed ⇢ Estrus

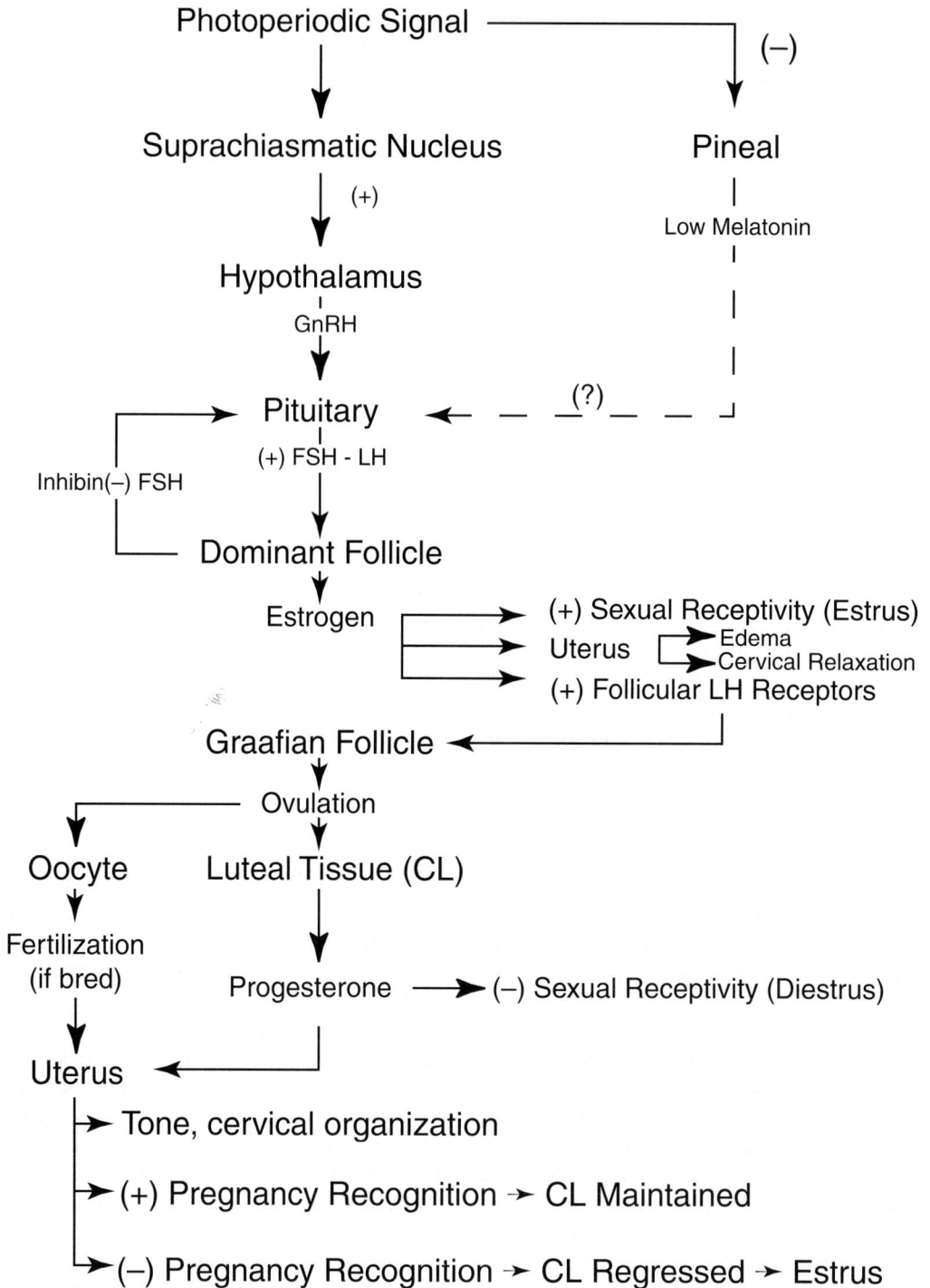

Fig. 13-1. Overview of the reproductive endocrinology of the mare, with emphasis on the follicular development leading to ovulation. (+) = stimulation; (−) = inhibition.

Puberty and Sexual Maturity in the Female

The onset of puberty, defined as the age at which a filly (young female horse) becomes reproductively active, begins to cycle, and ovulates, has not been investigated as extensively as for the age of puberty in females from other domestic species. Generally, young mares are not bred as soon as they become sexually active. Most fillies are thought to undergo puberty between 12 to 24 months of age and yet they may not be bred until after 3 years of age.

There are several major factors known to influence puberty in the filly: Age, as in somatic maturation, including weight, breed, nutrition, and season. These elements can be combined into the following model for the establishing of puberty: As the immature filly ages, the hypothalamic-pituitary axis becomes functionally active, and upon stimulation by hypothalamic-releasing factors, the pituitary gland secretes significant levels of FSH during the Spring and Summer months. Secretion of FSH declines during the short light months of the Fall. In the period of high FSH secretion, there is a concurrent increase in follicular development resulting in the secretion of estradiol-17β. Also during this period, there are pulses of LH of low frequency and amplitude which are insufficient to complete follicular growth. However, as the filly progresses into the breeding season, frequency and amplitude of LH release increase, resulting in the completion of follicular growth, maturation, and ovulation.

As stated previously, age of puberty is also influenced by body weight, nutrition, and season. Based on information from other species, the ability of the hypothalamus and pituitary to secrete LH is negatively influenced by low nutritional levels, particularly energy restriction. Consequently, even though a filly may be approaching the age of puberty, the onset may be delayed if the filly is or has been previously exposed to significant dietary restrictions or imbalances.

The effect of season on the onset of puberty primarily relates to the amount of light stimulation. In considering limited information on the onset of puberty in the filly, normal pubertal development requires exposure to both long and short daylight. Animals stimulated by a series of long (16-hour) or short (9-hour) periods of light had delayed onset of puberty. As a result, if a filly is old enough, has adequate body development, and is in the long photoperiod season, puberty will ensue, leading to full reproductive cyclicity. If, however, her age or body development is not adequate during this time, puberty will be delayed until the Spring or Summer of the next breeding season.

Estrous Cycle

The interestrous interval or duration of the estrous cycle is on the average 21 days during the breeding season with a range of 19 to 26 days. Mares express for each cycle during the breeding season the phases of **proestrus, estrus, metestrus,** and **diestrus;** however, from a clinical perspective, it is customary to divide the estrous cycle of the mare only into two phases:

1. **Estrus** or the follicular phase (duration 5 to 7 days).
2. **Diestrus** or the luteal phase (duration 14 to 16 days).

During this clinical phase of estrus, which also includes **proestrus**, the regression of the corpus luteum (CL) of the previous cycle is completed, and follicles rapidly grow under gonadotropin stimulation. In mares, the initial recruitment of follicles from the follicular cohort that will develop and ovulate begins 12 to 14 days prior to ovulation, while the progesterone levels are still greater than 1 ng/ml. Then, the selection of the dominant follicle from the cohort for further maturation takes place 6 to 7 days prior to ovulation. Subsequent to the initial secretion of prostaglandins from the uterus at day 14 of the estrous cycle, the CL rapidly regresses so that progesterone levels are at baseline levels in approximately 24 to 48 hours. The final maturation of the dominant follicle then takes place during the period of low levels of blood progesterone. The mare is quite sensitive, however, to the effects of estrogens from the dominant follicle or to estrogens from exogenous sources. With the sharp decline in progesterone secretion while the levels of estrogens are rising rapidly, mares initiate and display estrous behavior very quickly. The behavioral characteristics of estrus in mares are fully discussed in the section Estrus Detection of this chapter. Because the mare ovulates 24 to 48 hours prior to the end of estrus, the period of **metestrus**, defined as the postovulatory period during which the CL forms and begins to secrete progesterone, is contained within the last two 2 days of estrus. Estrous cyclicity generally begins in the Spring and continues during the Summer months and early Fall. The remainder of the year is typically divided into the Fall or Autumn transition leading into Winter anestrus, which is subsequently followed by Vernal or Spring transition.

Fall Transition and Winter Anestrus

The Fall-Winter transition or Autumn transition is poorly defined because mares either do not express overt estrus or are not typically bred at this time; research efforts have concentrated on the periods of seasonal breeding. At the end of the breeding season there is a final phase of follicular development and maturation, but these follicles do not ovulate. The failure to ovulate is presumed to be generated by the lack of an ovulatory surge of LH. This results in the persistence of nonovulated 'Autumn' follicle(s), which can be palpated or detected ultrasonographically for variable periods of time during the Autumn transition. During Winter anestrus, the hypothalamic-pituitary axis is quiescent. It has been postulated that increased secretion of melatonin from the pineal gland during the short light periods of late Fall and Winter block the synthesis and/or release of hypothalamic-releasing hormones.

Spring Transition

Spring transition is characterized by follicular development and regression over a time span of about 40 to 60 or more days. During the Spring transition, overt sexual behavior is erratic, particularly in reference to the expression of stand-ing estrus. As the pineal-hypothalamic-pituitary axis is reactivated by the increased photoperiod, FSH is released from the pituitary, and follicular growth ensues. Luteinizing hormone levels, however, remain at baseline, so the follicles do not fully mature and ultimately undergo atresia. This pattern of initial follicular development followed by regression continues throughout the Vernal transition until a fully developed and mature follicle is present in the ovary to secrete large amounts of estradiol-17β. In turn, the increasing levels of estradiol promote LH synthesis and secretion, leading to the ovulatory surge of LH followed by ovulation, and in nonmated mares, by the resumption of estrual cyclicity. In mares, as in other domestic species, LH is the luteotropic hormone needed to stimulate progesterone secretion by the corpus luteum. Hence, the postovulatory levels of progesterone are used clinically to confirm ovulation and that the mare has initiated normal ovulatory estrual cycles.

Follicular Dynamics

During the breeding season, which is the portion of the year in which mares exhibit overt, standing estrous cycles, the initial follicular development takes place in a single wave of follicular growth, beginning in mid-diestrus. This follicular wave develops during the FSH surge. In the majority of cases, all the follicles except for the dominant follicle are destined to undergo degenerative processes and atresia.

Follicular maturation involves endocrine as well as local regulation, which influences the granulosa and thecal cell layers (see Chapter 9). With the advent of ultrasonic imaging, it is now possible to anticipate and identify which is the dominant follicle selected for ovulation. A follicle reaching a mean diameter greater than 22 mm becomes dominant and continues to increase in diameter at a rate of approximately 2.5 mm/day. When the mean diameter exceeds 35 mm, this dominant follicle can be induced to ovulate by treatment with gonadotropins. Hence, follicular size is one component used as a timing aid for breeding. In about 20% of the time, a synchronous or asynchronous second follicle matures and ovulates. However, due to the embryo reduction phenomenon in mares (see Chapter 9), fewer than 0.5% of double ovulations result in the gestation to term of twins.

The tubular portion of the mare's reproductive tract is extremely sensitive to ovarian steroids. During the follicular phase of the cycle, estradiol-17β causes secretion of fluid by the uterus. This results in an edematous texture of uterine tissue on palpation and in a typical echogenic pattern of endometrial fold on ultrasonic evaluation. The cervix becomes shorter and more relaxed, which facilitates the intrauterine deposition of the ejaculate.

Ovulation

As with the other domestic species, ovulation in the mare is associated with an ovulatory surge of LH. However, the mare is peculiar in that ovulation occurs while the levels of LH are still rising. Thus, maximal or peak levels of LH are reached after ovulation has occurred. As stated previously, mares generally ovulate 24 to 48 hours prior to the cessation of estrus. Based on rectal palpation and ultrasonic imaging of the ovaries, most preovulatory follicles become softer and change shape from round to pear-like along with a slight increase in follicular wall thickness. In addition, the estrogenic echotexture of the uterus decreases shortly before ovulation. As previously indicated, ovulation normally takes place only through the ovulation fossa. The preovulatory follicle becomes hyperemic with vascular fenestrations resulting in an edematous theca interna layer. Most of the follicular fluid is emptied from the antrum within 1 minute after the ovulatory rupture of the follicular wall. Some mares, however, retain residual intrafollicular fluid for several more minutes. The bulk of the follicular fluid does not accompany the oocyte into the oviduct. Most of the fluid released from the follicle at time of ovulation flows into the peritoneal cavity.

Luteal Function

Following ovulation, the follicular wall collapses into apposition. It seems that in the mare, unlike the other domestic species, the granulosa cells develop into both large and small luteal cells, which are responsible for the secretion of progesterone, while the theca interna degenerates before ovulation and apparently does not contribute luteinized cells to the corpus luteum.[22] Levels of progesterone become detectable within 24 hours of ovulation. Growth of the granulosa luteal cells continues for approximately 9 days after ovulation, which also coincides with the point of maximal progesterone secretion. In cycling mares or mares that did not become pregnant, luteal regression begins as early as the 12th day of diestrus. By day 16 of diestrus, progesterone concentration in the blood becomes undetectable. Oxytocin and prostaglandin $F_{2\alpha}$ ($PGF_{2\alpha}$) induce regression of the corpus luteum only when mares have functionally active luteal tissue. If still within the breeding season, the mare will return to estrus within 3 to 4 days after treatment with prostaglandins.

During the luteal phase, the tubular reproductive tract has a palpably distinctive character and ultrasonic image due to the effects of progesterone. Progesterone causes the uterus to become turgid, and this turgidity is important during early pregnancy for attachment of the conceptus and gestation. The ultrasonic uterine cross-sectional image during diestrus appears uniform because of the progesterone dominance. The cervix also elongates and is tightly closed during diestrus or during pregnancy.

Breeding Management

Official Date of Birth for Purebred Racing Horses

Because of the arbitrary official date of birth for many breeds, established as the first of January of a given year, horse breeders demand treatment and management schemes of mares to advance the breeding season so the foals are born as close as possible to the first of January. For instance, a foal born in May is considered 1 year of age on January first of the following year, just as is for a foal born in February instead of May of that year. This group aging, at least in theory, gives the older, more mature foal a competitive performance advantage. Considering the average length of gestation of a mare, she could be bred as early as February 15th to produce a foal shortly after January 1st of the next year. This requirement for an official date of birth is not applied to all breeds of horses.

Estrus Detection

Detection of the onset of estrus in mares is important for the successful timing of breeding. Particularly, in view that the mare is in estrus for 5 to 7 days or longer and that she ovulates during the last 2 days of estrus. Daily hand matings in an attempt to ensure a high rate of pregnancy can be devastating for the average stallion because of overuse. As a conservative rule of thumb, a stallion can naturally breed 50 mares per breeding season (February 15th to June 15th), which represents about 100 ejaculations, without depressing his fertility from overuse. Also, overbreeding can contribute to uterine infections and to the development of infertility in mares. In well-managed breeding programs and to obtain maximal pregnancy rates, the follicular development is monitored and the mare is bred shortly prior to the projected time of ovulation (Table 13-1). If the mare fails to ovulate at the anticipated time, she is rebred 48 hours after the first breeding. This regimen typically requires only one to two breedings per estrous cycle. Initial pregnancy rates are not essentially different when mares are bred or artificially inseminated from 3 days prior to ovulation and up to 12 hours after ovulation. There is, however, a decrease in pregnancy rate due to an increase in early embryonic death in pregnancies resulting from breedings more than 6 hours postovulation.

The behavioral characteristics of estrus frequently become more intense and peak around the time of ovulation. These characteristic include, as positive signs, ear, neck, and foreleg posturing, eversion of the labia, squatting on the rear legs, tail elevation, and urination, particularly if the stallion is nearby. Some mares will display all of the above signs, while other mares only display a few and weaker signs of estrus. Typically, when a mare is first detected in estrus, she is examined by rectal palpation to evaluate the status of the tubular reproductive tract. The ovaries are then examined by ultrasound to ascertain the stage of follicular development. The position of the maturing follicle(s) in the ovary is recorded and then monitored sequentially at 24- to 48-hour intervals to estimate growth, preovulatory shape, and consistency in order to estimate the time of ovulation.

As mares approach the end of estrus, they keep the ears back, squeal, and kick or strike. As a general rule, signs of standing estrus predominate during estrogenic dominance, and these signs begin to diminish and finally vanish during the changeover from estrogenic to progesterone dominance.

Estrus Cycle Control

There are three main approaches applied to the control of the estrous cycle in mares: (a) to induce mares to initiate estrous cycles earlier in the year by shifting the Vernal transition; (b) increase; or (c) decrease the length of diestrus during the breeding season. All of these approaches, individually or in combination, may

Table 13-1   Relationship Between Time of Insemination with Fresh, Extended Semen and Conception Rates

	Day of Insemination with Respect to the Day of Ovulation							
	Days Before Ovulation						Day of Ovulation	Day After Ovulation
							0 (0 to 24 hrs)	1 (24 to 48 hrs)
	−6	−5	−4	−3	−2	−1		
No. of mares	9	8	12	12	21	8	69	43
Detected pregnant (%)	44	63	33	75	71	88	55	7

Adapted from: J. Woods, et al., Equine Vet. J. *22*:410, 1990.

be used to synchronize estrus in individual or in a group of mares (see Chapter 19). Some horse breeders, however, prefer to breed most of their mares during their naturally occurring breeding season. Except for special situations, this is the most cost- and labor-effective way to manage a horse population.

Alteration of the photoperiod is the simplest and possibly the most effective approach to stimulate estrous cyclicity. The high levels of melatonin associated with Winter anestrus can be functionally lowered by exposing the mare to an artificial source of light at a minimum intensity of 10 to 12 footcandles for at least 14.5 hours per day. There is a wide variation in the response of individual mares to lighting procedures. Some will respond relatively faster than others, so each animal must be dealt with individually. The light source may be incandescent or fluorescent bulbs which are controlled by timers. These light sources can be used in individual box stalls up to paddocks for group stimulation as long as the light intensity is adequate. As transition from anestrus to estrus progresses, there is an increasing rate of follicular development, but these follicles generally do not ovulate, possibly because LH is not released from the adenohypophysis or is released in insufficient amounts. Eventually, several follicles will develop and initiate steroidogenic pathways and secrete estradiol-17β, which brings about the psychic signs of estrus and stimulates the ovulatory surge of LH, which causes final follicular maturation and ovulation. This first estrus is frequently prolonged and may last for 10 to 20 days or longer. This prolonged estrus eventually terminates with the first ovulation of the season, which is then followed by the resumption of estrous cyclicity.

Augmented photostimulation does not change or shorten the events of Vernal transition; rather, it moves them earlier into the year. This necessitates that the mare be exposed to a program of increased artificial lighting for at least 2 months before the desired breeding time. Concurrently with the exposure of mares to an increased artificial lighting, mares should be provided with the nutritional requirements of an adequate and balanced diet. Also, photostimula-

tion by itself will not enhance fertility; rather, it provides the opportunity for the horse breeder to increase the number of breedings per season. As an example, if the anticipated fertility rate of a group of normal mares is about 50%, to increase the percentage of pregnant mares to 90%, some of the mares will require four breedings, which uses almost 3 months of the limited breeding season. The fertility of mares which are undergoing the first ovulation of the breeding season may be less fertile than the same mares in subsequent ovulations. As a result, some owners prefer to breed the mares during the second estrus rather than on the first estrus of the breeding season.

Another approach to further modify the transitional period from anestrus to estrus is to feed mares oral progestins for a minimum of 14 to 15 days during the mid to late part of the Vernal transition, after the mare had developed multiple follicles >20 mm in diameter and had displayed estrous behavior during teasing. Some mares ovulate upon withdrawal of treatment with progestins.

Once a mare had initiated estrous cycles during the breeding season, it is possible to modify the length of her estrous cycle by manipulating the duration of diestrus. This is done by giving prostaglandin $PGF_{2\alpha}$ 4 to 5 days after ovulation to induce regression of the corpus luteum. Luteal regression is followed by increased follicular development, estradiol secretion and release, and an early return to estrus.

Progestins are also used to inhibit estrus in order to synchronize a group of cycling mares which will cycle after withdrawal of treatment with progestins. Progestins are also used to block estrus in mares for exhibition or performance shows.

Breeding

Modern equine breeding programs are designed to minimize the number of services or artificial inseminations needed per conception. As previously mentioned, part of the rationale is to prevent overusing the stallion to decrease the number of oligospermic ejaculates containing too few spermatozoa for normal fertility. This approach also has the advantage of limiting the exposure of the female reproductive tract to potential pathogens and antigenic substances from the ejaculate. Artificial insemination helps to control pathogen exposure, but since semen itself is antigenic, the uterine stress cannot be completely eliminated. As a mare ages, the cumulative amount of uterine stress from breeding and foaling can result in decreased reproductive performance in older mares. Uterine insult is evidenced by the formation of periglandular fibrosis and/or by the delay in clearing out the postbreeding uterine contamination.

To establish the onset of estrus, mares are teased daily by a stallion. Then, mares found in estrus are examined by rectal palpation and by ultrasound to estimate follicular development and changes in the tubular tract. Breeding is recommended when the dominant follicle reaches a mean diameter of at least 35 mm. Although stallion spermatozoa from a natural breeding or from semen collected with an artificial vagina, then extended and inseminated, can remain viable in the oviducts of the mare for as long as 7 to 8 days, mares that fail to ovulate are generally rebred 48 hours later to increase the likelihood of fertilization. The use of cooled or frozen equine semen for AI requires different insemination times than those described above (see Chapter 10). Additionally, human chorionic gonadotropin (hCG) or GnRH implants can be used effectively, particularly early in the breeding season, to enhance the likelihood of a timely ovulation. Mares that had developed a follicle of 30–35 mm in diameter usually ovulate within 24 to 36 hours after the intravenous injection of hCG. Repeated administrations of hCG, however, may induce the formation of antibodies to hCG, which could be potentially harmful due to an anaphylactic response. Antibodies to hCG could also neutralize the biological activity of hCG by binding to the antigen. This, in turn, may result in the need of administering progressively higher doses of hCG. On these bases, hCG should not be used in any given mare more that twice during the breeding season.[25]

Pregnancy

In the mare, oocytes are ovulated as either primary oocytes, before the extrusion of the first polar body, or as secondary oocytes in metaphase II, with the first polar body already extruded (see Chapters 7 and 9). Upon ovulation, the oocyte displaces into the *ampulla* of the oviduct, where fertilization occurs. If the oocyte has been fertilized, it becomes an embryo and enters the uterus by day 6 postovulation. Unfertilized oocytes, however, are retained for months in the oviducts of the mare and undergo degeneration and lysis (see Chapters 7 and 9). Once in the uterus, the developing embryo displaces over the entire uterine internal surface until about day 16 and then fixes at the base of one uterine horn. The early migration is essential to the maternal recognition of pregnancy, probably by inhibiting the release of $PGF_{2\alpha}$ from the endometrial cells. If the embryonic mobility does not occur, the endometrial cells will produce and release $PGF_{2\alpha}$, the corpus luteum will regress, and, as a consequence, the pregnancy will be terminated.

As the embryo develops, trophoblastic cells from the chorionic girdle invade the maternal endometrium after day 35 of gestation, forming endometrial cryptae or endometrial cups. These cups are the source of the equine chorionic gonadotropin (eCG) also known as pregnant mare serum gonadotropin (PMSG), which has predominantly FSH- and also LH-like activities when given to another species. However, in the mare that is pregnant and producing eCG, the endogenous placental eCG or PMSG has predominantly LH-like activity. The endometrial cups are functional for up to 120 to 140 days with peak secretory activity around days 55 to 70 of gestation. Embryonic death after the development of the endometrial cryptae lowers but does not suppress the secretion of eCG. This results in a state of pseudopregnancy, producing a false positive immunological test for pregnancy in mares.

The mare is also unique when compared to the female of the other domestic species in that the mare develops accessory or secondary corpora lutea while the mare is in gestation. Once the signal of pregnancy is given, the corpus luteum of the cycle does not regress in the mare that became pregnant. This corpus luteum, which is called the primary corpus luteum, develops following ovulation and secretes progesterone up to about day 40 of pregnancy. At this time, possibly under the influence of the FSH-like activity of eCG and of pituitary FSH, new follicles develop and either ovulate or simply luteinize without ovulation to form the characteristic accessory, or also called secondary corpora lutea, of the equine species. The formation and functioning of the accessory corpora lutea is reflected in an increase in circulating levels of progesterone. The role of eCG in the maintenance of pregnancy is not completely understood. Perhaps a major role of eCG in the pregnant mare is to stimulate the primary and accessory corpora lutea to secrete progesterone in amounts sufficient for the maintenance of pregnancy. The pregnant mare is highly sensitive and responsive to low levels of progesterone in the blood, which is promptly followed by abortion.

Primary and secondary corpora lutea secrete progesterone up to days 180 to 220 of gestation, and by this time, their progesterone-secreting activity is replaced by progesterone secreted by the placenta. The placenta has the enzymatic machinery to secrete progesterone, as early as day 50 of pregnancy, when challenged by bilateral ovariectomy. Many mares will not abort when the bilateral ovariectomy is done after days 50 to 70 of pregnancy. Hence, the mare has an auto-sufficient placenta. The ovarian secretion of progesterone declines after day 150 of gestation, which results in significantly lower blood levels of progesterone until about day 220 of pregnancy. The placenta then takes over as the primary source of progesterone secretion until parturition.

Blood levels of estrogen, produced by the fetoplacental unit, rise at about 90 days of gestation, peak around 210 days, and gradually decline until parturition. Dehydroepiandrosterone produced by both the male or female fetal gonads is metabolized to estrogens. The role of estrogens during pregnancy in the mare remains unclear but can be monitored as an indicator of fetal viability.

The length of gestation is variable in the mare, with a modal range of 335 to 342 days. Gestations as short as 305 and as long as 400 days which resulted in the birth of viable foals have been reported, but these extreme ranges are very unusual. Factors which affect the length of pregnancy include sex of the fetus (male) and foaling early in the year which increase gestation length an average of 3 and 10 days, respectively. The majority of mares foal in the evening hours, between 10 PM and 2 AM. As mentioned previously, approximately 20% of the estrous cycles result in the ovulation of two oocytes, and about half of the time, both oocytes are fertilized and enter the uterus. In the majority of cases (70%), both embryos attach to the endometrium next to each other at the base of the same horn. However, only one embryo has sufficient endometrial contact for survival, while the other embryo is prevented to implant through a natural embryo-reduction phenomenon (see Chapter 9). Very rarely, both embryos may survive and implant, resulting in the establishment of a twin pregnancy. Typically, twinning leads to abortion because the maternal-placental interface becomes insufficient for fetal support as both fetuses grow in size. The rare occasional birth of two live foals is also undesirable because the mare does not produce sufficient nutritional milk to support both of the undersized foals.

Pregnancy can be diagnosed very early in gestation by ultrasonography. Some mares can be diagnosed as pregnant by day 11 of gestation. Early diagnosis of pregnancy allows the nonpregnant or open mare to be identified as such and rebred on her subsequent estrus. Also, ultrasonography allows for the identification and monitoring of twin pregnancies. If ultrasound equipment is not available, an experienced operator can usually determine whether a mare is pregnant or not via rectal examination after 25 to 30 days of gestation. Pregnancy can also be determined by immunological detection of equine chorionic gonadotropin in the serum using commercially available test kits from day 40 up to about 120 to 140 days of gestation. A potential false positive, however, occurs when the fetus dies after formation of the eCG-producing endometrial cryptae or cups.

Parturition

Parturition is the culmination of the gestational events and in mares is largely controlled by the fetoplacental unit. Classic signs of impending parturition are development of the udder, changes in mammary gland secretions, and relaxation of the sacrosciatic ligament and labia. The best predictive indicator is related to changes in the mammary gland. The mammary gland frequently engorges 24 to 48 hours prior to parturition with the concurrent appearance of colostrum. Many mares 'wax,' which is extruded colostrum that hangs down from the paired teat orifices approximately 24 hours prior to foaling. The calcium concentration of the mammary secretions increases, although variability exists in peak values. The commercially available calcium test strips, as a result, may better indicate which mares will not immediately foal (low calcium levels) rather than those that will.

Parturition is initiated by contractions of the myometrium, which culminate in the expulsion of the fetus followed shortly by the expulsion of the placenta. The endocrinological aspects of pregnancy and parturition, as well as the peculiarities among species, are presented in Chapters 12–18.

Stages of Labor

Three stages of labor are recognized: **Stage 1,** which is the period of cervical dilation and fetal repositioning; **Stage 2,** which is the period of parturition and delivery of the young; and **Stage 3,** which refers to the time elapsed from birth to detachment and expulsion of the placenta. During **Stage 1,** myometrial contractions displace the fetus and the chorionic membranes against the cervix, which initiates cervical dilation. Almost concurrently, the fetus repositions itself from a dorso-pubic position with the front legs flexed to a dorsosacral position with the legs extended. Approximately 98% of foals are delivered head first. **Stage 2** begins when the chorioallantoic membrane of the placenta ruptures followed by vaginal stimulation as the fetus is pushed through the birth canal. This results in the pressing contraction of the abdominal skeletal muscles, also called Ferguson's reflex, which adds to the net pressure caused by the uterine contractions. Typically **Stage 2** lasts less that 30 minutes and concludes with the birth

of the fetus. Most mares deliver the fetus while lying down and remain recumbent for about 15 minutes. Placental blood continues to be transferred to the neonate through the umbilical vessels during this time. **Stage 3** of parturition refers to the time elapsed from the birth of the foal and time required for placenta detachment and expulsion, which is completed within 6 hours from birth of the foal. Placental retention beyond this time is considered abnormal and may necessitate medical attention.

Uterine Involution

The mare is unique among the domestic species by having both the fastest rate of uterine involution and also a potentially fertile first postpartum estrus, termed foal heat. Most mares display foal heat between 5 to 12 days after parturition with an average range of ovulation between 8 to 12 days postpartum. Although breedings during the foal heat usually result in an overall pregnancy rate 10 to 20% lower than during subsequent breedings, some horse breeders consider this potential as an opportunity to produce foals on a yearly basis. However, breeding during the foal heat should be used with caution and only in healthy mares which have had a normal parturition and are projected to ovulate on or after day 10 postpartum.

Lactation

Lactation is an important physiological event for two reasons. First, early in the postpartum period, the mare's milk meets all nutritional requirements that the foal needs for survival, normal growth, and development. Second, the colostrum supplies immunoglobulins necessary for the immune protection of the foal because in horses there is no in-utero transfer of maternal antibodies across the epitheliochorial placenta to the fetus.

The quality of the colostrum varies depending on the immune status of the dam. Colostral antibodies are derived from the maternal blood and concentrated in the mammary secretions. As a result, it is important to maintain the dam's immune status at a high level by acclimating her to environmental pathogens and through a comprehensive prepartum vaccination program. Occasionally, a dam may undergo premature lactation before foaling, which results in the loss of colostrum and the subsequent failure of immunoglobulin transfer to the neonate. In this situation, colostrum from another mare, if available, should be administered.

The foal's intestine can absorb colostral antibodies over the first 24 hours of life, but the rate is maximal during the first few hours after birth. The special adsorptive cells, or enterocytes, are replaced within the first day by nonabsorptive cells. Foals which do not receive any or receive an insufficient amount of immunoglobulin in the colostrum are extremely susceptible to neonatal, infectious diseases.

THE MALE

Reproductive Tract of the Stallion

The reproductive organs of the stallion (Fig. 13-2) consists of two testes within a non-pendulous scrotum, the associated *epididymides,* and *vasa deferentia* which widen at their terminal portion, forming the *ampulla.* In addition, the stallion has a prostate gland, paired vesicular glands, and bulbourethral glands, and the penis. Testicular descent into the inguinal canal occurs in the male fetus at approximately 270 to 300 days of gestation. Testes descend into the scrotum shortly before or after birth. At birth, ap-

proximately 40 to 45% of colts may have the two testes in the scrotum. Stallion testes are ovoid in shape and are compressed side to side with their long axis being horizontal. The size of the testes remains relatively unchanged until approximately 10 to 12 months of age, at which time the testes begin to grow. Maximal testicular size is reached during the breeding season when the stallion is about 5 years of age (Table 13-2), with both testes of similar size and with one testis usually lying slightly cranial to the other. In the adult stallion, the testis is composed of 58 to 72% seminiferous tubules, with the remaining 28 to 42% made up of interstitial tissue.[106]

Puberty and Sexual Maturity in the Male

Puberty in the stallion, defined as the age at which the stallion releases spermatozoa in the ejaculate, commonly occurs during the second year of life and is preceded by an increase in LH and FSH concentrations in the blood. In the colt, breed and season of the year at birth can influence the time of onset of puberty. Furthermore, it is generally assumed that the stallion reaches sexual maturity from 2 to 4 years after the onset of puberty. Reproductive senescence, which is characterized in the stallion primarily by a progressive decrease in quality of ejaculates, occurs approximately after 20 years of age.

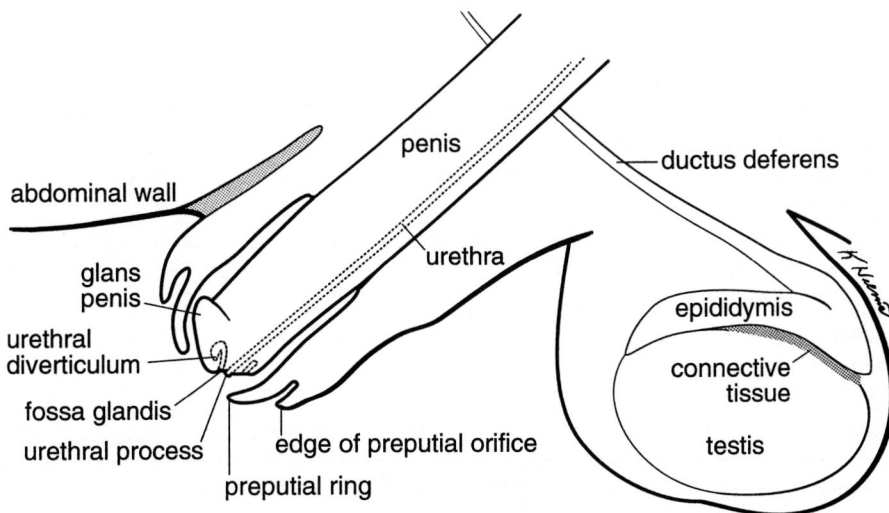

Fig. 13-2. Stallion reproductive organs.

Testicular size in the sexually mature stallion is influenced by season of the year. As the breeding season approaches, the testes increase in size due to the proliferation of both Leydig and Sertoli cells. The stallion reacts to shorter periods of daylight with a concomitant decrease in testis size. Unlike the mare, which enters into anestrus during periods of short daylight, the stallion still displays libido and produces ejaculates containing spermatozoa (Table 13-2).

The inguinal rings close by 14 days of age in a normal colt. If the testes have not descended into the scrotum prior to closure, they become retained in either the abdomen or inguinal canal. Stallions with one or both testes retained are termed unilateral or bilateral cryptorchids, respectively, and horse breeders call them 'ridgling' or rigs. Because the retained testes are exposed to high abdominal temperature, spermatogonia and Sertoli cells are negatively affected and spermatogenesis is minimal or does not occur. Production of testosterone by the Leydig cells is apparently not affected by the ectopic location of the testes. Cryptorchid stallions secrete testosterone and will display undesirable stallion-like behavior including vocalizing, herding mares, and challenging other stallions. Stallions are usually castrated to make them more manageable. It is unethical to remove only the descended testis from a unilateral cryptorchid

stallion because the animal will appear gelded but will still exhibit stallion-like behavior.

The epididymis lies on the dorsal surface of the testes with the head or *caput epididymidis* facing cranially, the body or *corpus epididymidis* runs along the dorsolateral surface of the testis, and the tail or *cauda epididymidis* is located at the caudal pole of the testis. Each *caput* of the *epididymis* is firmly attached to the cranial pole of the testis, but the *corpora* and *caudae epididymides* are loosely attached to the testes by connective tissue. Because of this loose attachment, when castrating a horse, one may inadvertently leave a portion of the epididymis behind if not cognizant of this unique anatomy. Stallions in which a portion of the epididymis was left behind during castration have been called 'proud cut' horses. Folklore dictates that 'proud cut' horses still retain their stallion-like behavior; documentation in the scientific literature, however, fails to support this belief.

The duration of spermatogenesis is approximately 57 days in the stallion (4.7 cycles of the seminiferous epithelium times 12.2 days, which is the duration of the cycle of the seminiferous epithelium). An additional 3 to 7 days are required for semen maturation and transport through the epididymis. Hence, injury or toxic exposure of spermatogonia will be reflected by

Table 13-2   Effect of Season on Characteristics of Stallion Testes[a]

Endpoint	Breeding Season	Nonbreeding Season
Parenchyma weight, paired testes (g)	154.0	116.0
Leydig cells (10^6/g testis)	22.0	20.0
(10^9/2 testes)	7.3	4.7
Sertoli cells		
(10^6/g testis)	24.2	23.6
(10^9/2 testes)	3.7	2.5
Daily sperm production		
(10^6/g testis)	19.1	14.6
(10^9/2 testes)	6.0	3.5
Serum concentrations		
FSH (ng/ml)	108.0	81.0
LH (ng/ml)	36.0	22.0
Testosterone (ng/ml)	0.36	0.27

[a] Data is compiled across studies and is presented as the mean for stallions 4 to 20 years of age. Not all data are from the same stallions. For most values n ≥ 48.

Adapted from: R. P. Amann, Functional anatomy of the adult male. *In:* Equine Reproduction, 1st ed., edited by A. O. McKinnon and J. L. Voss. Philadelphia, PA, Lea & Febiger, p. 650, 1993.

the presence of abnormal spermatozoa in the ejaculate approximately 59 to 64 days after the injury or toxic exposure. The time for migration through the epididymis is reduced to a total of 2 to 3 days if the stallion is naturally mated or semen is collected frequently. However, sufficient numbers of spermatozoa are stored in the caudae epididymides for several ejaculates. Normally, a stallion's libido will decline before the spermatozoal reserves are depleted. Daily spermatozoal production during the nonbreeding season is approximately only 50% of that which occurs during the breeding season. The decrease in daily spermatozoal (sperm) production, DSP, is believed to be due to a decrease in Sertoli cell numbers and germinal cell degeneration, which would occur gradually during the transition from the breeding to nonbreeding seasons.

The *vasa deferentia,* also called *ductus deferentes,* are conduits for the displacement of spermatozoa from the caudae epididymides to the urethra. The terminal portion of each *vas deferens* (*ductus deferens*) is located in the pelvic area and widens to form the *ampulla.* The *ampullae* of the stallion are well developed and easily identified during rectal palpation. The *ampullae* contains many cryptae and glands, with a lumenal size of approximately 3 to 4 times that of the *vas deferens.* Historically, it was wrongly believed that the *ampulla* functioned as a major site of storage of spermatozoa. Indeed, some stallions develop an abnormal 'ampullar plug' of caseated spermatozoa, which blocks the ampullar lumen. Rectal massage is usually needed to dislodge this plug.

In addition to the *ampullae,* the vesicular, prostate, and bulbourethral glands are accessory sex glands present in the stallion. The vesicular glands are hollow in the stallion, like in the human, and are sometimes termed seminal vesicles in these two species. The vesicular glands dramatically increase in size during sexual stimulation, contributing the gelatinous portion of the stallion ejaculate. The vesicular gland excretory ducts empty with the *ductus deferens* on the dorsal part of the urethra, craniad to the colliculus seminalis. In some stallions, the duct of the seminal vesicles and the *ampullae* of the *vasa deferentia* may empty into the urethra through a common orifice. The prostate lies caudal to the vesicular glands and consists of a prominent body with two narrow lobes. The prostate is a firm, nodular structure which can be palpated rectally and is similar in size in both the sexually rested and aroused stallion. The prostate produces a thin, watery secretion which can make up a significant portion of the volume of a stallion's ejaculate. The bulbourethral glands are located caudad to the prostate near the ischial arch. These glands have multiple ducts, which empty their secretion into the pelvic urethra. The bulbourethral glands increase in size, both length and width, during sexual stimulation. The secretions of the bulbourethral glands, however, make up a small fraction of the entire ejaculate.

The penis, under sympathetic innervation, is normally retracted back in the preputial sheath except during sexual arousal, voluntary relaxation, or in response to some pharmacologic agents. The stallion penis is musculocavernous, consisting mainly of the *corpus spongiosum* and the *corpus cavernosum penis.* During sexual excitement, parasympathetic innervation allows for the pooling of blood in these two erectile tissues, increasing the pressure in the corpus cavernosum to about 1,500 mm of Hg (see Chapter 8). This engorgement, when fully erect, enlarges by 50% the length and diameter of the penis over that of its normal relaxed state. During ejaculation, the glans penis achieves full engorgement (300 to 400% greater than its normal size) and is sometimes referred to as being 'mushroomed'. This mushrooming of the glans penis aids in dilating and positioning the mare's cervix in such a way as to help ensure ejaculation directly into the uterus. The urethra terminates into a tubular urethral process at the tip of the penis (Fig. 13-2). The urethral process is surrounded by a fossa. In the dorsal portion of the fossa, a blind pouch is present and is termed the urethral diverticulum. The fossa and urethral diverticulum accumulate glandular secretions and desquamated epithelial cells, termed smegma. The smegma can become concretous, especially in gelded males, and may need to be manually removed periodically to prevent irritation.

As one might expect, secretion and release of pituitary gonadotropins is maximal during the breeding season. Consequently, testosterone and estradiol-17β are at their highest levels in the blood during this time.

Interestingly, in free-ranging horses, a dominant stallion will collect and maintain a 'harem' of mares. The remaining subordinate stallions peacefully coexist in stable bachelor groups. The testosterone levels of the harem stallion are significantly higher than those of the bachelor group. If the harem stallion is removed, a bachelor takes over the harem and his testosterone levels increase. The removed former harem stallion has a subsequent sharp decline in testosterone levels. This suggests that housing and handling systems may also have a significant endocrinological effect on the stallion.

During the breeding season, mature stallions approximately 5 years of age or older have higher blood levels of LH, FSH, and prolactin than their younger counterparts. Unlike the changes in blood levels of LH that occur between breeding and nonbreeding seasons, FSH secretion varies little throughout the year. As with the mare, artificial light can be used to improve the seminal quality of the stallion during the transitional period between the nonbreeding and breeding seasons. Typically, when the stallion is evaluated for breeding soundness, semen is collected twice with an artificial vagina, 1 hour apart. The second ejaculate generally has about one-half as many spermatozoa as the first ejaculate. The influence of season has shown a significant effect on the seminal parameters from these paired ejaculates. During the peak of the breeding season, the total ejaculate and gel-free volumes, concentration of spermatozoa per ml, and total semen per ejaculate are maximal. There does not not appear, however, to be an influence of season on sperm motility estimates.

Breeding in the equine industry is done by either pasture mating, hand breeding, or artificial insemination. During natural mating under either pasture- or hand-breeding situations, the mare is teased for receptivity by the stallion. The stallion approaches the mare and tests her receptivity by licking, nipping, vocalizing, hoof stomping, and holding or pulling her tail with his teeth. Stallions will also sniff feces, urine, and the perineal area of the mare, which is frequently followed by a Flehman stance. The Flehman response, however, does not appear to be a routine part of the courtship sequence and may only allow identification of specific mares by the male.[102] Mares in estrus will stand to be mounted by the stallion, which then intromits his erected penis into the vagina. Ejaculation usually occurs 15 to 30 seconds after intromission. Some stallions, however, will mount with a nonerect penis and obtain a full erection only after they are positioned on the mare. Ejaculation in the stallion involves a series of 6 to 10 urethral contractions, which occur in synchrony with the 'flagging' of the stallions tail, and lasts for less than 1 minute. Stallions which run constantly with a band of mares rarely suffer breeding injuries. However, when hand breeding stallions, the mare and the operator are exposed to injury. Animal restraint, human interference with precopulatory interactive behavior, and the fact that the stallion trained to ejaculate in an artificial vagina follows the cues of the human handler rather than that of the mare appear to contribute to a higher incidence of breeding injuries during handling.

EQUINE HYBRIDS

Over thousands of years, male donkeys (jacks) have been bred to mares to produce mules. Mules have been used as beasts of burden because of the mule's endurance and agility. There are other less common interspecies crosses or hybrids such as the hinny, product of crossing a stallion × female donkey (jenny), and also a variety of combinations of crosses between female horses or donkeys and wild asses or zebra males (Fig. 13-3, zebrorse or zebronkey, respectively).

Not all interspecies crosses result in pregnancy and birth of offspring. Typically, the most successful crosses involve a mare which is inseminated by the interspecies male.

The hybrids themselves are sterile due to the inability to successfully complete meiosis because of differences in chromosomal numbers (Fig. 13-3; see also Chapter 7). There have been a few reported cases in the literature describing apparently successful reproduction by mules.

Karyotype of male zebronkey
n=53

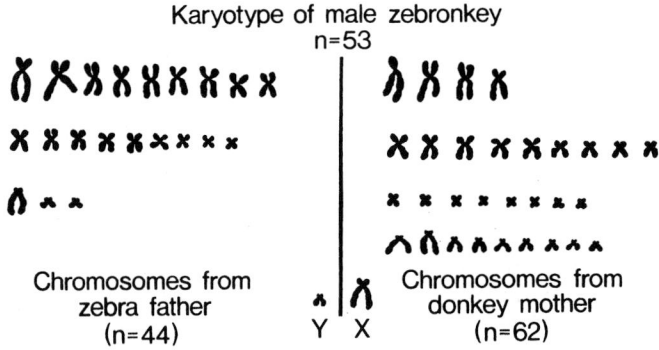

Chromosomes from
zebra father
(n=44)

Chromosomes from
donkey mother
(n=62)

Y   X

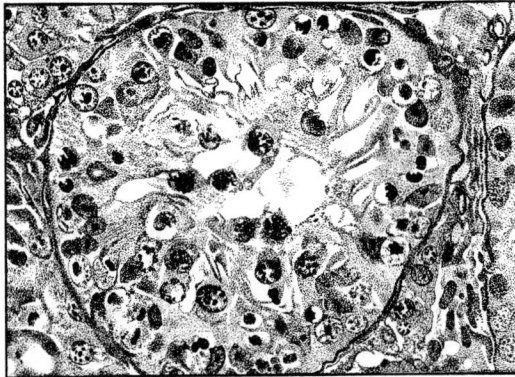

Zebronkey testis

Fig. 13-3. Karyotype of male zebronkey, (**top**) showing chromosomes contributed by each of the parents, illustrating the lack of pairs of homologous chromosomes. Failure of spermatogenesis in testis of male zebronkey (**bottom**). The large cells near the center of the seminiferous tubule are primary spermatocytes, arrested at the pachytene stage of meiosis as they try in vain to pair homologous chromosomes in preparation for the first reduction division. (From: C. R. Austin and R. V. Short, Reproduction in Mammals, Book 4, Reproduction Patterns. New York, NY, Cambridge University Press, 1972).

Under close scrutiny, none of these reports have unequivocally demonstrated that the reported offspring was in fact produced by the mule.[87]

As a result of investigations concerning the production and reproductive failure of the equine hybrids, in addition to using hybrids as embryo recipients, new ideas concerning equine pregnancies and the effect of fetal genotype have emerged and stimulated research. Most donkey embryos transferred to recipient mares develop an inadequate chorionic girdle. The cells of the trophoblastic girdle fail to invade the maternal endometrium and to produce eCG. Many of these pregnancies fail before 100 days of gestation; however, few continue to term.

This suggests that, at least for those donkey embryos that develop to term after transfer to mares, eCG and potentially the secondary corpora lutea may not be required for the maintenance of pregnancy in mares, but also may imply that the primary corpus luteum produces sufficient amounts of progesterone to maintain pregnancy. When horse embryos are transferred to donkey recipients, however, the endometrial cups develop, become prominent, and actively secrete eCG. The donkey's ovaries become extremely enlarged due to the presence of numerous secondary corpora lutea. The level of progesterone secretion by these ovaries is also greatly enhanced.

REFERENCES

1. Allen, W. R. (1982): Immunological aspects of the equine endometrial cup reaction and the effect of xenogeneic extraspecies pregnancy in horses and donkey. J. Reprod. Fertil. (Suppl. 31):57.
2. Amann, R. P. (1981): A critical review of methods for evaluation of spermatogenesis from seminal characteristics. J. Androl. *2*:37.
3. Amann, R. P., Thompson, D. L., Jr., Squires, E. L., et al. (1979): Effects of age and frequency of ejaculation on sperm production and extragonadal sperm reserves in stallions. J. Reprod. Fertil. (Suppl. 27):1.
4. Anderson, W. S. (1939): Fertile mare mules. J. Hered. *30*:549.
5. Bazer, F. W., Vallet, J. L., Roberts, R. M., et al. (1986): Role of conceptus secretory products in establishment of pregnancy. J. Reprod. Fertil. *76*:841.
6. Bergfelt, D. R. (2000): Anatomy and physiology of the mare. *In:* Equine Breeding Management and Artificial insemination, edited by J. C. Samper. W B Saunders, Philadelphia, PA, p. 141.
7. Bergin, W. C., Gier, H. T., Marion, G. B., et al. (1970): A developmental concept of equine cryptorchism. Biol. Reprod. *3*:82.
8. Berndtson, W. E., Squires, E. L., and Thompson, D. L., Jr. (1983): Spermatogenesis, testicular composition and the concentration of testosterone in the equine testis as influenced by season. Theriogenology 20:449.
9. Berndtson, W. E., Pickett, B. W., and Nett, T. M. (1974): Reproductive physiology of the stallion. IV. Seasonal changes in the testosterone concentration of peripheral plasma. J. Reprod. Fertil. *39*:115.
10. Betteridge, K. J., Renard, A., and Goff, A. K. (1985): Uterine prostaglandin release relative to embryo collection, transfer procedures and maintenance of the corpus luteum. Equine Vet. J. *3* (Suppl.):25.
11. Caraty, A., Antoine, C., Delaleu, B., et al. (1995): Nature and bioactivity of gonadotropin-releasing hormone (GnRH) secreted during the GnRH surge. Endocrinology *136*:3452.
12. Chandley, A. C. (1988): Fertile mules. J. Royal Soc. Med. *81*:2.
13. Chandley, A. C., Short, R. V., and Allen, W. R. (1975): Cytogenetic studies of three equine hybrids. J. Reprod. Fertil. (Suppl. 23):365.
14. Chevalier, F. and Palmer, E. (1982): Ultrasound echography in the mare. J. Reprod. Fertil. (Suppl. 32):423.
15. Clay, C. M., Squires, E. L., Amann, R. P., et al. (1988): Influences of season and artificial photoperiod on stallions: Luteinizing hormone, follicle-stimulating hormone and testosterone. J. Anim. Sci. *66*:1246.
16. Clay, C. M. and Squires, E. L. (1987): Influences of season and artificial photoperiod on stallions: Testicular size, seminal characteristics and sexual behavior. J. Anim. Sci. *64*:517.
17. Cleaver, B. D. and Sharp, D. C. (1995): LH secretion in anestrous mares exposed to artificially lengthened photoperiod and treated with estradiol. Biol. Reprod. Monograph Series *1*:449.
18. Cleaver, B. D. and Sharp, D. C. (1993): Does melatonin play a role in the secretion of LH and FSH in the mare? Proc. Soc. Theriogenology, Annu. Meeting, August 12–14, 1993, Jacksonville, FL, p. 148.
19. Cuoto, M. A. and Hughes, J. P. (1985): Intrauterine inoculation of a bacteria-free filtrate of *Streptococcus zooepidemicus* in clinically normal and infected mares. J. Equine Vet. Sci. *5*:81.
20. Danet-Desnoyers, G. H. (1994): Regulation of endometrial prostaglandin synthesis by phospholipases and interferon tau and characterization of endometrial prostaglandin synthesis inhibitor in the bovine. University of Florida, Gainesville, FL (Ph. D. Thesis).
21. de Kresta, D. M. and Kerr, J. B. (1988): The cytology of the testis. *In:* The Physiology of Reproduction, edited by E. Knobil and J. Neill. New York, NY, Raven Press, p. 837.
22. Discafani, C. M. (1995): Functional state of primary and secondary corpora lutea during mid-gestation in the mare. Colorado State University Fort Collins, CO (Ph. D. Thesis).
23. Doig, P. A. and Waelchli, R. O. (1993): Endometrial biopsy. *In:* Equine Reproduction, edited by A. O. McKinnon and J. L. Voss. Philadelphia, PA, Lea & Febiger, p. 225.
24. Douglas, R. H. and Ginther, O. J. (1975): Effects of prostaglandin F$_{2\alpha}$ on the oestrus cycle and pregnancy in mares. J. Reprod. Fertil. (Suppl. 23):257.
25. Duchamp, G., Bour, B., Combarnous, Y., et al. (1987): Alternative solutions to HCG induction of ovulation in the mare. J. Reprod. Fertil. (Suppl. 35):221.
26. Ellis, R. N. W. and Lawrence, T. L. J. (1978): Energy undernutrition in the weanling filly foal. Br. Vet. J. *134*:205.
27. Evans, M. J. (1977): Equine endocrinology: Studies on gonadotrophin releasing, sex steroid and thyroid hormones in mares. Lincoln College, University of Canterbury, Christchurch, New Zealand (Ph. D. Thesis).
28. Evans, M. J., Hamer, J. M., Gason, L. M., et al. (1987): Factors affecting uterine clearance of inoculated materials in mares. J. Reprod. Fertil. (Suppl. 35):327.
29. Fitzgerald, B. P., Affleck, K., Barrows, S. P., et al. (1987): Changes in LH pulse frequency and amplitude in intact mares during the transition into the breeding season. J. Reprod. Fertil. *79*:485.
30. Fitzgerald, B. P., Meyer, S. L., Affleck, K. J., et al. (1993): Effect of constant administration of a gonadotropin-releasing hormone agonist on reproductive activity in mares: Induction of ovulation during seasonal anestrus. Am. J. Vet. Res. *54*:1735.
31. Fitzgerald, B. P., Peterson, K. D., and Silvia, P. J. (1993): Effect of constant administration of a gonadotropin-releasing hormone agonist on reproductive activity in mares: Preliminary evidence on suppression of ovulation during the breeding season. Am. J. Vet. Res. *54*:1746.
32. Freeman, D. A., Woods, G. L., Vanderwall, D. K., et al. (1992): Embryo-initiated oviductal transport in mares. J. Reprod. Fertil. *95*:535.
33. Ganjam, V. K. and Kenny, R. M. (1975): Androgens and oestrogens in normal and cryptorchid stallions. J. Reprod. Fertil. (Suppl. 23):67.
34. Ganjam, V. K., Kenney, R. M., and Flickinger, G. (1975): Plasma progestagens in cyclic, pregnant and postpartum mares. J. Reprod. Fertil. (Suppl. 23):441.
35. Gebauer, M. R., Pickett, B. W., and Swierstra, E. E. (1974): Reproductive physiology of the stallion. III. Extra-gonadal transit time and sperm reserves. J. Anim. Sci. *39*:737.

36. Ginther, O. J. and First, N. L. (1971): Maintenance of the corpus luteum in hysterectomized mares. Am. J. Vet. Res. *32*:1687.

37. Ginther, O. J. and Pierson, R. A. (1983): Ultrasonic evaluation of the reproductive tract of the mare; principles, equipment and techniques. J. Equine Vet. Sci. *3*:195.

38. Ginther, O. J. and Pierson, R. A. (1984): Ultrasonic evaluation of the reproductive tract of the mare: Ovaries. J. Equine Vet. Sci. *4*:11.

39. Ginther, O. J. and Pierson, R. A. (1984): Ultrasonic anatomy and pathology of the equine uterus. Theriogenology *21*:505.

40. Goff, A. K., Pontbriand, D., and Sirois, J. (1987): Oxytocin stimulation of plasma 15-keto-13, 14-dihydroprostaglandin F2α during the oestrous cycle and early pregnancy in the mare. J. Reprod. Fertil. (Suppl. 35):253.

41. Goff, A. K., Sirois, J., and Pontbriand, D. (1993): Effect of oestradiol on oxytocin-stimulated prostaglandin F2α release in mares. J. Reprod. Fertil. *98*:107.

42. Harris, J. M., Irvine, C. H. G., and Evans, M. J. (1983): Seasonal changes in serum levels of FSH, LH and testosterone and in semen parameters in stallions. Theriogenology *19*:311.

43. Hinrichs, K., Cummins, M. R., Sertich, P. L., et al. (1988): Clinical significance of aerobic bacterial flora of the uterus, vagina, vestibule, and clitoral fossa of clinically normal mares. J. Am. Vet. Med. Assoc. *193*:72.

44. Hoagland, T. A., Mannen, K. A., Dinger, J. E., et al. (1986): Effects of unilateral castration on serum luteinizing hormone, follicle stimulating hormone, and testosterone concentrations in one-, two-, and three-year-old stallions. Theriogenology *26*:407.

45. Hurtgen, J. P. and Whitmore, H. L. (1978): Effects of endometrial biopsy, uterine culture, and cervical dilatation on the equine estrous cycle. J. Am. Vet. Med. Assoc. *173*:97.

46. Inoue, J., Cerbito, W. A., Oguri, N., et al. (1993): Serum levels of testosterone and oestrogens in normal and infertile stallions. Int. J. Androl. *16*:155.

47. Irvine, C. H. G. (1981): Endocrinology of the estrous cycle of the mare: Applications to embryo transfer. Theriogenology *15*:85.

48. Irvine, C. H. G. and Alexander, S. L. (1991): Effect of sexual arousal on gonadotrophin-releasing hormone, luteinizing hormone and follicle-stimulating hormone secretion in the stallion. J. Reprod. Fertil. (Suppl. 44):135.

49. Johnson, L. (1985): Increased daily sperm production in the breeding season of stallions is explained by an elevated population of spermatogonia. Biol. Reprod. *32*:1181.

50. Johnson, L. (1991): Seasonal differences in equine spermatocytogenesis. Biol. Reprod. *44*:284.

51. Johnson, L. and Neaves, W. B. (1981): Age-related changes in the Leydig cell population, seminiferous tubules and sperm production in stallions. Biol. Reprod. *24*:703.

52. Johnson, L. and Nguyen, H. B. (1986): Annual cycle of the Sertoli cell population in adult stallions. J. Reprod. Fertil. *76*:311.

53. Johnson, L. and Thompson, D. L., Jr. (1983): Age-related and seasonal variation in the Sertoli cell population, daily sperm production and serum concentrations of follicle-stimulating hormone, luteinizing hormone and testosterone in stallions. Biol. Reprod. *29*:777.

54. Johnson, L., Warner, D. D., Tatum, M. E., et al. (1991): Season but not age affects Sertoli cell number in adult stallions. Biol. Reprod. *45*:404.

55. Kastelic, J. P., Adams, G. P., and Ginther, O. J. (1987): Role of progesterone in mobility, fixation, orientation and survival of the equine embryonic vesicle. Theriogenology *27*:655.

56. Kenney, R. M. (1978): Cyclic and pathologic changes of the mare endometrium as detected by biopsy, with a note on early embryonic death. J. Am. Vet. Med. Assoc. *172*:241.

57. Kotilainen, T., Huhtinen, M., and Katila, T. (1994): Sperm induced leukocytosis in the equine uterus. Theriogenology *41*:629.

58. Leadon, D., Jeffcott, L., and Rossdale, P. (1984): Mammary secretions in normal spontaneous and induced premature parturition in the mare. Equine Vet. J. 16:259.

59. LeBlanc, M. M., Neuwirth, L., Asbury, A. C., et al. (1994): Oxytocin enhances clearance of radiocolloid from the uterine lumen of reproductively normal mares and mares susceptible to endometritis. Equine Vet. J. 26:279.

60. Ley, W. B., Bowen, J. M., Purswell, B. J., et al. (1993): The sensitivity, specificity and predictive value of measuring calcium carbonate in mares' pre-partum mammary secretions. Theriogenology *40*:189.

61. Lofstedt, R. M. (1988): Control of the estrous cycle in the mare. Vet. Clin. North Am., Equine Pract. *4*:177.

62. Lofstedt, R. M. and Patel, J. H. (1989): Evaluation of the ability of altrenogest to control the equine estrous cycle. J. Am. Vet. Med. Assoc. *194*:361.

63. Long, S. E. (1988): Chromosome anomalies and infertility in the mare. Equine Vet. J. *20*:89.

64. McCue, P. M., Figuierdo, E., and Lasley, B. L. (1992): Estrogen dynamics during the transition period in the mare. Biol. Reprod. *46* (Suppl. 1):157.

65. McDowell, K. J., Sharp, D. C., Peck, L. S., et al. (1985): Effect of restricted conceptus mobility on maternal recognition of pregnancy in mares. Equine Vet. J. (Suppl. 3):23.

66. McDowell, K. J., Sharp, D. C., Grubaugh, W. R., et al. (1988): Restricted conceptus mobility results in failure of pregnancy maintenance. Biol. Reprod. *39*:340.

67. McDowell, K. J., Sharp, D. C., Fazleabas, A. T., et al. (1990): Two dimensional polyacrylamide gel electrophoresis of proteins synthesized and released by conceptuses and endometria from pony mares. J. Reprod. Fertil. *89*:107.

68. McKinnon, A. O., Nobelius, A. M., del Marmol Figueroa, S. T., et al. (1993): Predictable ovulation in mares treated with an implant of the GnRH analogue deslorelin. Equine Vet. J. *25*:321.

69. McKinnon, A. O., Squires, E. L., Harrison, L. A., et al. (1988): Ultrasonographic studies on the reproductive tract of mares after parturition: Effect of involution and uterine fluid on pregnancy rates in mares with normal and delayed first postpartum ovulatory cycles. J. Am. Vet. Med. Assoc. *192*:350.

70. Michel, T. H. and Rossdale, P. D. (1986): Efficacy of hCG and GnRH for hastening ovulation in Thoroughbred mares. Equine Vet. J. *18*:438.

71. Naden, J., Amann, R. P., and Squires, E. L. (1990): Testicular growth, hormone concentrations, seminal characteristics and sexual behavior in stallions. J. Reprod. Fertil. *88*:167.

72. Neely, D. P. (1979): Studies on the control of luteal function and prostaglandin release in the mare. Ph. D. Thesis, University of California, Davis, CA.

73. Neely, D. P., Kindahl, H., Stabenfeldt, G. H., et al. (1979): Prostaglandin release patterns in the mare: Physiological, pathophysiological and therapeutic responses. J. Reprod. Fertil. (Suppl. 27):181.

74. Neely, D. P., Stabenfeldt, G. H., Kindahl, H., et al. (1979): Effect of intrauterine saline infusion during the late luteal phase on the estrous cycle and luteal function of the mare. Am. J. Vet. Res. *40*:665.

75. Nickel, R., Schummer, A., Seiferle, E., et al. (1973): The Viscera of the Domestic Mammals, edited by O. Schaller, R. E. Hael, and J. Frewein. New York, NY, Springer-Verlag, p. 139.

76. Oriol, J. C., Sharom, F. J., and Betteridge, K. J. (1993): Developmentally regulated changes in the glycoproteins of the equine embryonic capsule. J. Reprod. Fertil. *99*:653.

77. Ousey, J., Delclaux, M., and Rossdale, P. (1989): Evaluation of three strip tests for measuring electrolytes in mares' pre-partum mammary secretions and for predicting parturition. Equine Vet. J. 21:196.

78. Oxender, W. D., Noden, P. A., and Hafs, H. D. (1977): Estrus, ovulation, and serum progesterone, estradiol, and LH concentrations in mares after an increased photoperiod during Winter. Am. J. Vet. Res. *38*:203.

79. Peaker, M., Rossdale, P. D., Forsyth, I. A., et al. (1979): Changes in mammary development and the composition of secretion during late pregnancy in the mare. J. Reprod. Fertil. (Suppl. 27): 555.

80. Pearson, H. and Weaver, B. M. Q. (1978): Priapism after sedation, neuroleptanalgesia and anaesthesia in the horse. Equine Vet. J. 10:85.

81. Peltier, M. R. and Sharp, D. C. (1994): LH secretion during vernal transition in pony mares. Biol. Reprod. *50* (Suppl.):67.

82. Pierson, R. A., Kastelic, J. P., and Ginther, O. J. (1988): Basic principles and techniques for transrectal ultrasonography in cattle and horses. Theriogenology *29*:3.

83. Pycock, J. F. (1993): Cervical function and uterine fluid accumulation in mares. Proc. J. P. Hughes Int. Workshop on Equine Endometritis. Summarized by W. R. Allen. Equine Vet. J. *25*:191.

84. Rodriguez, H. and Bustos-Obregon, E. (1994): Seasonal and epididymal maturation of stallion spermatozoa. Andrologia *26*:161.

85. Rong, R., Chandley, A. C., Song, J., et al. (1988): A fertile mule and hinny in China. Cytogenet. Cell Genet. 47:134.

86. Roser, J. F., McCue, P. M., and Hoye, E. (1994): Inhibin activity in the mare and stallion. Domestic Anim. Endocrinol. *11*:87.

87. Ryder, D. A., Chemmick, L. G., Bowling, A. T., et al. (1985): Male mule qualifies as the offspring of a female mule and jack donkey. J. Hered. *76*:379.

88. Scraba, S. T. and Ginther, O. J. (1985): Effects of lighting programs on onset of the ovulatory season in mares. Theriogenology *24*:667.

89. Sharp, D. C. (1993): Maternal recognition of pregnancy. *In:* Equine Reproduction, edited by J. L. Voss

and A. O. McKinnon. Philadelphia, PA, Lea and Febiger, p. 486.

90. Sharp, D. C., Davis, S. D., and Cleaver, B. D. (1993): Photoperiod. *In:* Equine Reproduction, edited by J. L. Voss and A. O. McKinnon. Philadelphia, PA, Lea and Febiger, p. 179.

91. Sharp, D. C., Garcia, M. C., and Ginther, O. J. (1979): Luteinizing hormone during sexual maturation in pony mares. Am. J. Vet. Res. *40*:584.

92. Sharp, D. C., Salute, M. E., Thatcher, M-J, et al. (1994): Temporal relationship between oxytocin receptor (OTR), oxytocin (OT) and prostaglandin F2((PGF) release in response to cervical/uterine stimulation during the estrous cycle and early pregnancy in pony mares. Biol. Reprod. *50* (Suppl. 1):60.

93. Sherman, G. B., Wolfe, M. W., Farmerie, T. A., et al. (1992): A single gene encodes the β-subunits of equine luteinizing hormone and chorionic gonadotropin. Mol. Endocrinol. *6*:951.

94. Shore, M. D., Macpherson, M. L., Combes, G. B., et al. (1998): Fertility comparison between breeding at 24 hours or at 24 and 48 hours after collection with cooled equine semen. Theriogenology *50*:693.

95. Silberzahn, P., Zwain, I., Guerin, P., et al. (1988): Testosterone response to human chorionic gonadotropin injection in the stallion. Equine Vet. J. *20*:61.

96. Silver, M. (1992): Parturition: Spontaneous or induced preterm labour and its consequences for the neonate. Anim. Reprod. Sci. *28*:441.

97. Silvia, P. J., Squires, E. K., and Nett, T. M. (1986): Changes in the hypothalamic-hypophyseal axis of mares associated with seasonal reproductive recrudescence. Biol. Reprod. *35*:897.

98. Squires, E. L., Douglas, R. H., Steffenhagen, W. P., et al. (1974): Ovarian changes during the estrous cycle and pregnancy in mares. J. Anim. Sci. *38*:330.

99. Squires, E. L., McClain, M. G., Ginther, O. J., et al. (1987): Spontaneous multiple ovulation in the mare and its effect on the incidence of twin embryo collections. Theriogenology *28*:609.

100. Stabenfeldt, G. H., Hughes, J. P., and Evans, J. W. (1972): Ovarian activity during the estrous cycle of the mare. Endocrinology *90*:1379.

101. Stabenfeldt, G. H., Hughes, J. P., and Evans, J. W. (1974): Spontaneous prolongation of luteal activity in the mare. Equine Vet. J. *6*:158.

102. Stahlbaum, C. C. and Houpt, K. A. (1989): The role of the Flehmen response in the behavioral repertoire of the stallion. Physiol. Behav. *45*:1207.

103. Steffenhagen, W. P., Pineda, M. H., and Ginther, O. J. (1972): Retention of unfertilized ova in uterine tubes of mares. Am. J. Vet. Res. *33*:2391.

104. Sullivan, J. J., Parker, W. G., and Larson, L. L. (1973): Duration of estrus and ovulation time in nonlactating mares given human chorionic gonadotropin during three successive estrous periods. J. Am. Vet. Med. Assoc. *162*:895.

105. Swierstra, E. E., Pickett, B. W., and Gebauer, M. R. (1975): Spermatogenesis and duration of transit of spermatozoa through the excurrent ducts of stallions. J. Reprod. Fertil. (Suppl. 23):53.

106. Swierstra, E. E., Gebauer, M. R., and Pickett, B. W. (1974): Reproductive physiology of the stallion I. Spermatogenesis and testis composition. J. Reprod. Fertil. *40*:113.

107. Thompson, D. L., Jr., Johnson, L., St. George, R. L., et al. (1986): Concentrations of prolactin, luteinizing hormone and follicle stimulating hormone in pituitary and serum of horses: Effect of sex, season and reproductive state. J. Anim. Sci. *63*:854.

108. Thompson, D. L., Jr., Pickett, B. W., Berndtson, W. E., et al. (1977): Reproductive physiology of the stallion. VIII. Artificial photoperiod, collection interval and seminal characteristics, sexual behavior and concentrations of LH and testosterone in serum. J. Anim. Sci. *44*:656.

109. Thompson, D. L., Jr., Pickett, B. W., and Nett, T. M. (1978): The effect of season and artificial photoperiod on serum levels of estradiol-17β and estrone in stallions. J. Anim. Sci. *47*:184.

110. Thompson, D. L., Jr., Pickett, B. W., Squires, E. L., et al. (1979): Testicular measurements and reproductive characteristics in stallions. J. Reprod. Fertil. (Suppl. 27):13.

111. Thompson, D. L., Jr., Pickett, B. W., Squires, E. L., et al. (1980): Sexual behavior, seminal pH and accessory sex gland weights in geldings administered testosterone and (or) estradiol-17 beta. J. Anim. Sci. *51*:1358.

112. Thompson, D. L., Jr., St. George, R. L., Jones, L. S., et al. (1985): Patterns of secretion of luteinizing hormone, follicle stimulating hormone and testosterone in stallions during the Summer and Winter. J. Anim. Sci. *60*:741.

113. Troedsson, M. H. T. (1995): Uterine response to semen deposition in the mare. Proc. Soc. Theriogenology Annu. Meeting, September 13–15, 1995, San Antonio, TX, p. 130.

114. Troedsson, M. H. T. and Liu, I. K. M. (1991): Uterine clearance of non-antigenic markers (^{51}Cr) in response to a bacterial challenge in mares potentially suscepti-ble and resistant to chronic uterine infection. J. Reprod. Fertil. (Suppl. 44):283.

115. Voss, J. L., Squires, E. L., Pickett, B. W., et al. (1982): Effect of number and frequency of inseminations on fertility of mares. J. Reprod. Fertil. (Suppl. 32):53.

116. Webel, S. K. and Squires, E. L. (1982): Control of the oestrus cycle in mares with altrenogest. J. Reprod. Fertil. (Suppl. 32):193.

117. Williamson, P., Munyua, S., Martin, R., et al. (1987): Dynamics of the acute uterine response to infection, endotoxin infusion and physical manipulation of the reproductive tract in the mare. J. Reprod. Fertil. (Suppl. 35):317.

118. Witherspoon, D. M. and Talbot, R. B. (1970): Ovulation site in the mare. J. Am. Vet. Med. Assoc. *157*:1452.

119. Woods, J., Bengfelt, D. R., and Ginther, O. J. (1990): Effects of time of insemination relative to ovulation in pregnancy rate and embryonic loss rate in mares. Equine Vet. J. *22*:410.

References Added in Proof

120. Macpherson, M. L. and Reimer, J. M. (2000): Twin reduction in the mare: Current options. Anim. Reprod. Sci.*60–61*:233.

121. Nagy, P., Guillaume, D., and Daels, P. (2000): Seasonality in mares. Anim. Reprod. Sci. *60–61*:245.

122. Squires, E. L., McCue, P. M., and Vanderwall, D. (1999): The current status of equine embryo transfer. Theriogenology *51*:91.

123. Troedsson, M. H., Liu, I. K., and Crabo, B. G. (1998): Sperm transport and survival in the mare: A review. Theriogenology *50*:807.

Reproductive Patterns of Sheep and Goats*

M. H. PINEDA

14

*Much information concerned with reproduction in sheep and goats has been presented in Chapter 2 (Pituitary Gland), Chapter 7 (The Biology of Sex), Chapter 8 (Male Reproductive System), Chapter 9 (Female Reproductive System), Chapter 10 (Artificial Insemination), and Chapter 11 (Patterns of Reproduction). The reader is encouraged to refer to these chapters in order to permit conciseness.

SHEEP

INTRODUCTION

The domestic ewe is seasonally polyestrous with interestrous intervals averaging 16 to 17 days during the breeding season. Most estrous cycles in the Northern Hemisphere occur during the Fall and early Winter, from September to January. In the absence of fertile matings, ewes cycle six to nine times during the breeding season. In temperate climates, the breeding season is longer and sheep tend to approach a non-seasonal pattern of breeding.

Most of the estrous cycle of the sheep is occupied by the luteal phase. The luteal phase, which includes metestrus and diestrus, lasts 12 to 14 days. Proestrus is short, lasts 2 to 3 days, and is not a readily distinguishable phase of the cycle. Estrus lasts an average of 26 hours, with a range of 20 to 36 hours. Ovulation is spontaneous and occurs by the end of estrus. Double and triple ovulations are common in sheep, particularly in those breeds selected for twinning.

After puberty, the ram produces spermatozoa and is capable of fertile matings throughout the year. Rams tend to show seasonality in their libido as well as in their spermatogenesis and quality of ejaculates. Rams are more sexually active and produce better ejaculates during the breeding season in the Fall and early Winter. Their libido and seminal quality declines noticeably during late Winter, Spring, and Summer. A castrated ram is called a **wether.**

BREEDING SEASON

The breeding season varies considerably within and between breeds. Most domestic breeds such as the Hampshire, Southdown, Shropshire, Romney, and Rambouillet developed in colder climates and are distinctly seasonally polyestric. Breeding during the Fall with delivery in the Spring of the year, when climatic conditions are more favorable, increases the survival of the newborn lambs. Mediterranean breeds, such as the Merino, Karakul, Persian Blackhead, and to some extent the Dorset, developed in moderate climates. These breeds tend to be nonseasonal in their breeding patterns, but may revert to shorter seasonal patterns of breeding when exposed to adverse climates or restricted in either the availability or quality of feed. The most important regulator of the onset of the breeding season is the shortening of the daylight period. This begins after June 21 (summer solstice) in the Northern Hemisphere or December 21 in the Southern Hemisphere. Estrus and ovulation will trail these dates by 60 to 120 days. Ewes will reverse their seasons readily if transferred from one hemisphere to the other.

Ambient temperatures also affect the breeding season; extremely high temperatures of the Summer often delay the onset of the first estrus, while the presence of the ram hastens the onset of the breeding season. Refer to the discussion on breeding season regulation in Chapter 11.

Theoretically, it is possible for nonseasonal breeding ewes to have two lamb crops a year.

Under ideal climatic and husbandry conditions, this pattern is sometimes approached, but since ewes seldom come into estrus while nursing lambs, it is difficult, from the practical point of view, to have two gestation periods of approximately 5 months each and two nonpregnant periods of only 1 month within a year. A more practical compromise usually is three lamb crops in 2 years. However, this leads to lack of uniformity of the lambs since there is considerable variation in the lambing time under such conditions of management.

PUBERTY AND SEXUAL MATURITY IN THE MALE

The age of puberty in the ram-lamb, or he-lamb, as is also called, is affected by breed and by nutritional and environmental influences. Puberty and attainment of sexual maturity is earlier for rams of fast-growing breeds. Male lambs born early in the lambing season may reach puberty by 4 months of age during the first Fall, while the onset of puberty may be delayed 9 to 12 months for rams born late in the lambing season, particularly for those lambs exposed to poor feeding and adverse climatic conditions. Fertility is fairly low in these young males, and it is recommended that they be used sparingly. By the next Fall, the ram will be sexually mature and can be used to capacity.

PUBERTY AND SEXUAL MATURITY IN THE FEMALE

Ewe-lambs reach puberty by 6 to 7 months of age, but the age of puberty is greatly influenced by breed, nutritional, and environmental factors. Ewe-lambs from fast-growing breeds, such as Suffolk, Finnsheep, and Hampshire, tend to have an earlier onset of puberty than ewe-lambs from slower-growing breeds (Merino). The time of the year at which lambs are born is particularly influential on the age of puberty for lambs of both fast- and slow-growing breeds. Ewe-lambs born early in the lambing season tend to reach puberty at 5 months of age and also reach sexual maturity at a younger age than ewe-lambs born late in the lambing season. Ewe-lambs born late in the lambing season will reach puberty and display estrous cycles during the breeding season of the following year when they are 12 to 15 months of age.

At the time of puberty, the ewe lamb undergoes one or two ovulations without expressing behaviorally overt signs of estrus (silent estrus; see Chapter 9). Similarly, ewes which had cycled the previous year undergo silent estruses at the beginning of the breeding season.

A low plane of nutrition delays the onset of puberty in both female and male lambs, whereas lambs fed properly during their growing period attain development of their reproductive organs, puberty, and sexual maturity at an earlier age. Breeding ewe-lambs during the Fall breeding season of their first year is not recommended unless they have reached a body weight that is at least 50% of their expected adult weight. It is better to breed them the next breeding season, as yearlings. In temperate climates, those bred during the first Fall will probably produce more lambs during their lifetime, but the economic feasibility of such a practice in colder climates is questionable, since conception in ewe-lambs bred earlier is rather poor, with a 50% lamb crop being average.

THE ESTROUS CYCLE

The stages of the estrous and reproductive cycles of the ewe are depicted in Figure 14-1, and the changes in levels of reproductive hormones during the estrous cycle are shown in Figure 14-2.

Proestrus

Proestrus lasts for 2 to 3 days in the ewe and is characterized by rapid follicular growth and estrogen secretion under the stimulation of pituitary gonadotropins. Progressively increasing levels of estradiol-17β in the blood during proestrus are associated with changes in the reproductive organs including increased blood supply to the tubular genital tract. The ewe does not display overt signs during proestrus. However, as estrus approaches, the vulva swells, the vestibule becomes hyperemic, and the glands of

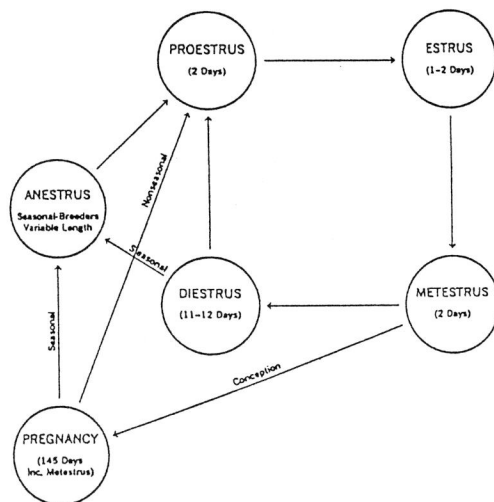

Fig. 14-1. The estrous cycle of the ewe.

the cervix and vagina secrete a serous or a mucous secretion which appears as a vaginal discharge.

Estrus and Sexual Behavior

Estrus is difficult to detect in the ewe when the detection is based solely on behavioral changes. Overt signs of estrus are less pronounced in the ewe than in mares, sows, cows, or even in goats. Estrous ewes may 'seek out the ram', but generally they tend to be passive. Other than vulvar swelling and an occasionally visible mucous discharge from the vulva, the standing of the ewe for mating is the most easily noticed sign of estrus. Successful reproductive management of ewes requires the use of teaser rams. Vasectomized or aproned rams are commonly used to detect estrous ewes. Marking ink can be placed on the ram's brisket (see Chapter 10, Fig. 10-18) to identify estrous ewes by the ink mark left on the rump of the ewe during mounting.

Estrus lasts an average of 26 hours, but may range from 20 to 36 hours during the breeding season. The duration of estrus is influenced by the photoperiod, age of the ewe, and by the presence of rams in the flock. The duration of estrus

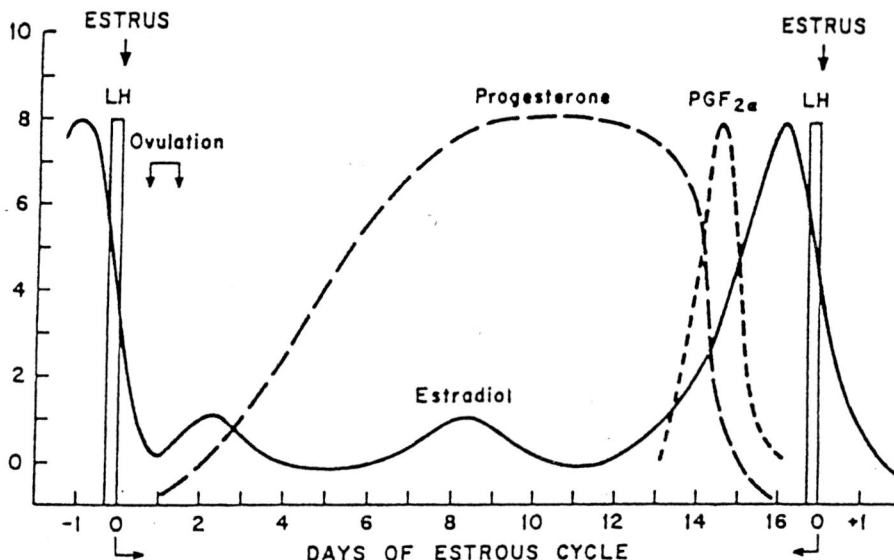

Fig. 14-2. A model of the sheep estrous cycle, indicating the relationship between hormonal levels, sexual receptivity, time of ovulation, and the key role played by $PGF_{2\alpha}$ in producing the demise of the corpus luteum. (Reproduced with permission from: B. V. Caldwell, S. A. Tillson, et al., Prostaglandins *1*:217, 1972).

is shorter and may last as little as 3 to 6 hours at the beginning or end of the breeding season. Estrus is also shorter in ewe-lambs displaying their first overt estrus, whereas the duration of estrus in yearling ewes approaches that of adult ewes. Rams exert an estrous synchronizing effect in ewes. The onset of estrus and breeding season are hastened in ewes exposed to rams before the beginning of the breeding season. Ewes maintained with rams tend to display shorter estruses than ewes not exposed or exposed only periodically to rams.

Ovulation

Ovulation is spontaneous and occurs toward the end of estrus. Continued visual and olfactory exposure of ewes to, or mating with, rams hastens ovulation by facilitating the release of GnRH and subsequently, the ovulatory surge of gonadotropins. The wool of rams, but apparently not the urine, contains pheromones that stimulate ovulation.

Double and triple ovulations are common in ewes. These ovulations occur within 2 hours after the first ovulation, and the right ovary of the ewe is more active than the left ovary. Approximately 62% of single ovulations and 56%

of double or triple ovulations occur from the right ovary.

The first ovulation of the breeding season in adult ewes or the first ovulation at the onset of puberty is silent, not associated with overt signs of behavioral estrus. This is due to the lack of a functional (CL) and of progesterone, which is needed for the full expression of behavioral estrus in ewes. In the ewe-lamb, the progesterone needed to establish postpubertal estrous cyclicity is provided by short-lived corpora lutea (see Chapter 9). In the adult ewe, due to the prolonged anestrus and lack of ovulations in the nonbreeding season, corpora lutea are not present. The progesterone needed for cyclicity and for the expression of behavioral estrus in pubertal lambs is provided by corpora lutea formed during the first silent ovulation.

Metestrus

The period of metestrus is only of academic significance in the ewe because ovulation occurs by the end of estrus. Metestrus, defined as the period of formative stage of the corpus luteum, is for all practical purposes included within diestrus. The corpus luteum forms rather rapidly in sheep, and significant increases in blood levels of progesterone are detectable within 3 days after ovulation (Fig. 14-2).

Diestrus

The luteal phase lasts for 12 to 14 days and is the dominant phase of the estrous cycle of the ewe. Viable embryos must be present in the uterus to provide luteotropic signals no later than day 13 of diestrus (day of estrus = day 0). If viable embryos are not present at this time, the corpus luteum regresses rapidly under the influence of prostaglandin $PGF_{2\alpha}$, the uterine luteolysin in sheep, and the ewe undergoes another estrous cycle (Fig. 14-2). If the ewe does not become pregnant, this process is repeated during subsequent estrous cycles until the end of the breeding season.

The $PGF_{2\alpha}$ released from the endometrium of the cycling, nonpregnant animal reaches the ovary and causes luteolysis through the local utero-ovarian, veno-arterial pathway discussed in Chapter 9. In the sheep, about 99% of exogenous prostaglandins are metabolized during a single passage through the lungs, regardless of the stage of the cycle.[20]

The length of the cycle based on the interestrous interval averages 17 days, with a modal range of 14 to 19 days for most domestic breeds of sheep. The length of the cycle tends to increase toward the end of the breeding season.

Endocrinology of the Cycle

Figure 14-2 depicts the hormonal patterns of LH, estradiol, progesterone, and $PGF_{2\alpha}$ during the estrous cycle of the ewe.

The corpus luteum is the main source of progesterone in the cycling ewe. Blood levels of progesterone are low (less than 1.0 ng/ml) during estrus and remain low until day 3 of diestrus. Progesterone levels increase rapidly from day 3 of diestrus, reaching maximal levels by day 8, and remain elevated until days 11 to 12 (Fig. 14-2). If embryos are not present in the uterus by day 13 of diestrus, progesterone levels decline rapidly due to the luteal regression induced by the endometrial $PGF_{2\alpha}$. Ovarian and posterior pituitary oxytocin stimulates endometrial secretion and release of prostaglandins (see Chapter 9, Fig. 9-27). Progesterone levels in the peripheral blood decrease to less than 1.0 ng/ml of blood by the last 2 days of diestrus.

Progesterone exerts a blocking effect on the release of pituitary gonadotropins, and since estrogens in sheep are secreted by large antral follicles, blood levels of estrogens remain low for most of the luteal phase of the cycle. There appear to be two waves of follicular growth during diestrus in sheep. These are reflected in the increased blood levels of estrogens on days 2 and 8 of diestrus (Fig. 14-2). As the levels of progesterone are declining by the end of diestrus, the levels of estrogens in the peripheral blood rise rapidly due to the rapid proestrual follicular growth and secretion. Estrogen levels peak about day 16 of the cycle, just prior to the next behavioral estrus.

The development and secretory activity of the corpus luteum of the sheep depends on the gonadotropic stimulation provided by LH and possibly, prolactin. Luteinizing hormone is released from the pituitary gland in episodic pulses at intervals of approximately 3.2 hours for most of diestrus. Due to the low magnitude of these pulses, LH remains at basal levels until the preovulatory surge of LH, which occurs approximately within 10 hours from the onset of estrus. During proestrus and estrus, prior to ovulation, the frequency of these episodic pulses of LH increases to intervals of about 1.0 hour. These LH pulses are followed by significant rises in blood levels of estradiol, which is associated with the changes in the reproductive organs and behavior that characterize estrus.

Photoperiod seems to be the major factor controlling the anestrous period during the nonbreeding season that follows the breeding season of sheep. This photoperiodic influence seems to be exerted through hypothalamic modulation of the pulsatile release of gonadotropins from the pituitary. During anestrus, the frequency and magnitude of the LH pulses are low.

ANATOMIC CHANGES OF THE REPRODUCTIVE ORGANS

During the nonbreeding season, the ovaries of the ewe undergo follicular development to the antral stages, but ovulation fails to occur, and the ewe does not express behavioral estrus. As the breeding season approaches, gonadotropic hormones stimulate the ovarian follicles to mature, secrete estrogens, and ovulate. Estrogens secreted by the maturing follicles in turn stimulate the macro- and microscopic changes in the oviducts, uterus, and vagina described in Chapter 9, Female Reproductive System. Follicular growth proceeds rapidly during proestrus and is completed during the preovulatory period of estrus. In the ewe, mature preovulatory follicles reach a diameter of approximately 1.0 cm.

The ovary of adult ewes may contain as many as 86,000 primordial follicles and 100 to 400 growing follicles, of which 10 to 40 follicles are visible on the surface of the ovary.[24] Single ovulating breeds tend to develop a single follicle at each ovulation, while the other growing follicles undergo atresia. In multiple ovulating breeds, such as the Booroola, several follicles develop and ovulate. It appears that the selection and emergence of a follicle or follicles for ovulation is completed about day 14 of the cycle. The mechanisms for the selection of those follicles which will ovulate while the other growing follicles undergo atresia are not known.

The oviducts of the ewe are approximately 15 to 20 cm long and have well-developed mucosal thickening at their junction with the uterine horns. These mucosal thickenings act like valves and control the passage of spermatozoa from the uterus into the oviduct. The fimbriated end of the sheep's oviduct is well developed and surrounds the ovary at the time of ovulation, increasing the chances of oocyte entrance into the oviduct.

The uterus of the sheep is bipartite, and the uterine mucosa, as in the cow, forms a septum that separates the uterine horns. The endometrium of the ewe is highly glandular and contains **caruncles,** which are nonglandular projections arranged in four rows extending from the uterine body to the horns. Externally, the horns are bound by an intercornual ligament.

Ewes grazing on pastures containing estrogenic (phytoestrogens) plants develop either acute, which is temporary and resolves within a month after exposure to phytoestrogens, or chronic reproductive deficiencies conducive to permanent infertility (see Chapter 9) that becomes progressively more intense with continued exposure. Low level or intermittent but for prolonged periods of exposure to phytoestrogens may be conducive to a subclinical infertility due to transdifferentiation of the cervix. This chronic form is expressed by low lambing rates.

FERTILIZATION

As for the other domestic species, ram spermatozoa need to be capacitated in the female tract to acquire the capability to fertilize the ewe's oocytes. Fertilization takes place in the ampullary region of the oviduct. After natural or artificial insemination, ram spermatozoa are displaced rather rapidly through the cervix and uterus. The cervix of the ewe controls spermatozoal displacement and possibly also exerts a selective effect on the population of spermatozoa deposited in the anterior vagina. Only a fraction of the spermatozoa deposited in the vagina enter the uterus. The cervical canal is both tortuous and contains nonaligned mucosal folds. Disalignment of these cervical folds prevents the routine intracervical and intrauterine inseminations in the ewe.

The utero-tubal junction further selects spermatozoa entering the oviduct from the uterus. Once in the oviduct, most ram spermatozoa are restricted to the caudal isthmus until ovulation. Two phases of spermatozoal transport within the oviduct have been described for the ewe:

1. a rapid phase within 15 minutes after mating that results in the entry of relatively few spermatozoa into the oviducts and

2. a more prolonged phase of transport which results in the slow accumulation of a functional population of spermatozoa within the ampullary region of the oviduct.

The fertilizable life of the oocyte is considered to be about 10 to 12 hours in the ewe, but may extend up to 24 hours after ovulation. The chances for oocyte aging and associated embryonic losses are reduced in sheep because ovulation occurs in most ewes by the end of estrus and insemination through matings are likely to occur early in estrus. In addition, ram spermatozoa maintain their fertilizing capability in the ewe's oviduct for periods extending up to 48 hours.

Ewe oocytes are released into the oviducts surrounded by cumulus cells. These cumulus cells break down rapidly after ovulation, and by the time of fertilization, the oocyte is practically free of cumulus cells. Cleavage of the fertilized oocyte to the two-cell stage occurs within 16 hours after fertilization or approximately 20 hours after ovulation. Sheep oocytes have been fertilized *in vitro,* and live offspring have been obtained after transfer of these *in vitro* fertilized oocytes. However, the rate of success has been low, and this technology needs to be improved to become profitable. Technological advancements have made it possible to apply micromanipulation to the sheep embryo (see Chapter 19), including embryo splitting, gene injection, nuclear transplantation and cell fusion, and cryopreservation.

PREGNANCY

Sheep embryos enter the uterus at the blastocyst stage by day 3 after ovulation. They remain spherical up to day 4 but undergo rapid elongation prior to attachment to the endometrium. Intrauterine migration of embryos begins after maternal recognition of pregnancy on day 13 and is associated with embryonic elongation and synthesis of estradiol-17β by the embryo. Transuterine migration of embryos occurs frequently in ewes with two or more ovulations from the same ovary and may occur occasionally in ewes with a single ovulation. Transuterine migration results in better spacing of the embryos and optimal utilization of the uterus for successful pregnancy. Endometrial attachment of these elongated blastocysts begins about the 16th day and is completed by 22 days after mating.

It has long been assumed that placentation in the ewe occurs only between the cotyledons of the chorioallantois and the uterine caruncles. Now it is evident that apposition and attachment occurs over the entire uterine surface,[54] although attachment at the intercaruncular spaces may be tenuous. The placenta of the sheep is diffuse for the first month. As gestation progresses, the attachment is reinforced by the placentomes, which interlock the chorionic villi into the crypts of the caruncles. In the sheep, the placental syncytium is formed from fetal cells and is syndesmochorial in structure, lacking a uterine epithelial component.[107] The number of placentomes formed by the fetal cotyledon and the maternal cotyledon or caruncle averages about 90 but may vary from 60 to 100. The placenta of the sheep produces relaxin and also a placental lactogen with prolactin-like activity.

Pregnancy lasts an average of 148 days but may range from 140 to 159 days when calculated from the time of mating or artificial insemination to parturition or lambing. The length of pregnancy in sheep is influenced by breed, and plane of nutrition, as well as by environmental conditions. Fast-growing breeds such as the Hampshire tend to have shorter gestations, averaging 145 days. Slow-growing breeds such as the Merino have longer gestations, averaging 151 days. A low plane of nutrition or twin pregnancies also shortens the length of gestation.

Cervical and vaginal stimulations by the lambs at the time of parturition elicit the onset of maternal behavior and selective bonding between mother and lamb. Acceptance of alien lambs can be induced by stimulating the vagina and cervix of nonpregnant ewes previously treated with estrogens and progesterone.[53]

Most ewes do not display estrous behavior during pregnancy. However, ewes that become pregnant early in the breeding season may, on occasion, display some degree of sexual activity.

Lactational anestrus is the norm in sheep. Some ewes display postpartum estrus within 30 hours after parturition when lambing occurs early in the breeding season. Pregnancy seldom results from matings which occur during the postpartum estrus. In general, ewes do not return to estrus until after the lambs are weaned, and in most cases, estrus is delayed until the next breeding season.

The regression of the corpus luteum of pregnancy proceeds at a lower rate than the regression of the corpus luteum of the cycle. The progesterone secreted by the corpus luteum is needed for the first 50 days of pregnancy in the sheep. If bilateral ovariectomy is performed after day 50 of pregnancy, placental secretion of progestagens is sufficient to prevent abortion.

Pregnancy Diagnosis

The nonreturn to estrus after a recorded mating is a relatively accurate sign of pregnancy in well-managed flocks, but is not accurate in free-mating conditions since ewes may not cycle for a variety of reasons and remain in a nonpregnant anestrus for the duration of the breeding season.

The use of ultrasound is particularly useful for early pregnancy diagnosis in ewes. It allows for accurate diagnosis of pregnancy from the third to fifth week by detection of the embryonic heart beat. Through the use of echonographic ultrasound equipment, accurate diagnosis of pregnancy can be made as early as day 35 after mating.

Determination of blood levels of progesterone is also a useful means for the early diagnosis of pregnancy in high-priced ewes that have not returned to estrus by day 18 after mating. High blood levels of progesterone indicate that luteal regression has not occurred, and in the majority of cases, this is due to the luteotropic signals provided by embryos in the uterus. Detection of chorionic-somatotropin in the blood after day 40 of gestation is also indicative of pregnancy.

Operators with thin arms can rectally palpate large ewes and diagnose pregnancy without harm to the ewe. Rectal-abdominal palpation, using rods introduced in the rectum to displace the fetus against the abdominal wall, also is used for pregnancy diagnosis in ewes. However, the use of these procedures should be discouraged because they are associated with a high incidence of perforated recta, peritonitis, and abortion, particularly frequent when performed by untrained individuals.

CONTROL OF REPRODUCTIVE EFFICIENCY

A fertile ewe is customarily defined as an ewe capable of producing at least one lamb per pregnancy. A crop of one lamb per ewe per year is considered the minimal fecundity or prolifi-

Table 14-1 Fecundity in Sheep

Breed	Lamb Crop, %
Cheviot	89
Scottish Blackface	93
Heath	103
Karakul	110
Corriedale, in Canada	114
Corriedale, in U.S.	118
Southdown	119
Rambouillet, in U.S.	122
Rambouillet, in Canada	124
American Shropshire	124
Oxford Down	127
Columbia	127
Dorset	127
Romney Marsh	128
Navaho	129
Targhee	129
Hampshire Down	132
Dorset Horn	137
Lincoln	140
Suffolk	144
Shropshire	162
Leicester	163
Wensleydale	172
Border Leicester	181
East Friesian Milch Sheep	205
Romanov	238
Finnsheep	300 to 600

From: S. A. Asdell, Patterns of Mammalian Reproduction, 2nd ed., Ithaca, NY, Comstock Publishing Associates, 1964.

cacy for the ewe and is referred to as a 100% lamb crop. Sheep breeders seek a prolificacy averaging at least 1.5 lambs per ewe, which represent a lamb crop of 150%.

Many factors, including environment, plane of nutrition, age, breed, and selection for high lambing influence prolificacy. The quantity as well as the quality of feed influences the incidence of estrus, ovulation rates, embryonic survival to term, and the lamb crop. Once the general daily requirements in dietary ingredients, especially in proteins and energy, are met, a detrimental influence of the plane of nutrition becomes dependent on the lack or excess of a particular component in the diet. Unfortunately, the dietary needs to meet specific requirements for each stage of the reproductive processes of sheep, including pregnancy, are not yet determined.

Breed differences in the fecundity of sheep are shown in Table 14-1. Selection within

Table 14-2 Effect of the Number of Offspring Born on the Subsequent Fecundity of Romanov Sheep

Ewes Born as	Average Number of Lambs Produced
Singleton	2.17
Twins	2.36
Triplets	2.63
Quadruplets	3.01

Adapted from: A. P. Belogradskii, Sov. Zooteh. *7*:88, 1940.

breeds for higher prolificacy can also be a factor contributing to higher lamb crops (Table 14-2). The ovulation rate, defined as the number of oocytes released at each ovulation, is a heritable trait affecting fecundity and the lambing crop. Repeatability of ovulation rate both within a season and between years is high for those ewes which tend to have a high lambing crop. Booroola ewes release 4 to 5 oocytes at each ovulation. The high ovulation rate and fecundity of the Booroola ewe is due to a gene which influences the rate of ovulation, probably by enhancing the sensitivity of follicular cells to pituitary gonadotropins. The trait for high ovulation rate is dominant in the F1 generation of crosses between the Booroola and other breeds.

The influence of the age of the dam on the lamb crop is shown in Table 14-3. The lamb crop per year was greater in ewes that were not bred until 1.5 years of age (effect of age of dam). This

Table 14-3 Fecundity of Hampshire Ewes

	Bred and Conceived as Lambs	Bred and Conceived as 1½-Year Olds
Breeding Season	Lamb Crop %	Lamb Crop %
First	106	–
Second	157	195
Third	176	202
Fourth	177	175
Fifth	200	208

Adapted from: D. A. Spencer et al., J. Anim. Sci. *1*:27, 1942.

superiority existed for the next 3 years, but the overall number of lambs produced by the ewe first bred when she was a lamb was still greater. Notice that the lamb crop continued to increase through the fifth season in both groups. Prolificacy peaks when the ewe is 4 to 6 years of age.

Because of the restricted breeding season of most breeds of sheep and the economical significance of increasing the lamb crop for the sheep breeder, several schemes have been developed to prolong the breeding season in order to produce lambs at any time of the year or to increase the crop of lambs by selecting breeds with high ovulation rates.

Induction of Estrus before the Breeding Season

Stimulation of the ovaries of sheep out of the breeding season using gonadotropins such as PMSG (also eCG) has produced satisfactory results, particularly when the gonadotropin is given shortly before the normal breeding period and after pretreatment of the ewes with progestagens. Attempts to produce two lamb crops per year by exogenous gonadotropic stimulation during the deep anestrus of the nonbreeding season, although possible under ideal conditions of feeding and management, has in general produced unsatisfactory results when applied in large scale. Most failures are attributed to fertilization failure or increased embryonic mortality.

Pretreatment of the out-of-the-breeding-season ewe with natural or synthetic progestagens is needed to initiate the cyclic release of endogenous gonadotropins (see Chapter 9). Progestagens are usually given for periods of 12 to 16 days, either as subcutaneous implants or in the form of vaginal pessaries. Gonadotropin treatment is given after the withdrawal of the implants or pessaries. Other experimental approaches include improved superovulatory treatments, embryo bisection, and the transfer of split, half-, or demi-embryos. These procedures, when applied under controlled conditions, produce lambs crops reaching 120%.

Artificial lighting to alter the natural ratio of light to dark or alterations between short and long lighting periods with melatonin treatment can also be used to advance the breeding season for ewes maintained in barns. This approach is generally more expensive and difficult to use on a large scale. Treatments combining artificial lighting with gonadotropic stimulation have also been used.

The social interaction of lambs and ewes with rams is an important component for the reproductive management of sheep. Exposure of ewes and prepubertal ewe-lambs to rams early in the breeding season hastens the onset of puberty and seasonal estrus. Pheromones from the ram's wool act as primers and stimulate LH release and ovulation in the ewe. The hair from the billy goat contains pheromones that, surprisingly, also effectively stimulate the ewe. Reproductive management of a flock should incorporate management schemes as well as building design to meet the needs for protection, feeding, and social interaction.

Other experimental approaches, such as the use of GnRH to induce surges of LH and cause ovulation in anestrous ewes, active immunization of ewes against androgens to increase ovulatory rates, and hastening the onset of puberty of ewe-lambs by treatment with progestagens and gonadotropins or by active immunizations against inhibin-enriched preparations, although successful, are not yet proven to be economically feasible under field conditions.

Estrus Synchronization

Two basic approaches are used to synchronize estrus in ewes:

1. treatment of ewes with progestagens for periods of 12 to 16 days or longer to inhibit the release of gonadotropins and prevent the initiation of the cycle or

2. treatment with $PGF_{2\alpha}$ in single or double treatments with or without progestagens (see Chapter 19, Embryo Transfer in Domestic Animals).

THE MALE

The growth of horns is apparently under the influence of gonadal hormones. In some breeds such as the Dorset, both sexes have horns, though the ewes have horns smaller than those of the ram. In Merinos and Rambouillets, only rams have horns. In English breeds, neither sex has horns.

Rams reach puberty, as determined by the presence of spermatozoa in their ejaculates, by 5 to 8 months of age. During the prepubertal period, there is pulsatile release of pituitary gonadotropins beginning as early as 1 week of age. Later, as the he-lamb approaches puberty, a temporal relationship develops between the pulsatile release of gonadotropins, mainly LH, and episodic increases of testosterone production by the testes. These lead to the onset of puberty and the establishment of the adult pattern of gonadotropin secretion (see Chapter 8, Male Reproductive System).

The duration of the cycle of the seminiferous epithelium, spermatogenesis, daily sperm production, and output of rams are discussed in Chapters 7 and 8. Rams are capable of spermatogenesis and produce fertile ejaculates throughout the year. The ram's endocrine system responds to photoperiodic changes, and the quality of the ejaculates is lower during the nonbreeding season. As the photoperiod decreases, rams of all breeds respond with an increased frequency of LH pulses and testosterone secretion.

Scrotal volume, circumference, and mean testicular diameter correlate relatively well with spermatozoal production. These parameters are often used as an indication of the breeding capacity of a male to establish ewe-to-ram ratios for the flock.

Collection of Semen

Semen is usually collected from the ram with an artificial vagina (AV) or by electroejaculation (EE). The AV method resembles natural mating, but requires training of rams to ejaculate in the AV. In addition, estrous ewes are needed during the period of training to stimulate the ejaculatory responses. Sexually inexperienced rams learn to copulate by observing experienced rams. In general, one or two exposures of sexually naive rams to estrous ewes establishes the reproductive patterns of detecting, approaching, and copulating with estrous females. The EE method is particularly useful to collect semen from untrained rams for soundness of breeding examination at the beginning of the breeding season. Several electroejaculation protocols have been developed. In general, electroejaculation produces larger volumes of ejaculate than when semen is collected with an AV and tends to produce less total numbers of spermatozoa. Refinements in the protocols of electrical stimulation, number and voltage of stimuli to be given, as well as improvements in the design of rectal probes, make electroejaculation a suitable procedure for the collection of semen from rams.

Spermatogenesis is affected by the temperature of the testes. When wool covers the scrotum of animals, there may be a temporary infertility during the hot summer months. Even in the absence of a wool covering, environmental temperatures above 90°F will usually interfere with spermatogenesis and lower the quality of the ejaculate.

Coitus is rapid, with one or two thrusts by the ram causing ejaculation and deposition of semen in the cranial end of the vagina. Rams will copulate frequently with estrous ewes. As many as 26 ejaculations have been recorded for a ram in a single day. In pasture, free-breeding conditions, particularly at the beginning of the breeding season, rams tend to copulate frequently with the first few ewes in estrus, which is conducive to wastage of spermatozoa.

Libido, mounting behavior, penial intromission, and ejaculatory reflex may be restored and maintained in wethers castrated before and after puberty by daily intramuscular injections of 4.0 to 6.0 mg of testosterone propionate. Wethers usually begin to respond with mounting and intromission behavior by the 4th week of treatment. Testosterone-treated wethers may be used as teasers to detect estrous ewes for hand-controlled matings or for artificial insemination.

Clearance of Spermatozoa from the Ejaculates of Vasectomized Rams

Rams of lesser genetic quality are commonly vasectomized and used as teasers to detect estrous ewes. Bilaterally vasectomized rams can be used as teasers 7 to 10 days after vasectomy due to the rapid clearance of most spermatozoa from the ejaculates. However, spermatozoal remnants, including a few intact, nonmotile spermatozoa may be found in ejaculates obtained months after vasectomy. As a precautionary measure, it is recommended to flush the *vasa deferentia* at the time of vasectomy to decrease the chances of undesired pregnancies. This approach reliably produces early azoospermic, postvasectomy ejaculates in dogs and cats.

With time, vasectomized rams show decreased libido, probably because of damage to the Leydig cells caused by the increased intratesticular and intraepididymal pressures which develop after vasal ligation. Treatment of vasectomized rams with testosterone before and during the breeding season stimulates their teasing activities.

Retrograde Flow of Spermatozoa into the Bladder

There is considerable retrograde flow of spermatozoa into the bladder of rams during electroejaculation (see Chapter 8, Table 8-5). The retrograde flow of spermatozoa into the bladder of rams averaged 28% and 20% during the nonbreeding and breeding seasons, respectively, is not affected by the method of seminal collection (AV vs. EE), and should be taken into account when evaluating the breeding soundness of rams. The determination of the total number of spermatozoa in the ejaculate and in the first postejaculation micturition should serve as a noninvasive method to accurately monitor the daily sperm production over extended periods for the selection of rams for breeding or in artificial insemination programs. Retrograde flow of spermatozoa into the bladder may be induced during sexual rest or prior to ejaculation by the administration of xylazine[42] to rams.

Ram Evaluation and Breeding Management

The examination of rams for breeding soundness prior to their introduction into the flock at the beginning of the breeding season is fundamental to ensure a high lambing crop and financial success for the producer. Rams of high fertility will settle more ewes within a shorter time and produce more lambs over time than rams of low fertility. It is estimated that to obtain maximal conception rates with one mating, at least

60×10^6 spermatozoa need to be naturally inseminated by the ram. However, conception rates and lamb crops are higher when at least a total of 500×10^6 spermatozoa were inseminated during several matings. It is not clear whether the effect is due to the higher total number of spermatozoa, to a stimulatory effect caused by multiple matings with the ram, or both.

A pubertal ram of 6 months of age or older, used sparingly, can serve up to 10 ewes. Yearling rams may serve up to 30 ewes, and adult rams, which may ejaculate up to three times daily without depleting their spermatozoal reserves, are usually stocked in a ratio of two to three rams per 100 ewes. These general recommendations are for pasture breeding and can be modified to achieve maximal breeding efficiency for a given flock. Rams tend to congregate around estrous ewes. The dominant ram copulates frequently and prevents the mating of the other rams. In hand-breeding programs, only estrous ewes are presented to the rams. Thus, the stocking ratio of rams to ewes can be reduced to one ram for 60 to 80 ewes.

GOAT

INTRODUCTION

Domestic goats are also seasonally polyestrous, and their breeding activity is influenced by the photoperiod. Although there are many similarities in the reproductive patterns of sheep and goats, there are distinct genetic and anatomical differences as well as differences in the physiology of their reproductive processes.

The female goat is usually called a doe or a nanny, the male, is called a buck or billy goat, and the offspring, kids.

SHEEP-GOAT MATINGS

The diploid number of chromosomes is 60 for the goat as compared to 54 for the sheep. Goats and sheep may have evolved from a common ancestor, which probably had 60 chromosomes. The Barbary sheep, thought to represent an intermediate link between sheep and goats, has 58 chromosomes (see Chapter 7, Table 7-1).

Matings between rams and does or between billy goats and ewes do occur when sheep and goats are together, and fertilization and early embryonic development may occur; however, the so-generated intergeneric embryos do not develop to term due to chromosomic and placental incompatibility and abnormal feto-maternal interactions. Sheep oocytes are resistant to fertilization by goat spermatozoa. However, intergeneric hybrid pregnancies may occur from the mating of ewes by billy goats or by experimental artificial insemination of ewes with billy goat semen. These hybrid concepti are aborted by about the 4th to the 6th week of gestation. Does will conceive when mated to a ram, but again, the resulting hybrids are aborted by the 8th week of pregnancy. Similarly, the intergeneric transfer of embryos between sheep and goats is not successful due to maternal rejection, which occurs as the placenta begins to develop. Chimeric, man-made sheep-goat embryos resulting from the combination of blastomeres obtained from sheep and goat embryos at different stages of embryonic development or from chronologically similar blastomeres will develop to term and produce live offspring when the embryonic trophoblasts have developed from blastomeres that were from the same species to which the embryos are transferred (see Chapter 19). Man-made sheep-goat chimeric hybrids, called Geeps, exhibit estrous cycles and the sexual behavioral characteristics of the species whose gonads are prevailing, such as those of ewes or goats, or may exhibit estrous cycle characteristics of both species, such as short 6- to 8-day cycles, though the sheep behavior seems to dominate.

The ovaries of a chimeric hybrid may ovulate either ovine or caprine oocytes and may even ovulate both species' oocytes if germinal cells from both species populated the ovaries. Geeps may become pregnant when back-crossed to a ram, and ovine embryos can implant successfully to term when transferred to a chimeric uterus. Transfer of man-made intergeneric embryos to chimeric animals has not resulted in pregnancies to term. However, ovine concepti may occasionally implant in the chimeric uterus. Placental production of progesterone may be a factor in interfering with pregnancy in the chimeric animal with a goat placenta. Because the placenta of the goat does not secrete progesterone to maintain pregnancy, the ovarian secretion of progesterone by the corpus luteum of the goat is required throughout gestation. The ewe, however, needs the ovarian secretion of progesterone only up to day 50 of pregnancy because the ewe's placenta produces sufficient progesterone to maintain pregnancy to term.

Male interspecies, sheep-goat chimeras may produce fertile sheep and goat spermatozoa derived from XY sheep and XY goat germinal cells in the same gonad.

BREEDING SEASON

The breeding season extends from late Summer to early Winter for most goat breeds in the continental United States. Swiss breeds, such as Toggenburg and Saanen, concentrate their breeding activity between late August and early February. Nubian goats tend to concentrate their breeding activity to the early Fall. Mediterranean breeds, such as the Creole and Shiba meat goats, do not have a definite breeding season. These breeds cycle year round in tropical areas or in geographic areas with temperate climates. The median month of conception in the continental United States is October, and the median month of kidding is March for Nubian, Toggenburg, Saanen, Alpine, and Lamancha breeds. There are minor variations among breeds according to the geographic location, probably due to influences caused by the photoperiod of the region. For instance, in the southern and south-western states, the median months of conception and kidding for the breeds mentioned above are September and February, respectively.

The length of the estrous cycle averages 21 days, with a range of 19 to 24 days. Estrus in goats lasts an average of 28 hours, with a range of 1 to 3 days. Most breeds of goats apparently do not undergo silent ovulations at the beginning of the breeding season, as is the case for the sheep. However, goats display short cycles with interestrous intervals of about 8 days at the be-

ginning, and occasionally during, the breeding season.

Double and triple ovulations are common to goats, and the kidding rate is usually greater than 200%.

The male goat is capable of producing fertile ejaculates year around, but, as for the ram, the seminal quality as well as the libido of billy goats is affected by the photoperiod. Billy goats exert estrous initiating and synchronizing effects in does at the interface of anestrus and the breeding season. Does tend to cycle earlier and more regularly when exposed to a buck.

PUBERTY AND SEXUAL MATURITY IN THE MALE

Bucks usually reach puberty between 5 and 6 months of age, but in some breeds, puberty may occur as early as 4 months of age. The onset of puberty is affected by breed, plane of nutrition, and season of the year.

PUBERTY AND SEXUAL MATURITY IN THE FEMALE

Does reach puberty around 6 months of age, but as for the ewe-lamb, the onset of puberty is variable and affected by the plane of nutrition, body weight, and month of birth. Puberty in does, as in ewe-lambs, is a gradual and interactive process involving maturation of the hypothalamic-pituitary-gonadal axis (see Chapter 9). Neither the blocking affect of estradiol-17β on the maturing hypothalamus nor the need for progesterone to initiate and establish the cyclic pattern, which is characteristic for the ewe-lamb, has been conclusively established for the goat. However, both pubertal and adult goats at the beginning of the breeding season display a short cycle of about 8 days, due to a short luteal phase lasting only 5 to 6 days. The second estrous cycle is usually a cycle of normal length, particularly when the does are exposed to and teased by a buck. This suggests that the hypothalamic-pituitary-gonadal axis of goats, as for sheep, may require progesterone for the initiation of regular cyclic activity subsequent to the first postpubertal estrus and also at the onset of the breeding season.

THE ESTROUS CYCLE

The interestrous interval averages 21 days in goats. The incidence of short, 8-day cycles is relatively high at the beginning of the breeding season, during lactation, particularly in dairy goats, and occasionally during the breeding season in nonlactating goats. Melatonin also appears to control frequency of LH pulses, maintaining blood levels of LH during the breeding season in the goat. Short cycles are due to a shorter luteal phase, lasting only for 5 to 6 days. These short cycles are apparently induced by the teasing activity of the billy goat, stimulated by pheromones produced by the buck. The typical sex odor of the buck is most pronounced during the breeding season. A high percentage of goats ovulate within 8 days after exposure to the male and cycle again, on the average, 19 days after this first estrus. Short cycles less than 17 days may also occur during the breeding season, particularly when does are continuously exposed to bucks. Apparently, the presence and teasing activity of the male goat induces luteolysis in the cycling doe, shortening the luteal phase of the cycle. Blood levels of progesterone fall below detectable levels 5 to 6 days after mating. When matings with fertile bucks are allowed during these male-induced, short cycles, the kidding rates remain within normal ranges. The mechanisms involved in this male-induced luteolysis remain to be determined.

Estrus

Estrus lasts an average of 28 hours, with a range of 1 to 3 days. Bucks show interest and will follow does 3 to 5 days before standing estrus occurs, suggesting proestrual activity. Behavioral signs of estrus are more pronounced in goats than in ewes. Riding and mounting of other goats is not common unless the goats are exposed to a billy goat or billy goat odor, particularly to the scent, probably pheromones, from glands located in the back of the head between the horns. Estrus detection is usually done by observation of does which stand and mate with a fertile buck or by using teasing males painted in their briskets with chin-ball marking ink. In addition, the swelling and reddening of the vulva, in conjunction with rapid flagging of the tail and vocalization, are signs that help to detect estrous goats.

Ovulation

Ovulation occurs 30 to 36 hours after the onset of estrus and is spontaneous, although it may be facilitated by the presence and mounting of the buck. The average ovulation rate is one to three oocytes, but may range from one to five oocytes depending upon the breed and management conditions. As for the ewe, the right ovary of the goat is more active than the left ovary.

The Corpus Luteum

The day of diestrus by which embryos must be present in the uterus to prevent regression of the corpus luteum has not been precisely determined for the goat. However, the corpora lutea of goats regress if viable embryos are not present by day 16 or 17 of diestrus, and the doe undergoes a subsequent cycle. As for the ewe, the lifespan of corpora lutea of goats is prolonged, for periods approaching those of pregnancy, by bilateral hysterectomy during mid-cycle.

There are no reported studies related to the utero-ovarian architecture or to the effects of unilateral hysterectomy in the goat. A local uterine luteolytic effect of the nonpregnant horn on the ipsilateral ovary may not exist in the goat. The available experimental evidence suggests that the transfer of uterine luteolytic activity is either systemic or through routes other than the venous drainage from the ipsilateral horn. Intrauterine devices exert a general rather than a local, unilateral shortening effect on the cycle of goats (see Chapter 9).

The corpus luteum is the major, if not the only source of progesterone for pregnancy in the goat. Bilateral ovariectomy, luteal enucleation, or induced luteolysis invariably results in abortion at any stage of gestation. In contrast to the ewe, the placenta of the goat does not produce progesterone.

The uterine prostaglandin $PGF_{2\alpha}$ appears to be the natural luteolysin for the goat, as in the ewe, and ovarian oxytocin plays a role in the uterine secretion of $PGF_{2\alpha}$. Administration of indomethacin, a prostaglandin synthetase inhibitor, or immunization against oxytocin suppresses the synthesis of $PGF_{2\alpha}$ and prolongs the lifespan of the corpora lutea of goats.

As demonstrated by studies on hypophysectomized goats, the corpus luteum depends on pituitary gonadotropic stimulation for development and maintenance of secretory activity during both the luteal phase of the cycle and pregnancy. Luteinizing hormone appears to be the major luteotropic gonadotropin for the goat and, in contrast to the ewe, prolactin does not appear to play any significant role.

Endocrinology of the Cycle

There is little information regarding the patterns of secretion of reproductive hormones during the estrous cycle of the goat.

Blood levels of progesterone are low, below 1.0 ng/ml during anestrus and early estrus, but increase rapidly after ovulation to reach peak values of 6 to 10 ng/ml by mid-cycle and decline rather abruptly by the end of diestrus. Blood levels of progesterone remain elevated if the doe becomes pregnant and may reach values of 10 to 12 ng/ml by day 21 of pregnancy. Levels of progesterone in milk from dairy goats parallel those of the blood but at higher concentrations. Levels of 2 to 4 ng/ml of milk are common during anestrus or estrus, when the levels of progesterone in the blood are below 1.0 ng/ml.

The ovulatory surge of LH is relatively prolonged, lasting for 9 hours, and blood levels of LH may reach peak values of 70 ng/ml. LH remains at basal levels for most of the cycle.

Blood levels of prolactin undergo circannual rhythms in the goat, reaching their highest levels during the breeding season to decline to basal levels during the nonbreeding season.

To date, there are no reported values for levels of estrogens during the estrous cycle of the goat.

ANATOMIC CHANGES OF THE REPRODUCTIVE ORGANS

The anatomic changes of the reproductive organs of the goat resemble those of the ewe. Since double or triple ovulations are common in breeds with high ovulatory rates, the ovary of

the doe tends to resemble a cluster of grapes due to either the large follicles or the corpora lutea protruding from the surface of the ovary.

The uterus of the goat has 115 to 120 caruncles, arranged in definite rows. The cervix has concentric mucosal folds which, in contrast to the ewe, are aligned. Alignment of these folds allows for deep intracervical or intrauterine insemination.

Polled Mutation

The polled mutation of goats is characterized by the absence of horns (polledness) associated with abnormal differentiation of the sexual organs. Phenotypically male polled goats, homozygous for the absence of horns, are genetically 60/XX individuals. They display testicular hypoplasia, enlarged clitoris, and different degrees of development of Wolffian structures. Genetically 60/XY polled goats may also display various degrees of intersexuality, including epididymal aplasia. Apparently, the lack of sry genes (see Chapter 7) or an XX/XY chimerism, in a freemartin-like situation, are not factors associated with the hermaphroditic intersexuality displayed by polled-mutant goats.

PREGNANCY AND PREGNANCY DIAGNOSIS

Gestation lasts an average of 150 days but may range from 146 to 155 days, depending upon breed, environmental conditions, and number of kids born. Singleton pregnancies, rare in most breeds of goats, tend to have longer gestations than pregnancy of twins or triplets.

Intrauterine migration of embryos is common in goats, and in cases of twin, triple, or quadruple pregnancies, serves the purpose of a better distribution of the fetuses and utilization of the uterine environment.

Placentation in goats, as in the sheep, is cotyledonary-syndesmochorial. The placentome is formed by apposition of the fetal and maternal cotyledons.

As indicated previously, progesterone secretion by the corpora lutea is needed throughout gestation because the placenta of the goat does not produce progesterone in amounts sufficient to maintain pregnancy. The placenta of the goat, however, is a rich source of a placental lactogen with prolactin-like activity. This placental lactogen, detectable in the blood from about day 60 of pregnancy, increases progressively throughout the second half of pregnancy to reach concentrations measurable in micrograms per milliliter of blood by the end of pregnancy.

Levels of pituitary prolactin also increase to maximal levels during the second half of gestation and remain high throughout the remainder of gestation, coinciding with the development of the mammary gland.

The nonreturn to estrus by 21 days after mating during the breeding season is a relatively reliable sign of pregnancy in goats. Other recommended diagnostic procedures include use of ultrasound to detect embryonic heartbeat, accurate after day 40 of pregnancy abdominal ballottement of the fetuses against the abdominal wall, is effective by about day 120 of pregnancy.

CONTROL OF REPRODUCTIVE EFFICIENCY

Several schemes have been developed to extend the breeding season in order to increase the kidding crop or to produce kids, particularly from dairy goats, at any time of the year.

Induction of Estrus before the Breeding Season

The exposure of yearling does to a male usually advances the breeding season by 3 weeks. Mature does may begin to cycle within 3 to 9 days after exposure to teasing bucks during the onset of the breeding season, and mating with fertile males results in pregnancy. Manipulation of the photoperiod by exposing yearling does to artificial lighting during the Spring anestrus, followed by exposure to teaser bucks, results in advancing the breeding season by as many as 80 days.

Synchronization of Estrus

During the breeding season, cycling does can be successfully synchronized using $PGF_{2\alpha}$ or synthetic analogs, either alone or after treatment of does for 12 to 16 days with progestagen implants or vaginal pessaries.

In the goat, the corpus luteum of the cycle is sensitive to the luteolytic activity of exogenous prostaglandins as early as day 4 of diestrus. Double prostaglandin treatments given 10 days apart effectively synchronize estrus in groups of does for artificial insemination or timed matings.

Prostaglandin $PGF_{2\alpha}$ or synthetic analogs are effective abortifacient agents at any stage of gestation. Abortion usually occurs within 50 hours after prostaglandin treatment. However, abortion or induction of parturition with prostaglandins may be associated with undesirable side effects in goats. A high incidence of deaths by septicemia has been reported after abortion with prostaglandins.

THE MALE

There is little information regarding spermatogenesis, and no information regarding daily spermatozoal production is available for the buck. Young bucks reportedly have a spermatogenic cycle lasting 22 days. Table 14-4 depicts the body weight, scrotal circumference, and some seminal parameters for the African Red Sokoto and Angora goats.

Kids are born with the testes located in the scrotum. Prepubertal development of the reproductive organs is rapid, and spermatozoa are present in the epididymides as early as 3.5 months of age. The penis is freed from the preputial sheath by 4 to 6 months of age, and fertile matings are possible at this age in most breeds. A diverticulum in the dorsal urethra, at the area of opening of the bulbourethral glands, prevents urethral catheterization in the buck.

Collection of Semen

Semen can be collected from the buck with an artificial vagina (AV) or by electroejaculation (EE). As for the ram, semen collected with an AV has a lower volume and higher spermatozoal concentration than semen collected by EE. However, semen collection by EE is suitable for breeding soundness examinations. Some bucks tend to ejaculate light yellow or yellow ejaculates due to pigmentation with riboflavin, while others produce white ejaculates.

Table 14-4   Body Weight, Scrotal Circumference, and Seminal Parameters[a] for the Red Sokoto African Goat and for the Angora Goat

| Endpoint | Red Sokoto | | Angora |
	Mean	Range	Mean ± SEM
Body weight, kg	17.80	---	---
Scrotal circumference, cm	21.80	20.90–22.50	--
Volume of ejaculate, ml	0.72	0.50–0.90	0.98 ± 0.52
Spermatozoal concentration per ml (10^9)	0.61	---	2.94 ± 0.45
Estimated total number of spermatozoa in ejaculate (10^9 vol. × concentration)	0.44	---	2.88
Total testicular spermatozoal reserves (10^9)	44.32	---	---
Epididymal spermatozoal reserves (10^9)	59.45	---	---

[a]Semen collected with an artificial vagina.

Adapted from: C. S. Daudu, Theriogenology, *21*:317, 1984 for Red Sokoto goats and from: G. Mendoza et al., Theriogenology, *32*:455, 1989 for Angora goats. See Chapter 8, Table 8-6, for other seminal parameters in goats.

Buck Evaluation and Breeding Management

Sexual behavior is established early in young bucks. Prepubertal kids display the Flehmen reaction and mounting behavior from about 1 month of age. These responses may be enhanced when the two sexes are reared together. As maturation progresses toward puberty, bucks develop the typical pungent odor of the billy goat. This characteristic odor, usually repugnant to man, is derived from the secretions from the sebaceous glands located between the horns and from the urine. As they grow older, bucks develop the habit of urinating on their own chin hair and forelegs. Sexually aroused bucks exhibit frequent self-enurination, Flehmen, and genital grooming. Self-enurination is a form of sexual stimulation. The billy goat odor exerts a powerful attractive and estrus-stimulating effect in does.

The buck is capable of fertile matings throughout the year, but both quality of semen and libido seem to be influenced by the photoperiod, particularly in geographic areas with pronounced seasonal fluctuations in daylight length and temperature. Serum levels of LH and testosterone increase with decreasing day length and reach maximal mean levels of 2.0 ng/ml of LH and 15 ng/ml of testosterone during the middle of the breeding season. In the nonbreeding season, billy goats may show depressed libido and seminal quality and a general lack of interest in does which have been artificially induced to cycle.

In general, the recommendations given for the breeding management of rams are applicable to the buck.

REFERENCES

Sheep

1. Adams, N. R. (1990): Permanent infertility in ewes exposed to plant oestrogens. Aust. Vet. J. *67*:197.
2. Adams, N. R. (1995): Detection of the effects of phytoestrogens on sheep and cattle. J. Anim. Sci. *73*:1509.
3. Al-Obaidi, S. A. R., Bindon, B. M., Hillard, M. A., et al. (1987): Reproductive characteristics of lambs actively immunized early in life with inhibin-enriched preparations from follicular fluid of cows. J. Reprod. Fertil. *81*:403.
4. Amann, R. P., Nett, T. M., and Niswender, G. D. (1978): Effects of LH, FSH, prolactin and $PGF_{2\alpha}$ on testicular blood flow and testosterone secretion in the ram. J. Anim. Sci. *47*:1307.
5. Baird, D. T. (1978): Pulsatile secretion of LH and ovarian estradiol during the follicular phase of the sheep estrous cycle. Biol. Reprod. *18*:359.
6. Bindon, B. M., Blanc, M. R., Pelletier, J., et al. (1979): Periovulatory gonadotrophin and ovarian

steroid patterns in sheep of breeds with differing fecundity. J. Reprod. Fertil. *55*:15.

7. Brinkley, H. J. (1981): Endocrine signaling and female reproduction. Biol. Reprod. *24*:22.

8. Burfening, P. J., Van Horn, J. L., and Blackwell, R. L. (1971): Genetic and phenotypic parameters including occurrence of estrus in Rambouillet ewe lambs. J. Anim. Sci. *33*:919.

9. Buttle, H. L. and Hancock, J. L. (1966): The chromosomes of goats, sheep, and their hybrids. Res. Vet. Sci, *7*:230.

10. Cameron, A. W. N., Tilbrook, A. J., Lindsay, D. R., et al. (1987): The number of spermatozoa required by naturally mated ewes and the ability of rams to meet these requirements. Anim. Reprod. Sci. *13*:91.

11. Carnegie, J. A., McCully, M. E., and Robertson, H. A. (1985): The early development of the sheep trophoblast and the involvement of cell death. Am. J. Anat. *174*:471.

12. Casida, L. E. and Warwick, E. J. (1945): The necessity of the corpus luteum for maintenance of pregnancy in the ewe. J. Anim. Sci. *4*:34.

13. Chemineau, P., Malpaux, B., Delgadillo, J. A., et al. (1992): Control of sheep and goat reproduction: Use of light and melatonin. Anim. Reprod. Sci. *30*:157.

14. Chesné, P., Colas, G., Cognié, Y., et al. (1987): Lamb production using superovulation, embryo bisection, and transfer. Theriogenology *27*:751.

15. Cottrell, W. O. (1985): Ram management for northeastern flocks. Cornell Vet. *75*:505.

16. Coulter, G. H., Senger, P. L., and Bailey, D. R. C. (1988): Relationship of scrotal surface temperature measured by infrared thermography to subcutaneous and deep testicular temperature in the ram. J. Reprod. Fertil. *84*:417.

17. Cran, D. G., Moor, R. M., and Hay, M. F. (1980): Fine structure of the sheep oocyte during antral follicle development. J. Reprod. Fertil. *59*:125.

18. Cumming, I. A., Baxter, R., and Lawson, R. A. S. (1974): Steroid hormone requirements for the maintenance of early pregnancy in sheep: A study using ovariectomized adrenalectomized ewes. J. Reprod. Fertil. *40*:443.

19. Cummins, L. J., O'Shea, T. O., Al-Obaidi, S. A. R., et al. (1986): Increase in ovulation rate after immunization of Merino ewes with a fraction of bovine follicular fluid containing inhibin activity. J. Reprod. Fertil. *77*:365.

20. Davis, A. J., Fleet, I. R., Harrison, F. A., et al. (1979): Pulmonary metabolism of prostaglandin $F_{2\alpha}$ in the conscious non-pregnant ewe and sow. J. Physiol. *290*:36P.

21. D'occhio, M. J. and Brooks, D. E. (1982): Threshold of plasma testosterone required for normal mating activity in male sheep. Hormones Behav. *16*:383.

22. D'occhio, M. J. and Suttie, J. M. (1992): The role of the pineal gland and melatonin in reproduction in male domestic ruminants. Anim. Reprod. Sci. *30*:135.

23. Driancourt, M. A., Cahill, L. P., and Bindon, B. M. (1985): Ovarian follicular populations and preovulatory enlargement in Booroola and control Merino ewes. J. Reprod. Fertil. *73*:93.

24. Driancourt, M. A., Gibson, W. R., and Cahill, L. P. (1985): Follicular dynamics throughout the oestrous cycle in sheep. A review. Reprod. Nutr. Dévélop. *25*:1.

25. Dunlop, A. A., Moule, G. R., and Southcott, W. H. (1963): Spermatozoa in the ejaculates of vasectomized rams. Aust. Vet. J. *39*:46.

26. Ellinwood, W. E., Nett, T. M., and Niswender, G. D. (1979): Maintenance of the corpus luteum of early pregnancy in the ewe. I. Luteotropic properties of embryonic homogenates. Biol. Reprod. *21*:281.

27. Ellinwood, W. E., Nett, T. M., and Niswender, G. D. (1979): Maintenance of the corpus luteum of early pregnancy in the ewe. II. Prostaglandin secretion by the endometrium *in vitro* and *in vivo*. Biol. Reprod. *21*:845.

28. Estes, R. D. (1972): The role of the vomeronasal organ in mammalian reproduction. Mammalia *36*:315.

29. Foster, D. and Ryan, K. (1979): Mechanisms governing onset of ovarian cyclicity at puberty in the lamb. Ann. Biol. Anim. Biochim. Biophys. *19*:1369.

30. Foster, D. L., Lemons, J. A., Jaffe, R. B., et al. (1975): Sequential patterns of circulating luteinizing hormone in female sheep from early postnatal life through the first estrous cycles. Endocrinology *97*:985.

31. García, A., Neary, M. K., Kelly, G. R., et al. (1993): Accuracy of ultrasonography in early pregnancy diagnosis in the ewe. Theriogenology *39*:847.

32. Garnier, D.-H., Cotta, Y., and Terqui, M. (1978): Androgen radioimmunoassay in the ram: Results of direct plasma testosterone and dehydroepiandrosterone measurement and physiological evaluation. Ann. Biol. Anim. Biochim. Biophys. *18*:265.

33. George, J. M. (1973): Post parturient oestrus in Merino and Dorset horn sheep. Aust. Vet. J. *49*:242.

34. Gerneke, W. H. (1965): Chromosomal evidence of the freemartin condition in sheep. J. S. Afr. Vet. Med. Assoc. *36*:99.

35. Ghannam, S. A. M., Bosc, M. J., and Du Mesnil-Du Buisson, F. (1972): Examination of vaginal epithelium of the sheep and its use in pregnancy diagnosis. Am. J. Vet. Res. *33*:1175.

36. Ginther, O. J. and Bisgard, G. E. (1972): Role of main uterine vein in local action of an intrauterine device on the corpus luteum in sheep. Am. J. Vet. Res. *33*:1583.

37. Ginther, O. J. and Del Campo, C. H. (1973): Vascular anatomy of the uterus and ovaries and the unilateral luteolytic effect of the uterus: Areas of close apposition between the ovarian artery and vessels which contain uterine venous blood in sheep. Am. J. Vet. Res. *34*:1387.

38. Ginther, O. J., Del Campo, C. H., and Rawlings, C. A. (1973): Vascular anatomy of the uterus and ovaries and the unilateral luteolytic effect of the uterus. A local venoarterial pathway between uterus and ovaries in sheep. Am. J. Vet. Res. *34*:723.

39. Hamon, M. H. and Heap, R. B. (1990): Progesterone and oestrogen concentrations in plasma of barbary sheep (Aoudad, *Ammotragus lervia*) compared with those of domestic sheep and goats during pregnancy. J. Reprod. Fertil. *90*:207.

40. Harding, C. F. (1981): Social modulation of circulating hormone levels in the male. Am. Zool. *21*:223.

41. Hauger, R. L., Karsch, F. J., and Foster, D. L. (1977): A new concept for control of the estrous cycle of the ewe based on the temporal relationships between luteinizing hormones, estradiol, and progesterone in

peripheral serum and evidence that progesterone inhibits tonic LH secretion. Endocrinology *101*:807.

42. Hernandez, F. I., Dooley, M. P., and Pineda, M. H. (1992): Effect of xylazine on the retrograde flow of spermatozoa into the urinary bladder of rams. *In:* 1992 Beef and Sheep Research Report, Iowa State University, Ames, IA, p. 160.

43. Hidiroglou, M. (1979): Trace element deficiencies and fertility in ruminants: A review. J. Dairy Sci. *62*:1195.

44. Hoagland, T. A. and Bolt, D. J. (1986): Serum follicle-stimulating hormone, luteinizing hormone, and testosterone in sexually stimulated intact and unilaterally castrated rams. Theriogenology *26*:671.

45. Hochereau-de Reviers, M.-T. and Courot, M. (1978): Sertoli cells and development of seminiferous epithelium. Ann. Biol. Anim. Biochim. Biophys. *18*:573.

46. Hogg, J. T. (1984): Mating in Bighorn sheep: Multiple creative male strategies. Science *225*:526.

47. Hollis, D. E., Frith, P. A., Vaughan, J. D., et al. (1984): Ultrastructural changes in the oviductal epithelium of Merino ewes during the estrous cycle. Am. J. Anat. *171*:441.

48. Hunter, R. H. F., Barbwise, L., and King, R. (1982): Sperm transport, storage and release in the sheep oviduct in relation to the time of ovulation. Br. Vet. J. *138*:225.

49. Hunter, R. H. F. and Nichol, R. (1983): Transport of spermatozoa in the sheep oviduct: Preovulatory sequestering of cells in the caudal isthmus. J. Exp. Zool. *228*:121.

50. Hunter, R. H. F., Nichol, R., and Crabtree, S. M., (1980): Transport of spermatozoa in the ewe: Timing of the establishment of a functional population in the oviduct. Reprod. Nutr. Devélop. *20*:1869.

51. Jindal, S. K. (1987): Studies on the gonadal and epididymal sperm reserves of Mujjafaranagri rams. J. Agr. Sci., Cambridge, England *108*:331.

52. Karsch, F. J., Foster, D. L., Legan, S. J., et al. (1979): Control of the preovulatory endocrine events in the ewe: Interrelationship of estradiol, progesterone, and luteinizing hormone. Endocrinology *105*:421.

53. Keverne, E. B., Levy, F., Poindron, P., et al. (1983): Vaginal stimulation: An important determinant of maternal bonding in sheep. Science *219*:81.

54. King, G. J., Atkinson, B. A., and Robertson, H. A. (1982): Implantation and early placentation in domestic ungulates. J. Reprod. Fertil. (Suppl. 31):17.

55. Kittok, R. J. and Britt, J. H. (1977): Corpus luteum function in ewes given estradiol during the estrous cycle or early pregnancy. J. Anim. Sci. *45*:336.

56. Knight, T. W. (1977): Methods for the indirect estimation of testes weight and sperm numbers in Merino and Romney rams. N. Z. J. Agric. Res. *20*:291.

57. Knight, T. W. and Lynch, P. R. (1980): Source of ram pheromones that stimulate ovulation in the ewe. Anim. Reprod. Sci. *3*:133.

58. Knight, T. W., Peterson, A. J., and Payne, E. (1978): The ovarian and hormonal response of the ewe to stimulation by the ram early in the breeding season. Theriogenology *10*:34.

59. Lacroix, M. C. and Kann, G. (1986): Aspects of the antiluteolytic activity of the conceptus during early pregnancy in ewes. J. Anim. Sci. *63*:1449.

60. Lees, J. L. (1978). Functional infertility in sheep. Vet. Rec. *102*:232.

61. Legan, S. J. and Karsch, F. J. (1983): Importance of retinal photoreceptors to photoperiodic control of seasonal breeding in the ewe. Biol. Reprod. *29*:316.

62. Legan, S. J., Karsch, F. J., and Foster, D. L. (1977): The endocrine control of seasonal reproductive function in the ewe: A marked change in response to the negative feedback action of estradiol on luteinizing hormone secretion. Endocrinology *101*:818.

63. Lewis, P. E. and Warren, J. E., Jr. (1977): Effect of indomethacin on luteal function in ewes and heifers. J. Anim. Sci. *46*:763.

64. Lincoln, G. A. (1976): Seasonal variation in the episodic secretion of luteinizing hormone and testosterone in the ram. J. Endocrinol. *60*:213.

65. Lindsay, D. R., Pelletier, J., Pisselet, C., et al. (1984): Changes in photoperiod and nutrition and their effect on testicular growth of rams. J. Reprod. Fertil. *71*:351.

66. Mapletoft, R. J., Lapin, D. R., and Ginther, O. J. (1976): The ovarian artery as the final component of the local luteotropic pathway between a gravid uterine horn and ovary in ewes. Biol. Reprod. *15*:414.

67. Mattner, E. and Voglmayr, J. K. (1962): A comparison of ram semen collected by the artificial vagina and by electroejaculation. Aust. J. Exp. Agric. Anim. Husb. *2*:78.

68. McNatty, K. P., Revfeim, K. J. A., and Young, A. (1973): Peripheral plasma progesterone concentrations in sheep during the oestrous cycle. J. Endocrinol. *58*:219.

69. McNatty, K. P., Gibb, M., Dobson, C., et al. (1981): Changes in the concentration of gonadotrophic and steroidal hormones in the antral fluid of ovarian follicles throughout the oestrous cycle of the sheep. Aust. J. Biol. Sci. *34*:67.

70. McNatty, K. P., Henderson, K. M., Lun, S., et al. (1985): Ovarian activity in Booroola X Romney ewes which have a major gene influencing their ovulation rate. J. Reprod. Fertil. *73*:109.

71. Mellin, T. N. and Bush, R. D. (1976): Corpus luteum function in the ewe: Effect of PGF2a and prostaglandin synthetase inhibitors. Theriogenology 12:303.

72. Murdoch, W. J. (1985): Follicular determinants of ovulation in the ewe. Domestic Anim. Endocrinol. *2*:105.

73. Nayak, R. K., Albert, E. N., and Kassira, W. N. (1976): Cyclic ultrastructural changes in ewe uterine tube (oviduct) infundibular epithelium. Am. J. Vet. Res. *37*:923.

74. Nephew, K. P., McClure, K. E., and Pope, W. F. (1989): Embryonic migration relative to maternal recognition of pregnancy in sheep. J. Anim. Sci. *67*:999.

75. Noordhuizen-Stassen, E. N., Charbon, G. A., de Jong, F. H., et al. (1985): Functional arterio-venous anastomoses between the testicular artery and the pampiniform plexus in the spermatic cord of rams. J. Reprod. Fertil. *75*:193.

76. O'Shea, J. D. and Wright, P. J. (1985): Regression of the corpus luteum of pregnancy following parturition in the ewe. Acta Anat., Basal, Switzerland *122*:69.

77. Parrot, R. F. and Baldwing, B. A. (1984): Sexual and aggressive behaviour of castrated male sheep after injection of gonadal steroids and implantation of androgens in the hypothalamus: A preliminary study. Theriogenology *21*:533.

78. Pelletier, J. (1986): Contribution of increasing and decreasing daylength to the photoperiodic control of LH secretion in the Ile-de-France ram. J. Reprod. Fertil. *77*:505.

79. Pineda, M. H., Dooley, M. P., Hembrough, F. B., et al. (1987): Retrograde flow of spermatozoa into the urinary bladder of rams. Am. J. Vet. Res. *48*:562.

80. Pineda, M. H. and Dooley, M. P. (1991): Effect of method of seminal collection on the retrograde flow of spermatozoa into the urinary bladder of rams. Am. J. Vet. Res. *52*:307.

81. Poulton, A. L. and Robinson, T. J. (1987): The response of rams and ewes of three breeds to artificial photoperiod. J. Reprod. Fertil. *79*:609.

82. Poulton, A. L., Symons, A. M., Kelly, M. I., et al. (1987): Intraruminal soluble glass boluses containing melatonin can induce early onset of ovarian activity in ewes. J. Reprod. Fertil. *80*:235.

83. Price, E. O., Estep, D. Q., Wallach, S. J. R., et al. (1991): Sexual performance of rams as determined by maturation and sexual experience. J. Anim. Sci. *69*:1047.

84. Ricketts, A. P., Sheldrick, E. L., Lindsay, K. S., et al. (1980): Induction of labour in sheep after fetal hypophysectomy: An investigation of the possible involvement of a fetal pituitary secretion in the activation of placental enzymes by fetal cortisol. Placenta *1*:287.

85. Rippel, R. H., Moyer, R. H., Johnson, E. S., et al. (1974): Response of the ewe to synthetic gonadotropin-releasing hormone. J. Anim. Sci. *38*:605.

86. Robertson, H. A., Dwyer, R. J., and King, G. J. (1985): Oestrogens in fetal and maternal fluids throughout pregnancy in the pig and comparisons with the ewe and cow. J. Endocrinol. *106*:355.

87. Robertson, H. A., Chan, J. S. D., Hackett, A. J., et al. (1980): Diagnosis of pregnancy in the ewe at midgestation. Anim. Reprod. Sci. *3*:69.

88. Sanford, L. M., Winter, J. S. D., Palmer, W. M., et al. (1974): The profile of LH and testosterone secretion in the ram. Endocrinology *96*:627.

89. Scaramuzzi, R. J., Davidson, W. G., and Van Look, P. F. A. (1977): Increasing ovulation rate in sheep by active immunization against an ovarian steroid androstenedione. Nature *269*:817.

90. Signoret, J. P. (1991): Sexual pheromones in the domestic sheep: Importance and limits in the regulation of reproductive physiology. J. Steroid Biochem. Mol. Biol. *39*:639.

91. Smith, J. F. (1988): Influence of nutrition on ovulation rate in the ewe. Aust. J. Biol. Sci. *41*:27.

92. Steger, K. and Wrobel, K.-H. (1996): Postnatal development of ovine seminiferous tubules: An electron microscopical and morphometric study. Ann. Anat. *178*:201.

93. Suttiyotin, P. and Thwaites, C. J. (1993): Evaluation of ram semen motility by a swim-up technique. J. Reprod. Fertil. *97*:339.

94. Thwaites, C. J. (1982): Semen quality after vasectomy in the ram. Livestock Prod. Sci. *8*:529.

95. Tilbrook, A. J. and Pearce, D. T. (1986): Time required for spermatozoa to remain in the vagina of the ewe to ensure conception. Aust. J. Biol. Sci. *39*:305.

96. Trapp, M. J. and Slyter, A. L. (1983): Pregnancy diagnosis in the ewe. J. Anim. Sci. *57*:1.

97. Trounson, A. O., Willadsen, S. M., and Moor, R. M. (1977): Reproductive function in prepubertal lambs: Ovulation, embryo development and ovarian steroidogenesis. J. Reprod. Fertil. *49*:69.

98. Tryphonas, L., Hidiroglou, M., and Collins, B. (1979): Reversal by testosterone of atrophy of accessory genital glands of castrated male sheep. Vet. Pathol. *16*:710.

99. Turnbull, K. E., Braden, A. W. H., and Mattner, P. E. (1977): The pattern of follicular growth and atresia in the ovine ovary. Aust. J. Biol. Sci. *30*:229.

100. Tyrrell, R. N. and Plant, J. W. (1979): Rectal damage in ewes following pregnancy diagnosis by rectal-abdominal palpation. J. Anim. Sci. *48*:348.

101. Van Wyk, L. C., Van Niekerk, C., and Belonje, P. C. (1972): Involution of the post-partum uterus of the ewe. J. South Afr. Vet. Assoc. *43*:19.

102. Walkley, J. R. W. and Smith, C. (1980): The use of physiological traits in genetic selection for litter size in sheep. J. Reprod. Fertil. *59*:83.

103. Wathes, D. C., Rees, J. M., and Porter, D. G. (1988): Identification of relaxin in the placenta of the ewe. J. Reprod. Fertil. *84*:247.

104. Wheeler, A. G. (1978): Comparisons of the ovulatory and steroidogenic activities of the left and right ovaries of the ewe. J. Reprod. Fertil. *53*:27.

105. Willadsen, S. M., (1986): Nuclear transplantation in sheep embryos. Nature *320*:63.

106. Willingham, T., Shelton, M., and Thompson, P. (1986): An assessment of reproductive wastage in sheep. Theriogenology *26*:179.

107. Wooding, F. B. P., Flint, A. P. F., Heap, R. B., et al. (1981): Autoradiographic evidence for migration and fusion of cells in the sheep placenta: Resolution of a problem in placental classification. Cell Biol. *5*:821.

References Added in Proof

108. Cognie, Y. (1999): State of the art in sheep-goat embryo transfer. Theriogenology *51*:105.

109. Kelk, D. A., Gartley, C. J., Buckrell, B. C., et al. (1997): The interbreeding of sheep and goats. Can. Vet. J. *38*:235.

110. Resko, J. A., Perkins, A., Roselli, C. E., et al. (1999): Sexual behaviour of rams: Male orientation and its endocrine correlates. J. Reprod. Fertil. (Suppl. 54):259.

111. Walkden-Brown, S. W., Martin, G. B., and Restall, B. J. (1999): Role of male-female interaction in regulating reproduction in sheep and goats. J. Reprod. Fertil. (Suppl. 54):243.

112. Wood, R. I. and Foster, D. L. (1998): Sexual differentiation of reproductive neuroendocrine function in sheep. Rev. Reprod. *3*:130.

Goats

1. Ali, B. H. and Mustafa, A. I. (1986): Semen characteristics of Nubian goats in the Sudan. Anim. Reprod. Sci. *12*:63.

2. Anderson, G. B., Anderson, D. L., Bon Durant, R. H., et al. (1995): Semen characteristics and production of germ cells in male sheep-goat chimeras. Anim. Reprod. Sci. *40*:31.

3. Anderson, G. B., Ruffing, N. A., BonDurant, R. H., et al. (1991): Preliminary observations on reproduction in a female sheep-goat chimaera. Vet. Rec. *129*:467.

4. Armstrong, D. T. and Evans, G. (1984): Hormonal regulation of reproduction: Induction of ovulation in sheep and goats with FSH preparations. Proc. 10th. Int. Congr. Anim. Reprod. A. I., Univ. Illinois, Champaign/Urbana, June 10–14, 1984, Vol. VII, p. 8.

5. Baril, G. and Vallet, J. C. (1990): Time of ovulations in dairy goats induced to superovulate with porcine follicle-stimulating hormone during and out of the breeding season. Theriogenology *34*:303.

6. Basrur, P. K. (1986): Goat-sheep hybrids. *In:* Current Therapy in Theriogenology 2, edited by D. A. Morrow. Philadelphia, PA, W. B. Saunders, Co., p. 613.

7. Basrur, P. K. and McKinnon, A. O. (1986): Caprine intersexes and freemartins. *In:* Current Therapy in Theriogenology 2, edited by D. A. Morrow. Philadelphia, PA, W. B. Saunders, Co., p. 596.

8. Battye, K. M., Fairclough, R. J., Cameron, A. W. N., et al. (1988): Evidence for prostaglandin involvement in early luteal regression of the superovulated nanny goat (*Capra hircus*). J. Reprod. Fertil. *84*:425.

9. Beckett, S. D., Reynolds, T. M., and Bartels, J. E. (1978): Angiography of the crus penis in the ram and buck during erection. Am. J. Vet. Res. *39*:1950.

10. Berger, T. (1989): Development of a zona-free hamster ova bioassay for goat sperm. Theriogenology *32*:69.

11. Berger, T., Drobnis, E. Z., Foley, L., et al. (1994): Evaluation of relative fertility of cryopreserved goat sperm. Theriogenology *41*:711.

12. Bon Durant, R. H. (1981): Reproductive physiology in the goat. Mod. Vet. Pract. *62*:525.

13. Bon Durant, R. H., Darien, B. J., Munro, C. J., et al. (1981): Photoperiod induction of fertile oestrus and changes in LH and progesterone concentrations in yearling dairy goats (*Capra hircus*). J. Reprod. Fertil. *63*:1.

14. Bretzlaff, K. N., Hill, A., and Ott, R. S. (1983): Induction of luteolysis in goats with prostaglandin $F_{2\alpha}$. Am. J. Vet. Res. *44*:1162.

15. Bretzlaff, K. N., Ott, R. S., Weston, P. G., et al. (1981): Dose of prostaglandin $F_{2\alpha}$ effective for induction of estrus in goats. Theriogenology *16*:587.

16. Buttle, H. L. (1978): The maintenance of pregnancy in hypophysectomized goats. J. Reprod. Fertil. *52*:255.

17. Cairoli, F., Tamanini, C., Bono, G., et al. (1987): Reproductive performance of female goats given progestagen associated with PMSG and/or HMG in deep anestrus. Reprod. Nutr. Dévélop. *27*:13.

18. Chemineau, P. (1983): Effect on oestrus and ovulation of exposing Creole goats to the male at three times of the year. J. Reprod. Fertil. *67*:65.

19. Chemineau, P. (1986): Sexual behaviour and gonadal activity during the year in the tropical Creole meat goat. I. Female oestrous behaviour and ovarian activity. Reprod. Nutr. Dévélop. *26*:441.

20. Chemineau, P. (1986): Sexual behaviour and gonadal activity during the year in the tropical Creole meat goat. II. Male mating behaviour, testis diameter, ejaculate characteristics and fertility. Reprod. Nutr. Dévélop. *26*:453.

21. Chemineau, P., Malpaux, B., Delgadillo, J. A., et al. (1992): Control of sheep and goat reproduction: Use of light and melatonin. Anim. Reprod. Sci. *30*:157.

22. Chemineau, P., Martin, G. B., Saumande, J., et al. (1988): Seasonal and hormonal control of pulsatile LH secretion in the dairy goat (*Capra hircus*). J. Reprod. Fertil. *83*:91.

23. Chemineau, P. and Xande, A. (1982): Reproductive efficiency of Creole meat goats permanently kept with males. Relationship to a tropical environment. Trop. Anim. Prod. *7*:98.

24. Claus, R., Over, R., and Dehnhard, M. (1990): Effect of male odour on LH secretion and the induction of ovulation in seasonally anoestrous goats. Anim. Reprod. Sci. *22*:27.

25. Cooke, R. G. and Homeida, A. M. (1983): Prevention of the luteolytic action of oxytocin in the goat by inhibition of prostaglandin synthesis. Theriogenology *20*:363.

26. Cooke, R. G. and Homeida, A. M. (1985): Suppression of prostaglandin $F_{2\alpha}$ release and delay of luteolysis after active immunization against oxytocin in the goat. J. Reprod. Fertil. *75*:63.

27. Cooke, R. G. and Knifton, A. (1980): Removal of corpora lutea in pregnant goats: Effects of intrauterine indomethacin. Res. Vet. Sci. *29*:77.

28. Crozet, N., Théron, M. C., and Chemineau, P. (1987): Ultrastructure of *in vivo* fertilization in the goat. Gamete Res. *18*:191.

29. Currie, W. B. (1974): Regression of the corpus luteum of pregnancy and initiation of labour in goats. J. Reprod. Fertil. *36*:481.

30. Currie, W. B. and Thorburn, G. D. (1974): Luteal function in hysterectomized goats. J. Reprod. Fertil. *41*:501.

31. Currie, W. B., Gorewit, R. C., and Michel, F. J. (1988): Endocrine changes, with special emphasis on oestradiol-17β, prolactin and oxytocin, before and during labour and delivery in goats. J. Reprod. Fertil. *82*:299.

32. Currie, W. B., Card, C. E., Michel, F. J., et al. (1990): Purification, partial characterization, and development of a specific radioimmunoassay for goat placental lactogen. J. Reprod. Fertil. *90*:25.

33. Daudu, C. S. (1984): Spermatozoa output, testicular sperm reserve and epididymal storage capacity of the Red Sokoto goats indigenous to Northern Nigeria. Theriogenology *21*:317.

34. Day, A. M. and Southwell, S. R. G. (1979): Termination of pregnancy in goats using cloprostenol. N. Z. Vet. J. *27*:207.

35. Dhingra, L. D. (1979): Angioarchitecture of the arteries of the testis of goat (*Capra aegagrus*). Zbl. Vet. Med. C. *8*:193.

36. D'occhio, M. J. and Suttie, J. M. (1992): The role of the pineal gland and melatonin in reproduction in male domestic ruminants. Anim. Reprod. Sci. *30*:135.

37. Erasmus, J. A., Fourie, A. J., and Venter, J. J. (1985): Influence of age on reproductive performance of the improved Boer goat doe. South Afr. J. Anim. Sci. *15*:5.

38. Forsyth, I. A., Byatt, J. C., and Iley, S. (1985): Hormone concentrations, mammary development and milk yield in goats given long-term bromocriptine treatment in pregnancy. J. Endocrinol. *104*:77.

39. Gadgil, B. A., Zala, P. M., Shukla, K. P., et al. (1969): Effect of intrauterine spirals on reproduction in goats. Ind. J. Exp. Biol. *7*:82.

40. Gustafson, R. A., Anderson, G. B., Bon Durant, R. H., et al. (1993): Failure of sheep-goat hybrid conceptuses to develop to term in sheep-goat chimeras. J. Reprod. Fertil. *99*:267.

41. Hamon, M. H. and Heap, R. B. (1990): Progesterone and oestrogen concentrations in plasma of barbary sheep (aoudad, *Ammotragus lervia*) compared with those of domestic sheep and goats during pregnancy. J. Reprod. Fertil. *90*:207.

42. Hayden, T. J., Thomas, C. R., Smith, S. V., et al. (1980): Placental lactogen in the goat in relation to stage of gestation, number of fetuses, metabolites, progesterone and time of day. J. Endocrinol. *86*:279.

43. Hinkle, R. F., Howard, J. L., and Stowater, J. L. (1978): An anatomic barrier to urethral catheterization in the male goat. J. Am. Vet. Med. Assoc. *173*:1584.

44. Humblot, P., De Montigny, G., Jeanguejot, N., et al. (1990): Pregnancy-specific protein B and progesterone concentrations in French alpine goats throughout gestation. J. Reprod. Fertil. *89*:205.

45. Jarrell, V. L. and Dziuk, P. J. (1991): Effect of number of corpora lutea and fetuses on concentrations of progesterone in blood of goats. J. Anim. Sci. *69*:770.

46. Li, R., Cameron, A. W. N., Batt, P. A., et al. (1990): Maximum survival of frozen goat embryos is attained at the expanded, hatching and hatched blastocyst stages of development. Reprod. Fertil. Develop. *2*:345.

47. Madani, M. O. K. and Rahal, M. S. (1988): Puberty in Libyan male goats. Anim. Reprod. Sci. *17*:207.

48. Martino, A., Mogas, T., Palomo, M. J., et al. (1994): Meiotic competence of prepubertal goat oocytes. Theriogenology *41*:969.

49. Meites, J., Webster, H. D., Young, F. W., et al. (1951): Effects of the corpora lutea removal and replacement with progesterone on pregnancy in goats. J. Anim. Sci. *10*:411.

50. Memon, M. A., Bretzlaff, K. N., and Ott, R. S. (1986): Comparison of semen collection techniques in goats. Theriogenology *26*:823.

51. Mendoza, G., White, I. G., and Chow, P. (1989): Studies of chemical components of Angora goat seminal plasma. Theriogenology *32*:455.

52. Mohammad, W. A., Grossman, M., and Vatthauer, J. L. (1984): Seasonal breeding in United States dairy goats. J. Dairy Sci. *67*:1813.

53. Mori, Y., Kano, Y., and Sawasaki, T. (1983): An application of culdoscopy to goats for serial observation of periovulatory ovary in the goats (sic). Jpn. J. Vet. Sci. *45*:667.

54. Muduuli, D. S., Sanford, L. M., Plamer, W. M., et al. (1979): Secretory patterns and circadian and seasonal changes in luteinizing hormone, follicle-stimulating hormone, prolactin, and testosterone in the male Pygmy goat. J. Anim. Sci. *49*:543.

55. Ott, R. S., Nelson, D. R., and Hixon, J. E. (1980): The effect of presence of the male on initiation of estrous cycle activity of goats. Theriogenology *13*:183.

56. Ott, R. S., Nelson, D. R., and Hixon, J. E. (1980): Fertility of goats following synchronization of estrus with prostaglandin F2 alpha. Theriogenology *13*:341.

57. Ott, R. S., Nelson, D. R., and Hixon, J. E. (1980): Peripheral serum progesterone and luteinizing hormone concentrations of goats during synchronization of estrus and ovulation with prostaglandin F2 alpha. Am. J. Vet. Res. *41*:1432.

58. Pailhoux, E., Cribiu, E. P., Chaffaux, S., et al. (1994): Molecular analysis of 60,XX pseudohermaphrodite polled goats for the presence of SRY and ZFY genes. J. Reprod. Fertil. *100*:491.

59. Price, E. O. and Smith, V. M. (1984/85): The relationship of male-male mounting to mate choice and sexual performance in male dairy goats. Appl. Anim. Behav. Sci. *13*:71.

60. Price, E. O., Smith, V. M., and Katz, L. S. (1986): Stimulus conditions influencing self-enuriration, genital grooming and Flehmen in male goats. Appl. Anim. Behav. Sci. *16*:371.

61. Refsal, K. R. (1986): Collection and evaluation of caprine semen. In: Current Therapy in Theriogenology 2, edited by D. A. Morrow. Philadelphia, PA, W. B. Saunders Co., p. 619.

62. Restall, B. J. (1992): Seasonal variation in reproductive activity in Australian goats. Anim. Reprod. Sci. *27*:305.

63. Riera, G. S. (1984): Some similarities and differences in female sheep and goat reproduction. Proc. 10th Int. Congr. Anim. Reprod. A.I., Univ. Illinois, Champaign/Urbana, June 10–14, 1984, Vol. VII, p. 1.

64. Ritar, A. J. (1991): Seasonal changes in LH, androgens and testes in the male Angora goat. Theriogenology *36*:959.

65. Ritar, A. J., Ball, P. D., and O'May, P. J. (1990): Examination of methods for the deep freezing of goat semen. Reprod. Fertil. Develop. *2*:27.

66. Ritar, A. J., Ball, P. D., and O'May, P. J. (1990): Artificial insemination of Cashmere goats: Effects of fertility and fecundity of intravaginal treatment, method and time of insemination, semen freezing process, number of motile spermatozoa and age of females. Reprod. Fertil. Develop. *2*:377.

67. Ritar, A. J. and Salamon, S. (1983): Fertility of fresh and frozen-thawed semen of the Angora goat. Aust. J. Biol. Sci. *36*:49.

68. Salamon, S. and Ritar, A. J. (1982): Deep freezing of Angora goat semen: Effects of diluent composition, method and rate of dilution on survival of spermatozoa. Aust. J. Biol. Sci. *35*:295.

69. Selgrath, J. P., Memon, M. A., Smith, T. E., et al. (1990): Collection and transfer of microinjectable embryos from dairy goats. Theriogenology *34*:1195.

70. Shelton, M. (1978): Reproduction and breeding of goats. J. Dairy Sci. *61*:994.

71. Sheldrick, E. L., Ricketts, A. P., and Flint, A. P. F. (1980): Placental production of progesterone in ovariectomized goats treated with a synthetic progestagen to maintain pregnancy. J. Reprod. Fertil. *60*:339.

72. Skalet, L. H., Rodrigues, H. D., Goyal, H. O., et al. (1988): Effects of age and season on the type and occurrence of sperm abnormalities in Nubian bucks. Am. J. Vet. Res. *49*:1284.

73. Staples, L. D., Fleet, I. R., and Heap, R. B. (1982): Anatomy of the utero-ovarian lymphatic network and the composition of afferent lymph in relation to the establishment of pregnancy in the sheep and goat. J. Reprod. Fertil. *64*:409.

74. Thibier, M., Pothelet, D., Jeanguyot, N., et al. (1981): Estrous behavior, progesterone in peripheral plasma and milk in dairy goats at onset of breeding season. J. Dairy Sci. *64*:513.

75. Thompson, F. N., Abrams, E., and Miller, D. M. (1983): Reproductive traits in Nubian dairy goats. Anim. Reprod. Sci. *6*:59.

76. Tokashiki, S. and Kawashima, Y. (1976): Histochemical changes in the endometrium of the goats during the course of estrous cycle and pregnancy. Jpn. J. Vet. Sci. *38*:639.

77. Wathes, D. C., Swann, R. W., Porter, D. G., et al. (1986): Oxytocin as an ovarian hormone. Current Topics Neuroendocrinol. *6*:129.

78. Williams, H. L. (1984): The effects of the physical and social environments on reproduction in adult sheep and goats. Proc. 10th Int. Congr. Anim. Reprod. A.I., Univ. Illinois, Champaign/Urbana, June 10–14, 1984, Vol. IV, p. 31.

References Added in Proof

79. Amoah, E. A. and Gelaye, S. (1997): Biotechnological advances in goat reproduction. J. Anim. Sci. *75*:578.

80. Cognie, Y. (1999): State of the art in sheep-goat embryo transfer. Theriogenology *51*:105.

81. Kawate, N., Monrita, N., Tsuji, M., et al. (2000): Roles of pulsatile release of LH in the development and maintenance of corpus luteum function in the goat. Theriogenology *54*:1133.

82. Kelk, D. A., Gartley, C. J., Buckrell, B. C., et al. (1997): The interbreeding of sheep and goats. Can. Vet. J. *38*:235.

83. Walkden-Brown, S. W., Martin, G. B., and Restall, B. J. (1999): Role of male-female interaction in regulating reproduction in sheep and goats. J. Reprod. Fertil. (Suppl. 54):243.

Reproductive Patterns of Swine*

L. E. EVANS

15

INTRODUCTION

The domestic female pig is polytocous and nonseasonally polyestrous, with estrus occurring at average intervals of 21 days. Proestrus lasts about 2 days, estrus 2 to 3 days, and metestrus for 1 or 2 days. The remainder of the cycle is diestrus. The corpora lutea are functional for about 16 days after ovulation. Ovulation occurs spontaneously, 36 to 44 hours after the onset of estrus or shortly beyond mid-estrus.

Pregnancy lasts 112 to 116 days, commonly resulting in litters of 8 to 10 pigs for pri-miparous young females, called **gilts**, or litters of 10 to 16 pigs for sows. During lactation, the sow may have an abbreviated estrus shortly after parturition but does not cycle normally and breed until after the pigs are weaned.

PUBERTY AND SEXUAL MATURITY

Several factors influence the onset of puberty in the gilt and continuance of regular estrous cycles. The most important of these include:

1. breed,
2. season of the year,
3. exposure to boars,
4. housing and degree of confinement,
5. nutrition, and
6. general health.

Under good management, puberty occurs in the gilt at approximately 6 to 7 months of age, when the gilt reaches a body weight of 100 to 110 kg.

The age of puberty is influenced by the breed and by selection within the breed. Generally, Landrace, the Large White breeds, and Hampshires have earlier first estrus than other common breeds in the United States. Within breeds, some genetic lines cycle at a younger age than others.

The percentage of gilts showing normal estrous cycles by 9 months of age is lower for those gilts reaching breeding age during the Summer than for gilts reaching breeding age during the other seasons. This effect is observed in both gilts reared in confinement and in nonconfinement conditions. Confinement reduces the number of gilts showing estrus at 7 to 9

*Additional information concerning reproduction in swine has been presented in Chapter 2 (Pituitary Gland), Chapter 7 (The Biology of Sex), Chapter 8 (Male Reproductive System), Chapter 9 (Female Reproductive System), Chapter 10 (Artificial Insemination), and Chapter 11 (Patterns of Reproduction). The reader is encouraged to refer to these chapters in order to permit conciseness.

months of age by 10 to 15% when compared to gilts housed in nonconfinement. Housing gilts in small groups of 2 to 3 per pen, or in large groups of 50 or more, also delays the first estrus. Other environmental factors such as lighting appear to have little effect on days to first estrus.

As the gilts approach puberty, exposure to a mature boar will shorten the interval to estrus and results in some synchronization of estrus. Puberty is often delayed if boar exposure is initiated when the gilts are only 3 to 4 months of age.

Under normal conditions of feeding and management, nutrition will have a minimal effect on puberty. A low-protein diet will delay growth and puberty, and a low-energy diet may depress ovulation rates. Likewise, unthriftiness due to disease can delay the first estrus.

The age at onset of puberty in the boar is earlier than that of the gilt. Primary spermatocytes first appear in the seminiferous tubules by 3 months, secondary spermatocytes at 4 to 5 months, and mature spermatozoa are present in the ejaculate at 5 to 6 months of age. At this age, the boar has limited fertility and should not be used on a regular basis for breeding until 8 months of age. Young boars should be selected for early sexual maturity because this characteristic is one of the heritable reproductive traits and may be reflected in age of puberty in his offspring. Boars raised without interaction with the opposite sex often have delayed behavioral development. A castrated male is called a **barrow**.

BREEDING SEASON

Postpubertal gilts or nonpregnant sows under ordinary environmental conditions are non-seasonally polyestrous, although cyclicity and fertility may be depressed in the late Summer and early Fall. Sows will show estrus approximately every 21 days until the age of 10 to 12 years, when senescence begins to affect ovarian function. Most sows are culled from the breeding herd for other reasons long before senescence sets in.

After parturition there is a period of anestrus characterized by quiescent ovaries. This quiescence generally lasts throughout lactation. Soon after weaning, which occurs at 2 to 5 weeks postpartum under present husbandry conditions,

there is a rapid growth of ovarian follicles, followed by estrus and ovulation within 3 to 7 days after weaning. It is desirable to breed the sow at this time since uterine involution is completed by 21 days postpartum and the sow's fertility is good. Weaning is often used as a means of achieving synchrony of estrus in a group of sows.

Most producers maximize sow productivity by rebreeding the sow as soon as possible after parturition. With a gestation period of 114 days and a lactational period of 21 days, sows which are bred 5 to 10 days after weaning can be expected to produce a litter every 5 months or an average of 2.4 litters and 22 to 26 pigs per year. However, due to other factors which reduce fertility, the average sow herd falls short of this potential level of production.

Utilizing a short lactational interval of 16 to 20 days, followed by a short weaning-to-estrus interval of 6 to 10 days and a high first service conception rates reaching 85 to 90%, herds may approach this level of productivity. The period when sows are not pregnant or lactating is termed nonproductive sow days. As the average for nonproductive sow days increase in the herd, the litters per sow per year will decrease.

THE ESTROUS CYCLE

The estrous cycle of the sow can be divided into events associated with the growth of the follicles and events associated with the growth and survival of the corpora lutea (Figs. 15-1 and 15-2). The histologic and secretory changes occurring in the tubular genital tract under the influence of rising levels of estrogens at the time of proestrus and estrus or rising progesterone levels during metestrus and diestrus are similar to those of other species (Fig. 15-2). The vaginal smear and electrical conductivity of vaginal secretions have been used to determine the stage of estrous cycle in the sow. However, neither method is used extensively in large production units; rather, most producers rely on teasing the sow with a boar to determine estrus and the proper time to mate.

Following ovulation at mid-estrus, cellular remnants from the follicular wall luteinize, resulting in the formation of progesterone-producing

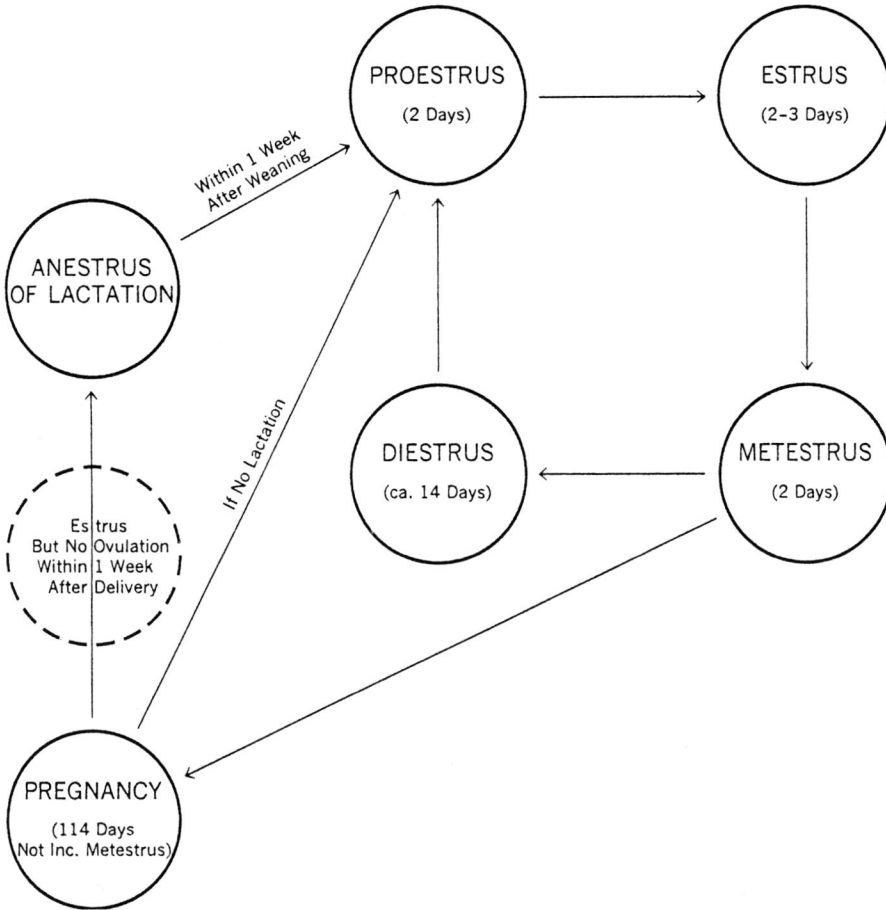

Fig. 15-1. The reproductive cycle of the sow with alternates.

corpora lutea (CL). Plasma progesterone levels rise to a peak of 25 to 30 ng/ml at 12 to 14 days of diestrus and are followed by a rapid decline, coincidental with luteolysis, 15 to 18 days after estrus. Prostaglandin $F_{2\alpha}$ is believed to be the natural luteolysin. Porcine corpora lutea are not responsive to a single dose of $PGF_{2\alpha}$ given before day 11 of the cycle, the time at which endogenous $PGF_{2\alpha}$ has already begun to induce irreversible, retrogressive changes on the corpora lutea. Hence, induction of luteolysis by a single treatment with prostaglandins is not of practical significance to induce estrus in the cycling sow or gilt. However, repeated injections of $PGF_{2\alpha}$ from days 5 to 10 of the cycle shorten the interestrous interval to 13 days[37] and histological examination of treated gilts[38] revealed evidence of

luteolysis by day 8. The fertility of gilts or sows induced to cycle with repeated doses of $PGF_{2\alpha}$ has not been reported.

As progesterone levels decline, the hypothalamo-hypophyseal axis responds by increasing the frequency of episodic release of LH. Ultimately, there is increased binding of gonadotropins by the cells of developing and mature follicles. An increase in circulating levels of estrogens, primarily estradiol-17β, occurs between days 15 and 20 of the estrous cycle. Circulating estrogens peak about 24 hours before the onset of behavioral estrus. LH levels peak at the beginning of estrus, and ovulation occurs 36 to 44 hours after the LH peak. The oocytes are shed from both ovaries over a range of 6 to 8 hours.

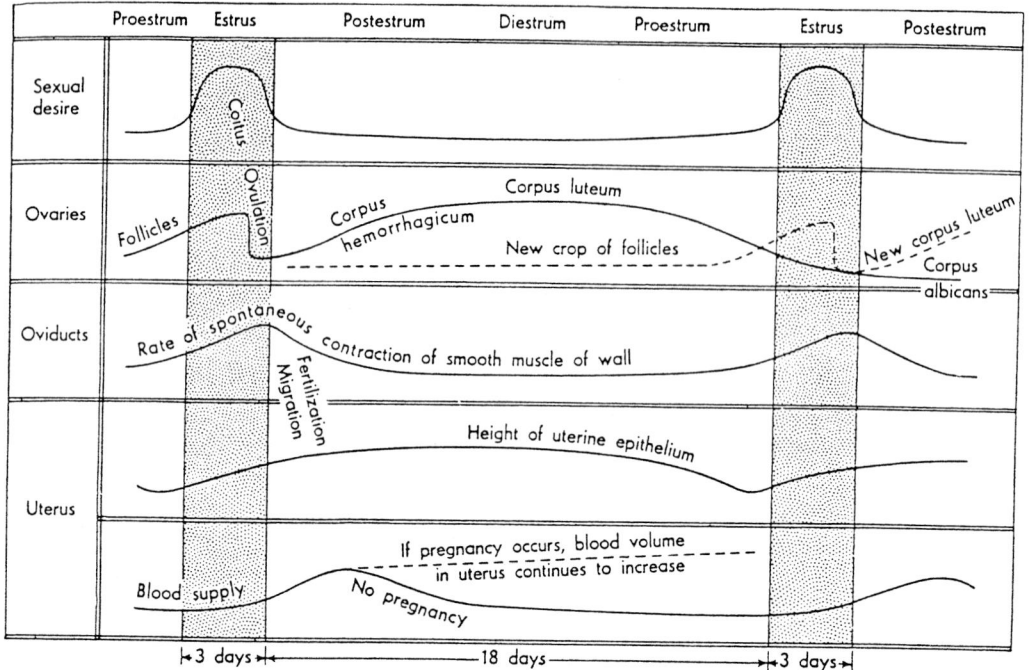

Fig. 15-2. Graph showing the behavioral responses and physiological changes within the reproductive tracts during the estrous cycle in the sow. Note the coincidence of the important events leading toward pregnancy (**coitus, ovulation, fertilization,** and the migration of the embryo through the oviduct to the uterus, and finally its attachment to the uterine mucosa) at the height of local activity as indicated by the curves. (From: B. M. Patten, *In:* Foundations of Embryology. New York, NY, McGraw-Hill Book Co., 1958).

Estrus and Sexual Behavior

Estrus in the sow lasts from 40 to 70 hours. Usually the sow seeks out the male when he is within sight. There may be nuzzling actions and attempts at mounting from both sows and the boar, but more commonly the female assumes a characteristic posture with elevation of the ears in response to the boar's vocalization and stands while the boar attempts to mount.

The boar will test sows for estrus by vocalizing, urinating, nuzzling, and attempting to mount. The boar will randomly seek the female with this pattern of courtship. Nasal-genital testing of the female is common in the boar, but boars do not display the Flehman reaction. Erection occurs after mounting. The boar has a corkscrew glans penis that penetrates and is anchored by the female's cervix during ejaculation. Mating commonly lasts from 5 to 8 minutes. Ejaculate volumes of 150 to 200 ml are common, and the ejaculate is deposited into the uterus through the penis anchored in the cervix.

With free access copulation may occur several times during estrus. However, matings can be limited by hand-mating. In this case, it is recommended that copulation be permitted once daily during estrus. Detection of estrus for hand-mating or artificial insemination generally requires a teaser boar. The standing response of the estrous sow to back pressure is often used by the herdsman. The swollen and red appearance of the vulva also provides a clue to an approaching estrus, especially in gilts.

Within 2 to 3 days after parturition, approximately one-fourth of sows will show a behavioral estrus in response to the elevated estrogen levels at farrowing. However, there is not a concomitant ovarian response, and normally ovulation does not occur.

Fertilization Time

The pregnancy rate is usually low for single breedings occurring either on the first day of estrus or after ovulation. Breeding 6 to 12 hours before ovulation results in the highest rate of pregnancy. Since estrus detection is not always accurate and ovulation time is even less predictable, it is a good practice to have the female bred on both the first and second days of estrus. Daily breeding during estrus is optimal and results in fertilization of nearly all of the ovulated oocytes.

EMBRYONIC MORTALITY

Under optimal breeding conditions, capacitated spermatozoa fertilize nearly 100% of the oocytes. Pig embryos enter the uterus at the four-cell stage, approximately 48 hours after ovulation. About 6 days after ovulation, the embryos have reached the stage of blastocyst and hatch from their zona pellucida. These embryos undergo intrauterine distribution into both horns, especially during the 9th to 11th days. By day 13, the embryos are evenly distributed within the horns as implantation begins. If the embryos are not distributed into both horns of the uterus at this time or if less than four embryos are present, the pregnancy will fail. Maternal recognition of pregnancy is completed primarily by day 14 after ovulation.

Embryonic losses within any one pregnancy may be as high as 25 to 40% of the oocytes ovulated. Nearly two-thirds of this loss occurs before pregnancy recognition by the female. The loss of the remaining one-third occurs before day 40 of pregnancy. If embryo death occurs before day 40 of gestation, resorption of the tissue will take place. If death occurs after bone calcification, then fetal mummification, abortion, or maceration will follow. The cause of this enormous loss of embryos during early pregnancy in the sow is not fully understood. However, embryos resulting from early ovulations appear to mature faster and survive at a higher rate than the embryos resulting from later ovulated oocytes. This loss cannot be fully compensated for by selecting for increased ovulation rates or by superovulation procedures. Thus, an innate limitation of litter size resides within the uterine functions of the sow.

Embryonic death may occur as the result of uterine pathology, infectious agents, or stress of the sow in early gestation. If the entire litter dies

before pregnancy recognition, the sow will recycle at the regular 21-day interval. Later deaths of the entire litter may cause pseudopregnancy or abortion with return to estrus at irregular intervals. If part of the litter survives, the pregnancy may go to term, resulting in a reduced litter size or mummified fetuses at parturition.

LITTER SIZE

Fecundity or **prolificacy** refers to the number of piglets in the litter. Litter size of the sow is dependent upon breed, age, days postpartum when bred, state of nutrition and, to a lesser extent, the environment and boar management at breeding.

Some breeds are more prolific than others. In general, the white breeds, Landrace, Large White, and bacon-type Yorkshires have a modest advantage in litter size. However, there is as much variation between genetic lines within a breed, as there is between breeds. In addition, improvement of litter size through genetic selection within the herd usually is very slow, 1 to 2% in each generation. The heritability of reproductive traits is apparently low; thus, genetic improvement of litter size in a given herd centers on selection of breeding stock from prolific herds and maximizing heterosis within the breed or utilizing a cross-breeding system.

Ovulation rate and litter size increase with advancing age or parity, stabilizing after 6 or 7 litters (Table 15-1). However, the rate of stillbirth increases slowly after the fourth parity, so the advantage of keeping older sows is gradu-

Table 15-1 Relationship Between Parity and Prolificacy in Pigs

Litter No.	Increase in No. of Young over First Litter
1	0
2	0.68
3	1.36
4	1.58
5	1.90
6	1.92
7	1.89
8	1.71
9	1.45

Data from: J. L. Lush and A. Molln, USDA Tech. Bull., 836, 1942.

ally lost. The size of the first litter increases with the number of estrous cycles that the gilt had prior to mating. Overall, and when later parities are considered, early-bred gilts perform as well as later-bred gilts.

Early weaning, resulting in a shorter interval from farrowing to the next breeding, will generally result in smaller litter sizes through all parities, but particularly following the first litter. Breeding sows at less than 21 days after farrowing will significantly reduce litter size. However, litter size will increase as the interval from farrowing increases up to about 35 days.

The nutritional status of the breeding herd may influence litter size, although these effects are minimal if a ration of adequate quality is fed. Nutritional deficiencies usually affect estrual cyclicity. Increasing feed intake (flushing) in gilts for 10 to 14 days before the expected time of breeding will increase ovulation rates, resulting in one or two more piglets per pregnancy. First and second parity sows are particularly vulnerable to energy and protein deficits, which lead to weight loss during lactation. These sows will benefit from full feeding during lactation and also after weaning. This results in better cyclicity and larger litters. However, a modest decrease in embryo survival may occur in sows or gilts that are overfed during early pregnancy.

High environmental temperatures may adversely affect the ovulation rate and increase embryonic mortality. Likewise, boar fertility may be depressed by extremely low or high environmental temperatures. Litter size and conception rate are also adversely affected by poor timing of the mating. Multiple matings help to avoid this problem. However, caution must be exercised because overuse of a boar results in a reduced impregnating dose of spermatozoa, which would adversely affect litter size and conception rates.

PREGNANCY DIAGNOSIS

Optimizing productivity in the breeding herd dictates that mated gilts or sows be examined for pregnancy so that any open females can be rebred or culled from the herd. This is particularly important for those breeding herds experiencing less than optimal conception (90–95%) or farrowing (85–90%) rates.

Since the normal open sow or gilt will recycle in 18 to 23 days post mating, boar exposure of females bred 18 to 23 days previously should detect the open/cycling female and give an indication of the potential farrowing rate for that group.

Several ultrasound devices are available for detection of pregnancy in the sow. Doppler ultrasound using a rectal probe will detect blood flow and fetal heartbeat fairly early, approximately 25–30 days of pregnancy. The A-mode ultrasound device has been used extensively in the past to detect fluid in the uterus of 30- to 70-day pregnant females using a transabdominal probe. More recently, real-time B-mode ultrasound via transabdominal probe (Fig. 15-3) has been shown to be effective at 22 days or more of pregnancy with 95–97% accuracy.[3] The advantage of real-time ultrasound is that electronic visualization of the fetus is possible. A few operators are currently attempting pregnancy detection with B-mode ultrasound at 18 days postbreeding so that open sows are detected before the expected 18–23 days return heat. At present, this procedure detects 75–80% of the pregnant sows as having fluid in the uterus (the embryo is not visualized). All sows which do not have signs of pregnancy are then subjected to boar exposure for the potential return to estrus and rebreeding if they are not pregnant.

PARTURITION

Parturition normally commences approximately 114 days after breeding. Filling of the mammary glands and vulvar swelling occur 2 to 3 days prior to parturition. Within a few hours of delivery, milk secretions may be expressed from the mammary glands. The sow shows restlessness, increased temperature and respiration rates, and nesting behavior during the hours preceding labor. Blood-stained fluids and small amounts of meconium usually appear in the vaginal secretions within 30 minutes of birth of the first pig.

Farrowing occurs with the sow in lateral recumbency and normally is completed within 2 to 4 hours, although this interval may be

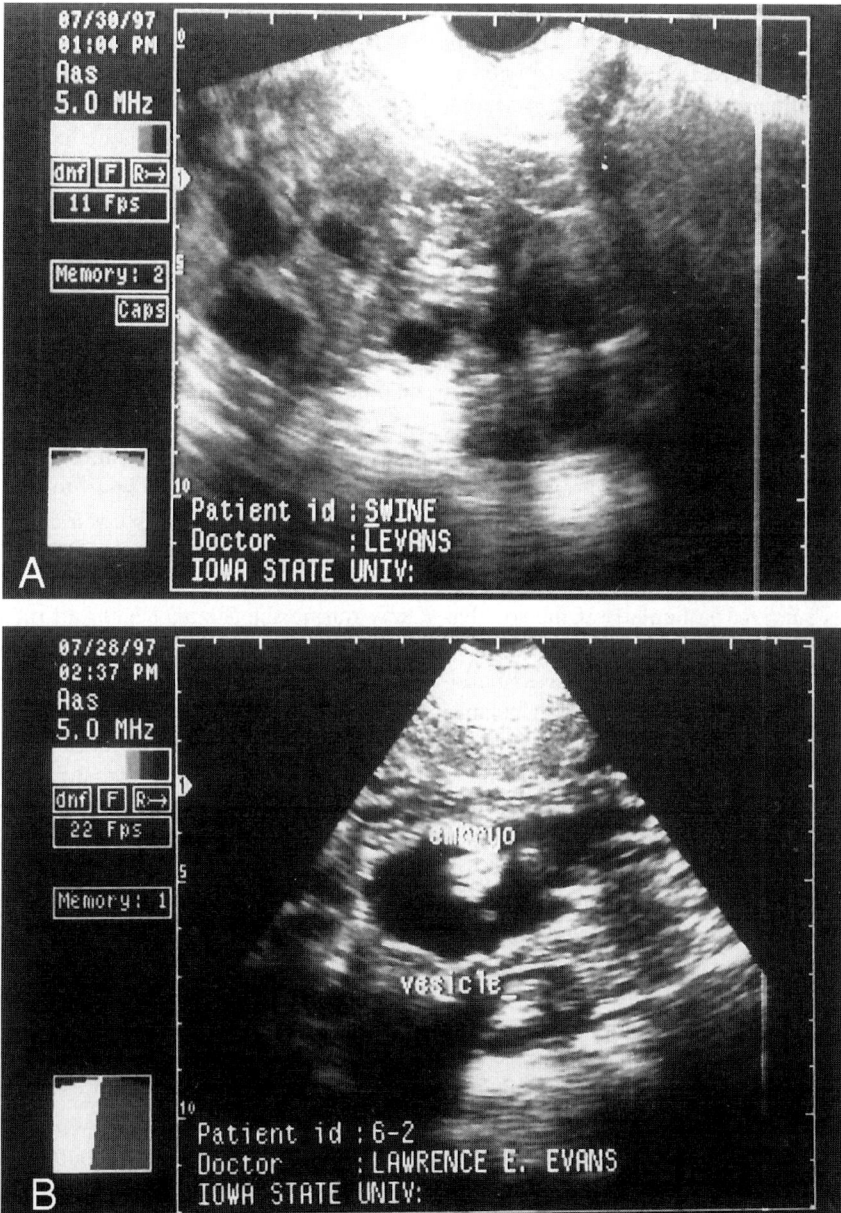

Fig. 15-3. Transabdominal real-time ultrasound images from pregnant sows using a 5.0 MHz Sector probe. Photograph **A** displaying small vesicles is from a sow on day 20 of pregnancy. Photograph **B** is from a sow on day 30 of pregnancy. Note the hypoechogenic fluid (dark vesicle) and echogenic embryo.

greatly extended if the sow is disturbed or dystocia occurs. The interval between pigs may range from a few minutes to 1 or 2 hours but averages about 15 minutes. In most instances, the pig is born with the umbilical cord attached. Pigs born with broken cords are usually in the last one-third of the farrowed litter and have a higher incidence of stillbirths. Pigs may be born head first with the forelegs under the chin or along the chest or rear feet first with the ventral part of the pig passing over the pubis of the sow. The fetal membranes are usually passed out after the delivery of the litter, but placentae may be passed out as the piglets are delivered. Retained fetal membranes are generally not a problem in the sow. When it occurs, this usually indicates retained pigs in the reproductive tract.

The neonatal pig is particularly susceptible to hazards of the environment, and up to one-fourth of the litter is often lost within the first 2 weeks. Newborn pigs require an environmental temperature of 28° to 30°C, which is normally supplied by supplemental heat. Piglets which get colostrum early after birth have the best chance for survival. The newborn pigs receive maternal antibodies via the colostrum. Colostrum also supplies the pig with a high-energy food source, a critical need, since the pig is born with very little energy reserves. Early success in obtaining this energy source often determines which pigs survive, particularly if the sow has fewer functional nipples than the number of pigs born. Cross-fostering is the process of allocating newborn pigs between sows to balance the number of available functional nipples among the litters. Once this maternal bond is established, individual pigs return to the same nipple. Cross-fostering or milk supplementation is necessary to save those smaller, weaker pigs which are in excess of available nipples.

Birth weight is the most important factor favoring survival of the neonate. Hence, good nutrition during late gestation, providing a favorable neonatal environment, and cross fostering of piglets are the major factors for improving neonatal survival.

POSTPARTUM RETURN TO ESTRUS

In order to maximize reproductive efficiency, it is important to minimize the weaning-to-breeding interval in the sow. Under optimum performance, estrus should occur 4 to 10 days after weaning in 85 to 90% of the sows. Return to estrus may be influenced by season, sow parity, nutritional status of the sow, boar exposure, litter size at weaning, duration of lactation, and stressful conditions following weaning.

The most common cause of a delay in the return to estrus after weaning (lactational anestrus) is insufficient dietary intake caused by higher demands of nutrients during lactation. This includes both caloric and protein intake and is particularly evident in sows weaning their first litters. Excessive weight loss during lactation or insufficient weight gain during late pregnancy often results in a post-weaning anestrus. Depressed feed consumption during the Summer months may result in excessive weight loss during lactation. This can be minimized by increasing the percent of fat in the diet to improve energy levels.

The stress associated with grouping sows or withholding feed after weaning will generally lengthen the return-to-estrus interval. Housing sows in small groups and maintaining them on a high energy intake for the first 7 to 10 days after weaning is beneficial. Exposure to a mature boar will also hasten the return to estrus in the weaned sow. Periods of reduced cyclicity in the sow during the Summer and Fall months may prolong the return to estrus in weaned sows. Maintaining adequate nutritional intake during lactation and post-weaning exposure to boars will help to reduce this problem.

The length of lactation also influences the return to estrus interval. Sows with short lactations—less than 16 days—usually require a slightly longer time to resume cyclicity. Weaning a portion of the litter, generally the largest pigs, at least 48 hours before the remaining pigs are weaned may shorten the time from weaning to estrus if delayed return to estrus is a problem in the herd.

OVARY

Since the sow is nonseasonal and polyestrous, the ovaries are cyclically active year-round after puberty. During the luteal and early follicular phases, there are up to 30 small follicles (less than 5 mm) per ovary. About half of these ovulate during estrus, and the others regress to be followed in a few days by a new wave of follicles, even though there are functional corpora lutea present on the ovary. Senescence eventually interrupts this pattern but, under practical farm conditions, the animal is usually slaughtered before senescence is reached. Following ovulation, the follicle collapses, there is slight hemorrhaging into the central cavity,

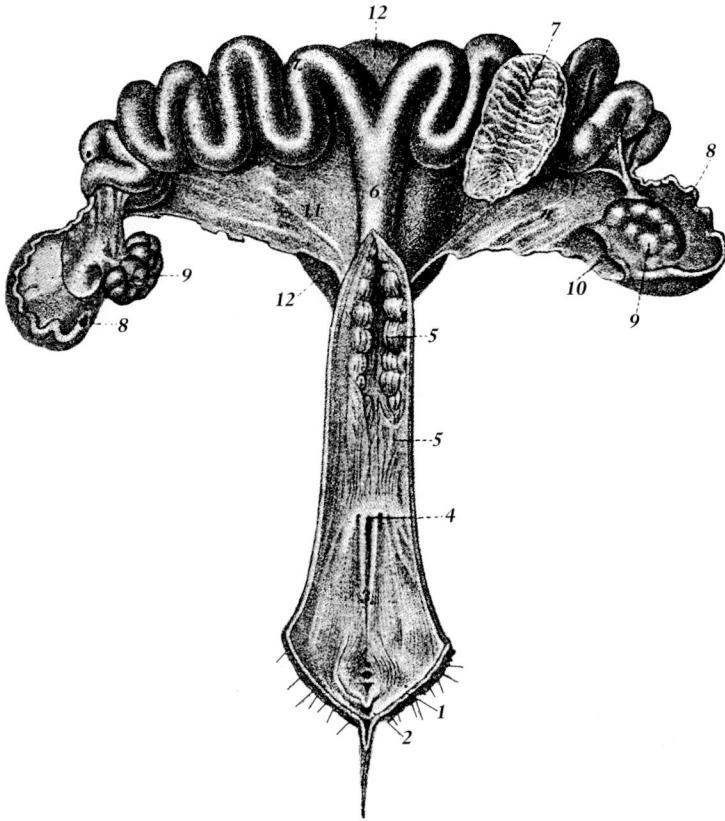

Fig. 15-4. Genital organs of the sow; dorsal view. The vulva, vagina, and cervix uteri are slit open. *1*, labium vulvae; *2*, glans clitoridis; *3*, vulva; *4*, external urethral orifice; *5*, vagina; *5'*, cervix uteri; *6*, corpus uteri; *7*, cornua uteri, one of which is opened at *7'*, to show the folds of mucous membrane; *8*, uterine tube; *8'*, abdominal opening of tube; *9*, ovaries; *10*, ovarian bursa; *11*, broad ligament of uterus; *12*, urinary bladder. (From: R. Getty, et al., Sisson and Grossman's: The Anatomy of Domestic Animals, 5th ed., Philadelphia, PA, W. B. Saunders Co. 2:1302, 1975).

and the granulosa cells begin to proliferate. The development of the corpus luteum is progressive and requires about 1 week for full development. Progesterone production begins to rise soon after ovulation. The corpora lutea are elevated above the surface of the ovary, giving an appearance of a cluster of grapes (see Figs. 9-24 and 15-4). If the sow becomes pregnant, the corpora lutea are maintained throughout pregnancy. If the animal does not become pregnant, irrecoverable luteolysis begins by the 14th day of the estrous cycle. The physiologic factors regulating the maintenance or regression of the corpus luteum are discussed in Chapter 9 (Female Reproductive System). The exterior of the newly formed corpora lutea are pink due to the

high vascularity, and the ovulation point remains visible on the corpus luteum until approximately day 12. By the end of diestrus, when the degenerative changes begin, the corpora lutea become yellowish-brown in color, especially on the cut surface.

The left ovary is more functional than the right ovary in the sow. Most studies indicate that about 55% of the oocytes released are from the left ovary. Intrauterine migration of the embryos before implantation is common. If one ovary of the sow is removed, there will still be a relatively equal distribution of embryos in both horns of the uterus before implantation. Thus, even though the left ovary is more functional than the right ovary, embryos usually distribute in equal numbers within each uterine horn. Bilateral ovariectomy causes abortion at any stage of pregnancy because of the ensuing drop in progesterone levels since the pig placenta does not produce this hormone.

A detailed description of morphologic changes of the sow ovary throughout the estrous cycle is provided in Chapter 9, Figure 9-24.

Estrous synchronization and embryo transfer in sows are discussed in Chapter 19.

OVIDUCTS

The oviduct has a columnar epithelium which reaches its peak height (25 μm) during estrus and then declines to approximately 10 μm near the end of diestrus. The uterotubal junction does not have a true sphincter, but the surrounding mucosa projects in fingerlike folds. These folds become edematous at the end of estrus and restrict the movement of fluids and oocytes through the junction to the uterus. This edema is thought to be caused by high levels of estrogen during estrus. Embryos are retained within the oviduct for 2 to 3 days, reaching the four-cell stage before entering the uterus. It has been suggested that the sow's multiple corpora lutea produce progesterone in sufficient amounts to override the estrogenic activity to reduce the edema and hasten the movement of the oocytes or embryos to the uterus.

UTERUS

Figure 15-4 depicts the macroscopic appearance of the genital organs of the sow. Cyclic changes in the histology and glandular secretions of the uterus of the sow are similar to those in other species. Hemorrhage from the uterus during the cycle, as it occurs in the cow or in the bitch, does not occur in the sow or gilt. As in other species, the endometrial glands secrete "uterine milk" for the nutrition of the developing preimplantation embryos. Because implantation of pig embryos does not occur until 15 to 18 days after conception, there is considerable need for nutrition during the preimplantation period. Myometrial activity is responsible for the spacing of embryos within the uterine horns during early pregnancy.

VAGINA AND VULVA

The vagina of the sow responds to rising levels of estrogens by a thickening of the layer of epithelial cells, hyperemia, congestion, and edema. During estrus, the internal portion of the vulva is congested and moistened by secretions from the vagina and other segments of the tract. Swelling of the vulva is intense and helps to identify those sows which are in estrus. There is an increase in the amount of vaginal mucus and an increase in number of leukocytes in the mucus during late estrus.

ANATOMIC ABNORMALITIES

A study of noninfectious infertility in swine[62] found that nearly half of the sterility of sows and gilts was due to ovarian cysts. The remaining infertility in that survey was primarily due to anatomic defects of the tubular genital tract of the female, especially hydrosalpinx. Unfortunately, little can be done to correct either condition. Therefore, early diagnosis of infertility is important so that affected females can be removed from the breeding herd.

A classification of ovarian cysts in swine is provided in Table 15-2. Figure 15-5 shows anatomic defects, including hydrosalpinx, multiple small and/or large ovarian cysts, and other abnormalities of the reproductive organs of the gilt or sow.

THE MALE

The boar produces fertile ejaculates year-round. Photoperiod or artificial lighting apparently have little effect on production of semen or age of puberty. However, adversely high or low environmental temperatures can result in oligospermic ejaculates and reduced seminal quality.

The limited use of boars may begin soon after puberty. However, intensive use of boars should be restricted until sexual maturity. Boars approaching 1 year of age should not be used for breeding more than once daily or five times per week. Mature boars, 18 months or older, can be used more than once daily if the breedings are spaced. Mature boars will produce 5 to 15 billion spermatozoa per day. An inseminating dose

Table 15-2 Classification of Swine Ovarian Cysts

Type of Cyst	Avg. No. Cysts per Ovary	Size	Effect on Cycle	Cyst Wall	Endometrium	Diagnosis and Treatment
Single or retention cyst (1–2 follicles fail to ovulate).	1–2	Slightly larger than normal follicles.	None: cycle continues normally.	Granulosa normal.	Depends on stage of estrous cycle.	Relatively unimportant and of low incidence. *Does not cause* **infertility**.
Multiple large cysts (see Fig. 15-5F).	5.6	Up to 10 cm.	Infrequent and irregular, intense heats. Prolonged anestrus; can be confused with pregnancy. Ovary contains less estrogen than normal.	Granulosa heavily luteinized, thick. Secretes progesterone.	Progestational type.	Irregular cycle. **Enlarged clitoris** (see Fig. 15-5) (do not confuse with enlarged clitoris of pregnancy). Few sows recover. Treatment useless, cannot clinically distinguish from multiple small cysts. Common cause of infertility.
Multiple small cysts (see Fig. 15-5C).	22.5	Only slightly larger than normal follicles, but more numerous.	Infrequent and irregular heats.	Granulosa normal. Secretes more estrogen than normal.	Estrogen type.	May recover spontaneously. Usually no enlargement of clitoris. No known treatment. Cannot distinguish clinically from cases of multiple large cysts.

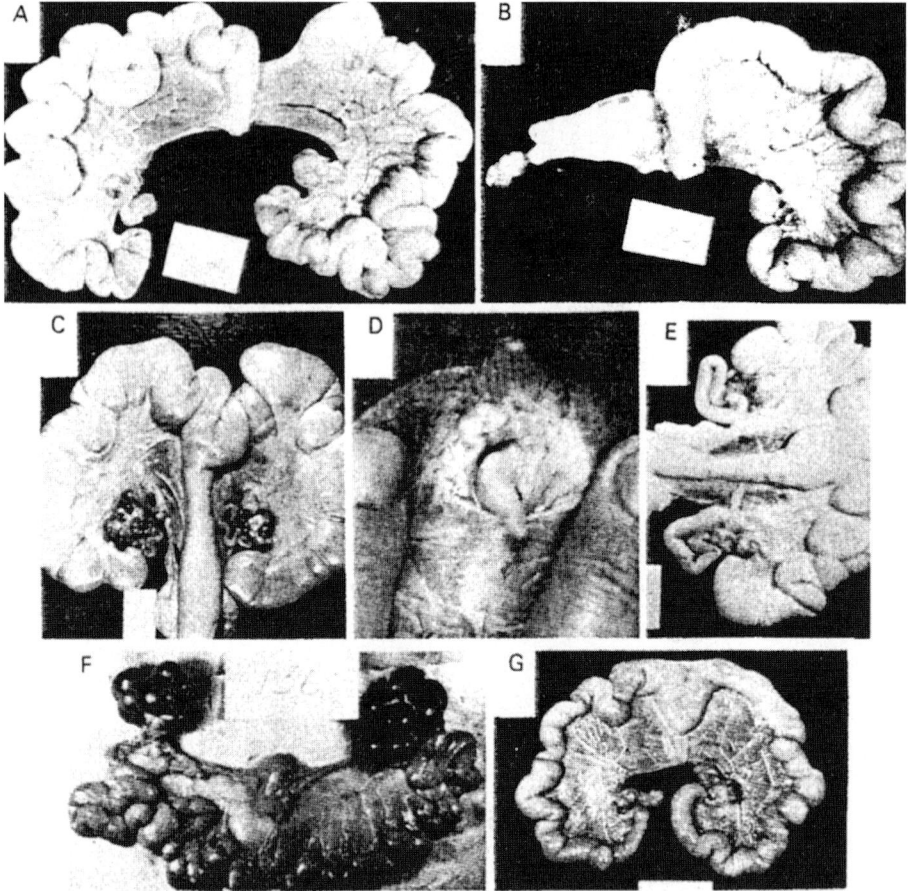

Fig. 15-5. Anatomic abnormalities in swine. **A.** Left uterine horn is 'blind'; right horn is patent. Note distension of blind horn due to to accumulation of fluid. **B.** Right uterine horn is missing, but both ovaries are present. **C.** 'Small' ovarian cysts. Compare with ovaries shown in F. **D.** Greatly enlarged clitoris frequently found in nonpregnant females with cystic ovaries. **E.** Bilateral hydrosalpinx, the most common anatomic cause of sterility in swine. **F.** 'Large' ovarian cysts, the most common physiologic cause of infertility in swine (compare with **C**). **G.** Cervix and vagina down to the vestibule are missing (compare with **C**). Ovaries, uterine body, and horns are normal. (From: A. V. Nalbandov, Fertil. Steril. *3:*100, 1952).

for the gilt or sow should have at least 2 billion spermatozoa.

The volume of ejaculate may vary from 70 to 500 ml. Most of the spermatozoa are released in the second fraction of the ejaculate. The gel fraction is produced by the Cowper's (bulbourethral) glands, while the gel-free fluid is derived primarily from the seminal vesicles and the prostate gland. The seminal vesicles provide most of the protein and fructose in the ejaculate, while the prostatic secretions are high in elec-

trolytes. These secretions enhance spermatozoal motility.

When exposed to a group of females, the boar randomly tests those females which are in close proximity. Sows in proestrus or estrus will actively seek the boar. Females in estrus will respond by standing to the boar's pheromones and smell, vocalization, nuzzling, and attempted mounting. Copulation normally lasts from 3 to 6 minutes. During ejaculation, the tip of the boar's penis is anchored in the cervix, enabling the ejaculate to be forcibly deposited into the uterus of the sow.

A few spermatozoa are present in the oviducts within 30 minutes after copulation, but the majority of the spermatozoa remain in the uterus and undergo capacitation. A small percentage of the capacitated spermatozoa are transported through the uterotubal junction and reach the *ampulla* of the oviduct, where they serve as a spermatozoal reservoir for about 24 hours. If capacitated spermatozoa are present in the oviduct, fertilization occurs within minutes of arrival of the oocytes.

Approximately 75–80% of sows in the United States are bred by artificial insemination (AI) with extended fresh or chilled semen, which may be collected on the farm or shipped to the farm. Use of AI in swine increases the utilization of genetically superior boars and significantly reduces the cost of labor (see Chapter 10, Artificial Insemination).

REFERENCES

1. Almond, G. W. and Richards, R. G. (1991): Endocrine changes associated with cystic ovarian degeneration in sows. J. Am. Vet. Med. Assoc. *199*:883.
2. Almond, G. W. (1992): Factors affecting reproductive performance of the weaned sow. *In:* Swine Reproduction, Vet. Clin. North Am., Large Anim. Pract., edited by R. C. Tubbs and A. D. Leman. Philadelphia, PA, W. B. Saunders Co., p. 503.
3. Althouse, G. C. (1998): Enhancement of Breeding Efficiency. Proc. 29th Annu. Meeting Am. Assoc. Swine Practitioners, March 7–10, 1998, Des Moines, IA, p. 341.
4. Baldwin, D. M. and Stabenfeldt, G. H. (1975): Endocrine changes in the pig during later pregnancy, parturition and lactation. Biol. Reprod. *12*:508.
5. Baltranena, E., Foxcroft, G. R., Aherne, F. X., et al. (1991): Endocrinology of nutritional flushing in gilts. Can. J. Anim. Sci. *71*:1063.
6. Bazer, F. W. (1989): Establishment of pregnancy in sheep and pigs. Reprod. Fertil. Develop. *1*:237.
7. Bazer, F. W. (1992): Mediators of maternal recognition of pregnancy in mammals. Proc. Soc. Exp. Biol. Med. *199*:373.
8. Benjaminson, E. and Karlberg, K.(1981): Postweaning oestrus and luteal function in primiparous and pluriparous sows. Res. Vet. Sci. *30*:318.
9. Bichard, M. and David, P. J. (1986): Producing more pigs per sow per year-genetic contributions. J. Anim. Sci. *63*:1275.
10. Bourn, P., Carlson, R., Lantz, B., et al. (1974): Age at puberty in gilts as influenced by age at boar exposure and transport. J. Anim. Sci. *39*:987.
11. Britt, J. H. (1986): Improving sow productivity through management during gestation, lactation and after weaning. J. Anim. Sci. *63*:1288.
12. Britt, J. H. (1996): Manipulation of porcine estrus cycle. Proc. Soc. Theriogenology Annu. Meeting Swine Symposium, August 15–17, 1996, Kansas City, MO.
13. Britt, J. H., Szarek, V. E., and Levis, D. G. (1983): Characterization of summer infertility of sows in large confinement units. Theriogenology *20*:133.
14. Britt, J. H., Armstrong, J. D., and Cox, N. M. (1985): Control of follicular development during and after lactation in sows. J. Reprod. Fertil. (Suppl. 33):37.
15. Britt, J. H., Day, B. N., and Webel, S. K. (1989): Induction of fertile estrus in prepuberal gilts by treatment with a combination of pregnant mare's serum gonadotropin and human chorionic gonadotropin (P. G. 600™). J. Anim. Sci. *67*:1148.
16. Cassar, G., Chapeau, C., and King, G. J. (1994): Effects of increased dietary energy after mating on developmental uniformity and survival of porcine conceptuses. J. Anim. Sci *72*:1320.
17. Caton, J. S., Jesse, G. W., Day, B. N., et al. (1986): The effect of duration of boar exposure on the frequency of gilts reaching first estrus. J. Anim. Sci. *62*:1210.
18. Christenson, R. K. (1981): Influence of confinement and season of the year on puberty and estrous activity of gilts. J. Anim. Sci. *52*:821.
19. Christenson, R. K. (1986): Swine management to increase gilt reproductive efficiency. J. Anim. Sci. *63*:1280.
20. Christenson, R. K. and Ford, J. J. (1979): Puberty and estrus in confinement-reared gilts. J. Anim. Sci. *49*:743.
21. Clark, L. K., Leman, A. D., and Morris, R. (1988): Factors influencing litter size in swine: Parity-one females. J. Am. Vet. Med. Assoc. *192*:187.
22. Claus, R., Schopper, D., Wagner, H. G., et al. (1985): Influence of light and photoperiodicity on pig prolificacy. J. Reprod. Fertil. (Suppl. 33):185.
23. Coffey, M. T. and Britt, J. H. (1993): Enhancement of sow reproductive performance by β-carotene or vitamin A. J. Anim. Sci. *71*:1198.
24. Cole, D. J. A. (1990): Nutritional strategies to optimize reproduction in pigs. J. Reprod. Fertil. (Suppl. 40):67.
25. Cox, N. M., Britt, J. H., Armstrong, J. D., et al. (1983): Effect of feeding fat and altered weaning schedule on rebreeding in primiparous sows. J. Anim. Sci. *56*:21.
26. Cronin, G. M., Hemsworth, P. H., and Winfield, C. G. (1982): Oestrous behaviour in relation to fertility and fecundity of gilts. Anim. Reprod. Sci. *5*:117.
27. Diekman, M. A. and Hoagland, T. A. (1983): Influence of supplemental lighting during periods of increasing or decreasing daylength on the onset of puberty in gilts. J. Anim. Sci. *57*:1235.
28. Dusza, L. and Tilton, J. E. (1990): Role of prolactin in the regulation of ovarian function in pigs. J. Reprod. Fertil. (Suppl. 40):33.
29. Dyck, G. W. (1988): The effect of housing, facilities and boar exposure after weaning on the incidence of postlactational anestrus in primiparous sows. Can. J. Anim. Sci. *68*:983.
30. Dyck, G. W. (1991): The effect of postmating diet on embryonic and fetal survival and litter size in gilts. Can. J. Anim. Sci. *71*:675.

31. Dyck, G. W. and Swierstra, E. E. (1987): Causes of piglet death from birth to weaning. Can. J. Anim. Sci. *67*:643.

32. Dziuk, P. J. (1970): Estimation of the optimum time for insemination of gilts and ewes by double-mating at certain times relative to ovulation. J. Reprod. Fertil. *22*:277.

33. Dziuk, P., Polge, J. C., and Rowson, L. E. (1964): Intrauterine migration and mixing of embryos in swine following egg transfer. J. Anim. Sci. *23:*37.

34. Einarsson, S. and Rojkittikhun, T. (1993): Effects of nutrition on pregnant and lactating sows. J. Reprod. Fertil. (Suppl. 48):229.

35. England, D. C. (1986): Improving sow efficiency by management to enhance opportunity for nutritional intake by neonatal piglets. J. Anim. Sci. *63:*1297.

36. Esbenshade, K. L., Britt, J. H., Armstrong, J. D., et al. (1986): Body condition of sows across parities and relationship to reproductive performance. J. Anim. Sci. *62:*1187.

37. Estill, C. T., Britt, J. H., and Gadsby, J. E. (1993): Repeated administration of prostaglandin F2 alpha during the early luteal phase causes premature luteolysis in the pig. Biol. Reprod. *49*:181.

38. Estill, C. T., Britt, J. H., and Gadsby, J. E. (1995): Does increased PGF2 alpha receptor concentration mediate PGF2 alpha-induced luteolys during early diestrus in the pig? Prostaglandins *49*:25..

39. Faillace, L. S. and Hunter, M. G. (1994): Follicle development and oocyte maturation during the immediate preovulatory period in Meishan and white hybrid gilts. J. Reprod. Fertil. *101*:571.

40. Fenton, F. R., Bazer, F. W., Robinson, O. W., et al. (1970): Effect of quantity of uterus on uterine capacity of gilts. J. Anim. Sci. *31:*104.

41. Friendship, R. (1989): Assessing the optimum weaning age. Compend. Cont. Educ. Pract. Vet. *10*:761.

42. Griffith, M. K. and Minton, J. E. (1992): Effect of light intensity on circadian profiles of melatonin, prolactin, ACTH, and cortisol in pigs. J. Anim. Sci. *70*:492.

43. Henricks, D. M., Guthrie, H. D., and Handlin, D. L. (1972): Plasma estrogen, progesterone and luteinizing hormone levels during the estrous cycle in pigs. Biol. Reprod. *6:*210.

44. Hilley, H. D., Dial, G. D., Hagan, J., et al. (1986): The influence of parity, season of the year, number of matings, and previous lactation length on the number of pigs born alive to multiparous sows. Proc. Int. Congr. Pig Vet. Soc., Barcelona, Spain, July 15th–18th, 1986, p. 24.

45. Hughes, P. E. (1993): The effect of food level during lactation and early gestation on the reproductive performance of mature sows. Anim. Prod. *57*:437.

46. Hunter, R. H. F. (1977): Physiological factors influencing ovulation, fertilization, early embryonic development and establishment of pregnancy in pigs. Br. Vet. J. *133*:461.

47. Jindal, R., Cosgrove, J. R., Aherne, F. X., et al. (1996): Effect of nutrition on embryonal mortality in gilts: Association with progesterone. J. Anim. Sci. *74*:620.

48. Johnston, L. J., Fogwell, R. L., Weldon, W. C., et al. (1989): Relationship between body fat and postweaning interval to estrus in primiparous sows. J. Anim. Sci. *67*:943.

49. King, G. J. (1993): Comparative placentation in ungulates. J. Exp. Zool. *266*:588.

50. Kirkwood, R. N., Mitaru, B. N., Gooneratne, A. D., et al. (1988): The influence of dietary energy intake during successive lactations on sow prolificacy. Can. J. Anim. Sci. *68*:283.

51. Ko, J. C. H., Evans, L. E., and Hopkins, S. M. (1989): Vaginal conductivity as an indicator for optimum breeding time in the sow after weaning. Theriogenology *32*:961.

52. Knox, R. V. and Althouse, G. C. (1999): Visualizing the reproductive tract of the female pig using real-time ultrasonography. Swine Health Prod. *7*:207.

53. Koketsu, Y. (2000): Productivity characteristics of high-performing commercial swine breeding farms. J. Am. Vet. Med. Assoc. *216*:376.

54. Lamberson, W. R., Johnson, R. K., Zimmerman, D. R., et al. (1991): Direct responses to selection for increased litter size, decreased age at puberty, or random selection following selection for ovulation rate in swine. J. Anim. Sci. *69*:3129.

55. Leman, A., Fraser, D., and Greenley, W. (1990): Factor affecting non-productive sow-days. Proc. Int. Congr. Pig Vet. Soc, Lausanne, Switzerland, July 1–5, p. 378.

56. Love, R. J., Evans, G., and Klupiec, C. (1993): Seasonal effects on fertility in gilts and sows. J. Reprod. Fertil. (Suppl. 48):191.

57. Lucia, T., Dial, G. D., and March, W. E. (1999): Estimation of lifetime productivity of female swine. J. Am. Vet. Med. Assoc. *214*:1056.

58. Mahan, D. C. (1994): Effects of dietary vitamin E on sow reproductive performance over a five-parity period. J. Anim. Sci. *72*:2870.

59. Mavrogenis, A. P. and Robison, O. W. (1976): Factors affecting puberty in swine. J. Anim. Sci. *42:*1251.

60. Molokwu, E. C. I. and Wagner, W. C. (1973): Endocrine physiology of the puerperal sow. J. Anim. Sci. *36:*1158.

61. Morbeck, D. E., Esbenshade, K. L., Flowers, W. L., et al. (1992): Kinetics of follicle growth in the prepubertal gilt. Biol. Reprod. *47*:485.

62. Nalbandov, A. V. (1952): Anatomic and endocrinologic causes of sterility in female swine. Fertil. Steril. *3:*100.

63. Napel, J., De Vries, A. G., Buiting, G. A. J., et al. (1995): Genetics of the interval from weaning to estrus in first-litter sows: Distribution of data, direct response of selection and heritability. J. Anim. Sci. *73*:2193.

64. Newton, E. A., Stevenson, J. S., and Davis, D. L. (1987): Influence of duration of litter separation and boar exposure on estrus expression of sows during and after lactation. J. Anim. Sci. *65*:1500.

65. Peacock, A. J., Evans, G., and Love, R. J. (1991): The role of melatonin in seasonal infertility of pig. Adv. Pineal Res. *6*:189.

66. Pearce, G. P. and Pearce, A. N. (1992): Contact with a sow in oestrus or a mature boar stimulates the onset of oestrus in weaned sows. Vet. Rec. *130*:5.

67. Polge, C. (1978): Fertilization in the pig and horse. J. Reprod. Fertil. *54:*461.

68. Rampacek, G. B., Kraeling, R. R., and Kiser, T. E. (1981): Delayed puberty in gilts in total confinement. Theriogenology *15:*491.

69. Reese, D. E., Peo, E. R., and Lewis, A. J. (1984): Relationship of lactation energy intake and occurrence of

postweaning estrus to body and backfat composition in sows. J. Anim. Sci. *58*:1236.

70. Robertson, H. A. and King, G. J. (1974): Plasma concentrations of progesterone, oestrone, oestradiol-17-β and oestrone sulphate in the pig at implantation, during pregnancy, and at parturition. J. Reprod. Fertil. *40:*133.

71. Rodgers, J. B., Sherwood, L. C., Fink, B. F., et al. (1993): Estrus detection by using vaginal cytologic examination in miniature swine. Lab. Anim. Sci. *43*:597.

72. Roseboom, D. W., Pettigrew, J. E., Moser, R. L., et al. (1996): Influence of gilt age and body composition at first breeding on sow reproductive performance and longevity. J. Anim. Sci. *74*:138.

73. Schmidt, W. E., Stevenson, J. S., and Davis, D. L. (1985): Reproductive traits of sows penned individually or in groups until 35 days after breeding. J. Anim. Sci. *60*:755.

74. Sesti, L. A. C. and Britt, J. H. (1993): Relationship of secretion of GnRH *in vitro* to changes in pituitary concentrations of LH and FSH and serum concentrations of LH during lactation in sows. J. Reprod. Fertil. *98*:393.

75. Shurson, G. C., Hogberg, M. G., DeFever, N., et al. (1986): Effects of adding fat to the sow lactation diet on lactation and rebreeding performance. J. Anim. Sci. *62*:672.

76. Stevenson, J. S., Cox, N. M., and Britt, J. H. (1981): Role of the ovary in controlling luteinizing hormone, follicle-stimulating hormone, and prolactin secretion during and after lactation in pigs. Biol. Reprod. *24:*341.

77. Stevenson, J. S., Pollmann, D. S., Davis, D. L., et al. (1983): Influence of supplemental light on sow performance during and after lactation. J. Anim. Sci. *56:*1282.

78. Svajgr, A. J., Hays, V. W., Cromwell, G. L., et al. (1974): Effect of lactation duration on reproductive performance of sows. J. Anim. Sci. *38*:100.

79. Szenci, O., Fekete, C., and Merics, I. (1992): Early pregnancy diagnosis with battery-operated ultrasonic scanner in sows. Can. Vet. J. 33:340.

80. Thompson, L. H. and Savage, J. S. (1978): Age at puberty and ovulation rate in gilts in confinement as influenced by exposure to a boar. J. Anim. Sci. *47:*1141.

81. Tokach, M. D., Richert, B. T., Goodband, R. D., et al. (1996): Amino acid requirements for lactating sows: New developments. Compend. Cont. Educ. Pract. Vet. *18* (Suppl.):127.

82. Tompkins, E. C., Heidenreich, C. J., and Stob, M. (1967): Effect of post-breeding thermal stress on embryonic mortality in swine. J. Anim. Sci. *26*:377.

83. Walker, N., Watt, D., MacLeod, A. S., et al. (1979): The effect of weaning at 10, 25, or 40 days on the reproductive performance of sows from the first to the fifth parity. J. Agric. Sci. Cambridge, England *92*:449.

84. Walton, J. S. (1986): Effect of boar presence before and after weaning on estrus and ovulation in sows. J. Anim. Sci. *62*:9.

85. Webel, S. K. and Dziuk, P. J. (1971): Pig fetal loss due to uterine space and fetal age. J. Anim. Sci. *33:*1165.

86. Wilson, M. R. and Dewey, C. E. (1993). The associations between weaning-to-estrus interval and sow efficiency. Swine Health Prod. *1*:10.

87. Wise, M. E., Allrich, R. D., Jones, A., et al. (1981): Influence of photoperiod (16L:8D) and size of rearing group (10 vs 30) on age at puberty in confinement-reared gilts. J. Anim. Sci. *53*:104.

88. Zimmerman, D. R. and Kopf, J. D. (1986): Age at puberty in gilts as affected by boar maturity, type of boar exposure and age of gilts when boar exposure is initiated. J. Anim. Sci. *63* (Suppl. 1):355.

References Added in Proof

89. Almeida, F.R.C.L., Novak, S., and Foxcroft, G. R. (2000): The time of ovulation in relation to estrus duration in gilts. Theriogenology *53*:1389.

90. Deaver, D. R. and Bryan, K. A. (1999): Effects of exogenous somatotropin (ST) on gonadal function in ruminants and swine. Domestic Anim. Endocrinol. *17*:287.

91. Hunter, M. G. (2000): Oocyte maturation and ovum quality in pigs. Rev. Reprod. *55*:122.

92. Kawarasaki, T., Matsumoto, K., Murofushi, J. et al. (2000): Sexing of porcine embryos by *in situ* hybridization using chromosome Y and 1-specific DNA probes. Theriogenology *53*:1501.

93. Peltoniemi, O. A., Tast, A., and Love, R. J. (2000): Factors effecting reproduction in the pig: Seasonal effects and restricted feeding of the pregnant gilt and sow. Anim. Reprod. Sci. *60-61*:173.

94. Zou, C.-X. and Yang, Z.-M. (2000): Evaluation on sperm quality of freshly ejaculated boar semen during *in vitro* storage under different temperatures. Theriogenology *53*:1477.

Reproductive Patterns of Dogs*

M. H. PINEDA

16

INTRODUCTION

The pattern of reproduction of the domestic male and female dog is remarkably different in several aspects from those of farm animal species. The female dog, called a bitch, is monoestric because she has only one estrus in each breeding season. This is followed by an extended period of anestrus. During each estrous cycle, the bitch has prolonged follicular and luteal phases compared to those of the cycling species of farm animals. Contrary to farm animal species, the bitch ovulates at the beginning of estrus and, at ovulation, releases primary oocytes. Oogenesis extends for about 2 months after birth, whereas in farm animals, oogenesis is completed to the dictyate stage of meiosis by the time of birth. The lifespan of the corpora lutea of the pregnant bitch is about the same as in the nonpregnant bitch. The uterus of the bitch does not seem to exert a discernible role in the maintenance or regression of the corpora lutea of the cycle. Furthermore, the vagina of the bitch has a dorsal median postcervical fold, which, together with the vaginal wall, contributes to the formation of a pseudocervix.

The male dog, called a dog, releases a large volume of ejaculate with a relatively low concentration of spermatozoa. About 97% of the volume of an ejaculate is contributed by the prostate gland, the only accessory sex gland present in the dog. The dog initiates copulation while the penis is only partially erected. Intromission of the dog's penis into the vagina of the bitch is facilitated by the support of the os penis. Full erection is achieved after intromission has been completed and ejaculation has begun. The dog's penis remains 'locked' in the bitch's vagina during ejaculation.

PUBERTY

Puberty, defined as the age at which the dog releases spermatozoa in his ejaculate or the bitch displays her first overt heat, occurs at 6 to 9 months of age for the male and between 9 to 16 months of age for the bitch. Puberty tends to occur earlier in smaller breeds than in larger breeds, and kenneled dogs tend to reach puberty

*Much information concerned with reproduction in dogs has been presented in Chapter 2 (Pituitary Gland), Chapter 7 (The Biology of Sex), Chapter 8 (Male Reproductive System), Chapter 9 (Female Reproductive System), Chapter 10 (Artificial Insemination), and Chapter 11 (Patterns of Reproduction). The reader is encouraged to refer to these chapters in order to permit conciseness.

later than free-roaming animals. The age of puberty is less predictable in the bitch than in the male dog. Age of puberty is probably influenced more in the bitch than in the dog by nutritional and environmental factors including social interactions with other dogs. Pubertal and maiden bitches often refuse mating, even though in heat, when exposed to young, sexually inexperienced dogs.

Prepubertal dogs respond with erection and coital movements when their penes are stimulated. These prepubertal dogs may ejaculate small volumes of seminal fluid, devoid of spermatozoa, weeks in advance of puberty. The response to penile stimulation is faster and the volume of seminal fluid produced increases as the dog approaches puberty. Some prepubertal dogs which produce azoospermic seminal fluid have significant numbers of spermatozoa in the urine collected by cystocentesis from the bladder after penile stimulation. This suggests that prepupertal dogs may have the capability to release spermatozoa into the urethra at an earlier age than previously anticipated. Once in the urethra, these spermatozoa retrograde into the bladder, probably following the path of least resistance. As the dog approaches puberty, it apparently acquires a more efficient ejaculatory mechanism to propel the spermatozoa through the penile urethra.

BREEDING SEASON

Although many dog breeders believe that there are two breeding seasons per year in the bitch, examination of available records does not substantiate this claim. Instead it appears that, under the controlled environmental conditions to which most pet dogs are now subjected, many of the seasonal breeding characteristics have been lost. Available records from dog colonies indicate that bitches cycle year-round with a higher incidence of estruses occurring in late Winter or early Spring. Table 16-1 shows the number of estruses per year for some breeds of dogs.

American Kennel Club records for Cockers, Setters, Great Danes, and Pekingese indicate an even distribution of periods of heat throughout the year. Kenneled Airedales and Beagles show estrus throughout the year, with a larger fre-

Table 16-1 Number of Estruses per Year in Some Breeds of Dogs[a]

Breed	Mean per Year
Basenji	1.0
Basset Hound	2.0
Beagle	1.5
Boston Terrier	1.5
Cocker Spaniel	2.0
German Shepherd	2.4
Pekingese	1.5
Toy Poodle	1.5

[a]Colony dogs. Compiled from information in: J. H. Sokolowski et al., J. Am. Vet. Med. Assoc. *171:*271, 1977.

quency in late Summer and the fewest periods occurring in the Fall. The Basenji has only one estrus each year, usually in the Fall. The tendency for a single breeding period each year in the Basenji is due to a single recessive gene. Crossing the Basenji with other breeds gives a variable response in the offspring, some with one season and others with two breeding periods. Dogs maintained in colonies show little or no seasonality, whereas a free-roaming dog may retain some seasonality. The household pet that roams may fall between these two extremes. Furthermore, there may be effects caused by latitude and climate similar to those in other domestic species.

LITTER SIZE

Litter size is extremely variable, especially between breeds. Some toy or miniature breeds have litters of 1 to 3 puppies, whereas larger bitches such as the Setters may have litters of 10 to 15 puppies. Considering all breeds, a litter of 5 to 8 puppies is average.

THE ESTROUS CYCLE

The bitch has only one estrous or estrual period in each reproductive cycle whether she is mated to fertile or infertile dogs or not mated at all. The interestrous interval is highly variable between breeds (Table 16-2) among bitches of the same breed, and probably is also influenced by environmental conditions and social interactions. After puberty, bitches cycle every 4 to 12 months. The average interestrous interval is about 7 months. The timing of estrus and onset of heat is determined from the first day of standing for the male and acceptance to mating. The bitch is considered to be in estrus as long as she accepts the male for mating.

Determination of the stages of the estrous cycle is facilitated by the use of vasectomized teaser dogs (Tables 16-3 and 16-4). When teaser dogs are not available, determination of the stages of the cycle, and particularly the timing

of estrus, is more difficult. Observation of the external signs and behavioral responses of the bitch as well as the examination of vaginal smears are acceptable and useful substitutes.

The stages of the estrous cycle of the bitch are associated with recognizable external signs. Figure 16-1 shows the stages and duration of the reproductive cycle of the bitch. The values indicated in Figure 16-1 are for the Beagle bitch, but are reasonably valid for other breeds.

For the bitch, proestrus is the beginning of the period of sexual activity. The onset of proestrus is gradually established in a series of sequential anatomic and behavioral changes induced by gonadotropic stimulation and subsequent follicular development, resulting in estrogenic influences exerted during late anestrus. For practical purposes, however, proestrus is considered to begin when the bitch discharges blood from the vulva. The first day of bloody discharge is generally agreed to represent the first day of proestrus. The blood discharged from the vulva at the time of proestrus is probably of uterine origin, and together with secretion from the uterine glands, is usually first detected and reported as "spotting" by the bitch's owner. As the bitch progresses through proestrus and approaches estrus, the vulva becomes distinctly swollen. During proestrus, the bitch tends to be excitable, restless, and may lose her appetite; water intake is usually increased, and the bitch tends to urinate frequently.

Bitches become attractive to males during proestrus. Pheromones released in the vaginal secretions and urine stimulate and attract males. Bitches in proestrus are inclined to roam and are

Table 16-2 Interestrous Intervals for Some Breeds of Dogs

Breed	Interval in Months
Basset Hound	5.8
Beagle	7.4
Boston Terrier	8.1
Boxer	8.0
Chihuahua	7.2
Cocker Spaniel	6.0
Dachshund	7.0
German Shepherd	5.0
Pekingese	7.7
Scottish Terrier	6.5
Toy Poodle	8.0

Compiled from different sources.

Table 16-3 Criteria to Determine the Length of Proestrus and Estrus in the Bitch with Teaser Dogs

Criteria	Stage of the Cycle
First day of discharge of blood from the vulva	Day 1 of Proestrus
First day of acceptance of the male for mating	Day 1 of Estrus
First day of refusal of the male for mating	Day 1 of Diestrus

Table 16-4 Patterns of Sexual Behavior in the Dog and Bitch

Dog Response	Bitch Response	Stage of the Cycle
Little or no interest for the bitch	Refuses advances of the male; barks or tries to bite	Anestrus
Shows interest and attempts to mount	Refuses male by retreating or hiding (no bloody discharge from vulva)	Late anestrus
Attempts to mount or sustained mounting with pelvic thrusting	Retreats or stands passively. Bloody discharge from the vulva	Proestrus
Sustained thrusting, intromission, and "locking" of the penis	Stands, displays vulva, and deviates tail for mating	Estrus

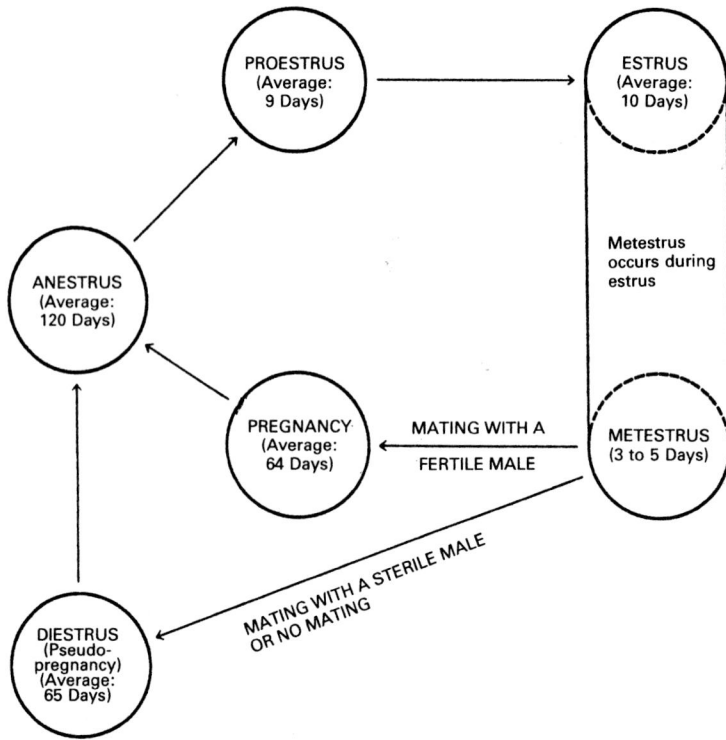

Fig. 16-1. The estrous and reproductive cycle of the bitch.

usually followed by a pack of dogs. During proestrus, the bitch will not accept the male for mating and may even be aggressive to the male. As the bitch approaches estrus, she becomes more receptive, and sexually experienced bitches may passively even allow mounting by the male.

Proestrus extends from the first day of bloody discharge from the vulva to the first day of acceptance of the male for mating; and lasts on the average 9 days but may range from 2 to 15 days.

Estrus, the period of sexual receptivity, is reliably determined by the bitch's acceptance of the male for mating. The bitch is considered to be in estrus when she accepts, stands, and successfully forms a copulatory tie with the male. Estrus lasts an average of 10 days, but may range from 3 to 12 days. The estrous bitch adopts a definite stance for mating, deviates and holds the tail to one side, and exposes the vulva by arching her back. Bitches in estrus actively seek males for mating. Since pheromonal release at this time is maximal, it is not unusual to

observe dogs, attracted from blocks away, in the yard waiting for the bitch. This attractiveness of the bitch to the dogs during late proestrus and estrus is undesirable to pet owners and the public in general because of damage to property and public hazards. Roaming bitches are often followed by a pack of dogs, usually barking, polluting the environment, and fighting. As estrus progresses, the edema of the vulva becomes less noticeable, and the bloody discharge becomes watery and reddish or yellowish in color.

Wild canidae (coyotes, dingoes, and wolves) have only one estrus per year. The estrous cycle is characterized, particularly in the coyote, by an extended proestrus lasting for 2 to 3 months.

Methyl p-hydroxybenzoate, which stimulates the mounting reaction in the male dog, was proposed as a pheromone released from the vagina of the bitch. Recent evidences, however, negate the pheromonal role of this compound.

Olfaction is the main determinant in communication between the canine sexes. Most of the courtship consists of the male seeking the female. Due to the lengthy proestrus and estrus, the period during which the male is attracted to the bitch is prolonged.

Interaction between the male and female during proestrus consists of frequent urination and attention shown toward each other. The male investigates and often licks the anogenital area of the female. The female may exhibit a bowing posture but does not allow mounting. Mounting may be discouraged by moving or by growling.

With the onset of estrus, the female lordoses for the male and allows mounting and intromission. Little courtship is involved during standing estrus, and receptiveness declines during late estrus.

Metestrus is the period of formation of the corpora lutea and beginning of secretion of progesterone. Since the bitch ovulates while in estrus, metestrus occurs in its entirety during the period of estrus. Based on blood levels of progesterone, metestrus lasts from 3 to 5 days and is only of academic interest in the bitch. However, some authors use the term metestrus to designate the stage of the cycle of the bitch that follows estrus and ovulation. In this chapter and throughout the text, metestrus is restricted to the short postovulatory period of corpus luteum development as indicated previously. The term diestrus is used to indicate that period which follows estrus, as applied to the other domestic species.

Diestrus begins with the bitch's refusal to mate and is the stage of the cycle in which the corpora lutea have grown to maximal size and are now fully functional. Toward the end of estrus, some bitches may refuse the male for mating on one day yet accept the male the following day. This is frequently observed in young bitches, particularly when the male is persistent and aggressive. Because of this dichotomous behavior, it is advisable to consider the bitch in diestrus when she refuses to mate on two consecutive days. Diestrus is considered to last for as long as blood levels of progesterone are greater than 1.0 ng/ml. Diestrus lasts an average of 65 days but may range from 55 to 90 days or more. Figures for the length of diestrus given in the literature vary considerably depending on the criteria used to define the end of diestrus. During the initial stages of diestrus, vulvar swelling and vaginal discharge decrease rapidly and the bitch becomes more relaxed as she progresses into diestrus.

If a fertile mating has occurred, pregnancy occupies most of diestrus. Bitches that are not mated or bitches that are mated with a sterile male may occasionally develop a false pregnancy (pseudopregnancy or pseudocyesis). Pseudopregnancy is characterized in some bitches by abdominal swelling, development of the mammary glands with light to full lactation, and profound behavioral changes.

Anestrus is the period of the estrous cycle that follows diestrus. This stage of the cycle in the bitch is characterized as a period of sexual quiescence and has been defined as the period of ovarian inactivity. That definition is no longer tenable since the ovaries of the bitch are quite active and responsive to endogenous gonadotropic stimulation weeks in advance of the next proestrus (see Chapter 9). Anestrus lasts an average of 120 days, but may vary from 40 to 270 days. The duration of anestrus determines the interestrous interval. The time elapsed from one cycle to the next varies considerably within an individual bitch or between bitches of the same breed.

OOGENESIS, OVULATION, AND FERTILIZATION

Oogenesis continues into the postnatal life of the bitch. At birth, the ovary of the pup does not contain primordial follicles, but oogonia are present and "pregranulosa" cells, forming irregularly shaped cords and lobules, are seen in apposition to or around oogonia. Oocytes entering the first meiotic prophase can be seen in the cortical area of the ovary by 5 days after birth, but oogonia continue mitotic divisions up to 14 days after birth. A few primordial follicles appear in the pup's ovary around days 17 to 22 after birth and continue to become more numerous until days 54 to 56 days, when oogenesis appears to be completed to the dictyate stage of meiosis (see Chapter 7 for further details). Polyovular follicles are frequent in young bitches, and their incidence decreases with age. Individual follicles containing up to nine oocytes have been reported. Spontaneous ovulation usually occurs within 5 days after the onset of estrus;

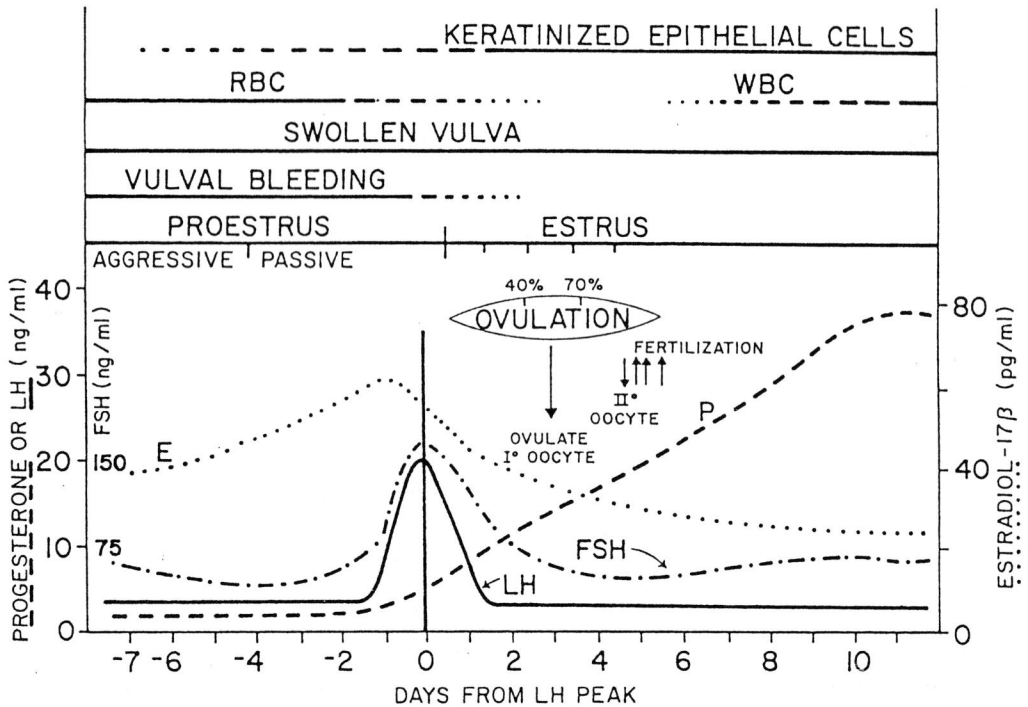

Fig. 16-2. Endocrine, cytological, and behavioral events during proestrus and estrus in the bitch. (**E**=estradiol-17β; **P**=progesterone; **RBC**=red blood cells; **WBC**=white blood cells).

40% of the bitches ovulate within the first 2 days and 70% or more ovulate within 3 days (Fig. 16-2). The bitch is peculiar with respect to farm animals in that she continues to accept the male for mating for several days after ovulation has occurred. Ovulation occurs 40 to 48 hours after the ovulatory surge of luteinizing hormone (LH), and all oocytes are discharged within 24 hours of the first ovulation. Variations reported in the day of ovulation in the bitch appear to be caused by the method used to determine the stage of the cycle. When teaser dogs are used daily to detect the onset and length of estrus, ovulation is remarkably constant and occurs within the first 3 days of standing estrus (Fig. 16-2). A blood level of progesterone higher than 5.0 ng/ml is considered a good indication that the bitch has ovulated.

In the bitch, each oocyte is released from the follicle before the completion of meiosis at the stage of primary oocyte. The release of primary oocytes appears to be a characteristic of canidae such as dogs and foxes. Extrusion of the first polar body and completion of meiosis occur during oviductal transport. In most species, the fertilizability of the oocyte decreases rapidly after ovulation. This is not the case in the bitch, where oocytes are viable for several days and do not become fertilizable until 2 or 3 days after ovulation. In the bitch, conception is possible whether breeding has occurred on the first day of standing estrus or on the last day of estrus. Pregnancy and conception rates are not different when bitches are mated only once, either on the first or on the seventh day of estrus. This prolonged fertilizable period is due to the long, postejaculatory survival of spermatozoa in the vagina and uterus of the bitch and the long survival of the oocytes in the oviducts.

Oviductal transport of unfertilized or fertilized oocytes is prolonged in the bitch. It has been estimated that more than 7 days are needed for the oocytes or embryos to complete oviductal transport and enter the uterus.

The exact timing of pregnancy is difficult in the dog because of the prolonged viability of spermatozoa and oocytes. Spermatozoa retain their viability and probably their fertilizing capability for 11 days within the genital tract of the bitch. The bitch's oocytes appear to require a period of maturation and extrusion of the first polar body in the oviduct before fertilization can actually occur. Thus, variable intervals from breeding to fertilization may contribute much of the variation observed in the length of gestation for the bitch.

ENDOCRINOLOGY OF THE REPRODUCTIVE CYCLE

Figure 16-2 depicts the changes in the blood levels of hormones and the associated changes in the reproductive organs during the follicular and the beginning of the luteal phases of the cycle in the bitch. Table 16-5 provides values for concentration of hormones during the reproductive cycle of the Beagle bitch. These values were compiled from different sources and were obtained using different radioimmunoassay systems. It is important to keep in mind that values for concentrations of hormones in the blood or tissues are greatly dependent on the assay system, the rate of secretion, and metabolic clearance rates for a given hormone as well as other variables. Therefore, the values provided in Table 16-5 are intended to serve only as a reference and should not be used to determine normality or abnormality.

Proestrus and the first days of estrus, prior to ovulation, form the follicular phase of the cycle. Concurrent with the growth and secretory activity of the follicles, levels of estrogens progressively increase from basal to peak levels during the last 2 days of proestrus. Follicle-stimulating hormone (FSH) and LH levels also increase progressively, in a relative synchrony, to reach peak values by the end of proestrus (Fig. 16-2). The changes in concentration of LH in the blood are more pronounced than those of FSH. Follicle-stimulating hormone levels tend to be suppressed during proestrus as compared to FSH levels during late anestrus. Recent evidence indicates that LH is released in a pulsatile fashion from the adenohypophysis of the bitch, whereas FSH release seems to be tonic. During proestrus, LH pulses, in synergy with FSH, stimulate the final maturation of the follicles. Estrogen secretion by the follicles probably

stimulates secretion of inhibin, and then both inhibin and the elevated blood levels of estrogens would feed back to inhibit the release of FSH by the adenohypophysis. The ovulatory surge of LH occurs in most bitches during the last 2 days of proestrus or first 2 days of standing estrus. However, there can be asynchrony between the behavioral responses of the bitch, corresponding with the stages of proestrus and standing estrus, and the ovulatory surge of LH. In some bitches, the ovulatory surge of LH may occur earlier in proestrus or during the first days of estrus. Most bitches ovulate within 48 hours after the ovulatory surge of LH, and LH levels rapidly decline to basal levels after the ovulatory surge.

As the blood levels of estrogens increase, the bitch develops the external signs and responses of the reproductive organs and of the nervous system associated with estrogenic stimulation. These include edema of the vulva, bloody discharge, increased receptivity to the male, and attraction of the male toward the bitch (Fig. 16-2). Toward the end of proestrus, increasing levels of LH promote follicular luteinization, and as a result, there is a progressive increase in the blood levels of progesterone. As the levels of progesterone produced by the luteinized follicles increase, blood levels of estrogens decline. The ovulatory surge of LH and ovulation bring about a further increase in progesterone secretion from the developing corpora lutea (Fig. 16-3). The behavioral transition of the bitch from the proestrous rejection to mating to standing and acceptance of the mating advances of the male is a relatively fast event. This often occurs within a 12- to 24-hour period, although in some bitches the transition may be more gradual.

As compared to farm animal species, the bitch is also peculiar in that behavioral estrus occurs when blood levels of progesterone are rapidly increasing while the levels of estrogens are rapidly declining. Concentration of receptors for progesterone and estradiol in the endometrium follow the same pattern as for concentration of progesterone and estradiol in the blood. In ovariectomized bitches, estrogens alone do not induce a full behavioral estrus. The ovariectomized bitch will respond to treatment with estrogens displaying edema and vulvar discharge of blood. She will become attractive to males but will not display standing estrus, even when estrogens are given in high doses. To induce standing estrus, ovariectomized bitches must be treated with progesterone after treatment with estrogens.

After ovulation, corpora lutea are formed and induced to secrete progesterone under the luteotropic stimulus of LH. The corpora lutea continue to secrete progesterone for 50 to 70 days from ovulation regardless of whether the bitch is pregnant or not (Figs. 16-3 and 16-4). This

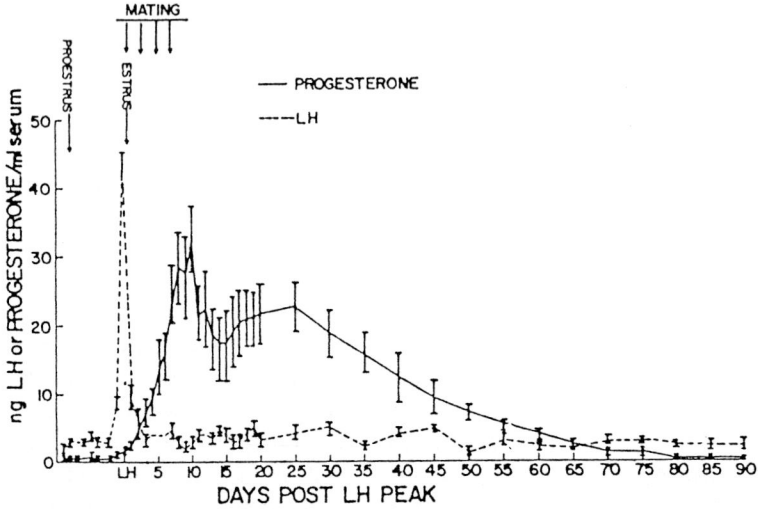

Fig. 16-3. Luteinizing hormone (**LH**) and **progesterone** concentrations in sterile-mated Beagles throughout the periods of proestrus, estrus, and diestrus. Vertical bars represent the standard error of the mean. **Mating** indicates the period of acceptance of the male for mating. (From: M. S. Smith and L. E. McDonald, Endocrinology *94*:404, 1974).

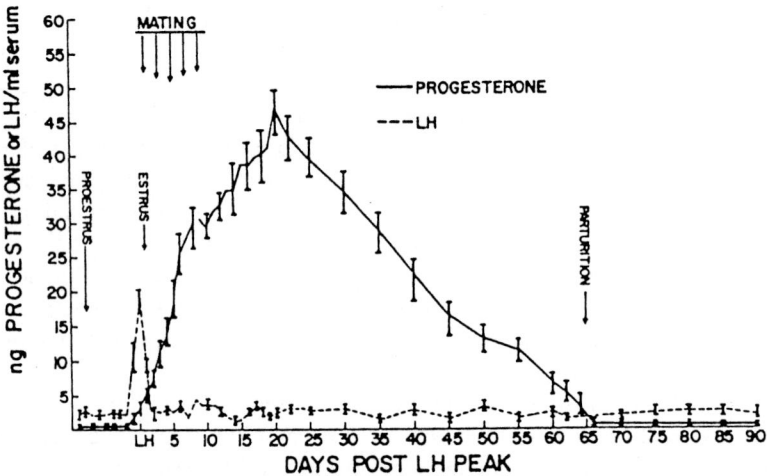

Fig. 16-4. Luteinizing hormone (**LH**) and **progesterone** concentrations during pregnancy in Beagles. Vertical bars represent the standard error of the mean. (From: M. S. Smith and L. E. McDonald, Endocrinology *94*:404, 1974).

peculiarity of the corpora lutea of the bitch will be discussed later in this chapter.

The luteal phase of the cycle includes the postovulatory, metestrual formative stage of the corpora lutea and the diestrual stage of the cycle. Based on the blood levels of progesterone, the duration of the luteal phase of the cycle in the nonpregnant bitch is variable. Progesterone declines to basal levels of 1.0 ng/ml or less by 70 to 80 days after the ovulatory LH surge (Fig. 16-3). If the bitch has undergone an intense pseudopregnant reaction including mammary gland development and secretion, this period may extend beyond 80 days. In the pregnant bitch, however, progesterone levels decrease rapidly at parturition and become undetectable by the day after parturition (Fig. 16-4).

Prolactin levels in the bitch remain relatively constant throughout the follicular and luteal phases of the cycle. The major role of prolactin is expressed during pregnancy or pseudopregnancy by forming the luteotropic complex with LH. The severity of several of the undesirable and overt manifestations of pseudopregnancy of the bitch, such as mammary gland secretion, can be controlled with bromocriptine (2-bromo-α-ergocryptine), a dopamine agonist, which selectively reduces prolactin secretion.

The endocrinology of anestrus in the bitch remained unexplored until recently. Researchers from Colorado State University demonstrated that neither the canine ovary nor the gonadotropic activity of the pituitary gland are quiescent during the last months of anestrus (Table 16-5). Mean concentrations of FSH were higher during the last month of anestrus than during proestrus. During this period, there were sporadic but significant increases in mean serum concentrations of LH. The mean concentration of prolactin also was elevated and variable during late anestrus, but no specific pattern could be detected. Estradiol-17β reached levels up to 46 pg/ml during late anestrus (Table 16-5), indicating that ovarian follicles developed and responded to gonadotropic stimulation. Progesterone levels, however, remained below 1.0 ng/ml of serum (Table 16-5). Even though it has not been determined whether similar adenohypophysial-ovarian responses occur throughout the duration of anestrus in the bitch, the long-held view that the ovary of the bitch is inactive during anestrus is no longer tenable. However, despite gonadotropic activity and estradiol secretion by the ovarian follicles during late anestrus, the bitch remains in a quiescent reproductive stage during this period. The external signs and vaginal smears are those typical for

Table 16-5   Hormonal Levels in the Blood of the Beagle Bitch

Reproductive Stage	LH (ng/ml)	FSH (ng/ml)	Prolactin (ng/ml)	Progesterone (ng/ml)	Estradiol-17β (pg/ml)
Proestrus	2.8 ± 0.1	59 ± 9	27	1.7 ± 0.3	58 ± 7
Estrus	36 ± 10	168 ± 37 297[a]	32	< 2.0	69 ± 11
Metestrus	---	69 ± 15	20	24 ± 3[a]	18 ± 3
Diestrus	4.2 ± 1.1	108 ± 19	20 to 35	18 ± 6	23 ± 7
Pregnancy	3.0 ± 0.2	197 ± 21 255 ± 28[a]	57 ± 14[b]	15 ± 10 3.8 ± 2.4[b] 1.2 ± 0.4[c]	19 ± 2
Anestrus	2.8 ± 0.3	---	---	0.6 ± 0.1	33 ± 15
Late anestrus	21 to 156	240 to 294	1.95 to 33.15	< 1.0	20 to 46

Data are mean ± standard deviation.
[a]Peak values.
[b]Days 55–58 of pregnancy.
[c]At parturition.
Compiled from different sources, including: T. M. Nett et al., Proc. Soc. Exp. Biol. Med. *148:*134, 1975; P. N. Olson et al., Biol. Reprod. *27:*1196, 1982; T. J. Reimers et al., Biol. Reprod., *19:*673, 1978.

Table 16-6   Concentration of Testosterone (pg/ml) in the Serum of Bitches

Stage of the Cycle		
Anestrus	Proestrus	At the Time of the Preovulatory Surge of LH
< 150	239 ± 113[a]	56 ± 225[a]

[a]Mean ± SEM.
Adapted from: P. N. Olson et al., Am. J. Vet. Res. *45*:145, 1984.

anestrus and thus were thought to represent inactive ovaries. The mechanisms by which the reproductive organs and the nervous system of the anestrous bitch fail to respond to the estrogenic stimulation, causing the bitch to fail to show estrous behavioral responses, have not been determined. During late anestrus, the blood progesterone remains below basal levels. Therefore, it is possible that follicles that develop during late anestrus are unable to luteinize and secrete progesterone. Because progesterone is needed for full expression of estrous behavior in the bitch, the low levels of progesterone may explain the absence of behavioral signs during anestrus.

The bitch has relatively high levels of testosterone in serum collected during late anestrus, proestrus, or early estrus. Blood levels of testosterone increase significantly during proestrus and decrease rapidly after the ovulatory surge of LH (Table 16-6). During diestrus, levels of testosterone remain at basal levels. The physiologic significance of these relatively high blood levels of testosterone in the bitch has not been determined. However, because the levels of testosterone are highest at the onset of estrus, this hormone may contribute to the libido and behavioral responses of the estrous bitch.

CORPORA LUTEA OF THE BITCH

The corpora lutea (CL) of the bitch and those of most of the farm animal species are chronically dependent on a pituitary luteotropic complex for maintenance and secretion. However, the concentration of receptors for LH in the canine corpora lutea remains relatively low and constant during most of diestrus, to then in-

crease after day 57 and remain constant thereafter until day 80 after estrus. Of this luteotropic complex, LH seems to play the major role, probably in synergy with prolactin. In bitches hypophysectomized on days 10 through 50 of the luteal phase of the cycle, progesterone secretion is rapidly impaired and ceases 3 to 17 days following hypophysectomy. Similarly, active immunization against LH or administration of antiserum containing antibodies which neutralize the biological activity of LH induces regression of the CL or severely impairs progesterone secretion by the bitch's corpora lutea. Prolactin also appears to be part of the luteotropic complex and is necessary for luteal maintenance and secretion. Treatment of diestrous bitches with bromocriptine or other dopamine agonists selectively reduces prolactin levels in the blood and causes an equally rapid decline in blood levels of progesterone.

The nonpregnant uterus does not appear to play any significant luteolytic role in the bitch. Either the nonpregnant uterus of the bitch does not produce luteolytic factors or the transfer of these factors from the uterus to the ovary does not occur. This could be due to the anatomic independence between the vein draining the bitch's uterus and the artery supplying the ovary. Recent studies on the effects of hysterectomy during diestrus in bitches indicate that neither the pregnant nor the nonpregnant uterus is an essential component of the regulatory mechanisms participating in luteal maintenance, secretion, and demise. During diestrus, blood levels of progesterone are not significantly different between nonpregnant and pregnant bitches. Blood levels of progesterone decline rapidly at parturition, whereas in the nonpregnant bitch, they persist at basal levels for extended periods. This suggests that the corpora lutea of the nonpregnant bitch are either resistant to luteolytic factors or simply that luteolytic factors are lacking and that the corpora lutea undergo retrogressive changes at the end of diestrus caused by their aging.

Exogenous prostaglandin $F_{2\alpha}$ or synthetic prostaglandin analogs can induce irreversible luteal regression during certain periods of diestrus or pregnancy in the bitch when given in a single high dose or in lower, but repeated, doses. The effective single dose of prostaglandin to cause irreversible luteolysis in the bitch approaches toxic levels. A lower single dose causes only a transient decline in the blood levels of progesterone. In addition, the corpora lutea of nonpregnant bitches are more sensitive to the luteolytic activity of exogenous prostaglandin $F_{2\alpha}$ after day 30 of diestrus than earlier in diestrus. Similarly, the corpora lutea of the pregnant bitch are more sensitive to exogenous prostaglandin $F_{2\alpha}$ in the second half of pregnancy. Several treatments with $PGF_{2\alpha}$ after day 30 of pregnancy cause a dramatic decrease in blood levels of progesterone, and abortion usually occurs 4 to 5 days after treatment.

VAGINAL CYTOLOGY

The vaginal smear can be a fairly good indicator of the stage of the estrous cycle in the bitch, particularly if a sequential series of daily smears are obtained. The smear represents secretions and cells from the uterus, cervix, and vagina. A smear that is quickly air dried and stained by the Giemsa technique is usually satisfactory for cytological examination. Table 16-7 summarizes the clinical signs, hormonal levels, and cytological changes in the vaginal smear of the bitch which are associated with the different stages of the cycle. Figure 16-5 shows the cellular changes observable in vaginal smears obtained during the phases of anestrus, proestrus, estrus, and diestrus. The anestrous smear con-

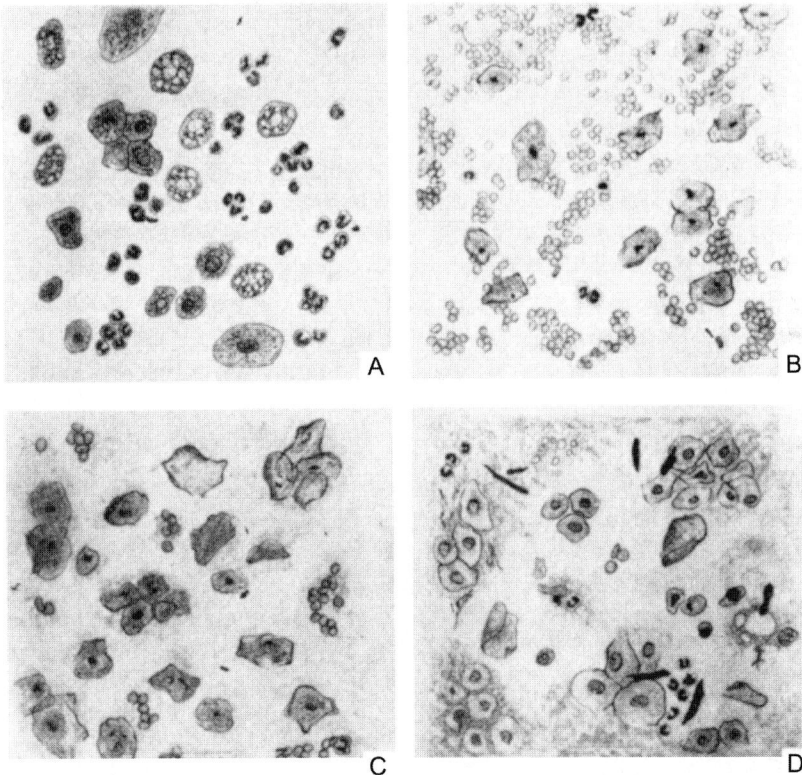

Fig. 16-5. Vaginal smears. **A.** Anestrus. Epithelial cells with cytoplasmic granules or vacuoles ("foam-cells") and varying numbers of the polymorphonuclear leukocytes. **B.** Proestrus. Erythrocytes are numerous. Cornified epithelial cells with pyknotic nuclei. Leukocytes are sparse. **C.** Estrus. Large number of cornified epithelial cells ("flakes"). Moderate number of erythrocytes. **D.** Diestrus. Epithelial elements varying in both size and staining characteristics, "boat-cells", leukocytes, and detritus. (From: H. H. Cole and P. T. Cupps, Reproduction in Domestic Animals. New York, NY, Academic Press, Inc., 1959).

Table 16-7   Clinical Signs, Vaginal Cytology, and Hormonal Levels in the Blood During the Estrous Cycle of the Bitch

Observation	Proestrus (Mean = 9 days; Range = 2–15 days)	Estrus (Mean = 10 days; Range = 3–12 days)	Diestrus (Mean = 65 days; Range = 55–90 days)	Anestrus (Mean = 120 days; Range = 40–270 days)
Clinical Signs	Enlargement of the vulva and bloody discharge; male is attracted to the bitch in late proestrus but is not accepted for mating.	Vulva is enlarged and swollen; reduced vaginal discharge; male is accepted for mating.	Refusal to mate; pregnancy or pseudo-pregnancy.	Sexual quiescence.
Vaginal Cytology	Number of cornified cells increases; numerous red blood cells but few leukocytes.	Mostly cornified cells.	Abrupt change from superficial to basal cells; number of leukocytes increases.	Foam cells; number of leukocytes is variable.
Hormonal Levels in Blood	Estrogens rise and peak; LH and FSH rise and may peak; slight rise in progesterone; testosterone increases to peak levels.	Estrogens decrease; progesterone rises; LH and FSH peak and decrease rapidly; testosterone decreases.	Progesterone peaks and decreases by the end of diestrus; LH declines to basal levels; FSH declines in non-pregnant bitches and increases in pregnant bitches. Testosterone remains at basal levels.	Late anestrus: LH, FSH, estrogens, and testosterone increase. Progesterone remains below basal levels.

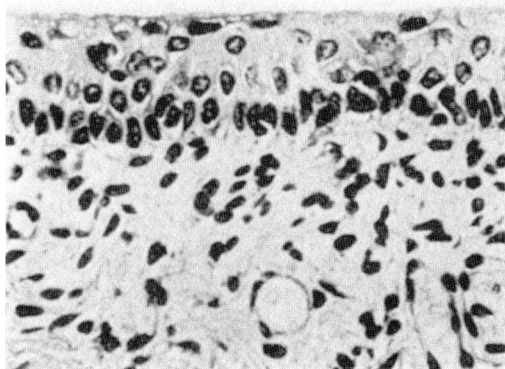

Fig. 16-6. The vaginal epithelium of the bitch at anestrus. The epithelium is low, tending toward a simple columnar type. (Reproduced by permission from: H. M. Evans and H. H. Cole, An Introduction to the Study of the Oestrous Cycle in the Dog, Memoirs of the University of California. Univ. California Press, Berkeley, CA, Vol. 9, No. 2, 1931).

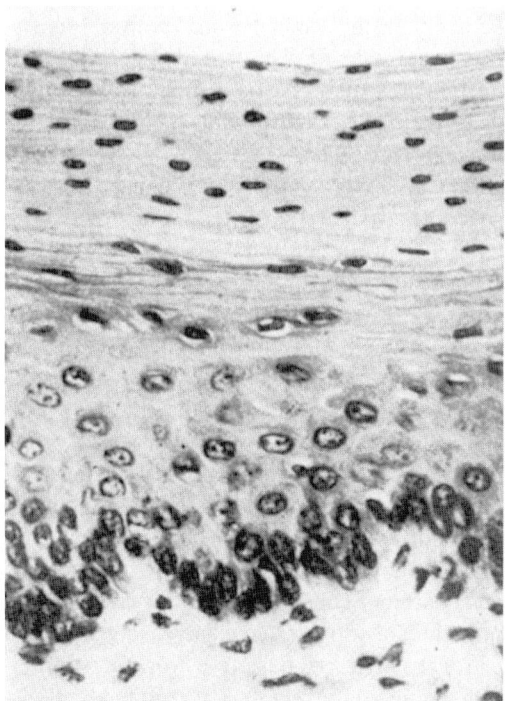

Fig. 16-7. The vaginal epithelium of the bitch at the beginning of proestrus shows the thickening and cornification of the surface layers. (Reproduced by permission from: H. M. Evans and H. H. Cole, An Introduction to the Study of the Oestrous Cycle in the Dog, Memoirs of the University of California. Univ. California Press, Berkeley, CA, Vol. 9, No. 2, 1931).

sists mainly of exfoliated epithelial cells and leukocytes (Fig. 16-5A). Red blood cells and cornified epithelial cells appear in vaginal smears early in proestrus. By the end of proestrus, large cornified epithelial cells are present (Fig. 16-5B), and most of the bleeding has ceased. Smears of mucus from the anterior vagina crystallize in a characteristic fern pattern like the cervical mucus of cows or humans. The ferning crystallization is more intense when the blood concentration of estrogens is at its peak. During estrus, the smear consists almost completely of keratinized superficial cells with pyknotic nuclei or anuclear cells. There are few erythrocytes (Fig. 16-5C). Toward the end of estrus, a few leukocytes begin to appear in the smear, and their number increases 2 or 3 days after the end of estrus (Fig. 16-5D).

The epithelial lining of the vagina during anestrus is only two or three layers thick (Fig. 16-6), but by the beginning of proestrus, it becomes stratified and increases to six to eight layers (Fig. 16-7). During proestrus, growth of the vaginal epithelium continues, and by the time estrus occurs, the epithelial lining may contain 12 to 20 cell layers. Desquamation of the epithelium begins by late estrus.

OVARY, OVIDUCTS, UTERUS, AND VAGINA

The ovary of the bitch is encapsulated by the bursa ovarica that has a ventrally located bursal slit. The ovary can be visualized through the slit during estrus using an endoscope. During anestrus, the bursal slit becomes closed. The ovaries of the newborn bitch contain an estimated 700,000 oocytes. This number of oocytes declines to 250,000 at puberty, 33,000 at 5 years of age, and only 500 remain by 10 years of age. Obviously, most of these follicles undergo atresia at different stages of follicular development, and the oocytes degenerate. After puberty, a wave of follicles develops with each estrus. Many follicles reach about 6 mm in diameter, but not all are destined to ovulate.

Canine oocytes are 90 to 110 μm in diameter. At ovulation, they are released from each follicle as a primary oocyte while the oocyte is at the dictyate stage of meiosis. The cytoplasm of the canine oocyte is rich in lipids, and the oocytes are opaque in appearance. Studies on the *in vitro* fertilization of canine oocytes indicate that dog spermatozoa require capacitation to penetrate the zona pellucida and fertilize the oocyte.

After ovulation, the granulosa luteal cells develop rapidly, and corpora lutea become functional before the end of estrus. Progesterone secretion by the corpora lutea throughout pregnancy is necessary for pregnancy maintenance in the bitch. Bilateral ovariectomy prior to day 56 of gestation is followed by abortion, indicating that the ovaries are the sole source of progesterone during most of pregnancy in the bitch. Pregnancy can be maintained in bilaterally ovariectomized bitches by daily administrations of progesterone.

The ovaries and uterus are attached to the dorsal abdominal wall by the broad ligaments,

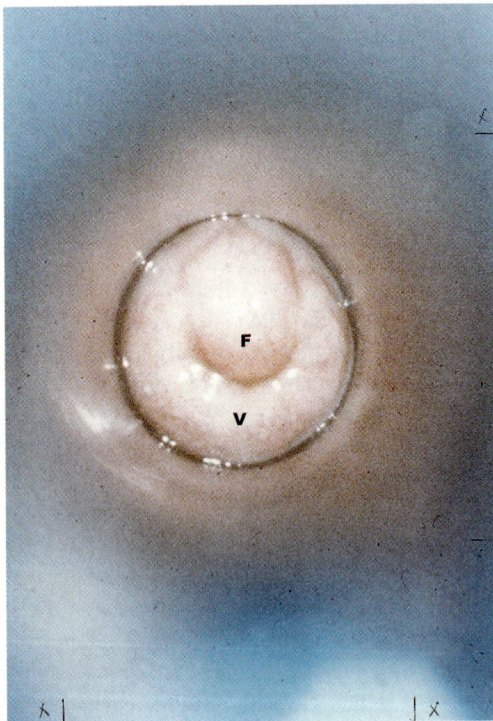

Fig. 16-8. Endoscopic view of the canine anterior vagina showing the pseudocervix (also called para-cervix) of the bitch, which simulates the external os of the cervix. **F**-dorsal medial cervical fold; **V**-vaginal wall. Readers interested in the pseudocervix of the bitch are addressed to references No. 120 and 156 for this chapter.

and the ovaries are attached to the dorsal aspects of the diaphragm by suspensory ligaments. They are attached to the anterior portion of the uterine horns by the proper ligament of the ovary. These attachments make it difficult to exteriorize the ovaries, oviducts, and anterior portion of the uterine horns at laparotomy. The infundibulum of the oviduct is attached to the bursa ovarica. The oviduct follows a convoluted course and encircles the ovary before reaching the uterine horn. The bicornuate uterus of the bitch is long and highly responsive to estrogenic and progestational stimulation. The cervix of the bitch is pendulous and the cervical canal is oblique in a dorsoventral direction, with the external os in close apposition to the ventral area of the vaginal fornix. The vagina of the bitch is bottle-shaped with the narrow end directed rostrally, and it has numerous folds or rugae in its mucosa. The vagina of the bitch contains a dorsal-medial postcervical fold,[156] which, together with the vaginal wall, forms a pseudocervix (Fig. 16-8). This pseudocervix is often mistaken as the cervix and cannulated as if it were the true cervix. In fact, the cervix of the bitch is difficult to visualize by vaginoscopy and generally is very difficult to cannulate unless specially designed catheters and endoscopic equipment are used. When the cervix is palpated transabdominally or observed during laparotomy, the anterior vagina, cervix, and pseudocervix of the bitch form a firm, long, cord-like, cylindrical structure. This structure is often mistaken to represent, as a unit, the external correspondent to the cervix of the bitch.

During anestrus and early proestrus, the adult bitch has a cuboidal epithelium and no cilia in the oviducts. The basal cells of the oviductal epithelium undergo differentiation into ciliated and secretory cells during proestrus, under the influence of progressively increasing levels of estrogens. The response to estrogenic stimulation is rapid; ciliogenesis and secretory cell differentiation can be observed in puppies within 3 days after treatment with exogenous estrogens. With the onset of proestrus, the endometrium responds rapidly to the rising levels of estrogen by becoming edematous, hyperemic, and hyperplastic. Consequently, the rapid development of the vascular system leads to the loss of blood into the uterine lumen by diapedesis. The uterine glands continue to develop, and serous secretion continues. As estrogen declines and progesterone rises, vaginal cornification decreases, noncornified cells reappear, and neutrophils are able to cross the epithelial lining.

The uterine response of the bitch to progesterone during pregnancy or pseudopregnancy is similar to that of other species, but it is more prolonged and exaggerated. The uterus of the bitch is particularly susceptible to both steroid hormones, progestagens and estrogens. Many steroids that have powerful progestagenic activity in the bitch are found to be weak progestagens in other species, and several estrogens that have relatively weak estrogenic activities in other species are powerful bone marrow depressors in the bitch. Exogenous progestagens in general, particularly when given for extended periods, induce hyperplasia of the endometrium in the bitch. This endometrial response is frequently conducive to a pathologic condition termed cystic hyperplasia or cystic hyperplastic complex of the endometrium. This complex is characterized by intense endometrial gland development and mucus secretion, which may develop first into mucometra and then into pyometra. The incidence of hyperplastic reaction increases and tends to become the cystic hyperplastic complex when the bitch has been primed with estrogens prior to the administration of progestagens. In addition to this undesirable endometrial reaction, progestagens stimulate mammary gland development, which in time tends to become nodular and often malignant.

Prolonged treatment with progestagens can induce electrolyte disturbances, affect water retention, and alter carbohydrate metabolism, promoting diabetogenic responses in bitches due to an associated increased pituitary secretion and release of growth hormone.

Myometrial reaction is pronounced, and a characteristic dose-dependent response, termed 'corkscrew', develops in bitches upon treatment with progestagens. The uterus normally enlarges (Fig. 16-9) and folds under the influence of progesterone. The reaction is more exagger-

ated when large doses of progesterone or progestagens are given and the uterine horns coil along their longitudinal axis, giving the 'corkscrew' appearance.

In addition to the myelotoxic, bone marrow-depressant activity of estrogens in dogs, treatment with estrogens frequently leads to a severe and often fatal aplastic anemia. Exogenous estrogens also induce proestrous signs in the bitch including hyperemia of the genital tract and bloody discharge from the vulva. However, estrogens alone do not induce estrous and standing behavior in bitches. Large doses and extended treatments with estrogens are associated with mammary gland hyperplasia, which can result in benign or malignant tumors in the bitch.

PSEUDOPREGNANCY

Pseudopregnancy, false pregnancy, or pseudocyesis can be defined as an exaggerated diestrous response of the bitch. Pseudopregnancy is a condition of considerable clinical importance and appears related to the extreme sensitivity of the canine endometrium and mammary gland to progesterone in synergy with other hormonal factors including prolactin. As previously discussed, the corpora lutea of the nonpregnant bitch remain functional for an extended period after ovulation. Development of the uterus is similar to that in early pregnancy in spite of the fact that no embryos are present in the uterus (Fig. 16-9). The uterus enlarges, and the abdomen may actually become relaxed. In most cases, diestrous bitches do not display external signs of pregnancy, and the progesterone-related enlargement of the uterus goes undetected. On occasion, however, the nonmated or the sterile-mated bitch develops a series of behavioral responses and external signs of pregnancy which has been termed 'overt pseudopregnancy'.

In overt pseudopregnancy, the mammary glands begin to develop in preparation for lactation. In addition, there is a relaxation of the pelvis and external genitalia similar to that during pregnancy. A maternal attitude develops toward her environment and associates. Pseudopregnancy often lasts as long as or longer than a

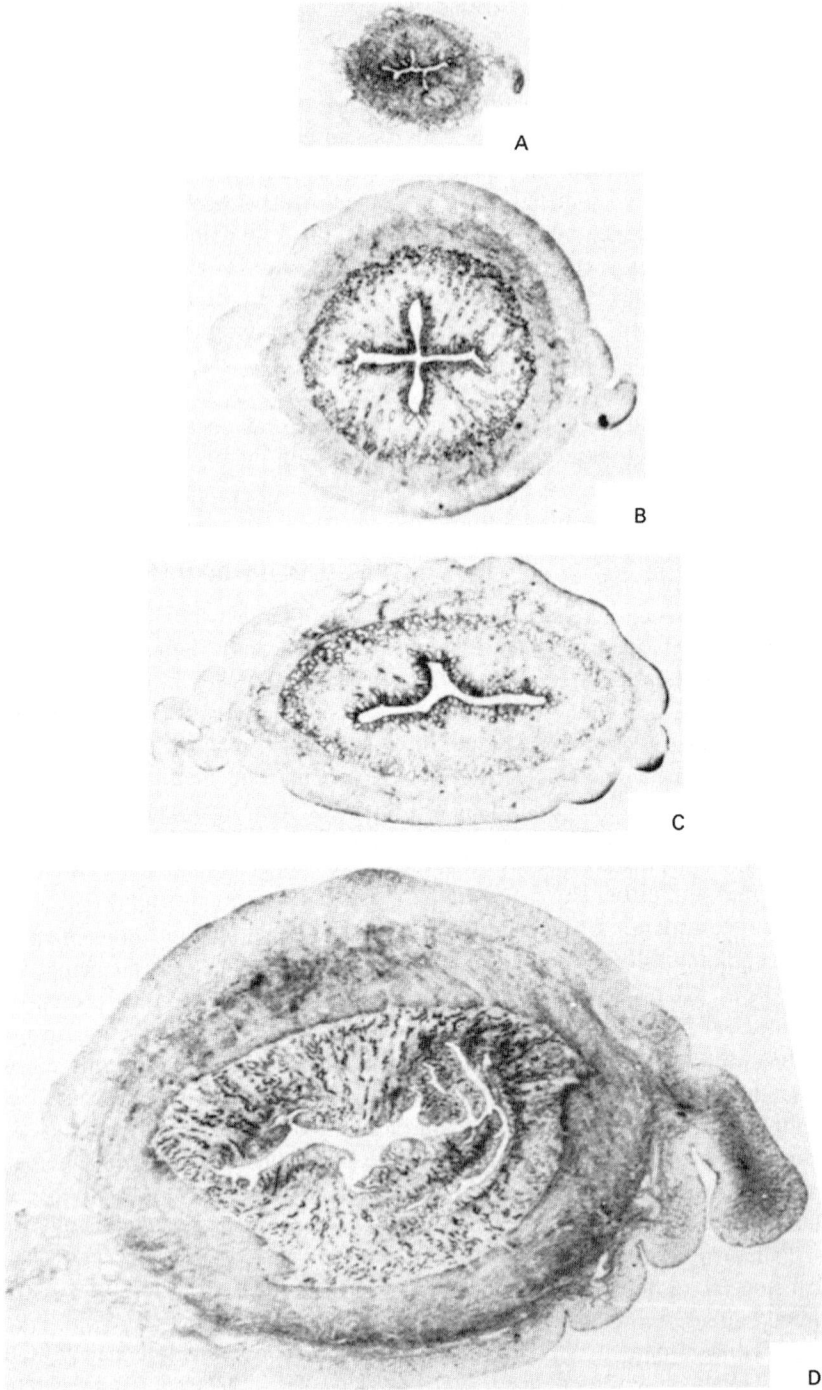

Fig. 16-9. Cross sections of the canine uterus. **A.** Anestrus. **B.** Proestrus. Note the increase in size and tubular appearance resulting largely from congestion and edema. **C.** Estrus. Note further enlargement due principally to hypertrophy of both myo- and endometrium. **D.** Diestrus. The increase in diameter is accompanied by a marked decrease in length of the cornu (Bouin's, nitrocellulose, hematoxylin, and eosin; section 12 microns thick. × 10). (From: H. H. Cole and P. T. Cupps, Reproduction in Domestic Animals. New York, NY, Academic Press, Inc., 1959).

normal pregnancy. With time, the psychological manifestations become intense, and the bitch may attempt to build a whelping nest in preparation for parturition. Occasionally the bitch may experience labor, although this is rare. The mammary glands may even develop to such an extent that lactation begins. Some pseudopregnant bitches can adopt and effectively nurse puppies from other bitches. Because the levels of progesterone in the blood are not different between pregnant and nonpregnant or pseudopregnant bitches, the determination of blood levels of relaxin, which increase in the pregnant but not in the nonpregnant bitch, offers a useful method to distinguish between pregnancy and pseudopregnancy in bitches.

In most cases, pseudopregnancy is so subtle in outward appearance that the owner is unaware of the condition. However, it is important for the veterinarian to understand and explain to the owner the known physiological processes involved. Administration of bromocriptine has proven to be effective to ameliorate the nesting behavior and other signs of overt pseudopregnancy, suggesting that increased pituitary prolactin secretion might contribute to these external manifestations of pseudopregnancy.

PREGNANCY AND PARTURITION

Even though conception is possible in the bitch, whether the breeding occurs once on the first day, subsequent days, or even on the last day of estrus without any apparent decrease in the pregnancy rate or the size of the litter, breeding on the first and either third or fourth days of estrus is recommended to increase the chance for pregnancy. Pregnancy lasts an average of 64 days when the length of pregnancy is calculated from the first day of standing estrus and breeding. Pregnancy may range between 56 to 68 days for bitches in dog colonies with controlled breeding programs. If the length of pregnancy is calculated from the first day that the bitch refuses to mate, that is, the first day of diestrus, the length of pregnancy is remarkably constant and lasts an average of 57 days. Most of the variation in the length of pregnancy reported in the literature for the bitch is likely due to the methods used to determine estrus and diestrus, particularly those solely based on interpreting the vaginal smear. Other contributing factors may include variations due to breed and time of ovulation, effects of single versus multiple matings, and false mounts of the male without actual genital lock and ejaculation. When teaser dogs are used to establish the onset

Table 16-8   Stages of Canine Prenatal Development for the Beagle

Stage of Development	Days Post Breeding	Size
Fertilized oocyte to blastocyst (in oviduct)	< 8	230 to 250 μm[a]
Spherical blastocyst (in uterus)	12	250 to 1250 μm[a]
Oval blastocyst (spaced in uterus)	16	1250 to 2500 μm[a]
Implantation; no primitive streak	17	>2500 μm[a]
Primitive streak	18	1 to 2 mm[b]
Neural groove; 1 to 4 somites	19	2 to 3 mm[b]
Cranial enlargement of neural groove; 5 to 9 somites	20	3 to 5 mm[b]
First limb buds; branchial arches	23	5 to 6 mm[b]
First appearance of eyes and hindlimb buds	24	6 to 14 mm[b]
Abdomen closes to umbilicus	25	10 to 15 mm[b]
Eyelids, facial vibrissae	27	12 to 15 mm[b]
Sexual differentiation	32	23 to 27 mm[b]
Closed eyelids; claws	35	28 to 41 mm[b]
Fully formed fetus	42	40 to 90 mm[b]
Appearance of hair	49	90 to 100 mm[b]

[a]Diameter.
[b]Length.
Adapted from: P. A. Holst and R. D. Phemister, Prenatal Canine Development. Description of Normal Development Stages. Annual Report. Collaborative Radiological Health Laboratory, Colorado State University, 1969.

of diestrus, variations in the estimated length of gestation are reduced considerably.

Preimplantation embryonic development begins in the oviduct, and the embryo enters the uterus of the bitch at the late morula or early blastocyst stage, 8 to 10 days after ovulation. Implantation sites are distinguishable by day 10 of diestrus. By day 16 of diestrus (approximately 23 days after the onset of estrus), the expansion of these implantation sites occurs, and the deep endometrial penetration of the trophoblast is completed by day 18 of diestrus. Table 16-8 displays the stages and time of appearance of prenatal development for the Beagle dog.

The uterine swellings at the implantation sites can be palpated transabdominally as early as day 20 and as late as day 31 of gestation. The detection of these swellings is not difficult in young, thin bitches, but becomes difficult or even impossible in obese bitches. Radiologic diagnosis of pregnancy is possible 42 to 46 days from the onset of estrus, when the bones of the fetus become radiopaque. Caution is imperative when performing radiologic examination of presumptively pregnant bitches. Excessive or prolonged exposure of the bitch and fetuses to X-rays may permanently alter the future reproductive function of both the mother and offspring because the ionizing radiation is detrimental to gametogenesis. Ultrasonographic diagnosis of pregnancy is another technique that has gained acceptance as a useful tool for pregnancy diagnosis in bitches. Even though embryos can be detected in the uterus using ultrasound by day 10 after breeding, it is recommended that another scan be performed 4 to 10 days later. By days 23 to 25 of gestation, the heartbeat can be detected in the developing fetus, and the number of fetuses can be determined between days 28 and 35 of gestation.

The placenta of the bitch is endotheliochorial and zonary because it attaches to the endometrium only at a central zone of the placenta. The yolk sac persists for most of the length of gestation, and the yolk sac may function as a supplementary liver during part of gestation.

An abrupt decline in progesterone levels 1 to 2 days before parturition is required for normal parturition in the bitch. This decline is probably in association with maturation of the pituitary-adrenal axis of the fetus. Exogenous progesterone delays parturition in the bitch. Androgens also decline at the time of parturition, but the role of androgens in the parturition of the bitch has not been determined. The elevation of maternal corticoid levels 1 to 4 days before parturition, at the time of maximal decline of blood levels of progesterone, may be due to fetal adrenal involvement in the parturition process.

Rectal temperature drops $1°$ to $1.5°F$ two days before parturition, a reflection of the disappearance of the thermogenic effect of progesterone. Rectal temperatures return to normal or remain slightly higher within 12 to 24 hours after parturition.

Bitches usually show increased restlessness and panting followed by nesting behavior 24 hours before parturition. Delivery or whelping is usually completed within a period of 8 to 10 hours but may take longer. Whelping time is influenced by the number of puppies to be born and varies among bitches. During whelping, there is an alternate expulsion of the puppies. The birth of the first pup, in relation to the left or right uterine horn, seems to be of random occurrence, but in most cases (78%) the second pup is born from the horn opposite to the one from which the first pup was born.

Lactation lasts from 6 to 9 weeks in the bitch, and during lactation the levels of prolactin are elevated. The mean interestrous interval does not seem to be different between pregnant and nonpregnant bitches, suggesting that lactational anestrus does not contribute to shorten or lengthen anestrus or the interval between consecutive estruses.

Relaxin in concentrations several folds above those present in the blood serum have been detected in the milk of nursing bitches. Suckling puppies may receive a high dose of relaxin and develop excessive laxity of the pelvic ligaments conducive to hip dysplasia in genetically predisposed puppies.

THE DOG

The testes of the dog pass through the inguinal canal on the third or fourth day after birth and reach their final scrotal location by 35 days after birth. Monolateral retention of a testis in the abdomen or inguinal canal is termed monorchidia or unilateral cryptorchidia. The bilateral retention of testes is termed bilateral cryptorchidia. Due to exposure of the retained testis to a higher temperature, monorchidia results in lack of spermatogenesis and atrophy of the retained testis and epididymis. Testosterone secretion does not seem to be significantly impaired in the cryptorchid testis whether in an abdominal or inguinal location when compared to testosterone produced by the scrotal testis. Bilateral cryptorchidism is associated with sterility.

Cryptorchidism is considered to be an autosomal recessive trait, expressed with more frequency in the right than in the left testis. Prevalence of cryptorchidism is greater in purebred (10%) than in mongrel (1%) dogs, suggesting an unplanned, undesired selection for this trait when dogs owners use inbreeding to select for other traits.

The average length of the cycle of the seminiferous epithelium (see Chapter 7) is estimated to be 13.6 days for the dog and coyote, and the duration of spermatogenesis lasts an average of 54.4 days. Each spermatogonium of the dog is thought to have the potential of producing 64 to 96 spermatozoa. The epididymal transit time (see Chapter 8, Table 8-1) is estimated to last 7 to 10 days.

After puberty, dogs are capable of mating and producing fertile ejaculates year-round. Mating in dogs is characterized by the genital lock between the male and the female (see Chapter 8, Fig. 8-19). Dogs attempting to mate mount the estrous bitch from the rear and perform several pelvic thrusts, releasing short bursts of presperm secretion while the penis is only partially erect. When the tip of the penis enters the bitch's vagina, the dog performs a deep thrust to introduce the penis, followed by a series of rapid thrusts with short penile displacement within the vagina until the penis becomes fully erect and anchored in the vagina. The *pars longa glandis* and the *bulbus glandis* expand during full erection to enlarge the length and the thickness of the penis. This is caused by the engorgement of the cavernous tissues due to occlusion of the venous return resulting from compression of the dorsal vein of the penis against the pelvis by contraction of the ischiourethralis and bulbospongiosus muscles. After the genital lock has been established, the dog dismounts and either turns away from the bitch or remains by her side facing in the same direction. When the dog dismounts the bitch, the root of the penis is twisted 180 degrees as the penis is reflected backwards between the hind legs of the dog without any apparent rotation of the glans penis and *bulbus glandis* within the vagina. This backward reflection and twisting at the base of the penis,[75] which truly constitutes a "paradox of flexible rigidity", compress the veins of the penis ensuring an extended erection and the genital lock that is essential due to the prolonged ejaculation and large volume of the dog's ejaculate. At mating, some bitches fall to the ground after the genital lock or even twist and turn vigorously while trying to bite the male. The genital lock of the penis within the vagina is firm enough to withstand those movements. Occasionally, dislodging of the penis from the vagina may occur when the male is unable to achieve or to keep a full erection or when the mating partners are frightened or disturbed. In this case, some dogs will continue to ejaculate, discharging the ejaculate on the ground. Pressure from the prepuce on the erect penis appears to be a sufficient stimulus to maintain this ongoing ejaculation.

The dog's ejaculate is delivered in three fractions (Table 16-9). The first, called the presperm fraction, is small in volume, clear, and usually contains only a few spermatozoa. Urethral, Littré glands were assumed to be the source of the presperm fraction of the dog's ejaculate. However,

Table 16-9   Fractions of the Dog's Ejaculate

Fraction	Volume (ml)	
	Mean	Range
Presperm	0.8	0.25– 2.8
Sperm-rich	0.6	0.40– 2.0
Postsperm	4.0	1.10–16.3
Total ejaculate	5.4	1.75–21.1

Adapted from: J. H. Boucher, et al., Cornell Vet. *48:*72, 1958.

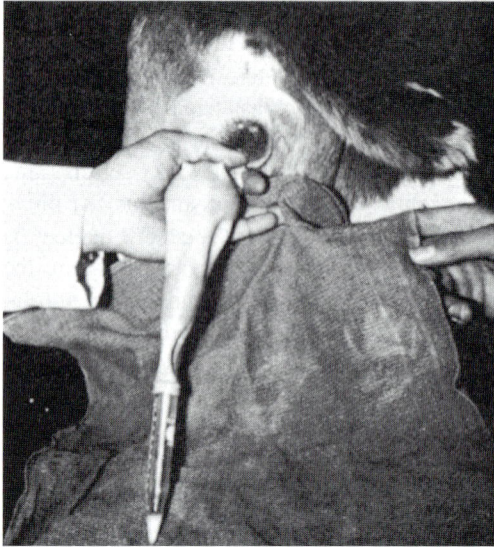

Fig. 16-10. Collection of dog semen by the cone method.[152]

Table 16-10   Physical Characteristics of Beagle Ejaculates Collected with an Artificial Vagina

Parameter	Mean	SD[a]	Range
Volume, ml	3.1	0.3	2.8–3.4
Motility (0 to 5)	3.0	0.3	2.2–3.9
Density (0 to 5)	1.5	1.1	0.0–4.2
Sperm concentration (10^6/ml)	111	22	57–164
Total sperm per ejaculate (10^6)	301	60	154–449
Percent sperm alive	90	2	84–95
Percent abnormal sperm	7	1	3–10

[a]SD = Standard deviation.
Adapted from: R. W. James et al., Vet. Rec. *104*:480, 1979.

Table 16-11   Daily Sperm Production (DSP), Daily Sperm Output (DSO), and Extra Gonadal Sperm Reserves (EGR) in the Beagle Dog

DSP (10^6)	DSO (10^6)	EGR (10^6)
594 ± 102	464 ± 16	479 ± 175

Data are mean ± standard error of the mean. Semen was collected by the digital manipulation method using a teaser bitch.
Adapted from: T. T. Olar, et al., Biol. Reprod., *29*:1114, 1983.

Littré glands have not been found in the urethra of dogs. Apparently, the presperm fraction is of prostatic origin. The second, sperm-rich fraction is small in volume, milky in appearance, and contains most of the spermatozoa released during ejaculation. The first two fractions are delivered within the first 2 or 3 minutes of ejaculation. The third, postsperm fraction is the most voluminous, may contain a few spermatozoa, and requires 3 to 40 minutes to be delivered. Most of the pre- and postsperm fractions are contributed by the prostate gland; thus, the collection of samples, particularly of postsperm fraction, can be very useful for studies on prostatic secretions and evaluation of prostatic diseases. After the completion of ejaculation, penile erection subsides and the dog separates from the bitch by withdrawing the penis.

Samples of semen can be collected from dogs with an artificial vagina or by digital manipulation using a rubber directing cone (Fig. 16-10). The method of digital manipulation is effective, easy to perform, and suitable for clinical practice, since little or no previous training of the dog is required. Semen can also be collected from the dog by electrical stimulation when dogs do not respond to the digital

stimulation of the penis. The process of inducing seminal emission by electrical stimulation is called electroejaculation, and the resulting product is an electroejaculate. Two to three series of 60 stimulations at 6.0V, 90-100 mA, at 30 Hz each produces electroejaculates suitable for evaluation of seminal qualities. Electroejaculation is particularly useful for the collection of semen from wild canidae such as coyotes, dingoes, and foxes. Dogs and wild canidae should be anesthetized prior to electroejaculation.

Table 16-10 displays some of the physical characteristics of ejaculates from Beagle dogs, and Table 16-11 shows the daily sperm production, output, and extragonadal sperm reserves for the Beagle dog. Seminal collections from dogs should not be performed more than once every 4 or 5 days. More frequent collections, especially for extended periods, result in a decreased output of spermatozoa per ejaculate. Depletion of spermatozoal reserves occurs when five or more ejaculates are obtained within 5 days.

In dogs, as well as in males of other species (see Chapter 8, Table 8-5), spermatozoa and possibly other seminal components can retrograde into the urinary bladder during ejaculation or during periods of prolonged sexual rest. The magnitude of spermatozoal losses in the urine of dogs during ejaculation induced by digital manipulation of the penis varies among dogs between 0% to 90% or more of the total number of spermatozoa displaced from the epididymides and vasa deferentia during the ejaculatory process. These urinary losses of spermatozoa result in severely oligospermic to azoospermic antegrade ejaculates. Retrograde flow of spermatozoa into the bladder of dogs also occurs when semen is collected by electroejaculation. The magnitude of retrograde flow or its association with the anesthetics used has not yet been established in systematic studies. Administration of xylazine, widely used in veterinary clinical practice as a tranquilizer and sedative for dogs, induces retrograde flow of spermatozoa into the bladder of sexually rested dogs. This retrograde flow-inducing effect of xylazine is prevented by pretreatment of dogs with yohimbine.[154]

Sertoli cell tumors have a relatively low incidence in dogs, though they are estimated to make up to about 5% of all testicular tumors in dogs. Only about 20% of Sertoli cell tumors in dogs are associated with a feminization syndrome, characterized by atrophy of the penile sheath, mammary gland development, symmetric alopecia, attractiveness to other dogs, and anemia. All of these symptoms have been traditionally ascribed to an increased secretion of estrogen by the Sertoli cell tumor. However, the peripheral concentrations of inhibin are increased and the levels of LH, FSH, and testosterone are decreased in dogs with Sertoli cell tumors, while the levels of estradiol-17β remain relatively constant. The feminization of dogs with Sertoli cell tumors is attributed to a significant increase in the estradiol/testosterone ratio rather than to a net increase in available peripheral concentration of estradiol-17β.

Persistent Müllerian Duct Syndrome, an autosomal recessive trait, has been reported for dogs with a karyotype of 78,XY. Affected dogs display a phenotype characterized by the persistence of a developed bicornuate uterus, oviducts, a blind-ending vagina, and bilaterally cryptorchid testes. The Sertoli cells of these dogs secrete Müllerian Inhibiting Hormone (MIH), but the oviducts and uterus fail to regress. Favored hypotheses are that dogs which are carriers of this trait have developed either a resistance to MIH during early fetal development or are deficient due to insufficient production of this hormone during the sensitive period of embryogenesis.

RESPONSE OF DOGS AND BITCHES TO EXOGENOUS HORMONES

The pituitary gland of dogs and anestrous or cycling bitches responds within minutes to the intravenous injection of GnRH by releasing both LH and FSH. Similarly, both prolactin and thyroid-stimulating hormone are released from the dog's pituitary gland following the injection of thyrotropin-releasing hormone. Dopamine agonists effectively suppress levels of prolactin in the blood.

An intramuscular dose of 3.0 mg of progesterone in oil per kg of body weight given once a day would maintain a concentration >10 ng/ml of progesterone in the blood, which is postulated as the minimal level of blood progesterone for maintenance of pregnancy in bitches.

Natural or synthetic estrogens, androgens, and progestagens effectively inhibit the release of gonadotropins from the pituitary of dogs and bitches. The influence of these reproductive hormonal steroids on gonadotropin release makes them useful as contraceptive steroids for the management and control of reproduction of dogs.

Although the pituitary of dogs and bitches is responsive to the stimulatory activity of releasing factors and to the inhibitory activity of steroids, the ovaries of anestrous bitches respond poorly and erratically to exogenous gonadotropic stimulation. Treatment of anestrous bitches with PMSG (also called eCG) or with FSH preparations to induce estrus often fails or results in only a small percentage of bitches responding with follicular development, standing estrous behavior, and ovulation. The ovulatory response to exogenous gonadotropins, particularly PMSG, is highly variable. The treatment of those bitches that respond to the treatment with FSH or FSH-like gonadotropins with hCG seems to improve their ovulatory response (Table 16-12). It is possible that the ovary of the bitch is similar to the ovary of the mare, which responds more reliably to homologous equine pituitary gonadotropins than to heterologous gonadotropins. Similarly, canine gonadotropins might allow for the reliable induction of estrus and ovulation in anestrous bitches. Unfortunately, canine pituitary gonadotropins are not commercially available, and they have not been used to induce estrus in anestrous bitches.

In dogs, the blood levels of LH and FSH increase dramatically after castration, whereas the levels of testosterone, progesterone, and estradiol-17β decrease significantly after castration (Table 16-13).

The pulsatile intravenous administration of 1.25 μg of GnRH every 90 minutes for up to 13 days induces estrous and ovulatory responses within 12 days from the last administration of GnRH. Mating bitches at this estrus produce successful pregnancies.

Treatment of the dog with GnRH significantly increases the levels of testosterone in the blood, and hCG increases testosterone secretion in perfused testes. Plasma concentration of androgens correlates with the plasma level of LH and the number of receptors for LH in the testes increase with age. Maximal rise in the number of LH receptors in the testes occurs when dogs are entering puberty, around 6 to 10 months of age.

The prostate gland, as other accessory male sex organs, depends on androgenic stimulation for developmental growth and function. However, the stroma and ductal epithelium of the dog's prostate contain receptors for estradiol and estrogens in general. The capability of these prostatic tissues to uptake estrogens is thought to play a role in the development of benign prostatic hyperplasia, common in aged dogs. The effectiveness of GnRH or of FSH, LH, and FSH- or LH-like hormones as treatment of reproductive problems of dogs, including their effects on libido, spermatogenesis, ejaculatory responses, and on the quality of ejaculate, have not been reported.

Table 16-12 Responses of Anestrous Bitches to Daily Injections of PMSG[a] Followed by a Single Treatment with HCG[b]

Response	Ratio	%
Estrous behavior[c]	5/8	63
Vulval bleeding	3/8	38
Vulval swelling	7/8	88
Bitches in standing estrus that ovulated	5/8	63

[a]PMSG, 250 IU/day, subcutaneous injections for 14 to 20 days until the bitch showed estrous vaginal smears.
[b]HCG, 500 IU, subcutaneous injection the first day of estrus after PMSG treatment was discontinued.
[c]Standing estrus, mating.
Adapted from: P. J. Wright, Aust. Vet. J. 59:123, 1982.

Table 16-13 Concentration in ng/ml (Mean ± SD) of LH, FSH, Testosterone, Progesterone, and Estradiol-17β in the Plasma of Intact and Bilaterally Castrated Dogs

Status	LH	FSH	Testosterone	Progesterone	Estradiol-17β
Intact	6.02 ± 5.2	89 ± 28	0.62 ± 0.35	1.15 ± 0.73	0.04 ± 0.02
Castrated					
12 hours post castration	---	---	0.08	0.59	0.008
6 months post castration	17.1 ± 9.9	858 ± 674	---	---	---

Calculated from data for steroid hormones in crossbred dogs from: K. Post, Can. Vet. J., *23*:98, 1982 and adapted from data for gonadotropic hormones in pet dogs from: P. N. Olson et al., Am. J. Vet. Res., *53*:762, 1992.

CONTRACEPTIVE STEROIDS FOR THE BITCH

The major aim of contraception is to prevent pregnancy by blocking or preventing estrus, ovulation, or any other appropriate interference with the reproductive processes. As stated previously, several natural or synthetic steroids effectively prevent estrus or inhibit the behavioral manifestations of estrus, thus preventing the bitch from accepting the male for mating. Unfortunately, most steroids also produce objectionable or undesirable side effects in the bitch.

Progestagens promote excessive endometrial and uterine growth and markedly stimulate the growth of the mammary gland in bitches. In addition, progestagens stimulate pituitary secretion of growth hormone, which may induce pronounced diabetogenic reactions in progestagen-treated bitches. Androgens masculinize the bitch and the fetus when given to pregnant bitches. Estrogens may induce irreversible aplastic anemia in dogs and bitches.

The demands created by the increasing population of pet animals prompted the search for safe and suitable steroids for use as contraceptives in dogs and cats. Of these, only two steroids have been approved by the United States Food and Drug Administration and are commercially available for canine contraception. These are megestrol acetate, a synthetic progestational compound, and mibolerone, a synthetic androgen derivative. Megestrol acetate, sold under the commercial name of Ovaban, is orally active and effective to block the progression from proestrus to estrus when given early in proestrus. Ovaban is also effective to postpone estrus when given during anestrus. Ovaban will not block behavioral estrus and should not be given to bitches in estrus because of the increased endometrial responses and abnormal uterine growth which is caused by this synthetic progestagen acting on an estrogen-primed uterus. Mibolerone, sold under the commercial name of Cheque, is an effective and apparently safe oral contraceptive for bitches. Mibolerone blocks the appearance of estrus when given daily to anestrous bitches. The drug is effective to postpone estrus while it is given

daily to the bitch. Daily administration of Mibolerone for periods as long as 2 years does not appear to cause detrimental effects to the bitch. Bitches return to estrus around 70 days after withdrawal of treatment.

Estrogens or estrogenic compounds such as tamoxifen have been used in the veterinary clinical practice for years as a replacement therapy in spayed bitches with urinary incontinence. Estrogens are also used to treat prostatic hypertrophy and perianal adenoma in dogs and to prevent pregnancies after mismatings or to terminate pregnancies. Recent evidences provided by carefully controlled studies indicate that the effectiveness of estrogen treatment to prevent or to terminate pregnancy needs to be re-evaluated in view of the inefficacy of some of the more widely used estrogens and the detrimental and myelotoxic effects of estrogens in dogs and bitches.

Two new products are emerging as potential contraceptives for bitches: Epostane and RU-486. Epostane is an androst-2-ene-2-carbonitrile compound that blocks progesterone synthesis by competitive inhibition of the enzyme 3β-hydroxysteroid dehydrogenase. As a result of Epostane activity, the pathway of synthesis of progesterone is blocked at the level of pregnenolone, resulting in high blood levels of pregnenolone, which is a biologically inactive steroid. As a consequence of this block, progesterone is not synthesized by the luteal tissue for lack of its natural precursor. Epostane induces abortion when given to pregnant bitches. Experimentally, Epostane appears to be safe when used to manage mismatings by terminating early pregnancy in bitches with daily doses of 2.5 to 5.0 mg/kg body weight for no longer than 7 days. Epostane does not have antiprogestational activity. Therefore, its effects are counteracted by the administration of progesterone. However, Epostane also blocks the steroid synthesis by the adrenal glands and placenta, which could be conducive to adrenal deficiencies in bitches and in other domestic animals when experimentally used to terminate pregnancy, induce parturition, or to synchronize estrus.

RU-486, also called mefipristone, is an antiprogesterone steroid used as an abortifacient contraceptive, or perhaps more properly, contragestive, for women. RU-486 binds competitively to progesterone and also glucocorticoid receptors. Thus, RU-486 excludes the binding of progesterone to receptors, resulting in progesterone deprivation, abortion, and potentially glucocorticoid deficiencies. RU-486 in a single subcutaneous dose of 20 mg/kg of body weight is effective to terminate pregnancy from days 20 to 55 in bitches and induces early parturition when given after day 55 of pregnancy. The effects of RU-486 are irreversible and cannot be prevented by the concurrent administration of progesterone.

REFERENCES

1. Abel, J. H., Jr., McClellan, M. C., Verhage, H. G., et al. (1975): Subcellular compartmentalization of the luteal cell in the ovary of the dog. Cell Tissue Res. *158*:461.
2. Abel, J. H., Jr., Verhage, H. G., McClellan, M. C., et al. (1975): Ultrastructural analysis of the granulosa-luteal cell transition in the ovary of the dog. Cell Tissue Res. *160*:155.
3. Al-Kafawi, A. A., Hopwood, M. L., Pineda M. H., et al. (1974): Immunization of dogs against human chorionic gonadotropin. Am. J. Vet. Res. *35*:261.
4. Allen, W. E. (1986): Pseudopregnancy in the bitch: The current view on aetiology and treatment. J. Small Anim. Pract. *27*:419.
5. Allen, W. E. and Meredith, M. J. (1981): Detection of pregnancy in the bitch: A study of abdominal palpation, A-mode ultrasound, and doppler ultrasound techniques. J. Small Anim. Pract. *22*:609.
6. Allen, W. E., Daker, M. G., and Hancock, J. L. (1981): Three intersexual dogs. Vet. Rec. *109*:468.
7. Anderson, A. C. and Simpson, M. E. (1973): The ovary and reproductive cycle of the dog (Beagle). Los Altos, CA, Geron-X, Inc.
8. Anderson, J. W. (1969): Ultrastructure of the placenta and fetal membranes of the dog. I. Placental labyrinth. Am. J. Anat. *165*:15.
9. Anderson, R. K., Gilmore, C. E., and Schnelle, G. B. (1965): Utero-ovarian disorders associated with use of medroxyprogesterone in dogs. J. Am. Vet. Med. Assoc. *146*:1311.
10. Arnold, S., Arnold, P., Hubler, M., et al. (1989): Urinary incontinence in spayed bitches: Prevalence and breed predisposition. Schweiz. Arch. Tierheilkd. *131*:259.
11. Aumuller, G., Stofft, E., and Tunn, U. (1980): Fine structure of the canine prostatic complex. Anat. Embryol. *160*:327.
12. Awoniyi, C., Hasson, T., Chandrashekar, V., et al. (1986): Regulation of gonadotropin secretion in the male: Effect of an aromatization inhibitor in estradiol-implanted, orchidectomized dogs. J. Androl. *7*:234.
13. Barrau, M. D., Abel, J. H., Jr., Torbit, C. A., et al. (1975): Development of the implantation chamber in the pregnant bitch. Am. J. Anat. *143*:115.

14. Barrau, M. D., Abel, J. H., Jr., Verhage, H. G., et al. (1975): Development of the endometrium during the estrous cycle in the bitch. Am. J. Anat. *142*:47.
15. Baumans, V., Dieleman, S. J., Wouterse, H. S., et al. (1983): Testosterone secretion during gubernacular development and testicular descent in the dog. J. Reprod. Fertil. *73*:21.
16. Baumans, V., Dijkstra, G., and Wensing, C. J. G. (1981): Testicular descent in the dog. Anat. Histol. Embryol. *10*:97.
17. Baumans, V., Dijkstra, G., and Wensing, C. J. G. (1983): The role of a non-androgenic testicular factor in the process of testicular descent in the dog. Int. J. Androl. *6*:541.
18. Baumans, V., Schoorl, M., Dijkstra, G., et al. (1988): Effect of simulated orchiopexy on spermatogenesis in the dog. Int. J. Androl. *11*:115.
19. Beach, F. A. (1970): Coital behavior in dogs. IX. Sequelae to "coitus interruptus" in males and females. Physiol. Behav. *5*:263.
20. Bell, E. T. and Christie, D. W. (1971): Duration of proestrus, oestrus and vulval bleeding in the Beagle bitch. Br. Vet. J. *127*:25.
21. Benhamou, B., Garcia, T., Lerouge, T., et al. (1992): A single amino acid that determines the sensitivity of progesterone receptors to RU486. Science *255*:206.
22. Bondestam, S., Alitalo, I., and Karkkainen, M. (1983): Real-time ultrasound pregnancy diagnosis in the bitch. J. Small Anim. Pract. *24*:145.
23. Bouchard, G. F., Solorzano, N., Concannon, P. W., et al. (1991): Determination of ovulation time in bitches based on teasing, vaginal cytology, and Elisa for progesterone. Theriogenology *35*:603.
24. Boucher, J. H., Foote, R. H., and Kirk, R. W. (1958): The evaluation of semen quality in the dog and the effects of frequency of ejaculation upon semen quality, libido, and depletion of sperm reserves. Cornell Vet. *48*:67.
25. Bowen, R. A., Olson, P. N., Behrendt, M. D., et al. (1985): Efficacy and toxicity of estrogens commonly used to terminate canine pregnancy. J. Am. Vet. Med. Assoc. *186*:783.
26. Bowen, R. A., Olson, P. N., Young, S., et al. (1988): Efficacy and toxicity of tamoxipen citrate for prevention and termination of pregnancy in bitches. Am. J. Vet. Res. *49*:27.
27. Boyden, T. W., Pamenter, R. W., and Silvert, M. A. (1980): Testosterone secretion by the isolated canine testis after controlled infusions of hCG. J. Reprod. Fertil. *59*:25.
28. Briggs, M. (1977): The Beagle dog and contraceptive steroids. Life Sci. *21*:275.
29. Briggs, M. H. (1980): Progestogens and mammary tumours in the Beagle bitch. Res. Vet. Sci. *28*:199.
30. Brodey, R. S., Fidler, I. J., and Howson, A. E. (1966): The relationship of estrous irregularity, pseudopregnancy, and pregnancy to the development of canine mammary neoplasms. J. Am. Vet. Med. Assoc. *149*:1047.
31. Cain, J. L., Cain, G. R., Feldman, E. C., et al. (1988): Use of pulsatile intravenous administration of gonadotropin-releasing hormone to induce fertile estrus in bitches. Am. J. Vet. Res. *49*:1993.
32. Capel-Edwards, K., Hall, D. E., Fellowes, K. P., et al. (1973): Long-term administration of progesterone to

the female Beagle dog. Toxicol. Appl. Pharmacol. *24*:474.

33. Cartee, R. E. and Rowles, T. (1984): Preliminary study of the ultrasonographic diagnosis of pregnancy and fetal development in the dog. Am. J. Vet. Res. *45*:1259.

34. Catling, P. C. (1979): Seasonal variation in plasma testosterone and the testis in captive male dingoes, *Canis familiaris dingo*. Aust. J. Zool. *27*:939.

35. Chakraborty, P. K. and Fletcher, W. S. (1977): Responsiveness of anestrous Labrador bitches to GnRH. Proc. Soc. Exp. Biol. Med. *154*:125.

36. Christiansen, Ib. J. (1984): Reproduction in the Dog and Cat. London, England, Bailliere Tindall.

37. Christie, D. W., Bailey, J. B., and Bell, E. T. (1972): Classification of cell types in vaginal smears during the canine oestrous cycle. Br. Vet. J. *128*:301.

38. Christie, D. W. and Bell, E. T. (1971): Some observations on the seasonal incidence and frequency of oestrus in breeding bitches in Britain. J. Small Anim. Pract. *12*:159.

39. Connell, C. J. (1980): Blood-testis barrier formation and the initiation of meiosis in the dog. *In:* Testicular Development, Structure, and Function, edited by A. Steinberger and E. Steinberger. New York, NY, Raven Press, p. 71.

40. Connell, C. J. (1984): An ultrastructural study of the cytoplasmic bridges between germ cells of the canine testis. Ann. N. Y. Acad. Sci. *438*:472.

41. Connell, C. J. and Donjacour, A. (1985): A morphological study of the epididymides of control and estradiol-treated prepubertal dogs. Biol. Reprod. *33*:951.

42. Crafts, R. C. (1948): The effects of estrogens on the bone marrow of adult female dogs. Blood *3*:276.

43. Daniels, T. J. (1983): The social organization of free-ranging urban dogs. I. Non-estrous social behavior. Appl. Anim. Ethol. *10*:341.

44. Daniels, T. J. (1983): The social organization of free-ranging urban dogs. II. Estrous groups and the mating system. Appl. Anim. Ethol. *10*:365.

45. De Coster, R., Beckers, J.-F., Beerens, D., et al. (1983): A homologous radioimmunoassay for canine prolactin: Plasma levels during the reproductive cycle. Acta Endocrinol. *103*:473.

46. Del Campo, C. H. and Ginther, O. J. (1974): Arteries and veins of uterus and ovaries in dogs and cats. Am. J. Vet. Res. *35*:409.

47. DePalatis, L., Moore, J., and Falvo, R. E. (1978): Plasma concentrations of testosterone and LH in male dog. J. Reprod. Fertil. *52*:201.

48. Doak, R. L., Hall, A., and Dale, H. E. (1967): Longevity of spermatozoa in the reproductive tract of the bitch. J. Reprod. Fertil. *13*:51.

49. Dooley, M. P., Pineda, M. H., Hopper, J. G., et al. (1990): Retrograde flow of spermatozoa into the urinary bladder of dogs during ejaculation or after sedation with xylazine. Am. J. Vet. Res. *51*:1574.

50. Doty, R. L. and Dunbar, I. (1974): Attraction of Beagles to conspecific urine, vaginal and anal sac secretion odors. Physiol. Behav. *12*:825.

51. Doty, R. L. and Mare, C. J. (1974): Color, odor, consistency and secretion rate of anal sac secretions from male, female, and early-androgenized female Beagles. Am. J. Vet. Res. *35*:669.

52. Drill, V. A. (1974): Some metabolic actions and possible toxic effects of hormonal contraceptives in animals and man. Acta Endocrinol. *75*:169.

53. Eigenmann, J. E. and Eigenmann, R. Y. (1981): Influence of medroxyprogesterone acetate (Provera) on plasma growth hormone levels and on carbohydrate metabolism. II. Studies in the ovario-hysterectomized, oestradiol-primed bitch. Acta Endocrinol. *98*:603.

54. Eigenmann, J. E. and Rijnberk, A. (1981): Influence of medroxyprogesterone acetate (Provera) on plasma growth hormone levels and on carbohydrate metabolism. I. Studies on the ovariectomized bitch. Acta Endocrinol. *98*:599.

55. England, G. C. W. and Allen, W. E. (1989): Crystallization patterns in anterior vaginal fluid from bitches in oestrus. J. Reprod. Fertil. *86*:335.

56. England, G. C. W. and Allen, W. E. (1990): An investigation into the origin of the first fraction of the canine ejaculate. Res. Vet. Sci. *49*:66.

57. Ewing, L. L., Berry, S. J., and Higginbottom, E. G. (1983): Dihydrotestosterone concentration of Beagle prostatic tissue: Effect of age and hyperplasia. Endocrinology *113*:2004.

58. Ewing, L. L., Zirkin, B. R., Cochran, R. C., et al. (1979): Testosterone secretion by rat, rabbit, guinea pig, dog, and hamster testes perfused *in vitro:* Correlation with Leydig cell mass. Endocrinology *105*:1135.

59. Falvo, R. E., Gerrit, M., Pirmann, J., et al. (1982): Testosterone pretreatment and the response of pituitary LH to gonadotropin-releasing hormone (GnRH) in the male dog. J. Androl. *3*:193.

60. Faulkner, L. C., Pineda, M. H., and Reimers, T. J. (1975): Immunization against gonadotropins in dogs. *In:* Immunization with Hormones in Reproduction Research, edited by E. Nieschlag. Amsterdam, Holland, North-Holland Publishing Co., p. 199.

61. Fernandez, P. A., Bowen, R. A., Kostas, A. C., et al. (1987): Luteal function in the bitch: Changes during diestrus in pituitary concentration of and the number of luteal receptors for luteinizing hormone and prolactin. Biol. Reprod. *37*:804.

62. Fernandez, P. A., Bowen, R. A., Sawyer, H. R., et al. (1989): Concentration of receptors for estradiol and progesterone in canine endometrium during estrus and diestrus. Am. J. Vet. Res. *50*:64.

63. Foote, R. H., Swierstra, E. E., and Hunt, W. L. (1972): Spermatogenesis in the dog. Anat. Rec. *173*:341.

64. Frank, D. W., Kirton, K. T., Murchison, T. E., et al. (1979): Mammary tumors and serum hormones in the bitch treated with medroxyprogesterone acetate or progesterone for four years. Fertil. Steril. *31*:340.

65. Frenette, M. D., Dooley, M. P., and Pineda, M. H. (1986): Effect of flushing the vasa deferentia at the time of vasectomy on the rate of clearance of spermatozoa from the ejaculates of dogs and cats. Am. J. Vet. Res. *47*:463.

66. Froman, D. P. and Amann, R. P. (1983): Inhibition of motility of bovine, canine and equine spermatozoa by artificial vagina lubricants. Theriogenology *20*:357.

67. Gerber, J. G., Hubbard, W. C., and Nies, A. S. (1976): Uterine vein prostaglandin levels in late pregnant dogs. Prostaglandins *17*:623.

68. Gill, H. P., Kaufman, C. F., Foote, R. H., et al. (1970): Artificial insemination of Beagle bitches with freshly collected, liquid-stored, and frozen-stored semen. Am. J. Vet. Res. *31*:1807.

69. Ginther, O. J. (1976): Comparative anatomy of utero-ovarian vasculature. Vet. Scope *20*:2.

70. Goldsmith, L. T., Lust, G., and Steinetz, B. G. (1994): Transmission of relaxin from lactating bitches to their offspring via suckling. Biol. Reprod. *50*:258.

71. Gonzalez, A., Allen, A. F., Post, K., et al. (1989): Immunological approaches to contraception in dogs. J. Reprod. Fertil. (Suppl. 39):189.

72. Goodwin, M., Gooding, K. M., and Regnier, F. (1979): Sex pheromone in the dog. Science *203*:559.

73. Graf, K.-J. (1978): Serum oestrogen, progesterone and prolactin concentrations in cyclic, pregnant and lactating Beagle dogs. J. Reprod. Fertil. *52*:9.

74. Graf, K.-J. and El Etreby, M. F. (1979): Endocrinology of reproduction in the female Beagle dog and its significance in mammary gland tumorogenesis. Acta Endocrinol. *90* (Suppl. 222):1.

75. Grandage, J. (1972): The erect dog penis: A paradox of flexible rigidity. Vet. Rec. *91*:141.

76. Grootenhuis, A. J., Van Sluijs, F. J., Klaij, I. A., et al. (1990): Inhibin, gonadotrophins and sex steroids in dogs with Sertoli cell tumours. J. Endocrinol. *127*:235.

77. Günzel-Apel, A. R., Hille, P., and Hoppen, H. O. (1994): Spontaneous and GnRH-induced pulsatile LH and testosterone release in pubertal, adult and aging male Beagles. Theriogenology *41*:737.

78. Hadley, J. C. (1975): Total unconjugated oestrogen and progesterone concentrations in peripheral blood during the oestrous cycle of the dog. J. Reprod. Fertil. *44*:445.

79. Hadley, J. C. (1975): Total unconjugated oestrogen and progesterone concentrations in peripheral blood during pregnancy in the dog. J. Reprod. Fertil. *44*:453.

80. Hadley, J. C. (1975): Unconjugated oestrogen and progesterone concentrations in the blood of bitches with false pregnancy and pyometra. Vet. Rec. *96*:545.

81. Hart, B. L. (1974): Gonadal androgen and socio-sexual behavior of male mammals: A comparative analysis. Physiol. Bull. *81*:383.

82. Hart, B. L. and Kitchell, R. L. (1966): Penile erection and contraction of penile muscles in the spinal and intact dog. Am. J. Physiol. *210*:257.

83. Hart, B. L. and Ladewig, J. (1979): Serum testosterone of neonatal male and female dogs. Biol. Reprod. *21*:289.

84. Hinsch, K.-D., Hinsch, E., Meinecke, B., et al. (1994): Identification of mouse ZP3 protein in mammalian oocytes with antisera against synthetic ZP3 peptides. Biol. Reprod. *51*:193.

85. Hinton, M. and Jones, D. R. E. (1977): Anemia in the dog: An analysis of laboratory data. J. Small Anim. Pract. *18*:701.

86. Hoffmann, B., Riesenbeck, A., and Klein, R. (1996): Reproductive endocrinology of bitches. Anim. Reprod. Sci. *42*:275.

87. Holst, P. A. and Phemister, R. D. (1971): The prenatal development of the dog: Preimplantation events. Biol. Reprod. *5*:194.

88. Holst, P. A. and Phemister, R. D. (1974): Onset of diestrus in the Beagle bitch: Definition and significance. Am. J. Vet. Res. *35*:401.

89. Holst, P. A. and Phemister, R. D. (1975): Temporal sequence of events in the estrous cycle of the bitch. Am. J. Vet. Res. *36*:705.

90. Holt, P. E. and Sayle, B. (1981): Congenital vestibulo-vaginal stenosis in the bitch. J. Small Anim. Pract. *22*:67.

91. Hopkins, S. G., Schubert, T. A., and Hart, B. L. (1976): Castration of adult male dogs: Effects on roaming, aggression, urine marking, and mounting. J. Am. Vet. Med. Assoc. *168*:1108.

92. Hutson, J. M., Baker, M., Masaru, T., et al. (1994): Hormonal control of testicular descent and the cause of cryptochidism. J. Reprod. Fertil. *6*:151.

93. Hyttel, P., Farstad, W., Mondain-Monval, M., et al. (1990): Structural aspects of oocyte maturation in the blue fox (*Alopex lagopus*). Anat. Embryol. *181*:325.

94. Ibach, B., Weissbach, L., and Hilscher, B. (1976): Stages of the cycle of the seminiferous epithelium in the dog. Andrologia *8*:297.

95. Ibach, B., Passia, D., Weissbach, L., et al. (1978): The effect of low-dose HCG on the testis of prepuberal dogs. Int. J. Androl. *6*:509.

96. Inaba, T., Matsuoka, S., Kawate, N., et al. (1994): Developmental changes in testicular luteinising (sic) hormone receptors and androgens in the dog. Res. Vet. Sci. *57*:305.

97. James, R. W., Crook, D., and Heywood, R. (1979): Canine pituitary-testicular function in relation to toxicity testing. Toxicology *13*:237.

98. James, R. W., Heywood, R., and Street, A. E. (1979): Biochemical observations on Beagle dog semen. Vet. Rec. *104*:480.

99. Jeffcoate, I. A. and Lindsay, F. E. F. (1989): Ovulation detection and timing of insemination based on hormone concentrations, vaginal cytology and the endoscopic appearance of the vagina in domestic bitches. J. Reprod. Fertil. (Suppl. 39):277.

100. Joby, R., Jemmett, J. E., and Miller, A. S. H. (1984): The control of undesirable behaviour in male dogs using megestrol acetate. J. Small Anim. Pract. *25*:567.

101. Johnson, A. N. (1989): Comparative aspects of contraceptive steroids-Effects observed in Beagle dogs. Toxicol. Pathol. *17*:389.

102. Johnston, S. D., Buoen, L. C., Weber, A. F., et al. (1985): X-trisomy in an Airedale bitch with ovarian dysplasia and primary anestrus. Theriogenology *24*:597.

103. Johnston, S. D., Kiang, D. T., Seguin, B. E., et al. (1985): Cytoplasmic estrogen and progesterone receptors in canine endometrium during the estrous cycle. Am. J. Vet. Res. *46*:1653.

104. Jordan, A., (1994): Toxicology of depot medroxyprogesterone acetate. Contraception *49*:189.

105. Kawakami, E., Tsutsui, T., Yamada, Y., et al. (1987): Spermatogenesis and peripheral spermatic venous plasma androgen levels in the unilateral cryptorchid dogs. Jpn. J. Vet. Sci. *49*:349.

106. Keister, D. M., Gutheil, R. F., Kaiser, L. D., et al. (1989): Efficacy of oral epostane administration to terminate pregnancy in mated laboratory bitches. J. Reprod. Fertil. (Suppl. 39):241.

107. Kennelly, J. J. (1969): The effect of mestranol on canine reproduction. Biol. Reprod. *1*:282.
108. Kennelly, J. J. (1972): Coyote reproduction. I. The duration of the spermatogenic cycle and epididymal sperm transport. J. Reprod. Fertil. *31*:163.
109. Kennelly, J. J. and Johns, B. E. (1976): The estrous cycle of coyotes. J. Wildlife Mngmt. *40*:272.
110. Kirdani, R. Y. and Sandberg, A. A. (1974): The fate of estriol in dogs. Steroids *23*:667.
111. Knol, B. W., Diekman, S. J., Bevers, M. M., et al. (1993): GnRH in the male dog: Dose-response relationships with LH and testosterone. J. Reprod. Fertil. *98*:159.
112. Krause, D., Hahmann, C. H., and Günzel-Apel, A.-R. (1989): Untersuchungen des Ejakulationsverhaltens des Hundes nach Verabreichung der α-bzw. β-Sympathomimetika Midodrin, Norepinephrin und Clenbuterol. Wien. Tierärztl. Monatschr. *76*:42.
113. Kruse, S. M. and Howard, W. E. (1983): Canid sex attractant studies. J. Chem. Ecol. *9*:1503.
114. Kumi-Diaka, J. and Badtram, G. (1994): Effect of storage on sperm membrane integrity and other functional characteristics of canine spermatozoa: *In vitro* bioassay for canine semen. Theriogenology *41*:1355.
115. Kwan, P. W. L., Merk, F. B., Leav, I., et al. (1982): Estrogen mediated exocytosis in the glandular epithelium of prostates in castrated and hypophysectomized dogs. Cell Tissue Res. *226*:689.
116. Lee, S. Y., Anderson, J. W., Scott, G. L., et al. (1983): Ultrastructure of the placenta and fetal membranes of the dog. II. The yolk sac. Am. J. Anat. *166*:313.
117. Lein, D. H. (1983): Examination of the bitch for breeding soundness. *In:* Current Veterinary Therapy, Vol. VIII, Small Animal Practice, edited by R. W. Kirk. Philadelphia, PA, W. B. Saunders Co., p. 909.
118. Lessey, B. A., Wahawisan, R., and Gorell, T. A. (1981): Hormonal regulation of cytoplasmic estrogen and progesterone receptors in the Beagle uterus and oviduct. Mol. Cell. Endocrinol. *21*:171.
119. Levine, B. N. (1984): Small animal pet population trends and demands for veterinary service. *In:* Proc. 8th Kal Kan Symp. for the Treatment of Small Animal Diseases, edited by E. van Marthens. Vernon, CA, Kal Kan, p. 49.
120. Lindsay, F. E. F. (1983): The normal endoscopic appearance of the caudal reproductive tract of the cyclic and non-cyclic bitch: Post-uterine endoscopy. J. Small Anim. Pract. *24*:1.
121. Lindsay, F. E. F. (1983): Endoscopy of the reproductive tract in the bitch. *In:* Current Veterinary Therapy, Vol. VIII, Small Animal Practice, edited by R. W. Kirk. Philadelphia, PA, W. B. Saunders Co., p. 912.
122. Lopate, C., Threlfall, W. R., and Rosol, T. J. (1989): Histopathological and gross effects of testicular biopsy in the dog. Theriogenology *32*:585.
123. Lunnen, J. E., Faulkner, L. C., Hopwood, M. L., et al. (1974): Immunization of dogs with bovine luteinizing hormone. Biol. Reprod. *10*:453.
124. Mahi, C. A. and Yanagimachi, R. (1976): Maturation and sperm penetration of canine ovarian oocytes *in vitro*. J. Exp. Zool. *196*:189.
125. Mahi, C. A. and Yanagimachi, R. (1978): Capacitation, acrosome reaction, and egg penetration by canine spermatozoa in a simple defined medium. Gamete Res. *1*:101.
126. Mahi, C. A. and Yanagimachi, R. (1979): Prevention of *in vitro* fertilization of canine oocytes by antiovary antisera: A potential approach to fertility control in the bitch. J. Exp. Zool. *210*:129.
127. Mahi-Brown, C. A., Yanagimachi, R., Hoffman, J. C., et al. (1985): Fertility control in the bitch by active immunization with porcine zonae pellucidae: Use of different adjuvants and patterns of estradiol and progesterone levels in estrous cycles. Biol. Reprod. *32*:761.
128. Mattheeuws, D. and Comhaire, F. H. (1989): Concentrations of oestradiol and testosterone in peripheral and spermatic venous blood of dogs with unilateral cryptochidism. Domestic Anim. Endocrinol. *6*:203.
129. McRae, G. I., Roberts, B. B., Worden, A. C., et al. (1985): Long-term reversible suppression of oestrus in bitches with nafarelin acetate, a potent LHRH agonist. J. Reprod. Fertil. *74*:389.
130. Myers, R. K., Cook, J. E., and Mosier, J. E. (1984): Comparative aging changes in canine uterine tubes (oviducts): Electron microscopy. Am. J. Vet. Res. *45*:2008.
131. Meyers-Wallen, V. N., Donahoe, P. K., Manganaro, T., et al. (1987): Müllerian inhibiting substance in sex-reversed dogs. Biol. Reprod. *37*:1015.
132. Meyers-Wallen, V. N., Donahoe, P. K., Ueno, S., et al. (1989): Müllerian inhibiting substance is present in testes of dogs with persistent Müllerian duct syndrome. Biol. Reprod. *41*:881.
133. Morton, D. B., Yaxley, R. E., Patel, I., et al. (1987): Use of DNA finger print analysis in identification of the sire. Vet. Rec. *121*:592.
134. Ninomiya, H. (1980): The penile cavernous system and its morphological changes in the erected state in the dog. Jpn. J. Vet. Sci. *42*:187.
135. Ninomiya, H. and Nakamura, T. (1981): Vascular architecture of the canine prepuce. Anat. Histol. Embryol. *10*:351.
136. Ninomiya, H., Nakamura, T., Niizuma, I., et al. (1989): Penile vascular system of the dog. An injection-corrosion and histological study. Jpn. J. Vet. Sci. *51*:765.
137. Oettle, E. E. and Soley, J. T. (1988): Sperm abnormalities in the dog: A light and electron microscopic study. Vet. Med. Rev. *59*:28.
138. Okkens, A. C., Dieleman, S. J., Bevers, M. M., et al. (1985): Evidence for the non-involvement of the uterus in the lifespan of the corpus luteum in the cyclic dog. Vet. Quart. *7*:169.
139. Okkens, A. C., Dieleman, S. J., Bevers, M. M., et al. (1986): Influence of hypophysectomy on the lifespan of the corpus luteum in the cyclic dog. J. Reprod. Fertil. *77*:187.
140. Olar, T. T., Amann, R. P., and Pickett, B. W. (1983): Relationships among testicular size, daily production and output of spermatozoa, and extragonadal spermatozoal reserves of the dog. Biol. Reprod. *29*:1114.
141. Olson, P. N., Bowen, R. A., Behrendt, M. D., et al. (1982): Concentrations of reproductive hormones in canine serum throughout late anestrus, proestrus, and estrus. Biol. Reprod. *27*:1196.
142. Olson, P. N., Bowen, R. A., Behrendt, M. D., et al. (1984): Validation of radioimmunoassays to measure prostaglandins $F_{2\alpha}$ and E_2 in canine endometrium and plasma. Am. J. Vet. Res. *45*:119.

143. Olson, P. N., Bowen, R. A., Behrendt, B. S., et al. (1984): Concentrations of testosterone in canine serum during late anestrus, proestrus, and early diestrus. Am. J. Vet. Res. *45*:145.

144. Olson, P. N., Bowen, R. A., Behrendt, M. D., et al. (1984): Concentrations of progesterone and luteinizing hormone in the serum of diestrous bitches before and after hysterectomy. Am. J. Vet. Res. *45*:149.

145. Olson, P. N., Mulnix, J. A., and Nett, T. M. (1992): Concentrations of luteinizing hormone and follicle stimulating hormone in the serum of sexually intact and neutered dogs. Am. J. Vet. Res. *53*:762.

146. O'Shea, J. D. and Jabara, A. G. (1967): The histogenesis of canine ovarian tumours induced by stilboestrol administration. Pathol. Vet. *4*:137.

147. Paisley, L. G. and Fahning, M. L. (1977): Effects of exogenous follicle-stimulating hormone and luteinizing hormone in bitches. J. Am. Vet. Med. Assoc. *171*:181.

148. Paradis, M., Post, K., and Mapletoft, R. J. (1983): Effects of prostaglandin $F_{2\alpha}$ on corpora lutea formation and function in mated bitches. Can. Vet. J. *24*:239.

149. Park, Y. S., Abe, M., Takehana, K., et al. (1993): Three-dimensional structure of dog Sertoli cells: A computer-aided reconstruction from serial semi-thin sections. Arch. Histol. Cytol. *56*:65.

150. Phemister, R. D., Holst, P. A., Spano, J. S., et al. (1973): Time of ovulation in the Beagle bitch. Biol. Reprod. *8*:74.

151. Picon, R., Picon, L., Chaffaux, S., et al. (1978): Effects of canine fetal testes and testicular tumors on Müllerian ducts. Biol. Reprod. *18*:459.

152. Pineda, M. H. (1977): A simple method for collection of semen from dogs. Canine Pract. *4*:14.

153. Pineda, M. H. (1986): Contraceptive procedures for the male dog. *In:* Current Therapy in Theriogenology, edited by D. A. Morrow. Philadelphia, PA, W. B. Saunders Co., p. 563.

154. Pineda, M. H. and Dooley, M. P. (1994): Yohimbine prevents the retrograde flow of spermatozoa into the urinary bladder of dogs induced by xylazine. J. Vet. Pharmacol. Therap. *17*:169.

155. Pineda, M. H. and Hepler, D. I. (1981): Chemical vasectomy in dogs. Long-term study. Theriogenology *16*:1.

156. Pineda, M. H., Kainer, R. A., and Faulkner, L. C. (1973): Dorsal median postcervical fold in the canine vagina. Am. J. Vet. Res. *34*:1487.

157. Pineda, M. H., Reimers, T. J., and Faulkner, L. C. (1976): Disappearance of spermatozoa from the ejaculates of vasectomized dogs. J. Am. Vet. Med. Assoc. *168*:502.

158. Pineda, M. H., Reimers, T. J., Faulkner, L. C., et al. (1977): Azoospermia in dogs induced by injection of sclerosing agents into the caudae of the epididymides. Am. J. Vet. Res. *38*:831.

159. Post, K. (1982): Effects of human chorionic gonadotrophin and castration on plasma gonadal steroid hormones of the dog. Can. Vet. J. *23*:98.

160. Reimers, T. J., Phemister, R. D., and Niswender, G. D. (1978): Radio-immunological measurement of follicle stimulating hormone and prolactin in the dog. Biol. Reprod. *19*:673.

161. Rodriguez-Gil, J. E., Montserrat, A., and Rigau, T. (1994): Effects of hypoosmotic incubation on acrosome and tail structure on canine spermatozoa. Theriogenology *42*:815.

162. Romagnoli, S. E., Camillo, F., Novellini, S., et al. (1996): Luteolytic effects of prostaglandin $F_{2\alpha}$ on day 8 to 19 corpora lutea in the bitch. Theriogenology *45*:397.

163. Roszel, J. F. (1975): Genital cytology of the bitch. Vet. Scope *19*:3.

164. Salmeri, K. R., Bloomberg, M. S., Scruggs, S. L., et al. (1991): Gonadectomy in immature dogs: Effects on skeletal, physical, and behavioral development. J. Am. Vet. Med. Assoc. *198*:1193.

165. Sankai, T., Endo, T., Kanayama, K., et al. (1991): Antiprogesterone compound, RU-486 administration to terminate pregnancy in dogs and cats. J. Vet. Med. Sci. *53*:1069.

166. Schardein, J. L., Reutner, T. F., Fitzgerald, J. E., et al. (1973): Canine teratogenesis with an estrogen antagonist. Teratology *7*:199.

167. Schnee, C. M. (1988): Untersuchungen zur Induktion retrograder Ejakulationen durch α-Rezeptorenblockade und fehlerhafte Samenentnahmemanipulationen beim Hund. d.m.v. Thesis, Tierärztliche Hochschule Hannover, pp. 1–112.

168. Schulze, H. and Barrack, E. R. (1987): Immunocytochemical localization of estrogen receptors in the normal male and female canine urinary tract and prostate. Endocrinology *121*:1773.

169. Schutte, A. P. (1967): Canine vaginal cytology. J. Small Anim. Pract. *8*:301.

170. Schwartz, E., Tornaben, J. A., and Boxill, G. C. (1969): Effects of chronic oral administration of a long-acting estrogen, quinestrol, to dogs. Toxicol. Appl. Pharmacol. *14*:487.

171. Scott-Moncrieff, J. C., Nelson, R. W., Bill, R. L., et al. (1990): Serum disposition of exogenous progesterone after intramuscular administration in bitches. Am. J. Vet. Res. *51*:893.

172. Selman, P. J., Wolfswinkel, J., and Mol, J. A. (1996): Binding specificity of medroxyprogesterone acetate and proligestone for the progesterone and glucocorticoid receptor in the dog. Steroids *61*:133.

173. Shille, V. M., Dorsey, D., and Thatcher, M.-J. (1984): Induction of abortion in the bitch with a synthetic prostaglandin analog. Am. J. Vet. Res. *45*:1295.

174. Shille, V. M., Thatcher, M. J., and Simmons, K. J. (1984): Efforts to induce estrus in the bitch, using pituitary gonadotropins. J. Am. Vet. Med. Assoc. *184*:1469.

175. Shille, V. M., Thatcher, M.-J., Lloyd, M. L., et al. (1989): Gonadotrophic control of follicular development and the use of exogenous gonadotrophins for induction of oestrus and ovulation in the bitch. J. Reprod. Fertil. (Suppl. 39):103.

176. Shimazu, Y., Yamada, S., Kawano, Y., et al. (1992): *In vitro* capacitation of canine spermatozoa. J. Reprod. Develop. *38*:67.

177. Silva, L. D. M., Onklin, K., and Verstegen, J. P. (1995): Cervical opening in relation to progesterone and oestradiol during heat in Beagle bitches. J. Reprod. Fertil. *104*:85.

178. Smith, M. S. and McDonald, L. E. (1974): Serum levels of luteinizing hormone and progesterone during the estrous cycle, pseudopregnancy and pregnancy in the dog. Endocrinology *94*:404.

179. Sokolowski, J. H. (1971): The effects of ovariectomy on pregnancy maintenance in the bitch. Lab. Anim. Sci. *21*:696.

180. Sokolowski, J. H. (1973): Reproductive features and patterns in the bitch. J. Am. Anim. Hosp. Assoc. *9*:71.

181. Sokolowski, J. H. and Geng, S. (1977): Effect of prostaglandin $F_{2\alpha}$-Tham in the bitch. J. Am. Vet. Med. Assoc. *170*:536.

182. Sokolowski, J. H. and Kasson, C. W. (1978): Effects of mibolerone on conception, pregnancy, parturition, and offspring in the Beagle. Am. J. Vet. Res. *39*:837.

183. Sokolowski, J. H. and Zimbelman, R. G. (1974): Canine reproduction: Effects of multiple treatments of medroxyprogesterone acetate on reproductive organs of the bitch. Am. J. Vet. Res. *35*:1285.

184. Sokolowski, J. H. and Zimbelman, R. G. (1976): Evaluation of selected compounds for estrus control in the bitch. Am. J. Vet. Res. *37*:939.

185. Sokolowski, J. H., Stover, D. G., and van Ravenswaay, F. (1977): Seasonal incidence of estrus and interestrous interval for bitches of seven breeds. J. Am. Vet. Med. Assoc. *171*:271.

186. Sokolowski, J. H., Zimbelman, R. G., and Goyings, L. S. (1973): Canine reproduction: Reproductive organs and related structures of the nonparous, parous, and postpartum bitch. Am. J. Vet. Res. *34*:1001.

187. Steinetz, B. G., Goldsmith, L. T., Harvey, H., et al. (1989): Serum relaxin and progesterone concentrations in pregnant, pseudopregnant, and ovariectomized, progestin-treated pregnant bitches: Detection of relaxin as a marker of pregnancy. Am. J. Vet. Res. *50*:68.

188. Taha, M. B. and Noakes, D. E. (1982): The effect of age and season of the year on testicular function in the dog, as determined by histological examination of the seminiferous tubules and the estimation of peripheral plasma testosterone concentrations. J. Small Anim. Pract. *23*:351.

189. Taha, M. B., Noakes, D. E., and Allen, W. E. (1982): Hemicastration and castration in the Beagle dog; the effects on libido, peripheral plasma testosterone concentrations, seminal characteristics and testicular function. J. Small Anim. Pract. *23*:279.

190. Telfer, E. and Gosden, R. G. (1987): A quantitative cytological study of polyovular follicles in mammalian ovaries with particular reference to the domestic bitch (*Canis familiaris*). J. Reprod. Fertil. *81*:137.

191. Teunissen, G. H. B. (1952): The development of endometritis in the dog and the effect of estradiol and progesterone on the uterus. Acta Endocrinol. *9*:407.

192. Thompson, D. L., Jr., Ewing, L. L., and Lasley, B. L. (1983): Oestrogen secretion by *in vitro* perfused testes: Species comparison and factors affecting short-term secretion. J. Endocrinol. *96*:97.

193. Thornton, D. A. K. (1967): Uterine cystic hyperplasia in a Siamese cat following treatment with medroxyprogesterone. Vet. Rec. *80*:380.

194. Thun, R., Watson, P., and Jackson, G. L. (1977): Induction of estrus and ovulation in the bitch, using exogenous gonadotropins. Am. J. Vet. Res. *38*:483.

195. Tyslowitz, R. and Dingemanse, E. (1941): Effect of large doses of estrogens on the blood picture of dogs. Endocrinology *29*:817.

196. Van der Weyden, G. C., Taverne, M. A. M., Okkens, A. C., et al. (1981): The intrauterine position of canine foetuses and their sequence of expulsion at birth. J. Small Anim. Pract. *22*:503.

197. Van Haaften, B., Dieleman, S. J., Okkens, A. C., et al. (1989): Timing the mating of dogs on the basis of blood progesterone concentration. Vet. Rec. *125*:524.

198. Varga, B. and Folly, G. (1977): Effects of prostaglandins on ovarian blood flow in the bitch. J. Reprod. Fertil. *51*:315.

199. Verhage, H. G., Abel, J. H., Jr., Tietz, W. J., Jr., et al. (1973): Development and maintenance of the oviductal epithelium during the estrous cycle in the bitch. Biol. Reprod. *9*:460.

200. Verhage, H. G., Abel, J. H., Jr., Tietz, W. J., Jr., et al. (1973): Estrogen-induced differentiation of the oviductal epithelium in prepubertal dogs. Biol. Reprod. *9*:475.

201. Vickery, B. and McRae, G. (1980): Effect of a synthetic prostaglandin analogue on pregnancy in Beagle bitches. Biol. Reprod. *22*:438.

202. Vincent, D. L., Kepic, T. A., Lathrop, J. C., et al. (1979): Testosterone regulation of luteinizing hormone secretion in the male dog. Int. J. Androl. *2*:241.

203. Wales, R. G. and White, I. G. (1965): Some observations on the chemistry of dog semen. J. Reprod. Fertil. *9*:69.

204. Watts, J. R. and Wright, P. J. (1995): Investigating uterine disease in the bitch: Uterine cannulation for cytology, microbiology and hysteroscopy. J. Small Anim. Pract. *36*:201.

205. Weikel, J. H., Jr. and Nelson, L. W. (1977): Problems in evaluating chronic toxicity of contraceptive steroids in dogs. J. Toxicol. Env. Health *3*:167.

206. Weissbach, L. and Ibach, B. (1976): Quantitative parameters for light microscopic assessment of the tubuli seminiferi. Fertil. Steril. *27*:836.

207. Wilson, M. S. (1993): Non-surgical intrauterine artificial insemination in bitches using frozen semen. J. Reprod. Fertil. (Suppl. 47):307.

208. Winter, M., Falvo, R. E., Schanbacker, B. D., et al. (1983): Regulation of gonadotropin secretion in the male dog. J. Androl. *4*:319.

209. Winter, M., Pirmann, J., Falvo, R. E., et al. (1982): Steroidal control of gonadotrophin secretion in the orchiectomized dog. J. Reprod. Fertil. *64*:449.

210. Woodall, P. F., Pavlov, P., and Tolley, L. K. (1993): Comparative dimensions of testes, epididymides and spermatozoa of Australian dingoes (*Canis familiaris dingo*) and domestic dogs (*Canis familiaris familiaris*): some effects of domestication. Aust. J. Zool. *41*:133.

211. Wright, P. J. (1980): The induction of oestrus and ovulation in the bitch using pregnant mare serum gonadotrophin and human chorionic gonadotrophin. Aust. Vet. J. *56*:137.

212. Wright, P. J. (1982): The induction of oestrus in the bitch using daily injections of pregnant mare serum gonadotrophin. Aust. Vet. J. *59*:123.

213. Wright, P. J. and Parry, B. W. (1989): Cytology of the canine reproductive system. Vet. Clin. North Am., Small Anim. Pract. *19*:851.

214. Yamada, S., Shimazu, Y., Kawaji, H., et al. (1992): Maturation, fertilization, and development of dog oocytes *in vitro*. Biol. Reprod. *46*:853.

215. Yeager, A. E., Mohammed, H. O., Meyers-Wallen, V., et al. (1992): Ultrasonographic appearance of the

uterus, placenta, fetus, and fetal membranes throughout accurately timed pregnancy in Beagles. Am. J. Vet. Res. *53*:342.

216. Zajc, I., Mellersh, C., Kelly, E. P., et al. (1994): A new method of paternity testing for dogs, based on microsatellite sequences. Vet. Rec. *135*:545.

217. Zirkin, B. R. and Strandberg, J. D. (1984): Quantitative changes in the morphology of the aging canine prostate. Anat. Rec. *208*:207.

References Added in Proof

218. Hoffmann, B. and Schuler, G. (2000): Receptor blockers - general aspects with respect to their use in domestic animal reproduction. Anim. Reprod. Sci. *60-61*:295.

219. Luvoni, G. C. and Grioni, A. (2000): Determination of gestational age in medium and small size bitches using ultrasonographic fetal measurements. J. Small Anim. Pract. *41*:292.

220. Melniczek, J. R., Dambach, D., Prociuk, U., et al. (1999): Sry-negative XX sex reversal in a family of Norwegian Elkhounds. J. Vet. Intern. Med. *13*:564.

Reproductive Patterns of Cats*

M. H. PINEDA

17

INTRODUCTION

Little is known about the reproductive biology of the domestic cat. In this regard, the domestic cat is a neglected species. In the last few years, considerable attention has been paid to the endocrinology of the reproductive cycle and to the mechanisms involved in the ovulatory process of the queen, the female domestic cat. The male cat, called a tom, has not yet received the same level of attention. Consequently, little is known about its reproductive physiology.

*Much information concerned with reproduction in cats has been presented in Chapter 2 (Pituitary Gland), Chapter 7 (The Biology of Sex), Chapter 8 (Male Reproductive System), Chapter 9 (Female Reproductive System), Chapter 10 (Artificial Insemination), and Chapter 11 (Patterns of Reproduction). The reader is encouraged to refer to these chapters in order to permit conciseness.

The queen will undergo a series of nonovulatory estruses in each breeding season. Although follicles will develop and secrete estrogens during each of these estruses, ovulation, in general, does not occur unless the queen is mated. The glans penis of the tom is covered with corneal spines and, during mating, these penile spines are essential to elicit the ovulatory surge of luteinizing hormone (LH) in the queen. However, queens exposed to visual and auditory contact with toms may ovulate spontaneously, even without coital or mechanical stimulation of the cervix. Toms mate frequently with the estrous queen. The number of matings determines the magnitude of the ovulatory surge of LH as well as the number of oocytes released by the queen.

PUBERTY AND SEXUAL MATURITY

The queen reaches puberty at 8 to 13 months of age (Table 17-1), but there is considerable variation between breeds. Puberty may be reached as early as 5 months or as late as 18 months of age depending on season and body weight. Queens heavier than 2.5 kg tend to have their first overt estrus at 5 to 6 months of age. Toms are thought to reach puberty at about the same age as the queen; however, the age of puberty of the tom cat has not been accurately determined, probably because of the difficulties in collecting semen with an artificial vagina from untrained, pubertal toms. The development of electroejaculation protocols for the collection of semen from the domestic cat in the late 1980s may promote and facilitate studies in this regard. Environmental factors may also influence the age of puberty in domestic cats, and it is

Table 17-1 Onset[a] of Puberty in the Queen

Breed	Average Age in Months
Abyssinian	11.3
Birman	11.3
Burmese	7.7
Colourpoint	13.0
Persian	10.4
Siamese	8.9
Long-haired domestic	11.0
Short-haired domestic	9.4

[a]Survey data.

Adapted from: J. E. Jemmett and J. M. Evans, J. Small Anim. Pract. *18*:31, 1977.

thought that free-roaming cats, because of exposure to the photoperiod, reach puberty earlier than animals confined in breeding colonies.

BREEDING SEASON

In the Northern Hemisphere, domestic cats have two main breeding seasons per year, one in late Winter and early Spring (January to March) and the other in late Summer or early Fall (August to early October). Environmental factors, particularly the amount of light, influence the length of the breeding season. The greatest incidence of estruses occurs in February and March in the Northern Hemisphere, while in temperate climates, matings may occur throughout the year. Cats maintained in colonies under controlled light schedules (12 hours of light:12 hours of darkness or 14 hours of light:10 hours of darkness) cycle throughout the year, yet exhibit peak periods of estruses in March, July, and October.

Female cats tend to have a definite nonbreeding season beginning in late October and extending through December. Household cats are more likely to behave, with regard to their breeding season, as cats kept within a colony.

After puberty, tomcats mate and ejaculate throughout the year without any discernible seasonal effect on the number of spermatozoa or fertility of the ejaculate.

THE ESTROUS CYCLE

The queen is seasonally polyestrous and an induced ovulator. As a consequence, the characteristics of the reproductive cycle of the queen are greatly influenced by mating (Fig. 17-1). The **nonmated queen** displays a series of nonovulatory estruses, each lasting an average of 7 days, with a range of 3 to 20 days. Each of these nonmated estruses is followed by an interestrous period of nonsexual receptivity, lasting an average of 10 days, with a range of 8 to 30 days (Table 17-2, Fig. 17-1). Values reported for the length of the nonmated estrus and interestrous intervals vary considerably, probably because it is difficult to accurately assess the onset and end of estrus solely by behavioral signs in the absence of a tom (see queen responses in Table 17-3). The length of the **nonmated** estrus and the interestrous interval are also influenced by breed, environmental conditions, and social interactions with other queens. Nonmated queens maintained under controlled light and temperature display an average of 13 estruses per year, with a range of four to 25 estruses. The average time elapsed from the onset of one nonovulatory estrus to the next is 17 days.

Follicular growth occurs rather rapidly during proestrus in the queen. Proestrus lasts from 1 to 3 days, before the onset of behavioral estrus, and it is associated with increased secretion of estradiol-17β and elevated blood levels of estrogens, which may reach peak values as high as 100 pg of estradiol-17β per ml. Due to the short period of follicular growth, the phase of proestrus is difficult to detect clinically.

Blood levels of estrogens decline during the first 5 days of estrus, as the follicles reach a mature stage. The follicles appear to retain their capability to respond to the ovulatory surges of LH should mating occur during the period of

Table 17-2 Length of the Reproductive Cycle of the Queen

Stage	Average (Days)	Range (Days)
Estrus	7	3 to 20
Interestrus		
Nonmated	10	8 to 30
Sterile-mated (pseudopregnancy)	45	30 to 70
Anestrus	90	30 to 210

Table 17-3   *Patterns of Sexual Behavior of the Queen and Tom*

Stage of the Cycle	Queen Response	Tom Response
Onset of proestrus (lasts for 1 to 3 days).	Rubbing of head and neck against objects; rolling on the floor. Refuses advances of the male; does not stand and does not allow intromission.	Shows interest, sniffs or attempts to sniff the female body, and in particular the anogenital region. Mounting is attempted.
Estrus	Responds by treading and crouching with her forequarters pressed to the ground. May vocalize for prolonged periods. When approached by the male or when stroked on the back shows lordosis, lateral deviation of the tail, and presentation of the perineal region with exposure of the vulva. Allows grasping the skin of the neck and mounting by the male. Minor vulvar discharge may be observed, but in general there are no conspicuous changes in the size or appearance of the external genitalia.	Intensely attracted to the queen; sniffing, scratching, and grooming. Bites the skin of the neck of the queen and mounts with vigorous pelvic thrusts leading to intromission. Licks the female's anogenital region.
Anestrus or interestrus	Ignores the male or shows defensive spitting, hisses, and fights the male with paw-swipes.	Little or no interest in the queen.

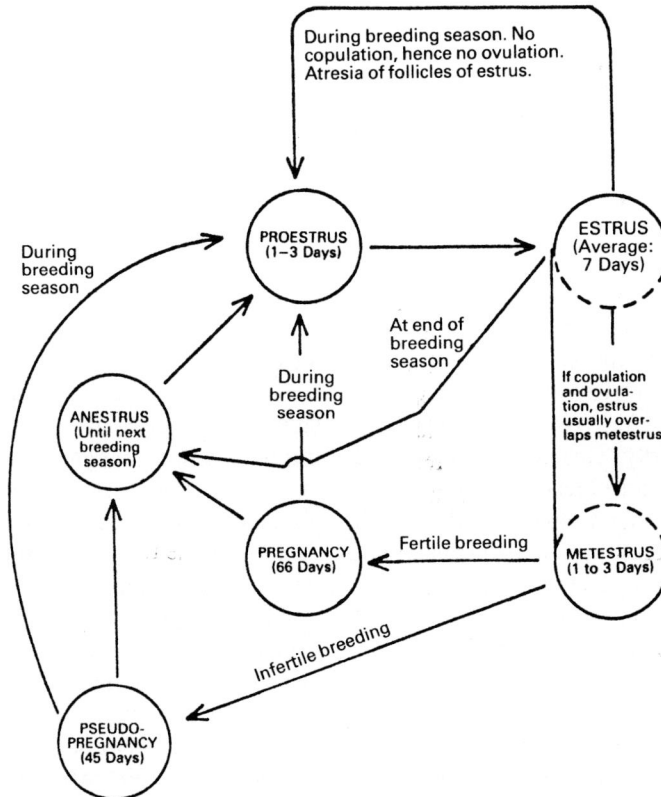

Fig. 17-1. The estrous cycle of the queen.

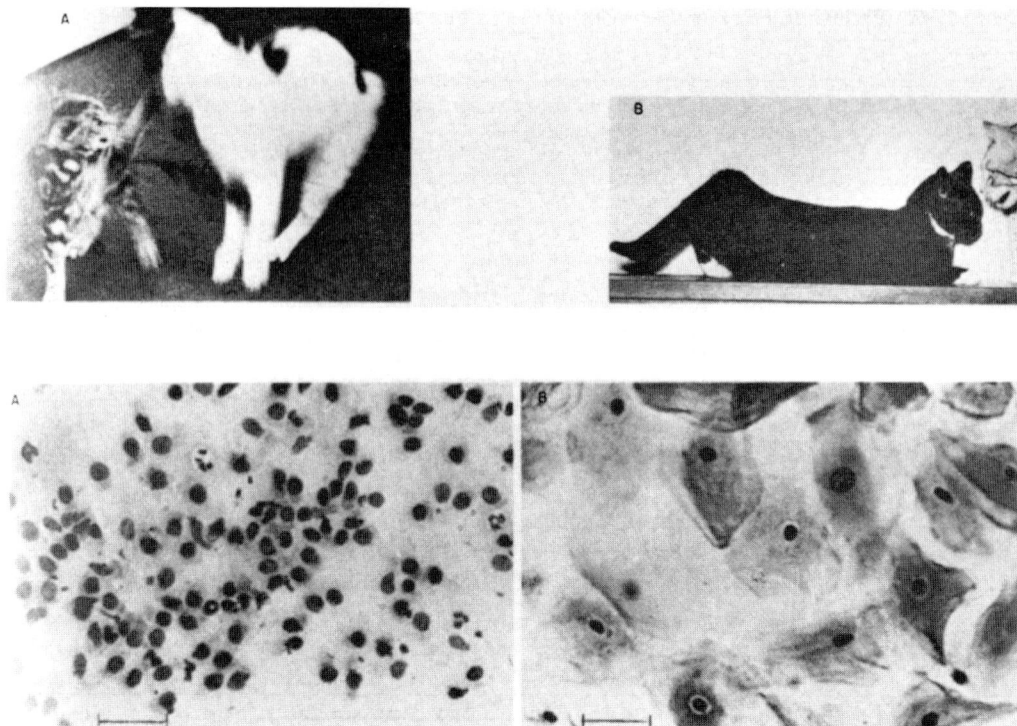

Fig. 17-2. **A.** Aggressive refusal reaction of anestrous or ovariectomized female cat. The queen is striking at the male, which is leaping away. **A′.** Typical anestrous vaginal smear. Only basal cells and leukocytes are seen. **B.** Receptive reaction by the queen when in estrus or when treated with estrogen. Estrual crouch and lordosis posture are adopted in presence of a male. **B′.** Estrous vaginal smear: Large cornified cells with pyknotic nuclei and perinuclear halos are seen. Scale 100 μm. (From: R. P. Michael, *In:* Handbook of Physiology, Section 7, Vol. II, Part I, edited by R. O. Greep and E. B. Astwood. Washington, D.C., American Physiological Society, 1973, p. 189).

sexual receptivity. The follicles that have reached the mature stage during a given estrus undergo atresia if the queen is not mated in that estrus, and the blood levels of estrogens, as well as the intensity of the associated behavioral signs, decline rapidly. This process is repeated several times during the breeding season if mating does not occur. A new wave of follicles will develop at each proestrus and the beginning of the subsequent estrus. Blood levels of progesterone remain at basal levels, less than 0.5 ng/ml of blood, during these nonovulatory estruses.

Mating Behavior

The behavioral responses of estrous queens are recognized with ease when the queen is exposed to the tom. The tom also displays a characteristic behavioral pattern when confronted with an estrous queen (Table 17-3, Fig. 17-2A and B). During the breeding season, the behavior of the male changes drastically. The male becomes aggressive and roams great distances, particularly at night, because cats are nocturnal. If a female in the neighborhood is in proestrus or estrus, males detect this by an olfactory mechanism involving pheromones. A male may guard a female for days or weeks, or sometimes several males are in intense competition for acceptance by the female. This may lead to destructive attacks by the males on each other. The owners of cats should be warned of this hazard, and if a female is to be bred, she should be housed with the male of choice and not allowed to run at will. If the male and female are to be housed together during the breeding period, the female should be brought to the male after he has had several days to become accustomed to his surroundings. Unfamiliar surroundings often prevent the mating response even in sexually experienced and active males.

The estrous queen readily stands and accepts mounting, neck biting by the male, and intromission. During intromission, particularly during thrusting by the male or during withdrawal of the penis from the vagina, the queen emits a loud, piercing cry, sometimes referred to as the 'mating cry'. Coitus is relatively brief and may

last up to half a minute. Experienced and vigorous males may intromit and thrust several times during a single copulation. If left unrestricted, as in free-mating situations, toms may attempt to copulate within minutes after penile withdrawal. Queens have been observed to allow multiple matings, 10 times or more in a few hours. It is not yet clear, however, whether the tom actually ejaculates each time that he copulates with the queen.

Copulation with either fertile or sterile vasectomized males induces the release of the ovulatory surge of LH in the queen. The magnitude of the surge and subsequent levels of LH in the blood are greatly influenced by the number of matings (Fig. 17-3, Table 17-4). In self-paced matings, maximal levels of LH are reached within 2 hours after six to eight matings. The corneal spines of the tom play an important role in eliciting the vaginal and possibly cervical stimulation, which results in the release of LH from the pituitary gland. The corneal spines of the penis of the adult tom are prominent, vary in length from 0.2 to 0.8 mm, and are directed caudally toward the base of the penis. The penile spines may also play a role in preventing the premature withdrawal of the penis from the vagina of queens that attempt to separate from the copulating male.

The ovary of the queen is richly innervated with predominantly adrenergic nerves and relatively few cholinergic fibers. This substantial intrinsic innervation of the ovary, particularly with the sympathetic, adrenergic innervation, apparently is not directly involved in follicular growth and ovulation in the queen. However,

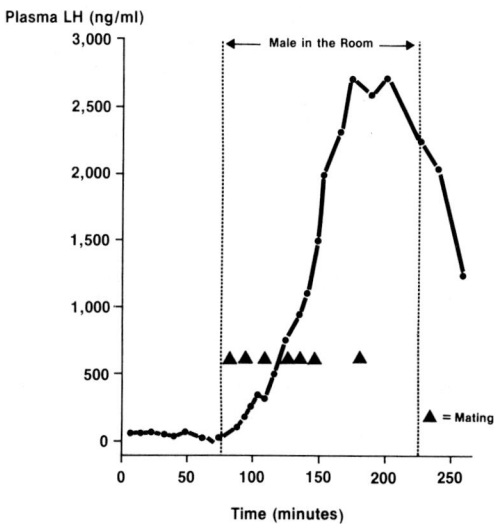

Fig. 17-3. Mean cumulative plasma levels of luteinizing hormone (LH) in two estrous queens permitted self-paced matings. Ovine-ovine LH radioimmunoassay system using ovine and rat purified LH preparations and cat pituitary extract as reference. (Drawn from data in: L. M. Johnson and V. L. Gay, Endocrinology *109*:247, 1981).

Table 17-4   Incidence of Ovulation and Serum LH Peak in Cats Following Single or Multiple Copulations on Day 3 of Estrus

Treatment	Ratio of Queens Ovulating (%)	LH Peak (ng/ml)[a]
Exposed but not mounted by the male	0/2 (0)	1.0 ± 0.8
Mounted without intromission	0/4 (0)	4.1 ± 1.1
One copulation	9/18 (50)	23.9 ± 5.8
Four copulations in a 4-hr period	23/23 (100)	88.9 ± 14.8
Eight to 12 copulations in a 4-hr period	13/13 (100)	120.5 ± 23.8

[a]Mean ± SEM.
Adapted from: P. W. Concannon et al., Biol. Reprod. *23*:111, 1980.

adrenergic innervation seems to play a role in the control of progesterone secretion.

Ovulation occurs 24 to 50 hours after mating. The number of follicles that ovulate and the number of oocytes released are dependent upon the number of matings and may be related to the day of estrus, since ovulation is more likely to occur after the second day of estrus. Mounting by the male without intromission is not a sufficient stimulus to induce the ovulatory surge of LH (Table 17-4). A single mating induces ovulation in only 50% of the queens, yet increasing the number beyond four copulations within a 4-hour period does not improve the ovulatory response of the queen (Table 17-4).

Ovulation in the queen can also be induced by repeated mechanical stimulation of the cervix via the vagina, but the ovulatory response is erratic. The administration of hCG in doses of 250 IU on the first and second days of estrus reportedly induces ovulation in more than 85% of queens. Ovulatory responses can also be induced in estrous queens by exogenous GnRH (Table 17-5) and may occur spontaneously in estrous queens caged in proximity to one another or when exposed to males in the same room.

Blood levels of estradiol-17β decline rapidly from about 50 pg/ml of serum at the time of the ovulatory surge of LH to less than 20 pg/ml by 96 hours after coitus (Fig. 17-4). Corpora lutea form within 1 to 3 days (metestrus) after coitus and progesterone levels in the blood rise rapidly from baseline levels of less than 1.0 ng/ml to

reach 2 to 3 ng/ml (Fig. 17-4). Blood levels of progesterone reach peak levels of 15 to 90 ng/ml 15 to 25 days after coitus. The period of metestrus, only of academic significance in the cat, is partially included within the period of estrus.

Pseudopregnancy

Queens that are induced to ovulate by mechanical stimulation of the vagina, exogenous hormones, or by matings with sterile males become pseudopregnant. Pseudopregnancy lasts an average of 45 days, with a range of 30 to 70 days. Up to about day 30, levels of progesterone in the blood of pseudopregnant queens are similar to that of pregnant queens. Progesterone levels then decline in the pseudopregnant queen and become significantly lower than those found in the pregnant cat. Progesterone levels return to baseline levels of less than 1.0 ng/ml of blood by about day 40 of pseudopregnancy. If pseudopregnancy is induced early in the breeding season, the queen may display one or more estruses during that breeding season. If the pseudopregnancy is induced late in the breeding season, the queen enters into a period of anestrus lasting until the next breeding season.

The corpora lutea of pseudopregnant and pregnant queens are resistant to the luteolytic actions of prostaglandins. Repeated treatments with prostaglandin $F_{2\alpha}$ cause a transient decline in blood levels of progesterone but do not induce abortion in pregnant queens or shorten the length of pseudopregnancy. Thus, the uterus does not appear to exert any control on the function of the corpora lutea of the queen. The anatomic features of the ovarian and uterine vasculature of the queen do not favor the transfer of luteolytic substances, if any, from the uterus to the arteries supplying the ovary. Furthermore, bilateral hysterectomy or ligation of uterine blood vessels does not alter the duration of functional activity of hormonally-induced corpora lutea of queens. Corpora lutea of pseudopregnant queens produce progesterone in comparable amounts to that of pregnant queens up to about day 30 of pseudopregnancy. Therefore, it is doubtful that the nonpregnant uterus influences luteal function in the pseudopregnant

Table 17-5 Ovulatory Response of Anestrous and Estrous Queens after a Single Intramuscular Injection of GnRH

Dose of GnRH (μg)	Number of Queens Ovulating (%)	
	Anestrous	Estrous
5	0/4 (0)	1/4 (25%)
10	0/4 (0)	2/4 (50%)
25	0/4 (0)	4/4 (100%)

Adapted from: P. K. Chakraborty, et al., *Lab. Anim. Sci.* *29:*338, 1979.

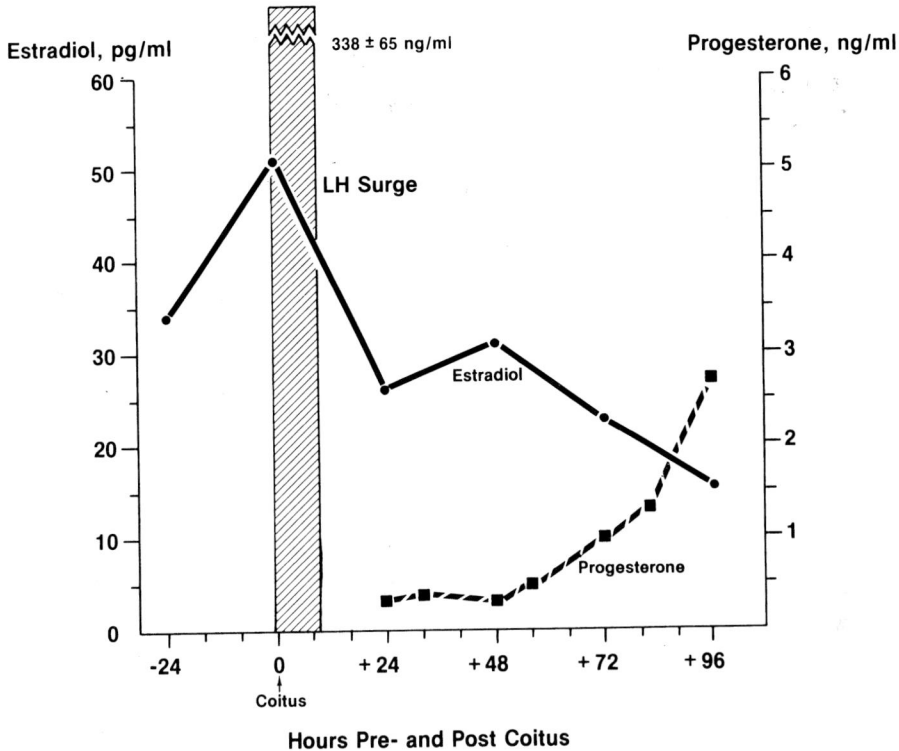

Fig. 17-4. Pre- and postcoital changes in **estradiol-17β** and postovulatory changes in **progesterone** in the blood of the queen. (Adapted from: D. H. Banks and G. Stabenfeldt, Biol. Reprod. *26:*603, 1982).

queen. However, the corpora lutea of the pseudopregnant queen undergo gradual retrogressive changes after day 40 of pseudopregnancy. It is possible then that the ovulatory surge of LH provides enough luteotropic support for the corpus luteum to remain functional for 30 days. In pregnant queens, the luteotropic stimulus from developing embryos may provide additional support for luteal maintenance beyond day 30 of pregnancy.

Pseudopregnancy in the queen is not associated with the profound, organic, and behavioral changes observed in the bitch (see Chapter 16) and seldom leads to lactation and nesting behavior. However, pseudopregnant queens undergo vaginal, uterine, and oviductal changes induced by the progesterone secreted by the corpora lutea.

The tubular genitalia of the queen respond to the gonadal hormones estradiol and progesterone in a manner similar to that described for the bitch. During anestrus, the oviductal and uterine epithelia are low cuboidal cells, and the uterine glands are straight and barely extend into the mucosa. At proestrus and estrus, rising levels of estrogens stimulate the development of the oviductal and uterine epithelia, which increase in both height and mitotic activity. The oviductal secretory and ciliated cells also differentiate under estrogenic stimulation. After ovulation, the endometrial glands increase in diameter and coil under the influence of progesterone secreted by the developing corpora lutea. As progesterone levels increase, endometrial glandular development continues, leading to the secretion of "uterine milk" to nourish the preimplantation embryos.

VAGINAL CYTOLOGY

The vaginal smear of the queen is less distinct and defined than in the bitch. During anestrus, the vaginal epithelium consists only of

Table 17-6 *Cytological Changes in the Vaginal Smear[a] of the Queen*

Follicular Phase (Proestrus and Estrus, Prior to Ovulation)	Luteal Phase and Interestrus (Estrus after Ovulation, Pregnancy, Pseudopregnancy)
Absence of noncellular debris (clearing of the vaginal smear) is the earliest sign of follicular activity.	A few anuclear cells may be found.
Increased proportion of **anuclear, cornified cells** (from 5 to 40% of total cell population), remaining around 40% through the first day of the luteal phase.	Superficial and intermediate cells are the dominant type (>80% of the total cell population).
Intermediate cells, partially cornified with intact nucleus, progressively decrease from 45 to 6% from the first to the fourth day of the follicular phase.	Parabasal cells are present; their relative percentage varies between 1% and 6%.
Superficial cells, partially cornified with signs of nuclear degeneration, remain at about 50% throughout estrus.	
Parabasal, noncornified cells are not found.	
Erythrocytes are rarely seen.	

[a]Cotton swabs moistened with saline solution were used to obtain material for the smears. Smears were fixed with 90% ethanol, air-dried, and stained with Giemsa.
Adapted from: V. M. Shille, et al., Biol. Reprod. *21*:953, 1979.

a few layers of cells. The anestrous smear contains nucleated basal epithelial cells and leukocytes. Cornified cells are absent or only present in small numbers (Fig. 17-2A'). Under the influence of estrogens, the vaginal epithelium thickens and becomes cornified in its superficial layers. During the follicular phase, prior to ovulation, the vaginal smear consists mainly of anuclear cornified cells and intermediate and superficial partially cornified cells (Fig. 17-2B', Table 17-6). After ovulation, during the luteal phase, the superficial and intermediate cells become predominant, although a few parabasal cells may be found (Table 17-6).

The mechanical stimulation exerted during the collection of vaginal samples for smears may induce ovulation in some queens. This possibility must be considered when repeated vaginal smears are to be taken from a queen.

OOGENESIS

Sexual differentiation occurs in the fetus around day 30 of pregnancy and continues in the newborn kitten until day 37 of age.[59] Oocytes in meiotic prophase can be observed in the fetal queen from day 50 of pregnancy to about day 40 of the postnatal period, when it appears that all of the oocytes have reached the dictyate stage of meiosis.[59] Frequency of polyovular follicles is relatively low for the queen.

FERTILIZATION AND OVIDUCTAL TRANSPORT

The oocytes of the queen are ovulated as secondary oocytes. As in the other domestic species, fertilization occurs in the ampullary region of the oviduct. The embryos or the unfertilized oocytes migrate toward the uterus over a 4- to 5-day period, reaching the uterus by day 6 after ovulation. Since ovulation in the queen is induced by mating, spermatozoa are usually in the oviducts by the time the oocytes are released from follicles. Thus, infertility due to aging of the gametes caused by asynchronous matings is seldom a problem in the queen. The ejaculated spermatozoa of the tom must be capacitated to fertilize the oocytes. Capacitation requires a 1- to 2-hour exposure to the fluids secreted by the genital tract of the queen. Epididymal spermatozoa are capable of fertilizing the queen's oocytes *in vitro*, suggesting that the accessory sex glands of the tom contribute a decapacitation factor or factors to the semen at the time of ejaculation (see Chapter 7, Table 7-5).

***Table 17-7   Reproductive Performance in a
Cat[a] Colony***

Mean gestation length, days	66
Range, days	62–70
Mean litter size	4.3
Mean percentage of kittens reared	84.0
Mean interval between litters, months	5.2
Average number of litters/cat per year	2.2
Average age of replacement of brood queen, years	6.0

[a]Controlled light (12-hour light/darkness, 150 Lux), humidity (55 ± 10%), and temperature (23 ± 2°C).
  Adapted from: H. Hurni, *Z. Versuchstierkd. 23:*102, 1981.

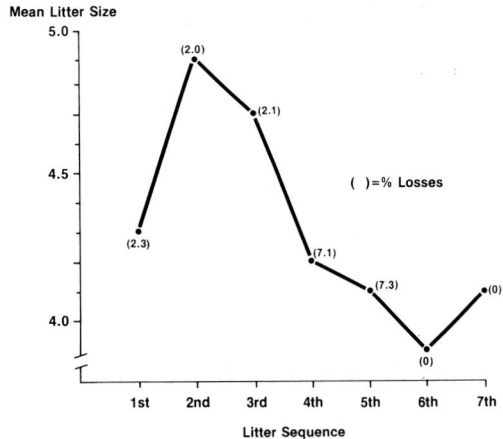

Fig. 17-5. Breeding performance of cats in a breeding colony. Queens were approximately 10 months old (n = 61 queens) when first introduced to the colony, and the total length of the observation period was 2.6 years. (Drawn from data in: H. Hurni, Z. Versuchstierkd. *23:*102, 1981).

Transuterine migration of embryos is frequent in the queen and serves the purpose of equalizing the number of developing fetuses by distributing embryos between the uterine horns prior to implantation.

PREGNANCY

Counting from the first mating of the queen, the length of pregnancy in cat colonies is 66 days on the average, with a range of 62 to 70 days (Table 17-7). Mean litter size in cat colonies is 4.3 and an average of 84% of the kittens are successfully reared. In breeding colonies, under controlled environmental conditions, the average number of litters per cat per year is 2.2, and the mean interval between litters is 5.2 months (Table 17-7). The average litter size varies over the reproductive life of the queen (Fig. 17-5).

In the cat, placentation is zonary or girdle in nature. By apposition of tissues, the queen's placenta is lamellar and chorioallantoic. By maternal-fetal blood flow, the queen's placenta represents a crosscurrent type.[55] Implantation is believed to occur between 13 to 14 days after the first fertile mating. The low aromatase activity in the trophoblasts of the cat embryo suggests that estrogens do not play a role in implantation. The levels of estradiol-17β and of progesterone in the blood of pregnant queens are not different from those of pseudopregnant queens up to about day 30 of pregnancy. After day 30 of pregnancy, levels of progesterone in the blood are higher in pregnant than in pseudopregnant queens. Levels of progesterone in the blood of pregnant queens begin to decline gradually during the latter stages of pregnancy, returning to a baseline of less than 1.0 ng of progesterone per ml of blood at the time of parturition. Prolactin levels remain relatively constant during pregnancy, increase several fold 2 to 3 days before parturition, and remain elevated during the first 4 weeks after parturition. Lactation and kitten's suckling appear to be powerful inhibitors of ovarian follicular development and of estrus in the queen. The interestrous interval for lactating queens is usually 120 days (66 days of gestation plus 54 days of lactation). On the average, estrus occurs 18 days after weaning of the kittens. However, there is considerable variation between queens in the time of return to estrus after weaning, particularly for queens not maintained in breeding colonies and, therefore, exposed to variable environmental conditions.

Luteal progesterone secretion is needed for the major part of pregnancy in the queen. Bilateral ovariectomy causes abortion when performed before day 49 of gestation. After day 50 of pregnancy, abortion does not occur following bilateral ovariectomy. Gestation continues to term, apparently without harmful effects to the kittens. Exogenous progesterone can maintain pregnancy in queens bilaterally ovariectomized prior to day 49 of pregnancy.

Relaxin has been detected in the blood of pregnant queens by day 25 of pregnancy. Relaxin levels plateau by day 35 of pregnancy, remain high during most of the gestation, and decline gradually beginning 10 days before parturition. Relaxin is undetectable in the blood within 24 hours after parturition. Determination of blood levels of relaxin may serve as a diagnostic tool to differentiate between pregnant and pseudopregnant queens because blood levels of relaxin are undetectable in pseudopregnant queens.

Pregnancy Diagnosis

Abdominal palpation allows the detection of fetuses from day 20 to 30 of pregnancy. Pregnancy can also be diagnosed in the queen by ultrasound or by X-ray examination. The same considerations described in Chapter 16 for the X-ray examination of the pregnant bitch are applicable to the pregnant queen. Increased levels of progesterone >5.0 ng/ml in the blood of queens 6 days after mating with a known fertile tom is accurate for diagnosis of timed pregnancies in the queen. The measurement of progesterone levels is of no value to distinguish between pregnant and pseudopregnant queens.

THE TOM

Other than scattered publications of studies on specialized aspects of spermatogenesis, such as on differentiation of spermatids, there is no published information concerning the duration of the cycle of the seminiferous epithelium and of spermatogenesis, daily sperm production, epididymal transport, spermatozoal reserves, or daily spermatozoal output for the domestic tom. The male kitten is born with the testicles already descended and located in the external inguinal ring or in the scrotum. After puberty, the tom is capable of mating and releasing fertile ejaculates year-round. Toms usually approach the queen cautiously, assessing her reactions. When the queen is receptive, the tom will approach her from the rear and grasp the skin of her neck with his teeth, positioning himself for mounting and

intromission. Ejaculation appears to be fast, lasting only a few seconds, and is nearly simultaneous with intromission. Toms tend to intromit the penis in the vagina several times during mating, but it is not clear whether or not they ejaculate during each intromission. Similar responses are observed in some toms when semen is collected with an artificial vagina. Frequency of intromission during mating and the number of copulations of the tom with the estrous queen may be an evolutionary trait. The small volume and relatively low numbers of spermatozoa in the tom's ejaculate may have evolved to prevent depletion of the spermatozoal reserves, in view of the frequent matings needed for ovulation of the queen. Multiple matings may ensure the release of sufficient amounts of GnRH conducive to an adequate ovulatory surge of LH in the queen.

The deposition of cat odor by urine spraying is a form of territorial marking pronounced in wild felids, but is also present in the domestic tom. Tom cat odor is androgen dependent and can be suppressed by castration. Urine spraying by the domestic tom may also have an estrous synchronizing effect on the queen. Pheromones produced by the convoluted tubules of the kidneys and possibly by the anal glands of the tom, which appear to be added to the urine during spraying, facilitate the expression of behavioral estrus in the queen. Valeric acid in the vaginal secretions from estrous queens has been suggested as a candidate pheromone which would synchronize estrus between queens. Valeric acid may also attract and stimulate mating behavior in the tom.

Toms and queens, when exposed to the smell of bruised leaves of catnip or cat mint (*Nepeta cataria L*), develop a characteristic behavioral response, which includes sniffing, licking, and cheek and body rubbing. An active compound, nepetalactone, has been isolated from catnip. This compound induces hallucinogenic effects in cats, which mimic the estrous-like responses induced by pheromones. The behavioral response of the cats to catnip is an autosomal dominant trait that appears not to be correlated with breed or color of the cat. The response to catnip intensifies with age and may not be evident until the kittens are 3-months or older. Cat owners buy catnip as dry leaves or as an extract in spray cans in supermarkets and pet shops, and they often provide the catnip as a treat to their pets. However, it is doubtful that catnip has any estrous-facilitating effects.

Little is known about the reproductive endocrinology and blood levels of reproductive hormones in the tom cat. Table 17-8 shows the concentration of testosterone and androstenedione in the blood of the domestic tom. Both testosterone and androstenedione decrease rapidly after castration.

Semen Collection

Semen can be collected from tom cats with an artificial vagina (AV) or by electroejaculation (EE). Although an AV can be easily assembled from inexpensive components (see Fig. 10-10A and B and Fig. 17-6A and B), the AV method is not practical for clinical use in veterinary medicine because toms are not easily trained to ejaculate in the AV and often require a prolonged period of training. Only 10 to 20% of toms can be trained to ejaculate in the AV. Furthermore, estrous queens, either naturally cycling or hormonally-induced, are needed to stimulate the mating behavior for training toms to ejaculate in the AV (Fig 17-6A and B).

A regimen of electrical stimulation has been developed[23] to collect semen from the anesthetized tom. Even though general anesthesia must be given prior to electrical stimulation, electroejaculation is the method of choice for the routine collection of semen from tom cats. Semen can be collected consistently and reliably from any tom by EE, and estrous queens are not needed to successfully complete the collection. These characteristics make the method of electroejaculation suitable for most clinical settings. Figure 17-7 shows semen collection by electroejaculation in an anesthetized tom cat. Table 17-9 displays the seminal characteristics of ejaculates obtained with an AV and by EE, when these two methods of seminal collections were applied to the same toms. The method of electroejaculation is safe and can be used repeatedly without apparent harmful effects to the tom.[72] Seminal samples obtained with an AV have lower volume and pH and tend to have more spermatozoa per ejaculate than semen collected by electroejaculation (Table 17-9). The larger volume of semen collected by electroejaculation is apparently due to the secretions contributed by the prostate and bulbourethral glands, the only accessory sex glands in the tom cat. However, through use of an appropriate regimen of electrical stimulation,[23] electroejaculation produces semen that is comparable to seminal samples obtained with an AV. An assay to evaluate spermatozoal viability based on the exclusion of a micromolar concentration of eosin B has been developed[23] for cat semen, but critical studies to correlate seminal parameters with the fertility of an ejaculate have not been done for the cat. Thus, there are no experimentally tested and reliable guidelines for the clinician to assess the potential fertility of an ejaculate and the breeding soundness of a given tom.

Insemination of queens which have been induced to ovulate with exogenous gonadotropins using freshly collected and diluted semen produces litters with numbers of kittens comparable to those obtained by natural matings. Ejacu-

---

Table 17-8   Testosterone and Androstenedione Concentrations in the Blood of the Domestic Cat

	Testosterone (ng/ml)	Androstenedione (ng/ml)
Intact[a]	6.33 ± 1.81	7.10 ± 2.98
Castrated[b]		
24 hours after castration	0.03 ± 0.19	1.16 ± 0.51
96 hours after castration	0.08 ± 0.11	0.29 ± 0.43

[a]Hourly samples over 24 hours during two seasons of the year from four intact males. Mean ± SD.
[b]From two castrated males.
Adapted from data in: I. P. Johnstone, et al., Anim. Reprod. Sci. *7*:363, 1984.

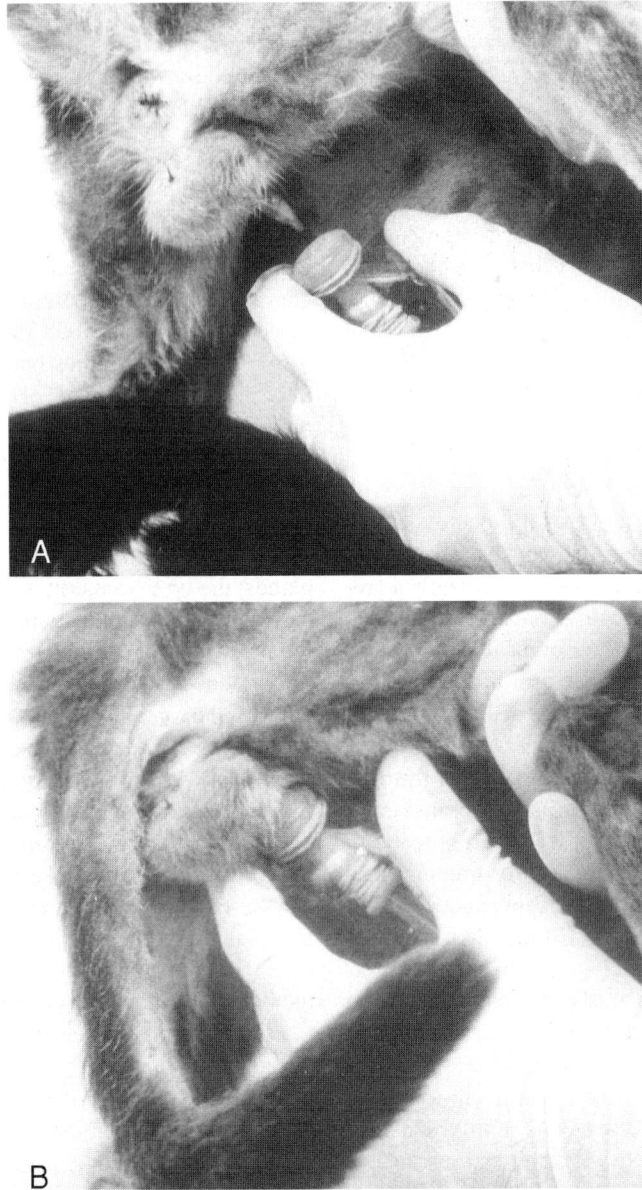

Fig. 17-6. Collection of semen from the tom with an artificial vagina (AV). Notice that the AV was constructed using a glass vial so that the semen could be visualized in the AV. The right leg of the tom is raised to facilitate the photography of the process. **A.** After the tom mounts and grips the queen's neck, the AV is placed over the erect penis. **B.** The tom is allowed to thrust and ejaculate in the AV.

lates collected from toms with an AV appear to have enough spermatozoa to inseminate several queens, and artificial insemination with frozen-stored semen has been reported. The rate of conception and litter size obtained with frozen semen is low, with decreased fertilization and embryonic cleavage rates. Thus, procedures for cryopreservation of cat semen need to be improved.

After vasectomy, the volume of ejaculate does not change significantly from the volume of ejaculate before vasectomy,[70] indicating that

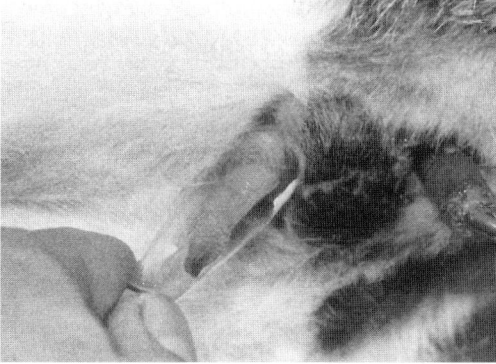

Fig. 17-7. Electroejaculation in an anesthetized tom cat. Notice the penile spines and the seminal fluid in the collecting tube.

in toms, most of the ejaculate volume is contributed by the secretion of the prostate and bulbourethral glands. Most of the spermatozoa present in a tom's ejaculate originate from the epididymides. Vasectomized toms become azoospermic 56 to 63 days after bilateral vasectomy, but intact spermatozoa are cleared from the ejaculate by day 49 postvasectomy. If pregnancies are to be prevented, a period of restraint of at least 49 days postvasectomy should be observed. Flushing the vasa deferentia at the time of vasectomy will dramatically decrease the time from vasectomy to the potentially safe uti-

lization of cats as teasers, from 63 days to 7 days.[30]

Variable but significant numbers of spermatozoa flow into the urinary bladder at the time of ejaculation in the tom cat. Retrograde flow into the urinary bladder occurs during natural mating, when semen is collected with an AV, or during electroejaculation, when seminal emission is induced by electrical stimulation in the anesthetized cat (see Chapter 8, Table 8-5 and Fig. 8-10). The total number of spermatozoa displaced from the sites of storage in the epididymides and vasa deferentia during ejaculation or electroejaculation can be estimated by adding the total number of spermatozoa in the ejaculate or electroejaculate to the total number of spermatozoa in the urine obtained from the bladder by cystocentesis after ejaculation. The percentage of the total number of spermatozoa displaced, which is found in the urine, is considered to represent the percentage of retrograde flow of spermatozoa. Table 17-10 displays the volume and concentration of spermatozoa in the urine obtained by cystocentesis before electroejaculation; the volume and total number of spermatozoa in the urine, also obtained by cystocentesis, after electroejaculation; the volume of the electroejaculate; the total number of spermatozoa in the electroejaculate; and the calculated

Table 17-9 Effect of Method of Collection on the Seminal Characteristics of the Domestic Cat

	Method of Collection					
	Artificial Vagina			Electroejaculation[a]		
Seminal Characteristic	Mean[b]	SD	Range	Mean[b]	SD	Range
Volume (ml)	0.06[c]	0.02	0.03–0.09	0.26	0.13	0.11–0.49
Number of spermatozoa (10^6)	60.97	31.05	21.50–117.00	42.70	20.51	11.10–65.96
Spermatozoal:						
Motility (%)	58	27	4–87	65	14	44–85
Viability (%)[d]	67	28	5–95	73	14	49–93
pH	8.32[c]	0.15	8.15–8.57	8.61	0.09	8.45–8.77
Osmolality (mOsm/kg)	324	31	274–368	339	22	317–390

[a]Spermatozoa and seminal fluid obtained during the application of 240 stimuli (four series of 60 stimuli) at 6V.
[b]Means for each method of collection were obtained from four cats with replication, n = 8 .
[c]Significantly different (P < 0.005) from the corresponding mean in the same row.
[d]Percentage of spermatozoa that were unstained after incubation for 15 minutes in a micromolar solution of eosin B.
Adapted from: M. P. Dooley and M. H. Pineda, Am. J. Vet. Res. *47*:286, 1986.

Table 17-10   *Total Number of Spermatozoa (10^6) in the Ejaculate and in the Urine Obtained by Cystocentesis Before and After Electroejaculation (EE) of the Domestic Cat*

| | Urine | | | | Ejaculate | | |
| | Pre-EE | | Post-EE | | | | |
Cat	Volume (ml)	Spermatozoal Concentration (10^6/ml)	Volume (ml)	Total No. Spermatozoa (10^6)	Volume (ml)	Total No. Spermatozoa (10^6)	Retrograde Flow (%)[a]
1	2.0	0	6.5	0.20	0.10	0.05	80.0
2	1.6	0.015	6.4	17.28	0.29	5.22	76.8
3	2.1	0	1.6	3.92	0.25	4.00	49.5
4	1.5	0	10.5	74.03	0.39	27.30	73.1
5	1.0	0	6.4	21.76	0.22	27.50	44.2
6	0.8	0.005	6.9	69.28	0.15	8.25	89.4
7	0.7	0.050	17.0	31.96	0.26	49.40	39.3
8	0.6	0.005	2.7	31.62	0.24	1.92	94.3

[a]The percentage of the total number of spermatozoa displaced during EE that were recovered in the urine. Adapted from: M. P. Dooley, et al., Proc. 10th Int. Congr. Anim. Reprod. A. I., Univ. Illinois, Champaign/Urbana, IL, Vol. III, Brief Commun. No. 363, 1984. For additional information, see also: M. P. Dooley, et al., Am. J. Vet. Res. *52*:687, 1991.

percentage of retrograde flow for each of eight cats. Notice that retrograde flow accounted for 39 to 94% of the estimated total number of spermatozoa displaced. These results indicate that urinary losses of spermatozoa, because of the retrograde flow of spermatozoa into the bladder of the tom cat during electroejaculation, are considerable and should not be ignored when performing breeding soundness examinations in cats. Retrograde flow of spermatozoa into the bladder of sexually rested tom cats has not been reported, but may also occur as it does in sexually rested dogs. The finding that the fluid used to flush the vasa deferentia of toms at the time of vasectomy retrograded into the bladder, instead of being eliminated through the penile urethra,[30] suggests that the passage of fluid from the urethra into the bladder follows the pathway of least resistance.

Male tortoiseshell cats are rare (1:3000) and infertile. The male tortoiseshell cat is infertile because of azoospermic ejaculates. The genes for orange or black hair are allelic on the X chromosome; consequently if the phenotype includes both colors, the tom would have two X chromosomes and one Y chromosome. In the presence of white spotting ('piebald', an autosomal dominant trait), the phenotype is often described as tortoiseshell and white, tortie and white, tricolor, or "calico".

RESPONSE OF CATS TO EXOGENOUS HORMONES

The pituitary gland of the cat responds to intravenous injections of GnRH by releasing LH. It is likely that FSH is also released, but to date there are no published data on this releasing effect.

The ovary of the queen is responsive to exogenous gonadotropins such as PMSG (eCG), FSH, LH, and human urinary FSH, highly purified porcine FSH, human menopausal gonadotropin (hMG), and hCG. These hormones are used to induce estrus in anestrous queens as well as superovulatory responses (see Chapter 20).

There is no published information regarding the effects of GnRH, pituitary, or placental gonadotropins on male libido, spermatogenesis, ejaculatory responses, or quality of ejaculates.

CONTRACEPTIVES FOR THE QUEEN

To date, there is no approved contraceptive for the queen in the United States. In other countries, synthetic progestagens, such as medroxyprogesterone acetate and megestrol ac-

Table 17-11 *Crown-rump Measurements of Cat Feti at Various Stages of Pregnancy*

Days after Mating	Crown-rump Length (mm)
17	6
19	7
21	10
23	14
25	19–20
27	23
29	26–28
31	35–36
33	37–38
35	45
38	58
42	80
45	86
48	95
52	106
56	120–122
60	136
At parturition	145–150

Adapted from: Ib. J. Christiansen, see reference no. 14, p. 276.

etate (Ovaban), are used to control estrus in queens. Also, synthetic progestagens, such as megestrol acetate, appear to control urine spraying in queens and toms. The queen seems to be less susceptible to the hyperplastic reactions of the endometrium and the nodular development of tumors of the mammary gland, which are associated with exogenous progestagens in the bitch. Nevertheless, treatment of queens with progestagens must be approached with caution, particularly when uterine infections are suspected. In addition, progestagens may induce a diabetogenic state in cats due to hypersecretion of growth hormone.

Mibolerone is an orally effective, synthetic androgenic compound. Mibolerone is sold under the commercial name of Cheque for blocking estrus in bitches and it also appears to be effective and safe to control estrus when given to anestrous queens. Mibolerone has not yet been cleared for use in queens in the United States.

Estrogens are reportedly effective in preventing pregnancies after mismatings in the queen, particularly when given about 40 hours after coitus. Exogenous estrogens appear to retard oviductal transport and delay passage of the developing embryos to the uterus. However, estrogens may be toxic to cats and, therefore, must be used with caution.

There are no reports on the use of Epostane (see Chapter 16), a 3β-hydroxysteroid dehydrogenase inhibitor that blocks progesterone synthesis, as a potential contragestive agent in queens. RU-486 is a progesterone analog that acts as a contragestive in humans and bitches. RU-486 is not effective as an abortifacient for queens,[76] possibly because the hormone-binding domain of the progesterone receptor of queens may lack the amino acid glycine[6] (see Chapter 9). Glycine is needed for the binding of RU-486 to the progesterone receptor.

The fetal growth expressed as crown-rump measurements for cat fetuses at various stages of pregnancy is presented in Table 17-11.

REFERENCES

1. Banks, D. H. and Stabenfeldt, G. (1982): Luteinizing hormone release in the cat in response to coitus on consecutive days of estrus. Biol. Reprod. *26*:603.
2. Banks, D. R., Paape, S. R., and Stabenfeldt, G. H. (1983): Prolactin in the cat: I. Pseudopregnancy, pregnancy and lactation. Biol. Reprod. *28*:923.
3. Bareither, M. L. and Verhage, H. G. (1981): Control of the secretory cell cycle in cat oviduct by estradiol and progesterone. Am J. Anat. *162*:107.
4. Beaver, B. V. (1977): Mating behavior in the cat. Vet. Clin. North Am. *7*:729.
5. Bellenger, C. R. and Chen, J. C. (1990): Effect of megestrol acetate on the endometrium of the prepubertally ovariectomized kitten. Res. Vet. Sci. *48*:112.
6. Benhamou, B., Garcia, T., Lerouge, T., et al. (1992): A single amino acid that determines the sensitivity of progesterone receptors to RU486. Science *255*:206.
7. Bland, K. P. (1979): Tom-cat odour and other pheromones in feline reproduction. Vet. Sci. Commun. *3*:125.
8. Boomsa, R. A. and Verhage, H. G. (1982): The uterine progestational response in cats: Ultrastructural changes during chronic administration of progesterone to estradiol-primed and nonprimed animals. Am. J. Anat. *164*:243.
9. Bowen, R. A. (1977): Fertilization *in vitro* of feline ova by spermatozoa from the ductus deferens. Biol. Reprod. *17*:144.
10. Burgos, M. H. and Fawcett, D. W. (1955): Studies on the fine structure of the mammalian testis. I. Differentiation of the spermatids in the cat (*Felis domestica*). J. Biophys. Biochem. Cytol. *1*:287.
11. Burke, T. J., Reynolds, H. A., and Sokolowski, J. H. (1977): A 180-day tolerance-efficacy study with mibolerone for suppression of estrus in the cat. Am. J. Vet. Res. *38*:469.

12. Chakraborty, P. K., Wildt, D. E., and Seager, S. W. J. (1979): Serum luteinizing hormone and ovulatory response to luteinizing hormone-releasing hormone in the estrous and anestrous domestic cat. Lab. Anim. Sci. *29*:338.

13. Chan, S. Y. W., Chakraborty, P. K., Bass, E. J., et al. (1982): Ovarian-endocrine-behavioural function in the domestic cat treated with exogenous gonadotrophins during mid-gestation. J. Reprod. Fertil. *65*:395.

14. Christiansen, Ib. J. (1984): Reproduction in the Dog and Cat. London, Baillierè Tindall.

15. Church, D. B., Watson, A. D. J., Emslie, D. R., et al. (1994): Effects of proligestone and megestrol on plasma adrenocorticotrophic hormone, insulin, and insulin-like growth factor-1 concentrations in cats. Res. Vet. Sci. *56*:175.

16. Cline, E. M., Jennings, L. L., and Sojka, N. J. (1980): Analysis of the feline vaginal epithelial cycle. Feline Reprod. *10*:47.

17. Cline, E. M., Jennings, L. L., and Sojka, N. J. (1980): Breeding laboratory cats during artificially induced estrus. Lab. Anim. Sci. *30*:1003.

18. Colby, E. D. (1970): Induced estrus and timed pregnancies in cats. Lab. Anim. Care *20*:1075.

19. Courrier, R. and Gros, G. (1932): Remarques sur la nidation de l'oeuf chez la chatte. Compt. Rend. Soc. Biol., Paris, France, *111*:787.

20. Dawson, A. B. (1981): The development and morphology of the corpus luteum of the cat. Anat. Rec. *79*:155.

21. Dederer, P. H. (1934): Polyovular follicles in the cat. Anat. Rec. *60*:391.

22. Del Campo, C. H. and Ginther, O. J. (1974): Arteries and veins of uterus and ovaries in dogs and cats. Am. J. Vet. Res. *35*:409.

23. Dooley, M. P. and Pineda, M. H. (1986): Effect of method of collection on seminal characteristics of the domestic cat. Am. J. Vet. Res. *47*:286.

24. Dooley, M. P., Murase, K., and Pineda, M. H. (1983): An electroejaculator for the collection of semen from the domestic cat. Theriogenology *20*:297.

25. Dooley, M. P., Pineda, M. H., Hopper, J. G., et al. (1984): Retrograde flow of semen caused by electroejaculation in the domestic cat. Proc. 10th Int. Congr. Anim. Reprod. A. I., Univ. Illinois, Champaign/Urbana, IL, June 10–14, 1984, Vol. III, Brief Commun. No. 363.

26. Dooley, M. P., Pineda, M. H., Hopper, J. G., et al. (1991): Retrograde flow of spermatozoa into the urinary bladder of cats during electroejaculation, collection of semen with an artificial vagina, and mating. Am. J. Vet. Res. *52*:687.

27. Dresser, B. L., Sehlhorst, C. S., Wachs, K. B., et al. (1987): Hormonal stimulation and embryo collection in the domestic cat (*Felis catus*). Theriogenology *28*:915.

28. Elcock, L. H. and Schoning, P. (1984): Age-related changes in the cat testis and epididymis. Am. J. Vet. Res. *45*:2380.

29. Foster, M. A. and Hisaw, F. L. (1935): Experimental ovulation and the resulting pseudopregnancy in anestrous cats. Anat. Rec. *62*:75.

30. Frenette, M. D., Dooley, M. P., and Pineda, M. H. (1986): Effect of flushing the vasa deferentia at the time of vasectomy on the rate of clearance of spermatozoa from the ejaculates of dogs and cats. Am. J. Vet. Res. *47*:463.

31. Gadsby, J. E., Heap, R. B., and Burton, R. D. (1980): Oestrogen production by blastocyst and early embryonic tissue of various species. J. Reprod. Fertil. *60*:409.

32. Goodrowe, K. L, Howard, J. G., Schmidt, P. M., et al. (1989): Reproductive biology of the domestic cat with special reference to endocrinology, sperm function and *in-vitro* fertilization. J. Reprod. Fertil. *39*:73.

33. Grognet, J. (1990): Catnip: Its uses and effects, past and present. Can. Vet. J. *31*:455.

34. Hammer, J. G. and Howland, D. R. (1991): Use of serum progesterone levels as an early, indirect evaluation of pregnancy in the timed pregnant domestic cat. Lab. Anim. Sci. *41*:42.

35. Hammner, C. E., Jennings, L. L. and Sojka, N. J. (1970): Cat (*Felis catus L.*) spermatozoa require capacitation. J. Reprod. Fertil. *23*:477.

36. Hart, B. L. (1980): Objectionable urine spraying and urine marking in cats: Evaluation of progestin treatment in gonadectomized males and females. J. Am. Vet. Med. Assoc. *177*:529.

37. Hart, B. L. and Cooper, L. (1984): Factors relating to urine spraying and fighting in prepubertally gonadectomized cats. J. Am. Vet. Med. Assoc. *184*:1255.

38. Henderson, R. T. (1984): Prostaglandin therapeutics in the bitch and queen. Aust. Vet. J. *61*:317.

39. Howard, J. G., Barone, M. A., Donoghue, A. M., et al. (1992): The effect of pre-ovulatory anesthesia on ovulation in laparoscopically inseminated domestic cats. J. Reprod. Fertil. *96*:175.

40. Hughes, B. J., Bowen, J. M., Campion, D. R., et al. (1983): Effect of denervation or castration on ultrastructural and histochemical properties of feline bulbocavernosus muscle. Acta Anat. *115*:97.

41. Hurni, H. (1981): Daylength and breeding in the domestic cat. Lab Anim. *15*:229.

42. Hurni, H. (1981): SPF-cat breeding. Z. Versuchtierkd. *23*:102.

43. Jemmett, J. E. and Evans, J. M. (1977): A survey of sexual behaviour and reproduction of female cats. J. Small Anim. Pract. *18*:31.

44. Jewgenow, K. and Göritz, F. (1995): The recovery of preantral follicles from ovaries of domestic cats and their characterisation before and after culture. Anim. Reprod. Sci. *39*:285.

45. Johnson, L. M. and Gay, V. L. (1981): Luteinizing hormone in the cat. I. Tonic secretion. Endocrinology *109*:240.

46. Johnson, L. M. and Gay, V. L. (1981): Luteinizing hormone in the cat. II. Mating-induced secretion. Endocrinology *109*:247.

47. Johnston, S. D., Hayden, D. W., Kiang, D. T., et al. (1984): Progesterone receptors in feline mammary adenocarcinomas. Am. J. Vet. Res. *45*:379.

48. Johnstone, I. P., Brancroft, B. J., and McFarlane, J. R. (1984): Testosterone and androstenedione profiles in the blood of domestic tomcats. Anim. Reprod. Sci. *7*:363.

49. Jones, T. C. (1969): Sex chromosome anomaly, Klinefelter's syndrome. Comp. Pathol. Bull. *1*:1.

50. Kelly, R. E. and Verhage, H. G. (1981): Hormonal effects on the contractile apparatus of the myometrium. Am. J. Anat. *161*:375.

51. Legay, J.-M. and Pontier, D. (1985): Relation age-Fecondite dans les populations de chats domestiques, *Felis catus*. Mammalia *49*:395.

52. Lawler, D. F., Evans, R. H., Reimers, T. J., et al. (1991): Histopathologic features, environmental factors, and serum estrogen, progesterone, and prolactin values associated with ovarian phase and inflammatory uterine disease in cats. Am. J. Vet. Res. *52*:1747.

53. Lawler, D. F., Johnston, S. D., Hegstad, R. L., et al. (1993): Ovulation without cervical stimulation in domestic cats. J. Reprod. Fertil. (Suppl. 47):57.

54. Lein, D. H. and Concannon, P. W. (1983): Infertility and fertility treatments and management in the queen and tom cat. *In:* Current Veterinary Therapy. VIII. Small Animal Practice, edited by R. W. Kirk. Philadelphia, PA, W. B. Saunders Co., p. 936.

55. Leiser, R. and Koob, B. (1993): Development and characteristics of placentation in a carnivore, the domestic cat. J. Exp. Zool. *266*:642.

56. Lengwinat, T. and Blottner, S. (1994): *In vitro* fertilization of follicular oocytes of domestic cat using fresh and cryopreserved epididymal spermatozoa. Anim. Reprod. Sci. *35*:291.

57. Levine, B. N. (1984): Small animal population trends and demands for veterinary service. *In:* Proc. 8th Kal Kan Symp. for the Treatment of Small Animal Disease, edited by E. Van Marthens. Vernon, California, Kal Kan, p. 49.

58. Manwell, E. J. and Wickens, P. G. (1928): The mechanisms of ovulation and implantation in the domestic cat. Anat. Rec. *38*:54.

59. Mauleon, P. (1967): Cinétique de l'ovogenèse chez les mammifères. Arch d'Anat. Microsc. Morphol. Exp. *56*:125.

60. Michael, R. P. (1961): Observations upon the sexual behavior of the domestic cat (*Felis catus L.*) under laboratory conditions. Behavior *18*:1.

61. Michael, R. P. (1973): The effects of hormones on sexual behavior in female cat and Rhesus monkey. *In:* Handbook of Physiology, Section 7, Vol. II, edited by R. O. Greep and E. B. Astwood. Washington, D. C., American Physiological Society, pp. 187–221.

62. Michel, C. (1993): Induction of oestrus in cats by photoperiodic manipulation and social stimuli. Lab. Anim. *27*:278.

63. Motta, P. and Van Blerkom, J. (1979): Morphodynamic aspects of the ovarian superficial epithelium as revealed by transmission, scanning and high voltage electron microscopy. Ann. Biol. Anim. Biochim. Biophys. *19*:1559.

64. Neville, P. F. and Remfry, J. (1984): Effect of neutering on two groups of feral cats. Vet. Rec. *114*:447.

65. Ninomiya, H., Fukase, T., and Nakamura, T. (1984): Scanning electron microscopy of celluloid replicas of the penile spines of the domestic cat. Exp. Anim. *33*:525.

66. Niwa, K., Ohara, K., Hosoi, Y., et al. (1985): Early events of *in vitro* fertilization of cat eggs by epididymal spermatozoa. J. Reprod. Fertil. *74*:657.

67. Oikawa, H. (1987): Fluorescence-positive body in the spermatozoa of domestic cat (*Felis catus*). Jpn. J. Vet. Sci. *49*:942.

68. Orosz, S. E., Morris, P. J., Doody, M. C., et al. (1992): Stimulation of folliculogenesis in domestic cats with human FSH and LH. Theriogenology *37*:993.

69. Paape, S. R., Shille, V. M., Seto, H., et al. (1975): Luteal activity in the pseudopregnant cat. Biol. Reprod. *13*:470.

70. Pineda, M. H. and Dooley, M. P. (1984): Surgical and chemical vasectomy in the cat. Am. J. Vet. Res. *45*:291.

71. Pineda, M. H. and Dooley, M. P. (1984): Effects of voltage and order of voltage application on seminal characteristics of electroejaculates of the domestic cat. Am. J. Vet. Res. *45*:1520.

72. Pineda, M. H., Dooley, M. P., and Martin, P. A. (1984): Long-term study on the effects of electroejaculation on seminal characteristics of the domestic cat. Am. J. Vet. Res. *45*:1038.

73. Rees, H. D., Swite, G. M., and Michael, R. P. (1980): The estrogen-sensitive neural system in the brain of female cats. J. Comp. Neurol. *193*:789.

74. Remfry, J. (1978): Control of feral cat populations by long-term administration of megestrol acetate. Vet. Rec. *103*:403.

75. Robinson, R. and Cox, H. W. (1970): Reproductive performance in a cat colony over a 10-year period. Lab. Anim. *4*:99.

76. Sankai, T., Endo, T., Kanayama, K., et al. (1991): Antiprogesterone compound, RU486 administration to terminate pregnancy in dogs and cats. Jpn. J. Med. Sci. *53*:1069.

77. Schmidt, P. M., Chakraborty, P. K., and Wildt, D. E. (1983): Ovarian activity, circulatory hormones and sexual behavior in the cat. II. Relationships during pregnancy, parturition, lactation and the postpartum estrus. Biol. Reprod. *28*:657.

78. Shille, V. M., and Stabenfeldt, G. H. (1979): Luteal function in the domestic cat during pseudopregnancy and after treatment with prostaglandin $F_{2\alpha}$. Biol. Reprod. *21*:1217.

79. Shille, V. M., Kerstin, E., Lundstrom, E., et al., (1979): Follicular function in domestic cats as determined by estradiol-17β concentrations in plasma: Relation to estrous behavior and cornification of exfoliated vaginal epithelium. Biol. Reprod. *21*:953.

80. Shille, V. M., Munro, C., Farmer, S. W., et al. (1983): Ovarian and endocrine responses in the cat after coitus. J. Reprod. Fertil. *68*:29.

81. Sojka, N. J., Jennings, L. L., and Hamner, C. E. (1970): Artificial insemination in the cat (*Felis catus L.*) Lab. Anim. Care *20*:198.

82. Stabenfeldt, G. H. (1974): Physiologic, pathologic and therapeutic roles of progestins in domestic animals. J. Am. Vet. Med. Assoc. *164*:311.

83. Stewart, D. R. and Stabenfeldt, G. H. (1985): Relaxin activity in the pregnant cat. Biol. Reprod. *32*:848.

84. Stover, D. G. and Sokolowski, J. H. (1978): Estrous behavior of the domestic cat. Feline Pract. *8*:54.

85. Strasser, H., Brunk, R., and Baeder, C. (1971): Studies in the sexual cycle of the cat. Berl. Munch. Tierärztl. Wochenschr. *84*:253.

86. Telfer, E. and Gosden, R. G. (1987): A quantitative cytological study of polyovular follicles in mammalian ovaries with particular reference to the domestic bitch (*Canis familiaris*). J. Reprod. Fertil. *81*:137.

87. Thuline, H. C. and Norby, D. E. (1961): Spontaneous occurrence of chromosome abnormality in cats. Science *134*:554.

88. Tsutsui, T., Amano, T., Shimizu, T., et al. (1989): Evidence for transuterine migration of embryos in the domestic cat. Jpn. J. Vet. Sci. *51*:613.

89. Van der Stricht, R. (1911): Vitellogenese dans l'ovule de chatte. Arch. Biol. *26*:365.

90. Verhage, H. G., Beamer, N. B., and Brenner, R. M. (1976): Plasma levels of estradiol and progesterone in the cat during polyestrus, pregnancy and pseudopregnancy. Biol. Reprod. *14*:579.

91. Verstegen, J. P., Onclin, K., Silva, L. D. M., et al. (1993): Superovulation and embryo culture *in vitro* following treatment with ultra-pure follicle-stimulating hormone in cats. J. Reprod. Fertil. (Suppl. 47):209.

92. Watson, A. D. J., Church, D. B., Emslie, D. R., et al. (1989): Comparative effects of proligestone and megestrol acetate on basal plasma glucose concentrations and cortisol responses to exogenous adrenocorticotrophic hormone in cats. Res. Vet. Sci. *47*:374.

93. West, N. B., Verhage, H. G., and Brenner, R. M. (1976): Suppression of the estradiol receptor system by progesterone in the oviduct and uterus of the cat. Endocrinology *99*:1010.

94. Whalen, R. E. (1963): Sexual behavior of cats. Behavior *20*:321.

95. Wheeler, A. G., Walker, M., and Lean, J. (1987): Influence of adrenergic receptors on ovarian progesterone secretion in the pseudopregnant cat and oestradiol secretion in the oestrous cat. J. Reprod. Fertil. *79*:195.

96. Wheeler, A. G., Walker, M., and Lean, J. (1988): Function of hormonally-induced corpora lutea in the domestic cat. Theriogenology *29*:971.

97. Wyckoff, J. T. and Ganjam, V. K. (1979): Successful termination of pregnancy in cats by the administration of a combination of adrenocorticotrophic hormone and prostaglandin $F_{2\alpha}$-Tris (hydroxymethal) amino-methane salt. Fed. Proc. *38*:1189 (Abstract).

98. Younglai, E. V., Belbeck, L. W., Dimond, P., et al. (1976): Testosterone production by ovarian follicles of the domestic cat (*Felis catus*). Hormone Res. *7*:91.

References Added in Proof

99. Axner, E., Linde-Forsberg, C., and Einarsson, S. (1999): Morphology and motility of spermatozoa from different regions of the epididymal duct in the domestic cat. Theriogenology *52*:767.

100. Heyn, R., Muglia, U., and Motta, P. M. (1997): Microarchitecture of the cat testis with special reference to Leydig cells: A three-dimensional study by alkali maceration method and scanning electron microscopy. Arch. Androl. *39*:135.

101. Jewgenow, K., Rohleder, M., and Wegner, I. (2000): Differences between antigenic determinants of pig and cat zona pellucida proteins. J. Reprod. Fertil. *119*:15.

102. Tanaka, A., Kuwabara, S., Takagi, Y., et al. (2000): Effect of ejaculation intervals on semen quality in cats. J. Vet. Med. Sci. *62*:1157.

103. Say, L., Pontier, D., and Natoli, E. (1999): High variation in multiple paternity of domestic cats (*Felis catus* L.) in relation to environmental conditions. Proc. Royal Soc., [B], London, England *266*:2071.

Reproductive Patterns of Alpacas and Llamas, with Reference to the Vicuña and Guanaco

P. A. MARTIN

18

INTRODUCTION

Camelidae are classified into 2 groups, the camels or Old World camelids and the New World camelids which include the alpaca, llama, guanaco, and vicuña. Camels are indigenous to the arid and semi-arid regions of central and southwestern Asia and northern Africa and are well-adapted to desert conditions. There are 2 species of camels, the Arabian or 1-humped camel (*Camelus dromedarius*) and the 2-humped camel (*Camelus bactrianus*). New World or South American camelids are indigenous to the high plains of the Andes Mountains and are well-adapted to high altitudes. South American camelids tolerate large fluctuations in daily temperature, wet and dry seasons, and are able to forage on a wide variety of vegetation. Four species of South American camelids are recognized. Two species are domesticated, the alpaca (*Lama pacos*) and the llama (*Lama glama*) and 2 species are wild, the vicuña (*Vicugna vicugna*) and guanaco (*Lama guanacoe*).

Despite their evolution under markedly different environments and on two separate continents, an estimated 11 million years of reproductive isolation apparently does not preclude hybrids between Old and New World camelids. Thus, molecular data revealing that Old and New World camelids are related[118] is consistent with the reported[103] birth of a live offspring, resulting from the artificial insemination of a guanaco female with camel (dromedary) semen. Though the male hybrid is not expected to be fertile, attempts to form hybrids between camels (dromedary) and camelids (guanaco) resulted in 6 pregnancies in guanaco females (9 females; 34 breeding cycles) and 2 pregnancies in dromedary females (30 females; 50 breeding cycles). For those females known to be pregnant, embryos were resorbed *in utero* (n = 2), the fetus was aborted (n = 3), delivered stillborn (n = 2), or born alive (n = 1).

Interspecific matings are common among New World camelids and the hybrid offspring are fertile. Hence, the classification[62] of the alpaca, llama, guanaco, and vicuña as separate species (see Chapter 7) is controversial. Based on DNA hybridization profiles specific to South American camelids,[117,118] hereafter referred to as camelids, it was proposed that the llama is a domesticated form of the guanaco and that the hybridization profile for DNA from the alpaca appeared to be intermediate to that of the guanaco and vicuña. These authors[118] suggested the phylogenetic origin of the alpaca to be a crossbred of the guanaco and the vicuña.

The largest concentrations of alpacas, llamas, and vicuñas are found at altitudes from 2,300 to 4,600 meters above sea level in Peru, western Bolivia, and near the northern border of Argentina and Chile. For centuries, alpacas and llamas have played a major role in the lives and economy of the indigenous populations of Peru and Bolivia. The llama is the largest (100 to 175 kg) of the 4 camelids and has been the major beast of burden in the high plains of the Andes. Llamas also serve as a source of meat and coarse wool used to make bags, carpets, blankets, and rope.

In South America, alpacas are primarily used as a source of high quality wool and pelts and, secondarily, as a source of meat. The quality of the wool and pelt of the alpaca is superior to that of sheep and, since the 1970s, major efforts have been made in Peru to develop the alpaca industry and to improve the quality of the animals.

The vicuña is the smallest (35 to 45 kg) of the South American camelids, and has the highest quality wool and pelt. For this reason, these animals were nearly hunted to extinction by 1970. Since then, the number of vicuñas has increased rapidly due to governmental programs to protect the species and to support the commercial production of vicuñas for their wool and pelts. Today, up to 90 to 95% of the vicuñas in South America may be in captive herds.

The guanaco is the larger of the 2 wild camelids and, of the 4 camelids, is the one with the broadest geographic distribution and can adapt to a range of habitats. Guanacos are found from Peru to the southern tip of South America, however, the largest numbers are located in Argentina and Chile.[62] Guanaco populations range from sea level to an altitude of 4,600 meters or more. Guanacos are also highly prized for their wool and pelts and by 1970 their numbers were also seriously depleted.

The use of domestic camelids in South America is markedly different than in the United States. In the United States, alpacas and llamas are primarily raised and used as pets and show animals. Some llamas are also used as recreational pack animals for carrying camping equipment and supplies in the Rocky and Appalachian mountains. Demand for alpacas and llamas as pets during the last 2 to 3 decades has resulted in a significant increase in their numbers in the United States.

Very little was known about the reproduction of camelids before 1970. Since then, considerable information has been amassed about the reproduction of alpacas and llamas. Nevertheless, their reproductive processes are poorly understood compared to that of our common livestock species. The impetus for reproductive research on alpacas was driven largely by the need to improve the reproductive efficiency of these animals for the developing, government-supported, alpaca industry in South America, whereas, reproductive research in llamas has primarily been driven by the needs of the llama industry in the United States.

It is important to remember that the habitat and management practices of alpacas and llamas in South America are markedly different from those in the United States and other countries. The extent to which these factors affect the reproduction of camelids has not been determined. However, it is known that many male alpacas and llamas in the United States are infertile during the Summer, whereas they are fertile throughout the year in South America.

ANATOMICAL CHARACTERISTICS OF REPRODUCTIVE ORGANS

Male

Camelids are born with testes in the scrotum. The scrotum is located in the perianal region in a position similar to that of dogs and boars. The size of the testes is positively correlated with fertility. The testes are small before puberty and, as for other species, they begin to grow more rapidly during the peripubertal period and attain their adult size in alpacas and llamas at approximately 30 months of age.

Camelids have a fibroelastic penis with a sigmoid flexure (Fig. 18–1) as do ruminants and boars. Hence, the increase in the diameter of the penis due to engorgement during erection is minimal due to the limited amount of erectile tissue in these species. In adult males the tapered tip of the penis has a clockwise curve to which is attached a unique cartilaginous process (Fig. 18–1) that also has a clockwise curve. The cartilaginous process is believed to facilitate the threading of the penis through the clockwise folds or rings of the cervix during mating. In camelids, the bulk of the ejaculate is deposited in the uterine horns.

The prepuce of camelids is also peculiar. It is oriented caudally, rather than cranially, so that during micturition the stream of urine is discharged caudally between the hind legs. The protractor preputial muscles pull the prepuce cranially to allow forward projection of the penis when the male is sexually aroused.

The penis of neonates does not have a cartilaginous process and the glans penis is firmly attached to the prepuce by adhesions. Consequently, extrusion of the penis from the prepuce is not possible. Formation of the cartilaginous process and breakdown of penile adhesions begin during the peripubertal period. These events are believed to be androgen-dependent because penile adhesions fail to breakdown completely in males that are castrated before puberty. Few male alpacas are free of penile adhesions by 1 year of age and it usually takes another 2 years before all males are completely free of penile adhesions. Postpubertal males with penile adhesions are seldom successful breeders because the semen cannot be deposited into the uterine horns. Hence, breeding males should be selected for early breakdown of penile adhesions.

Camelids have a prostrate and 2 bulbourethral glands, but do not have vesicular glands (Fig. 18–1). The *vas deferens* does not have a defined ampulla.

Female

The dominant feature of the ovaries of adult, nonmated alpacas and llamas is the presence of follicles that are 2 to 12 mm in diameter. The large, mature follicle destined for ovulation is called the dominant follicle. Follicles are also present on ovaries which have a corpus luteum (CL, Fig. 18–2A and B). Camelids are induced ovulators, hence, a CL develops following sterile or fertile matings. The CL is large and may constitute half of the ovarian tissue (Fig. 18–2A and B).

Unlike most domestic species, the ovary is enveloped by the *bursa ovarica*. The posterior end of the oviduct empties on a papilla at the tip of the uterine horn. In alpacas and llamas, as for swine and horses, it is not possible to flush fluid from the uterus into the oviduct to recover embryos (see Fig. 19–1A).

Camelids have a bicornuate uterus with a short body. Unlike other species, there is a disparity in the size of the uterine horns, the left being larger than the right uterine horn (Fig. 18–2A) in most alpacas and llamas.[51] Until recently, it was believed that the large size of the left uterine horn was due to the fact that approximately 95% of term pregnancies occur in the left uterine horn (Fig. 18–2B). It now seems that the disparity in the size of the 2 uterine horns in camelids is attributable to a peculiar angioarchitecture[51] which provides a greater flow of blood to the left uterine horn. Unlike ruminants, the uterus of camelids does not have caruncles.

The cervix has 2 or 3 clockwise, ringlike folds which can make cannulation of the cervix difficult. The remainder of the reproductive organs are unremarkable except there may be a narrowing or constriction at the vestibulovaginal junction.[105]

Camelids have 2 mammary glands each of which has a nipple rather than a teat as in ruminants and horses. The nipples of alpacas are small and each has 1 to 5 orifices.[61]

PUBERTY AND SEXUAL MATURITY IN THE MALE

Puberty in the male is defined as the age at which spermatozoa are released in the ejaculate (see Chapter 8). The age of puberty in camelids has not been determined with accuracy because of the difficulties in obtaining semen from untrained males, the adhesions between the penis and prepuce in young camelids, and the lack of defined methods for the collection of semen by electroejaculation. Although some males produce spermatozoa at 12 months of age, the mean age of puberty may be closer to 18 to 24 months.

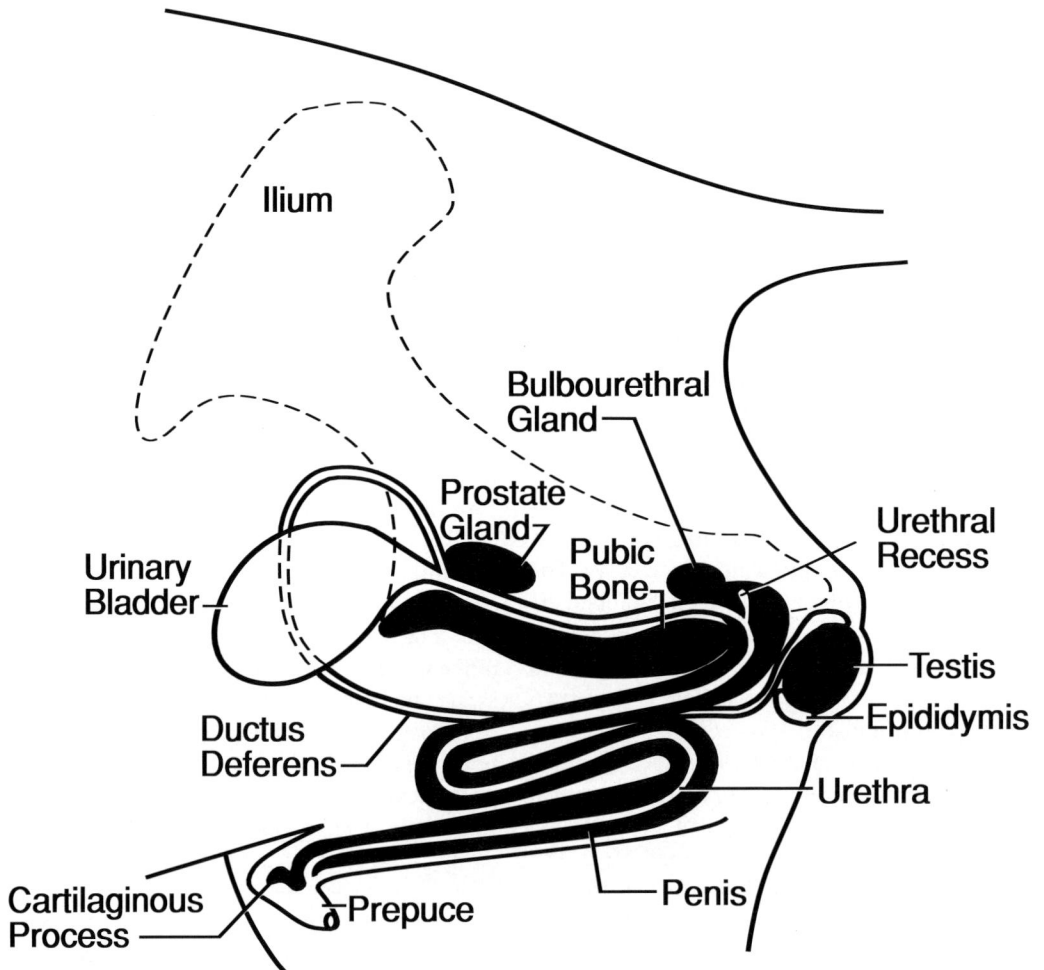

Fig. 18–1. Illustration of the genitalia of the male camelid. Note the cartilaginous process at the tip of the penis, the sigmoid flexure, and the prepuce which is directed caudally. During arousal, the protractor preputial muscles contract to pull the prepuce cranially to facilitate extension of the penis and intromission. (Adapted and redrawn from: M. E. Fowler and P. W. Bravo,[68] 1998 and J. Kubicek,[82] 1974).

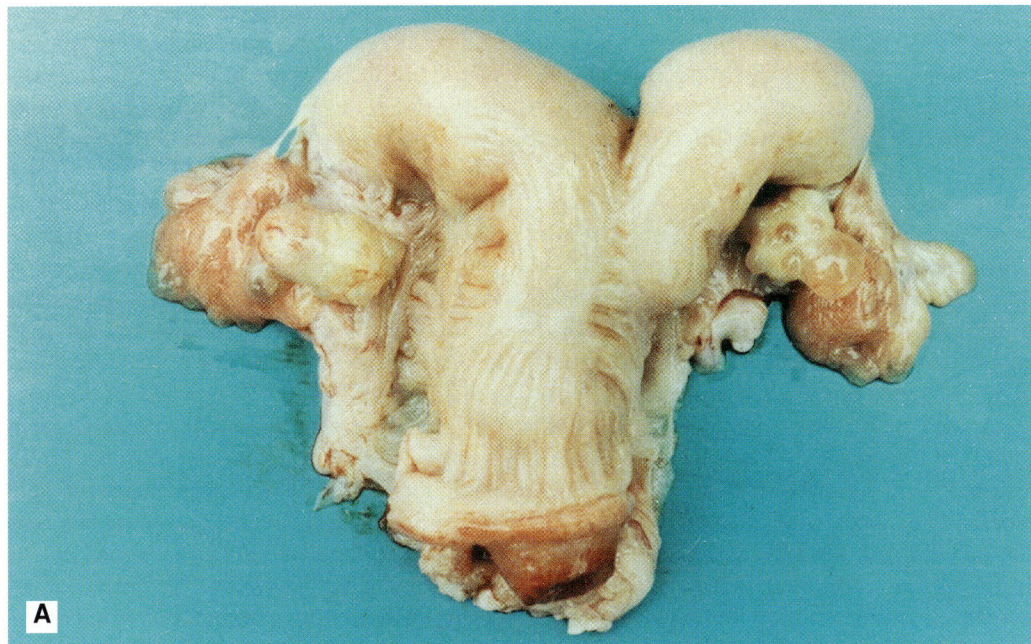

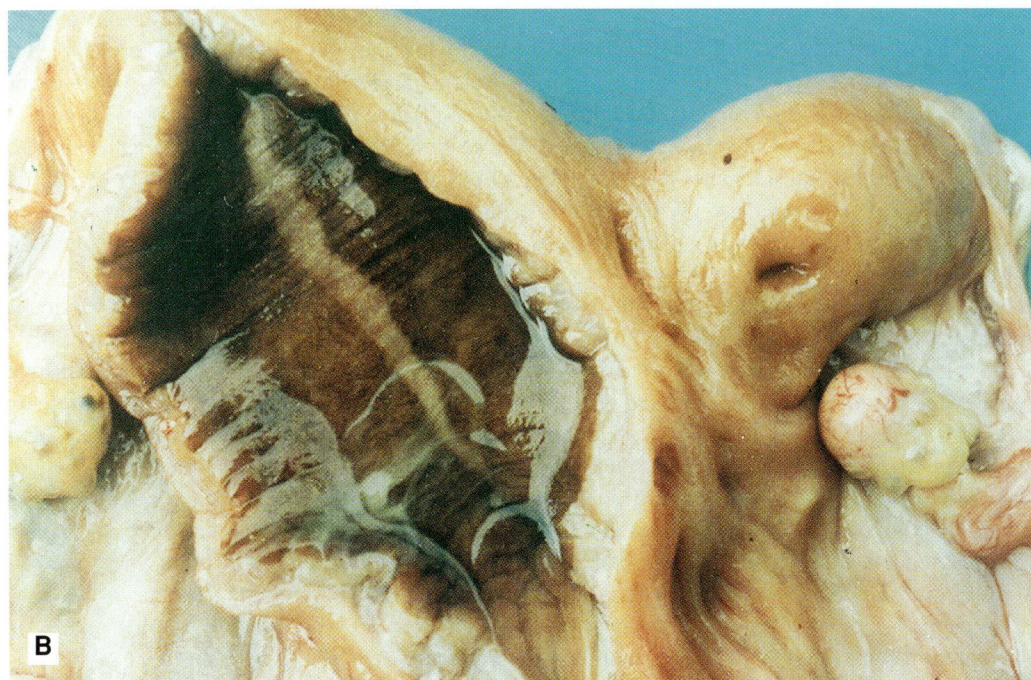

Fig. 18–2. A. Dorsal view of the ovaries, oviducts, uterus, and cervix of an adult, nulliparous llama in estrus at the time of euthanasia. Note the large, dominant follicle ➤ on the right ovary and several smaller follicles on the right and left ovaries. A regressing corpus luteum (CL) is located on the left ovary ➤ . **B.** Early pregnancy in a llama. Small follicles are evident on the left and right ovaries and the CL of pregnancy is located on the right ovary. Note the conceptus attached to the left uterine wall and the reflection of light from the embryonic membranes. [Courtesy: Drs. C. H. Del Campo and M. R. Del Campo. Proyecto Fondecyt # 09–41–91 funded by the Comisión Nacional de Investigación Científica y Technológica (CONICYT), Valdivia, Chile].

Testes in alpacas and llamas grow rapidly between 6 to 30 months of age and reach a plateau by 30 months in alpacas and after 36 months in llamas. The size of the testes in alpacas and llamas is positively correlated with fertility. Currently, there is heavy selection pressure in South America for alpaca breeding males that have large testes and are pubertal and free of penile adhesions by 12 months of age.

Testosterone levels have been determined, from birth to 4 years of age in male llamas. Levels of testosterone remain low (40–100 pg/ml) until 19 months of age after which testosterone levels increase rapidly to adult levels (520–980 pg/ml) by 24 months of age. The increase in testosterone is correlated with an increase in libido and the appearance of spermatozoa in the seminal fluids collected during electroejaculation. In contrast to llamas, testosterone levels in male alpacas attain adult levels by 12 months of age.

PUBERTY AND SEXUAL MATURITY IN THE FEMALE

The age of onset of puberty in female alpacas and llamas has not been accurately determined. If nutrition is adequate, most females reach puberty between 5 and 9 months of age. By 6 months of age, most llamas have intermittent increases in estrone sulfate, a metabolite of estrone, and by 10 months of age, the ovarian follicular cycle resembles that of adult females. Estradiol-17β and estrone sulfate levels in the blood and urine of adult female alpacas and llamas are correlated with the size of ovarian follicles.

The onset of puberty in female alpacas and llamas is markedly influenced by nutritional status. Depending on the quality and quantity of feedstuffs, the age of onset of puberty can be as short as 5 months or as long as 24 months or more. Females usually become pubertal when they attain approximately 60% of their adult body weight.

BREEDING SEASON

Alpacas and llamas breed throughout the year. However, for herds in the high plains of South America in which males are free-roaming with the females, at least 75% of the offspring or **crias** are born during the rainy season (December to April), when feeding conditions and survival of the crias are optimal. The nadir occurs during the winter months. Under free-mating systems in zoos in the northern hemisphere, the crias of most llamas are also born during the late Spring and Summer (June to October) which is an offset of 6 months compared to the birthing season in South America. However, the proportion of llamas born during late Spring and Summer in zoos of the northern hemisphere is lower (55%) than for free-roaming herds in South America (>75%).

The guanaco and vicuña, in contrast to their domestic relatives, are definite seasonal breeders. In their native habitat most vicuñas are born in late Spring and Summer; crias are not born during the winter months. Guanacos, on the other hand, have 2 peaks for the birth of crias, during the late Spring and early Summer (December and January) and again in mid-winter (August). The reasons for these 2 peaks are not clear, but may be related to the broader geographic distribution of guanacos and differences in climatic and environmental conditions. In zoos in the northern hemisphere, guanacos breed throughout the year and approximately 75% of the crias are born between May and October. The year-round breeding of captive guanacos has been attributed to differences in the quality and quantity of feed and, perhaps, to more favorable environmental and climatic conditions.

In their natural habitat, postpubertal, wild and domestic camelids can ejaculate and release semen throughout the year. However, the effects of season and associated environmental changes on the quality and fertility of the ejaculates have not been determined. As indicated earlier, male alpacas and llamas in the United States are frequently infertile during the Summer.

THE ESTROUS CYCLE

Estrus and Nonreceptivity

All 4 camelids are induced ovulators whose nonmated, nonovulatory cycle is characterized by repetitive waves of follicular growth and regression. In the absence of mating, spontaneous ovulations are reported for 3 to 10% of animals randomly selected for laparotomy. The duration of estrus or receptivity, and the period of nonreceptivity to mating in alpacas and llamas are unpredictable and highly variable. During the breeding season, estrus may be as short as 2 days or longer than 36 and 90 days in alpacas and llamas, respectively. Factors that markedly influence the duration of estrus and nonreceptivity in llamas include:

1. Time of the year,
2. whether females are exposed to males before the breeding season, and
3. the number of days that females are exposed to males before mating is allowed (Table 18–1).

The relationship between the mating behavior of female alpacas and llamas and the associated ovarian follicular dynamics, including secretion and levels of ovarian steroid hormones, have not been established.

Mating Behavior

Male alpacas and llamas search for receptive females (Fig. 18–3). Alpacas and llamas in estrus are very submissive and, frequently, when the female is approached by the male, she immediately lays down in sternal recumbency and raises the pelvis to facilitate intromission. The male straddles the recumbent female during mating and ejaculates while in a 'sitting position' (Fig. 18–4A). Some estrous females remain standing when approached by the male and will not become recumbent until mounted by the male. Other estrous females may approach a mating pair and assume the mating position (Fig. 18–4A) or mount other recumbent females that are in estrus. Timid, nonreceptive females may also lie down when approached by dominant or aggressive males and allow mating (Fig. 18–4B). Dominant males may also mount standing, nonreceptive females and, frequently, these females become recumbent and mate. Aggressive males have even been reported to

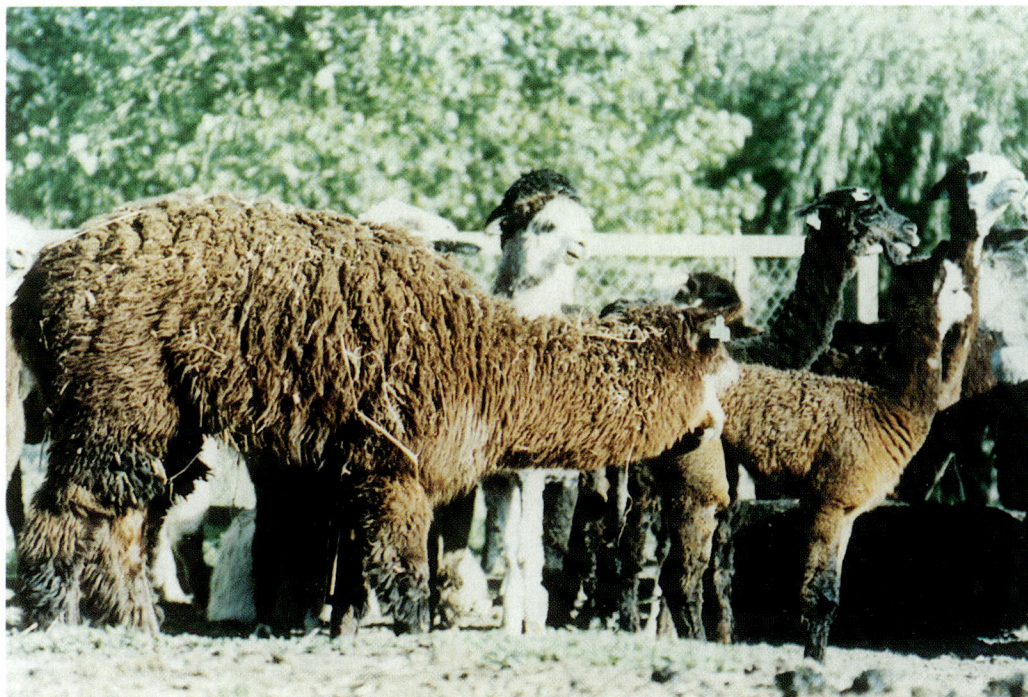

Fig. 18–3. Alpaca herd in northern Chile. The brown male alpaca in the foreground is testing the female for receptivity. [Courtesy: Drs. C. H. Del Campo and M. R. Del Campo. Proyecto Fondecyt # 09–41–91 funded by the Comisión Nacional de Investigación Científica y Technológica (CONICYT), Valdivia, Chile].

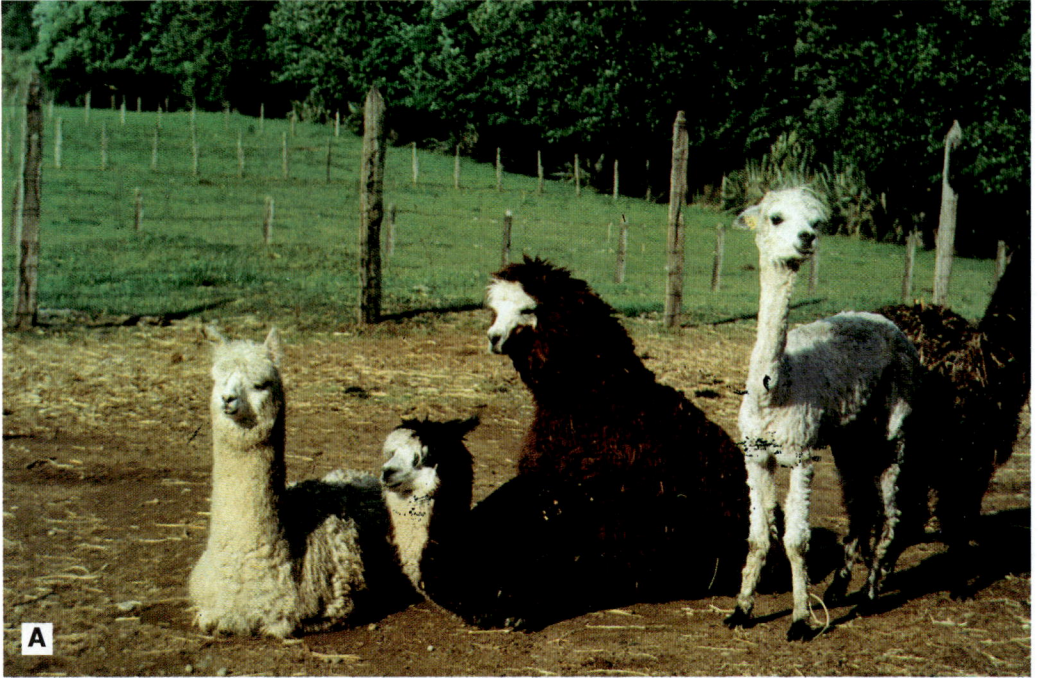

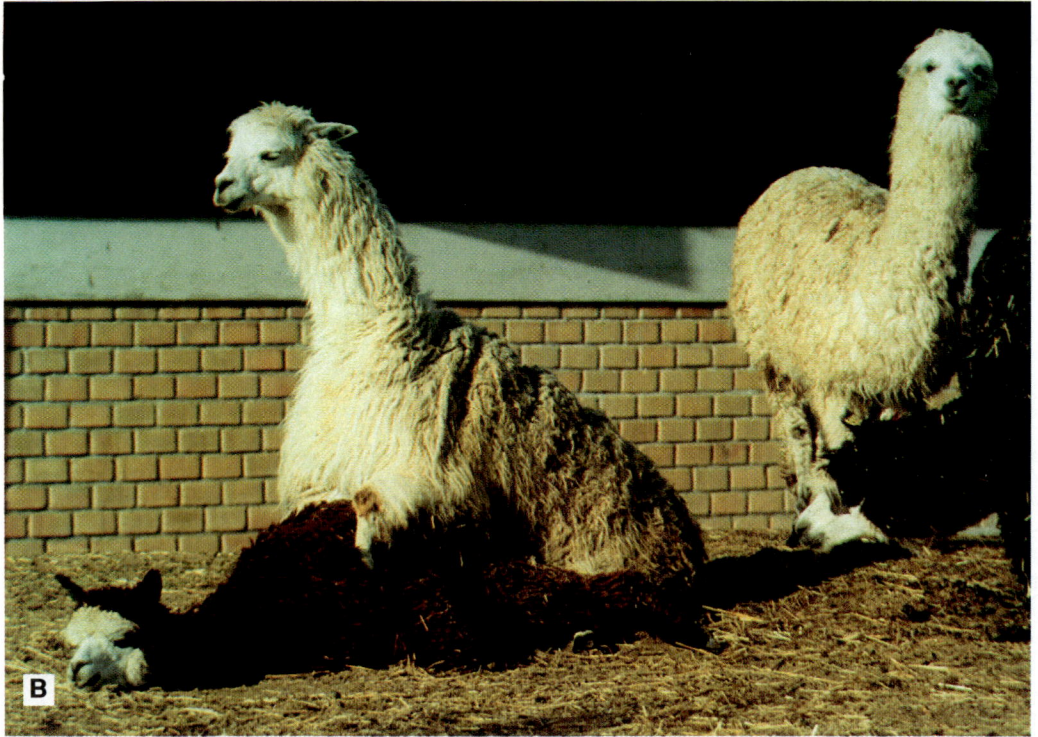

Fig. 18–4. Mating in camelids. **A.** A female in estrus has adopted the mating position adjacent to the mating pair. **B.** Notice the submissive posture of the female during mating. [Courtesy: Drs. C. H. Del Campo and M. R. Del Campo. Proyecto Fondecyt # 09–41–91 funded by the Comisión Nacional de Investigación Científica y Technológica (CONICYT), Valdivia, Chile].

Table 18-1 **Influence of Exposure to Males on the Sexual Receptivity of Female Llamas**

No. Days of Pre-exposure to Males[a]	No. of Females	Receptivity[b] of Females Expressed as Percentage (%) of Days Receptive to the Male				Overall Mean
		1–25	26–50	51–75	76–100	
0	9	100	63	60	34	61
36	4	86	72	58	51	56
69	5	59	20	14	26	30

[a]Females were separated from males for several months and then exposed to males twice daily for 0, 36, or 69 days before the first day of assessment for receptivity to mating. Tests for receptivity were performed at the Patacamaya Experiment Station (Bolivia) in the high plains of the Andes mountains starting in January. Daily assessment of receptivity was continued for a period of 100 days and was completed in April.
[b]A female was considered to be sexually receptive if the mating position was assumed within 4 minutes after the male showed interest in the female. Adapted from: B. G. England et al.,[59] 1971.

"rape" pregnant females.[68] Consequently, the periods of estrus and nonreceptivity do not necessarily coincide with ovarian status and levels of estradiol-17β and progesterone, as for other livestock and companion animal species. Furthermore, some alpacas and llamas may refuse to mate, regardless of ovarian status.

The duration of mating for the alpaca and llama is approximately 15 to 20 minutes, with a range of 5 to 60 minutes. However, in the presence of other breeding males, matings are shortened to approximately 8 minutes. Male vicuñas may temporarily suspend mating to chase away intruding males. Ejaculation occurs throughout the mating period[82] and the bulk of the semen is deposited in the uterine horns. Males reposition themselves during mating and this may facilitate the distribution of spermatozoa between the uterine horns.[29]

The cartilaginous appendage with clockwise curve attached to the tapered tip of the glans penis is believed to facilitate the dilation of the cervix and threading of the penis through the folds of the camelid cervix. However, thrusting of the male during mating may traumatize the uterus, causing inflammation, edema, and hyperemia.[29]

Ovulation

Camelids are induced ovulators and nonmated females display repeated waves of follicular activity that result in the growth, maturation, and regression of the dominant follicle. Spontaneous ovulation occurs in a small propor-

tion of females.[108] In alpacas and llamas, ovulatory responses are dependent on the stage of the follicular cycle at the time of mating (Table 18–2). Only females with mature follicles or follicles in the final stage of growth ovulate following mating. Matings that occur while follicles are small and immature do not cause ovulation or affect ovarian functions and structures, when compared to nonmated females. Matings can also occur while follicles are regressing and undergoing atresia, however, those follicles do not ovulate but may luteinize and secrete progesterone (Table 18–2). The lifespan of the luteinized follicle is 5 days compared to a lifespan of approximately 10 days for the CL that forms spontaneously or following a sterile mating.

In llamas, the regression of the dominant follicle and the next wave of follicular growth overlap.[10,16,25] The interwave interval, or the time required for successive dominant follicles to emerge or reach maximal size ranges from 11 to 18 days for llamas, 8 to 12 days for alpacas, and 9 to 10 days for the vicuña. Approximately 80% of the time, the next wave of follicular growth and formation of the dominant follicle occurs on the opposite ovary in alpacas, whereas in llamas, each ovary has an equal chance of forming the dominant follicle that results from the next wave of follicular growth.

The CL induced by the mating of llamas, alpacas, and vicuñas with vasectomized males attains maximal size 8 to 9 days after mating and then regression begins. Two days later, progesterone levels in alpacas and llamas return to baseline levels, though the CL is not fully regressed until Day 12 to 13.

In alpacas, the interval between mating and ovulation is 26 hours with a range of 24 to 48 hours. In contrast, llamas ovulate 48 hours after mating. Approximately 85 to 90% of females with mature follicles ovulate after a single mating. The effect of various stimuli on the proportion of alpacas that ovulate is shown in Table 18–3. Multiple matings do not increase the proportion of alpacas that ovulate (Table 18–4) or the number of oocytes released by the ovaries. In this regard, alpacas and llamas differ from queens, which are also induced ovulators. Multiple matings in queens increase the percentage of queens that ovulate and the total number of ovulated oocytes (see Chapter 17). Furthermore, interrupting the mating of alpacas 5 minutes after the onset of mating has little, if any, effect on the proportion of alpacas that ovulate when compared to the number that ovulate following uninterrupted matings.[108]

Table 18-2   Relationship Between the Stage of Follicular Development and the Proportion of Alpacas and Llamas to Ovulate after a Single Mating

	Stage of Follicular Development[a]			
Species	Small (4 - 5 mm)	Growing (6 - 7 mm)	Mature (8 - 12 mm)	Regressing[b] (10 - 7 mm)
Alpaca	0/4 (0)	3/4 (75)	4/4 (100)	0/3 (0)
Llama	0/4 (0)	4/4 (100)	4/4 (100)	0/4 (0)
Overall	0/8 (0)	7/8 (88)	8/8 (100)	0/7 (0)

Data for llama (n = 16) and alpaca (n = 15) females mated to intact males. The ratio of mated alpacas and llamas to ovulate is shown for each stage of follicular development. The percentage of females that ovulated is shown in parentheses.
[a]Ovarian status was monitored daily by ultrasonography and by measurement of metabolites of progesterone in urine.
[b]For each of the mated females, the follicle luteinized without ovulation.
Adapted from: P. W. Bravo, et al.,[37] 1991.

Table 18-3   Ovulatory Response of Alpacas to Various Stimuli

	Number of Females	
Stimulus	Total	Ovulating (%)
Unstimulated control	20	1 (5)
Mounted; no intromission	13	2 (15)
Mounted; no intromission + AI	9	3 (33)
Mating limited to 5 minutes	10	6 (60)
Mated to vasectomized male	22	17 (77)
Mated to vasectomized male + AI	21	18 (86)
Mated once to intact male	44	36 (82)
Mated 3 times to intact male	10	7 (70)
Treated with hCG	10	10 (100)
Treated with hCG + AI	18	18 (100)

AI = Artificial insemination.
For alpacas treated with human chorionic gonadotropin (hCG), a single injection containing 750 international units (IU) was administered.
Adapted from: J. Sumar,[108] 1994.

Endocrinology of the Cycle

The major ovarian structures in the adult, nonmated alpaca and llama are follicles.

The size of the follicles varies throughout the estrous cycle and the dominant ovarian hormone is estradiol-17β. Blood levels of estradiol-17β and estrone sulfate and urinary levels of estrone sulfate are correlated with the size of the ovarian follicles. It appears that for camelids, as for other species, the concentration of estradiol-17β is critical for triggering the ovulatory surge of luteinizing hormone (LH). Immature and small, growing follicles secrete estrogens, but not in amounts sufficient to induce the ovulatory surge of LH. Matings that occur during the final stages of follicular growth or when the follicle is mature induce the ovulatory surge of LH and cause ovulation (Table 18–5). The blood level of LH increases within 15 minutes from the onset of mating.

Alpacas and llamas that are mated while follicles are regressing fail to ovulate despite the release of a surge of LH that is equivalent to the LH surge that causes ovulation of the mature follicle. However, the regressing follicles can luteinize and secrete progesterone. These observations suggest that regressing follicles secrete levels of estradiol-17β that can stimulate a surge of LH to cause the regressing follicles to luteinize without ovulation.[37]

The profiles of the basal levels of LH and of the ovulatory surge of LH are the same whether

Table 18-4 Relationship Between the Number of Matings and the Ovulatory Response and Fertility of Lactating Alpacas

Number of Matings[a]	Number Bred	Number and Percentage (%) to Ovulate	Number and Percentage (%) Pregnant on:	
			Day 21[b]	Day 40[c]
1	62	43 (69)	32 (74)	27 (63)
2	58	42 (72)	35 (83)	32 (76)
3	56	47 (84)	40 (85)	35 (74)

[a]Mated 10, 20, or 30 days postpartum with an interval of 24 hours between successive matings.
[b]Proportion of ovulating females classified as pregnant on Day 21 was based on a concentration of progesterone >1 ng/ml in plasma.
[c]Proportion of ovulating females classified as pregnant on Day 40 was based on physical examination by rectal palpation and a concentration of progesterone >1 ng/ml in plasma.
Adapted from: P. W. Bravo, et al.,[31] 1995.

Table 18-5 Number of Animals and the Relationship Between the Size of Ovarian Follicles and the Average Concentration of Luteinizing Hormone (LH) in Blood[a] Collected after Mating of Alpacas and Llamas with an Intact Male

	Alpaca		Llama	
Follicular Status	Number	LH (ng/ml)	Number	LH (ng/ml)
4-5 mm (small)	4	28	4	31
6-7 mm (growing)	4	56	4	69
8-12 mm (mature)	4	38	4	72
10-7 mm (regressing)	3	42	4	86

[a]Blood samples were collected at 15-minute intervals during a 6-hour period after mating. Samples were collected from animals shown in Table 18-2.
Adapted from: P. W. Bravo, et al.,[37] 1991.

alpacas and llamas are mated once or twice. A second mating, either 6 or 24 hours after the initial mating, does not cause an increase in the level of LH (Table 18–6). Hence, the camelid pituitary appears to be refractory to the release of significant amounts of LH for at least 24 hours following the initial mating. Similar refractoriness occurs after multiple injections of gonadotropin releasing hormone (GnRH) in llamas, alpacas, sheep, and swine. In contrast, multiple matings in queens augment the secretion and release of LH by significant amounts until the day after the initial mating (see Chapter 17).

Progesterone levels in alpacas and llamas are almost nondetectable unless ovulation is induced by a fertile or sterile mating or occurs spontaneously. Progesterone levels increase within 3 to 4 days after mating and maximal levels are attained by 7 to 8 days after mating. The serum concentration of progesterone declines to basal levels approximately 12 days after a sterile mating. Following a fertile mating, progesterone levels remain elevated until several days before parturition. While progesterone levels remain elevated, females usually refuse to mate. The levels of progesterone in the circulation are correlated with the size of the CL which can be visualized by ultrasonography from the time an increase in serum progesterone is detected and until the concentration of progesterone returns to basal levels.

Prostaglandin $F_{2\alpha}$ ($PGF_{2\alpha}$) appears to be the luteolytic factor in camelids. Measurements of a metabolite, 15-keto-13, 14-dihydro-$PGF_{2\alpha}$, have been used to monitor prostaglandin levels. The demise of the CL and rapid decline in progesterone levels in nonpregnant alpacas, llamas, and the vicuña coincide with large surges of 15-keto-13, 14-dihydro-$PGF_{2\alpha}$ on Day 9 and 10, after which the levels of this $PGF_{2\alpha}$ metabolite and progesterone decline slowly and attain basal levels when the CL has completely regressed. The uterus of the alpaca and llama is the source of the luteolysin. Uterine $PGF_{2\alpha}$ is known to be the luteolysin in other livestock species and its secretion coincides with the regression of CL (see Chapter 9).

THE OVARIES AND TUBULAR REPRODUCTIVE TRACT

Utero-ovarian Relationships

The utero-ovarian relationships in alpacas and llamas are different from that of other livestock species. This was demonstrated[66] in alpacas that were induced to ovulate by mating to vasectomized males followed by the removal of one uterine horn. Removal of the left uterine horn in females with a CL on the left ovary prolonged the lifespan of that CL for at least 70 days. However, when the right uterine horn was removed in females with the CL on the right ovary, the lifespan of that CL was not increased and the CL regressed approximately 11 days after mating. Furthermore, both corpora lutea regressed when a CL was present on each ovary and the right uterine horn was removed, whereas, removal of the left uterine horn prolonged the lifespan of the CL on the left ovary but had no effect on the lifespan of the CL on

Table 18-6 Number of Animals and the Average Concentration of Luteinizing Hormone (LH) in Blood[a] Collected Following a First and a Second Mating with an Intact Male

Mating	Alpaca		Llama	
	Number	LH (ng/ml)	Number	LH (ng/ml)
First	18	31	18	31
Second[b]	14	4	14	5
Not mated	4	4	4	4

[a]Blood samples were collected at 30-minute intervals during a 5-hour period after each mating.
[b]The second mating of the female with an intact male was allowed at 6 hours or 24 hours after the first mating.
Adapted from: P. W. Bravo, et al.,[35] 1992.

the right ovary. It was postulated[66] that the right uterine horn of the alpaca exerted a local effect on the CL of the right ovary, whereas, the left uterine horn exerted local (left ovary) and systemic (right ovary) effects on the CL. More recently, a detailed study[51] of the vascular anatomy of the uterus, oviducts, and ovaries of the alpaca and llama has revealed that most camelids have a large cross-over branch of the right artery which is the major blood supply for much of the left uterine horn and that a large branch of the left uterine vein crosses over to the right uterine horn (Fig. 18–5). These cross-over vessels are clearly visible in the uterus of feti re-

covered at mid-gestation (Fig. 18–6). On these anatomical bases, it appears that the cross-over branch of the left uterine vein allows luteolysin from the left uterine horn to exert control over the CL of the right ovary. Furthermore, both the ovarian arteries and the utero-ovarian veins are tortuous, highly intertwined, and in close apposition to each other, providing the anatomical basis for transfer of luteolysin by a **local veno-arterial pathway,** as is the case for sheep[73] and cattle[72,74] which also have a local utero-ovarian relationship. See Chapter 9 for the physiological implications of this peculiar vascular arrangement on the regulation of ovarian activity.

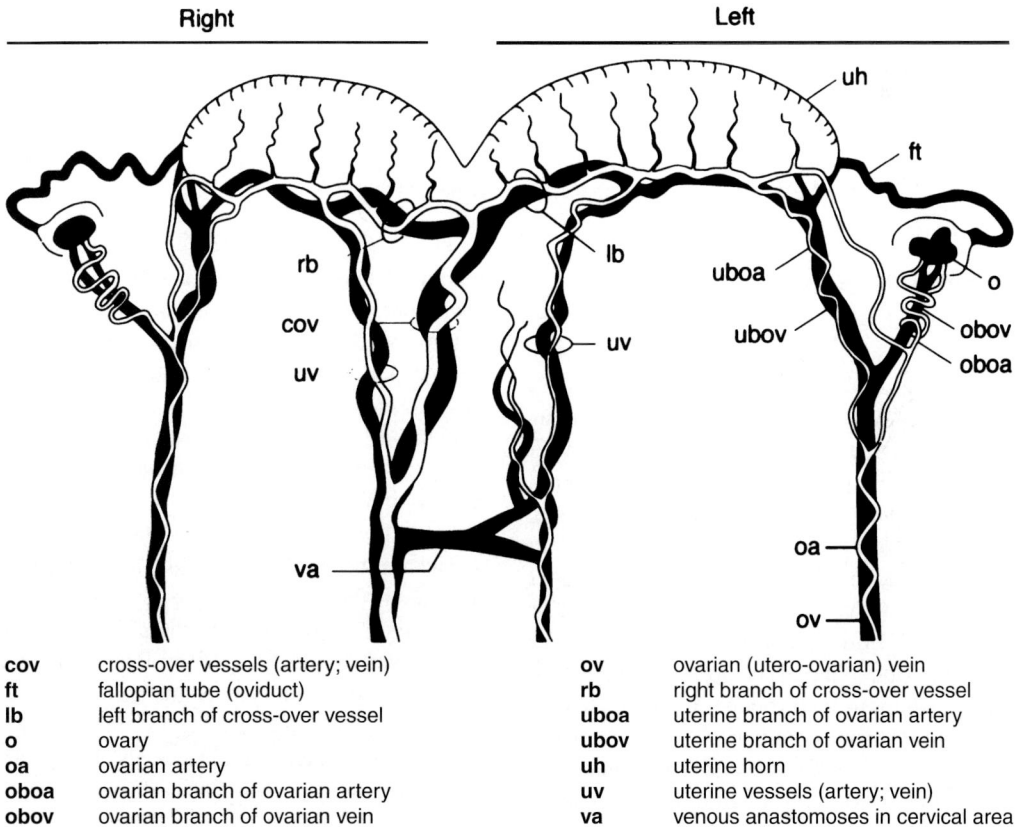

cov	cross-over vessels (artery; vein)	**ov**	ovarian (utero-ovarian) vein
ft	fallopian tube (oviduct)	**rb**	right branch of cross-over vessel
lb	left branch of cross-over vessel	**uboa**	uterine branch of ovarian artery
o	ovary	**ubov**	uterine branch of ovarian vein
oa	ovarian artery	**uh**	uterine horn
oboa	ovarian branch of ovarian artery	**uv**	uterine vessels (artery; vein)
obov	ovarian branch of ovarian vein	**va**	venous anastomoses in cervical area

Fig. 18–5. Diagrammatic representation of the angioarchitecture of the ovaries, oviducts, and uterus of alpacas and llamas. In this diagram, arteries are depicted as light (white) vessels and the veins are black. The right uterine artery is the major supply of blood to the right and left uterine horns, whereas the right uterine vein drains the right uterine horn and receives much of the blood from left uterine horn via anastomoses of the right and left uterine veins within the cervical region. [Courtesy: Drs. C. H. Del Campo and M. R. Del Campo. Proyecto Fondecyt # 09–41–91 funded by the Comisión Nacional de Investigación Científica y Tecnológica (CONICYT), Valdivia, Chile and Theriogenology 46:983, 1996].

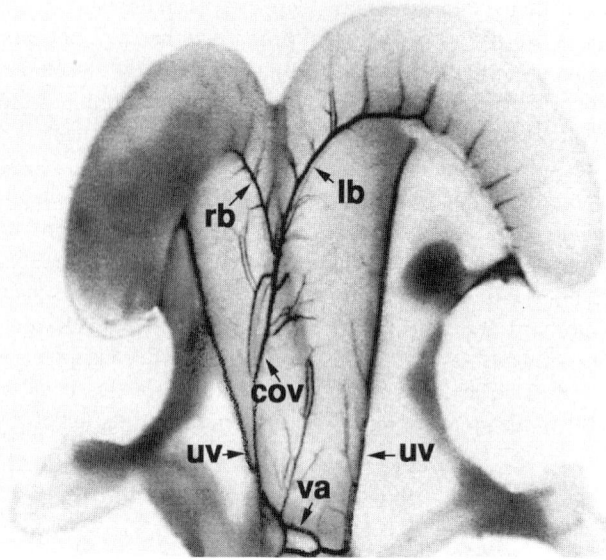

Fig. 18–6. Ventral view of the vasculature of a fluid-filled uterus of a fetal llama. The specimen was transillumi-nated to reveal the outline of the uterine vessels (**uv**) which supply the left and right horns, the anatomical loca-tion of the arterial and venous cross-over vessels (**cov**), the right (**rb**) and left (**lb**) branches of the cross-over vessels, and the venous anastomoses (**va**) in the cervical area. [Courtesy: Drs. C. H. Del Campo and M. R. Del Campo. Proyecto Fondecyt # 09–41–91 funded by the Comisión Nacional de Investigación Científica y Tech-nológica (CONICYT), Valdivia, Chile and Theriogenology 46:983, 1996].

Tubular Reproductive Tract

Under estrogenic dominance, the uterus of the alpaca and llama is edematous, turgid, and longi-tudinal uterine folds or rugae can be palpated. The cervix and the cervical folds are soft and pli-able. The vagina is slippery due to the presence of a thin, watery fluid and appears shiny and pink.

If ovulation occurs, the CL forms and proges-terone becomes the dominant hormone. The uterus of the nonpregnant alpaca and llama, under progesterone dominance, is no longer ede-matous and turgid and the uterine folds are no longer palpable. The cervix closes, becomes firm, and penetration is difficult. Vaginal changes under progesterone dominance are also dramatic. The mucosa becomes pale and the vagina is dry and sticky, making it difficult to insert nonlubri-cated instruments for examination purposes.

FERTILIZATION RATES AND THE ESTABLISHMENT OF PREGNANCY

The time required for the transport of sper-matozoa to the utero-tubal junction and the isth-mus in alpacas is slow compared to other live-stock species. This may be attributable to the extreme viscosity of the semen which inhibits the transport of spermatozoa until the coagulum of the semen liquefies. This is likely to be the case for all camelids because their semen is highly viscous. The average time required for liquefaction of the coagulum is approximately 23 hours for alpaca semen maintained at 37°C.

The number of oocytes available for fertiliza-tion is contributed equally by each ovary. Fertil-ization likely takes place in the *ampulla* of the oviduct, but the exact site of fertilization and the amount of time embryos reside in the oviduct has not been determined. Because fewer than 2 to 5% of pregnancies in alpacas and llamas are established in the right uterine horn, embryos originating from the right oviduct must migrate to the left uterine horn to survive. Transuterine migration has also been reported in guanacos.

Regardless of the ovary that releases the oocyte, an embryo must be present in the left uterine horn to counteract the local luteolytic effect of the left horn on the CL that forms, either on the left or right ovary. The time when embryos migrate from the right to the left uterine horn and the last day by which the embryo must migrate to the left uterine horn for pregnancy to be maintained has not been determined. However, it seems likely that the embryo must migrate from the right to the left uterine horn no later than 8 to 9 days after mating. Otherwise, it would be too late for the embryo or embryonic factors to rescue the CL which begins to regress on Day 9 to 10 in females mated to sterile males. Fertilization and embryonic survival rates for vicuñas and guanacos have not been reported.

In their native habitat, the fertilization rate for alpacas 3 days after mating is approximately 70 to 80%. However, during the next 4 weeks 40 to 50% of those embryos perish, a mortality rate comparable to that of swine and horses, but greater than that of domestic ruminants. The reason for the high rate of embryonic death in the alpaca, and presumably for the other camelids, is unknown but could be due to the fertilization of immature or aged oocytes, reduction of the number of embryos in females with twin embryos, failure of embryos to migrate from the right to the left uterine horn, the harsh environment, or a combination of these factors.

Although it is not unusual for alpacas and llamas to ovulate 2 oocytes following mating, these animals rarely give birth to twins. This phenomenon may be similar to that of horses and is sometimes referred to as the "killer" embryo effect (see Chapters 9 and 13) in which, by unknown mechanisms, 1 of the 2 embryos causes the demise of the other. It has been suggested that in alpacas and llamas this phenomenon usually occurs before attachment of the embryo. Attachment occurs 21 to 27 days after mating but the precise time has not been determined.

PREGNANCY

Pregnancy ranges from 330 to 368 days in camelids. The mean duration of pregnancy for alpacas is reported as 342 to 345 days in their South American habitat and 350 days for llamas in the United States.

Camelids have a simple epitheliochorial placenta. In the llama, numerous, small, thin, semi-circular domes of epithelial and vascular tissue that fit into depressions on the surface of the uterus are evident on the surface of the chorion by the third month of pregnancy. These 2 structures, as for the entire interface between the chorion and the uterus, are loosely attached and do not interlock as occurs in the placentomes of ruminants.

The placentation of camelids is unique. Camelids have an extra fetal membrane which consists of a thin layer of epithelium and keratin that forms between the fetus and the amnion. This epidermal membrane develops at midpregnancy and is attached to the umbilicus, feet, and to the periphery of the anus, urogenital organs, and nostrils and mouth such that the membrane does not affect fetal swallowing, excretion of waste into the amniotic sac, or the cria's breathing while in the birth canal and after parturition. The cria is usually delivered with an intact epidermal membrane.

The wet, epidermal membrane is very slippery and is believed to serve an important role in facilitating the delivery of the fetus. The amnion of camelids contains a minimal amount of thin, watery fluid rather than mucoid fluid that serves as the lubricant for the birth canal during parturition in other species.

Endocrinology of Pregnancy

Much of the endocrinology of pregnancy in alpacas and llamas is similar to that of livestock species. Four to 5 days after mating, progesterone in the blood increases rapidly from basal to high levels by Day 8 to 9. Thereafter, levels of progesterone decline slowly until Day 12 to 13 and then increase again. This period of decline in progesterone coincides with the presumed maternal signal of pregnancy and a temporary increase in metabolites of $PGF_{2\alpha}$. However, the levels of 15-keto-13, 14-dihydro-$PGF_{2\alpha}$ are lower than for temporal levels of 15-keto-13, 14-dihydro-$PGF_{2\alpha}$ in nonpregnant alpacas and llamas with a regressing CL. In contrast, the progesterone levels of ruminants do not decline during the maternal recognition of pregnancy.

During the remainder of pregnancy, levels of progesterone in the blood are elevated (Table 18–7) and remain high until 2 weeks before parturition when progesterone levels begin to decline, before dropping sharply to low levels during the last 2 days of pregnancy. The major source of progesterone is the corpus luteum and bilateral ovariectomy, when performed between early pregnancy and 1 to 2 weeks before parturition leads to abortion. Hence, as is the case for sows and goats, the CL of alpacas and llamas is required throughout gestation for the maintenance of pregnancy.

The concentration of relaxin during pregnancy in alpacas and llamas is biphasic. Relaxin remains at basal levels for the first 2 months before they begin to increase. The first peak of relaxin occurs at $3\frac{1}{2}$ months and the nadir is between the fifth and eighth months of pregnancy (Table 18–7). Relaxin peaks again approximately 1 week before parturition.

The concentration of estrogens, as estimated from the concentration of estrone sulfate in the blood and urine (Table 18–7), is elevated during the third week of pregnancy and levels then decline. However, during the last third of pregnancy the levels of estrogens begin to increase again, peak one week before parturition, then decline and drop precipitously during the last 24 hours of pregnancy. The source of estrogens during pregnancy has not

been determined although, as for other species, it is likely to originate from the placenta or the fetoplacental unit.

Diagnosis of Pregnancy

Various methods are available for the diagnosis of pregnancy in camelids and all of them have advantages and disadvantages such as cost, reliability, ease of method, skills required to administer and interpret the tests, stage of pregnancy when the accuracy of the test is the highest, and whether or not the results of the test are immediately available.

Traditional methods to determine whether camelids are pregnant include the use of males to test the female's receptivity or willingness to mate and ballottement. Tests for receptivity must be done periodically and are time consuming. This test is unreliable in alpacas and llamas when done during the first month of pregnancy because nonpregnant females with a functional CL resist mating and the embryonic death rate during the first month of pregnancy is high (40–50%). The reliability of the test for receptivity increases if it is repeated on Day 30, 60, and 90 of pregnancy. The accuracy of the test for receptivity in alpacas and llamas is esti-

Table 18-7   *Concentration (ng/ml) of Progesterone, Relaxin, and Estrone Sulfate in the Blood and Estrone Sulfate in the Urine[a] of Pregnant Alpacas and Llamas*

Hormone	Time of Gestation	Alpaca	Llama
Progesterone	Mating	0.5	0.4
	First Month	2.5	3.3
	Three Months	2.9	3.1
	Six Months	2.7	2.6
	Last Month	1.9	2.3
Relaxin	First Month	0.4	0.3
	Three Months	21.9	20.7
	Six Months	4.7	3.7
	Last Month	21.2	24.9
Estrone Sulfate	Mating	0.2 (8)[a]	0.2 (6)[a]
	Day 21	48.1 (73)	44.5 (81)
	Three Months	0.6 (3)	0.3 (3)
	Six Months	0.4 (14)	0.2 (11)
	Last Month	38.6 (889)	42.3 (1,087)

[a]Values within parentheses are levels of estrone sulfate in the urine and are expressed as ng/mg of creatinine.
Adapted from: P. W. Bravo, et al.,[38] 1996.

mated to be 85% when performed 70 to 75 days after mating and 88 to 95% when performed 125 days after mating.

Ballottement is one of the most widely used tests of pregnancy in the high plains of South America and the method is accurate after the 10th month of pregnancy, when done by experienced personnel.

Rectal palpation is possible in most llamas and in 70 to 80% of alpacas, provided the examiner has a small hand and thin forearm. With this method it is possible to detect pregnancy as early as Day 30 to 35 and the accuracy of diagnosis approaches 100% when done 45 to 60 days after mating. At approximately 90 days of pregnancy, the fetus and uterus become abdominal rather than pelvic and palpation of the fetus is not possible. After the fifth or sixth month of pregnancy the fetus enters the pelvic canal and can be palpated again.

More recently, ultrasonography and tests for levels of hormones have been used for the diagnosis of pregnancy in alpacas and llamas. Ultrasound equipment is expensive and considerable skill is required to accurately interpret ultrasonograms. With this technology, embryos can be detected 9 to 15 days after mating. However, if only a single ultrasonogram for the diagnosis of pregnancy is to be done, the test should be delayed until after the first month of pregnancy due to the high rate of embryonic mortality before this time. The accuracy of pregnancy diagnosis using ultrasound has been estimated to be 92% for the alpaca on Day 80 and 100% for the llama on Day 75.[12] Thereafter, the accuracy declines to 84% and 65% on Day 165 in alpacas and llamas, respectively. Ultrasound can also be used to estimate the age of the fetus.

Estrogens, including estradiol-17β and estrone sulfate, progesterone, and relaxin are hormones that can serve as indicators of pregnancy. Levels of estrogens can be estimated indirectly by measuring a metabolite, estrone sulfate. However, the reliability of estrone sulfate as a test for the diagnosis of pregnancy has not been determined. Estrone sulfate levels in the blood and urine of alpacas and llamas increase rapidly from 19 to 22 days after mating and return to baseline values by Day 28. The source of this estrone sulfate is believed to originate from the embryo and/or placental membranes rather than from the dam.

Levels of progesterone in the blood and milk are also used as an indicator of pregnancy in alpacas and llamas. This test should be performed after the first month following mating to increase the accuracy of the diagnosis.

Levels of relaxin in the blood of the alpaca and llama are low throughout the first 2 months of pregnancy. Levels of relaxin then increase rapidly and remain elevated for the remainder of pregnancy. The ideal time to determine pregnancy based on levels of relaxin would likely be 3 to 4 months after mating, when the reliability of this test would likely be expected to be very high.

Parturition

Predicting the time of parturition for alpacas and llamas is very difficult. The enlargement of the abdomen and mammary glands may not even be apparent because they are obscured by a thick coat of wool. Furthermore, the enlargement of the abdomen during pregnancy is small compared to other species.

The mammary glands of nulliparous females show little growth before parturition whereas the mammary glands of multiparous females usually begins to increase in size 2 to 3 weeks before parturition. However, neither the onset of the increase in size or the degree of enlargement of the mammary gland is related to the day of parturition. Three to 4 days before parturition nipples may increase in size and 'wax' as occurs in horses.

Before the onset of parturition the female isolates herself from the herd. The duration of labor is only 2 to 3 hours in multiparous females and is slightly longer for nulliparous females. The reported incidence of dystocia is low, 1.6%. In South America, 94% of alpaca crias are born between 0700 and 1300 hours but the range is more variable in North America. Most llamas, guanacos, and vicuñas are also born in the morning. Morning births are advantageous in the high plains of South America because crias become ambulatory and are dry before nightfall when, even in the Summer, temperatures commonly drop to below freezing.

Camelids do not lick their crias nor do they ingest the placenta. Because they do not receive help from the dam, crias free themselves of the epidermal membrane and the other placental membranes by rolling on the ground.

The survival rates[44] of alpaca crias in South America is surprisingly high despite the harsh environmental conditions. The survival rate of crias born to 3 year-old dams is 78%. Thereafter, survival rates increase steadily to a peak of 91% for crias born to 9 to 11 year-old dams but survival rates decrease to 85% for 15 year-old dams.

The Postpartum Period

Involution of the uterus is rapid in alpacas and llamas. Twelve to 24 hours after parturition there is a marked decrease in the size of the uterus and within another 9 days there is a 6 to 7 fold decrease in the weight of the uterus. Involution of the uterus is completed 17 to 21 days after parturition.

The CL of alpacas and llamas regresses within 1 to 3 days after parturition and progesterone returns to basal levels of less than 1 ng/ml. Follicles begin to grow and the female becomes receptive to mating within 2 to 3 days after parturition. However, mating at this time is not recommended because, as for horses bred at the 'foal heat' or first postpartum estrus, involution of the uterus is incomplete and conception rates are low. The pregnancy rate of alpacas mated 10 to 12 days after parturition is lower (31%) than for matings 20 to 22 days (60%) or 30 to 32 days (71%) postpartum. The rapid return to estrus and involution of the uterus are critical if camelids are to produce crias on a yearly basis.

CONTROL OF REPRODUCTIVE EFFICIENCY

Induction of Estrus and Estrous Synchronization

Regimens to efficiently induce estrus or to synchronize estrus for routine use in breeding programs for camelids have not been developed. Perhaps, the primary reasons for the lack of interest in developing regimens for the control of reproduction of camelids may be related to the fact that alpacas and llamas breed successfully at very young ages (12 months) and nonpregnant females are usually receptive and can be bred throughout the year. In addition, artificial insemination services are not available and the economical return does not warrant the wide application of these procedures.

Embryo Transfer

Regimens to synchronize estrus and to induce ovulation and superovulatory responses in camelids have been reported. Ovulation can be induced and synchronized reliably in alpacas and llamas with mature follicles by mating or by injections of human chorionic gonadotropin (hCG) or gonadotropin-releasing hormone (GnRH). Progestagen treatments for 7 to 12 days in combination with follicle-stimulating hormone (FSH) or equine chorionic gonadotropin (eCG) have been used to induce superovulation in alpacas and llamas. In most cases, 2 to 6 ovulations are induced with a range of 0 to 12.[49] Because most pregnancies are established in the left uterine horn, embryos should be transferred to this horn. The demand for this technology in the United States and other countries has prompted an increase in research related to embryo transfer in camelids.

Breeding Regimens

In most herds of llamas in South America, males and females are joined throughout the year. With this management practice, crias may be born at any time of the year but most (> 75%) are born in the late Spring and Summer.

In many alpaca herds, males and females are separated between breeding seasons. The stocking rate in these herds is 1 breeding male for every 15 to 35 females. Approximately 70% of these females mate within 4 to 5 days after they are joined with the male. However, only one-half of these matings result in the birth of a cria. This low rate of birth has been attributed to matings which occur while follicles are still growing or are regressing, to the high rate of embryonic loss, and to mating with infertile males.

By 12 days after alpaca males and females are joined, there is a dramatic drop in the breeding activity of males, despite the presence of receptive females. At this time the nonpregnant females also exhibit a decreased interest in males. To reduce the impact of these phenomena, breeding males are replaced every 7 to 14 days. This practice maximizes breeding activity and conception rates and also assures that most crias are born within a relatively short time.

THE MALE

Collection of Semen

The collection of ejaculates from camelids for seminal evaluation or for artificial insemination is not a common practice. Attempts to collect semen from vaginal sacs and sponges inserted into the female before mating are unreliable. The collection of semen by electroejaculation does not require the aid of an estrual female or training of the male, however, a high proportion of electroejaculates are contaminated with urine which is harmful to spermatozoa and precludes the valid assessment of seminal quality. Hence, further improvement of the method is needed, particularly in relation to the design of rectal probes, optimal voltage and amperage, and the duration and number of electrical stimuli necessary to obtain a representative ejaculate.

Ejaculates can be obtained from alpacas trained to ejaculate in an artificial vagina.[22] The amount of time males copulate with the dummy or with females is comparable. Of course, males must be trained to accept the dummy and ejaculate in the artificial vagina, whether the ejaculate is used for the examination of breeding soundness, artificial insemination, or other assisted reproductive technologies.

The common method for obtaining semen samples for clinical examination is to aspirate semen from the anterior floor of the vagina of the recently mated female. Unfortunately this approach precludes the accurate determination of the volume of ejaculate, concentration of spermatozoa, or total number of spermatozoa released during ejaculation. Therefore, under these conditions, the examination of the semen is limited to observations on the motility and morphology of spermatozoa and on the ratio of live and dead spermatozoa.

Seminal Characteristics

Temperature has a marked effect on the motility of spermatozoa. Consequently, it is imperative to maintain the semen at 37°C during the examination of spermatozoal motility. Camelid spermatozoa, in contrast to spermatozoa from ruminants, do not exhibit swirling motions or progressive motility due to the high viscosity of the camelids' ejaculates.

The morphological defects in the spermatozoa of alpacas and llamas are similar to those seen in other species. Norms have not been established for the proportion of morphologically normal and abnormal spermatozoa and for the percentage of live spermatozoa in the ejaculate. The percentage of normal spermatozoa in the semen of alpacas collected with an artificial vagina ranges from 70 to 85% for most males and the percentage of live spermatozoa ranges from 60 to 85% (Table 18–8). There is little information on the effects of season on the quality of semen except that ejaculates from alpacas and llamas may be azoospermic when collected during the summer months in the southern and southwestern parts of the United States. Characteristics of semen from alpacas and llamas collected with an artificial vagina are shown in Table 18–8.

In alpaca breeding herds in South America, males are rotated every 7 to 14 days. Despite this management practice, oligospermia results in some males, particularly if the male ejaculates more than 2 to 3 times per day. Because males may mate up to 18 times on the day they are joined with females, the depletion of spermatozoal reserves may account for the high proportion of infertile males (20%) in traditional breeding herds.

Vasectomized alpacas may have motile spermatozoa present in their ejaculates 20 to 30 days after vasectomy.[40]

Breeding Soundness Examination

Breeding soundness examinations should include the evaluation of semen whenever possi-

Table 18-8 Characteristics of Semen Collected from Alpacas and Llamas Using an Artificial Vagina

Parameter	Species	
	Alpaca	Llama
Volume (ml)	1.9	3.5
Spermatozoal concentration (10^6/ml)	148	84.7
Total number of spermatozoa (10^6)	281	296
Motility (%)	79	25
Normal spermatozoa (%)	76	32
Live spermatozoa (%)	76	83

Adapted from: P. W. Bravo, et al.,[22,23] 1997, M. E. Fowler and P. W. Bravo,[68] 1998, A. B. Lichtenwalner, et al,[85] 1996, and L. von Baer and C. Hellemann,[119] 1998.

ADDITIONAL REFERENCES ON THE SEMINAL CHARACTERISTICS OF CAMELIDS:

1) Garnica, J., Achata, R., and Bravo, P. W. (1993): Physical and biochemical characteristics of alpaca semen. Anim. Reprod. Sci. *33*:85-90. NOTE: Authors do not report data for spermatozoal concentration but report spermatozoa were 11.5% of seminal volume after centrifugation.

2) Garnica, J., Flores, E., and Bravo, P. W. (1995): Citric acid and fructose concentrations in seminal plasma of the alpaca. Small Ruminant Research *18*:95-98. NOTE: Spermatozoal concentration (10^6) for the alpaca ranged from 0.085 to 0.195 per milliliter (ml) with a mean concentration of 0.150 x 10^6 per ml for repeated collections from 6 animals.

3) Graham, E. F., Schmell, M. K. L., Eversen, B. K., et al. (1978): Semen preservation in nondomestic mammals. Symp. Zool. Soc., London, England *43*:153-173. NOTE: Authors report spermatozoal concentration for the llama was 460 x 10^6 per ml following seminal dilution at a ratio of 1:8.

4) Kubicek, J. (1974): Samenentnahme beim Alpaka durch eine Harnröhrenfistel. Z. Tierzüchtg. Züchtgsbiol. *90*:335. NOTE: Seminal volumes ranged from 1 to 21 ml and the spermatozoal concentration ranged from 5 to 4,708 x 10^6 per ml in semen collected from males with an urethral fistula.

5) McEvoy, T. G., Kyle, C. E., Young, P., et al. (1992): Aspects of artificial breeding and establishment of pregnancy in South American camelids. Proc. 12th Internat. Cong. Anim. Reprod. *4*:1963-1965. NOTE: The concentration of spermatozoa in semen collected from llamas by electroejaculation or using an intravaginal sheath ranged from 17 to 20 x 10^6 per ml.

ble. When performed, the clinician should observe the male's libido, sexual behavior, and whether or not the male experiences any difficulties during copulation.

Procedures for examining the reproductive organs is similar to that of other livestock species and should include a rectal examination whenever possible. The prepuce, scrotum, testes, and epididymides should be examined for swellings and injuries and possible signs of trauma due to fighting and biting among breeding males. Testicular size should be considered when selecting males for breeding. It is particularly important in North America to carefully examine the testes, penis, and other reproduc-

tive organs, because there is a high incidence of hypogonadism, cryptorchidism, persistent adhesions between the prepuce and glans penis, small and malformed penises, intersexism, and other congenital anomalies. Hence, the use of affected animals for breeding is strongly discouraged.

REFERENCES

1. Aba, M. A., Bravo, P. W., Forsberg, M., et al. (1997): Endocrine changes during early pregnancy in the alpaca. Anim. Reprod. Sci. *47*:273.
2. Aba, M. A. and Forsberg, M. (1995): Heterologous radioimmunoassay for llama and alpaca luteinizing hormone with a monoclonal antibody, an equine standard and a human tracer. Acta Vet. Scand. *36*:367.

3. Aba, M. A., Forsberg, M., Kindahl, H., et al. (1995): Endocrine changes after mating in pregnant and non-pregnant llamas and alpacas. Acta Vet. Scand. *36:*489.

4. Aba, M. A., Kindahl, H., Forsberg, M., et al. (2000): Levels of progesterone and changes in prostaglandin F (2 alpha) release during luteolysis and early pregnancy in llamas and the effect of treatment with flunixin meglumine. Anim. Reprod. Sci. *59:*87.

5. Aba, M. A., Quiroga, M. A., Auza, N., et al. (1999): Control of ovarian activity in llamas (*Lama glama*) with medroxyprogesterone acetate. Reprod. Domestic Anim. *34:*471.

6. Aba, M. A., Sumar, J., Kindahl, H., et al. (1998): Plasma concentrations of 15-ketodihydro-PGF$_{2\alpha}$, progesterone, oestrone sulfate, oestradiol-17β and cortisol during late gestation, parturition and the early postpartum period in llamas and alpacas. Anim. Reprod. Sci. *50:*111.

7. Adam, C. L., Bourke, D. A., Kyle, C. L. et al. (1992): Ovulation and embryo recovery in the llama. Proc. First Int. Camel Conf., Dubai, United Arab Emirates, Feb. 2–6, 1992, p. 125.

8. Adam, C. L., Moir, C. E., and Shiach, P. (1989): Plasma progesterone concentrations in pregnant and non-pregnant llamas *(Lama glama)*. Vet. Rec. *125:*618.

9. Adams, G. P., Griffin, P. G., and Ginther, O. J. (1989): *In situ* morphologic dynamics of ovaries, uterus, and cervix in llamas. Biol. Reprod. *41:*551.

10. Adams, G. P., Sumar, J., and Ginther, O. J. (1990): Effect of lactational and reproductive status on ovarian follicular waves in llamas *(Lama glama)*. J. Reprod. Fertil. *90:*535.

11. Adams, G. P., Sumar, J., and Ginther, O. J. (1991): Form and function of the corpus luteum in llamas. Anim. Reprod. Sci. *24:*127.

12. Alarcón, V., Sumar, J., Riera, G. S., et al. (1990): Comparison of three methods of pregnancy diagnosis in alpacas and llamas. Theriogenology *34:*1119.

13. Bader, H. (1982): An investigation of sperm migration into the oviducts of the mare. J. Reprod. Fertil. (Suppl. *32*):59.

14. Banks, D. H. and Stabenfeldt, G. H. (1982): Luteinizing hormone release in the cat in response to coitus on consecutive days of estrus. Biol. Reprod. *26:*603.

15. Basu, S. and Kendahl, H. (1987): Development of a continuous blood collection technique and a detailed study of prostaglandin F$_{2\alpha}$ release during luteolysis and early pregnancy in heifers. J. Vet. Med. Series A *34:*487.

16. Bourke, D. A., Adam, C. L., and Kyle, C. E. (1992): Ultrasonography as an aid to controlled breeding in the llama *(Lama glama)*. Vet. Rec. *130:*424.

17. Bourke, D. A., Adam, C. L., Kyle, C. E., et al. (1992): Superovulation and embryo transfer in the llama. Proc. First Int. Camel Conf., Dubai, United Arab Emirates, Feb. 2–6, 1992, p. 183.

18. Bourke, D. A., Kyle, C. E., McEvoy, T. G., et al. (1995): Superovulatory responses to eCG in llamas *(Lama glama)*. Theriogenology *44:*255.

19. Bravo, P. W. (1994): Reproductive endocrinology of llamas and alpacas. Vet. Clin. North Am., Food Anim. Pract. *10:*265.

20. Bravo, P. W., Bayan, P. J., Troedsson, M. H. T., et al. (1996): Induction of parturition in alpacas and subsequent survival of neonates. J. Am. Vet. Med. Assoc. *209:*1760.

21. Bravo, P. W., Ccallo, M., and Garnica, J. (2000): The effects of enzymes on semen viscosity in Llamas and Alpacas. Small Ruminant Res. *38:*91.

22. Bravo, P. W., Flores, U., Garnica, J., et al. (1997): Collection of semen and artificial insemination of alpacas. Theriogenology *47:*619.

23. Bravo, P. W., Flores, D., and Ordoñez, C. (1997): Effect of repeated collection on semen characteristics of alpacas. Biol. Reprod. *57:*520.

24. Bravo, P. W., Fowler, M. E., and Lasley, B. L. (1994): The postpartum llama: Fertility after parturition. Biol. Reprod. *51:*1084.

25. Bravo, P. W., Fowler, M. E., Stabenfeldt, G. H., et al. (1990): Ovarian follicular dynamics in the llama. Biol. Reprod. *43:*579.

26. Bravo, P. W., Fowler, M. E., Stabenfeldt, G. H., et al. (1990): Endocrine responses in the llama to copulation. Theriogenology *33:*891.

27. Bravo, P. W. and Johnson, L. W. (1994): Reproductive physiology of the male camelid. Vet. Clin. North Am., Food Anim. Pract. *10:*259.

28. Bravo, P. W., Mayta, M. M., and Ordonez, C.A. (2000): Growth of the conceptus in alpacas. Am. J. Vet. Res. *61:*1508.

29. Bravo, P. W., Moscoso, J., Ordóñez, C., et al. (1996): Transport of spermatozoa and ova in female alpaca. Anim. Reprod. Sci. *43:*173.

30. Bravo, P. W., Pacheco, C., Quispe, G., et al. (1999): Degelification of alpaca semen and the effect of dilution rates on artificial insemination outcome. Arch. Androl. *43:*239.

31. Bravo, P. W., Pezo, D., and Alarcón, V. (1995): Evaluation of early reproductive performance in the postpartum alpaca by progesterone concentrations. Anim. Reprod. Sci. *39:*71.

32. Bravo, P. W., Skidmore, J. A., and Zhao, X. X. (2000): Reproductive aspects and storage of semen in camelidae. Anim. Reprod. Sci. *62:*173.

33. Bravo, P. W., Solis, P., Ordonez, C., et al. (1997): Fertility of the male alpaca: Effect of daily consecutive breeding. Anim. Reprod. Sci. *46:*305.

34. Bravo, P. W., Stabenfeldt, G. H., Fowler, M. E., et al. (1991): Urinary steroids in the periparturient and postpartum periods through early pregnancy in llamas. Theriogenology *36:*267.

35. Bravo, P. W., Stabenfeldt, G. H., Fowler, M. E., et al. (1992): Pituitary response to repeated copulation and/or gonadotropin-releasing hormone administration in llamas and alpacas. Biol. Reprod. *47:*884.

36. Bravo, P. W., Stabenfeldt, G. H., Fowler, M. E., et al. (1993): Ovarian and endocrine patterns associated with reproductive abnormalities in llamas and alpacas. J. Am. Vet. Med. Assoc. *202:*268.

37. Bravo, P. W., Stabenfeldt, G. H., Lasley, B. L. et al. (1991): The effect of ovarian follicle size on pituitary and ovarian responses to copulation in domesticated South American camelids. Biol. Reprod. *45:*553.

38. Bravo, P. W., Steward, D. R., Lasley, B. L., et al. (1996): Hormonal indicators of pregnancy in llamas and alpacas. J. Am. Vet. Med. Assoc. *208:*2027.

39. Bravo, P. W. and Sumar, J. (1989): Laparoscopic examination of the ovarian activity in alpacas. Anim. Reprod. Sci. *21:*271.

40. Bravo, P. W. and Sumar, J. (1991): Evaluation of intra-abdominal vasectomy in llamas and alpacas. J. Am. Vet. Med. Assoc. *199:*1164.

41. Bravo, P. W., Tsutsui, T., and Lasley, B. L. (1995): Dose responses to equine chorionic gonadotropin and subsequent ovulation in llamas. Small Ruminant Res. *18:*157.

42. Bravo, P. W. and Valera, M. H. (1993): Prenatal development of the alpaca *(Lama pacos).* Anim. Reprod. Sci. *32:*245.

43. Brown, B.W. (2000): A review on reproduction in South American camelids. Anim. Reprod. Sci. *58:*169.

44. Bustinza, A. V., Burfening, P. J., and Blackwell, R. L. (1988): Factors affecting survival in young alpacas *(Lama pacos).* J. Anim. Sci. *66:*1139.

45. Chakraborty, R. K., Reeves, J. J., Arimura, A., et al. (1973): Serum LH levels in prepubertal female pigs chronically treated with synthetic luteinizing releasing hormone/follicle stimulating releasing hormone (LHRH/FSHRH). Endocrinology *92:*55.

46. Concannon, P., Hodgson, B., and Lein, D. (1980): Reflex LH release in estrous cats following single and multiple copulations. Biol. Reprod. *23:*111.

47. Del Campo, C. H. and Ginther, O. J. (1973): Vascular anatomy of the uterus and ovaries and the unilateral luteolytic effect of the uterus: Horses, sheep, and swine. Am. J. Vet. Res. *34:*305.

48. Del Campo, C. H. and Ginther, O. J. (1973): Vascular anatomy of the uterus and ovaries and the luteolytic effect of the uterus: Angioarchitecture in sheep. Am. J. Vet. Res. *34:*1377.

49. Del Campo, M. R., Del Campo, C. H., Adams, G. P., et al. (1995): The application of new reproductive technologies to South American camelids. Theriogenology *43:*21.

50. Del Campo, M. R., Del Campo, C. H., Donoso, M. X., et al. (1994): *In vitro* fertilization and development of llama *(Lama glama)* oocytes using epididymal spermatozoa and oviductal cell co-culture. Theriogenology *41:*1219.

51. Del Campo, M. R., Del Campo, C. H., and Ginther, O. J. (1996): Vascular provisions for a local uteroovarian cross-over pathway in New World camelids. Theriogenology *46:*983.

52. Del Campo, M. R., Del Campo, C. H., Mapletoft, R. J., et al. (1995): Morphology and location of attached follicular cumulus-oocyte complexes in horses, cattle and llamas. Theriogenology *43:*533.

53. Delhon, G. A. and Von Lawzewitsch, I. (1987): Reproduction in the male llama *(Lama glama),* a South American camelid. 1. Spermatogenesis and organization of the intertubular space of the mature testis. Acta Anat. *129:*59.

54. Delhon, G. and Von Lawzewitsch, I. (1994): Ductus epididymidis compartments and morphology of epididymal spermatozoa in llamas. Anat. Histol. Embryol. *23:*217.

55. Drew, M. L., Alexander, B. M., and Sassen, G. (1995): Pregnancy determination by use of pregnancy-specific protein B radioimmunoassay in llamas. J. Am. Vet. Med. Assoc. *207:*217.

56. Drew, M. L., Meyers-Wallen, V. N., Acland, G. M., et al. (1999): Presumptive Sry-negative XX sex reversal in a llama with multiple congenital anomalies. J. Am. Vet. Med. Assoc. *215:*1134.

57. Ebel, S. (1989): The llama industry in the United States. Vet. Clin. North Am., Food Anim. Pract. *5:*1.

58. England, B. G., Cardozo, A. G., and Foote, W. C. (1969): A review of the physiology of reproduction in the New World Camelidae. Int. Zoo Yearbook *9:*104.

59. England, B. G., Foote, W. C., Cardozo, A. G., et al. (1971): Oestrous and mating behaviour in the llama *(Llama glama).* Anim. Behav. *19:*722.

60. England, B. G., Foote, W. C., Matthews, D. H., et al. (1969): Ovulation and corpus luteum function in the llama *(Lama glama).* J. Endocrinol. *45:*505.

61. Escobar, R. C. (1984): The alpaca. *In:* Animal Breeding and Production of American Camelids. Lima, Peru, Talleres Gráficos de Abril, p. 59.

62. Fernández-Baca, S. (1990): Llamoids or new world camelidae: Llama, alpaca, guanaco and vicuña. Chapter 10. *In:* An Introduction to Animal Husbandry in the Tropics, 4th edition, edited by W. J. A. Payne. New York, NY, John Wiley & Sons, Inc., p. 557.

63. Fernández-Baca, S. (1993): Manipulation of reproductive functions in male and female New World camelids. Anim. Reprod. Sci. *33:*307.

64. Fernández-Baca, S., Hansel, W., and Novoa, C. (1970): Embryonic mortality in the alpaca. Biol. Reprod. *3:*243.

65. Fernández-Baca, S., Hansel, W., and Novoa, C. (1970): Corpus luteal function in the alpaca. Biol. Reprod. *3:*252.

66. Fernández-Baca, S., Hansel, W., Saatman, R., et al. (1979): Differential luteolytic effects of right and left uterine horns in the alpaca. Biol. Reprod. *20:*586.

67. Fernández-Baca, S., Madden, D. H. L., and Novoa, C. (1970): Effect of different mating stimuli on induction of ovulation in the alpaca. J. Reprod. Fertil. *22:*261.

68. Fowler, M. E. and Bravo, P. W. (1998): Reproduction. *In:* Medicine and Surgery of South American Camelids Llama, Alpaca, Vicuña, Guanaco, 2nd ed., edited by M. E. Fowler. Ames, IA, Iowa State University Press, p. 381.

69. Fowler, M. E. and Olander, H. J. (1990): Fetal membranes and ancillary structures of llama *(Lama glama).* Am. J. Vet. Res. *51:*1495.

70. Garnica, J., Achata, R., and Bravo, P. W. (1993): Physical and biochemical characteristics of alpaca semen. Anim. Reprod. Sci. *32:*85.

71. Garnica, J., Flores, E., and Bravo, P. W. (1995): Technical note. Citric acid and fructose concentrations in seminal plasma of the alpaca. Small Ruminant Res. *18:*95.

72. Ginther, O. J. (1981): Local versus systemic uteroovarian relationships in farm animals. Acta Vet. Scand. (Suppl.) *77:*103.

73. Ginther, O. J. and Del Campo, C. H. (1973): Areas of close apposition between the ovarian artery and vessels which contain uterine venous blood in sheep. Am. J. Vet. Res. *34:*1387.

74. Ginther, O. J. and Del Campo, C. H. (1974): Vascular anatomy of the uterus and ovaries and the unilateral luteolytic effect of the uterus. Am. J. Vet. Res. *35:*193.

75. Ginther, O. J., Garcia, M. C., Squires, E. L., et al. (1972): Anatomy of vasculature of uterus and ovaries in the mare. Am. J. Vet. Res. *33:*1561.

76. Haibel, G. K. and Fung, E. D. (1991): Real-time ultrasonic biparietal diameter measurement for the pre-

diction of gestational age in llamas. Theriogenology *35:*683.

77. Hinrichs, K., Buoen, L.C., and Ruth, G. R. (1999): XX/XY chimerism and freemartinism in a female llama co-twin to a male. J. Am. Vet. Med. Assoc. *215:*1140.

78. Hunter, R. H. F. (1980): Transport and storage of spermatozoa in the female tract. Proc. 9th Int. Cong. Anim. Reprod. A. I., Madrid, Spain, June 16–20, 1980, *2:*227.

79. Hunter, R. H. F. (1981): Sperm transport and reservoirs in the pig oviduct in relation to the time of ovulation. J. Reprod. Fertil. *63:*109.

80. Johnson, L. W. (1989): Llama reproduction. Vet. Clin. North Am., Food Anim. Pract. *5:*159.

81. Knight, T. W., Death, A. F., and Wyeth, T. K. (1995): Photoperiodic control of the time of parturition in alpacas *(Lama pacos)*. Anim. Reprod. Sci. *39:*259.

82. Kubicek, J. (1974): Samenentnahme beim Alpaka durch eine Harnröhrenfistel. Z. Tierzüchtg. Züchtgsbiol. *90:*335.

83. Leipold, H. W., Hiraga, T. H., and Johnson, L. W. (1994): Congenital defects in the llama. Vet. Clin. North Am., Food Anim. Pract. *10:*401.

84. Leon, J. B., Smith, B. B., Timm, K. I., et al. (1990): Endocrine changes during pregnancy, parturition and the early post-partum period in the llama *(Lama glama)*. J. Reprod. Fertil. *88:*503.

85. Lichtenwalner, A. B., Woods, G. L., and Weber, J. A. (1996): Seminal collection, seminal characteristics and pattern of ejaculation in llamas. Theriogenology *46:*293.

86. Lichtenwalner, A. B., Woods, G. L., and Weber, J. A. (1998): Male llama choice between receptive and non-receptive females. Appl. Anim. Behav. Sci. *59:*349.

87. Loy, R. G. (1980): Characteristics of postpartum reproduction in mares. Vet. Clin. North Am., Large Anim. Pract. *2:*345.

88. Mattner, P. E. and Braden, A. W. H. (1963): Spermatozoa in the genital tract of the ewe. I. Rapidity of transport. Aust. J. Biol. Sci. *16:*473.

89. Merkt, H., Böer, M., Rath, D., et al. (1988): The presence of an additional fetal membrane and its function in the newborn guanaco *(Lama guanacoë)*. Theriogenology *30:*437.

90. Morton, W. R. M. (1960): The full-term fetal membranes of some camelidae. Anat. Rec. *136:*247.

91. Morton, W. R. M. (1961): Observations on the full-term foetal membranes of three members of the camelidae *(Camelus dromedarius L., Camelus bactrianus L.* and *Lama glama L.)*. J. Anat. *95:*200.

92. Novoa, C. (1970): Reproduction in Camelidae. J. Reprod. Fertil. *22:*3.

93. Paolicchi, F., Urquieta, B., Del Valle, L., et al. (1999): Biological activity of the seminal plasma of alpacas: Stimulus for the production of LH by pituitary cells. Anim. Reprod. Sci. *54:*203.

94. Paul-Murphy, J., Tell, L. A., Bravo, W., et al. (1991): Urinary steroid evaluations to monitor ovarian function in exotic ungulates: VIII. Correspondence of urinary and plasma steroids in the llama *(Lama glama)* during nonconceptive and conceptive cycles. Zoo Biol. *10:*225.

95. Pollard, J. C., Littlejohn, R. P., and Moore, G. H. (1995): Seasonal and other factors affecting the sexual behaviour of alpacas. Anim. Reprod. Sci. *37:*349.

96. Pollard, J. C., Littlejohn, R. P., and Scott, I. C. (1994): The effects of mating on the sexual receptivity of female alpacas. Anim. Reprod. Sci. *34:*289.

97. Pugh, D. G. and Montes, A. J. (1994): Advanced reproductive technologies in South American camelids. Vet. Clin. North Am., Food Anim. Pract. *10:*281.

98. Raggi, L. A., Ferrando, G., Parraguez, V. H., et al. (1999): Plasma progesterone in alpaca *(Lama pacos)* during pregnancy, parturition, and early postpartum. Anim. Reprod. Sci. *54:*245.

99. Ripple, R. H., Johnson, E. S., and White, W. F. (1974): Effect of consecutive injections of synthetic gonadotropin releasing hormone on LH release in the anestrous and ovariectomized ewe. J. Anim. Sci. *39:*907.

100. San-Martin, M., Copaira, M., Zuniga, J., et al. (1968): Aspects of reproduction in the alpaca. J. Reprod. Fertil. *16:*395.

101. Schmidt, C. R. (1973): Breeding seasons and notes on some other aspects of reproduction in captive camelids. Int. Zoo Yearbook *13:*387.

102. Schwarzenberger, F., Speckbacher, G., and Bamberg, E. (1995): Plasma and fecal progestin evaluations during and after the breeding season of the female vicuna *(Vicuna vicuna)*. Theriogenology *43:*625.

103. Skidmore, J. A., Billah, M., Binns, M., et al. (1999): Hybridizing Old and New World camelids: *Camelus dromedarius* x *Lama guanicoe*. Proc. Royal Soc., [B], London, England *266:*649.

104. Smith, B. B., Timm, K. I., Reed, P. J., et al. (2000): Use of cloprostenol as an abortifacient in the llama *(Lama glama)*. Theriogenology *54:*497.

105. Smith, C. L., Peter, A. T., and Pugh, D. G. (1994): Reproduction in llamas and alpacas: A review. Theriogenology *41:*573.

106. Stewart, D. R. (1986): Development of a homologous equine relaxin radioimmunoassay. Endocrinology *119:*1100.

107. Sumar, J. (1988): Removal of the ovaries or ablation of the corpus luteum and its effect on the maintenance of gestation in the alpaca and llama. Acta Vet. Scand. (Suppl.) *83:*133.

108. Sumar, J. (1994): Effects of various ovulation induction stimuli in alpacas and llamas. J. Arid Environ. *26:*39.

109. Sumar, J. B. (1999): Reproduction in female South American domestic camelids. J. Reprod. Fertil. Suppl. *54:*169.

110. Sumar, J. and Bravo, P. W. (1991): *In situ* observation of the ovaries of llamas and alpacas by use of laparoscopic technique. J. Am. Vet. Med. Assoc. *199:*1159.

111. Sumar, J., Bravo, P. W., and Foote, W. C. (1993): Sexual receptivity and time of ovulation in alpacas. Small Ruminant Res. *11:*143.

112. Sumar, J., Fredriksson, G., Alarcón, V., et al. (1988): Levels of 15-keto-13, 14-dihydro-PFG$_{2\alpha}$ (sic), progesterone, and oestradiol-17β after induced ovulations in llamas and alpacas. Acta Vet. Scand. *29:*339.

113. Tibary, A. and Memon, M.A. (1999): Reproduction in the male South American Camelidae. J. Camel Pract. Res. *6:*235.

114. Urquieta, B., Cepeda, R., Cáceres, J. E., et al. (1994): Seasonal variation in some reproductive parameters of male vicuña in the High Andes of northern Chile. J. Arid Environ. *26:*79.

115. Urquieta, B. and Rojas, J. R. (1990): An introduction to South American camelids. *In:* Livestock Reproduction in Latin America. Proc. Final Research Co-ordination Meeting of the FAO (Food and Agriculture Organization)/IAEA (International Atomic Energy Agency)/ARCAL III Regional Network, Bogota, Colombia, September 19–23, 1988, p. 389.

116. Urquieta, B. and Rojas, J. R. (1990): Studies on the reproductive physiology of the vicuña (*Vicugna vicugna) In:* Livestock Reproduction in Latin America. Proc. Final Research Co-ordination Meeting of the FAO (Food and Agriculture Organization)/IAEA (International Atomic Energy Agency)/ARCAL III Regional Network, Bogota, Colombia, September 19–23, 1988, p. 407.

117. Vidal-Rioja, L., Semorile, L., Bianchi, N. O. et al. (1987): DNA composition in South American camelids. I. Characterization and *in situ* hybridization of satellite DNA fraction. Genetica *15:*137.

118. Vidal-Rioja, L., Zambelli, A., and Semorile, L. (1994): An assessment of the relationships among species of Camelidae by satellite DNA comparisons. Hereditas *121:*283.

119. von Baer, L. and Hellemann, C. (1998): Variables seminales en llama (*Lama glama*). Archivos de Medicina Veterinaria *2:*171, 1998.

120. von Baer, L. and Hellemann, C. (1999): Cryopreservation of llama (*Lama glama*) semen. Reprod. Domestic Anim. *34:*95.

121. Wiepz, D. W. and Chapman, R. J. (1985): Nonsurgical embryo transfer and live birth in a llama. Theriogenology *24:*251.

122. Wildt, D. E., Seager, S. W. J., and Chakraborty, P. K. (1980): Effect of copulation stimuli on incidence of ovulation and on serum luteinizing hormone in the cat. Endocrinology *107:*1212.

Embryo Transfer in Domestic Animals

R. A. Bowen

19

INTRODUCTION

Embryo transfer refers to the techniques by which embryos are collected from a female called the **donor** and transferred, for development to term, to another female called the **recipient.** At its simplest, the chain of events in the process of embryo transfer includes management of the donor for production of a suitable number of viable oocytes, mating or artificial insemination, collection, evaluation, and short-term storage of embryos from the donor, and finally, the transfer of these embryos to suitable recipients. Also associated with embryo transfer are a number of ancillary procedures, including maintenance of a rigorous health program for both donors and recipients and the keeping of a detailed series of records for every aspect of the program. Like other complex tasks, this chain of events is only as strong as its weakest link.

For simplicity and consistency in nomenclature, the term **embryo** will be used in this chapter to refer to any stage of embryonic development from the **cytula,** the one-cell fertilized oocyte, to the preattachment blastocyst.

The main objective of embryo transfer is the improvement of animal populations through increased utilization of superior females. Artificial insemination in several mammalian species, and especially in dairy cattle, has substantially contributed to the dissemination of superior genetic material from the male, allowing acceleration of genetic selection at a much greater rate than could be hoped for with natural matings. Theoretical arguments have been developed which imply that embryo transfer will never be a tool for genetic improvement as efficient as artificial insemination, primarily because of the comparatively small number of oocytes obtained even in superovulated animals. However, there is no doubt that embryo transfer allows for the dissemination of genetic material from the female and for the expansion of desirable genetic pools for breed and herd improvement.

547

The expansion of genetic pools provided by embryo transfer is especially important for monotocous species, such as cattle and horses, which have long gestation periods and low rates of reproduction. In these animals, the intensity of selection that can be applied and the natural rate of genetic improvement are limited by this relatively low reproductive efficiency. Even under ideal conditions of health and management, a highly productive cow may produce only 8 to 12 calves in her reproductive lifetime. However, it has been estimated that the ovaries of a prepubertal heifer contain more than 100,000 oocytes. Using current technology for superovulation and embryo transfer, it is feasible to obtain 30 to 40 calves from a single cow over a period of a year. The intensity of genetic selection of females is thus facilitated by embryo transfer since it is possible–even assuming a 50% sex ratio–to obtain more daughters, all of the same age, from a single mating of a superior dam by using recipients of a lesser genetic value as foster mothers. Due to the enhancement of reproductive potential, careful selection of embryo donors to avoid propagation of undesirable heritable traits is nearly as important as the selection of the sire.

The transfer of embryos offers other real or potential contributions to the livestock industry. The generation interval from birth to reproductive age can be shortened by obtaining and transferring embryos from prepubertal animals. The sex of embryos can be determined prior to transfer and the use of this technique, especially when coupled with low temperature preservation of sexed embryos, offers exciting possibilities. Reliable induction of twinning in cattle would be of benefit, and embryo transfer appears as the most promising of the available methods to induce twinning.

Infertility, especially in the older animal, is a wasteful and economically important problem in the livestock industry. In the majority of cases, infertile food-producing animals should be culled. There are, however, many genetically superior females which become infertile due to uterine or oviductal diseases or to old age. In many instances, embryo recovery and transfer techniques can be used to obtain additional progeny from such animals.

Embryo transfer offers new opportunities for assisting reproduction of domestic and nondomestic animals. There has been considerable interest in using embryo transfer as a tool for managing reproduction in endangered species and some zoo animals, and this has prompted the development of superovulatory and embryo transfer techniques for a variety of wild animals. Without doubt, embryo transfer could also be applied to companion animals, although it is unlikely that there would be a significant incentive to do so.

The application of embryo transfer has expanded rapidly in the last few decades. Only a few years ago, problems in development of technology for recovery, storage, and transfer of embryos, variability in results, and the high costs of performing embryo transfer precluded its extensive application to farm animals. As a result of stimulation for research in this field, prompted in large part by economic demand, embryo transfer is now utilized commercially throughout the world in cattle, sheep, and swine, and, to a lesser extent, in horses. Research and application of embryo transfer for cattle has far and away been the most intense. The first commercial bovine embryo transfers were performed in the early 1970s. Table 19-1 presents estimates, almost certainly underestimates, of the number of bovine embryos transferred throughout the world in 1994. In the United States and Canada, it is estimated that approximately 100,000 embryo transfer calves have been born each year since the mid-1980s.

Table 19-1   *Estimates of Bovine Embryo Transfer Activity in 1994*

Continent	Number of Embryos Transferred to Recipients		
	Fresh	Frozen	Total
North America	93,414	76,357	169,771
South America	25,556	13,445	39,001
Africa	6,743	3,158	9,901
Asia	13,420	39,066	52,486
Europe	48,402	54,485	102,887
Oceania	6,078	3,716	9,794
Total	193,613	190,227	383,840

Data from: M. Thibier, Embryo Transfer Newsletter, International Embryo Transfer Society, *13*:18, 1995.

In addition to commercial applications, embryo transfer technology is being used at an ever-increasing rate in research. Embryo transfer has been useful in investigations of spermatozoal physiology, fertilization, and embryonic differentiation. Investigations of viral infections of embryos and attempts to detect carriers of heritable diseases provide other applications for embryo transfer techniques. Finally, embryo transfer is the technology upon which all efforts at genetic engineering in mammals are based.

INCREASING THE AVAILABILITY OF EMBRYOS

The availability of embryos for transfer may be increased by inducing superovulation in adult and prepubertal animals or by using oocytes harvested directly from the ovarian follicles. Induction of twinning in monotocous species by transfer of two embryos or transfer of a single embryo to an animal already bred has been successful, but the higher abortion rate and other complications of twin pregnancy limit the routine use of this technique.

Superovulation in Adult Animals

Superovulation is a pharmacologic technique applied to increase the ovulatory response of a female. It is generated in an animal by the administration of exogenous gonadotropic hormones. The main objective of superovulatory treatment is to increase the number of oocytes released by an animal at ovulation above what would be expected to occur naturally, thereby increasing the potential number of embryos for transfer. The yield of viable embryos after superovulation is more important for a successful embryo transfer program than the total number of ovulations induced and oocytes released in each individual animal. Superovulatory treatment in the cow, ewe, goat, sow, and queen can generally increase the number of ovulations 2- to 10-fold over that occurring normally.

Pregnant mare serum gonadotropin (PMSG), also called equine chorionic gonadotropin (eCG), partially purified or recombinant follicle-stimulating hormone (FSH), human chorionic gonadotropin (hCG), and crude pituitary extracts containing both FSH and luteinizing hormone (LH) have been used to stimulate follicular growth and ovulation in domestic animals. Of these gonadotropins, FSH is currently the most widely used in cattle, sheep, and goats.

Superovulatory treatment can be applied to animals during a normal estrus cycle or can be combined with an estrus synchronizing treatment. In the former case, treatment with gonadotropins is generally begun 3 to 5 days prior to the expected onset of estrus, and estrus and ovulation are then allowed to occur naturally. A much more reliable and commonly used method of timing superovulation is based on the discovery that prostaglandin $F_{2\alpha}$ ($PGF_{2\alpha}$) induces luteolysis in several species. $PGF_{2\alpha}$ and a series of synthetic analogues are available to regulate the length of the estrous cycle when administered during the luteal phase of the cycle. The use of prostaglandins to synchronize the cycle in conjunction with superovulatory regimens allows for a more constant length of exposure to gonadotropins, and cows treated with $PGF_{2\alpha}$ during superovulation yield larger numbers of transferable embryos than cows superovulated without the use of $PGF_{2\alpha}$.

Superovulation of sheep and goats using gonadotropins in conjunction with prostaglandin treatment is also quite successful. Another means of synchronizing estrus that is commonly applied to these two species is treatment with a progestagen or progestins, as these synthetic progestagens are called, for 16 days or more, followed by withdrawal of treatment and mating when the animals come into estrus.

The cycling sow responds well to superovulatory treatments with PMSG and does not require supplementary treatment to induce ovulation, although hCG can be administered to time ovulation more precisely. Most sows come into estrus 3 to 7 days after weaning, and superovulating doses of PMSG can be administered to match that event. Also, superovulatory treatment can be initiated in pregnant or pseudopregnant sows 24 hours prior to $PGF_{2\alpha}$-induced luteolysis. Suppression of estrus by administration of progestagens, followed by their withdrawal, has been used to synchronize estrus in donor sows, but is associated with a relatively high incidence of ovarian cysts.

Even though follicular growth can be induced, the ovaries of both the mare and the bitch are resistant to ovulatory stimulation by exogenous gonadotropins. Cycling or seasonally anovulatory mares treated with crude or partially purified equine pituitary gonadotropins containing both FSH and LH activities typically ovulate only two to three oocytes. Also, pregnancy rates after transfer of embryos from superovulated mares have generally been lower than pregnancy rates obtained after the transfer of embryos recovered from normally ovulating mares. Thus, while some progress has been made in inducing superovulatory responses in the equine, it has not advanced to the point of routine use. Similarly, although some degree of success has been achieved in stimulating follicular growth and ovulation in the anestrous bitch, the results have been disappointing.

Porcine or ovine FSH has been successfully used to induce estrus in anestrous cats, followed by hCG treatment to induce ovulation. Pregnant mare serum gonadotropin in single or in multiple injections induces follicular growth in cats, but the ovulatory response to hCG treatment after PMSG seems more variable than the ovulatory response to hCG after FSH treatment.

The greatest problem with superovulation is the large degree of variation in response among individuals of the same species. At this time, there is no reliable way of predicting the number of oocytes that will be released from a given animal in response to exogenous gonadotropins. Much of this variability may be due to genetic differences among animals, but differences in potency, purity, and quality of commercially available gonadotropins, and also in the species of origin of the preparation, may also contribute to the variable response of animals to superovulatory treatment. Older cows appear to be less responsive to superovulatory treatments with gonadotropins than heifers. Other factors that may contribute to this variability include breed differences and seasonal effects. The general health, lactational status, and past reproductive performance of the donor certainly influence the response to superovulation. Cows that are "problem breeders" ovulate lower numbers of oocytes in response to superovulatory treatments, and fewer transferable embryos can be recovered from these cows than from reproductively healthy cows (Table 19-2).

It is desirable to superovulate valuable donors as many times as possible to obtain maximal numbers of embryos. However, repeated treatment with gonadotropins may induce the formation of antibodies to these gonadotropins, resulting in a lower number of oocytes ovulated with each successive treatment. Heterologous gonadotropins are more likely to induce antibodies than homologous gonadotropins. Experimentally, cattle and various laboratory animals produce antibodies to gonadotropins in response to superovulatory treatments, but the clinical effects of this response have not been adequately investigated. Another possible consequence of the immunogenicity of gonadotropins is the potential for development of high titers of antibodies and subse-

Table 19-2   Superovulatory Responses[a] of Reproductively "Healthy" and "Problem" Lactating Holstein Cows

	Reproductive Status	
End Point	Healthy	Problem
Number of cows superovulated	666	318
Total oocytes and embryos recovered	6,828	1,943
Mean number of embryos per donor cow	6.4	2.4
Percentage of donors with no embryos recovered	14	51
Number of embryos transferred to recipients	3,707	604
Percentage of recipients becoming pregnant	68	58

[a]Superovulation induced with porcine FSH.
Adapted from: J. F. Hasler, A. D. McCauley, E. C. Schermerhorn, et al., Theriogenology *19*:83, 1983.

quent anaphylaxis following the administration of additional gonadotropin. Clinically, however, this does not appear to be a common problem.

Superovulation in Prepubertal Animals

Follicular growth and ovulation can be induced in prepubertal animals of some species by treatment with exogenous gonadotropins. Although this technique has not been adopted for commercial use, the appeal of using such young animals as oocyte donors is that it would allow early progeny testing and shortening of the generation interval, which could significantly enhance the rate of genetic gain. However, the genetic implications of transferring embryos from young animals, which have not been proven for their production capabilities, need to be carefully evaluated. The age of the prospective donor appears to be a limiting factor in the response to superovulation and in the quality of oocytes recovered. Although there is species variation, sensitivity of the ovaries to stimulation with exogenous gonadotropins generally increases gradually from birth to puberty. The closer the animal is to puberty, the better the response to superovulatory treatments. More importantly, even though one can effectively superovulate animals well before puberty and fertilize such oocytes *in vitro,* many of the resulting embryos are not developmentally competent and fail to develop to term. The rate of success improves considerably as the animals approach puberty, and it is possible that prepubertal animals, particularly calves, will someday play an important role in programs for genetic improvement.

Utilization of Follicular Oocytes and In Vitro *Fertilization*

In vitro fertilization is the process by which oocytes are matured and fertilized outside of the female. The resulting embryos are then transferred back to the same or different females for development to term. Mature oocytes can be collected by flushing the oviducts shortly after ovulation or by aspiration of preovulatory follicles. Follicular oocytes can be recovered by aspiration from follicles visualized with a laparoscope, which avoids some of the disadvantages of major

abdominal surgery. Oocytes can also be aspirated from ovaries collected at slaughter; in this case, the number of oocytes available is, for practical purposes, limited only by desire, but the genetic merit of the donor is usually unknown.

Follicular oocytes are generally not yet mature at the time of aspiration, and must be cultured in sterile medium to allow for nuclear maturation prior to fertilization. Spermatozoa must be capacitated before they are capable of fertilizing the oocyte, although this process appears to be less stringent in some species (cattle) compared to others (rabbits). Capacitated spermatozoa can be recovered from another inseminated female or can be achieved by incubation for several hours in an appropriate 'capacitation medium'. Fertilization occurs several hours after mixing cultured oocytes and capacitated spermatozoa, and the resulting embryos are generally cultured *in vitro* for an additional period of time before transfer back to the recipient.

Transfer of *in vitro* fertilized oocytes has resulted in births in most species, but has been most widely investigated and applied to cattle. One application of this technology is to obtain additional offspring from females with certain types of acquired infertility such as periovarian adhesions. Frozen semen from valuable males, which may be long dead, can also be utilized much more efficiently. *In vitro* fertilization may also become a commonly used technique for assessing the fertility of both male and female gametes. Finally, fertilization *in vitro* is a valuable adjunct technology in efforts to apply genetic engineering techniques to domestic animals.

RECOVERY OF EMBRYOS

Embryo transfer evolved around the use of surgical techniques for the recovery of embryos. After the initial demonstration of the commercial feasibility of embryo transfer in cattle, the development and improvement of less costly and less traumatic methods of embryo recovery became a major goal in embryo transfer programs. As a result of the combined research efforts of several groups, techniques have been improved, and the recovery of embryos from cattle and horses is now carried out almost exclusively by nonsurgical means. Routine embryo recovery from sheep, goats, and swine remains a surgical procedure.

Surgical Methods

Even though there are minor differences in the techniques applied to each species, the basic approach for surgical recovery of embryos is similar for all species. Several variations in technique and equipment have been developed for surgical recovery of embryos, and this discussion is intended to serve only as a general guide.

The embryo donor is bred at estrus by natural service or, more commonly, by artificial insemination. Since superovulated animals tend to ovulate over an extended period of time, they are commonly inseminated more than once to ensure a high fertilization rate. In cattle, the donor is usually inseminated twice at approximately 12 and 24 hours after the onset of estrus.

Several factors influence the decision as to when the embryos should be recovered for transfer. Because the transfer of embryos to the uterus rather than to the oviducts generally is easier to perform and this approach results in higher pregnancy rates, the recovery of embryos should coincide with the time when the embryos would normally be in the uterus of the donor. The requirements of synchrony of the estrous cycle between the donor and recipient appear to be less critical for older embryos. However, the upper limit for recovery time is determined by the size and fragility of the developing embryos, and in some species, by implantation time. Large, elongating blastocysts, such as those found in the cow after day 13, are difficult to recover without damage. In general, embryos that are to be transferred are recovered between the 8-cell and blastocyst stages, while the embryo is still surrounded by the zona pellucida.

Surgical recovery of embryos is best carried out with the donor under general anesthesia. Feed and water should be withheld for 24 to 36 hours before the operation. This period of preoperative fasting is especially critical in ruminants, because they tend to bloat quickly, making exposure of the reproductive tract difficult and more traumatic. Anesthesia may be induced with a short-acting barbiturate given as an intravenous bolus.

After intubation, anesthesia is maintained with halothane or a similar agent. The ventral abdomen is clipped, disinfected, and draped for aseptic surgery. The ovaries and uterine horns are exteriorized through a midline incision for flushing. After recovery of the embryos, the reproductive tract is replaced into the abdominal cavity, and the incision is closed in a standard fashion.

The surgical recovery of embryos often reduces the fertility of the donor at subsequent inseminations by causing periovarian adhesions. The fimbriae, where even minor adhesions can greatly interfere with oocyte pick-up and transport, are the most critical sites for such problems. Consequently, surgical procedures should be carried out aseptically and as carefully as possible, making every effort to minimize trauma to the tissues. The exposed reproductive tract should be kept moist with saline solution and handled as little as possible.

Several basic techniques have been used for the actual recovery of embryos. In all procedures, a warm medium is flushed through the lumen of the reproductive tract and collected at some distal site. A variety of balanced salt solutions or complete cell culture media such as Medium 199 have been used for recovering embryos; one of the most widely used media is Dulbecco's phosphate-buffered saline (Table 19-3). These media are usually supplemented with serum or serum components to provide a source of protein and reduce the problem of embryos sticking to the recovery equipment.

A method for the recovery of embryos from the uterus and oviducts of cattle utilizes a glass or plastic cannula and a blunt hypodermic needle attached to a syringe containing the flushing

Table 19-3 Phosphate-buffered Saline[a] for Recovery and Storage of Embryos

Compound	Concentration (g/L)	mM
NaCl	8.00	136.9
$CaCl_2$	0.10	0.9
$MgCl_2 \cdot 6H_2O$	0.10	0.5
KCl	0.20	2.7
KH_2PO_4	0.20	1.5
$Na_2HPO_4 \cdot 7H_2O$	2.16	8.1

[a]Commonly supplemented with serum.

medium. The cannula is inserted in the fimbrial opening of the oviduct and maintained in position by finger pressure or with a small atraumatic clamp. The uterine horn is punctured at a site close to the intercornual bifurcation, and the medium is forced through the uterine horn and oviduct and out through the cannula into a collection dish (Fig. 19-1A). The surgeon should keep pressure on the uterus around the needle to prevent loss of medium. Passage of the medium through the tract is aided by gently milking the uterus. The volume of fluid to be infused depends on the size of the uterus but generally varies between 25 and 100 ml. This method cannot be used in the mare, sow, or queen due to valve-like papillae at the uterotubal junction which prevents fluid from being milked from the uterus into the oviduct and out through the cannula placed in the fimbrial opening. In these three species, the medium is usually flushed only through the uterine horns.

When embryos are expected to be located exclusively in the uterus, because of the elapsed time from ovulation, only the uterine horns need be flushed (Fig. 19-1B). An important advantage of this approach is that the oviducts are not handled, and fimbrial adhesions are less likely to be induced.

Nonsurgical Methods

To recover embryos nonsurgically, the donor cow is restrained in a standing position in a chute, and the perineal area is clipped of hair and disinfected. Epidural anesthesia is usually administered to prevent straining during the recovery. A variety of instruments have been used for nonsurgical recovery of embryos; one of the most successful of these is a soft rubber catheter such as the Foley catheter (Fig. 19-2A). This catheter is made of flexible latex and has three channels, one to inflate a balloon near the tip of the catheter and separate channels for the inflow and outflow of the flushing medium. In cows, the cervix is usually tightly closed at the time of embryo recovery, and a cervical dilator is required to open the cervical canal while the cervix is fixed with a hand. Once the cervix is dilated, the catheter is maneuvered through the cervix with the aid of a stiff metal stylet. The balloon of the

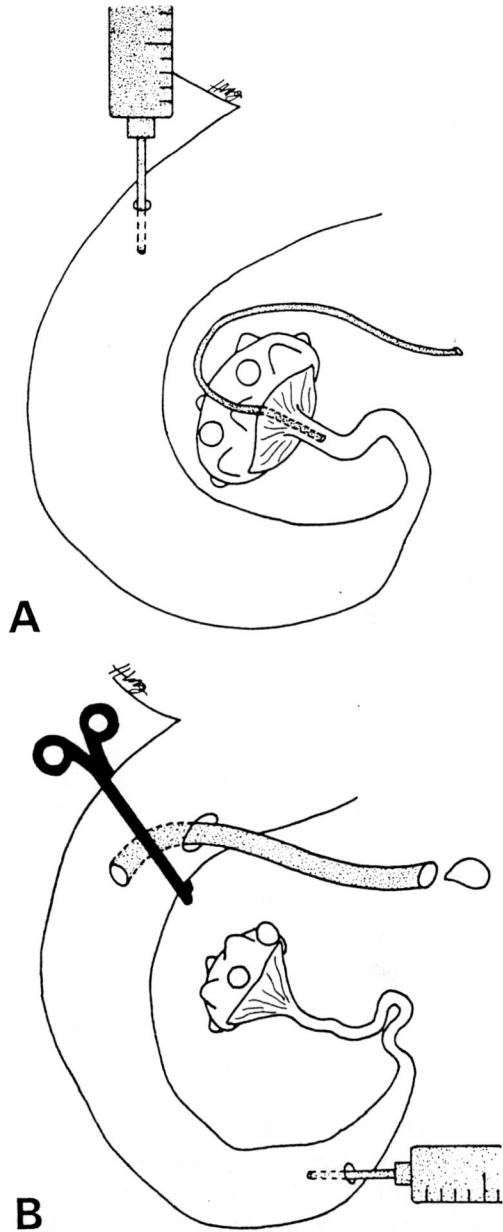

Fig. 19-1. Schematic representation of methods for surgical recovery of embryos. **A.** From the oviduct. **B.** From the uterus.

Foley catheter is inflated just proximal to the uterine bifurcation, and each uterine horn is flushed individually. After one horn is flushed, the balloon is deflated, the stylet is reinserted, and the catheter is placed in the other uterine

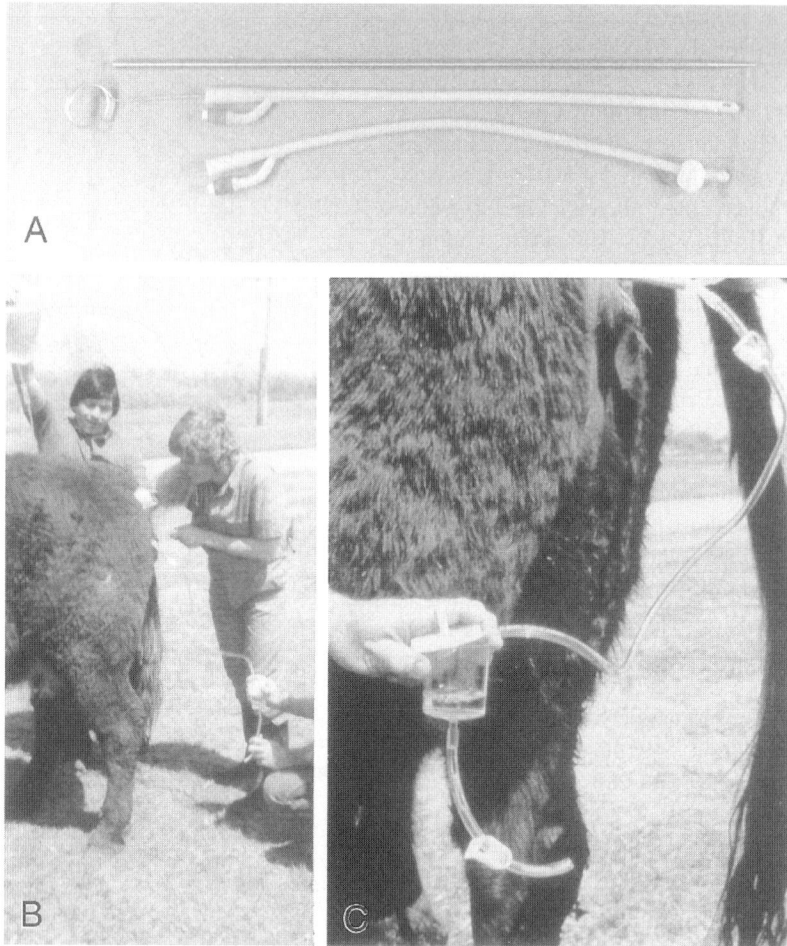

Fig. 19-2. Equipment and procedures used in nonsurgical bovine embryo recovery. **A.** Cervical dilator (**top**) and Foley catheters (with and without cuff inflated). **B.** Nonsurgical recovery of embryos from a cow with flushing medium delivered by gravity flow. **C.** Embryo collection funnel showing collection of fluid.

horn. The medium used for flushing is fed through the inflow channel of the catheter by gravity flow from a suspended reservoir, and the uterine horn is distended until it becomes turgid. The inflow is then interrupted, the out-flow channel is opened, and the accumulated fluid is allowed to drain into a collection container. The whole procedure is monitored by palpation per rectum and aided by gentle massage of the uterine horns. The flushing and recovery procedure is repeated until approximately one liter of medium has been flushed through each uterine horn. Few adverse effects of this type of nonsurgical recovery have been observed, and the fer-

tility of the donor subsequent to several nonsurgical recoveries appears to be normal.

Excluding primates, the mare is the only other animal for which a routine procedure for nonsurgical recovery has been developed. The methods used for mares are basically modifications of those developed for cattle. Passage of the catheter through the cervix is much easier in the mare, and the entire uterus is flushed at once.

The relative advantages and disadvantages of nonsurgical versus surgical methods for the recovery of embryos are compared in Table 19-4. The major disadvantage of surgical methods for the recovery of embryos is the virtually un-

Table 19-4   Comparison of Surgical and Nonsurgical Methods for Recovery of Embryos

End Point	Method of Recovery	
	Surgical	Nonsurgical
Anesthesia	General	Epidural
Fasting	Required	Helpful, but not required
Ability to recover embryos at any stage	Excellent	Limited
Ability to accurately assess number of ovulations	Excellent	Poor
Risk of acute complications to donor	Definite possibility	Virtually nil
Risk to future reproductive performance of donor	Yes	Probably none
Embryo recovery rate	Excellent	Good
Ability to assess and give prognosis for reproductive tract pathology	Good	Poor
Can be performed on the farm	No	Yes

avoidable induction of periovarian adhesions, which can reduce subsequent fertility. In addition, surgery under general anesthesia always carries the risks of anesthetic-related mortality, aspiration pneumonia from regurgitation, postoperative herniation, and other surgical complications. Even though these complications are actually rare, they do occur. Nonsurgical recovery, on the other hand, rarely results in acute complications and does not appear to be detrimental to long-term fertility. Two major disadvantages of nonsurgical recovery are:

1. the embryos which are still in the oviduct at the time of recovery cannot be collected, and
2. even a person skilled at palpation per rectum can gain only a rough idea of the number of corpora lutea on superovulated ovaries as an indication of the number of ovulations.

Finally, if a pathologic condition is present, such as oviductal obstruction or minor periovarian adhesions, rectal palpation of the genital tract alone, while performing nonsurgical recovery, cannot substitute for the direct visualization of such lesions, which is possible during surgical exposure of the reproductive tract.

HANDLING, EVALUATION, AND STORAGE OF EMBRYOS

After flushing the reproductive tract and collecting the flushing medium, the embryos must be located in the collection medium, recovered, and prepared for transfer or storage.

Location of Embryos after Recovery

The medium collected after flushing the reproductive tract is examined with a stereomicroscope to locate the embryos. A microscope is necessary due to the small size of the embryos and the presence of varying amounts of cellular debris in the recovered medium. The size of embryos from domestic animals changes little from fertilization to the onset of cavitation, the beginning of the blastocyst stage. The diameter across the zona pellucida in these embryos is approximately 150 microns. At later stages of embryonal development, the expanding blastocysts can be located without the aid of a microscope.

Finding embryos, even in large volumes of fluid collected in a nonsurgical recovery, is greatly facilitated by the fact that embryos have a density greater than that of the collection medium and therefore sink to the bottom of the recovery vessel. Occasionally, however, embryos may be found floating near the surface of the medium. Embryos are retrieved from the fluid by passing the medium, as it is being collected, through a nylon mesh filter that will retain embryos and large pieces of debris (Fig. 19-2B and C). At the end of the collection, the embryos are washed off the filter into a small dish for searching with the microscope. An alternative technique involves collecting the flushing fluid into a large cylinder, allowing the embryos to settle, then siphoning off the bulk of the liquid. When only a small amount of medium is flushed from the donor, as with surgical collections, it may be collected directly into the searching dish. Once located, embryos are transferred to another dish containing fresh, sterile medium. These and subsequent manipulations of the embryos are performed with small glass pipets or plastic catheters, which are attached to a syringe or operated by suction from a mouth-piece. The embryos are "washed" through several changes of fresh medium to remove contaminating debris and to dilute possible bacterial contamination. Mammalian embryos do not appear to be adversely affected by short-term exposure to room temperature, but the recovered medium and dishes containing the embryos are usually kept in an incubator at approximately 38°C. Exposure to cold drafts or especially to temperatures above body temperature should be avoided.

Short-term Storage of Embryos

A variety of media, ranging from simple balanced salt solutions supplemented with serum to complex cell culture media, have been used for maintenance of embryos between recovery and transfer. Most standard cell culture media are based on a bicarbonate buffer system, and these must be maintained in an atmosphere containing carbon dioxide (usually 5% CO_2 in air) to prevent a detrimental rise in pH. For short-term storage of embryos, a simple medium such as described in Table 19-3 appears to be adequate. The pH of the storage medium should be in the range of 7.2 to 7.4. Media buffered with phosphate or one of the organic buffers such as HEPES (N-2-hydroxyethyl-piperazine-N′-2-ethanesulfonic acid) allow for the media to be kept in room atmosphere. Another important variable in culture medium is osmolality. Media with an osmolality between 270 and 310 mOsm per kg are acceptable for embryo culture.

Placement of embryos from cows, ewes, or sows in the oviducts of a rabbit has been used for the short-term storage of embryos. Such embryos continue to develop normally for a period of 2 to 3 days in the temporary host, after which they can be recovered and retransferred to the original donor species. This technique has been used for long-distance transport of embryos and for a variety of experimental purposes, but is rarely used today.

Evaluation of Embryos

A preliminary assessment of embryonic viability and differentiation between embryos and unfertilized oocytes can be made by examina-

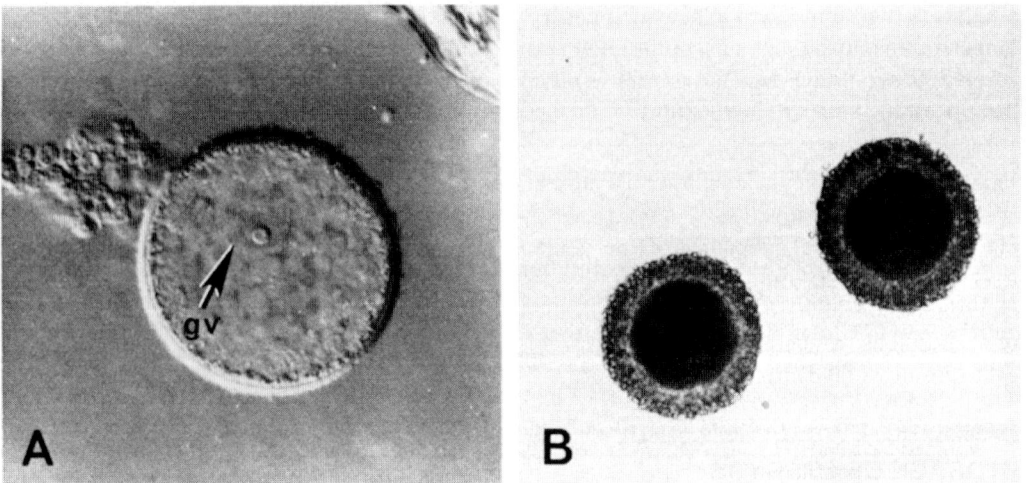

Fig. 19-3. Normal unfertilized oocytes. **A.** Follicular oocyte from a raccoon, showing germinal vesicle (**gv**). **B.** Recently ovulated canine oocytes surrounded by cumulus cells.

tion with a stereomicroscope. A more definitive evaluation, especially with embryos of questionable quality, is done by observation with a compound microscope (Fig. 19-3). An embryo is initially classified as being either transferable or nontransferable, according to whether it is judged to have a significant probability of establishing a pregnancy in the recipient. This can be a difficult judgment and is based primarily on how closely the recovered embryo corresponds with the expected stage of development normally found on that day of gestation (Table 19-5, Figs. 19-4 and 19-5). Unfertilized oocytes or an embryo whose development has been arrested early are generally easy to recognize as nontransferable (Fig. 19-6). However, cell fragmentation, which can give the false impression that a morula has been recovered, often occurs. Fragmented, nonviable embryos are often recognized because of large differences in the size of the various cellular fragments.

The next level of difficulty in classifying embryos occurs when the embryo is only moderately retarded in development. An example of this situation in cattle would be the recovery on day 7 of an early morula, generally seen on day 4 or 5, when one would expect an early blastocyst. Often, a mixture of embryos, some normal and some developmentally retarded, is recovered. The question that arises is whether the retarded embryo died at an earlier stage, or whether it is truly retarded in development, perhaps from being fertilized late, but still viable. Deciding whether an embryo is transferable rests primarily on economic considerations, and the probability of establishing a pregnancy from a retarded embryo must be weighed against the potential value of that offspring.

Sexing Embryos before Transfer

In many cases, especially in cattle and horses, the offspring of one sex are much more valuable than those of the opposite sex. A demand for transfer of 'presexed' embryos is thus created. Several approaches have been taken to fulfill this demand, but to date no technique has proven to be simple and reliable enough for routine use.

Direct examination of sex chromosomes from the embryonic cells has been used for sexing, but usually requires embryos at a stage more advanced than that of embryos usually transferred. The first step in such a procedure is to biopsy a group of cells from the embryo. Older embryos, such as day 13 or 14 blastocysts from cattle, tolerate the removal of small pieces of trophoblast relatively well. The biopsied embryo is then

Table 19-5　Cleavage and Hatching of Embryos

Stage of Development	Species					
	Cow[a]	Ewe[a]	Sow[a]	Mare[a]	Bitch[b]	Cat[a]
1-cell	0–2	0–1	0–1	0–1	1–8	0–1
2-cell	1–3	0–1	0–1	0–1	—	1–2
4-cell	2–3	1–2	1–2	1–2	—	1–3
8-cell	3–5	2–3	2–3	2–3	—	2–3
Morula	5–7	3–6	3–5	2–5	5–12	3–6
Pre-hatching blastocyst	7–10	5–8	4–6	5–8	8–20	6–7
Hatching or hatched blastocyst	9–11	8–9	5–7	8–9	17–20	7–9

[a]Days after ovulation.
[b]Days after onset of estrus.
Data for Cow: Seidel, G. E. and Seidel, S. M., Training Manual for Embryo Transfer in Cattle. FAO Animal
　　Production and Health Paper 77, 1991.
　Ewe: Moore, N. W. and Shelton, J. N., J. Reprod. Fertil. *7:*145, 1964; Rowson, L. E. A. and Moore, R.
　　M.: J. Anat. *100:*777, 1966.
　Sow: Hunter, R. H. F., Anat. Rec. *178:*169, 1974.
　Mare: Betteridge, K. J., Embryo Transfer in Farm Animals. Monograph No. 16, Canada Department of
　　Agriculture, 1977.
　Bitch: Holst, P. A. and Phemister, R. D., Biol. Reprod. *5:*194, 1971.
　Cat: Roth, T. L., Swanson, W. F., and Wildt, D. E., Biol. Reprod. *51:*441, 1994.

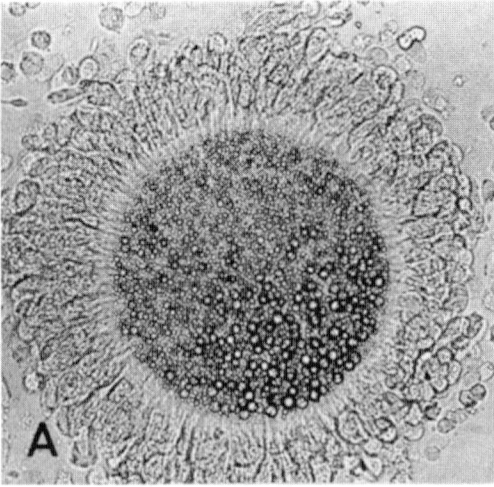

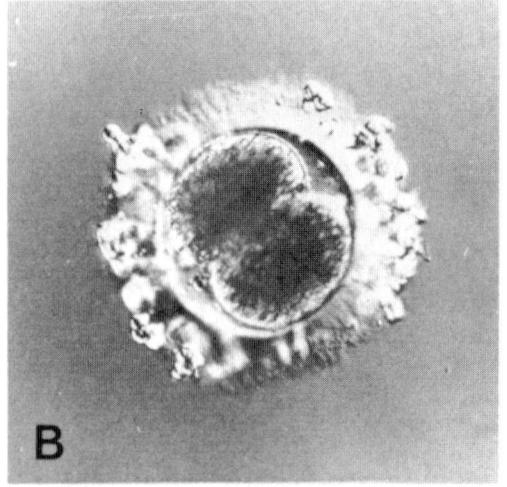

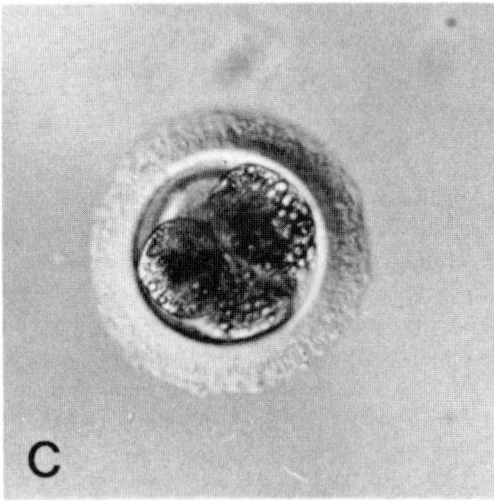

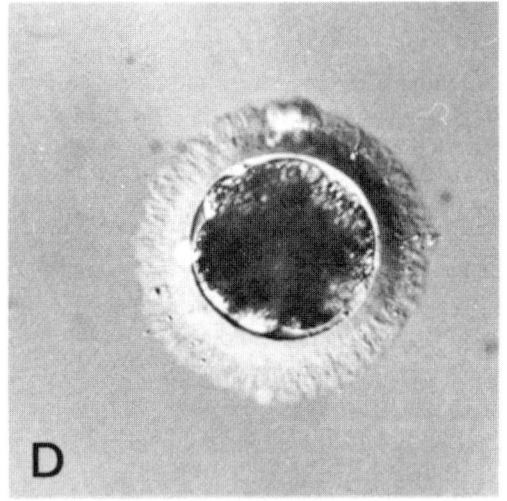

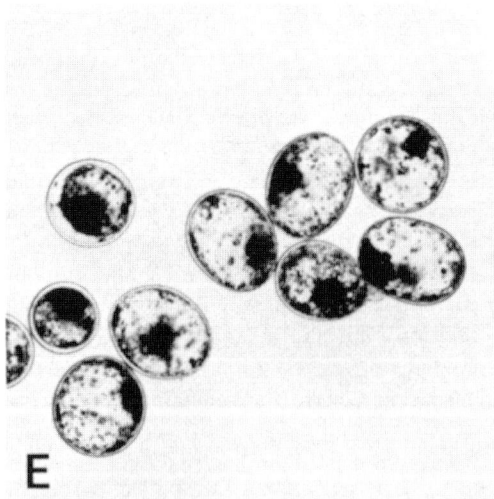

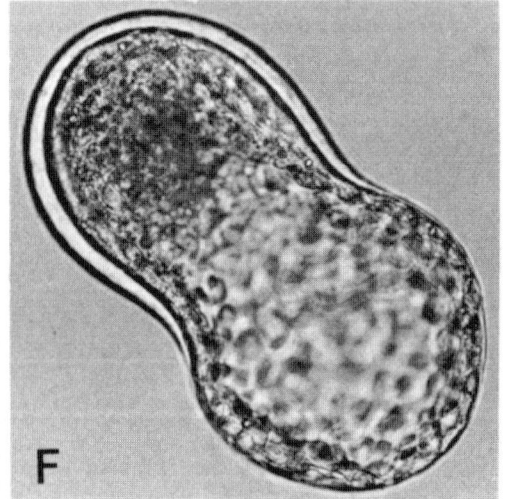

Fig. 19-4. Ovulated oocyte and early embryonic development in the domestic cat. **A.** Recently ovulated oocyte before fertilization, showing cumulus cells surrounding the zona pellucida. **B.** Two-cell embryo. **C.** Four-cell embryo. **D.** Early morula. **E.** Group of expanding blastocysts still within the zona pellucida. **F.** Hatching blastocyst.

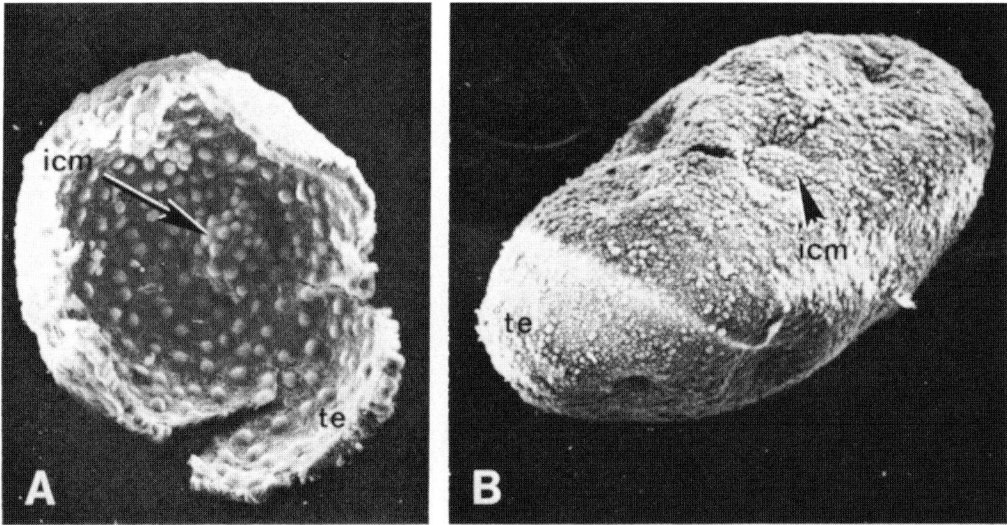

Fig. 19-5. Scanning electron micrographs of bovine blastocysts showing trophectoderm (**te**) and inner cell mass (**icm**). **A.** Ten days after the onset of estrus (broken open to show blastocoel). **B.** Thirteen days after the onset of estrus. At this time, the embryo is 3 to 4 mm long.

held in culture while the cells which have been removed are processed for cytogenetic analysis. Using this technique, the sex of approximately one-half to two-thirds of the embryos examined can be determined. The preparations from the remaining embryos are generally not of sufficient quality for accurate determination. An alternative and seemingly more useful method of sexing involves using fluorescently-labeled specific antibodies to detect the presence of the male-specific H-Y antigen (see Chapter 7) on the surface of male embryos. Finally, embryos can be sexed by the use of molecular probes for Y chromosome-specific DNA. Biopsy of even a single cell provides enough DNA to diagnose sex using polymerase chain reaction techniques, but that procedure requires the use of a micromanipulator and other equipment not generally available in the common laboratory. Improvements in accuracy and modifications of these techniques will provide valuable additions to the technology of embryo transfer.

Long-term Storage of Embryos

Advances in the theory and practice of low temperature preservation of mammalian cells led to the report in 1972 of the birth of mice which had been frozen as embryos. Within a short time, these cryobiological techniques had been successfully applied to embryos from cattle, sheep, mares, and goats. Cryopreservation of bovine embryos is now widely applied and quite successful. For example, of all the bovine embryos transferred during 1994 in North America, roughly 45% of them had been frozen. Piglets have also been born from frozen embryos, but the porcine embryo is extremely sensitive to cooling damage, and the field application of embryo freezing for that species is problematic.

Frozen storage of embryos from farm animals offers several practical applications. The time for which embryos can be stored *in vitro* limits the distance over which embryos can be transported from donors in one area to recipients in another. These time limitations are abolished by low temperature preservation. The establishment of banks of frozen embryos has already begun with valuable laboratory animals and may in the future be useful for livestock improvement programs. If large numbers of embryos are obtained from a donor, the excess embryos can be frozen and then transferred at some later time, avoiding the need of excess numbers of synchronous recipients at each collection.

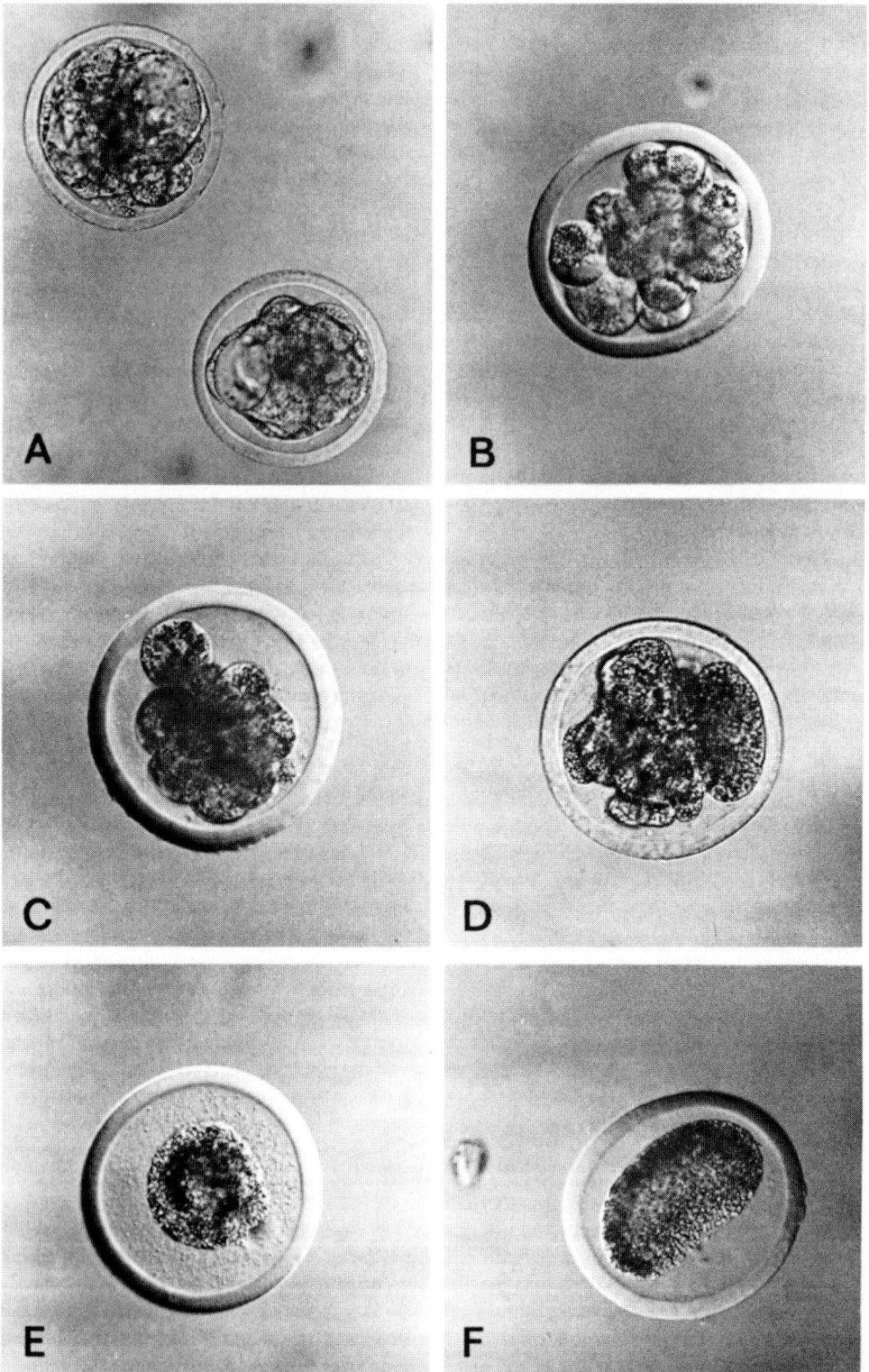

Fig. 19-6. Oocytes and embryos recovered from cattle 7 days after the onset of estrus. **A.** Early blastocysts. **B, C,** and **D.** Embryos with varying degrees of developmental retardation or fragmentation; classified as having a low probability of establishing a pregnancy if transferred. **E** and **F.** Degenerate, unfertilized oocytes.

MANAGEMENT OF RECIPIENTS AND TRANSFER OF EMBRYOS

The methods for transferring embryos to recipient females have followed a similar developmental pattern as with recovery of embryos. Surgical transfer was developed first, nonsurgical transfer later.

Surgical and Nonsurgical Transfer

Different techniques have been successfully applied for the actual process of transferring embryos surgically. The original method for embryo transfer in cattle, sheep, and goats required general anesthesia and a midline laparotomy to expose the reproductive tract of the recipient. More recently, many centers have begun transferring embryos using a paralumbar incision under local anesthesia. There appears to be no significant difference in success rates between these two methods. In either case, the uterine horn ipsilateral to the corpus luteum is exteriorized through the incision, and a probe or the blunt end of a suture needle is used to puncture the uterine wall. A small quantity of medium containing the embryo or embryos to be transferred is taken up into a slender glass pipet, and after insertion of the pipet into the uterine lumen, the embryos are gently expelled. Before expulsion of the embryos, one must be certain that the tip of the pipet is indeed in the lumen rather than embedded in the subendometrial tissues.

Surgical transfer of embryos in the sow is carried out in a similar fashion, and many embryos are transferred to each recipient. Because transuterine migration of embryos readily occurs in the sow, all of the embryos can be transferred to one uterine horn.

Surgical transfer of embryos in the mare has been performed basically as outlined for cattle. Work on embryo transfer in dogs and cats has been extremely limited, and only a small number of offspring have been obtained by embryo transfer in these species.

Perhaps more work has been done to develop a successful system for nonsurgical transfer of embryos in cattle than was necessary for the development of nonsurgical recovery. Initially, success rates following the nonsurgical transfer of embryos were disappointing. This lack of success was thought to be due to stimulation of uterine contractions as a consequence of invading the cervix. However, many groups have now reported a high pregnancy rate using transcervical transfer of embryos in the cow. Straws, such as those for freezing semen, are used to carry the embryos through the cervix to be deposited into the uterine lumen. A similar technique has been used successfully in mares, but the rate of success in this species is generally lower than with surgical transfer. Nonsurgical transfer also requires considerable skill and experience, but if done correctly, pregnancy rates are similar to those achieved with surgical transfer. Today, virtually all commercial bovine embryo transfer is conducted using nonsurgical transfer because it entails fewer personnel, less time and expense, and can be conducted on the farm.

Regardless of method of transfer, one of the primary factors affecting success in transferring embryos is the degree of estrous cycle synchrony between donor and recipient. In cattle and sheep, in which the bulk of the work with embryo transfer has been done, it has been clearly demonstrated that the highest degree of success is achieved when the donor and recipient are in estrus at the same time or within a day of each other (Fig. 19-7). When normal embryos are transferred to recipients with this synchrony, 60 to 75% of the recipients usually become pregnant. Pregnancy rates generally fall precipitously when asynchrony between donor and recipient is greater than 2 days.

Synchronization and Induction of Estrus

Reliable methods for the artificial regulation of the estrous cycle have long been sought for the purpose of increasing productivity and decreasing costs in food-producing animals. The widespread application of artificial insemination to cattle, and more recently to other species, has prompted interest in developing methods for the artificial regulation of estrous cycles in order to inseminate maximal numbers of animals on a single day.

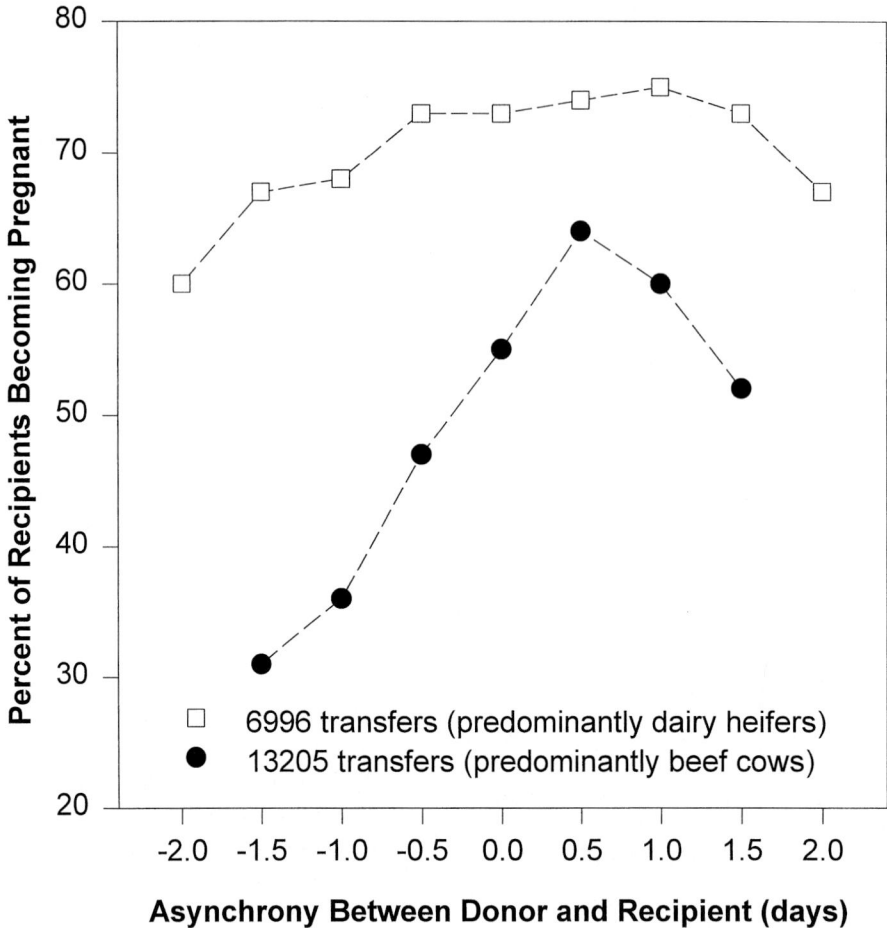

Fig. 19-7. Effect of donor-recipient synchrony on pregnancy rate in bovine embryo transfer. Positive asynchrony refers to recipient being in estrus before the donor. Data represented by open squares (□) represent transfers predominantly into Holstein heifers synchronized with $PGF_{2\alpha}$ (Hasler, J. F., McCauley, A. D., Lathrop, W. F., et al., Theriogenology 27:139, 1987), whereas data represented by closed circles (●) represent transfers predominantly into naturally-cycling beef cows (Putney, D. J., Thatcher W. W., Drost, M., et al., Theriogenology 30:905, 1988).

Methods that were first developed often resulted in acceptable synchronization of estrus, but were associated with poor fertility at the first postsynchronization insemination. Techniques are now available to predictably alter the time of estrus within the breeding season (**estrous synchronization**) and to induce estrus during periods of anestrus (**estrous induction**) while maintaining a high level of fertility. Two basic approaches are used for synchronization of estrus:

1. administration of prostaglandins to cause regression of the corpus luteum, with a subsequent return to estrus or

2. administration of progesterone, or more commonly progestagens, to temporarily suppress ovarian activity while the animals are under treatment.

Prostaglandin-induced synchronization treatments were based on the finding that $PGF_{2\alpha}$ is luteolytic in several species. Several synthetic analogues of $PGF_{2\alpha}$ have been developed which have greater potency and in some cases fewer undesirable side effects than $PGF_{2\alpha}$. It is important to keep in mind that pregnant animals will often abort upon treatment with prostaglandins. Moreover, these agents are effective only in animals with a functional corpus luteum. Because of this requirement, prostaglandins are ineffective for estrous synchronization in animals that are not cycling due to age, poor nutrition, postpartum or lactational anestrus, or other causes.

In cattle, $PGF_{2\alpha}$ is effective in causing luteolysis only between days 5 and 16 of the estrous cycle. When the stage and day of the cycle is known, synchronization of estrus can be induced by a single injection of $PGF_{2\alpha}$, but when a large group of cows is to be synchronized, a "double injection" schedule, with treatments 10 to 12 days apart, is often used. In this program, the first $PGF_{2\alpha}$ injection causes luteolysis and induces return to estrus in those cows that are in the stage of the cycle between days 5 and 16. At the time of the second injection, all cows should have a functional corpus luteum which can then be induced to regress. Synchronization treatments with $PGF_{2\alpha}$ in cattle are successful and are accompanied in most instances by good fertility. The luteolytic dose of $PGF_{2\alpha}$ in the cow is dramatically influenced by route of administration. Intrauterine instillation of only a small fraction of the dose required for subcutaneous or intramuscular injection will induce luteolysis. However, intrauterine treatment may be followed by uterine infection if administration is not done aseptically. Synchronization of estrus with prostaglandins in sheep and goats during the breeding season is similar to that in cattle.

In the cycling sow, $PGF_{2\alpha}$ effectively induces luteolysis but only on days 11 and 12 of the estrous cycle, which is very close to the time at which natural luteal regression takes place. Therefore, it is not practical to use prostaglandins to synchronize estrus in the normally cycling sow. However, the use of prostaglandins for estrous synchronization becomes practical and effective if the cycling sow is first treated with estrogens to pharmacologically prolong the lifespan of the corpora lutea or when gilts or sows are treated with gonadotropins to induce follicular development, ovulation, and formation of accessory corpora lutea. Estrus can also be synchronized in mated sows by inducing abortion with prostaglandins during early gestation, with good post-abortion rates of conception.

The corpus luteum of the mare is sensitive to $PGF_{2\alpha}$-mediated luteolysis after approximately day 5 of diestrus, and synchronization with normal fertility can be induced by administration of small doses of $PGF_{2\alpha}$. Groups of mares can be synchronized by a 'double injection' schedule with $PGF_{2\alpha}$ treatments given 14 days apart. Human chorionic gonadotropin is given 6 days after each treatment with $PGF_{2\alpha}$ to induce and synchronize ovulation in mares that return to estrus after treatment with $PGF_{2\alpha}$. Prostaglandin treatment also appears to be of benefit in the treatment of anestrus in the nonpregnant mare due to a persistent corpus luteum. Horses are more susceptible to the side effects of $PGF_{2\alpha}$ such as sweating and colic; these are less of a problem with some of the prostaglandin analogues than with $PGF_{2\alpha}$ itself.

Synchronization of estrus by treatment with progestagens is based on the finding that progestagens suppress follicular activity by preventing release of gonadotropins from the pituitary. If treatment is continued for a period equal to or longer than the life span of the corpus luteum, all progestagen-treated animals should have regressed corpora lutea at the end of treatment. Thus, follicular growth is reinitiated in a relatively synchronous manner upon withdrawal of the progestagen treatment. Several routes for the administration of a progestagen are available:

1. oral administration in feed,
2. daily injections,
3. vaginal pessaries or coils, and
4. subcutaneous implants.

Several of the schedules for synchronization of estrus with progestagens also involve administration of estrogens at the termination of treatment with progestagens.

In cattle, the most successful programs for synchronization of estrus with progestagens have utilized subcutaneous implants. Implants are also used in sheep, but pessaries are perhaps in more widespread use. Estrus and ovulation can be induced during the nonbreeding season in sheep and goats through gonadotropic treatment, generally PMSG, in combination with progestagens and withdrawal. In cycling sows, oral administration of progestagens, such as Altrenogest, results in effective synchronization of estrus.

Treatments for synchronization of estrus are used in embryo transfer programs for the regulation of the estrous cycles of both the donors and recipients. An almost universal practice in programs for the transfer of bovine embryos is to combine superovulation induced by gonadotropins and estrous synchronization induced by prostaglandins. There are two major reasons for this practice. First, in programs in which embryos are recovered from a significant number of donors, it is advantageous to be able to reliably schedule when embryos will be recovered from each donor, both for the sake of convenience and for optimal use of the recipient herd. Secondly, induced luteolysis allows for a more consistent superovulatory response and results in the recovery of more transferable embryos than from gonadotropic treatment alone. As an example, a typical regimen for inducing superovulation without prostaglandin treatment is to inject FSH 4 to 5 days before the anticipated onset of estrus. Without artificial control of luteal regression, cows will return to estrus anytime between 1 and 10 days after FSH treatment. This results in either a short or an extended period of superovulation for many of the cows, and as a consequence, the recovery of transferable embryos is reduced. Embryo recovery in sheep is also commonly carried out with donors that have been synchronized by either progestagens or prostaglandin treatment. In mares, estrus is commonly synchronized either by feeding oral progestagens or by parenteral administration of progesterone and estradiol. Superovulation and embryo recovery in wild ruminants, an area only recently explored, is an endeavor in which synchronization of estrus of the donor and recipient is mandatory because of the difficulty in detecting estrus in these animals.

Synchronization of estrus in the recipients of a large embryo transfer program is used to a lesser extent than the synchronization of donors. When dealing with large numbers of recipients, the costs of labor and drugs for repeated synchronization of estrus can become prohibitory. In addition, the high degree of variability in the number of embryos recovered causes many of the synchronized recipients to go unused, and

when large numbers of embryos are recovered, not enough recipients may have been synchronized. However, estrous synchronization of recipients can be a useful tool in small programs of embryo transfer when limited numbers of embryos are to be recovered or when the owner of the donor desires to use his own recipients.

Relatively little research has been devoted to the induction or synchronization of estrus in dogs and cats. Attempts to induce estrus in anestrous bitches with exogenous gonadotropins frequently fail. At best, the results are erratic and unpredictable (see Chapter 16). Follicular growth can be induced in the queen by treatment with PMSG or FSH, and many of these queens come into a fertile estrus (see Chapter 17). As in naturally cycling queens, seasonal influences play a role in natural or artificial induction of estrus. Administration of estrogen and testosterone has also been reported to induce behavioral estrus in the queen, but fertility following these treatments has not been adequately investigated.

OTHER APPLICATIONS OF EMBRYO TRANSFER TECHNOLOGY

Control of Disease Transmission

Many genetically valuable animals are isolated and restricted from international trade because of the risk of transmitting infectious diseases. Also, a large number of animals, particularly swine, are maintained in specific pathogen-free, closed herds that will eventually require the introduction of new genetic material. Today, livestock germplasm can be dispersed by movement of live animals, semen, or embryos. Of these procedures, transfer of embryos appears to be the one that offers the least risk of transmitting agents causing infectious diseases. There are several arguments to support this contention:

1. Early embryos at the stages used for embryo transfer appear to be relatively resistant to viral infection because the zona pellucida that encases them has been shown to prevent contact with most, but not all classes of viruses.

2. If viruses were present in the maternal environment, the embryo and thus the medium used to recover them would also be contami-

nated with viruses. However, the standard procedure of washing the embryos several times in sterile medium prior to transfer serves to greatly diminish the quantity of infectious agent present, probably to a level that would not establish an infection in the recipient.

3. Embryos can be frozen and the transfer postponed until sufficient time has elapsed to assure that the donor was not in the incubation stage of a particular disease at the time of embryo recovery. A limited number of studies have indicated that embryos can be recovered and transferred from animals infected with viruses such as those causing bovine leukemia, bluetongue, pseudorabies, and bovine rhinotracheitis without transmission of these agents to either the embryo or the recipient. Many more trials will have to be conducted to conclusively prove that embryo transfer is virtually free of the danger of transmitting a given disease.

Embryo Transfer in Exotic and Endangered Species

Many animal species are now endangered or extinct in their native habitats, with only small populations residing in zoos. Reproductive management of endangered animals in captivity is thus of critical importance in attempts either to prevent extinction or to return populations of these animals to the wild. Recently, embryo transfer techniques have successfully been applied to several species of exotic animals. As with embryo transfer in domestic animals, the goal of this work is to maximize the reproductive performance of a valuable female (the endangered animal) by superovulation and transfer of her embryos to compatible but less valuable recipients. The recipients in this case are from a different species that is not threatened or is less endangered. For most of the exotic species, there is a relative paucity of data concerning basic reproductive physiology, which makes successful embryo transfer particularly challenging.

Intergeneric transfer of embryos has been unsuccessful in a number of attempts. Often, as is seen with goat-sheep transfer, the transferred embryo develops normally for a time, but then, as the placenta begins to develop, the fetus is resorbed or aborted. In certain instances, a recipi-

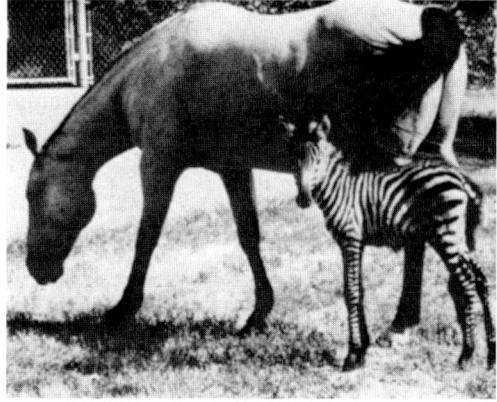

Fig. 19-8. Grant's zebra carried to term after transfer of the embryo to a domestic mare (Courtesy of the Louisville Zoo, Louisville, KY).

ent from one genus can carry the fetus of another genus to term if the transferred embryo is chimeric (see below). Transfer between different species in the same genus has been much more successful. Thus, recipient Elands have given birth to Bongo antelopes, domestic mares to donkeys and zebras (Fig. 19-8), a domestic cow to a gaur, and domestic ewes to Mouflon sheep. Many other possibilities exist for interspecific embryo transfer of exotic animals, and this technique will likely be utilized more in the future.

Production of Identical Multiplets and Chimeras

A recent advance in technology to manipulate embryos is the ability to reliably produce identical twins by splitting embryos. It has long been known that the cells of the early embryo are totipotent; that is, if one blastomere of a two-cell embryo is destroyed, the other blastomere can continue to develop to a normal adult. If, instead of destroying one blastomere, the two blastomeres are separated and allowed to develop independently, identical twins can result. Separation of blastomeres has resulted in the production of identical twin, triplet, and quadruplet lambs. A more common practice, and one that is used commercially, is to surgically divide a morula or early blastocyst into two parts, and then transfer both half-embryos (demi-embryos) to one or preferably two recipients. The microsurgical

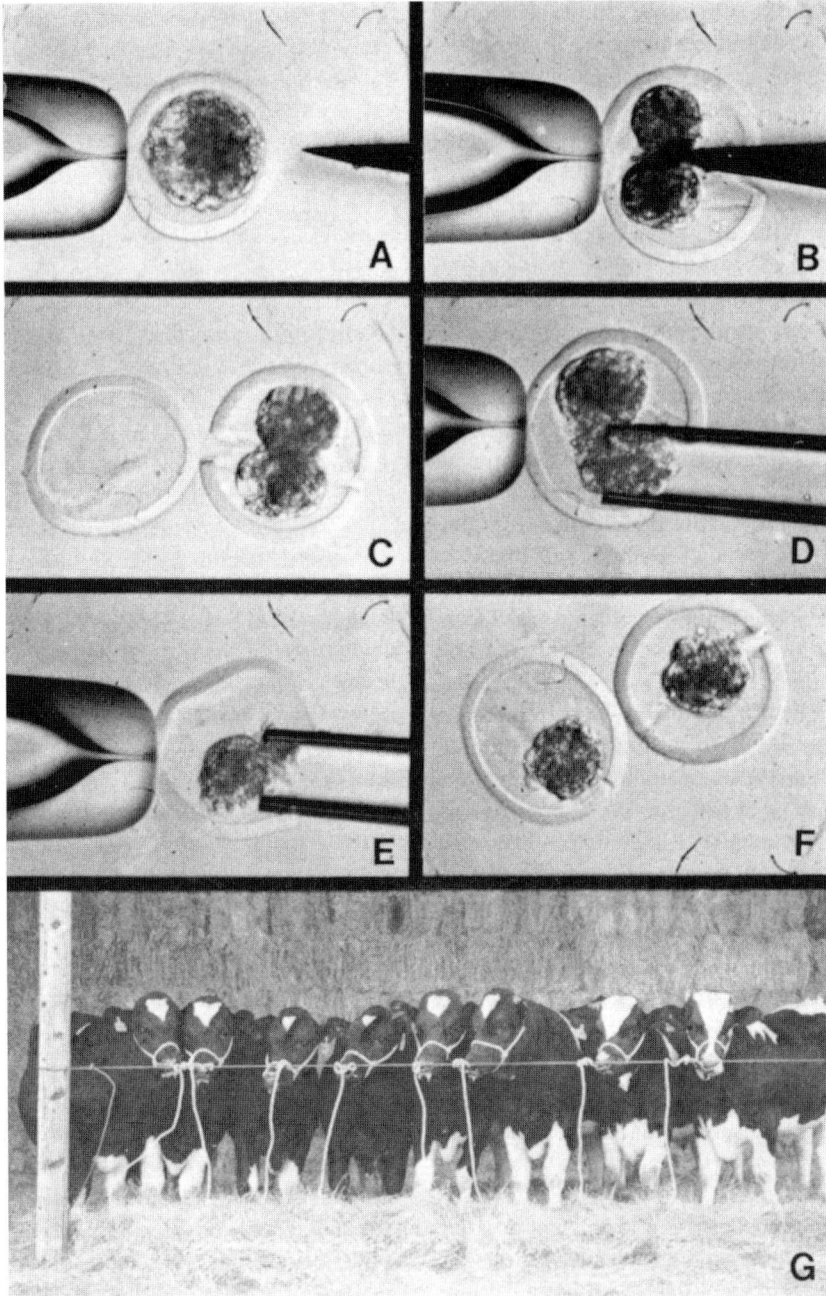

Fig. 19-9. Procedure for producing identical twin calves by bisecting embryos. **A.** Early blastocyst held by suction pipet. **B.** Bisection of embryo. **C.** Bisected embryo and empty surrogate zona pellucida. **D.** Removal of the demi-embryo from original zona pellucida. **E.** Placement of demi-embryo into surrogate zona pellucida. **F.** Two demi-embryos ready for transfer. **G.** Four pairs of identical twin Holstein bulls produced by embryo splitting and transfer of demi-embryos (Courtesy of G. E. Seidel, Jr. and R. P. Amann, Colorado State University, Fort Collins, CO).

dissection of the embryo is conducted with the microscope and the aid of a micromanipulator, an instrument that translates relatively large movements of the operator's hand into small movements of the microsurgical tool. In cattle, this seemingly crude technique works remarkably well, and in many cases, 50 to 65% of the half-embryos develop into calves (Fig. 19-9). Embryo splitting is an extremely valuable tool for producing identical twins for research studies. Commercial interest in this technique occurs not only because it produces identical twins, but also because it allows pregnancy rates to exceed 100%. If 60% of these half embryos develop into calves, then each original embryo will yield 1.2 calves, whereas with transfer of intact embryos, one can rarely expect more than a 75% pregnancy rate. A number of interesting applications exist with embryo splitting. For example, one-half of the split embryo can be frozen while the other half is transferred; and then, if the transferred embryo is of the desired sex and has an outstanding phenotype as an adult, the twin can be thawed to double that genetic material.

If whole embryos or blastomeres from different embryos are isolated and then combined, a chimeric embryo is formed which can often develop into a viable offspring after transfer. Chimeras can be produced by combining blastomeres from two or more cleavage-stage embryos in a common zona pellucida or by microinjecting blastomeres or an inner cell mass from one embryo into the blastocoel of another embryo. If cells from each original embryo survive and populate the resulting fetus, the offspring is said to be a **chimera.** This technique has proven to be extremely valuable in a number of research settings, particularly in studies on immunogenicity and immune tolerance. Because each chimeric animal is unique and not reproducible by breeding, production of chimeras has limited commercial potential. However, one possible application of the chimeras is to allow successful intergeneric embryo transfers. As mentioned above, when embryos from one genus are transferred to recipients of another genus, the embryos almost inevitably fail to develop to term. This incompatibility can be circumvented by making chimeras with cells from embryos from the two different genera. If chimeric sheep-goat embryos are produced such that the placenta is derived exclusively from sheep cells and the fetus from goat cells (see Chapter 14), a recipient ewe can give birth to a normal goat kid.

Cloning by Nuclear Transfer

The efficiency of producing identical multiplets by embryo splitting declines precipitously past twins. However, much larger groups of genetically identical animals can be generated by nuclear transfer. In this technique, a cleavage stage embryo is disaggregated into individual blastomeres, which are then fused individually to enucleated oocytes. The resulting zygotes are then cultured and transferred to recipient females for development to term. This procedure has been most avidly pursued with cattle and, although rates of success are quite variable, up to 30 cloned calves have been produced from a single donor embryo. Potentially, larger groups of clones can be generated by using cloned embryos as donors for subsequent rounds of nuclear transfer.

Production of Transgenic Animals

A recent development in embryo transfer technology and genetic engineering involves transferring a selected gene into an embryo so that the resulting offspring carry and express that gene later in life. This procedure, like embryo splitting, is conducted with the aid of a micromanipulator. The solution containing the DNA sequence of interest is drawn into a fine pipet, and a small volume, measured in picoliters, is injected into one of the pronuclei of the recently fertilized oocyte. In some of these microinjected embryos, the introduced DNA will become integrated into the genome of the embryo, and because the DNA was introduced at the one-cell stage, the gene will be present in each of the cells of the resulting offspring. Animals that carry a copy of a foreign gene are referred to as being **transgenic.** In a now classical demonstration of this technique, the gene for growth hormone was isolated from rats, linked to the regulatory sequences from another gene, and then was introduced into the pronuclei of mouse embryos. In some of those embryos, the rat gene was integrated into the mouse's genome, and the transgene was expressed in large quantities after birth, leading to "giant mice" that displayed rapid growth and a large body size. The prospect of engineering strains of domestic livestock that display rapid growth, resistance to disease, or other desirable characteristics is obviously of great interest.

Quite a number of transgenic pigs, goats, and sheep have been produced, as well as a few transgenic cattle. The pigs and sheep transgenic for growth hormone generally have not shown accelerated growth, and most manifest infertility and sometimes musculoskeletal disease. In contrast, one transgenic strategy involving farm animals that may prove to be of exceptional value is "molecular pharming." If the transgene consists of a milk protein promoter fused appropriately to a sequence encoding a pharmaceutical or vac-

cine protein, the transgenic animal will secrete that protein into milk (Fig. 19-10). Ruminants are prodigious milk producers and if only a fraction of milk protein is from the transgene, huge amounts of recombinant protein can be harvested from milk. Several companies have established programs to generate this type of transgenic animal (usually goats or sheep), and the technology continues to look promising; some transgenic sheep have been shown to secrete up to 30 g of recombinant protein per liter of milk.

Another technology with great potential for producing transgenic farm animals involves generating chimeras with embryonic stem cells. These cells are derived from early embryos and are totipotent. When injected into the blastocoele or aggregated with early embryos, they can be-

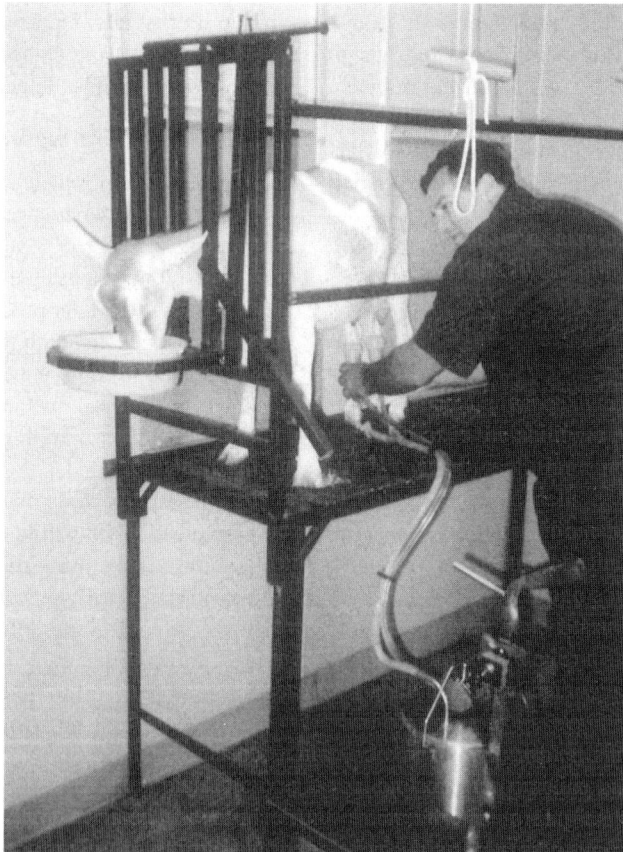

Fig. 19-10. Transgenic goat that secretes large quantities of human antithrombin III in her milk (Courtesy of Genzyme Transgenics, Inc., Framingham, MA).

come incorporated into the embryo and become part of the resulting adult. Germ cells derived from stem cells are thus capable of transmitting the stem cell genome to offspring, and if the stem cells are genetically engineered, the offspring, as well as the chimera, will be transgenic. The potential advantage of this procedure is that very sophisticated genetic manipulations can first be performed on embryonic stem cells in culture and thereby be introduced back into whole animals. This technology has been widely applied to mice and very recently to swine.

Transgenic animals, particularly mice, have already contributed enormously to our understanding of gene expression and molecular mechanisms of disease. Much additional work will be required before this technology has a practical impact on animal agriculture.

REFERENCES

Introduction

1. Betteridge, K. J. (1981): A historical look at embryo transfer. J. Reprod. Fertil. *62*:1.
2. Hasler, J. F. (1992): Current status and potential of embryo transfer and reproductive technology in dairy cattle. J. Dairy Sci. *75*:2857.
3. Lohuis, M. M. (1995): Potential benefits of bovine embryo manipulation technologies to genetic improvement programs. Theriogenology *43*:51.
4. Mapletoft, R. J., Johnson, W. H., and Miller, D. M. (1980): Embryo transfer techniques in repeat breeding cows. Theriogenology *13*:103.
5. Squires, E. L. and Seidel, G. E., Jr. (1995): Collection and Transfer of Equine Embryos. Animal Reproduction and Biotechnology Laboratory Bulletin no. 8, Colorado State University, Fort Collins, CO.
6. Stringfellow, D. A. and Seidel, S. M. (1990): Manual of the International Embryo Transfer Society. Champaign, IL, International Embryo Transfer Society.
7. Van Vleck, L. D. (1981): Potential genetic impact of artificial insemination, sex selection, embryo transfer, cloning and selfing in dairy cattle. *In:* New Technologies in Animal Breeding, edited by B. G. Brackett, G. E. Seidel, Jr., and S. M. Seidel. New York, NY, Academic Press, Inc., p. 221.

Increasing the Availability of Embryos

8. Armstrong, D. T. and Evans, G. (1983): Factors influencing success of embryo transfer in sheep and goats. Theriogenology *19*:31.
9. Armstrong, D. T. (1993): Recent advances in superovulation of cattle. Theriogenology *39*:7.
10. Bowen, R. A., Reed, M. L., Schnieke, A., et al. (1994): Transgenic cattle resulting from biopsied embryos: Expression of c-ski in a transgenic calf. Biol. Reprod. *50*:664.

11. Brackett, B. G., Bousquet, D., Boice, M. L., et al. (1982): Normal development following *in vitro* fertilization in the cow. Biol. Reprod. *27*:147.
12. Christenson, R. K., Pope, C. E., Zimmerman-Pope, V. A., et al. (1973): Synchronization of estrus and ovulation in superovulated gilts. J. Anim. Sci. *36*:914.
13. Donoghue, A. M., Johnston, L. A., Munson, L., et al. (1992): Influence of gonadotropin treatment interval on follicular maturation, *in vitro* fertilization, circulating steroid concentrations, and subsequent luteal function in the domestic cat. Biol. Reprod. *46*:972.
14. Duby, R. T., Damiani, P. I., Looney, C. R., et al. (1996): Prepubertal calves as oocyte donors: Promises and problems. Theriogenology *45*:121.
15. Ebert, K. M. and Schindler, J. E. S. (1993): Transgenic farm animals: Progress report. Theriogenology *39*:121.
16. Fortune, J. E. and Kimmich, T. L. (1993): Purified pig FSH increases the rate of double ovulation in mares. Equine Vet. J. *15* (Suppl.):95.
17. Hasler, J. F., McCauley, A. D., Schermerhorn, E. C., et al. (1983): Superovulatory responses of Holstein cows. Theriogenology *19*:83.
18. Lambert, R. D., Sirard, M. A., Bernard, C., et al. (1986): *In vitro* fertilization of bovine oocytes matured *in vivo* and collected at laparoscopy. Theriogenology *25*:117.
19. Logan, J. S. and Martin, M. J. (1994): Transgenic swine as a recombinant production system for human hemoglobin. Methods Enzymol. *231:* 435.
20. Looney, C. R., Lindsey, B. R., Gonseth, C. L., et al. (1994): Commercial aspects of oocyte retrieval and *in vitro* fertilization (IVF) for embryo production in problem cows. Theriogenology *41*:67.
21. McCue, P. M. (1996): Superovulation. Vet. Clin. North Am., Equine Pract. *12*:1.
22. Nagai, T. (1994): Current status and perspectives in IVM-IVF of porcine oocytes. Theriogenology *41*:73.
23. Yamada, S., Shimazu Y., Kawaji, H., et al. (1992): Maturation, fertilization and development of dog oocytes *in vitro*. Biol. Reprod. *46*:853.
24. Woods, G. L. and Ginther, O. J. (1983): Ovarian response, pregnancy rate and incidence of multiple fetuses in mares treated with an equine pituitary extract. J. Reprod. Fertil. (Suppl. 32):415.
25. Zhang, J. J., Muzs, L. Z., and Boyle, M. S. (1990): *In vitro* fertilization of horse follicular oocytes matured *in vitro*. Mol. Reprod. Develop. *26*:361.

Recovery of Embryos

26. Brand, A. and Drost, M. (1977): Embryo collection by non-surgical methods. *In:* Embryo Transfer in Farm Animals. A Review of Techniques and Applications, edited by K. J. Betteridge. Monograph 16, Canada Department of Agriculture, Station H, Ottawa K2H8P9, Canada, p. 16.
27. Elsden, R. P., Hasler, J. F., and Seidel, G. E., Jr. (1976): Non-surgical recovery of bovine eggs. Theriogenology *6*:523.
28. Greve, T., Lehn-Jensen, H., and Rasbeck, N. O. (1977): Non-surgical recovery of bovine embryos. Theriogenology *7*:239.
29. Imel, K. J., Squires, E. L., Elsden, R. P., et al. (1981): Collection and transfer of equine embryos. J. Am. Vet. Med. Assoc. *179*:987.

30. Davis, D. L. and Day, B. N. (1978): Cleavage and blastocyst formation by pig eggs *in vitro.* J. Anim. Sci. *46*:1043.
31. Hasler, J. F., Henderson W. B., Hurtgen, P. J., et al. (1995): Production, freezing and transfer of bovine IVF-embryos and subsequent calving. Theriogenology *43*:141.
32. Holst, P. A. and Phemister, R. D. (1971): The prenatal development of the dog: Preimplantation events. Biol. Reprod. *5*:194.
33. Hunter, R. H. F. (1974): Chronological and cytological details of fertilization and early embryonic development in the domestic pig, *Sus scrofa.* Anat. Rec. *178*:169.
34. McKinnon, A. O., Squires, E. L., Voss, J. L., et al. (1988): Equine embryo transfer-a review. Compend. Cont. Educ. Pract. Vet. *10*:343.
35. Newcomb, R. and Rowson, L. E. A. (1975): Conception rate after uterine transfer of cow eggs in relation to synchronization of oestrus and age of eggs. J. Reprod. Fertil. *43*:539.
36. Wright, J. M. (1985): Commercial freezing of bovine embryos in straws. Theriogenology *23*:17.

Management of Recipients and Transfer of Embryos

37. Allen, W. R. (1982): Egg transfer in the horse. *In:* Mammalian Egg Transfer, edited by C. E. Adams. Boca Raton, FL, CRC Press, p. 135.
38. Carney, N. J., Squires, E. L., Cook, V. M., et al. (1991): Comparison of pregnancy rates from transfer of fresh versus cooled, transported equine embryos. Theriogenology *36*:23.
39. Christenson, R. K., Pope, C. E., Zimmerman-Pope, V. A., et al. (1973): Synchronization of estrus and ovulation in superovulated gilts. J. Anim. Sci. *36*:914.
40. Del Campo, M. R., Rowe, R. F., Chaichareon, D., et al. (1983): Effect of the relative locations of embryo and corpus luteum on embryo survival in cattle. Reprod. Nutr. Develop. *23*:303.
41. Donaldson, L. E. (1985): Matching of embryo stages and grades with recipients oestrus synchrony in bovine embryo transfer. Vet. Rec. *117*:489.
42. Iuliano, M. F., Squires, E. L., and Cook, V. M. (1985): Effect of age of equine embryos and method of transfer on pregnancy rate. J. Anim. Sci. *60*:258.
43. Kraemer, D. C. (1983): Intra- and interspecific embryo transfer. J. Exp. Zool. *228*:363.
44. Kraemer, D. C., Flow, B. L., Schriver, M. D., et al. (1979): Embryo transfer in the non-human primate, feline and canine. Theriogenology *11*:51.
45. Moore, N. W., Rowson, L. E. A., and Short, R. V. (1960): Egg transfer in sheep. Factors affecting the survival and development of transferred eggs. J. Reprod. Fertil. *1*:332.
46. Pope, W. F. and First, N. L. (1985): Factors affecting the survival of pig embryos. Theriogenology *23*:91.
47. Pope, W. F., Maurer, R. R., and Stormshak, F. (1982): Survival of porcine embryos after asynchronous transfer. Proc. Soc. Exp. Biol. Med. *171*:179.
48. Rowson, L. E. A., Lawson, R. A. S., Moor, R. M., et al. (1972): Egg transfer in the cow: Synchronization requirements. J. Reprod. Fertil. *28*:427.
49. Wilmut, I., Sales, D. I., and Ashworth, C. J. (1985): The influence of variation in embryo stage and maternal hormone profiles on embryo survival in farm animals. Theriogenology *23*:107.

Other Applications of Embryo Transfer Technology

50. Allen, W. R. and Pasken, R. L. (1984): Production of monozygotic (identical) horse twins by embryo micromanipulation. J. Reprod. Fertil. *71*:607.
51. Bondioli K. (1992): Embryo sexing: A review of current techniques and their potential for commercial application in livestock production. J. Anim. Sci. *70* (Suppl 2):19.
52. Bowen, R. A., Reed, M. L., Schnieke, A., et al. (1994). Transgenic cattle resulting from biopsied embryos: Expression of c-ski in a transgenic calf. Biol. Reprod. *50*:664.
53. Boyle, M. S., Allen, W. R., Tischner, M., et al. (1985): Storage and international transport of horse embryos in liquid nitrogen. Equine Vet. J. *3* (Suppl.):36.
54. Campbell, K. H. S., McWhir, J., Ritchie, W. A., et al. (1996): Sheep cloned by nuclear transfer from a cultured cell line. Nature *380*:64.
55. Curnock, R. M., Day, B. N., and Dziuk, P. J. (1975): Embryo transfer in pigs: A method for introducing genetic material into primary specific-pathogen-free herds. Am. J. Vet. Res. *37*:97.
56. Donoghue, A. M., Johnston, L. A., Seal, U. S., et al. (1990): *In vitro* fertilization and embryo development *in vitro* and *in vivo* in the tiger (*Panthera tigris*). Biol. Reprod. *43*:733.
57. Dresser, B. L., Pope, C. E., Kramer, L., et al. (1985): Birth of Bongo antelope (*Tragelaphus euryceros*) to Eland antelope (*Tragelaphus oryx*) and cryopreservation of Bongo embryos. Theriogenology *23*:190.
58. Durrant, B. S., Oosterhuis, J. E., and Hoge, M. L. (1986): The application of artificial reproduction techniques to the propagation of selected endangered species. Theriogenology *25*:25.
59. Fehilly, C. B., Willadsen, S. M., and Tucker, E. M. (1984): Interspecific chimaerism between goat and sheep. Nature *307*:634.
60. Hammer, R. E., Pursel, V. G., Rexroad, C. E., et al. (1985): Production of transgenic rabbits, sheep and pigs by microinjection. Nature *315*:680.
61. Loskutoff, N. M., Bartels, P., Meintjes, M., et al. (1995). Assisted reproductive technology in nondomestic ungulates: A model approach to preserving and managing genetic diversity. Theriogenology *43*:1.
62. Meinecke-Tillmann, S. and Meinecke, B. (1984): Experimental chimaeras-removal of reproductive barrier between sheep and goats. Nature *307*:637.
63. Singh, E. L. and Hare, W. C. D. (1986): Embryo pathogen interactions in relation to disease transmission. *In:* Current Therapy in Theriogenology, 2nd ed., edited by D. A. Morrow. Philadelphia, PA, W. B. Saunders Co., p. 84.
64. Stice, S. L. and Keefer, C. L. (1993): Multiple generational bovine embryo cloning. Biol. Reprod. *48*:715.
65. Thibier, M. (1995): Embryo Transfer Newsletter, Int. Embryo Transf. Soc. *13*:18.
66. Thibier, M. and Nibart, M. (1995): The sexing of bovine embryos in the field. Theriogenology *43*:71.

67. Wall, R. J. (1996): Transgenic livestock: Progress and prospects for the future. Theriogenology *45*:57.
68. Westhusin, M. E., Pryor, H. H., and Bondioli, K. R. (1991): Nuclear transfer in the bovine embryo: A comparison of 5-day, 6-day, frozen-thawed, and nuclear transfer donor embryos. Mol. Reprod. Develop. *28*:119.
69. Williams, T. J., Elsden, R. P., and Seidel, G. E., Jr. (1984): Pregnancy rates with bisected bovine embryos. Theriogenology *22*:521.
70. Wrathall, A. E. (1995): Embryo transfer and disease transmission in livestock: A review of recent research. Theriogenology *43*:81.

References Added in Proof

71. Cognie, Y. (1999): State of the art in sheep-goat embryo transfer. Theriogenology *51*:105.
72. Hunter, M. G. (2000): Oocyte maturation and ovum quality in pigs. Rev. Reprod. *55*:122.
73. Kawarasaki, T., Matsumoto, K., Murofushi, J. et al. (2000): Sexing of porcine embryos by *in situ* hybridization using chromosome Y and 1-specific DNA probes. Theriogenology *53*:1501.
74, Lewis, I. M., Peura, T. T., and Trounson, A. O. (1998): Large-scale applications of cloning technologies for agriculture: An industry perspective. Reprod. Fertil. Develop. *10*:677.
75. Squires, E. L., McCue, P. M., and Vanderwall, D. (1999): The current status of equine embryo transfer. Theriogenology *51*:91.

Index

Page numbers in *italics* indicate figures. Page numbers followed by a "t" refer to tables.